D0225386

ALEXANDER'S

CARE OF

THE PATIENT IN SURGERY

ALEXANDER'S

CARE OF THE PATIENT IN SURGERY

BARBARA J. GRUENDEMANN, RN, BS, MS
Director of Education, Operating Room,
Centinela Hospital Medical Center,
Inglewood, California

MARGARET HUTH MEEKER, RN, BSN, CNOR
Director of Nursing, O.R./R.R.,
The Ohio State University Hospitals,
Columbus, Ohio

SEVENTH EDITION

with **1880** illustrations
including **1** color plate

THE C. V. MOSBY COMPANY

ST. LOUIS • TORONTO • LONDON 1983

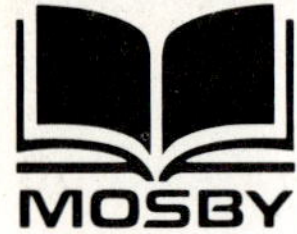

A TRADITION OF PUBLISHING EXCELLENCE

Editor: Julie Cardamon
Assistant editor: Bess Arends
Manuscript editor: Jeanne L. Heitman
Designer: Kay M. Kramer
Production: Sue Soehngen, Carolyn Biby

SEVENTH EDITION

Printed in the United States of America

The C.V. Mosby Company
11830 Westline Industrial Drive, St. Louis, Missouri 63141

Library of Congress Cataloging in Publication Data

Alexander, Edythe Louise.
Alexander's Care of the patient in surgery.

Bibliography: p.
Includes index.
1. Operating room nursing. I. Gruendemann, Barbara J. II. Meeker, Margaret Huth. III. Title. IV. Title: Care of the patient in surgery. [DNLM: 1. Nursing care. 2. Surgical nursing. WY 161 A375o]
RD32.3.A43 1983 617'.0024613 82-8212
ISBN 0-8016-4147-0

C/VH/VH 9 8 7 6 5 4 3 2 1 03/A/306

Contributors

AUDREY N. BELL, RN

Supervisor, Operating Suite, Children's Medical Center, Dallas, Texas

CATHERINE A. BROWN, RN, CNOR

Manager, Nursing Communications, Anthony J. Jannetti, Inc., Pitman, New Jersey; Formerly Supervisor, O.R., R.R., C.S.R., Scottish Rite Hospital for Crippled Children, Atlanta, Georgia

EDWARD CARDEN, MD, FRCP (C)

Associate Clinical Professor, University of California Medical Center, Los Angeles; Staff Anesthesiologist, Centinela Hospital Medical Center, Inglewood, California

MARGARET R. GALLAGHER, RN

Nursing Education Instructor, Operating Room, Western Pennsylvania Hospital, Pittsburgh, Pennsylvania

BARBARA J. GRUENDEMANN, RN, BS, MS

Director of Education, Operating Room, Centinela Hospital Medical Center, Inglewood, California

CYNTHIA C. HAYES, RN, MN

Director, Operating Room Services, Shands Hospital, University of Florida, Gainesville, Florida

JOAN S. KOEHLER, RN

Surgical Nurse Practitioner, Phoenix, Arizona

JUNE LORIG, RN, BSN

Clinical Supervisor, Operating Rooms, University Hospitals of Cleveland, Cleveland, Ohio

MARGARET HUTH MEEKER, RN, BSN, CNOR

Director of Nursing, O.R./R.R., The Ohio State University Hospitals, Columbus, Ohio

MARY G. NOLAN, RN, MN

Director of Nursing, Surgery, and Post Anesthesia Recovery; Vice President, Patient Care Services, Memorial Hospital Medical Center, Long Beach, California

ELIZABETH A. REED, RN, CNOR

Operating Room Supervisor, University of California, San Francisco, San Francisco, California

ADELE RILEY, RN, BSN, MSN

Formerly Head Nurse, O.R., Bellevue Hospital Center, New York, New York

ROSEMARY A. ROTH, RN, MS

Senior Associate Nursing Faculty, University of Rochester; Assistant Director of Nursing Practice, O.R., R.R., A.S.U., The Genesee Hospital, Rochester, New York

JOANNE SAUTER, RN

Staff Nurse, Main Operating Rooms, Cook County Hospital, Chicago, Illinois

CAROL TYLER, RN, BS, CNOR

Staff Development Coordinator, O.R., Evanston Hospital, Evanston, Illinois

CHRISTINE LARSON WEBER, RN

Staff Nurse, Operating Room, Henry Mayo Newhall Memorial Hospital, Valencia, California

Preface

The seventh edition of *Alexander's Care of the Patient in Surgery* has been revised to reflect changes in nursing practice and operating room technology that have occurred since the last edition. The goal in presenting this text remains the same: to provide a basic reference for the humane and technological nursing care of the patient during surgical intervention. Inclusion of material from contributors located in various parts of the United States provides a broad range of experience and technological information.

The text is written primarily for professional nurses but is also useful for nursing students, operating room technologists, and licensed vocational nurses. Nuring considerations for patients undergoing specific surgical procedures have been expanded to emphasize the importance of assessing needs and planning quality perioperative nursing care.

Part One, General Considerations, presents fundamental principles and concepts employed in all surgical suites. A new chapter on anesthesia discusses the various agents used and the nurse's responsibility during their administration, the maintenance of airways, and the use of endotracheal tubes.

Part Two, Surgical Interventions, provides pertinent information on general and specialty surgical procedures. In Chapter 15, new material has been added on cesarean sections, and Chapter 20 now contains information on amputations. Indications for specific operations, the preparation of the patient, the instruments and equipment required, and the more common operations in the specialty area are included. Although complete lists of instruments preferred in any given hospital cannot be included, we hope that the description of basic and special trays will be adequate guides for every hospital.

We would like to acknowledge the valuable assistance of reviewers, photographers, illustrators, and secretaries who have contributed their time and expertise to facilitate the revision of this text.

Alexander's Care of the Patient in Surgery is written by and for operating room nursing personnel and is dedicated to excellence in care for each patient who experiences surgical intervention.

Barbara J. Gruendemann
Margaret Huth Meeker

Contents

PART ONE

GENERAL CONSIDERATIONS

1 Concepts basic to operating room nursing

Probably no other area of nursing requires the broad knowledge base, the instant recall of facts and past experiences, the diversity of thoughts and actions, the stamina, and the pliability needed in operating room endeavors. Whether a generalist or specialist, the operating room nurse stores away pertinent anatomy and physiology, as well as ''tricks'' and ''clues'' that are unwritten but successful ways of communicating that lead to desired actions, and brings them to bear in a minute's notice.

The size of this mental repertoire is staggering and points out the constant discipline and presence of mind demanded in operating room nursing. However, the greater the requirements, the more satisfactory and indelible are the joys that come to the operating room nurse, truly an expert!

Operating room nursing is a purposeful, dynamic, professional process. Through planned interventions and actions, surgical patients are assured safe scientific care when undergoing surgery. Operating room nurses are responsible for providing a safe, efficient, and caring operating room environment, one in which the surgical team can function and in which the outcome for the patient is as positive as possible.

This textbook is by nature technical because a large portion of operating room nursing is technical. Knowledge of skills, procedures, setups, and instruments aids the operating room nurse in preparation, anticipation of the steps in the surgical procedure, and in functioning as a solid team member. Needs of patients and surgeons can be foreseen best by nurses who are well versed in the detailed technical components contained in this text. Techniques are at the heart of operating room nursing.

But all of operating room nursing is not technical; some is conceptual, some behavioral. If this were not so, operating room nurses could be replaced by mechanized robots, programmed to deliver correct instruments and sutures at precise moments during operations. Since the emphasis in this text is technical, refer to the suggested readings at the end of this chapter for more in-depth sources on behavioral care.

In this chapter, operating room nursing is considered in toto. The purpose is to place operating room nursing in perspective, spelling out the place for and details of some of the behavioral components. It sets the scene, so to speak, for the remainder of the book. A fundamental assumption is that operating room nursing is a blend of the technical and behavioral; it is thinking as well as doing, people-caring as well as instrument-handling.

PERIOPERATIVE NURSING

Perioperative nursing, a new term describing the scope and depth of operating room nursing, is gaining wide acceptance. Emanating from work of the Association of Operating Room Nurses (AORN), the term helps define the role of the operating room nurse during three patient phases: preoperative, intraoperative, and postoperative. A model depicting the role illustrates a continuum on which the nurse functions, from basic competency to excellence.

The perioperative role concept brings together the traditional and expanded nursing activities during the intraoperative period with the newer preoperative and postoperative patient teaching, counseling, assessment, and evaluation functions. This text presents a significant discussion of perioperative nursing but is not a comprehensive treatise on the subject.

The practice of perioperative nursing is a goal of operating room nurses. Until this concept is universally practiced, however, the well-understood terms ''operating room nurse'' and ''operating room nursing'' will continue to be used, as is true in this text. Support of perioperative nursing stipulates continuity of teaching and care throughout the total surgical patient experience. It mandates the use of talking, touching, doing, and teaching skills, and it directs the operating room nurse to focus all efforts on the patient and the surgery.

Above all, perioperative nursing care ensures a smooth course for the patient before, during, and after surgery, obviating piecemeal, assembly-line treatment.

Perioperative nursing describes a total package of hand and head skills performed by the operating room nurse. It provides a schema whereby operating room nursing is viewed in professional perspective and the nursing process is a pervasive thread.

NURSING PROCESS

Operating room nursing is a planned process, or a series of integrated steps. If viewed only as ''setting up cases,'' operating room nursing becomes nothing more than rote equipment preparation and paper shuffling. If, rather, it is viewed as *patient care,* it becomes a scientific process and an exciting stimulus for the nurse to perform optimally.

The process of nursing is a way of looking at nursing and bringing it into perspective as *a methodical thought process that guides actions.* This is in contrast to considering nursing as only a set of cookbook rituals and procedures to be learned. The focus of nursing process is on the patient, and nursing interventions prescribed are those which meet patient needs. Operating room nursing is particularly vulnerable to being considered only a conglomeration of rote techniques and a carrying out of surgeon's orders. By using the nursing process, operating room nurses can focus on the patient and, at the same time, put skills and know-how in dealing with patients *and* implementing procedures in proper perspective.

In its simplest form, the nursing process consists of four phases: assessment, planning, intervention, and evaluation (Fig. 1-1). The process is circular and continuous.

Assessment is the collection of relevant data about the patient. Sources of data may be a preoperative interview with the patient and the patient's family by an operating room or unit nurse; the nursing care plans, Kardex, and patient's chart; and the surgeon and anesthesiologist, unit nurses, or other personnel.

These data are collected and interpreted. Based on this information, the nursing diagnosis or patient problem identification is recorded.

The operating room nurse now has some knowledge of the patient, which helps in (1) planning the operating room nursing care, (2) viewing the patient as an individual and not as a "case," and (3) gaining more satisfaction because the *person* having the surgery is now considered *as well as* the tools, setups, and environmental controls needed to perform the surgery. If operating room nursing care fails to put its main emphasis on the human being having the operation, it can no longer be labeled professional nursing.

For an operating room nurse, assessment often means a thoughtful, quick scan of the patient and chart, the surgical procedure, and the resources and knowledge necessary to successfully direct the patient through an operative course. At other times, there are thorough assessments of all aspects of the patient and his condition, along with preoperative and postoperative reviews.

In a discussion of assessment, the question of whether operating room nurses should perform preoperative interviews invariably arises. Preoperative interviews, or visits, are standard procedure in many institutions. In others, these interviews are neither done nor supported by the administration because of reasons such as shortages of time and personnel.

Preoperative visits by operating room nurses are neither an end in themselves nor a panacea for "getting operating room nurses in touch with their patients." However, if planned properly to fill the needs of both patients and nurses, visits can be extremely beneficial (Fig. 1-2); evidence abounds to support this concept.

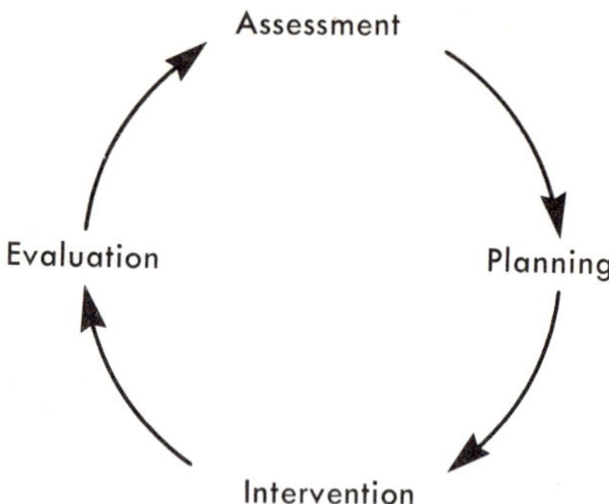

Fig. 1-1. Four phases of nursing process.

When thinking about preoperative interviewing and teaching, consider the following: Is relevant, concise patient information already being transmitted to the operating room nursing staff? Is enough information available to allow operating room nurses to consider patient peculiarities when setting up the room (special equipment, supports, instruments, sutures)? Is there sufficient time to initiate a meaningful nurse-patient interaction before time of induction? Are surgical patients satisfied with their operating room nursing care (do they express feelings of comfort and satisfaction regarding their care in the operating room), and do they have knowledge of the operating room nurse's role? Is there continuity of care between the operating room and the surgical units?

It is helpful when unit and operating room nurses can exchange information about their patients by face-to-face meetings or telephone or written messages (Fig. 1-3). A thorough assessment, made and recorded by the unit nurses, can accompany patients to the operating room and serve as a useful guide to operating room personnel. Often, however, this is not done or is not useful to the nurses in the surgical suite. Then it is up to the operating room nurse to do some form of preoperative patient assessment.

Individual sessions may be the answer. In some hospitals, group preoperative classes not only serve the purpose of getting to know the patients, but also that of imparting information on common routines, reactions, sensations, and nursing procedures that will take place preoperatively, intraoperatively, and postoperatively. The important point is that some form of assessment and teaching be done. How it is accomplished is up to the particular hospital and nursing staff.

Assessment, then, is knowing and understanding the patient as a person and as a candidate for a surgical procedure.

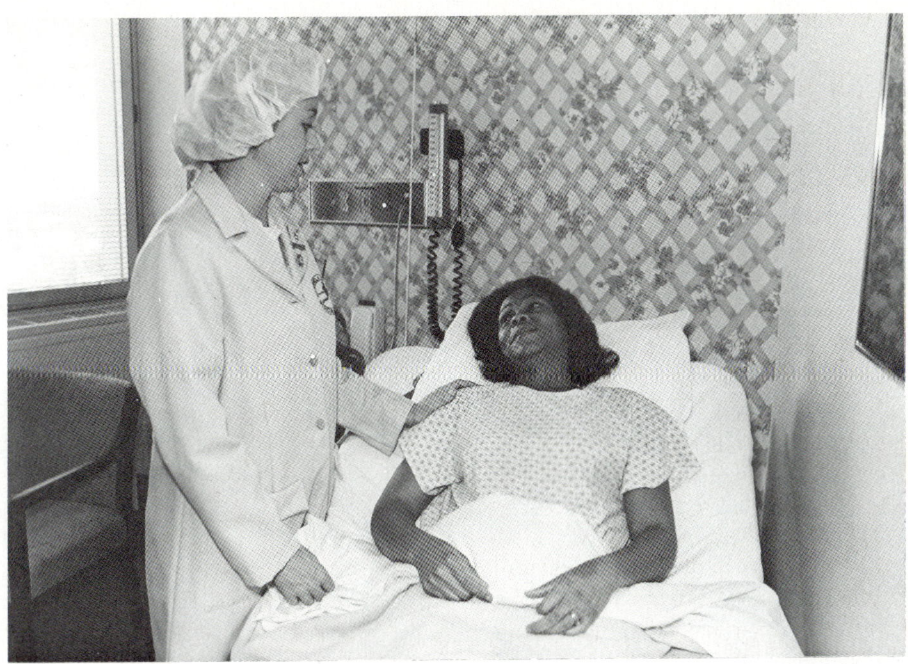

Fig. 1-2. Operating room nurse interviews surgical patient. Purpose of visit is to assess patient needs, to obtain information about patient and family, and to teach patient regarding common routines, sensations, and nursing care.

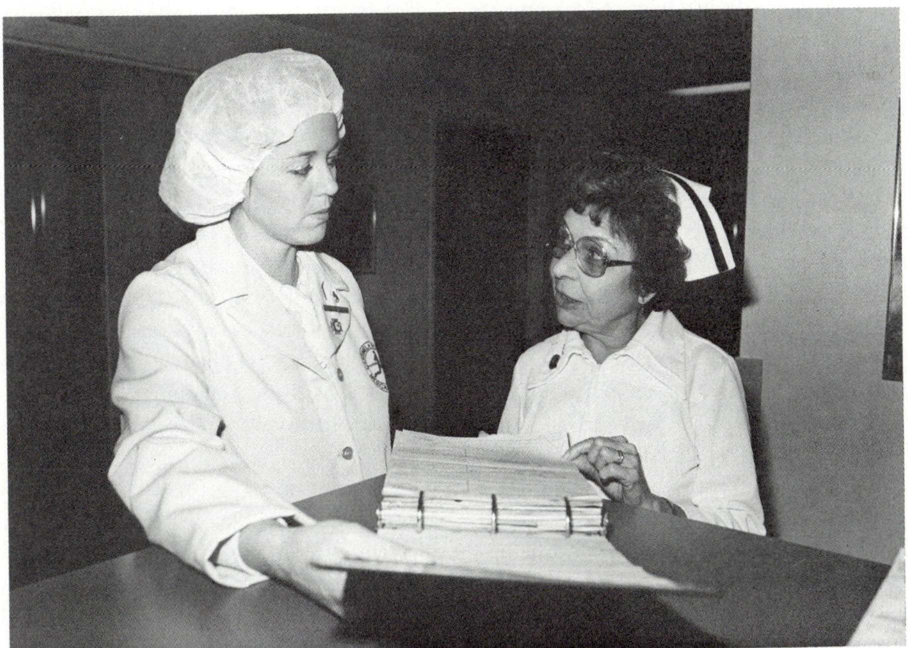

Fig. 1-3. Operating room nurse and unit nurse discuss and plan patient care and preparation for surgery by sharing findings and relevant data.

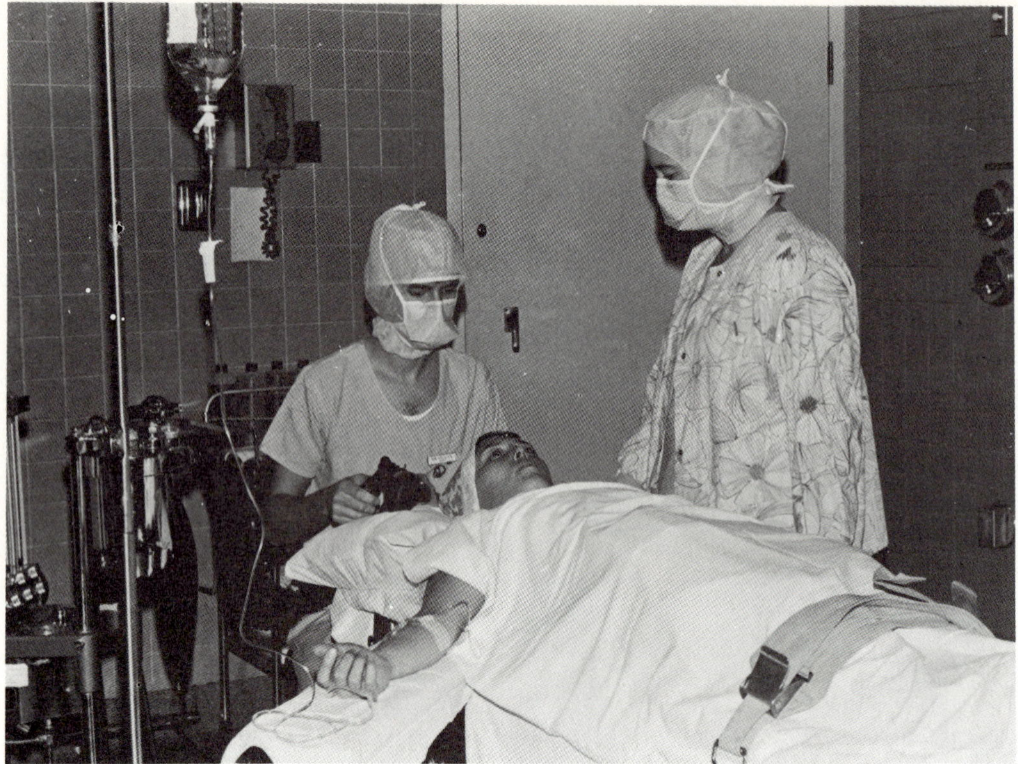

Fig. 1-4. Critical time for each surgical patient is preinduction phase.

The second step in the nursing process is *planning*. Planning means that operating room nurses use their nursing knowledge and information about the patient to accurately prepare the operating room environment. It means checking equipment, having unusual and usual supplies ready, and using knowledge of body area anatomy to have proper instruments and sutures ready. It means knowing the common steps in a procedure and using the surgeon's preference cards and nursing care guides to have the room and equipment ready for the patient.

Planning is knowing ahead of time what is going to happen and being prepared. Planning also requires some knowledge of the patient's reaction to the proposed operation, so that an extra, needed explanation or a comforting hand grasp can be provided during that critical preinduction stage (Fig. 1-4).

Planning also involves a broad understanding of operating room nursing. This means participating in continuing education programs (Fig. 1-5), reading journals, and keeping up to date in the rapidly advancing world of operating room nursing.

Implementation is performing the nursing care that was planned and responding to changes in routine or emergencies with calmness and orderly thinking. It is employing established standards of nursing care and other guidelines developed and maintained by the nursing profession (see suggested readings at end of chapter).

Implicit in implementation is teamwork (Fig. 1-6). Nowhere is a smoothly functioning team of more importance to the patient than in the operating room. Respect for others' expertise, the ability to work harmoniously, and the art of communicating effectively are all necessary ingredients for a well-functioning team. Implementation is being the patient's advocate and carrying out nursing care as a part of a well-defined team in the operating room.

Evaluation, the fourth phase of the nursing process, is checking and appraising the results of what was done. Evaluation of operating room nursing care can be performed through on-the-spot correction of deficiencies and through education to keep personnel up to date on new procedures and equipment. It is also accomplished through quality assurance activities, notably audit, peer review, and problem solving. Resources are available to assist in initiation of these processes.

Many hospitals now have quality assurance programs, which involve many ways of evaluating and improving care, including that given to surgical patients. An operating room nursing audit, for example, should be a part of the hospital's program of quality assurance and should have input from non–operating room personnel, as well as from those directly involved in operating room nursing care. Quality assurance programs identify problems in patient care, propose solutions, and evaluate specified actions in solving the problems.

Evaluation must also include interviews and checks

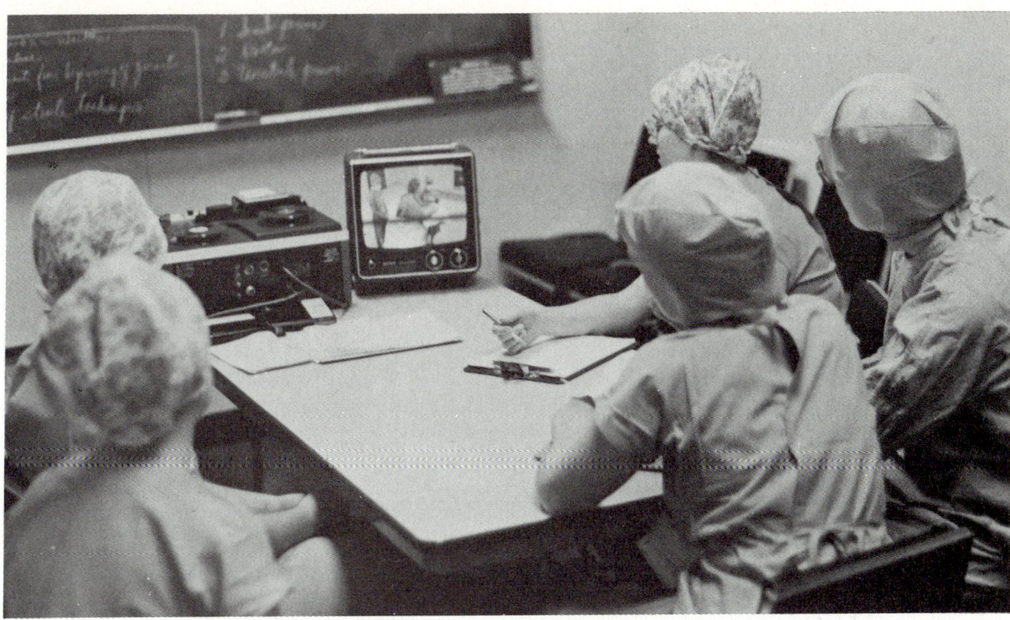

Fig. 1-5. Continuing education is necessary for all operating room nurses. Self-instruction, conferences, and informal discussions are examples.

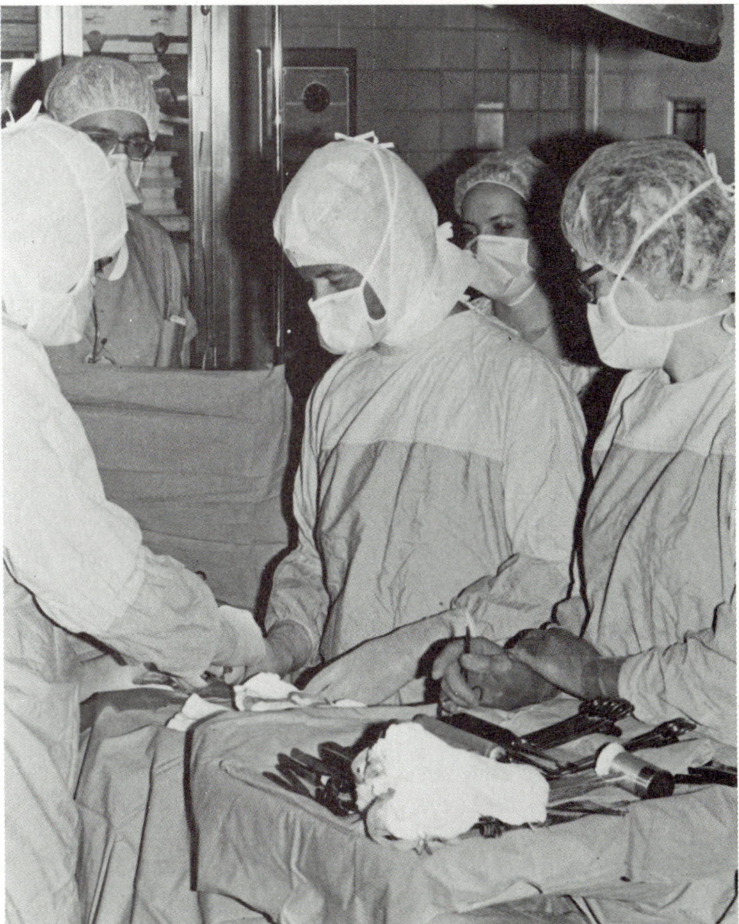

Fig. 1-6. Teamwork in operating room implies collegial relationships, skills, knowledge, and effective communication among members (surgeons, anesthesiologists, and scrub and circulating nurses).

of patients to determine outcomes and reactions to their surgical experiences. Evaluation, then, is a learning process in which both strengths and weaknesses are exposed and examined.

The nursing process is continuous in that evaluation may lead back to assessment. Changes in patient care patterns may require new assessments and plans. The nursing process is never a dead end. It is continuous and always leads to better quality care.

NURSING ROLES

The profession of nursing is in a state of self-evaluation, renewal, and emergence as a strong force on the health scene. Nurses, in addition to many others outside the profession, are incisively questioning the profession's identity, status, and reward system. The triad of nurse-physician-administrator is under positive scrutiny. New roles, new definitions, and new parameters of practice are being explored and tested. Regardless of title and function, every nurse working in the operating room is assuming greater responsibilities and is becoming a colleague of physicians in patient care.

With greater responsibility always comes accountability. Operating room nurses are accountable to their patients and are demonstrating this by the use of standards and auditing and by constantly strengthening their professional skills through education.

As perioperative nursing progresses, new roles will emerge. All of these roles, however, whether staff nurse, clinician, or administrator, will make use of the nursing process and will still mean humanized care for surgical patients and their families. Perhaps a future operating room nurse practitioner role will include assisting during the operation or consulting more with the patients' families. Each new function must be tested with time and integrated into the profession only if it enhances the patients' overall care.

The operating room nurse teaches staff and patients and counsels those who need help in adjusting to a new diagnosis or a changed body image. The operating room nurse always works collaboratively with surgeons and anesthesiologists to plan the best course of action for each patient.

"Scrubbing" and "circulating" may, in the future, become obsolete terms; already we know that these terms define two well-circumscribed functions that are only a part of the operating room nurse's total sphere. The future may bring new names and functions but will never erase the critical function in surgical patient care that every operating room nurse fills.

With this perspective, consider the remainder of this book as one part of the operating room nurse's total knowledge bank. The remaining chapters are intentionally technical and contain vital, basic information needed to function in a surgical setting.

SUGGESTED READINGS

Alexander, C., Schrader, E., and Kneedler, J.: Preoperative visits: the OR nurse unmasks, AORN J. **19:**401, 1974.

American Nurses' Association Division on Medical-Surgical Nursing Practice and Association of Operating Room Nurses: Standards of perioperative nursing practice, Kansas City, Mo., 1981, American Nurses' Association.

Atkinson, L.J., and Kohn, M.L.: Berry and Kohn's introduction to operating room technique, ed. 5, New York, 1978, McGraw-Hill Book Co.

A better way to calm the patient who fears the worst, RN **40:**47, April 1977.

Brooks, S.M.: Fundamentals of operating room nursing, ed. 2, St. Louis, 1979, The C.V. Mosby Co.

Coates, L.: Nursing by assessment, AORN J. **19:**1091, 1974.

Crabtree, M.: Application of cost-benefit analysis to clinical nursing practice: a comparison of individual and group preoperative teaching, J. Nurs. Admin. **8:**11, Dec. 1978.

Dziurbejko, M.M., and Larkin, J.C.: Including the family in preoperative teaching, Am. J. Nurs. **78:**1892, 1978.

Groah, L.: Do patients value preoperative assessments? AORN J. **29:**1250, 1979.

Gruendemann, B.J.: Preoperative group session part of nursing process, AORN J. **26:**257, 1977.

Gruendemann, B.J., and others: Nursing audit: challenge to the operating room nurse, Denver, 1974, Association of Operating Room Nurses, Inc.

Gruendemann, B.J., and others: The surgical patient: behavioral concepts for the operating room nurse, ed. 2, St. Louis, 1977, The C.V. Mosby Co.

Hansen, A.E.: Planning to implement preoperative interviews, AORN J. **30:**792, 1979.

Hoopes, N.M., and McConnell, M.: An approach to preoperative visits, AORN J. **26:**1048, 1977.

Jasmin, S., and Trygstad, L.N.: Behavioral concepts and the nursing process, St. Louis, 1979, The C.V. Mosby Co.

Kneedler, J.A.: Perioperative role in three dimensions, AORN J. **30:**859, 1979.

Koehler, J.S.: Perioperative nursing can be cost effective, AORN J. **32:**1068, 1980.

Lang, N.M.: Quality assurance in nursing, AORN J. **22:**180, 1975.

LeMaitre, G.D., and Finnegan, J.A.: The patient in surgery: a guide for nurses, ed. 4, Philadelphia, 1980, W.B. Saunders Co.

Marriner, A.: The nursing process: a scientific approach to nursing care, ed. 2, St. Louis, 1979, The C.V. Mosby Co.

Nicholls, M.E., and Wessells, V.G., editors: Nursing standards and nursing process, Wakefield, Mass., 1977, Contemporary Publishing, Inc.

Nursing care of the patient in the O.R., Somerville, N.J., 1972, Ethicon, Inc.

Operating room nursing: perioperative role, AORN J. **27:**1156, 1978.

Pesetski, J.D.: A practical guide for perioperative practice, AORN J. **32:**1049, 1980.

Saylor, D.E.: Understanding presurgical anxiety, AORN J. **22:**624, 1975.

Schrankel, D.P.: Preoperative teaching, Superv. Nurse, **9:**82, May 1978.

Walters, J.: Four practical questions to ask when organizing preoperative classes, Am. J. Nurs. **78:**1892, 1978.

Yura, H., and Walsh, M.B.: The nursing process: assessing, planning, implementing, evaluating, ed. 3, New York, 1979, Appleton-Century-Crofts.

2 Administration of operating room nursing services

Operating room nursing care should be administered within the parameters of professional nursing standards. Consumers have the right to quality care within the framework of a contemporary health care system. With the ever-increasing advances in medical, nursing, and technological research and the spiraling of health care costs, operating room nursing personnel are obligated to implement new approaches in the provision of patient care. They should continually develop knowledge and skills associated with new surgical concepts in patient care. Sound administrative practices should facilitate quality care.

The administration of operating room nursing services should be consistent with that of the nursing department and the hospital. Professional management guidelines allow for the establishment and maintenance of good interdepartmental and intradepartmental relationships.

STANDARDS FOR OPERATING ROOM NURSING PRACTICE

The Association of Operating Room Nurses has established standards for operating room nursing practice that can serve as guidelines for measuring the quality of patient care. They are sound principles that are broad in scope, attainable, definitive, and relevant for the operating room. The standards represent a comprehensive approach to meeting the health needs of surgical patients.

AORN and the American Nurses' Association (ANA) have jointly published *Standards of Perioperative Nursing Practice*. These standards pertain to operating room nursing practice and are based on the nursing process. In August 1981, AORN published revised *Standards of Administrative Nursing Practice: OR* to provide guidance for professionals in administrative roles (pp. 9 to 13). Both sets of standards should be used in conjunction with the AORN recommended technical and aseptic practices that are optimum achievable goals toward which operating room nursing personnel should strive.

STANDARDS OF ADMINISTRATIVE NURSING PRACTICE: OR

The Association of Operating Room Nurses believes that professions must regulate themselves and demonstrate accountability to the consumer and other health care professionals. As a professional association, AORN is committed to the development of mechanisms that establish accountability and measure the quality and effectiveness of health care.

Standards are an effective tool for identifying activities that are appropriate in the development of a contemporary health care system. Implementation of professional standards creates an environment that is beneficial to the consumers of health care and to the professionals rendering care. Standards are established through the collaboration of experts in the field of practice, consumers, and other health care professionals.

These administrative standards should be used in conjunction with the Standards of Nursing Practice: Operating Room and the recommended technical and aseptic practices established by AORN. The Standards of Nursing Practice: Operating Room are based on the nursing process and encompass nursing activities of preoperative assessment and preparation, intraoperative intervention, and postoperative evaluation. The recommended technical and aseptic practices are based on principles of microbiology and research and are directed toward providing a safe operating room environment for the patient.

The Standards of Administrative Nursing Practice: Operating Room were developed to guide professionals in administrative roles and to provide a model for evaluating practice. The standards are broad in scope, definitive, relevant, attainable, and subject to ongoing evaluation and revision.

These standards have been developed by the Standards of Administrative Nursing Practice: Operating Room Committee and are intended to assist agencies in establishing administrative practice in their settings. Compliance with these standards is voluntary.

Continued.

Standard I. A philosophy, purpose, and objectives shall be formulated to guide operating room services.

Criteria

1. The philosophy, purpose, and objectives are based on those of the agency and nursing department.
2. The philosophy explains the beliefs of the operating room personnel and determines how operating room personnel will accomplish the purpose.
3. The purpose is a statement that describes the reason for operating room services, and is based on the philosophy.
4. The objectives are realistic and are used to measure the accomplishment of the purpose.
5. Operating room personnel share in the formulation, implementation, and periodic review and revision of the philosophy, purpose, and objectives.
6. The philosophy, purpose, and objectives are distributed and interpreted to the agency administration and medical staff.

Interpretive statement

Realistic, easily understood, and functional statements of philosophy, purpose, and objectives serve as guidelines for operating room services.

Standard II. An organizational plan for the operating room shall be developed and communicated.

Criteria

1. The plan reflects the philosophy, purpose, and objectives of operating room services.
2. The plan identifies the lines of formal authority, responsibility, accountability, and communication within the operating room.
3. The plan describes the relationship of the operating room to administration, medical staff, and other departments.
4. The plan depicts relationships between people and/or functions.
5. The plan is a tool for developing descriptions of functions within the operating room.

Interpretive statement

The organizational plan is an arrangement of functions and resources that contribute to the achievement of the objectives of the operating room.

Standard III. A registered nurse shall be authorized with administrative accountability and responsibility for the operating room services.

Criteria

1. The registered nurse administrator has experience and expertise in perioperative nursing practice. Perioperative nursing is professional operating room nursing during preoperative, intraoperative, and postoperative phases of the patient's surgical experience.
2. The registered nurse administrator is prepared in management and leadership skills through education and experience.
   a. Management skills include but are not limited to the ability to plan, organize, direct, control, and evaluate.
   b. Leadership skills include but are not limited to flexibility, effective communication, and the ability to establish a climate to facilitate group effort.
3. The registered nurse administrator maintains competencies in management practices through participation in continuing education offerings.
4. The administrative responsibilities must be delegated to another registered nurse in the registered nurse administrator's absence.

Interpretive statement

The registered nurse administrator is responsible for the interpretation, direction, and evaluation of nursing practice and the coordination of operating room services through the use of clinical, management, and leadership skills. Registered nurses with these skills must be the managers of operating room suites. They must have the authority to negotiate with other health care disciplines on policy matters.

Standard IV. The registered nurse administrator shall be accountable and responsible for developing mechanisms that assure optimal patient care.

Criteria

1. The registered nurse administrator has responsibility for the identification, interpretation, and implementation of the standards of nursing care.
2. The registered nurse administrator has responsibility for
   a. fiscal management
   b. policy development, implementation, and revisions
   c. integration and coordination of the activities of other health care disciplines in the operating room
   d. management of human, material, and environmental services.
3. The registered nurse administrator interacts with other departments and serves on hospital committees.

Interpretive statement

The registered nurse administrator is accountable and responsible for the integrated management of multifaceted services. Operating room services require management of human resources, fiscal resources, facilities, and material. Optimal patient care is assured through collaboration, communication, coordination, and effective interdepartmental relationships.

Standard V. The operating room management team shall develop and manage the budget for operating room services.

Criteria

1. The budget is developed.
   a. Assessment factors include but are not limited to
      historical data
      changes in patient population
      changes in services offered
      changes in composition of medical staff
      changes in delivery of health care services
      changes in nursing practice
      impact of regulatory agencies.
   b. Fiscal impact of trends is forecast.
   c. The budget is submitted and appropriate approval obtained.
2. The budget is implemented.
   a. An action plan is developed, which should include but is not limited to setting priorities and schedules for the procurement of human resources, equipment, and supplies.
   b. The budget is communicated to operating room personnel, medical staff, and supportive service departments.
3. The budget is monitored and investigated for variances, and corrective action is taken as necessary.
   a. Periodic review of comparative data, including human

resources, equipment, and supply costs related to revenue, is carried out.

b. Results of the periodic review are shared with staff for their contributions to corrective action.

c. Corrective action is taken.

Interpretive statement

Fiscal management is a major administrative nursing responsibility in the operating room. Budget preparation, implementation, and monitoring are paramount to sound fiscal management of the unit. Fiscal management assures the consumer of management's commitment to a balance between cost and quality.

The operating room management team must be aware of current and future technological changes that will have a fiscal impact. Input must be obtained from the agency administration, medical staff, operating room personnel, and supporting departments about trends that could affect the preparation or implementation of the budget for the operating room.

Standard VI. The operating room service shall have written standards of nursing practice.

Criteria

1. The standards are based on accepted standards of nursing practice.
2. Operating room nursing personnel share in the formulation of the standards of nursing practice and interpretation to other disciplines.
3. The standards are implemented, periodically reviewed, and revised to reflect change in nursing practice.

Interpretive statement

The standards provide guidelines for measuring the quality of patient care. They are a means of establishing accountability for care.

Standard VII. The operating room services shall have written policies and procedures that serve as operational guidelines.

Criteria

1. Policies and procedures are written, dated, and enforceable.
2. Operating room personnel share in formulation of policies and procedures and yearly review and revision.
3. Obsolete policies and procedures are removed from the manual. One copy is filed for reference.
4. Policies and procedures for the operating room shall include but are not limited to
   a. operative and special consents
   b. fire and disaster plans
   c. environmental control
   d. visitor and traffic control
   e. safety regulations
   f. infection control
   g. care and disposition of surgical specimens, cultures, and foreign bodies
   h. care of special equipment including preventive maintenance contracts and records where necessary
   i. emergency actions, such as cardiopulmonary resuscitation.
   j. orientation of all personnel entering the operating room.
5. Policies and procedures are approved and interpreted to all appropriate persons.
6. All deviations from established policy shall be documented as directed by the agency.
7. Policy and procedure manuals available to operating room personnel should include but are not limited to
   a. operating room policy manual
   b. operating room procedure manual
   c. personnel policies
   d. agency policies and rules and regulations
   e. anesthesia policies
   f. medical staff rules and regulations.

Interpretive statement

The registered nurse administrator is accountable and responsible for assuring there are clear, concise, and current written policies and procedures. They are used to standardize practices, assist staff, and minimize risk factors.

Standard VIII. The operating room management team shall be responsible for establishing staffing requirements, selecting personnel, and planning for appropriate utilization of human resources.

Criteria

1. Staffing requirements and patterns are determined by
   a. philosophy, purpose, and objectives
   b. complexity of consumer acuity
   c. scope of services
   d. fiscal resources.
2. Selection of personnel is determined by
   a. philosophy and objectives guiding the quality of care to be delivered
   b. hiring policies of the agency and department
   c. job requirements
   d. vacancies
   e. qualifications
   f. availability.
3. The utilization of human resources is consistent with needs of the consumer, the nature of support functions, and agency requirements.
   a. Clinical assignments are based on consumer needs and the competence of the categories of human resources.
   b. Use of personnel is based on identified levels of competency.

Interpretive statement

Staffing is an administrative function. Staffing patterns, selection, and utilization have a direct bearing on the well-being of the consumer, the effectiveness and efficiency of the agency, and the cost of health care. Staffing depends on the size of the agency and the scope of its services.

Standard IX. Staff development programs shall be provided for operating room personnel.

Criteria

1. Orientation programs are established and required for all personnel. Content includes but is not limited to
   a. philosophy, mission, and role of the agency
   b. philosophy, purpose, and objectives of operating room services
   c. policies and procedures of agency and operating room
   d. job descriptions and performance standards
   e. skills assessment.
2. Technical and professional programs and experiences are scheduled based on
   a. identified learning needs of the personnel
   b. need to communicate agency and OR directives, policies, and procedures

c. need to maintain and promote clinical and management competencies.
3. There should be planned learning experiences designed to promote clinical competence.
4. Involvement in career development activities is encouraged and facilitated.
5. Involvement in professional activities is encouraged. This includes but is not limited to
   a. participation in professional organizations
   b. reading professional journals
   c. participation in educational programs and meetings
   d. collegial interchange.

Interpretive statement

Orientation programs assist employees to adjust to the organization, environment, and duties. Staff development programs enhance performance and foster professional and personal growth. Basic or advanced technical and professional programs are designed to develop job knowledge, skills, and attitudes as they affect direct patient care.

Standard X. A safe operating room environment shall be established, controlled, and consistently monitored.

Criteria

1. Technical and aseptic practice guidelines are established, maintained, and periodically reviewed and revised in accordance with AORN recommended practices of technical and aseptic practice for the operating room.
2. Electrical safety is maintained, consistent with accepted agency, regional, and national standards.
3. Occupational safety for personnel is maintained by
   a. safety programs and surveillance
   b. infection control program and surveillance
   c. radiation monitoring and protection
   d. minimizing exposure to toxic substances, infectious wastes, and other hazards
   e. employee health programs.
4. Physical facilities are maintained by
   a. temperature control within acceptable ranges
   b. humidity control within acceptable ranges
   c. adequate air circulation and filtration system
   d. proper maintenance of air filtering system
   e. fire alert systems
   f. constantly monitored gas systems
   g. constantly monitored vacuum system
   h. automatic auxiliary power system
   i. electrical safety monitors.
5. Guidelines and regulations not limited to the following are used in determining and monitoring operating room safety
   a. governing boards
   b. licensing agencies
   c. National Fire Protection Association
   d. Joint Commission on Accreditation of Hospitals
   e. Occupational Safety and Health Administration
   f. US Department of Health and Human Services
   g. Environmental Protection Agency
   h. American National Standards Institute
   j. manufacturers' equipment manuals.

Interpretive statement

A safe, comfortable, therapeutic operating room environment is maintained for patients and health care providers.

Standard XI. The operating room management team shall promote the discovery and integration of new knowledge by encouraging development of and use of nursing research.

Criteria

1. Operating room nursing management recognizes its professional responsibility to expand the knowledge base in perioperative nursing.
2. Operating room nursing management affirms the value of nursing research by encouraging staff to initiate, promote, and support nursing research projects.
3. Research studies are conducted in accordance with the American Nurses' Association ethical standards of nursing research.
4. Operating room nursing management facilitates the application of research findings to perioperative nursing practice, education and administration.

Interpretive statement

Research is increasingly important in perioperative nursing. Continual development of a scientific body of knowledge is fundamental to improving practice and the quality of service offered to clients.

Standard XII. The operating room staff shall maintain appropriate documentation related to OR activities.

Criteria

1. Perioperative nursing care is documented on the patient record as outlined in *Recommended Practices for Documentation of Perioperative Nursing Care.* (See recommended practices in the March 1982 *AORN Journal.)*
2. An operative record is maintained for each patient that includes but is not limited to
   a. patient's name
   b. patient's agency number
   c. date and times
   d. surgeon(s)
   e. anesthetist
   f. assistant(s) to surgeon
   g. scrub person and circulating nurse
   h. preoperative and postoperative diagnosis
   i. operative procedure
   j. wound status
   k. implants
   l. specimen and disposition
   m. complications.
3. Records are maintained to provide statistical data that include but are not limited to
   a. the numbers, types, and duration of operative procedures
   b. utilization of operating room, manpower, supplies, and equipment
   c. environmental controls
   d. infection control.
4. The operating room administration and medical record department maintain and control records for the length of time required by the agency and legal statute.
5. Minutes of meetings are maintained.
6. Current personnel performance records are maintained.
7. Confidentiality of records is established by the agency and legal statute.

Interpretive statement

The responsibility of the operating room management team includes the assurance of appropriate documentation of activities. A record of perioperative care, which becomes a part of the patient's permanent record, is documented. Records maintained for statistical data are used to determine increases or decreases in speciality activity for future budget and special agency requirements. Personnel records are maintained for current employees that include staff development activities and pertinent chronological entries regarding the individual's achievement of established performance standards.

Standard XIII. The operating room management team shall recognize a professional responsibility to promote, provide, and participate in a learning environment for students in health care disciplines.

Criteria

1. A written agreement is made, as appropriate, with each educational provider seeking to use the agency or staff.
2. There is ongoing collaboration with faculty and the learner to facilitate the achievement of educational objectives.
3. The safety and welfare of the consumer must be maintained while providing a controlled learning experience for students.

Interpretive statement

The operating room offers health care students a clinical laboratory where they can experience a variety of activities not performed elsewhere. This experience is essential to their understanding the trauma of surgery, the care required to ensure the safety of the anesthetized patient, the necessity for proper patient preparation, interdisciplinary team functioning, stress management, and the application of medical-surgical asepsis. Use of the operating room for these student experiences must be controlled. This experience will broaden the competencies of the beginning health care practitioner, promoting higher quality patient care.

Standard XIV. There shall be a quality assurance program for operating room services.

Criteria

1. An ongoing review process of nursing practice in the operating room is established and documented. The goal of this review is to assure optimal achievable care for the consumer.
2. Continued competence in meeting performance standards is assured by ongoing personnel performance appraisal.
3. The safety and cost effectiveness of purchased goods and services are assured by ongoing multidisciplinary product evaluation.
4. A safe, comfortable, and therapeutic environment is assured the consumer and personnel through
   a. adherence to guidelines and regulations established for operating room safety.
   b. ongoing monitoring of the facility.
5. The optimal use of human, facility, and fiscal resources is assured through periodic evaluation of
   a. staffing patterns
   b. scheduling methodology
   c. case load distribution
   d. provisions for emergency care
   e. facilities utilization
   f. budget review.
6. The plan of action is developed, implemented, and monitored.
7. The quality assurance program for the operating room interfaces with and supports the agency's quality assurance program.
8. A confidentiality policy guides how quality assurance information is reported and stored and which qualified individuals will have access to it.

Interpretive statement

The quality assurance program in the operating room is flexible and encourages innovative approaches to patient care. The activity begins with the identification of real or potential problems. The identification may be accomplished through many activities, such as audit procedures, peer review, committee meetings, staff meetings, review of incident reports, and patient or staff surveys or comments. The problems are resolved through a plan of action. This plan of action includes an assessment of the problems through data collection, comparison of findings to acceptable standards, and recommended changes. Following the assessment, problems are ranked according to their impact on patient care. Once implemented, the change is closely monitored through a review process. A positive outcome is permanently incorporated into standard operating procedures. Negative outcomes warrant identifying and selecting other alternatives to correct the problem.

PHILOSOPHY, PURPOSE, AND OBJECTIVES OF OPERATING ROOM NURSING

Philosophy

A written statement of operating room nursing philosophy describes values and beliefs that pertain to nursing practice in the operating room department and serves as the basis for choosing the means to accomplish objectives. It formalizes nurses' visions of what practice is believed to be. Philosophy statements are certain value statements about people as patients or workers, about work that will be performed by nurses for patients, about nursing as a profession, about education as it pertains to competence of nurses, and about the setting in which nursing services are provided. The philosophy of operating room nursing should blend with that of the hospital and the department of nursing, the general and specialty surgical programs, and appropriate educational and research programs.

One philosophy of operating room nursing service may be summarized as follows:

1. Operating room nursing is a dynamic, behavioral, and highly technical process directed toward provision of quality patient care during surgical intervention.
2. Operating room nursing service comprises distinct functions concerned with a safe physical environment and protection of patients, with continuous awareness of the dignity of humans and their physical and spiritual needs.

3. Operating room nursing service promotes knowledge and skills of its members as a means of meeting scientific and technological progress in the health care field.
4. Operating room nursing service continually adjusts its organization and functions in accordance with current health and educational programs.

The philosophy defined by the professional operating room nursing staff should be approved by the department of nursing.

Purpose

Every nursing department exists for a reason. The reason for existence is the purpose or mission of the department. Just as the department of nursing has a purpose, so should the operating room. The purpose should be stated in writing and be developed or revised in participation with operating room nursing personnel who are governed by it. It should be known and understood by them. A meaningful statement of purpose indicates the relationships between the operating room nursing service and patients, personnel, the nursing department, and the hospital.

A statement of purpose of operating room nursing might include the following:

1. To plan and provide perioperative nursing care that is consistent with standards for professional nursing practice as defined by the professional nurses of the staff and by the ANA/AORN *Standards of Perioperative Nursing Practice*
2. To collaborate and cooperate with other members of the health care team in meeting the emergency, restorative, and preventive health needs of patients in a safe, comfortable, and therapeutic environment

Objectives

The objectives of operating room nursing service should be practical, specific, and measurable for the persons performing nursing functions. They should be detailed statements supporting the defined philosophy and employing the nursing process. Effective objectives are developed and changed in accordance with overall institutional policy through the cooperative efforts of the director, supervisors, and other members of the staff. Frequently, difficulties arise in the delegation, coordination, and establishment of standards in the absence of unified objectives.

In developing objectives, the professional nursing service group should consider the following factors:

1. Overall objectives of the department of nursing should be the core around which the operating room nursing staff members work.

2. Objectives should be written in positive "doing" terms to help all staff members achieve them. For example, the operating room department may initiate a nurse internship program or an open heart surgical program. The objectives should clearly state the overall functions of the groups concerned, the limits of authority, and the managerial and training functions of the various group members.

3. Objectives should provide for assignment of duties to permit personnel to perform at the highest potential and provide a means for the staff members to broaden their knowledge base.

4. Objectives should be reasonable, attainable, and measurable in the light of existing and foreseen conditions, such as availability of trained personnel, facilities, operating time scheduled, and operational costs.

5. Overlapping of objectives within the institution should promote cooperation between group members and coordination between departments. From the institutional aspects of operating room nursing, the housekeeping department has similar objectives concerning the prevention and control of infection.

6. Objectives should be written for, freely available to, and understood by all personnel. A positive attitude on the part of the administrator, supervisors, head nurses, and employees is essential to the fulfillment of the objectives. The nursing staff should be encouraged through daily conferences and training programs to help set measurable goals to meet the objectives.

7. Objectives should be reviewed and revised periodically.

Following are sample objectives of operating room nursing:

1. To provide quality intraoperative nursing care that is professionally planned and implemented
2. To provide nursing personnel who are knowledgeable, effective, and efficient in meeting the individual needs of the patient during surgical intervention
3. To provide a safe and therapeutic environment for patients and personnel
4. To provide proper equipment and supplies for all operative procedures
5. To evaluate and revise nursing standards in accordance with current nursing practice
6. To provide educational opportunities that encourage individual motivation and growth

PURPOSE OF ORGANIZATION

An organization may be defined as a framework within which people in various groups perform certain jobs. Formal organization theory rests on several major principles: that the division of work is essential for efficiency, that coordination is a primary responsibility of management, that the formal structure is the main network for organizing and managing the various activities of the institution, and that the span of supervision sets outside limits on the number of subordinates a manager can effectively supervise. One of the responsibilities of an institution is to advance the level of managerial performance.

Centralization or decentralization

Evidence seems to indicate the need for both centralization and decentralization in fitting the parts of an organization together. The balance between them becomes a managerial decision. Trends influencing centralization are the size of the units, capital costs of consolidating expensive equipment in one area, operational costs (locating specialized services in one unit rather than in several functional areas), and use of mechanized administrative tools such as computers.

The advantages of decentralization are quicker decisions, administrative development, reduced levels of organization, and the freeing of supervisors to concentrate on broader responsibilities. Decentralization provides for flexibility and better communication within the group involved.

Specialization in medicine, nursing, and administration also affects the organizational structure. Because of expanding specialization in surgery, nursing personnel must select certain independent functions and delegate other functions to the allied health group members. For both management and professional roles, specialization involves learning one thing in depth. Surgeons achieve excellence of performance through intensive training in narrow segments of their potentialities. In the same vein, nursing personnel achieve excellence of performance through intensive training in their particular specialties. Thus the dynamic content of an organization is provided by people who have the capacity to function as generalists, by people who are specialists, by other combinations of internal groups, and by external environmental forces.

In dealing with the processes of change, it is important that nursing supervisors accept the concept that not everything is controllable. In adopting this principle, one can begin to gain a proper perspective of the managerial aspects of the position. This is done by asking what is controllable and by seeking to discover what has to be controlled.

A dynamic nursing department provides for the following: (1) safe, continuous, and therapeutic patient care; (2) an effective communication system to facilitate flow of instructions and information through the vertical and horizontal lines of the organizational structure; (3) a system for collecting and recording current facts concerning the quality and the quantity of services rendered; (4) a smooth, economical, effective procedure of operation; and (5) a demarcation of responsibilities and authority that states in detail the *line* and *staff* responsibilities of groups for obtaining instructions, reporting facts, appraising situations, and taking decision-making actions.

Organizational chart

An organizational chart is a static diagnostic statement of formal relationships between groups who act to achieve the established objectives in a specific situation. The chart should show the pattern of administrative control in an orderly manner, linking together the different levels of responsibility and authority (Fig. 2-1).

The most common format for hospital organizational charts reflects the hierarchical chain of command from the top down. The levels of authority are shown vertically. Each employee has an immediate superior who is delegated to give orders and guidance. The organizational chart is meaningful only if the depicted system is a reality.

The term *line responsibility* stems from the chain of command that is transferred from the top administrator down the line of assistants, supervisors, head nurses, and staff nurses to other individual employees. Line functions consist of action-producing duties on the job.

The term *staff responsibility* within the diagonal structure may be advisory in nature, or it may be a direct responsibility delegated by the controlling body to a committee, to an administrative professional group, or to an individual within the organization. The medical, administrative, and nursing groups have both line and staff functions within an organization. For example, the director of surgery has professional supervisory relations and direct responsibility relations for the care of patients. Through staff responsibilities, the professionals work as a team to meet the needs of patients and to elevate the standards of patient care. In appraising care, they may make recommendations for improvement of patient care services to the infection control committee, to the director of a service, to the administration, or to the faculty curriculum committee of an educational program. It is extremely important to clarify the position of all staff advisors; otherwise confusion within the organization will arise. This confusion will tend to negate the usefulness of their advice.

Committees

Horizontal coordination of activities results between departments and other professional groups within the hospital hierarchy.

The *committee* or *conference* structure of the hospital and department should not perform functions that can be performed by established departments for which individuals can be held accountable.

There are advantages and disadvantages of committee action. Advantages of committees are that they (1) disseminate information and ideas, (2) provide for integration of ideas, (3) deter quick decision-making actions, (4) provide for coordinated action by individuals having line and staff responsibilities, and (5) broaden individual viewpoints pertaining to a specific problem or plan. The disadvantages of committee action are (1) difficulty in achieving control of action, (2) time consumed to achieve general agreement of the group, (3) difficulty in getting members to attend, especially when emergency decision-making action is needed, (4) difficulty in appraising results because of diffusion of responsibilities within the group, and (5) decreased quality of decisions because of compromised consensus.

Within a department in the hospital, committees—administrative, advisory, judicial, executive, and others—combine a number of functions and characteristics. Organizationally, a committee may have line or staff responsibility. A line or staff committee may be delegated decision-making or enforcement responsibilities established by the governing board. For example, the administrative supervisor of the operating room department, as a member of the steering (executive) nursing service committee, has a staff responsibility for decision-making in accordance with the established functions of the committee. The administrative supervisor of the operating room, because of line responsibility, may become a staff advisor as a member of the operating room committee.

A formal or standing committee has a permanent place in the organizational structure of the hospital and department. The informal, temporary, or special ad hoc committee does not have a permanent place in the organizational chart. It is appointed to collect and analyze data and make recommendations. When the charge is completed, the ad hoc committee is discharged. In developing or revising the committee structure, the following factors should be considered: (1) establishment and statement of the purposes of each committee, (2) determination of the rules and regulations pertaining to selection and tenure of members and their responsibilities to provide effective functioning, and (3) approval of the committee structure by the governing board.

Meetings

The three major types of meetings are informational, advisory, and problem-solving. Before a meeting is scheduled, several decisions must be made regarding (1) the purpose of the meeting; (2) who should attend, always considering their responsibility and authority; (3) who should conduct the meeting; and (4) how it should be conducted.

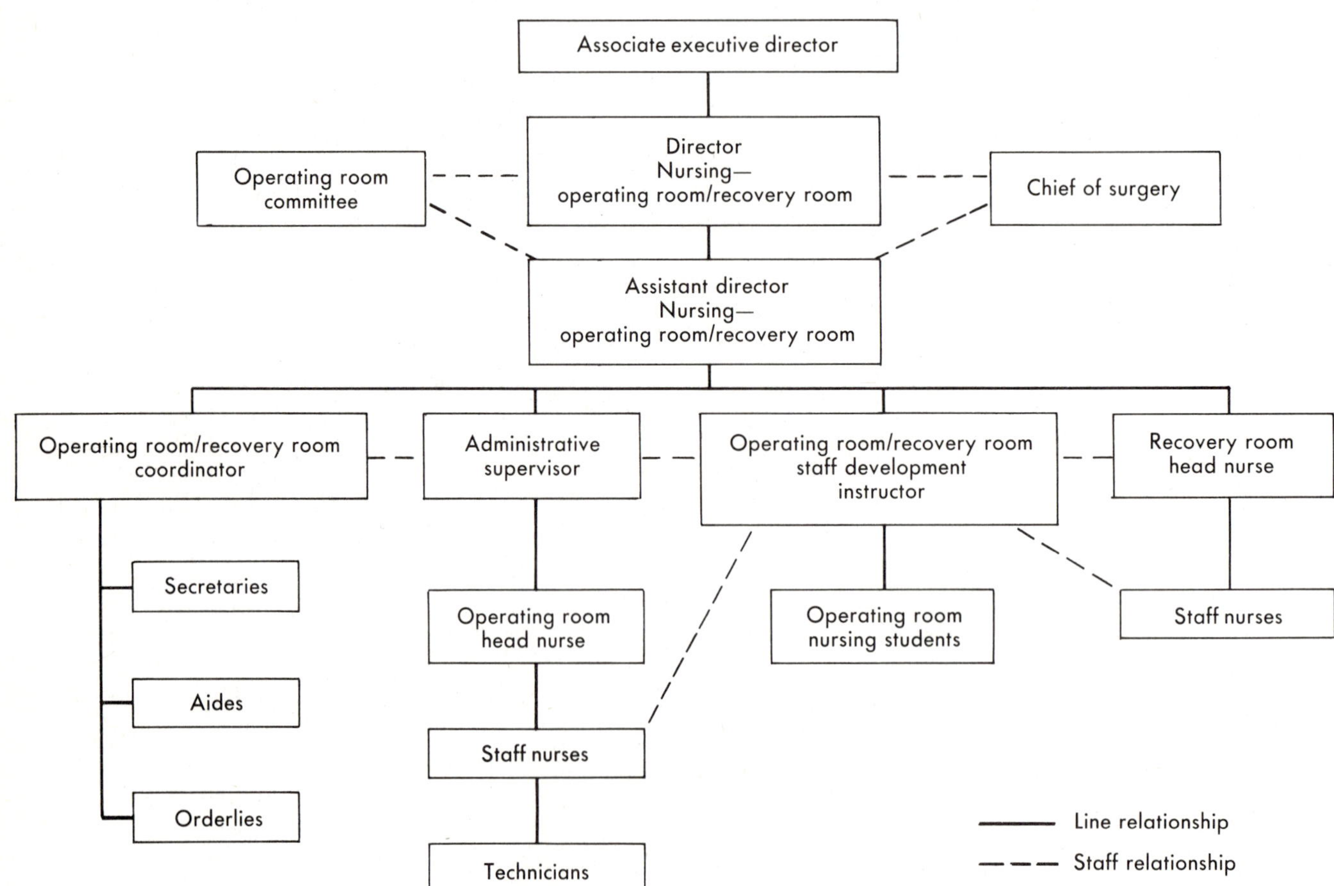

Fig. 2-1. Organizational chart of operating and recovery rooms, demonstrating line and staff responsibility in decentralized nursing department.

ELEMENTS OF PROFESSIONAL MANAGEMENT

The highest efficiency in organized nursing services is obtained by providing the necessary quantity of nursing staff of the desired quality, at the required time, and in the most economical way.

Management is a process of actions with a common goal. It is the process of planning, organizing, directing, and controlling all activities of the department. The integrated function of management is coordination.

Planning is the process of formulating in advance the direction a department intends to follow in fulfilling its stated objectives. It is largely conceptual, but there is visual evidence that it occurred. Planning includes the prior determination of who is to do a task and when and where it is to be done. It is within this management function that proper selection and training of a staff takes place.

Organizing involves arranging the various components of any unified effort—the people, tasks, and materials necessary for putting plans into operation. The purpose of the organizing function is to correlate these elements so that they are oriented toward executing plans and meeting objectives. For managers to successfully fulfill the function of organizing, six essential steps in the process must be considered: (1) establishment of objectives, (2) identification of tasks, (3) logical grouping of tasks, (4) assignment of employees, (5) delineation of authority and responsibility, and (6) establishment of authority and responsibility relationships. Organizing enables a manager to develop order, promote cooperation among personnel, and foster productivity.

Directing is the complex managerial function concerned with the supervision of employees as they perform their assignments. Directing is doing things through others. A manager is actively involved with the human factor in the directing process. To accomplish the objectives of the department, the nursing manager must deal with conflict and motivate and discipline staff. All these tasks require good communication skills, assertive behavior, and positive motivation.

Controlling is seeing that plans that have been developed are carried through to completion. The basic steps in this management function are (1) setting standards, (2) measuring performance against these standards, (3) reporting the results, and (4) taking corrective action.

Coordinating requires that the manager possess the ability to integrate the functions of planning, organizing, directing, and controlling into a unified process. It is appropriately described as the overall function of management (Fig. 2-2) and, as such, requires effective leadership skills.

The nursing manager should be knowledgeable regarding the range of leadership behavior available, the

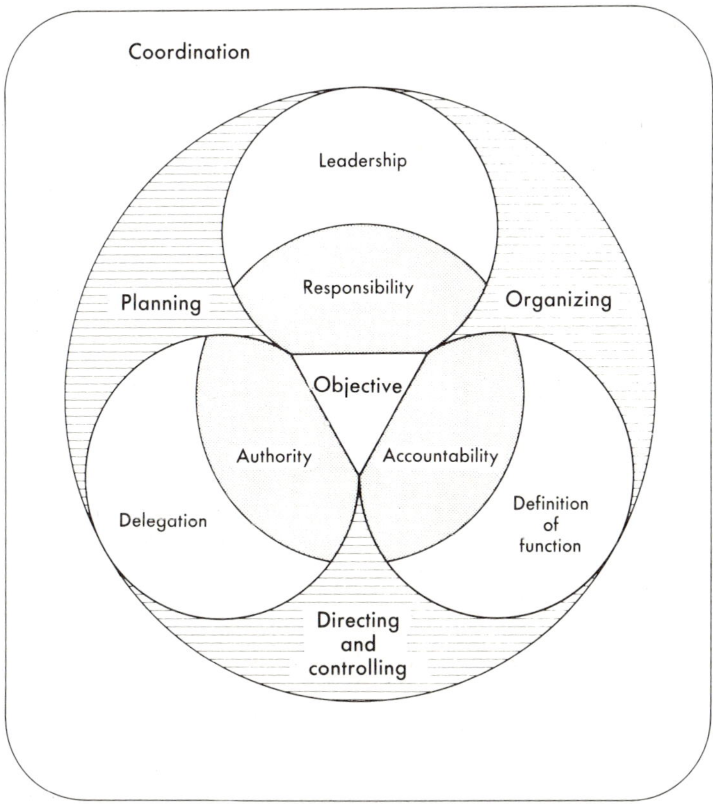

Fig. 2-2. Management functions. (From Arndt, C., and Huckabay, L.M.D.: Nursing administration: theory for practice with a systems approach, ed. 2, St. Louis, 1980, The C.V. Mosby Co.)

priority responsibilities of the management role, and the nature of the forces influencing action. Leadership should not be stereotyped as either forceful or permissive but viewed as a process consisting of a range of possible alternative behaviors. The effective manager chooses a behavioral alternative appropriate to the demands of each task encountered.

The executive level in the professional nursing hierarchy determines the time and resources to be spent in different functions. Many lesser decisions should be made at the first-line supervisory level because this is the level at which the details of a situation are known.

DEVELOPING JOB DESCRIPTIONS FOR OPERATING ROOM NURSING POSITIONS

Terminology

In preparation for job analysis and the resultant job description, the staff should know common definitions and understand terminology.

A *task,* or duty, is a unit of work or human effort exerted to achieve a specific purpose. Examples are checking identification bands of patients, checking patient charts to ensure the safety of each patient, and assembling surgical instruments in a metal sterilizer tray. When a sufficient number of similar tasks have developed, a position is created for one person.

A *function* is a group of closely related tasks (duties) that logically fall into a unified unit of work for the accomplishment of a responsibility delegated to a staff member or a department. An example is to plan, organize, and control the staffing pattern to ensure effective use of personnel in meeting the nursing care needs of a group of patients. This function comprises several tasks performed by the clinical nursing supervisor or head nurse.

A *position* is a collection of tasks and responsibilities rendered by one staff member who is delegated to perform specific functions.

A *job* refers to a group of positions that involve the same duties, skills, knowledge, and responsibilities.

A *job description* is a written statement of the requirements, major duties and responsibilities, and organizational relationships of a given position.

The *job specification* sets forth clearly and specifically the qualification requirements. It includes the degree of education, the amount of previous experience in similar work, and the skill required, as well as physical requirements.

Job relationships refer to the interrelatedness of other staff members within and outside the department who have similar duties or joint responsibilities to achieve specific objectives.

Job analysis is the study of a position to determine knowledge, skills, aptitude, and personal characteristics needed to successfully perform the responsibilities. Ultimately, the job analysis determines minimum job requirements and sets standards for such factors as education, experiences, and personality. An effective job analysis program is dependent on several important factors, as follows:

1. The individual who performs the job analysis should have the ability to get along with people and be able to express ideas effectively in an analytical manner.
2. The program must be planned in detail, as much as is possible.
3. The program must be approved and supported by the administration.
4. The personnel concerned must understand the purpose and mechanics of the program.
5. The supervisory staff must review the collected data.
6. The analyst must observe and interview the personnel, write the first draft, review it with the supervisory staff, and then revise the draft until it is accepted by the department head.

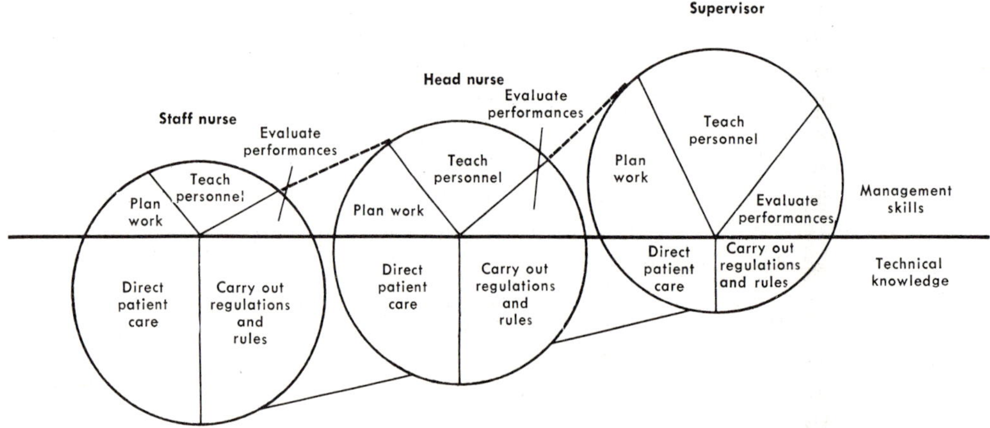

Fig. 2-3. Allocation of functions and responsibilities of staff nurse, head nurse, and supervisor in relation to planning of work, teaching, direct patient care, and rules and regulations.

Job descriptions

Job descriptions should be current, accurate, and realistic. The title of the job indicates the major responsibilities and sets the job apart from others. The job description should be a complete but not detailed summary of primary job duties. Duties should be arranged in a logical order and stated concisely in action terms. Job descriptions help prevent overlapping of duties and subsequent conflict and frustration. They play an important part in performance evaluations and in decisions concerning promotions and salary rates.

The professional nurse, regardless of position in the nursing service hierarchy, performs clinical, managerial, and operational nursing duties. In the upward progression of the hierarchy, clinical leadership duties increase and operational (performance) duties decrease (Fig. 2-3). The functions of the administrative supervisor involve almost entirely clinical leadership duties. Many operating room nursing departments have implemented a manager/coordinator program to coordinate nonnursing functions.

The number and type of positions required to meet the nursing care needs of patients in the operating room depend on the size and complexity of the surgical services offered to patients.

POLICIES AND PROCEDURES

The governing board of the institution delegates to the medical board the responsibility for the medical treatment of patients and to the hospital personnel, through the executive administrative staff, clearly defined functions and lines of authority concerned with meeting the needs of patients.

A policy may be defined as a written statement that explains how goals will be achieved and defines the general course and scope of activities permissible for goal achievement. A procedure may be defined as a guide to action that enumerates the chronological sequence of steps needed to accomplish a task.

Medical staff policies

Policies pertaining to dependent functions of the medical staff are formulated by a representative committee and are recommended to the administrative staff for approval by the governing board. Many policies and rules relate to the interdependent functions of medicine and nursing. The medical, hospital, and nursing administrative staffs have joint responsibilities in formulating overall policies related to therapeutic aspects of patient care.

Administrative policies and procedures

The objectives of administrative policies and procedures are to protect patients and personnel from injury and to meet medical and sanitation codes; local, state, and federal government laws; and the Standards for Hospital Accreditation of the Joint Commission on Accreditation of Hospitals. The laws concerning negligence, legal obligations, and grounds for liability may vary from state to state. The policies should interpret the existing laws that affect the hospital, patient, and personnel.

Nursing administrative manual

The nursing administrative manual should include the philosophy and objectives of nursing, the qualitative nursing standards to meet patient care needs, procedures for the control of equipment and supplies, quantity standards, budgetary information (costs and expenditures), organizational chart, committee structure of the department and related departments, and personnel policies. In some hospitals, the personnel policies, including job descriptions, master staffing plan, and performance appraisal format, may be in a separate personnel policies manual.

The in-service education manual should include the purpose, content, methods of instruction, hours, and length of the program for orientation of various categories of personnel; on-the-job training; and leadership staff development.

Operating room policies and procedures

Written policies and procedures must be available to all personnel who provide patient care in the operating room. This information should be maintained in a readily accessible manual that will facilitate uniform interpretation and administration of policies and procedures. The manual should be reviewed annually and revised as often as needed to meet the changing standards of practice.

Policies and procedures affecting operating room personnel should be formulated by representatives of the groups concerned with the delivery of patient care in this area. The operating room committee (surgical committee) serves in a staff capacity and recommends policies and procedures affecting the therapeutic aspects of patient care. The membership of the committee should consist of representatives from the following departments: surgery, anesthesia, hospital administration, operating room nursing, and others appropriate to the individual hospital.

The operating room policy and procedure manual should include but not be limited to the following:

1. Safety of patients and personnel
   a. Fire regulations
   b. Safety regulations
   c. Infection control
   d. Incident reports
   e. Disaster procedures
   f. Handling of nuclear materials
2. Admission of patients
   a. Identification of patient
   b. Laboratory tests and other diagnostic procedures
   c. Consent for surgical procedures

3. Records
    a. Operative record
    b. Anesthesia record
    c. Tissue examination request form
4. Surgical and aseptic techniques
5. Care and handling of instruments and equipment
6. Sponge, needle, and instrument counts
7. Administration of narcotics
8. Care and disposition of surgical specimens
9. Postmortem care
10. Visitor and traffic control
11. Surgical staff privileges
12. Personnel policies
    a. Dress code
    b. Attendance
    c. Vacation
    d. Performance appraisals
    e. Promotion
    f. Sick leave, maternity leave of absence, and personal leave of absence
13. Public relations

Most operating rooms have separate procedure manuals or cards that enumerate surgeons' preferences of instruments, sutures, supplies, and equipment for each type of operation.

Operating room personnel should participate as members of committees or conference groups to improve operating room nursing practices and their own knowledge and skills. They should also serve as representatives on nursing and hospital committees.

Scheduling policies and procedures

Clearly defined scheduling policies and procedures promote effective and economical services to patients and provide all surgeons with equitable opportunity to use the facilities. Factors affecting scheduling include the following:

1. Scheduling of operations should be under the control of one scheduler.
2. A deadline for scheduling elective operations should be strictly adhered to.
3. Specific facts must be obtained:
    a. Patient's name and age
    b. Surgeon's name
    c. Type and classification of procedure (elective or urgent)
    d. Estimated operative time
    e. Units of blood required
    f. Type of anesthesia
    g. Date and time requested

A system of measurements and controls should be initiated to enhance the daily effectiveness of the scheduling policies. Data should be collected at periodic intervals concerning the following: (1) the variations of actual numbers of operations per week from predicted scheduling policies; (2) the total hours of actual operating room time used, showing the range between maximum and minimum hours used each week; (3) the average setup time and the average terminal cleanup time; and (4) the unused operating room time, resulting from variations in the schedule or improper observance of rules.

Collection and analysis of data assist management personnel in determining methods by which to decrease excessive expenditures for staffing and equipment that result from the practice of staffing based on maximum for existing case load rather than on the expected demand for services.

SUGGESTED READINGS

Alexander, E.L.: Nursing administration in the hospital health care system, ed. 2, St. Louis, 1978, The C.V. Mosby Co.

American Nurses' Association Division on Medical-Surgical Nursing Practice and Association of Operating Room Nurses: Standards of perioperative nursing practice, Kansas City, Mo., 1981, American Nurses' Association.

Armstrong, D.M.: Nursing administration expectations of O.R. leader, AORN J. **25:**859, 1977.

Arndt, C., and Huckabay, L.M.D.: Nursing administration: theory for practice with a systems approach, ed. 2, St. Louis, 1980, The C.V. Mosby Co.

Association of Operating Room Nurses: Standards of administrative nursing practice: OR, AORN J. **34:**268, 1981.

Brockenshire, A., and Hattstaedt, M.J.: Revising job descriptions: a consensus approach, Superv. Nurse **11:**16, March 1980.

Carter, K.A.: Managerial role development in the nursing supervisor, Superv. Nurse **11:**26, July 1980.

Cox, C.L.: Decentralization: uniting authority and responsibility, Superv. Nurse **11:**28, March 1980.

Creighton, H.: Law every nurse should know, ed. 4, Philadelphia, 1981, W.B. Saunders Co.

Douglass, L.M.: The effective nurse: leader and manager, St. Louis, 1980, The C.V. Mosby Co.

Grubb, R.D., and Ondov, G.: Operating room guidelines: an illustrated manual, St. Louis, 1979, The C.V. Mosby Co.

Marriner, A., editor: Current perspectives in nursing management, St. Louis, 1979, The C.V. Mosby Co.

Marriner, A.: Guide to nursing management, St. Louis, 1980, The C.V. Mosby Co.

Mauksch, I.G., and Miller, M.H.: Implementing change in nursing, St. Louis, 1981, The C.V. Mosby Co.

Phippen, M.L.: Power: what nursing schools never taught, AORN J. **33:**650, 1981.

Stevens, B.J.: The nurse as executive, Wakefield, Mass., 1980, Nursing Resources, Inc.

Swansburg, R.C.: Planning: a function of nursing administration (pt. 1), Superv. Nurse **9:**25, April 1978.

Swansburg, R.C.: Planning: a function of nursing administration (pt. 2), Superv. Nurse **9:**76, May 1978.

3 Design of the surgical suite

Although the renovation of old hospitals and the building of new ones continue, the restraints by federal control are a fact of current hospital planning. These restraints are imposed to contain costs, to avoid duplication of services, and to maximize use of operating rooms and all other hospital facilities.

Surgeons and operating room personnel are frequently requested to provide advice on a new surgical suite. The purpose of this chapter is to outline an approach to a thoughtful analysis of surgical suite design by operating room nursing personnel. It includes consideration of systems analysis, suite and operating room configuration, environmental control, and safety. The end result of these factors must be an operating room suite that will effectively facilitate provision of quality patient care. However, too often it is a compromise because costs, prejudices, and outdated building codes cause the best plans to be altered. Health Systems Agencies (HSA) established under Public Law (PL) 94-370 have become a determining factor in planning all new facilities by controlling expenditures and number of operating rooms and imposing regulations with respect to methods and specifications of construction.

Approach to the analysis

The request for an analysis by operating room nursing personnel is usually initiated by the architect through the hospital and nursing administrators. However, the nursing division may be consulted only after the fact, for example, after plans have been drawn by the architect and approved by the hospital administration or renovation and building committees. This is unwise. It is crucial that operating room nursing management be involved in the planning from inception. Few surgeons or administrators are familiar with all aspects of the daily process by which the operating suite functions. Initiative, assertion of the right to advise, and well-defined proposals promptly submitted are necessary if a functional, technologically efficient, and cost-effective new surgical suite is to meet patient and nursing needs.

To begin the analysis, consider the following: Is any major demographic shift within the community anticipated? Is the local health systems agency considering restrictions on specific functions and services, such as open heart surgery? What new surgical technology is expected during the next 10 to 15 years? Will certain services require additional surgical beds to accommodate growth? Will additional surgical specialties be added? What changes can be anticipated in relation to the provision of inpatient versus outpatient surgery? What is the total of planned or present acute care beds? About 2.5% of the total number of acute care beds is a reasonable estimate of the number of operating rooms required. Using this information, determine the requirements necessary to perform the type and number of surgical operations anticipated.

The second consideration is the materials-handling systems in use. If a renovation of existing facilities is planned and the central supply section will be unchanged, the flow and work patterns of personnel may be dictated, in part, by the way materials enter and leave the suite. Include an analysis of instrument processing, sterilization systems, storage of supplies and equipment, decontamination methods, and delivery systems.

The third consideration is the needs of the persons involved: patients, nursing personnel, surgeons, anesthesiologists, and ancillary staff. Lack of in-depth analysis of the characteristics of surgical personnel, actual human activity patterns, and time-efficiency data has resulted in dissatisfaction with new or renovated facilities. Analysis depends, in part, on the organization of surgical suite nursing personnel. If personnel are assigned to specific surgical services in which duties and responsibilities are fairly constant and well defined, suggestions should come up the line through each head nurse to the administrative supervisor and then to the director of the surgical suite. Studies should be made of the activity patterns of each operating room team. Inefficient movement results in slower case turnover and increased costs.

OPERATING ROOM SYSTEMS

Once the general requirements for the performance of surgery in the community and hospital have been considered, the analysis may be carried into more detail and specificity by reducing the surgical suite activities into four major systems: traffic and commerce (activities), surgical support systems (physical environment), communication and information (record), and administration (management). These systems are discussed throughout the remainder of this chapter.

Traffic and commerce

Specific traffic patterns for patients and personnel must be determined. These are dependent on the entrances and exits to the suite. Renovation planning of existing facilities should consider renovation of central supply and storage areas to bring these as close to the point of utilization as possible. Where entirely new wings, buildings, or hospital complexes are being considered, there is opportunity to design traffic patterns, materials-handling, and storage systems around the requirements of the surgical suite.

Traffic control design should address movement into and out of the suite, as well as movement within the suite. A three-zone concept clearly designates one area from another. The three zones are the unrestricted area, the semirestricted area, and the restricted area. Individuals in street clothes (outside traffic) are permitted in the unrestricted area. This zone permits limited access for communication with department personnel, hospital personnel, and patients' families. The semirestricted area may have a blend of inside and outside traffic, mixing individuals in street clothes with personnel in scrub attire. The locker rooms, the surgical scheduling office, and the operating room supervisor's office are examples of this intermediate zone. Places at which inside and outside traffic meet are often designed with a barrier. For example, in the scheduling office, contact may be limited to visual and auditory interaction by a window or Dutch door. Operating room attire is required in the restricted zone, which is limited to inside traffic. This area includes the operating rooms, substerile rooms, scrub rooms, instrument processing area, and supplies storage area. The operating room control office may be in any one of the three zones but should be adjacent to the locker rooms to aid in monitoring personnel traffic into and out of the restricted area. This point is often used for collecting messages and transmitting information between operating room personnel and outside areas.

Patients should be transported into, through, and out of the surgical suite by the most direct route that prevents cross-contamination and protects them from potentially upsetting sights and sounds. Patients are transported from their rooms on carts or beds and may be transferred to a clean or "inside" cart on entry into the restricted area. Several problems are inherent with this transfer. The safe transfer of certain patients, such as one immobilized by traction, would be impossible. A logistical problem occurs when several patients arrive at the transfer point at the same time. When a patient is being transported out of the suite immediately after surgery, the additional movement could be painful or hazardous. Undoubtedly, keen assessment of the patient and good judgment must determine if the transfer can be safely and expeditiously accomplished. A meaningful decrease in environmental contamination has not been documented with the transfer process. A scheduled program of frequent floor cleaning and cleaning of stretcher wheels and frames should diminish any threat of environmental contamination from "outside" carts.

Commerce in the surgical suite refers to the movement of reusable and disposable supplies, equipment, laundry, and trash. The location of the instrument and supplies processing area must be determined before any other planning for a new or renovated surgical suite takes place. Transfer of processing to a central area outside the surgical suite is occurring more frequently in hospital design. It is essential to study the patterns of instruments and supplies usage at the onset. The original concept of central processing suggested that all surgical instruments be removed from the surgical suite. However, many hospitals that have instituted this process have revised the system and, by necessity, have returned certain types of instruments to be processed and stored within the surgical suite.

An efficient materials-handling system is critical to effective use of the surgical suite. Materials-handling systems are often difficult to integrate into the desired traffic pattern. Three options are available: a horizontal system in which all materials-handling is on the same floor, a stacked or vertical system in which materials travel by elevator or dumbwaiter or a combination of the two. The decision as to which system to use may be determined by vertical versus horizontal construction costs, the degree of automation of the material delivery systems that will be employed, and the cost of storage of disposables as opposed to reusable items. Conveyor systems can be time saving and cost effective, even though mechanical problems may occur.

Traffic patterns for clean and sterile supplies and equipment should be separated by space or time from those employed for soiled items and waste. External packing containers must be removed before materials are transported to the surgical suite. Sterile and clean supplies should be delivered to and transported within the surgical suite in containers or vehicles that protect the integrity of the items. Soiled materials and equipment should be handled according to the AORN recommended practices for operating room sanitation.

The proximity of ancillary services within the hospital to the operating room suite can have a significant impact on the amount of time a patient is in the operating room. Such services include those of the x-ray and pathology departments, the various laboratories, and the blood bank. Careful planning of physical facilities should facilitate expeditious movement between the operating room suite and these areas.

Surgical suite design

Suite design is dictated in part by the number of operating rooms required. In hospitals with 100 beds or less,

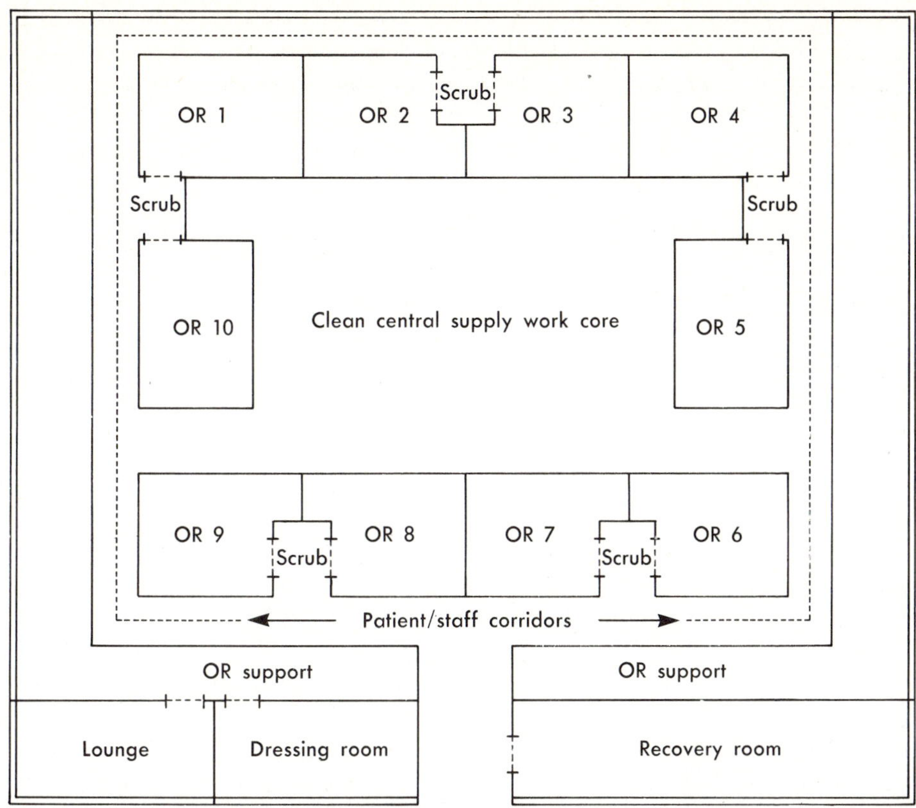

Fig. 3-1. Peripheral corridor design. (Adapted from Chvala, C.: OR supervisor's role in planning the surgical suite, AORN J. **23:**1242, 1976.)

many functions (sterilization, storage, delivery) can be carried on within the same area of the surgical suite. The single-corridor or L-shaped designs are applicable for two or three operating rooms and support areas. In hospitals with a capacity of from 500 to 600 beds, twelve to fifteen operating rooms will be required, and the double-corridor, U- or T-shaped suites are more suitable. In larger hospitals, all these have been used, as well as the cluster, circular, or rectangular patterns with either central core and radial distribution or the peripheral corridor plan. However, the peripheral corridor scheme tends to be more expensive because of excessive corridor space. The large passageway becomes a storage area for movable equipment. Two designs are illustrated (Figs. 3-1 and 3-2). The peripheral corridor design incorporates the operating rooms around a central supply area with a patient/staff corridor around the outer perimeters. The basic modular design has four operating rooms with a system of peripheral patient/staff corridors and a central supporting internal core. This modular approach is the most flexible because identical modules can be added with little disruption.

In both these designs, the flow of supplies is from the clean core area through the operating rooms to the peripheral corridor. Soiled materials should not reenter the clean core area. Soiled linen and trash collection areas should be separate from personnel and patient traffic, if possible. If instruments and other supplies are partially or totally reprocessed within the surgical suite, a unidirectional traffic pattern should ensure movement from decontamination area to processing and storage. Work areas for each task should be clearly identified to eliminate crossover or mixing of soiled and cleaned instruments or supplies. When planning a central processing system for operating room instruments and supplies, it is wise to keep fragile instruments and high-cost, low-volume items within the surgical suite. To facilitate appropriate processing of these items, a decontamination area and a processing area must be located in the suite.

Three basic faults frequently found in newly constructed surgical suites are poorly designed traffic patterns, inefficient materials handling, and insufficient, poorly organized storage space. A common misconception among hospital and operating room designers is that a large central supply area negates the need for storage within the surgical suite. A quick perusal of any suite reveals multiple pieces of equipment that must be kept within the department. With ever-continuing technological advances in surgery, an increased volume of equipment can be anticipated. Concurrently, backup supplies and instruments must be available in the suite for unanticipated needs that arise in even the best planned system of surgical supplies

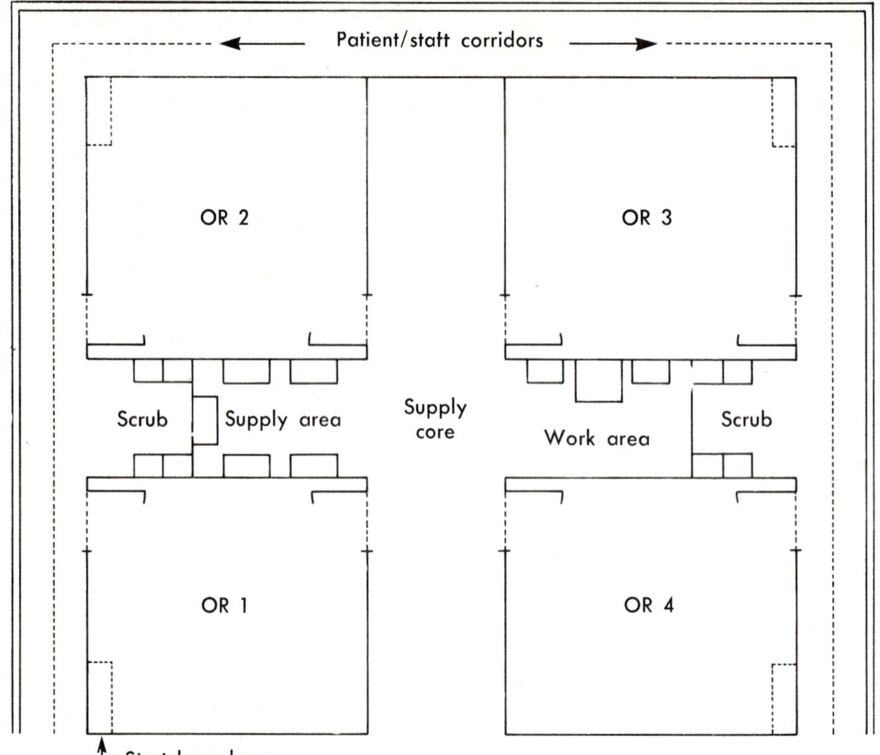

Fig. 3-2. Basic modular design. (Adapted from Chvala, C.: OR supervisor's role in planning the surgical suite, AORN J. **23:**1243, 1976.)

management. These supplies and equipment should be stored as closely as possible to the point of use to facilitate quick retrieval. Specialty service carts containing unique and frequently needed specialty items provide a convenient, easily accessible mode of storage. In-depth analysis of operating room functioning and thoughtful planning can eliminate or reduce the problems that frequently occur in newly constructed surgical suites.

A preoperative patient holding area should be provided in the design of a new or renovated suite. It should be located near the main entrance of the suite and have a quiet, restful atmosphere. Here the patient receives preoperative medications and the incisional site is shaved, if required. Intravenous therapy is initiated, and the chart is checked to ascertain that all requested diagnostic tests have been completed and results recorded. The proximity of the holding area enables the operating room nurse to perform an immediate preoperative assessment of the patient and alter the plan of intraoperative care if warranted. The surgeon and anesthesiologist visit the patient and, in many suites, transport the patient to the operating room. Use of a holding area is psychologically advantageous to the patient and reduces preparation time in the operating room.

Outpatient surgery facilities

Large-volume outpatient surgery facilities are becoming increasingly more common because of escalating costs of inpatient hospital care, limited numbers of beds, and the convenience to patients and their families. Careful consideration of present and future community needs and direction of hospital growth must be made before planning such a facility. Outpatient surgery facilities have been integrated into major operating room facilities or have been built as separate, economically self-sustaining units. The advantages of the integrated suite are the consolidation of staff, equipment, and supplies; the delivery of quality care and sterile technique by a knowledgeable staff; the convenience to the surgeon of being able to go from surgical outpatients to inpatients without changing clothes and violating traffic flow; and the use of these outpatient operating rooms for inpatient surgery when there are no outpatients.

Outpatient surgery facilities require special considerations because most patients are fully awake on entering the facility. Traffic design is highly important; the most successful facilities have a one-way traffic pattern. The outer clerical and waiting area should have a warm and friendly atmosphere that provides a sense of security. A patient preparation room should be provided in a clean area. This room should have privacy and should permit changing of clothes, skin washing, and access to toilet facilities. Entrance to the operating room should be direct and protective, so that the previous patient is not seen. After the operation, the patient is taken to a recovery, or observation, room. Some independent facilities provide overnight rooms. When ready for discharge, the patient dresses and leaves the facility without retracing any steps. Double-doored lockers that open on one side in the admission dressing room and on the other in the discharge dressing room facilitate one-way traffic flow. Special attention must be given to the psychological aspects of surgical care by consideration of color, excessive noise, privacy, music, and conduct of operating room and recovery room personnel.

Operating room design

Operating rooms have been built in a myriad of shapes, but the rectangle or square remains the most practical and flexible and the least expensive. Ovoid and multifaceted rooms have not offered significant advantages over simpler designs that lend themselves to modular and prefabricated constructional techniques.

There is controversy about the ideal size of an operating room. A 400–square foot area is satisfactory except when procedures require extensive peripheral equipment such as a heart-lung machine. Open heart procedures may require as much as 600 square feet of usable space. Similarly, endoscopy, cystoscopy, and outpatient minor surgical rooms require half the floor space. Thus a modular unit system can be devised that will accommodate each need by halving or doubling the basic unit for special applications.

The interior of the operating room has specific requirements for environmental control. Ceilings and walls should be nonporous, smooth, easy to clean, waterproof, and fire resistant. Soundproofing is preferable. Ceiling heights should be approximately 10 feet to accommodate ceiling-mounted surgical lighting fixtures. Where possible, there should be a 4-foot space between the ceiling and the next floor to facilitate maintenance. Room lighting should be flush-mounted in the ceiling and should have prismatic lenses and fixtures solidly grounded for elimination of transient radio frequency interference.

High-impact vinyl materials and flexible wall coverings, together with new adhesives, permit completely sealed wall, ceiling, and floor joints so that the surfaces may be washed with microbicidal cleaning solutions. Tile walls are not desirable because most grout lines are porous and can harbor microorganisms.

All cabinets, view boxes, and receptacles should be recessed. Wall-mounted shelves and cabinets and freestanding storage cabinets are being used less and less because of difficulty in cleaning and maintaining supplies. The trend is toward a cart system by which mobile units may be easily supplied and cleaned on a consistent basis.

No windows should be installed in the operating rooms because of critical need for precise illumination during surgery and energy-saving requirements. However, personnel should have access to natural light in corridors or lounges. Several authors have reported that persons confined in an artificially lighted environment for an extended period of time may become fatigued more readily, lose vitality, and be less attentive.

Floor coverings must have the same requirements as the wall surfaces but, in addition, must be highly wear resistant. Conductive flooring is not required where flammable anesthetic gases are prohibited.

Sliding doors should be used in the operating room to eliminate air turbulence caused by swinging doors. A marked increase in microbial counts is noted when swinging doors are opened or closed. Doors should be of the surface-sliding type, if possible, so that all surfaces may be washed. Fire regulations require that the doors be capable of being swung open if necessary. All door frames should be a minimum of 5 feet in width.

Color requirements of the ceiling, walls, doors, and floors are few. Obviously, the chosen hue must be generally acceptable. Most new surgical suites are using warmer tones rather than the cool white or green traditionally used. Similar or the same color hues throughout give a sense of increased space.

Certain surgical specialties require consideration of special needs. For example, flush-mounted snap-lock water connections for the heart-lung machine, x-ray facilities, space for neurocryosurgery, and special outlets for air-powered equipment may be required. Some specialties use fiberoptics, a laser apparatus, or special built-in television or cine cameras. Each service should be consulted for any anticipated specific needs that require preparation, operation, or maintenance by nursing personnel.

An increasing number of operating room suites are being designed to facilitate the use of computers in the monitoring of patients, in obtaining diagnostic data and calculations, in surgical scheduling, and in the ordering of supplies. Hospital designers plan for computer terminals to be directly accessible to specially trained individuals who can interpret the data in the operating room.

Surgical support systems

Environmental design aids in the control of surgical infections. Temperature should be controlled at between 20° and 24° C (68° and 75° F) and humidity at a minimum of 50% to aid in the control of bacterial growth and the suppression of static electricity. New operating rooms should have at least twenty-five room air exchanges per hour, five changes of which should be fresh air. High-efficiency particulate air (HEPA) filters are being used routinely in many conventional operating room ventilation systems. Dispersion of inlet air should come from vents in the central portion of the ceiling, and return air exhaust ducts should be located in one or more walls. Slightly less air is exhausted than is introduced to create positive pressure within the room. Positive pressure is created to prevent potentially contaminated air from entering the operating room from adjacent areas. This mandates keeping the doors to the operating room closed at all times other than patient entry and exit. Without the use of HEPA filters, conventional operating room air may contain as many as 10 to 15 bacteria per cubic foot and as many as 250,000 particles per cubic foot. The level of airborne bacterial contamination increases as the number of personnel in the operating room increases.

High-flow unidirectional ventilation

The use of laminar airflow systems in the operating room has been a source of controversy since its implementation by the aerospace industry in the early 1960s. Laminar airflow is described as the flowing of air at a uniform velocity along parallel flow lines within a confined area. The term *laminar flow system* is actually a misnomer when applied to operating rooms because of the air turbulence created by the operating room team and objects in the room. A more accurate description is *high-flow unidirectional ventilation system*. In designing a clean air system, it is essential to properly plan the use of the surgical area so that turbulence of airflow is reduced and does not occur over the surgical site. A volume of 500 to 600 room air changes per hour may be achieved through an entire wall or ceiling covered with HEPA filters. When the filters are not plugged or damaged, they will filter out all particles down to 0.3 microns, or macrovirus size. Although a definitive relationship between airborne contamination and surgical infections is not universally agreed on, there is little question that clean air systems reduce bacterial contamination of the surgical wound at the time of operation. It is known that wound infections are directly related to the type and number of organisms that are deposited in the wound and the host's ability to combat infection. Airborne contamination plays a more important role when a prosthesis is implanted into a surgical wound than when no foreign body is implanted.

In summary, high-flow unidirectional ventilation systems provide a cleaner operating room environment and may reduce the potential for infection in certain procedures in which prosthetic materials are employed. Of far greater importance in the control of wound infections is meticulous surgical technique, strict maintenance of sterile technique, preoperative elimination of clinical and subclinical infection in the patient, containment of the surgical team through the use of barrier gowns and proper operating room attire, reduction of activity within the operating room, and control of traffic into and out of the room.

Operating room lighting

Lighting is an important aspect of the operating room environment. An effective lighting system should provide ambient room lighting that complements the operating task light. General room illumination should be a minimum of 200 foot-candles uniformly distributed with provision for reducing the level. To minimize eye fatigue, the ratio of task light intensity to general room lighting should range from 3:1 to 5:1. These light levels should also be maintained in the adjacent corridor and scrub rooms to facilitate more rapid visual accommodation as the surgical team approaches the surgical field.

A variety of surgical task lights are available today; most are designed for use by all surgical specialties. Since different surgeons may perform various procedures in the same operating room, each surgeon should review the specifications of a lighting system to see if individual requirements are met. The Illuminating Engineering Society recommends that a surgical lighting system provide a minimum of 2500 foot-candles at the center of a 10-inch circle on the illuminated surgical field that is 42 inches from the lower edge of the lamp cover or reflector. At the periphery of the circle 500 foot-candles is desirable.

Diverse surgical exposures require that the main beam of light be capable of coming from a variety of directions. Gimbal-mounted lights appear to have more versatility and mobility than do track-mounted lights. Movement of track-mounted lights may shower dust on the surgical field, since the tracks are difficult to clean thoroughly. The direction of many surgical lights can be controlled either by the circulating nurse or by the surgeon by way of a sterile handle. The latter practice is subject to criticism because of the questionable maintenance of sterility of the handle.

Shadow reduction is an important consideration when choosing a surgical light. Theoretically, the shadowing effect can be minimized by providing a sufficiently diffuse number of light sources to bypass the heads and hands of the surgical team. Surgical lights produce heat at the source and at the point where the light strikes. Some lighting systems reduce the heat problem through multilayer reflectors or glass lenses.

Perception of the color of tissue is determined by the character of the tissue as well as the light reflected from it. Although no tests have documented the color of light that is best for the performance of surgery, most surgeons prefer light at about 5000° K, which is approximately the color of noon sunlight. Other factors to consider when evaluating a surgical light are mobility, stability, and memory.

An increasing number of surgeons are employing fiberoptic head lights to enhance surgical task lighting, especially in small or deep incisions.

Safety design

Safety design incorporates features that prevent or control the potential of infection, flame, explosion, and electrical hazards. Methods for infection control have already been detailed. Well-devised traffic patterns, materials-handling systems, and disposal systems; strict adherence to aseptic technique; containment of shedding through proper attire; positive-pressure and well-dispersed clean ventilation; and high-flow unidirectional ventilation systems for special applications all contribute to a safe surgical environment. Flame and explosion hazards have decreased significantly in recent years as a result of the use of nonflammable anesthetics. Electrical hazards continue to be a problem.

Currently, problems revolve about the grounding systems and the increasing use of electronic monitoring. If a voltage exists between any two electrical conductors touching the patient, an electrical current will flow. This can lead to ventricular fibrillation and sudden death. Although they are no longer required, some operating rooms have isolated electrical systems referenced to a common ground. The maximum point-to-point resistance of the systems should be less than 50 milliohms. Each isolated power system must have a continually operating line isolation monitor that indicates possible leakage or fault currents. Most monitors have a green signal lamp that remains lighted when the system is isolated from ground. A red signal lamp and an audible warning signal are energized when a ground fault is detected.

The static electricity hazard is greatly reduced with control of the humidity at a minimum of 50% and the use of nonflammable anesthetics. The extensive use of electronic monitoring for cardiac patients has led to wider application of its use in all surgical specialties. The electrocardiogram is electively monitored in most routine operations. Electronic measurement of vascular pressures requires the use of voltage in most pressure transducers. Damaged transducers can cause current flow in the patient and result in disaster. Thus special attention must be directed to rooms that will require special engineering to yield a safe environment for the surgical patient.

Communications system

The third system to consider in design is the communications system. An analysis of the number of telephone lines required both to the control desk and to the surgical suite administrative offices is necessary. A reliable intercommunications system is required from each operating room to the control desk and from there to the blood bank, operating room director's office, recovery room, intensive care unit, and surgical pathology, x-ray, and central supply departments. Pneumatic tube systems have been of value as an accessory supply and communications network in some suites, although there is potential hazard of environmental contamination.

Administration

The last major system in the delineation of surgical suite activities—administration—is discussed in Chapter 2.

SUMMARY

An approach to analysis of the requirements of a surgical suite in terms of systems, materials, and human needs has been outlined. Specificity of design can be determined with consideration of the four major surgical suite systems: traffic and commerce, surgical support systems, communication and information, and administration. Specific suite design depends on the number of operating rooms involved. Single-corridor and L-shaped configurations are most applicable to suites with two or three operating rooms, whereas the double-corridor T and U shapes are more appropriate for twelve to fifteen operating rooms. The peripheral corridor-modular design has become popular in large suites. The principal faults found in newly constructed surgical suites have been poorly designed traffic patterns, insufficient storage areas, and inefficient materials-handling systems. The rectangular- or square-shaped operating room has been found most useful; an average unit size of 400 square feet is required. Specialty rooms may require half to twice the unit size. Uniform size and shape aid in cost control in construction. All interior surfaces must be washable. Conventional tile walls are not recommended. Doors should be of the sliding type, and floors need not be conductive if flammable gases are not used. The unique needs of specialty operating rooms are emphasized. Environmental design includes consideration of highly filtered center ceiling air distribution with at least twenty-five room air changes per hour. Relative humidity should be closely controlled at a minimum of 50% with the temperature between 20° and 24° C (68° and 75° F). The effectiveness of high-flow unidirectional ventilation systems in the prevention of surgical wound infections has not been proven. Gimbal-mounted surgical lights are suggested, as is appropriate room illumination to prevent sharp contrast of lighting zones. Safety design has been emphasized to reduce the potential of electrical hazards to the patient.

The most important concepts in renovating or designing an operating room suite are infection control, safety, flexibility and efficiency of operation, capability of expansion, and accessibility to ancillary hospital services. Operating room nursing management, the architect, surgeons, anesthesiologists, and administrators should all be part of the team who designs the suite.

SUGGESTED READINGS

Association of Operating Room Nurses: Proposed recommended practices for operating room sanitation, AORN J. **33**:1263, 1981.

Association of Operating Room Nurses: Recommended practices for traffic patterns in the surgical suite, AORN J. **35**:750, 1982.

Beck, W.C.: Choosing surgical illumination, Am. J. Surg. **140**:327, 1980.

Beck, W.C.: Lighting systems. In Laufman, H., editor: Hospital special care facilities, New York, 1981, Academic Press, Inc.

Beck, W.C.: Operating room illumination: the current state of the art, Bull. Am. Coll. Surg. **66**(5):10, 1981.

Department of Health, Education, and Welfare: Minimum requirements of construction and equipment for hospitals and medical facilities, DHEW publication no. (HRA) 79-14500, Washington, D.C., 1978, U.S. Government Printing Office.

Doody, L., and Payne, W.P.: Revamping surgical suites to latest standards, Dimens. Health Serv. **57**(3):13, 1980.

Hinshaw, J.R.: The art and the science of O.R. management, Bull. Am. Coll. Surg. **66**(5):6, 1981.

Kapsar, P.P.: Case cart systems: yea or nay? AORN J. **30:**58, 1979.

Kaufman, J., editor: Illuminating Engineering Society handbook, New York, 1981, The Society.

Keep, P.J.: Stimulus deprivation in windowless rooms, Anaesthesia **32:**598, 1977.

Klebanoff, G.: Operating room design: an introduction, Bull. Am. Coll. Surg. **64**(11):6, 1979.

Laufman, H.: Airflow effects in surgery, Arch. Surg. **114:**826, 1979.

Laufman, H., editor: Hospital special care facilities, New York, 1981, Academic Press, Inc.

National Fire Protection Association: National electric code, NFPA code no. 70-1978, Boston, 1978, The Association.

National Fire Protection Association: Safe use of electricity in patient care areas of hospitals, NFPA code no. 76B, Boston, 1980, The Association.

National Fire Protection Association: Standard for the use of inhalation anesthetics, NFPA code no. 56A, Boston, 1980, The Association.

Nelson, C.: Environmental bacteriology in the unidirectional (horizontal) operating room, Arch. Surg. **114:**778, 1979.

Schneiderman, H.B.: Building a new surgical suite, AORN J. **30:**35, 1979.

Schultz, J.K.: Does windowless O.R. environment affect behavior? AORN J. **30:**26, 1979.

Schultz, J.K.: O.R. wall material: is there a choice? AORN J. **29:**1222, 1979.

Schultz, J.K.: Traffic and commerce in the surgical suite. In Laufman, H., editor: Hospital special care facilities, New York, 1981, Academic Press, Inc.

Thomas, R.: Unidirectional flow vs. traditional system, AORN J. **31:**722, 1980.

Tornello, J.: When I build my O.R.: dream and reality, AORN J. **30:**44, 1979.

4 Procedural and environmental safety

The increase in the number and size of health care facilities, the overlapping of departmental functions, the complexity of organizational structures, and the current stress on professional standards have all emphasized the need for a complete policy and procedure manual. Numerous intrinsic hazards can be prevented, reduced, and controlled through this method of consolidated guidelines. This manual will assist personnel in the delivery of quality health care.

Policies and procedures are designed to ensure the safety of patients and personnel and to provide a setting in which all activities of the surgical team and ancillary personnel fit together, resulting in an efficient course of action for the benefit of each patient. Organizational structure, delegation of responsibilities, and authority of staff members are considered in Chapter 2.

SAFE ENVIRONMENT

People, rather than equipment, are the real obstacles to the creation and maintenance of a safe environment. Incidental to this factor is the architecture of a hospital and surgical suite. The design of a surgical suite in terms of systems, materials, and human needs is described in Chapter 3. The design incorporates physical and mechanical means of reducing and controlling infection in the suite.

The cause and effect of infectious microorganisms and basic principles of sterilization, disinfection, and aseptic technique are described in Chapter 5.

Administrative control measures

The operating room nursing staff actively participates with the hospital administrative and medical staffs in creating and maintaining standards, usually through scheduled meetings with the operating room, infection control and safety committees.

Each nurse should understand the professional, legal, and ethical responsibilities to each patient as established by the Nurse Practice Act of each state.

Records and forms

The operating room policy and procedure manual should contain current and accurate directions to protect patients and personnel. Protection of patients' personal, moral, and legal rights begins at the time of admission. The course of action involves correctly identifying patients, safeguarding their right to privacy, and keeping confidential all records and reports. Conditions of admission to the hospital and consent forms for treatment or operations are important records that protect both the patients and the persons who render care to them.

The hospital administration provides appropriate forms that are legally acceptable. Personnel who obtain consents or witness them should be aware of the conditions that ensure validity and their personal responsibility to appear in a court of law if necessary. It should be recognized that a signed consent must also be an informed consent, which implies adequate communication with the patient regarding the procedure for which the consent is being signed. No surgical procedure should be performed without a signed and witnessed informed consent. The surgeon is responsible for informing the patient about the proposed operation, inherent risks, and complications. The ultimate responsibility for obtaining consent is the surgeon's. All consent forms must be signed before the administration of preoperative medications. On the patient's arrival in the operating room, it is the responsibility of the circulating nurse and the anesthesiologist to ensure that the consent is on the chart, is correct, and is properly signed and witnessed.

Special permits for specific operations, such as sterilization, therapeutic abortion, disposal of severed members of the body, and autopsy, provide additional safeguards for patient, staff, and hospital. In case of a death in the operating room or recovery room, the nursing policy manual should state the course of action to be carried out in regard to informing the hospital authorities, notifying physicians and family, referring to the medical examiner, and so forth.

The Joint Commission on Accreditation of Hospitals requires that a record be kept of each operation, including the nature of the surgery performed, the preoperative and postoperative diagnoses, and the name of the personnel participating in the patient's care. The record should also indicate the results of sponge, needle, and instrument counts and the presence of drains. The operative and anesthesia records become a permanent part of the patient's chart.

Admission of the patient

The operating room policy and procedure manual should contain the admission procedure and delegation of responsibilities. The major facts of the admission procedure should include the following:

1. The operating room nurse should review the patient's identification and chart. Information on the patient's identification band, the chart, and the tag on the stretcher or bed should be accurate and identical with patient's name, hospital number, room number, and physician's name.

2. The operative consent form, history, and physical and laboratory examination results should be complete. The controlling body of the institution determines which examinations are mandatory as part of the patient's preoperative preparation. These usually include completed records for physical examination, health history, recent determinations of blood and urine, and chest x-ray examination. The administration should provide a checklist of required medical admission records for reference by the staff in the admission of patients. This tool aids in preventing oversights and omissions in routines designed to protect patients and staff. A preoperative checklist is also helpful for intramural reporting when a patient is transferred from his room to the operating room department. Any allergies or previous unfavorable reactions to anesthesia or blood transfusions must be carefully noted.

3. The patient should be examined for personal effects, including clothing, money, jewelry, wigs, religious symbols, and prostheses such as dentures, lenses, glass eyes, and hearing aids. The nurse is responsible for ensuring their proper disposition and safety.

4. The operating room nurse should review the orders and results concerning nutrition and elimination, such as enema given and amount of urine voided or catheterized. It is important to determine the condition of an infusion and whether preoperative dietary and fluid restrictions have been maintained. Aspiration of gastric contents during anesthesia induction is a danger. Every precaution should be taken to prevent such an accident by ensuring that the suctioning apparatus is functional and by having personnel present to assist the anesthetist.

5. The nurse should chart meticulously any fluids, blood, or plasma administered as ordered during the immediate preoperative period.

6. The nursing staff should apply side rails and/or restraint straps on beds, carriers, and operating tables to prevent falls and injury to the patient during transportation, transfer, and positioning.

7. Peace of mind and reassurance are within the gift of nursing personnel in their care of and concern for the patient. By judicious use of *directions* and *self*—assuming a calm, confident manner and a quiet voice; using gentle, precise movements in execution of activities; and providing spiritual assistance on request—the nursing staff member can help the patient face surgery with some equanimity.

Safety measures

All operating room and recovery room personnel participate in the hospital safety program. At least one member of the operating room department should be a member of the hospital safety committee. Each staff member should be prepared to carry out special duties in the care of patients in an emergency situation and in natural or man-made disasters. Periodic review of duties, fire drills, and safety education programs should be initiated. All personnel should be aware of the daily hazards peculiar to operating room activities and working conditions.

Minimizing human error helps eliminate hazardous conditions. In the operating room, where the patient is relatively helpless, nursing personnel must be always alert.

The failure to communicate vital medical information to the surgical team members could be dangerous to the patient. An allergy identification band prevents the administration of drugs or the use of materials that would evoke a sensitive reaction in the patient. Pertinent data on the chart alone may not be sufficient, since the chart is often read by various members of the surgical team.

Preoperative medication errors can happen if both the surgeon and the anesthesiologist write orders; therefore orders should be written by only one of them. These orders should be time dated. All medications must be checked three times: (1) when removed from the drug cabinet, (2) before being drawn up in the syringe, and (3) before being given to the patient.

The patient's hearing tends to become more acute after the administration of the preoperative medication and in the induction stage of anesthesia. A quiet environment is essential for all patients awaiting surgery. A sudden loud noise can be distorted and frightening. High noise levels interfere with accurate communication among members of the surgical team and may increase the likelihood of error. Most noise in the operating room can be controlled and kept to a minimum.

Beds, stretchers, and operating room tables must be stabilized by locking the wheels and by personnel actions when a patient is moving from one to the other. The patient should be instructed and assisted to prevent injury or a fall. One person should stabilize the stretcher while another stands on the opposite side of the table to receive the patient. All safety devices on stretchers, operating tables, and the like must be in proper working order. These devices—locking mechanisms, side rails, knee straps, intravenous standards, hydraulic controls, and arm boards—should be used whenever and wherever necessary.

Electrical and fire hazards

General electrical and fire safety regulations should be approved by the operating room committee and hospital administration. Operating room nursing management should be delegated the responsibility and authority to see that the regulations are put into effect by all operating room staff members. The regulations may include the following:

1. The biomedical technician or electrical safety officer should determine whether electrical apparatus, cameras, lights, and cauteries are safe for use in a given situation.
2. Neither smoking nor the use of any apparatus or device producing an open flame is permitted.
3. Preliminary evaluation of all new equipment should ensure optimum safety and performance.
4. All equipment, regardless of source, should be inspected for safety and proper functioning before use.
5. Inventory control, regular inspection, preventive maintenance, and safety approval systems should be established.
6. Personnel must receive instruction in the safe usage of all equipment. Satisfactory return demonstration is mandatory. A standard procedure for care and use of electrical equipment should include the following:
   a. All electrical equipment must be checked before a surgical procedure begins.
   b. Kinks and curls should be removed from electrical cords before plugging into wall outlets.
   c. In plugging into or removing from outlets, the plug should be handled, not the cord. Pulling on the cord causes it to break at the point where the wire is attached to the plug.
   d. Wires and connections should be handled in accordance with their delicacy. They cannot withstand pulling or rough treatment.
   e. Cords should not be wrapped tightly around equipment. This causes the protective covering to wear and also breaks the wires inside the covering.
   f. Cords should always be removed from pathways before rolling in equipment such as beds or machines.
   g. Cord breakage is inconvenient, dangerous, and extremely expensive.
7. All personnel must be familiar with the procedure for prompt repair of defective equipment.
8. A qualified electrician should make monthly or as requested inspections of electrical outlets and equipment and should file written reports with the director of operating rooms.

Most potentially hazardous situations are caused by the combination of electrical equipment and combustible materials found in every surgical suite. Since flammable anesthetics are rarely used today (for example, in very limited teaching situations), environmental safety precautions associated with their use are not presented in this chapter.

Departments in which only nonflammable inhalation anesthetic agents are used must post signs at all entrances to the area indicating this. Conductive flooring and footwear are not required in the area. However, if conductive flooring exists, annual testing of conductivity must be performed and test reports kept on file.

Isolated power system. An isolated power system may be provided in anesthetizing locations. This may reduce the hazard of shock or burn from electric current flowing through the body to ground. Each isolated power system must be provided with a continually operating line isolation monitor that indicates possible leakage or fault currents to ground. Most monitors are designed with green and red signal lamps. The green lamp remains lit when the system is isolated from ground. When the monitor detects a ground fault, the red light and an audible warning signal are activated. All operating room personnel must know the procedure to follow when this occurs:

1. The last electrical device to be plugged in must be shut off and unplugged.
2. If the red light remains lit, each piece of nonessential equipment must be systematically unplugged until the defective device is found.
3. A replacement must be obtained and the defective device removed from service and sent to the appropriate department for inspection and repair.
4. If a defective device cannot be identified and the red light remains lit, the operating room must be shut down following the completion of that patient's surgery until the situation is corrected.
5. Appropriate electrical safety individuals must be notified.

Volatile liquids. Solutions that are flammable must be properly stored. Volatile liquids such as acetone and aerosol sprays are prohibited for cleaning and incidental use in hazardous locations. Skin preparation solutions should be applied with care, since pooling beneath the patient may lead to a chemical burn. In addition, the solution may be ignited by a spark from the active electrode of the electrosurgical unit. Ignition can occur from the vapors as the solution evaporates. All solutions used for skin preparation should be nonflammable whenever an electrosurgical unit is used.

Electrosurgery

High-frequency current from an electrosurgical unit is frequently used to cut tissue and to coagulate bleeders. Advanced technology has dramatically improved electrosurgical capabilities with the development of solid-state generators and isolated systems (Fig. 4-1). These units significantly decrease the potential of burns and shock hazards that were inherent in the original spark gap units. It is essential that personnel understand the proper use of electrosurgical equipment.

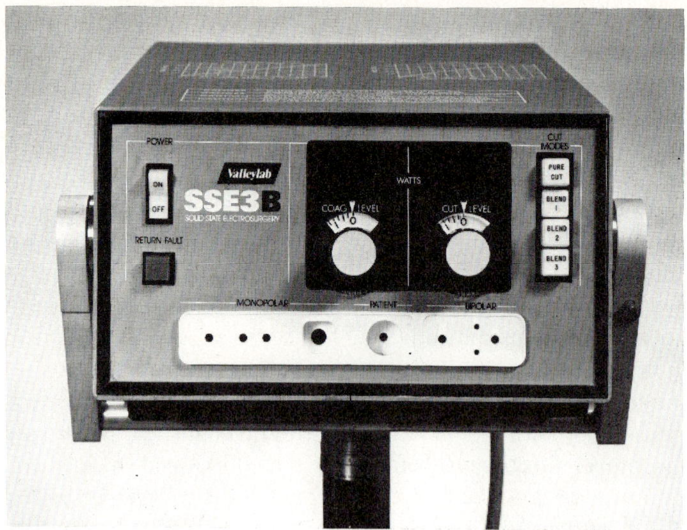

Fig. 4-1. Solid-state electrosurgical unit.

The desired connection between the patient and the unit is established by placing a plate or pad (the inactive electrode) in good contact with the patient's skin. This plate must be adequately lubricated with an electrosurgical gel and placed on a fleshy, nonhairy body surface, close to the operative site. Ground plates should not be placed directly over bony prominences. The grounded pathway returns the electrical current to the unit after the surgeon delivers it to the operative site through the electrosurgical pencil (active electrode). In a nonisolated system, failure of this electrical pathway can result in current traveling in alternate pathways, causing burns in the area of contact.

A faulty return pathway should be suspected if the surgeon requests higher settings because of inadequate cutting or coagulating results. The connection from the patient to the machine should be checked immediately. A faulty return pathway may result from the following:

1. Inadequate patient contact with the plate
2. Poor placement of the plate (it should be placed as close to the operative site as is possible; for example, abdominal surgery patients should be grounded in the buttock or upper thigh area)
3. Inadequate connection of the cable to the plate
4. Inadequate connection at the unit

Electrosurgical burns may result from the unit's action on other electrical equipment. When the electrocardiogram monitor is used, the electrodes should be placed on the patient's shoulders and upper chest. Distant positioning will minimize the alternate flow of electrosurgical current through the electrodes and monitor to the ground.

Some contemporary electrosurgical units possess a patient return electrode monitoring system. Current flowing from the active electrode is measured and compared with current returning from the patient return electrode. If the currents are not balanced, the circuit determines that the patient return electrode is not functioning properly and the unit is deactivated. The most recent innovation in electrosurgical safety is the expanded capability of the return electrode monitoring system to measure the potential for current concentration that may result in a burn at the return electrode site. It identifies inadequate electrode application or reduction of electrode contact area. It also measures the continuity of the entire electrical circuit, patient-pad-cord, for safe current flow. This represents a vital patient safety feature.

Prevention of accidents and infections

All personnel should be instructed in the use of good body mechanics to avert common falls and strains when reaching, stretching, lifting, or moving heavy patients or articles. Good body mechanics and application of work simplification principles conserve human energy and protect the worker, thereby promoting good performance.

All personnel should be instructed and supervised in the proper use of equipment to prevent injury such as cuts from knife blades, burns from autoclaves and electrical equipment, and abrasions from contact with metal accessory levers and swinging doors.

Steam, electrical, vacuum, hydraulic, ventilation, and plumbing systems should be inspected by the maintenance or engineering departments according to an established schedule.

The maintenance and cleaning program should be clearly defined and understood by the nursing staff. Prompt attention to spillage, prompt drying of wet floors, use of warning signs in danger areas, and keeping the corridors and all traffic areas clear of obstacles are important housekeeping duties.

Cleaning, disinfection, and sterilization of equipment, control of airborne contaminants, and application of aseptic techniques are basic to an effective infection control program. Breaks in asepsis may also result from the intrusion of pests, vermin, insects, noxious substances, chemicals, gases, and infectious body fluids and wastes into the protected areas.

Effective disposal procedures for soiled materials and debris are essential to render the area safe for patients and personnel.

The professional nursing staff has a responsibility to work with the infection control committee in the establishment of regulations and the reporting of incidents.

ROUTINE PROCEDURES

Administration of local anesthetics

Local anesthesia refers to the administration of an anesthetic agent to one part of the body by topical application, local infiltration, or subcutaneous injection (see also Chapter 9). It is usually administered by the surgeon. Local anesthesia is preferred if the patient's cooperation is necessary or the patient's physical condition warrants its use. The patient does not lose consciousness and is aware of the surroundings. Local anesthesia is economical and eliminates the undesirable effects of general anesthesia. However, it too may be hazardous. Adverse reactions may occur from large amounts of local agents. If the agent used enters the bloodstream, circulatory and respiratory distress, cardiovascular collapse, or even death can result.

The topical agent may be cocaine hydrochloride, tetracaine, or lidocaine applied to the mucous membranes of the nose, throat, or trachea, or it may be ethyl chloride sprayed onto a specific area of the skin. Procaine, 1%, and 0.5% to 2% lidocaine, with or without epinephrine, are the drugs commonly used for infiltration and local injection anesthesia. Epinephrine, a vasoconstrictor, acts to control bleeding and prolong the local anesthetic effects. It is contraindicated in patients with hypertension, diabetes, or heart disease. All local anesthetic containers or syringes must be labeled when on the sterile table.

Patients must be carefully observed for drug reactions, and emergency drugs, suction apparatus, and resuscitation equipment should be readily available. Symptoms to be observed include diaphoresis, complaints of nausea, palpitation, disturbed respiration, pallor or flushing, syncope, and convulsive movements.

Setup

Anesthetic drugs as ordered
Sterile local anesthesia tray that includes the following items:
- 2 Luer-Lok syringes, 10 ml
- 1 Luer-Lok syringe, 2 ml
- 1 Needle, 25 gauge, ½ inch
- 1 Needle, 25 gauge, 1½ inches
- 1 Needle, 22 gauge, 1½ inches
- 1 Medicine cup, graduated, 2 oz
- 1 Cup, metal, 6 oz
- 1 Basin, metal, 4-inch diameter
- Medication labels

Procedure

The patient should be attended by a registered nurse or an anesthesiologist when a local anesthetic is used. A general recommendation is that no more than 50 ml of 1% solution or 100 ml of 0.5% solution of an anesthetic drug such as lidocaine or procaine be injected per hour for local anesthesia.

In the absence of an anesthesiologist or anesthetist, the circulating nurse or an additional ''monitor nurse'' is responsible for monitoring the patient's vital signs, cardiac readings, and intravenous infusion. These data as well as the total amount of anesthetic and supplementary drugs administered to the patient should be documented. Psychological support must be given to the patient throughout the operation.

Procedure for handling blood

Maintenance of circulating blood volume is imperative during surgical procedures in which excessive blood loss may occur. Appropriate precautions must be taken to reduce the hazards of administration of blood and blood components.

When requesting blood or blood components, the appropriate institutional ''blood grouping Rh'' requisition sheet should be sent to the blood bank. Attached to this sheet should be the number of units desired. If the patient is sent to the operating room directly from the emergency room without a chart, all patient information must be plainly printed on a piece of paper. The blood bank should be contacted by the nurse in charge to explain the situation. Proper communication facilitates release of the needed units.

Before the administration of blood, the circulating nurse and the anesthesiologist or anesthetist should confirm the following:

1. That the number on the unit of blood corresponds with the number on the blood requisition
2. That the name and number on the patient's identification band agrees with the name and number on the unit of blood
3. That the patient's name on the unit of blood corresponds with the name on the requisition
4. That the blood group indicated on the unit of blood corresponds with that of the patient
5. That the date of expiration has not been reached

When it becomes apparent that more blood will be needed than was originally anticipated, the blood bank should be requested to stay ahead a specific number of units. This allows the blood bank to cross-match the units on a routine basis without jeopardizing the patient. Cross-match requisitions should be sent for the additional units requested. A new, properly labeled sample with a blood grouping requisition may also be needed to have adequate serum for cross matching.

The need for rapid blood transfusion necessitates the

warming of blood to prevent hypothermia, which may induce cardiac arrest. Methods of warming blood vary from the simple immersion of the administration tubing in warm water to various types of heaters. The method chosen must not affect the physical characteristics of whole blood or blood components. It must be simple to use, dependable, and consistent in its performance.

The probability of a transfusion reaction increases in direct proportion to the number of units transfused. The circulating nurse should be alert to any signs of reaction. If any suspicious reactions occur, the circulating nurse should assist the anesthesiologist with the following:

1. Stopping the transfusion
2. Reporting the reaction to the surgeon and the blood bank
3. Returning the unused blood and a sample of the patient's blood to the blood bank
4. Sending a urine sample to the laboratory as soon as possible
5. Completing an incident report covering the details of the reaction

Unused blood should be returned as soon as the patient leaves the operating room suite. This allows for maximum use of the supply.

Autotransfusion, the reinfusion of a patient's own blood, is being used with increasing frequency (see Chapter 13). The blood may be collected days or weeks before surgery. Intraoperative autotransfusion facilitates recovery of blood as it is lost during the surgical procedure and retransfusion to the patient. Special sterile equipment simultaneously suctions, filters, anticoagulates, defoams, and returns blood from the operative site to the patient. This technique can be lifesaving in emergency situations such as major trauma.

Procedure for estimating blood loss

Estimation of blood loss is a vital procedure in the surgical management of infants, critically ill or elderly patients, and patients undergoing complex, extensive surgery. The gravimetric method of weighing sponges provides a reliable means of judging the amount of blood to be replaced. The weight of the unit of dry sponges and the plastic bag for the soiled sponges must be known. Grams are converted to milliliters on a one-to-one basis.

Setup

Blood loss record
Gram scale
Plastic bags and twisters to hold soiled sponges

Procedure

1. Allowing for the weight of the unit of dry sponges and the plastic bag, the scale is adjusted to register at zero.
2. Bagged sponges are placed on the scale.
3. The scale reading is recorded: 1 gm equals 1 ml of blood loss.
4. The blood loss is noted on the record.
5. The new weight is added to the preceding weight each time sponges are weighed so that a current total blood loss from sponges is available.
6. Blood in the suction bottles is measured at regular intervals, and the amount of blood loss is added to the total recorded from sponges. Allowances must be made for any irrigating solutions that may have been used.

Procedure for sponge, needle, and instrument counts

Every operating room should establish specific written policies and procedures for sponge, needle, and instrument counts that define materials to be counted, the times when counts must be done, and the documentation required. Certain general guidelines pertain to counting all three types of items. The scrubbed person and the circulating nurse should count all items in unison and aloud, quietly, as the scrubbed person touches each item. Counting should not be interrupted. If there is any uncertainty about a count, it should be repeated. The circulating nurse should immediately record the count for each type of item on the count record or worksheet. If additional items are dispensed during the procedure, the circulating nurse should record the number and initial it. The names of the circulating nurse and the scrubbed person should be recorded as soon as each total count is completed. Linen or waste containers should neither be emptied nor their contents removed from the operating room until the procedure is completed and the patient has left the room. Extreme patient emergencies sometimes necessitate omission of counts, the occurrence of which should be documented on the operative record.

Sponge counts

All types of sponges should be counted on all procedures. The scrubbed person and the circulating nurse should count them before the beginning of the operation, before closure begins, and when skin closure is started. Additional counts may be indicated according to individual hospital policy and circumstance. Additional counts should always be taken before a cavity within a cavity is closed, for example, when the uterus is closed during a cesarean section. Types and sizes of sponges used should be kept to a minimum. It is imperative that all soft goods that are used within a wound and that are not intended to be left in the wound after closure contain an x-ray–detectable element. This facilitates finding any item that may be presumed lost or left in the cavity when an incorrect count occurs. Along the same line, x-ray–detectable sponges should never be used for dressings to eliminate the possibility of a seemingly foreign body appearing on postoperative x-ray studies that may be taken.

Each type and size of sponge should be kept separate

from the other types. Sponges must be kept away from other supplies such as towels and drapes to prevent a sponge from being carried inadvertently into the wound or misplaced. Counted sponges should never be taken from the operating room for any reason during surgery.

If an incorrectly numbered package of sponges is dispensed to the field, it should be handed off the field, marked as not included in the count, and placed in an isolated spot. This reduces the potential for error by using only standard multiples of sponges.

During surgery, the scrubbed person should discard soiled sponges into a plastic-lined bucket or receptacle. The circulating nurse transfers the discarded sponges into impermeable plastic bags or other appropriate containers, according to type and prescribed number after counting with the scrubbed person. The bag is then closed, secured, and labeled with the type and number of sponges and the initials of the persons who counted them. The bag can be set aside, and, unless there is a discrepancy, the sponges need not be taken out and counted again at the time of the closure sponge counts. Bagging of sponges reduces the possibility of airborne contaminants arising from the sponges as they become dry and enables the anesthesiologist to visually assess the patient's blood loss.

The circulating nurse should tally the numbers of each type of sponge dispensed, as recorded on the count worksheet, before the closure counts are taken. At the beginning of the first line of closure sutures, the scrubbed person and the circulating nurse should count all sponges consecutively, proceeding from the sterile field to the back table and off the field. At the completion of the count, the circulating nurse should inform the surgeon of the results of the count. The same procedure should be repeated as skin closure is begun.

Needle counts

Needles should be counted on all procedures by the scrubbed person and the circulating nurse at the same times as sponges. When needles are counted before surgery begins, it is not necessary to open every package of suture dispensed onto the field. The needles may be counted according to the number indicated on the package. If a package indicates that three needle sutures are contained within, three needles should be documented on the worksheet. It is the responsibility of the scrubbed person to verify the number of needles at the time the package is opened. Scrubbed personnel should continually count needles during the procedure and hand them to the surgeon on an exchange basis.

It is helpful to collect used needles on a needle pad or container to ensure their containment on the table. On procedures in which a high volume of needles may be used, the scrubbed person can count any filled needle pads with the circulating nurse and hand them off the field. The circulating nurse should then bag them and label them with the number of needles contained and the initials of the individuals who counted them.

Needles broken during the procedure must be accounted for in their entirety. Like sponges, needles should never be taken from the room for any reason during a procedure. Closure counts are conducted in the same format as that for sponges.

Instrument counts

It is recommended that instrument counts be taken on all procedures. However, the policy of some hospitals specifies that instrument counts be taken only when a major body cavity is entered or when the depth and location of the wound is such that an instrument could accidentally be left in the patient. Individual hospital policy must be followed without deviation. Instrument sets should be standardized for ease in counting, with the minimum number and type of instruments in each set. Instruments should be counted in the instrument room as they are being set up, in the operating room by the scrubbed person and the circulating nurse before the beginning of the operation, and before closure begins. Additional counts may be indicated according to hospital policy or individual circumstance. Instruments that are broken or disassembled during the procedure must be accounted for in their entirety. No instruments should be taken from the operating room during a procedure. Printed instrument count sheets with the names of all items to be counted help expedite the count procedure.

Incorrect counts

If any closure count is incorrect, it should be repeated immediately. If it remains incorrect, the circulating nurse should notify the surgeon and a search should be made for the item. All personnel should direct their immediate attention to locating the missing item. If it is not found, an x-ray film is taken. If the x-ray study is negative, the count is recorded as incorrect and the x-ray results noted. An incident report should be initiated according to hospital policy.

Accurate counting and recording of sponges, needles, and instruments are essential for the protection of the patient, personnel, and the hospital.

Procedure for preservation of skin

A skin graft is a temporary measure in which a harvested piece of skin is used to cover a denuded area. The skin can be obtained from the patient on whom it is to be grafted (autograft) or from a donor (homograft). Whatever the source, the skin must be preserved until it is used.

Setup

The setup should include the skin specimen and the following items:

Sterile 3-inch roller gauze
Basin with normal saline solution
Sterile jar with screw cap
Adhesive tape for sealing and labeling jar

Procedure

1. The skin should be kept on the instrument table until it is ready for storage.
2. The skin must be kept moist with saline at all times.
3. The skin is gently flattened, smoothed out, and placed on a piece of saline-moistened roller gauze, with its external surface facing downward.
4. The scrubbed person rolls the gauze/skin loosely, places the roll in the sterile jar, and screws on the cap.
5. The circulating nurse labels the jar with the patient's name and hospital number, location of donor site, and date of operation.
6. If the surgeon anticipates using the preserved skin within 72 hours, it is stored in a refrigerator at 4.5° C (40° F) until it is used.
7. If the skin is unused within 72 hours, or if the surgeon does not anticipate using the skin within 72 hours, it is frozen in the skin bank.

Procedure for emergency signals

Every operating room suite must have an emergency system that can be activated from within each operating room proper. A light outside the door of the room involved should appear, and a buzzer or bell should sound in a central nursing or anesthesia area. The signals should remain on until the light is turned off at the source. All personnel should be familiar with the system and should know both how to send a signal and how to respond to it. Such a system, restricted to use in life-threatening emergencies, saves invaluable time in bringing additional assistance.

Procedure for cardiopulmonary resuscitation

Cardiopulmonary resuscitation is the immediate restoration of circulatory and respiratory functions by means of manual and mechanical methods and administration of drugs to provide for ventilation and conversion of the heartbeat to normal sinus rhythm.

Cardiac arrest, standstill, or fibrillation may occur in patients undergoing surgery because of the hazards of surgery such as blood loss and shock or unfavorable reactions to anesthesia such as hypoxia and poor ventilation.

For survival of the patient, all body organs and tissues must receive sufficient oxygen through the circulatory system. The circulating blood must carry the oxygen supplied by pulmonary ventilation. Ventilation may be reestablished by mouth-to-mouth breathing or by other means of artificial respiration, such as oxygen apparatus, face mask, and intubation (artificial airway and endotracheal tube). Cardiac compression is directed toward reestablishment of circulation.

A well-defined written protocol should be posted in a designated area in each operating room and should be clearly understood by all personnel. Periodic practice sessions in relation to delegated duties should be scheduled as part of the safety program.

Setup

A movable emergency cardiopulmonary arrest cart containing all items that may be needed should be immediately available. The operating room committee, the surgical staff, and the anesthesiology staff should determine the equipment needed and the plan of treatment to be initiated, stressing the team approach. The equipment should include the following items:

Emergency thoracotomy kit

1 Scalpel handle no. 4 with blade no. 20
1 Rib retractor
1 Finochietto or Harken self-retaining retractor

Ventilation and resuscitation equipment

Ambu resuscitator, anesthesia machine, or Kreiselmann resuscitator
Airways—oral and nasal
Endotracheal equipment
Laryngoscope
Suctioning apparatus

Syringes (Luer-Lok) and needles

3 Syringes, 3 ml
4 Syringes, 5 ml
4 Syringes, 10 ml
2 Syringes, 20 ml
2 Syringes, 50 ml
5 Needles, 25 gauge, ⅝ inch
5 Needles, 20 gauge, 1½ inches
5 Needles, 18 gauge, 1½ inches
2 Needles, 20 gauge, 3 inches (intracardiac)

Emergency drugs

Where available, commercially prefilled syringes should be used.
Sodium bicarbonate
Lidocaine
Epinephrine
Calcium chloride
Dopamine
Dobutamine
Isoproterenol (Isuprel) hydrochloride
Methylprednisolone sodium succinate (Solu-Medrol)
Atropine
Propranolol hydrochloride (Inderal)
Levarterenol bitartrate (Levophed)
Procaine amide (Pronestyl)
Lanatoside C (Cedilanid)
Aminophylline

Sodium chloride for injection
Water for injection

Infusion equipment

Fluids for intravenous infusion
Venesection tray
Infusion administration sets
Cutdown tray and intracatheters
Stopcocks
Alcohol sponges
Prep swabs
Tourniquets
Infusion pump
Blood sampling kit
Blood tubes
Heparinized syringes

Cardiac support equipment

Defibrillator
Cardiac monitoring equipment

Cardiac arrest board (for use if patient is in a bed)

A *thoracotomy setup* (Chapter 17) should be available in case open heart massage is attempted. Open heart massage is rarely performed today unless the chest is already open and a thoracic surgeon is present. Closed chest massage is considered equally effective with fewer inherent hazards.

Procedure

1. The emergency alarm should be activated to alert the operating room supervisor and appropriate surgical and anesthesia personnel. The exact time of arrest is recorded, and additional assistance procured as required.

2. In the absence of an anesthetist or resuscitative equipment, an airway should be established and ventilation of the patient begun by means of mouth-to-mouth resuscitation or other artificial respiration to restore and maintain oxygenation.

3. Closed chest massage is applied to maintain circulation and provision of oxygen to vital tissues.

4. Nursing personnel responding to the alarm should bring the cardiopulmonary arrest cart to the room.

5. As soon as additional personnel arrive, one person should be designated as the charge person (usually the anesthesiologist) and another as recorder. The recorder should maintain ongoing documentation of all medications given and procedures performed.

6. Medications are prepared and administered as ordered.

7. Infusions or transfusions are procured and prepared as ordered.

8. The surgeon and anesthesiologist are assisted as needed.

9. At the conclusion of the procedure, the event and care given are documented.

10. Appropriate administrative services are notified as the situation requires. Included would be a request to the service supplying religious rites and notification to the proper services of the change in the patient's conditon and the need to inform the patient's family.

SUGGESTED READINGS

Association of Operating Room Nurses: Standards for technical and aseptic practice, Denver, 1978, The Association.

Board of Commissioners of Joint Commission on Accreditation of Hospitals: Accreditation manual for hospitals, Chicago, 1982, The Commission.

Chambers, J.J., and Saha, A.K.: Electrocution during anaesthesia, Anaesthesia **34:**173, 1979.

Gendron, F.: Burns occurring during lengthy surgical procedures, J. Clin. Engin. **5:**19, Jan.-March 1980.

Grubb, R.D., and Ondov, G.: Operating room guidelines: an illustrated manual, St. Louis, 1979, The C.V. Mosby Co.

Harvey, C.K., and others: Nonflammable germicides and electrosurgical unit (Q & A), AORN J. **30:**85, 1979.

Kuhn, P.A., editor: Massachusetts General Hospital Department of Nursing—operating room procedure manual, Reston, Va., 1981, Reston Publishing Co., Inc.

Lawson, B.N.: A nurse's guide to electrosurgery, AORN J. **25:**314, 1977.

LeMaitre, G., and Finnegan, J.: The patient in surgery: a guide for nurses, ed. 4, Philadelphia, 1980, W.B. Saunders Co.

Liechty, R.D., and Soper, R.T.: Synopsis of surgery, ed. 4, St. Louis, 1980, The C.V. Mosby Co.

Manuel, B.J.: Reporting and documenting patient care: operating room, Denver, 1980, Association of Operating Room Nurses, Inc.

Marriner, A.: Guide to nursing management, St. Louis, 1980, The C.V. Mosby Co.

McLain, N.B.: Risk management in the operating room, AORN J. **31:**692, 1980.

National Fire Protection Association: National electric code, NFPA code no. 70-1978, Boston, 1978, The Association.

National Fire Protection Association: Safe use of electricity in patient care areas of hospitals, NFPA code no. 76B, Boston, 1980, The Association.

National Fire Protection Association: Standard for the use of inhalation anesthetics, NFPA code no. 56A, Boston, 1980, The Association.

Phipps, W.J., Long, B.C., and Woods, N.F.: Medical-surgical nursing: concepts and clinical practice, St. Louis, 1979, The C.V. Mosby Co.

5 Principles and procedures of asepsis

The term *asepsis* means the absence of any infectious agents. Asepsis is directed at cleanliness and the elimination of all infectious agents. Aseptic techniques exclude microorganisms present in the environment and prevent those living harmlessly within or on the body from reaching the open wound, so that healing may take place by first intention.

Aseptic technique is the foundation on which contemporary surgery is built. It is difficult to envision surgery without the basics known today, but it is only during the last 150 years that surgery has developed into a science. Some concepts of surgical sepsis and aseptic technique are evident in history as early as 460 BC. Hippocrates, the father of surgery, used wine or boiled water to irrigate wounds. Galen, a Roman who lived during the second century AD, supposedly boiled his instruments before use.

Although various forms of surgery were probably practiced throughout the centuries, the first period of surgical prominence was during the 1500s when Ambrose Pare developed the use of ligatures to control bleeding. In that same era, Fracastorius, the world's first epidemiologist, proclaimed that diseases were spread in three ways: by direct contact, by handling articles that infected people had handled previously, and by transmission from a distance.

In the middle of the nineteenth century, a new era began that greatly expanded the horizons of the world of surgery. Anesthesia became a beneficial tool of the surgeon, permitting pain-free operations and decreasing the need for speed during surgery. Interest in surgical techniques and the development of new operations flourished. The preservation of life, however, was still not being fulfilled. Wound infections were so common that they were considered normal. When pus appeared in the incision, it was thought to be a healthy sign, signaling the beginning of clinical improvement. Unfortunately, this septic wound often ruined the surgical procedure, lengthened the patient's hospital stay, and even threatened the patient's life.

About the same time, Semmelweis made a simple but great contribution to infection control by advocating that hands be washed between examinations of patients.

In the 1850s, Louis Pasteur theorized that fermentation was caused by particles of living matter so small that they could not be seen but could be carried freely in the air. He referred to these microorganisms as *germs* and found that heat killed these germs. Not being a physician, Pasteur did not grasp the relationship between the fermentation process and the putrefaction of tissue. In 1860, Joseph Lister learned about Pasteur's work, recognized the analogous relationship between the two processes, and set out to investigate the relationship of the germ theory to the process of infection. By 1867, Lister was advocating carbolic soaks and sprays for hands, wounds, dressings, sutures, and the operating room itself. Even though Lister's antiseptic methods and principles were crude and undeveloped, their use resulted in a drop in the surgical mortality rate from 45% to 15%.[5] This marked the beginning of the antiseptic era and the modern age of surgery.

CAUSE AND PREVENTION OF INFECTIONS

How can the surgical patient be assured of a bacteria-free operating room? How can surgical asepsis be maintained? How can the patient be protected against hospital-acquired infection? The answers to these questions are based on extensive scientific information and principles of microbiology and bacteriology.

Effective hospital and operating room infection control programs must be carried out by all persons who help care for patients. Control programs involve methods of housekeeping and maintenance of the facilities; cleanliness of the air in the suite and of the skin and apparel of patients, surgeons, and personnel; sterility of surgical equipment; strict aseptic technique; and careful observance by all the staff of well-defined written procedures, rules, and regulations.

An infection control program is based on a knowledge of the nature and characteristics of microorganisms that are capable of producing infection in the surgical patient and an understanding of their transmission in the environment and wound. An ongoing and up-to-date control program requires study and critical analysis of the latest accepted information to provide effective methods that will destroy or inhibit specific microorganisms in particular situations.

Definitions of terms should be agreed on and clarified. It is important that each member of the surgical team have some understanding of the nature and characteristics of pathogenic and nonpathogenic microorganisms.

Terms related to infection and infecting agents

Pathogens are microorganisms that are capable of producing disease under certain conditions. In humans, a satisfactory balance may be reached between the invading pathogens and the host, resulting in no noticeable ill effects. The aggressiveness and virulence of pathogens, the size and composition of the microbial population, the physical environment, and the susceptibility of the host determine the occurrence of an infection.

Most pathogenic bacteria are capable of leading a parasitic or saprophytic existence. Some pathogens reside naturally on or within humans without producing disease until the opportunity arises. For example, the enteric microorganisms are a large group of gram-negative, non–spore-forming bacilli whose natural habitat is within the lumen of the intestine of humans and animals. *Escherichia coli,* one of the enteric bacilli, is capable of producing infection on entrance into the peritoneal cavity.

Parasites are microorganisms that reside on or within the bodies of living organisms called *hosts* in order to find the environment and food they require for life and reproduction. Some microorganisms are obligatory parasites, meaning that they are dependent on their hosts for survival and reproduction. Other microorganisms are facultative parasites, meaning that they normally reside on dead matter but may receive nourishment from living matter. All disease-producing microorganisms are parasites; however, not all parasites are disease producing.

Saprophytes are microorganisms that reside on dead or decaying organic matter. They are found in water, soil, and debris—wherever the process of decay occurs. They reduce decaying matter to simple soluble compounds, which in turn become available to bacteria. For example, *Clostridium tetani,* which causes tetanus (lockjaw), cannot survive in healthy tissue but requires dead (necrotic) material. Some microorganisms are facultative saprophytes, meaning that they usually obtain their nourishment from living matter but may obtain it from dead organic matter.

Certain bacteria, members of the genera *Bacillus, Clostridium,* and *Sporozoa,* form and develop specialized structures called *spores* (endospores) within the cell under specific conditions. One cell generally produces one spore. The specific environment that starts sporulation is still unknown. When conditions are again favorable for growth, the spore germinates to produce one vegetative cell. The spore appears to possess a large number of active enzymes and is especially resistant to heat, chemicals, and drying.

So-called *transient microorganisms* are those having a very short span of life, such as the normal flora present on the skin surface of humans.

Resident microorganisms are those which habitually live in the epidermis, deep in the crevices and folds of the skin.

Most bacteria produce one or more poisonous materials known as *toxins*. The term *exotoxin* refers to specific injurious toxins that are formed by certain microorganisms and diffuse freely from the microorganisms into the environment. *C. tetani, C. botulinum,* the sporulating anaerobes isolated from gas gangrene such as *C. perfringens, Streptococcus pyogenes,* and *Staphylococcus aureus* are some of the microorganisms with this property.

Endotoxins are toxins that are part of the cell wall of some microorganisms. Endotoxic substances are not secreted to a significant degree into the parasites' environment but are released after death and dissolution of the microorganisms. Their poisonous effect depends on the species. *Salmonella typhosa* and *Neisseria meningitidis* are endotoxic pathogens.

Bacteria differ from one another in their relationship to molecular oxygen. The strictly *aerobic* (obligatory-type) bacteria are unable to live and produce without access to free atmospheric oxygen. *Mycobacterium tuberculosis, Vibrio comma* (agent of Asiatic cholera), *Bacillus subtilis,* and *Corynebacterium diphtheriae* are aerobic bacteria. The strictly *anaerobic* bacteria can live only in the absence of air; atmospheric oxygen is poisonous to them. The pathogenic bacteria, such as *Clostridium tetani, C. botulinum,* and *C. perfringens,* are anaerobic bacteria. However, many facultative bacteria have enzyme systems that permit them to live and produce with, without, or with a very small amount of free oxygen.

The term *infectious agent* refers to a microorganism (bacterium, spirochete, fungus, virus, or any other type of organism) that is capable of producing infection. Infection is the process by which living pathogenic microorganisms enter the body of the host under conditions favorable for their growth and by the production of toxins may act injuriously on the tissues of the host.

The term *source* refers to the object, substance, or individual from which an infectious agent passes to a host. In some cases, transfer is direct from the reservoir, or source, to the host. The source may be at any point in the chain of transmission. For example, the nose of an individual may be the reservoir, or source; hands, clothing, or mask may become the intermediate mechanism for the transfer of the agent to the host.

Nosocomial infections are infections that occur in patients during hospitalization, with confirmation of diagnosis by clinical or laboratory evidence. The infective microorganisms may originate from endogenous sources, as from one tissue to another within the patient (self-infection), or from exogenous sources, as acquired from objects or other patients within the hospital (cross-infection) (Fig. 5-1). Nosocomial infections, which are often referred to as *hospital-acquired infections,* may not become apparent until after the patient has left the hospital. Factors that influence the development of nosocomial in-

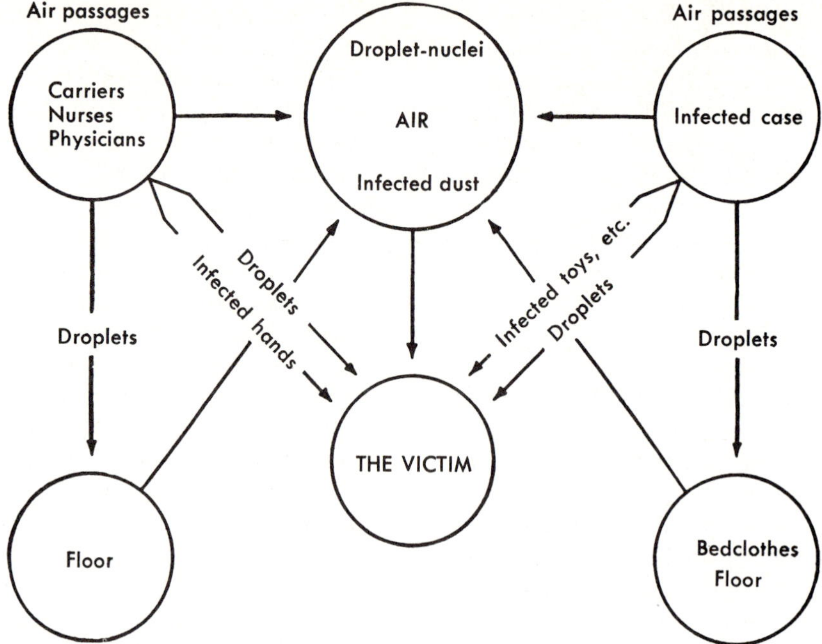

Fig. 5-1. Diagram showing how infections may be accidentally spread in hospitals. (From Medical Research Council War Memorandum no. 11. Reproduced by permission of the Comptroller of His Britannic Majesty's Stationery Office.)

fections are the source of infection, the microbial agent, the route of transmission, the susceptibility of the host, and the environment.

A *carrier* is a person who harbors one or more specific pathogens in the absence of discernible clinical disease. Carriers may be classified into three groups: convalescent carriers who continue to harbor or shed microorganisms for variable periods during recovery from the disease, chronic or permanent carriers who harbor microorganisms usually for the duration of life, and transitory or temporary carriers who, without a recognized attack of the disease, harbor microorganisms for short periods.

The term *contamination* refers to the presence of pathogenic microorganisms on or in an animate or inanimate vector. It generally is used in reference to a specific object, substance, or tissue that contains microorganisms, especially disease-producing microorganisms. For example, a person's skin or an instrument may be contaminated by contact with pathogenic microorganisms, but it is not infected.

Inflammation is a defense reaction by the body to an injury or abnormal stimulation caused by a physical, chemical, or biological agent. Frequently, the tissue of the host cells, assisted by phagocytes, localize and destroy the pathogenic invader. This reaction is observed as a local inflammation. Nature provides many barriers for protection against disease-producing microorganisms, such as intact skin and mucous membranes.

A *local* infection is one in which the causative agent is limited to one locality of the body and becomes circumscribed in a boil or abscess. *Primary* infection is the first infection that develops after microbial invasion. In *secondary* infection the microorganisms invade tissues in which there is an existing primary infection. When the infectious agents spread throughout the body tissues, the condition is termed a *systemic* infection. A *bacteremia* is the result of a singular or intermittent dissemination of microorganisms from a primary focus of infection into the bloodstream. In *septicemia,* the microorganisms and/or their toxins are distributed more or less constantly and are continually present in the blood.

Sepsis is a generalized reaction to pathogenic microorganisms, their poisons, or both. The septic condition may be evident clinically by the signs of inflammation and the systemic manifestations of the patient.

Normally the leukocytes (white blood cells) remove debris, including bacteria, from the blood by devouring these foreign particles. This process is called *phagocytosis,* and the devouring cells are called *phagocytes*. In some cases the white cells are killed in the process and accumulate at the site of the infection. This accumulation of decayed cells and serum is called *pus*. The inflammatory battle is an overall reaction of the body to injury. The action of the phagocytes, the bactericidal substances in the blood, and the desire of the tissues to localize the infection result in production of the cardinal inflammatory signs of redness, heat, swelling, and pain.

An *antigen* is a foreign substance in the body that encourages specific immunity by production of specific substances called *antibodies*. General antibodies, which are proteins, appear to be produced mainly in the spleen, lymph glands, and bone marrow.

MICROORGANISMS THAT CAUSE INFECTION

Staphylococci

There are two recognized species of staphylococci: *Staphylococcus aureus and S. epidermidis.*

Numerous disease processes are associated with *S. aureus*. There are several portals of entry: the skin, the respiratory tract, and the genitourinary tract. Staphylococci survive for long periods in the air, in dust, in debris, in bedding, and in clothing. Pathogenic staphylococci grow in the sweat, urine, tissue, and skin of humans. They are resistant to heat and chemicals, including high concentrations of sodium chloride. They are more difficult to destroy than many other non–spore-forming microorganisms.

Staphylococci are called *coagulase-positive* (pathogenic) when they are capable of clotting plasma and, conversely, are called *coagulase-negative* (usually nonpathogenic) where there is clumping by the plasma. *S. aureus* is hemolytic, parasitic, pathogenic, and coagulase-positive. *S. epidermidis* is parasitic, less pathogenic, and coagulase-negative.

In studying the response of staphylococci to various bacteriophages, it was found that certain strains have epidemic potentials and that some are particularly virulent and drug resistant. Two strains classified in this manner that are known to be highly virulent are 80/81 type and 77 type. In the past there were only one or two epidemic strains, whereas today there are several. Staphylococci vary in their resistance to antibiotics. For example, resistance of staphylococci to penicillin differs from their resistance to other antibiotics. Many strains formerly nonpathogenic are now disease-producing microorganisms.

Pathogenic staphylococci are capable of causing rapid suppuration. In many cases the staphylococci have a tendency to remain localized as an abscess and then break through to the outside. Eventually healing occurs. Wound sepsis is not the only manifestation of staphylococcal infection. Patients may suffer staphylococcal pneumonia, enterocolitis, urinary tract infection, or skin infection. Patients who undergo operations on the heart and great vessels seem to be particularly susceptible to coagulase-negative staphylococci.

Staphylococcal pneumonia may develop in patients who contract influenza in the hospital, especially surgical patients with advanced chronic bronchitis, uremia, or some other type of debilitating disease. If the pneumonia has been classified as caused by an epidemic strain of staphylococci, the patient may become a potent source of infection for other persons. A patient with enterocolitis may suffer an acute onset of tachycardia, fever, and profuse diarrhea after surgery. For this reason, terminal disinfection and zoning environmental principles, including adequate air changes, are important factors in an infection control program.

The skin surface is the most common site of staphylococci. Studies indicate that 30% to 70% of persons carry staphylococci on their skin, which may lead to contamination of clothing and dispersal of the microorganisms.

For no known reason, persons who are skin carriers of staphylococci differ in their ability to shed the microorganisms. There appears to be no obvious difference in hygiene and skin condition between light and heavy shedders, and no other contributing factor is apparent. Heavy shedders appear to be in normal good health.

The nasal and throat cavities are the most important reservoirs that continually replenish the external environment. Studies indicate that 40% of adults and 60% of persons under 20 years of age are carriers. Colonization of staphylococci occurs within 8 days after birth in 80% of infants. Among hospital personnel, the carrier rate may vary from 10% to 70%. The potential for patient infection increases greatly as the personnel carrier rate increases. Up to 70% of hospital personnel are intermittent carriers; 15% to 20% are permanent or long-term carriers; 15% never become carriers. At least 50% of nasal carriers are also skin carriers.[1] Carriers usually harbor either coagulase-positive (pathogenic) or coagulase-negative (nonpathogenic) staphylococci, seldom both types, and rarely more than one strain. Since an individual may be a carrier of staphylococci one day and a noncarrier the next day, frequent swab testing of the nose as a check to the spread of the microorganisms is impractical. Cleanliness of the environment, proper handling and sterilization of linens and equipment, and adherence to adequate washing techniques are important controls to prevent transmission of infection.

The severity of a staphylococcal infection in human beings is determined by many factors: type and size of the invading population, route of transmission, properties of the toxic products, and previous exposure and susceptibility of the host. Other contributing factors are the amount of physical trauma, the general health and nutritional state of the patient, the possibility of allergic states, and the presence of uncontrollable diabetes or toxemia.

Streptococci

Most streptococci are generally gram-positive nonmotile, non–spore-forming microorganisms. Streptocci are classified according to their action on red blood cells (alpha, beta, or gamma hemolysis), their resistance to physical and chemical factors (for example, growth at 45° C, growth in 6.5% NaCl), and biochemical tests (for example, group-specific C carbohydrates). Alpha-hemolytic streptococci produce a number of toxic substances resulting in partial hemolysis of red blood cells. When alpha-hemolytic streptococci are present, a greenish discoloration surrounds the colony. Beta-hemolytic streptococci produce toxins that completely hemolyze red cells; when they are cultured on blood agar plates (preferably containing sheep blood), a colorless, clear zone surrounds the colony. Gamma-hemolytic streptococci do not hemolyze blood.

According to immunological differentiation proposed by Lancefield, group A hemolytic streptococci are primarily pathogens of humans, whereas group C hemolytic microorganisms are occasionally pathogens of humans. Other species are entirely saprophytic for humans. Virulent streptococci are more serious invaders than are staphylococci because the former tend to involve wide areas of tissue and to cause necrosis without localization. However, this is partially counterbalanced by the fact that, whereas these virulent streptococci are usually sensitive to penicillin, this may not be the case with staphylococci. Streptococci also occur in mixed infections with other pathogens.

In wounds, a streptococcal infection is introduced through the skin and spreads by way of the lymph vessels and nodes, resulting in inflammation, cellulitis, and sometimes suppuration. Alpha-hemolytic, or viridans-type, streptococci, which normally reside in the respiratory tract or throat of humans, may produce a localized infection such as an abscess in the gums or teeth or subacute bacterial endocarditis. Alpha-hemolytic streptococci may also produce meningitis, although they are not very virulent in contrast to pyogenic beta-hemolytic streptococci. Nonhemolytic streptococci or enterococci occasionally may produce atypical pneumonia, endocarditis, or urinary tract infection.

Transmission of streptococci from the infected person to the susceptible host is accomplished in part by direct contact and in part by contamination of the environment. Direct contact may be by inhalation of infectious droplets expelled from the nose and mouth or by hand-to-hand contact. Indirect contact is by means of infected air and dust in the environment. Most upper respiratory tract infections appear to be caused by airborne microorganisms. By far the most dangerous is the nasal carrier, who contributes large numbers of streptococci to the environment (Fig. 5-1).

Prevention of streptococcal infections, via persons and via wounds, can be accomplished by adherence to aseptic techniques, including proper handling of contaminated clothing and masks, adequate ventilation with frequent air changes, exclusion from patient contact of personnel with acute sinusitis, and effective sterilization of supplies and instruments.

Streptococcus (Diplococcus) pneumoniae is a nonmotile, generally gram-positive, non–spore-forming diplococcus that produces no toxins of real significance. Pneumococci are the normal inhabitants of the upper respiratory tract of humans. Between 20% and 70% of persons are at some time carriers of pneumococci.[7] The carrier state is not permanent but sporadic and intermittent. A majority of carriers tend to carry the less virulent types of microorganisms. An individual may carry two or more types simultaneously. A healthy carrier is more important in dissemination of infection than is an infected patient.

Pneumococci are the primary cause of lobar pneumonia in humans. In this disease, pneumococci do not remain in the lung but migrate from the source of infection through the nasal passages or are distributed by means of the vascular system to other parts of the body, appearing as a localized infection. Sinusitis, parotitis, conjunctivitis, peritonitis, and pyogenic infection such as arthritis are frequently caused by pneumococci.

Pneumococci are transmitted primarily by direct contact with and by inhalation of droplets expelled into the air from the throat of the infected person or the carrier. Indirect transmission by way of contaminated objects is also possible. Prevention of pneumococcal infection is accomplished through environmental sanitation, exclusion of carriers from the operating room, effective care of patients, strict adherence to surgical and medical asepsis, and use of chemotherapy.

Neisseria

Neisseria species are gram-negative, nonmotile, non–spore-forming diplococci. *N. catarrhalis* is found frequently in the nasopharynx of healthy persons and in persons with colds and other respiratory infections. *N. sicca* is present on the mucous membrane of the respiratory tract and may be a causative agent of kidney infection.

N. gonorrhoeae usually gains entrance to the tissues after being deposited on and by burrowing through the mucous membranes, from which it is spread by the lymphatic or blood vessels. It may invade the bloodstream by means of local lesions. Gonorrheal vulvovaginitis is transmitted by bedding, clothing, and other inanimate vectors, whereas gonorrhea is spread by direct contact. Prophylaxis and control are accomplished by environmental sanitation and chemotherapy.

N. meningitidis, the meningococcus, is a pathogenic organism capable of producing acute meningitis in humans. Meningococci may gain access to the central nervous system via the nasopharynx. The method whereby the meningococci leave the nasopharynx, invade the bloodstream, and reach the central nervous system is not known. Meningococcal meningitis is disseminated by direct contact and by droplet infection from secretions of the mouth, nose, and throat. Some persons are temporary carriers, whereas others are chronic meningococcal carriers.

Clostridium

Members of the genus *Clostridium* are anaerobic, spore-forming bacilli, many of which are pathogenic for humans. The species include *C. tetani, C. perfringens, C. novyi, C. histolyticum, C. septicum,* and *C. botu-*

linum. *C. sporogenes* is one of the nonpathogenic species.

C. tetani produces tetanus (lockjaw) in humans. The bacilli normally reside in the soil and in the intestinal contents of some animals and humans. Tetanus toxin is a potent poisonous substance to humans. Tetanus is characterized by spasms of the voluntary muscles, particularly those of the jaw and neck—thus the name lockjaw. The bacilli gain entrance to the tissues by way of a deep, dirty wound and set up a localized infection. The toxin is disseminated throughout the body; when it reaches the nervous system, lockjaw occurs. Surgical tetanus may occur postoperatively and usually results from faulty sterilization of equipment or dressings. Puncture wounds provide anaerobic conditions that facilitate multiplication of tetanus bacilli. Injection-related tetanus in narcotic addicts is a contemporary public health problem. Tetanus of the newborn (tetanus neonatorum) may follow infection of the umbilicus. Treatment includes the use of antitoxin and an active immunization program.

Gaseous gangrene is produced by spores of *Clostridium* species present in contaminated wounds, especially those involving fracture or extensive tissue necrosis. Although usually associated with traumatic injuries, it sometimes develops in hospitalized patients in situations in which necrosis, vascular insufficiency, and possible fecal contamination occur. Accidental injuries, puerperal sepsis, and ruptured appendix may be accompanied by gaseous gangrene. It is usually caused by anaerobic, toxin-producing, spore-forming bacilli. The gangrenous process results from the activity of the sporulating obligate anaerobes and the exotoxins they produce. Several species of *Clostridium* may infect wounds and produce gaseous gangrene. The most common are *C. perfringens, C. novyi,* and *C. septicum*. *C. sporogenes,* although considered nonpathogenic, is found in many cases.

C. perfringens is an anaerobic pathogen capable of producing gaseous gangrene alone or with other anaerobic microorganisms in a closed abscess in uterine, gastrointestinal, genitourinary, or biliary infections. This microorganism is a normal inhabitant of the intestinal tract of humans. Entrance of *C. perfringens* into a wound does not always produce gaseous gangrene. The pathogenicity of a *Clostridium* species depends on the amount of powerful exotoxins it produces either within the body or in circumscribed tissues. In gaseous gangrene, the gas in the tissues causes them to expand. This creates pressure, thereby decreasing the flow of blood to the tissues, and necrosis results. The powerful exotoxins also weaken the general condition of the patient.

Pseudomonas

The best-known pathogenic, aerobic species of *Pseudomonas* for humans is *P. aeruginosa*. It is frequently found in soil, water, sewage, debris, and air and occasionally in the normal flora of the skin and intestines. Its incidence increases in the intestine when the coliform microorganisms are suppressed. Until recently, it was considered a harmless saprophyte or possibly a microorganism of slight pathogenic power. It is now known that this bacillus may be associated with a great many suppurative infections in humans. *P. aeruginosa* appears to be a pathogen only when it is introduced into areas devoid of normal defenses, when it is superimposed on staphylococcal infection, or when it is present in a mixed infection. It may attack a debilitated patient with extensive burns or traumatic injuries.

P. aeruginosa is resistant to most antimicrobial agents. Environmental sanitation and strict adherence to aseptic techniques are important preventive measures.

Salmonella

Salmonella species are members of a large general classification of microorganisms that are often called *enteric* (or coliform) bacilli because they inhabit the intestinal tract of humans. These microorganisms are gram-negative, non–spore-forming, aerobic bacteria. Other well-known members are *Shigella* species (the dysentery bacilli), *Escherichia* species, and *Proteus* species (the paracolon bacilli).

Salmonella species are all pathogenic to a greater or lesser degree and are non–spore-forming, gram-negative, motile bacteria. They do not form exotoxins, but all possess endotoxins. *Salmonella* infection in humans is acquired by ingestion of the microorganism, usually in contaminated food or water. These bacteria may produce either clinical or subclinical infection. The three major diseases for which they are causative microorganisms are enteric fever, gastroenteritis, and septicemia.

S. typhosa is the causative agent of typhoid fever. About 3% of patients with typhoid fever become carriers for some time. The bacteria remain in the gallbladder and intestine and occasionally in the urinary tract.

Escherichia

Escherichia coli is one of the most common causes of septicemia, inflammation of the liver, and gallbladder and urinary tract infections, especially when the host's defenses are inadequate, as in infants or elderly patients with terminal diseases. These microorganisms may also cause infection after radiation treatment and may escape through the wall of the bowel, causing secondary peritonitis. However, most strains of *E. coli* are nonpathogenic in the normal, healthy host.

Proteus

Proteus vulgaris is often associated with *Pseudomonas aeruginosa*. *Proteus* microorganisms are gram-negative, motile, aerobic bacilli, usually found free living in water, soil, dust, and sewage.

P. vulgaris is frequently found in the normal fecal flora of the intestinal tract. These bacilli also produce infection in humans only when they leave the intestinal tract. This species may become the causative agent of cystitis and is most resistant to heat and antimicrobial agents. Specific antibiotics are active agents against *Proteus*.

Mycobacterium

Mycobacterium tuberculosis is a non–spore-forming aerobic bacillus. Disease is produced by establishment and proliferation of virulent microorganisms and interactions with the host. Tubercle bacilli spread in the host by direct extension through the lymphatic channels and bloodstream and by way of the bronchi and gastrointestinal tract. These bacilli can infect almost any tissue, including skin, bones, lymph nodes, intestinal tract, and fallopian tubes.

Tubercle bacilli are transmitted directly by means of discharge from the respiratory tract, less frequently through the digestive tract, by inhalation of droplets expelled during coughing, or by kissing; and indirectly by means of contaminated articles and dust floating through the air.

Prevention and control programs include rigid environmental hygiene, disinfection and sterilization of contaminated equipment, and isolation of persons with active infections.

INFECTION CONTROL PRACTICES FOR OPERATING ROOM PERSONNEL

Statistics prove that the economics of wound infection are awesome. Large quantities of bacteria are present in the nose and mouth, on the skin, and on the attire of personnel who enter the restricted areas of the operating room suite. Proper design of facilities and regulations for use of operating room attire are important ways of preventing transportation of microorganisms into operating rooms, where they may infect the open wounds of patients.

Areas should be provided where staff members may remove personal clothing, don operating room attire, and enter the clean operating suite directly, without passing through a contaminated area.

Daily body cleanliness and clean, dandruff-free hair help prevent superficial wound infections. Hair is a fertile source of bacteria. The hair of the head and of other areas of the body may shed debris and dead cells that may be transported to an open wound. The person who is well rested and healthy is less subject to infectious diseases. It should be against regulations for personnel who have infections of the nose or throat, are known to be carriers, or have open sores to enter the operating room.

Proper operating room attire

Every operating room department should have a written policy and procedure regarding proper attire in the surgical suite. Many points should be considered in establishing regulations for proper operating room apparel.

Street clothes should never be worn within restricted areas of the surgical suite. There should be a point of demarcation past which no one may go unless properly attired. All persons who enter restricted surgical areas should be required to wear clean operating room apparel made of materials that meet the National Fire Protection Association standards. This apparel should include hat or hood, one-piece or two-piece pantsuit or dress, shoe covers, and face mask (Fig. 5-2). Apparel should cover as much skin as possible to protect against shedding and should be flame resistant, lint free, cool, and comfortable. All reusable apparel should be laundered within hospital facilities.

The first item of apparel donned should be a clean, lint-free surgical hat or hood that completely covers all possible head and facial hair. This eliminates the possibility of hair or dandruff being shed on the scrub suit. It is essential that all hair is *contained* as well as covered. Skull caps that fail to cover the side hair above the ears and hair at the nape of the neck should not be worn in the operating room. The cap should be of flame-resistant material that provides ventilation and comfort yet fits snugly, within the edges secured by elastic, fasteners, or drawstrings. Net or crinoline caps should not be used because they do not provide a barrier to dandruff and hair fallout.

Hair acts as a filter when left uncovered and collects bacteria, which are released into the air during activity. Hair attracts, harbors, and sheds bacteria in proportion to its length, curliness, or oiliness. Cleanliness of homemade caps becomes a debatable subject; therefore use of these caps should be prohibited unless hospital facilities are available for laundering daily. Disposable headgear should be discarded in a designated receptacle immediately after use. Headgear should not be worn outside the suite. It should always be worn in areas where equipment and supplies are processed and stored.

Scrub clothes should be designed so that personnel may don and remove them without passing them over the head. Care must be taken when donning scrub pants to avoid dragging the pant legs on the floor. If a scrub dress is worn, intact panty hose should be worn to contain bacterial shedding (Fig. 5-2, *C*). Clothing should be of good fit for comfort and appearance.

Scrub suits should be made of a closely woven fabric to prevent dispersal of body bacteria. The top of a scrub suit should be secured at the waist or tucked into the pants. The pants should have stockinette cuffs or ankle closures (Fig. 5-2, *A* and *B*). Loose, flapping folds or shirttails and baggy trousers are sources of possible contamination as personnel move; bacteria are freed by friction.

It is good practice for circulating personnel to wear warm-up jackets to prevent shedding from bare arms (Fig. 5-2, *D*). Jackets should be snapped at all times in the

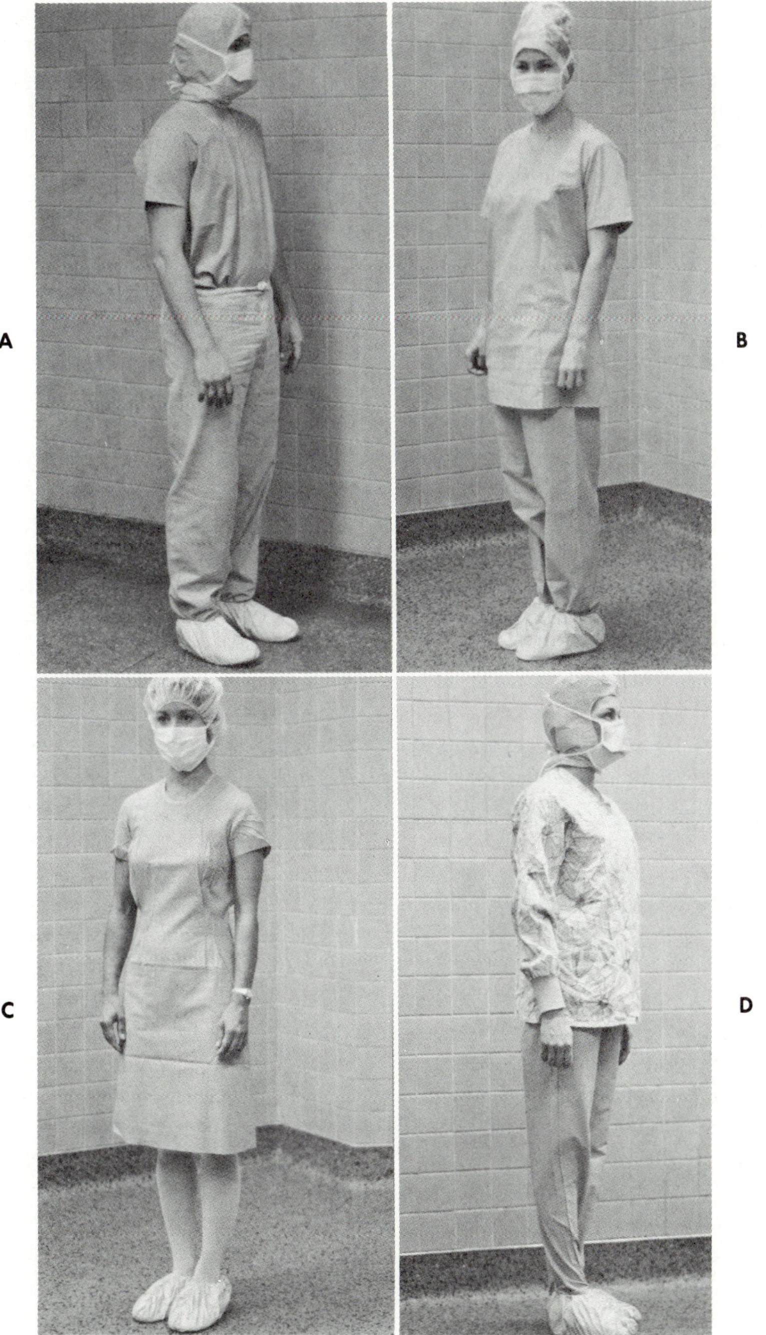

Fig. 5-2. Proper operating room attire. **A,** Scrub top should be tucked into pants or, **B,** should conform to waist to reduce dispersal of bacteria. Ankle closures on scrub pants ensure containment of potential contaminants. **C,** Scrub dress should be secured at waist. Advocates of scrub dresses believe that bacteria can be contained as effectively with panty hose as with pantsuits. **D,** Warm-up jacket worn over scrub suit provides maximum coverage of skin.

operating room to eliminate the possibility of the material brushing against a sterile field.

Absorbent cotton socks or hose help maintain healthy feet. Footwear should provide support for the feet. They should also be easy to clean. Shoe covers should be worn by all persons entering the restricted areas of the surgical suite. The primary reason for the use of shoe covers is sanitation because even the most conscientious person has difficulty keeping shoes clean all the time in a busy operating room. When the same shoes are worn for successive operations, they provide a very high bacterial count with the potential of cross-infection; therefore it is necessary to clean or change them between procedures. Shoe covers must be conductive in areas where static spark is a hazard. Care must be taken when donning most conventional shoe covers to make sure that the black carbon strip is placed inside the shoe between the sock or hose in good contact with the inner sole. Conductivity should be checked when first entering the restricted area and periodically throughout the day.

Logically, shoe covers should be located in an area adjacent to the restricted area entrance. Shoe covers should be removed on leaving the restricted area, and clean shoe covers should be put on when returning to that area. Cross-contamination from other areas of the hospital must be prevented. Bacterial protection is negated if the shoe covers are worn in the same area as street shoes or if the shoe covers are not intact. Clogs, sandals, and tennis shoes present a potential safety hazard and therefore are not acceptable types of footwear for use in the operating room.

Masking in the operating room is vital to prevention of infection. High filtration efficiency disposable masks should be worn at all times by all persons in the operating room. One mask is worn. Double masking provides a barrier rather than a filter and therefore is unacceptable. The physical aspects of the surgical suite determine additional areas where a mask should be worn.

Cloth or gauze masks are no longer acceptable for use in the operating room. They have a very low filtration efficiency and may become ineffective as a bacterial barrier within 30 minutes of wear. The wearer who breathes through a face mask that is thickly inoculated with expired bacteria may expel a higher number of microorganisms into the atmosphere than does the individual who breathes normally and quietly without a mask. Forceful expulsion of the breathing during talking, laughing, or sneezing propels large concentrations of microorganisms into the air.

When choosing a synthetic disposable mask, it is important to select one with a filtration efficiency of 95% or above. The most effective filter mask is relatively useless if worn incorrectly and can be dangerous if handled improperly. To handle or don a mask, the person should first wash his or her hands to prevent contamination of the mask. The mask must cover the mouth and nose entirely and be tied securely to prevent venting (Fig. 5-3, *A*). The strings should not be crossed when tied because the sides of the mask will gap. A pliable metal strip is inserted in the top hem of most masks to provide a firm contour fit over the bridge of the nose. This strip also helps prevent fogging of eyeglasses.

Air should pass only through the filtering system of the mask. Masks should be either on or off. They should not be saved from one operation to the next by allowing them to hang around the neck or by tucking them into a pocket. Bacteria that have been filtered by the mask will become dry and airborne if the mask is worn necklace fashion. Touching only the strings when removing the mask reduces contamination of the hands (Fig. 5-3, *B* and *C*). Masks should be changed between procedures and sometimes during a procedure, depending on the length of the operation and the amount of talking done by the surgical team.

To remove a mask, the wearer should handle only the ties. The facepiece, which is highly contaminated with droplet nuclei, should not come in contact with the hands of personnel. Immediately after removal, masks should be discarded directly into a designated, covered waste receptacle (Fig. 5-3, *D*). After discarding the mask, the wearer must wash and dry his or her hands thoroughly.

No jewelry, with the exception of pierced earring posts, should be worn in the operating room. If pierced earrings are worn, they must be contained within the scrub hat at all times.

Operating room attire should not be worn outside the operating room department. However, if this practice is not feasible, the scrub suit should be covered by a clean, buttoned laboratory coat when a person leaves the department. The head and shoe coverings should always be removed. When the person returns to the department, the scrub suit should be changed.

Basic aseptic technique

An object or substance is considered sterile when it is completely free of all living microorganisms and is incapable of producing any form of life. The basic principles of aseptic technique prevent contamination of the open wound, isolate the operative site from the surrounding unsterile physical environment, and create and maintain a sterile field in which surgery can be performed safely.

The surgical team is composed of scrub and circulating persons. The persons who scrub their hands and arms and don sterile gowns and gloves are referred to as the *scrub* persons; the persons who supply the needs of the scrubbed team members, coordinate room activities, and attend to patient needs are referred to as the *circulating* persons.

Proper adherence to aseptic technique eliminates or minimizes modes and sources of contamination. Certain basic principles must be observed during surgery to provide a well-defined margin of safety for the patient.

1. All materials in contact with the wound and used within the sterile field must be sterile. The inadvertent use of unsterile items may introduce contaminants into the wound. When using or dispensing a sterile item, personnel must be assured that the item is sterile and will remain sterile until used. The circulating nurse should check the package integrity, the expiration date, and the appearance of the sterilizer indicating tape before dispensing a sterile item.

2. Gowns of the operating team are considered sterile in front from chest to table level. The sleeves are also considered sterile to 2 inches above the elbow. Areas of the gown that must be considered unsterile are the neckline, shoulders, areas under the arms, and back. These areas may become contaminated by perspiration or by collar and shoulder surfaces rubbing together during head and neck movements. Wraparound gowns that completely cover the back may be sterile when first put on. The back of the gown, however, *must not* be considered

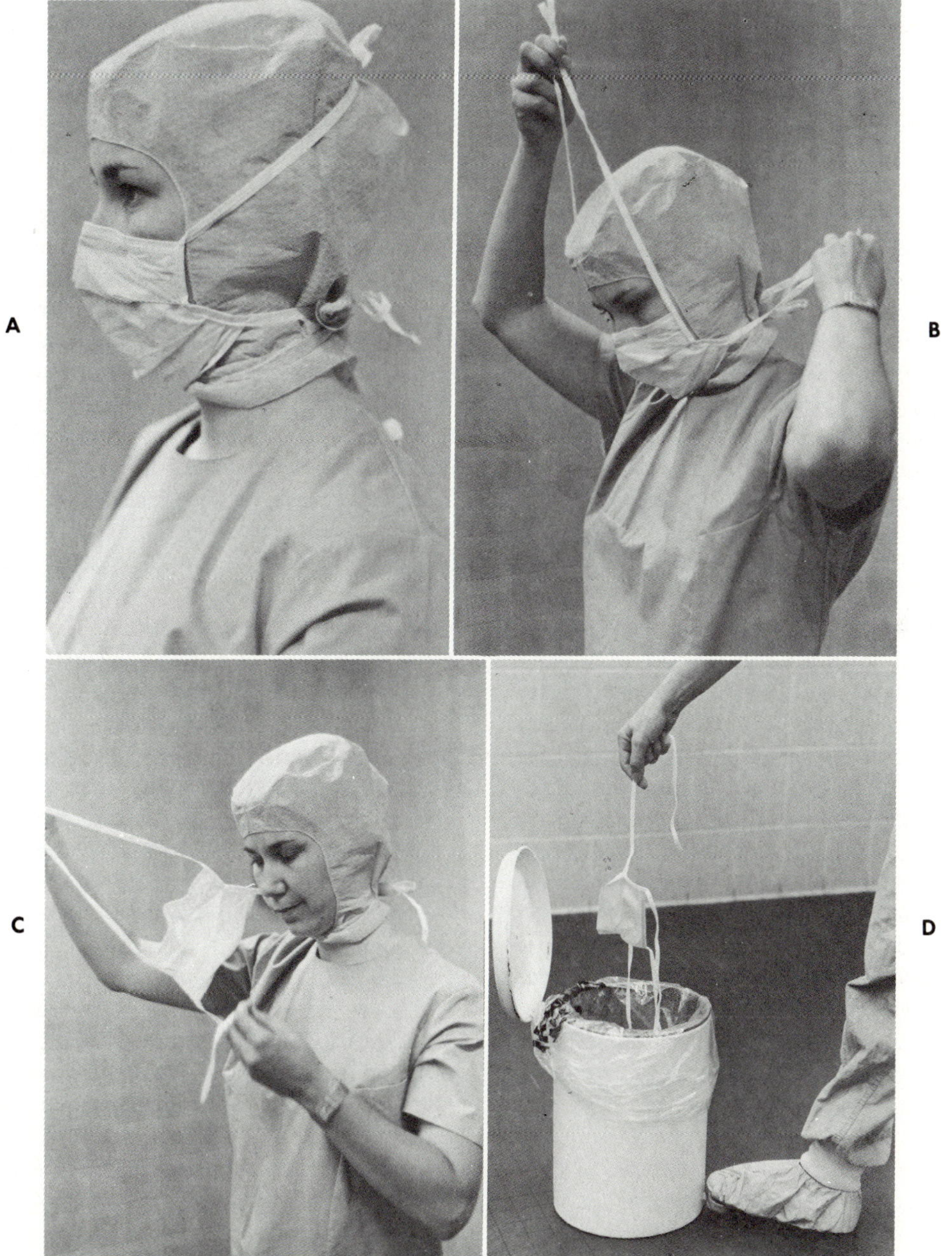

Fig. 5-3. Proper handling of mask. **A,** Edges of properly worn mask conform to facial contours when mask is applied and tied correctly. **B** and **C,** Personnel should avoid touching filter portion of mask when removing it. **D,** Use of covered waste container with foot-controlled lid opener reduces possibility of contamination during mask disposal.

sterile because it cannot be observed by the scrub person and protected from contamination.

The sterile area of the front of the gown extends to the level of the table because most scrubbed personnel work adjacent to a sterile table. For this reason, the scrub person should avoid changing levels as would occur while moving from footstool to floor. To maintain sterility, scrub persons should not allow their hands or any sterile item to fall below table level. Scrub persons should neither sit nor lean against unsterile surfaces because the threat of contamination is great. The only time scrub persons may sit is when the entire surgical procedure will be performed from the sitting position.

3. Only the top surface of a draped table is considered sterile. Although a bacterial barrier may be draped over the sides of a table, the sides cannot be considered sterile. Any item that extends beyond the sterile boundary is considered contaminated and cannot be brought back onto the sterile field. A contaminated item must be lifted clear of the operative field without contacting the sterile surface and must be dropped with minimum handling to an unsterile person, area, or receptacle. Interpretation of sterile areas versus unsterile areas on a draped patient requires astute observation and use of good judgment.

4. After a sterile package or container is opened, the edges are considered unsterile. Sterile and unsterile boundaries are often intangible. A 1-inch safety margin is usually considered standard on package wrappers, whereas the sterile boundary on a wrapper used to drape a table is at the table edge. On peel-back packages, the inner edge of the heat seal is the line of demarcation. Being hypothetical, these boundaries may not apply to every situation.

The edge of a bottle cap is considered contaminated once the cap has been removed from the bottle. The sterility of the bottle contents cannot be ensured if the cap is replaced on the bottle. Therefore, when sterile liquids are dispensed, the entire contents of a bottle must be poured or the remainder discarded. It is essential to use good judgment based on an understanding of aseptic principles when interpreting sterile boundaries.

5. Motions of the surgical team are from sterile to sterile areas and from unsterile to unsterile areas. Scrub persons and sterile items contact only sterile areas; circulating nurses and unsterile items contact only unsterile areas. All members of the surgical team must understand which areas are considered sterile and which are considered unsterile. All must maintain a continual awareness of these areas. Scrub persons must guard their sterile fields to prevent any unsterile item from contaminating the fields or them. The circulating nurses must neither touch or reach over a sterile field nor allow any unsterile item to contaminate the field.

When a circulating nurse opens a package, hand and arm motions are always from unsterile to unsterile objects. The hands are placed under the cuff to provide a protected wide margin of safety between the inside of the pack (sterile) and the hands (unsterile) (Fig. 5-4). When the circulating nurse opens a sterile article that is wrapped sequentially in two wrappers with the corners folded toward the center of the article, the corner farthest from the body is opened first, and the corner nearest the body last (Fig. 5-5, *A* and *B*).

When a scrub nurse opens a sterile wrapper, the side nearest the body is opened first. This portion of the drape then protects the gown, enabling the nurse to move closer to the table to open the opposite side (Fig. 5-6).

If a solution must be poured into a sterile receptacle on a sterile table, the scrub nurse holds the receptacle away from the table or sets it near the edge of a waterproof-draped table (Fig. 5-7, *A* and *B*). This eliminates the need for the circulating nurse to reach over the sterile field. Maintenance of a safe margin of space can help eliminate accidental contamination in passing items between sterile and unsterile fields. An instrument may be used as an extension of a team member's hands to ensure a safe margin between fields. The use of transfer forceps, however, is not acceptable. Maintenance of sterility of these forceps is questionable because there are so many variables, such as method of sterilization, type of container, and type and amount of soaking solution used. Incorrect handling of the forceps is always a problem. Transfer forceps have been replaced by a packaged sterile instrument that is used once and then considered contaminated.

6. Movement around a sterile field must not cause contamination of that sterile field. The patient is the center of the sterile field during an operation; additional sterile areas are grouped around the patient. If contamination is to be prevented, patterns of movement within or around this sterile grouping must be established and rigidly practiced. Scrub persons stay close to the sterile field. If they change positions, they turn face to face or back to back while maintaining a safe distance between. Accidental contamination is a threat to any scrub person who wanders into a traffic pathway or out of the clean area of the operating room.

Circulating persons approach sterile areas facing them and never walk between two sterile fields. Keeping sterile areas in view during movement around the area and maintaining at least a 1-foot distance from sterile fields helps prevent accidental contamination. Bacterial fallout from the body or clothing is a source of contamination when a circulating person leans over a sterile field. All operating room personnel must maintain a vigilant watch over sterile areas and point out any contamination immediately.

7. Whenever a sterile barrier is permeated, it must be considered contaminated. This principle applies to packaging materials as well as to draping and gowning mate-

rials. Obvious contamination occurs from direct contact between sterile and unsterile objects. Other less apparent modes of contamination are the filtration of airborne microorganisms through materials, the passage of liquids through materials, and the undetected perforations in materials. When moisture soaks through a drape, gown, or package, *strike-through* occurs, and the item must be considered contaminated. Potential contaminants can be curtailed by the use of effective barrier materials, the characteristics of which are discussed later in this chapter.

8. Items of doubtful sterility must be considered unsterile. In practice, the state of sterility is an absolute; items are either sterile or unsterile. Any item that falls on the floor or into any area of questionable cleanliness must be considered unsterile.

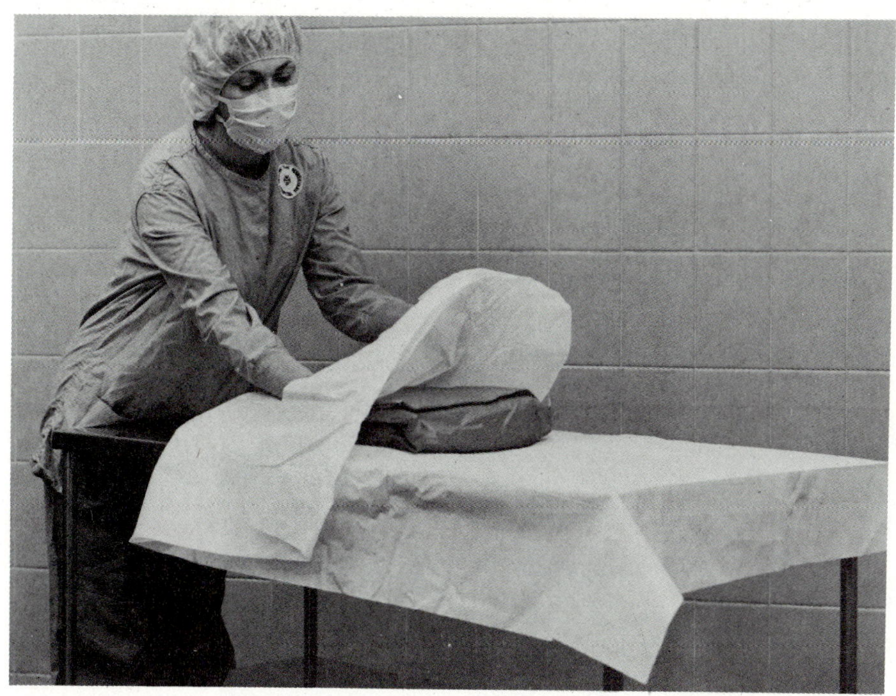

Fig. 5-4. Circulating nurse is shown opening outer cover of pack containing sterile drapes for surgery. Cover is cuffed to provide protection for sterile contents. Circulating nurse avoids contact with sterile area by keeping all fingers under cuff as cover is drawn back over table to expose inner pack.

Fig. 5-5. A, When opening sterile package, circulating nurse opens corner nearest body last to avoid potential contamination of inner pack. **B,** To prevent unsterile corners of outer wrapper from touching scrub nurse or sterile field, circulating nurse draws back corners of opened wrapper when presenting inner package.

A

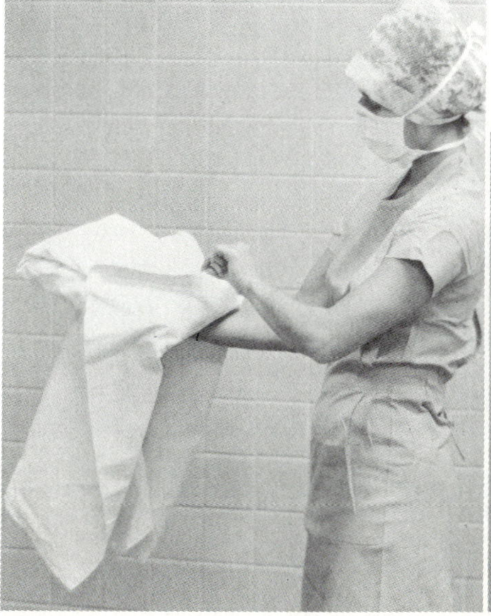

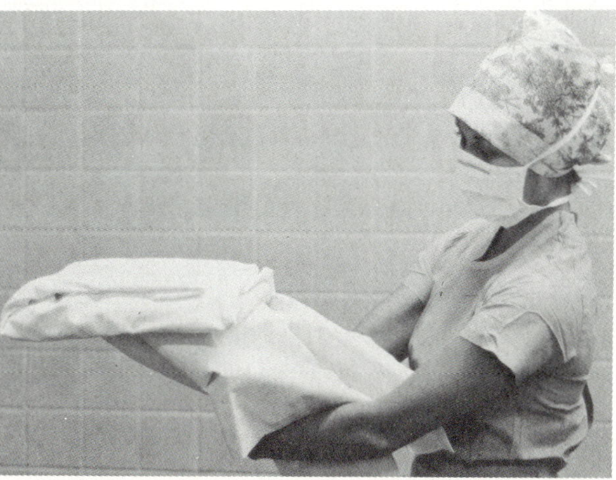

B

Preparation of sterile setups hours before needed and the subsequent covering of these setups with sterile sheets are not acceptable for two reasons: the setups are usually left unguarded and thus become prey to sources of contamination, and removal of the cover sheets without contaminating the sterile setups is almost impossible. Therefore sterile fields should be prepared as closely as possible to the scheduled time of use. If sterile setups are covered or left unguarded, they should be considered contaminated.

Close adherence to principles of asepsis and consistent observance of the boundaries established in the principles provide protection against infection. Application of the basic principles of aseptic technique depends primarily on the individual's understanding and conscience.

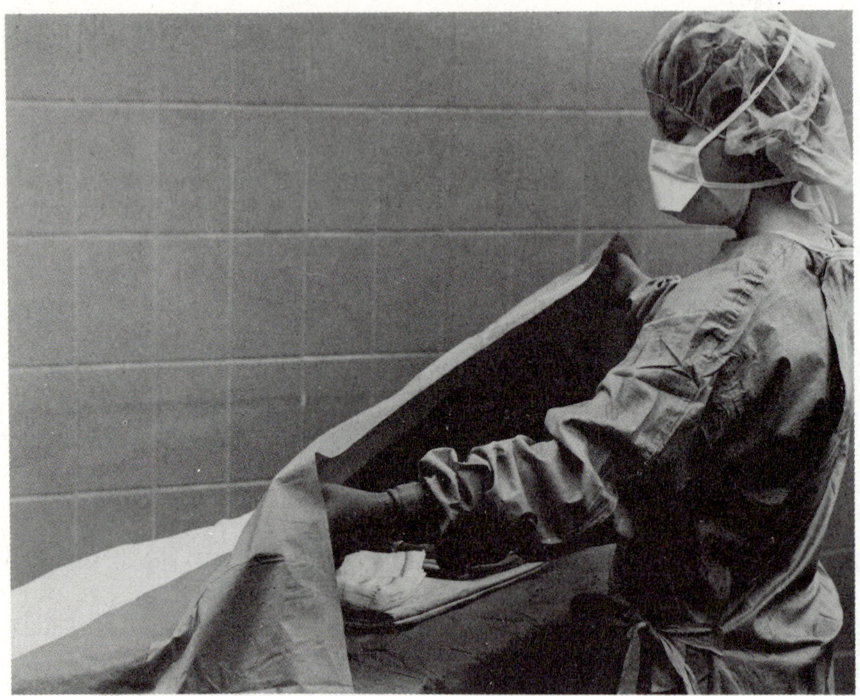

Fig. 5-6. Scrub nurse protects gloves with cuff of drape when opening inner wrapper of pack, which will serve as sterile table cover.

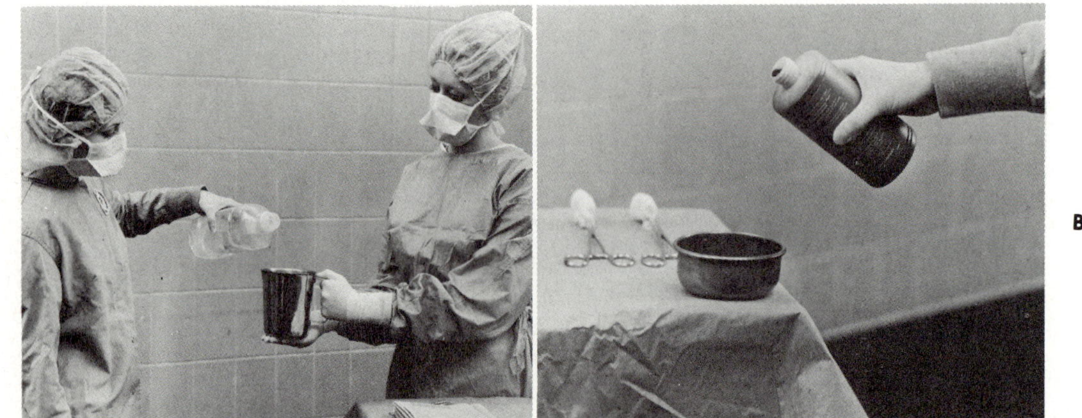

Fig. 5-7. A, When pouring solution into receptacle held by scrub nurse, circulating nurse maintains safe margin of space to avoid contamination of sterile surfaces. **B,** Care must be used when pouring solution into receptacle on sterile field. Placement of receptacle near edge of table permits circulating nurse to pour solution without reaching over any portion of sterile field.

INSTRUMENT CLEANING METHODS FOR PREVENTION OF INFECTION

To prevent infection in humans, specific microorganisms must be destroyed, removed, or inhibited by one of several methods, depending on the circumstances. Instruments, equipment, and supplies must be thoroughly cleaned before they can be sterilized. The cleaning method must be economical and must provide protection from cross-contamination, damage to the instrument, and injury to the worker. All instruments should be terminally washed and sterilized after use, before being returned to trays or storage.

Mechanical washing of instruments

Soiled instruments should be cleaned as soon as possible after use to prevent blood and other substances from drying on the surfaces or in the crevices. The horizontal type of pressure instrument washer-sterilizer (cabinet design) (Figs. 5-8 and 5-9) can be used to terminally wash and sterilize soiled instruments. Hinged instruments should be opened, and instruments with more than one part should be disassembled as they are placed in an instrument tray that has a wire mesh bottom. The tray of instruments should be placed in the washer-sterilizer and exposed to a complete wash and sterilize cycle.

When a washer-sterilizer is used, the instruments are cleaned by a mechanically agitated water bath containing a detergent, the water is removed from the washer-sterilizer, and the instruments are sterilized for 3 minutes at 132° C (270° F). Washer-sterilizers of this type help control the spread of microorganisms, reduce labor costs, and conserve time.

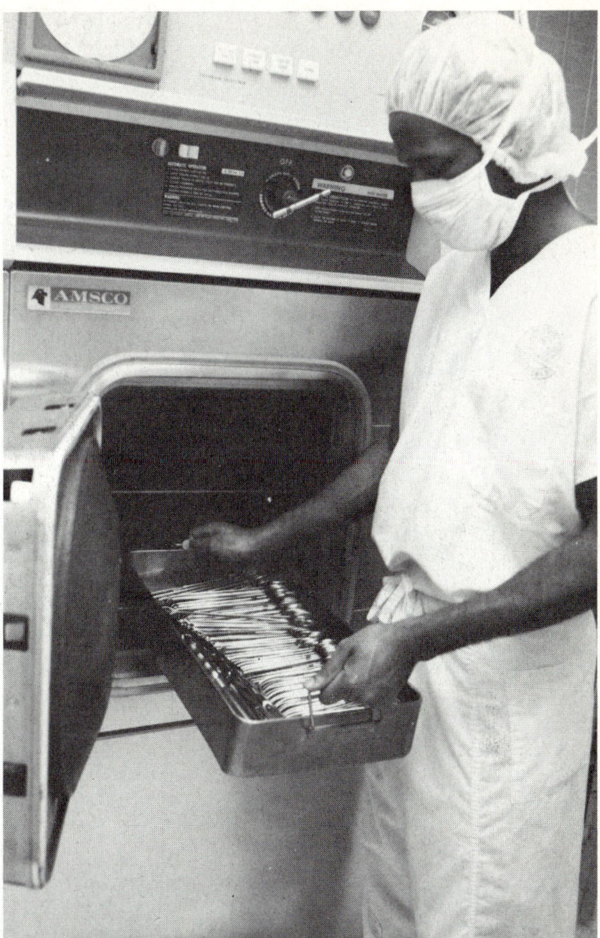

Fig. 5-8. Automatic washer-sterilizer. This type of sterilizer is used to clean and terminally sterilize instruments and utensils immediately after any surgical procedure to routinely protect personnel and to prevent cross-contamination. It is designed specifically for this function; however, it may be used in supplementary capacity for automatically programmed 3-minute and 10-minute sterilization of surgical instruments and utensils.

The efficiency of the process depends on the kind of foreign material present and the number of instruments in the load. Complete removal of all soil from the serrations and crevices of instruments depends on the construction of the instrument, the time of exposure, and the pH and efficiency of the detergent solution. Soiled grooved instruments such as intestinal anastomosis clamps and vascular clamps should be soaked in water immediately after use to prevent foreign material from drying in the grooves. They should be processed as soon as possible in the pressure instrument washer-sterilizer. The worker should always follow the operational instructions prepared by the manufacturer. If proper precautions are taken in using the equipment, questions about sterility should not arise.

If a washer-sterilizer is not available, either of two procedures can be used to ensure terminal decontamination of the instruments before they are handled by personnel:

1. The instruments should be rinsed carefully in a basin of water, placed in a perforated tray, and autoclaved for 3 minutes at 132° C (270° F) or 15 to 20 minutes at 121° C (250° F).

2. The instruments should be opened or disassembled, placed in a watertight basin, covered with a 2% solution of trisodium phosphate, placed in a pressure steam sterilizer, and sterilized for 30 minutes at 132° C (270° F) or 45 minutes at 121° C (250° F), using the fast exhaust cycle.[2]

Following terminal decontamination, the instruments can be transferred to the ultrasonic cleaner for final cleansing.

If an ultrasonic cleaner is not available, the instruments can be washed manually with a noncorrosive detergent to remove any remaining soil. If it is necessary to scrub the instruments with a brush, the brush and instruments must be kept beneath the water level to prevent aerosolization. The instruments should be rinsed in hot water, dried thoroughly, inspected, and returned to trays or storage.

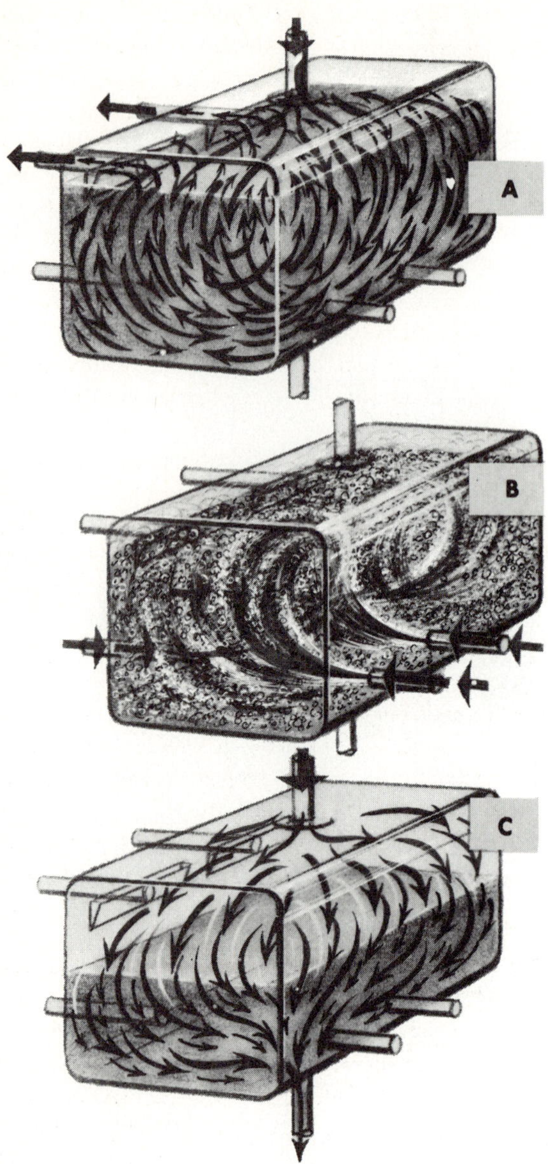

Fig. 5-9. Automatic washer-sterilizer. Washing action attained in washer-sterilizer is created by unique combination of high-velocity jet streams of steam and air, which develops violent underwater turbulence. **A,** Cold water fills chamber, covering load to overflow. This cold water, with aid of a detergent, begins to loosen and dissolve gross soil such as blood, tissue, and foreign matter. **B,** Four powerful jet streams of steam and air located near bottom of chamber drive water into violent turbulence to continue cleaning process. Water temperature rises to 62° to 69° C (145° to 155° F). This expanding water causes water level to rise; released soil and scum overflow into waste line. **C,** Steam is activated into top of chamber, thereby forcing wash water out through bottom drain. Steam under pressure floods chamber, and temperature holds at 132° C (270° F) for not less than 3 minutes. Then steam is exhausted through automatic condenser exhaust, and audible signal indicates that unit is ready for unloading. (Courtesy American Sterilizer Co., Erie, Pa.)

Ultrasonic cleaning

The ultrasonic cleaning process removes tenacious soil that remains on instruments after they have been mechanically or manually washed. This process is based on electronic engineering principles. An electric current, usually 230 volts and 60 cycles, is fed into an electronic generator, where the frequency is raised to a rate of 18,000 to 20,000 cycles per second. This electrical energy then flows into a magnetic device known as a transducer, which converts the electrical energy into mechanical energy. The ultrasonic waves pass through the fluid in the bath. When passing through the fluid of the bath, the ultrasonic waves form very small bubbles that expand until they are unstable and then collapse quickly, thus creating a negative pressure action on all surfaces of the instruments in the bath. By means of this pulling action, called the *cavitation process,* debris and material are removed from all surfaces of the instruments without damage to the instruments.

Ultrasonic cleaning plays a vital role in the care and processing of surgical instruments but must not be considered a substitute for terminal sterilization.

STERILIZATION METHODS FOR PREVENTION OF INFECTION

Modern surgery demands increasingly intricate and delicate instruments and more efficient dry goods, utensils, and fluids. Methods of sterilization of surgical items must result in complete destruction of all microbial life, including spores, and absence of toxic residue on the objects, as well as little or no deterioration or damage to heat- and moisture-sensitive instruments and other items.

Steam sterilization

Saturated steam under pressure is recognized as the safest, most practical means of sterilizing surgical dry goods, fluids, the majority of instruments, and other inanimate objects. Steam under pressure permits permeation of moist heat to porous substances by condensation and results in destruction of all microbial life.

Saturated steam exerts the maximum pressure for water vapor at a given temperature and pressure.

Theory of microbial destruction

It is believed that microorganisms are destroyed by moist heat through a process of denaturation and coagulation of the enzyme-protein system within the bacterial cell. Microorganisms are killed at a lower temperature when moist heat is used than when dry heat is used. This fact is based on the theory that all chemical reactions, including coagulation of proteins, are catalyzed by the presence of water.

Compressed steam results in effective sterilization because moisture and heat are always present. When steam comes in contact with a cold object, condensation takes place immediately. As the steam condenses, it gives off latent heat and results in heating and wetting of the object; in other words, both moisture and heat are provided.

Principles and mechanism

Pure steam at sea level atmospheric pressure has a temperature of 100° C (212° F). When water is boiled in a vessel from which the steam cannot escape, a higher temperature is reached. To attain steam under pressure, a vessel that can be closed tightly must be used. A home pressure cooker generates steam from the water inside the tightly closed vessel when it is placed over a gas flame or electric plate. In the hospital autoclave, the steam coming from the boilers is compressed, thus giving off latent heat.

The higher the steam pressure, the higher the temperature becomes. The steam is the sterilizing agent, not the compressed hot air. If steam is mixed with air at the same pressure, the temperature will be lower than pure steam at atmospheric pressure. For example, if the mixture is two thirds steam and one third air, the temperature at 15 pounds pressure per square inch (psi) will be 115° C (240° F) instead of 121° C (250° F). The air acts as a barrier to steam penetration.

Generally, the autoclave consists of two metal cylinders (the chamber and the shell), one within the other. Between the cylinders is an enclosed space (the jacket) in which steam and heat can be maintained. This steam jacket facilitates fast, efficient, and effective drying of the load following sterilization.

In the conventional steam sterilizer, the sterilization process may be divided into five distinct phases:

1. Loading phase, in which the objects are packaged and loaded in the sterilizer
2. Heating phase, in which the steam is brought to the proper temperature and allowed to penetrate around and through the objects in the chamber
3. Destroying phase, or the time-temperature cycle, in which all microbial life is exposed to the killing effects of the steam
4. Drying and cooling phase, in which the objects are dried and cooled, filtered air is introduced into the chamber, the door is opened, and the objects are removed and stored
5. Testing phase, in which the efficiency of the sterilizing process is checked

Phase 1

Packaging of surgical supplies and their arrangement in loads in the sterilizer are important factors that govern the effectiveness of steam sterilization.

The prime function of a package containing a surgical item is to permit sterilization of the contents and to ensure the sterility of the contents up to the time the package is intentionally opened. Provision must be made for the contents to be removed without contamination. Numerous factors should be considered in selecting an effective packaging material. It must be suitable for the method of sterilization used, permitting adequate air removal and steam penetration when steam sterilization is used, and adequate penetration and release of gas and moisture sterilants when gas sterilization is used. It should be durable so as to resist tearing or puncture and should be free of pinholes. It also should be moisture resistant. An effective wrapper should be flexible and memory free to allow easy aseptic presentation with assurance of no particulate contamination when the package is opened. It should establish a barrier to microorganisms or their vehicles.[4]

If textile wrappers are used, they must be laundered between sterilization exposures to ensure sufficient moisture content of the fibers, which prevents superheating and absorption of the sterilizing agent. Laundering also reduces the deterioration rate of woven materials. All wrappers must be checked for torn areas and holes before they are used.

Many inhospital packaging materials—woven and nonwoven, reusable and disposable—are marketed today. Available materials should be carefully evaluated before a product is chosen. The present standards for steam sterilization are based on a 140-thread–count muslin. Manufacturers of packaging materials should be able to show that sterilization can be achieved with practical sterilizer operating cycles.

The size and density of woven textile packs must be restricted to ensure uniform steam penetration. The size of the pack should not exceed 12 × 12 × 20 inches and should not weigh more than 12 pounds. In assembling the items in the pack, the lighter materials should be placed near the center of the pack. Each succeeding layer of dry goods should be placed crosswise on the layer below to promote free circulation of steam and removal of air. Pack density should not exceed 7.2 pounds per cubic foot. A chemical indicator that accurately reflects one or more of the physical parameters of sterilization should be inserted in the center of each pack. The parameters for steam sterilization include time, temperature, and moisture. The more parameters monitored, the greater the assurance that conditions necessary for sterilization have been met.

The pack should be wrapped sequentially in two double-thickness muslin wrappers or the equivalent in other types of wrappers. Wrappers are made in suitable dimensions for the various items that must be packaged. The familiar envelope wrap is made by placing the article diagonally in the center of the wrapper. The near corner, which should point toward the worker, is brought over the item, and the triangular tip is folded back to form a cuff. The two side flaps are folded to the center in like manner. The far corner of the wrapper is then folded on top of the other three and secured with autoclave indicator tape. The flaps at the corners are used to form a cuff over the worker's fingers and a safe barrier for the sterile goods. When the items are wrapped, the wrappers should not be folded tightly about the contents, but the package should be firm and sealed securely to prevent contamination in handling and storage.

Tubes, needles, and drains must have moisture in the lumen that can turn to steam and prevent trapping of air, which creates a barrier against effective sterilization. Their containers must be covered with a material that permits penetration of steam to all inside surfaces of the containers.

Pressure-sensitive autoclave tape should be used to hold wrappers in place on packages and to indicate that the packages have been exposed to the physical conditions of an autoclave cycle. When packages are opened, these tapes should be removed from reusable wrappers because they create laundry problems, such as stopping up screens and filters. In some cases, the tapes leave a dye on the wrappers that may cause deterioration of the material.

Every package intended for sterile use should be imprinted or labeled with a lot control number that identifies the date of sterilization, the sterilizer used, the cycle or load number, and the date of expiration. Dating of packages prepared in the hospital assists in inventory control and rotation of older goods into early use.

When the chamber of the sterilizer is loaded, the bundles and packages should be arranged so that there is little resistance to the passage of steam through the load from the top of the chamber toward the bottom of the sterilizer. All packages should be placed in the sterilizer on edge in a vertical, loose-contact position to allow free circulation and penetration of steam, enhance air elimination, and prevent entrapment of air or water. A second or upper layer may be placed crosswise on the first or lower layer.

All jars, tubes, canisters and other nonporous objects should be arranged on their sides with their covers or lids removed to provide a horizontal path for the escape of air and free flow of steam and heat.

Instruments should be placed in trays that have mesh or perforated bottoms. They may be autoclaved while unwrapped and then used immediately, or they may be wrapped and sterilized for later use.

To guard against superheating, the surgical packs should not be subjected to preheating in the sterilizer with steam in the jacket before sterilization.

Phase 2

When the steam enters the autoclave, it will be at the same pressure as that of the atmosphere. With closure of the valves and doors communicating with the outside, the pressure of the steam inside rises, resulting in an increase in the temperature of the steam.

Gauges on traditional autoclaves register the pressure in both the jacket and the chamber. Most vacuums are designated in terms of inches of mercury. A perfect vacuum is represented by a column of mercury 29.92 inches high. Standard gauges indicate vacuum starting with zero (at room or normal atmospheric pressure). As the air is removed, the gauge registers down to 30 inches.

Evacuation of air from the conventional sterilizer is necessary to permit proper permeation of steam. The most common method for removal of air is the downward or gravity displacement method. This method is based on the principle that air is heavier than steam. The steam that is piped into the sterilizer through a multiport valve is introduced into the chamber. The steam forces the heavier air ahead of it, down and forward, until all the air is discharged from a line at the front of the sterilizer. If a sterilizer is improperly loaded, mixing of air with steam acts as a barrier to steam penetration and prevents the attainment of the sterilization temperature.

Phase 3

The destruction period is based on the known time-temperature cycle necessary to accomplish sterilization in saturated steam. Authorities have shown that the order of death in a given bacterial population subjected to a sterilizing process is determined by definite laws. If the temperature is increased, the time may be decreased. The minimum time-temperature relationships in terms of sterilizing efficiency are as follows:

2 minutes at 132° C (270° F)
8 minutes at 125° C (257° F)
18 minutes at 118° C (245° F)

To provide a safety margin, the minimum estimated exposure is extended to cover the lag between the attainment of the selected temperature in the chamber and the temperature of the load. The length of exposure varies, depending on the composition of items to be sterilized.

In a gravity displacement sterilizer, instruments (metal only) in an unwrapped perforated tray should be exposed for 3 minutes at 132° C (270° F) or 15 minutes at 121° C (250° F). When metal instruments are combined with porous instruments or materials in an unwrapped perforated tray, they must be exposed for 10 minutes at 132° C or 20 minutes at 121° C. Instruments wrapped in four thicknesses of muslin should be exposed for 15 minutes at 132° C or 30 minutes at 121° C. All types of linen packs should be exposed for 30 minutes at 121° C. Bulk loads of supplies, with the exception of rubber gloves and solutions, can be sterilized safely and practically at 121° C for 30 minutes.

In a prevacuum sterilizer, supplies should be exposed for 4 minutes after the temperature reaches at least 132° C at the center of the pack.

The recording thermometer, not the pressure gauge, is the important guide to the sterilizing phase. The recording clock on the sterilizer gives information about the run of the load and to what temperature the goods were exposed. The temperature inside the chamber must be maintained throughout the determined time of exposure.

Phase 4

At completion of the sterilization cycle, the steam inside the chamber is removed immediately so that it will not condense and wet the packs. To assist in the drying process, the jacket pressure should be maintained to keep the walls of the chamber hot as the steam from the chamber is exhausted to zero gauge pressure. When chamber pressure has been exhausted, the door may be opened slightly to permit vapor to escape. Another method is to introduce clean, filtered air by means of a vacuum dryer (ejector) device in conjunction with the operating valve on the sterilizer. The minimum drying time for all methods is approximately 15 to 20 minutes.

Following removal from the sterilizer, freshly sterilized packs should be left on the loading carriage for 15 to 60 minutes or until adequately cooled. If a loading carriage has not been used, the packs should be placed on edge on wire mesh surfaces that are covered with several layers of muslin to absorb the sweating moisture. Freshly sterilized packages should not be placed on cold surfaces such as metal tabletops. The sweating that occurs on the cool table will form pools of water that may pick up contaminants and be reabsorbed by the dry goods. Since bacteria are capable of passing through layers of wet material, any packages that are wet must be considered unsterile.

Sterile packages must be handled with care and as little as possible. They should be stored in clean, dry, dustproof, and verminproof areas that are well ventilated and have controlled temperature and humidity. Closed cabinets are preferred to open shelves for sterile storage. If open shelves must be used, the lowest shelf should be 8 to 10 inches from the floor and the highest should be at least 18 inches from the ceiling. All shelves should be at least 2 inches from outside walls. Shelving should be smooth and well spaced, with no projections or sharp corners that might damage the wrappers. Sterilized packs should never be stacked in close contact with each other. Their arrangement on the shelves should provide for air circulation on all sides of each package. Excessive handling, crowding, dropping, and pummeling of sterile packs tend to force particles through the mesh or matrix of the wrapping material, which might contaminate the contents. For proper rotation, the most recently dated sterile packages should be placed behind those already on the shelves.

Shelf life refers to the length of time a pack may be considered sterile. It is actually event related, not time related. Variables that must be considered in determining shelf life are the type and number of layers of packaging material used, the presence or absence of dustcovers, the number of times a package is handled before use, and the conditions of storage. Double-wrapped muslin, nonwoven fabric, and paper-wrapped items can be considered sterile for 21 to 30 days. Plastic or plastic-paper combination wraps that are heat sealed will maintain sterility for 6 months to a year. Impervious plastic overwraps (dustcovers) will extend shelf life to 6 months or more, depending on the sealing method used. When dustcovers are used to protect sterilized items, they should be designated as such to prevent their being mistaken for a sterile wrap. They should be applied only to thoroughly cooled, dry packs at the time of removal from the sterilizer cart, following the required cooling period.

Many commercially prepared sterile disposable drapes, packs, and materials are sealed in nonwoven envelopes that are encased in plastic, sealed wrappers. They theoretically maintain sterility for indefinite periods; their sterility, however, is dependent on their exposure during storage, the amount of handling, and the kind and condition of the wrapper.

Supply standards should be planned to maintain adequate stock with prompt turnover. Appropriate volume and proper rotation of supplies reduces the need for concern about shelf life. The longer an item is stored, the greater the chances of contamination.

A written record of existing conditions during each sterilization cycle should be maintained. It should include the sterilizer number, the cycle or load number, the time and temperature of the cycle, the date of sterilization, the contents of the load, and the initials of the operator. These records should be retained for the length of time designated by the statute of limitations in each state.

Phase 5

All mechanical parts of sterilizers, including gauges, steam lines, and drains, should be periodically checked by a competent engineer. Reports of these inspections should be kept by the person responsible for the sterilizers. Temperature, humidity, and vacuum should be measured with control equipment, independently of the fixed gauges. There are several methods of keeping a constant check on the proper functioning of a sterilizer and ensuring the efficiency of the sterilizing process.

Mechanical controls such as thermometers and automatic controls assist in identifying and preventing malfunction of the sterilizing equipment and operational errors made by the personnel. Indicating thermometers, located on the discharge line of the sterilizer, indicate the temperature throughout the sterilizing cycle on a dial on the front of the sterilizer. The device indicates a drop in temperature, when and if it occurs, and can act as a warning of sterilizer failure. Because lowering of the temperature may be intermittent and is not recorded permanently, it must be seen by those responsible for operating the sterilizer. This device cannot detect air pockets within the load or pack. Air is a poor conductor of heat; therefore it is one of the greatest causes, other than human error, of sterilization failure.

Recording thermometers indicate and record the same temperature as the indicating thermometers. They record the time the sterilizer reaches the desired degree of temperature and the duration of each exposure. The recording thermometer can be helpful if several individuals are using the sterilizer or if the operator should forget to time the load. Its recordings act as daily proof that exposure time of loads has been correct, as well as show that proper temperature limits have been maintained. The daily record should show the number of the sterilizer, the number of cycles run, the time, and the date. This evidence can be used to correct discrepancies should error occur. Like the indicating thermometer, the recording thermometer does not detect cool air pockets; therefore additional controls are necessary for complete safety.

Automatic controls are devices that, by a predetermined plan, control all phases of the sterilizing process. The controls allow the steam to enter, time the sterilizing cycle, exhaust the steam, and allow drying. Some lock the door so that it cannot be opened until the cycle is complete.

A thermocouple may be placed within the pack or load to indicate whether the required degree of temperature has been reached and maintained within the contents throughout the sterilizing cycle.

Chemical controls or sterilizer indicators, such as sealed glass tubes, sterilizer indicating tape, and color-change cards or strips, can be used to detect cool air pockets inside the sterilizing chamber. They can be useful in checking packaging and loading techniques on a package-by-package or load-by-load basis, as well as the mechanical functioning of the sterilizer.

One chemical control is a sealed glass tube that contains a pellet that melts when favorable time and temperature conditions for sterilization are achieved. These tubes are placed in the center of each linen pack.

Chemical indicator cards and strips are impregnated with a dye that changes color when steam initiates a chemical reaction in the dye. Indicators that are sensitive to ethylene oxide are also available.

Tapes, labels, or legends printed on packaging materials may have lines, squares, or wording that changes color when exposed to the sterilizing agent for a certain time and temperature and identifies packages that have been exposed to the physical conditions of a sterilization cycle.

An external chemical indicator should be used on every package to be sterilized and should be sensitive to three factors: time, temperature, and moisture. However, these indicators do not *prove* sterilization because some of them react even when the temperature is inadequate for sterilization. A method of checking thermal controls is to expose them to steam in a sterilizer set at 115° C (240° F) for 30 minutes. This temperature is inadequate for sterilization; therefore the controls should not react.

A biological control is the most accurate method of checking sterilization effectiveness. Commercially prepared spore strips and ampules that have been approved by the biological division of the National Institutes of Health are available. They contain a known population of *Bacillus stearothermophilus,* a highly heat-resistant, spore-forming microorganism that does not produce toxins and is nonpathogenic. The spore strips or ampules should be placed in the largest density test packs of linen and in the areas of the sterilizer least accessible to steam. When spore strips or ampules are removed, they are sent to the bacteriology laboratory, a commercial laboratory, or the manufacturer for results.

Biological testing of steam sterilizer loads should be conducted at least weekly, on the first run of the day. The spore strips or ampules should be placed in a test pack that is positioned in the front bottom section of the steam sterilizer. The test pack for gravity displacement and prevacuum steam sterilizers should consist of three muslin gowns, twelve towels, thirty 4 × 4 gauze sponges, five 12 × 12 laparotomy sponges, and one muslin drape sheet. Two biological indicators and an internal chemical indicator are placed in the center of the pack, separated by a towel.

Following the sterilization cycle, the biological indicator is removed from the pack and incubated according to manufacturer's instructions. *Negative* reports indicate that wrapping techniques, loading procedures, and sterilizing conditions are correct and that the sterilizer is functioning properly. Results of these tests should be filed as a permanent record. If a positive report is received, the sterilizer should be taken out of service until it is operationally inspected and retested and the results of retesting are negative. All items produced in the suspect load should be considered unsterile. They should be retrieved if possible and washed, repackaged, and resterilized in another sterilizer.

Spore control ampules containing *B. stearothermophilus* are used for steam sterilization only and cannot be used in hot air (dry heat) sterilizers, since 121° C (250° F) would also sterilize them without sterilizing the load itself. In general, hot air sterilization is not as good as either steam or ethylene oxide and should be avoided whenever possible. Spore strips containing *B. subtilis* should not be used to check steam sterilizers because they are not sufficiently heat resistant. They may be used, however, to check ethylene oxide and dry heat sterilizers.

High-speed pressure sterilization

The high-speed pressure instrument steam sterilizer, commonly referred to as a *flash sterilizer,* is adjusted to operate at 132° C (270° F) and 27 psi (Fig. 5-10). Although it can be used for sterilizing packs and solutions, it is most frequently used in the operating room for the sterilization of instruments that are urgently needed. The operational process consists of the following steps:

1. Steam is maintained in the jacket of the sterilizer before and during the daily operating schedule.
2. Soiled instruments are cleaned with warm tap water containing a detergent and then rinsed thoroughly in a fat-solvent solution.
3. The opened instruments are placed in a perforated metal tray, the tray positioned in the sterilizer, and the door of the sterilizer closed and locked.
4. The chamber steam supply valve is opened, and the operating valve is turned to the sterilizing setting. Time exposure begins when the thermometer records 132° C (270° F). If the sterilizer is automatic, the timer is set for a 3-minute or 10-minute exposure period (based on the composition of the instruments), and the selector switch is turned to the fast exhaust setting.
5. On completion of the exposure period, the chamber steam valve is closed and the operating valve turned to exhaust.
6. The door is opened when the exhaust valve registers zero.
7. By aseptic technique, the instruments are removed and delivered to the operating table.

Prevacuum, high-temperature sterilization

The automatic prevacuum, high-temperature sterilization method has replaced, in many instances, the downward displacement method of sterilization. Prevacuum, high-temperature sterilization is usually accomplished by means of an air-blasted, oil-sealed rotary pump, protected by a condensor and coupled with an automatic control mechanism (Fig. 5-11).

Air removal is accomplished by means of a powerful vacuum pump that draws a near-absolute vacuum in the chamber in the first 5 minutes of the cycle, before the steam is introduced. This mechanism reduces the time necessary to accomplish all phases of the sterilizing process.

The prevacuum, high-temperature steam sterilizer provides a system that is automatically controlled and reduces the total cycle time to as little as 20 minutes. The cycle time will vary with the size of the sterilizer, the adequacy of the steam, and the supply of water. Faulty packaging and overloading or incorrect placement of objects in the chamber is not likely to interfere with air removal, and full heating of the load will take place more rapidly than with the downward displacement method. The prevacuum, high-temperature steam sterilizer will permit more supplies to be sterilized within a given time.

The Bowie-Dick type test should be used to evaluate the ability of a prevacuum steam sterilizer to effectively reduce air residuals from the chamber to prevent air reentrainment into the load and to detect the presence of air leaks. It should be used daily on the first run of the day or at a designated time each day if sterilizers are used 24 hours a day. The test is conducted by placing four strips of autoclave tape approximately 8 inches long on the surface of a huckaback towel in a crisscross manner. Towels folded no smaller than 9 × 12 inches are stacked one on top of another until the stack measures 10 to 11 inches. The towel with the crossed indicator tape or a commercially prepared Bowie-Dick type test sheet is placed in the center of the stack of towels, and a single wrapper is loosely applied. The pack is placed horizontally in the bottom front of the sterilizer rack near the door and over the drain. The cycle is then run according to the sterilizer manufacturer's directions. At the completion of the cycle, the test towel or sheet is removed from the pack and examined by a person trained in its interpretation. A uniform color change throughout the crossed indicator tape or test sheet indicates a satisfactory test. The Bowie-Dick type test does not measure the efficacy of the sterilization process.[3]

Boiling water (nonpressure)

Boiling does *not* sterilize instruments or other inanimate objects. The boiling point of water varies at different altitudes. For example, at sea level the boiling point of water is 100° C (212° F), at 5000 feet above sea level the boiling point is 94.5° C (202° F), and at 10,000 feet above sea level the boiling point is 89° C (192° F). Heat-resistant microorganisms, bacterial spores, and certain viruses can withstand boiling water at 100° C (212° F) for many hours.

Hot air (dry heat) sterilization

When the physical characteristics of certain materials such as powders, grease, and anhydrous oils do not permit permeation of steam, dry heat sterilization may be used. As the proteins become dry during exposure to dry heat, their resistance to denaturation increases. For this reason, at a given temperature, dry heat sterilization is much less effective then moist heat.

Dry heat sterilization is accomplished by means of a mechanical convection hot air sterilizer at a temperature of 160° C (320° F), for an exposure period of an hour or longer. The sterilizer should be equipped with a blower for forced air circulation. Overloading the sterilizer should be avoided because it delays heat convection and circulation.

An autoclave can be used on a temporary basis as a hot air sterilizer. It is important to remember that the maximum temperature that can be maintained in the chamber is 121° C (250° F) and the minimum exposure time is 6 hours, preferably longer. It is also difficult to determine the true temperature of the chamber because the thermometer on the autoclave does not record the temperature when moist heat is not present in the chamber.

Incineration, or actual burning of materials, is the most drastic application of dry heat. It is used for the disposal of contaminated gloves, dry goods, and other inorganic and organic wastes and materials.

Chemical sterilization

New materials that cannot be heat sterilized are continually being introduced for use in hospitals. This requires the use of other methods of sterilization. An effective alternate method is based on the use of chemical agents.

Sterilization can be achieved by many agents when only vegetative cells are present. If the microbial population is unknown, however, a sporicidal agent must be employed for sterilization assurance. An antimicrobial agent must exhibit a wide microbiological spectrum and sporicidal activity to qualify as a chemosterilizer. The use of chemosterilizers is governed by the U.S. Department of Agriculture and has been restricted to ethylene oxide (a gaseous chemosterilizer) and aqueous glutaraldehyde (a liquid chemosterilizer).

Chemical sterilization is frequently referred to as *cold sterilization*. This term refers to the maximum temperature of 54° C (130° F) to 60° C (140° F) of gaseous sterilization as compared with the 121° C (250° F) to 132° C (270° F) temperatures of steam sterilization.

Gaseous chemical sterilization

In recent years, gaseous chemical sterilization has had considerable application in sterilization of heat-labile and moisture-sensitive items, such as intricate, delicate surgical instruments, large pieces of equipment used in the hospital, plastic and porous materials, and electrical instruments—all of which are difficult to steam sterilize without deterioration and damage.

Ethylene oxide is the most frequently used gas. It is colorless at ordinary temperatures, has an odor similar to ether, and has an inhalation toxicity similar to that of ammonia gas. It is easily kept as a liquid that will boil at 10.73° C (51.3° F) and will freeze at −111.3° C (−168.3° F).

Ethylene oxide is highly explosive and very flammable in the presence of air. These hazards have been greatly reduced by diluting the ethylene oxide with inert gases such as carbon dioxide or fluorinated hydrocarbons (Freon). Neither of these two inert gases appears to affect the bactericidal activity of the ethylene oxide but serves only as an inert diluent that prevents the flammability hazard.

Several theories on how ethylene oxide kills bacteria have been proposed. It is generally believed that the killing rate of bacteria is relative to the rate of diffusion of the gas through their cell walls and the availability or accessibility of one of the chemical groups in the bacterial cell walls to react with the ethylene oxide. The killing rate is also dependent on whether the bacterial cell is in a vegetative or spore state. Destruction takes place by alkylation through chemical interference and probably inactivation of the reproductive process of the cell.

Sterilizers range in size from small tubular devices

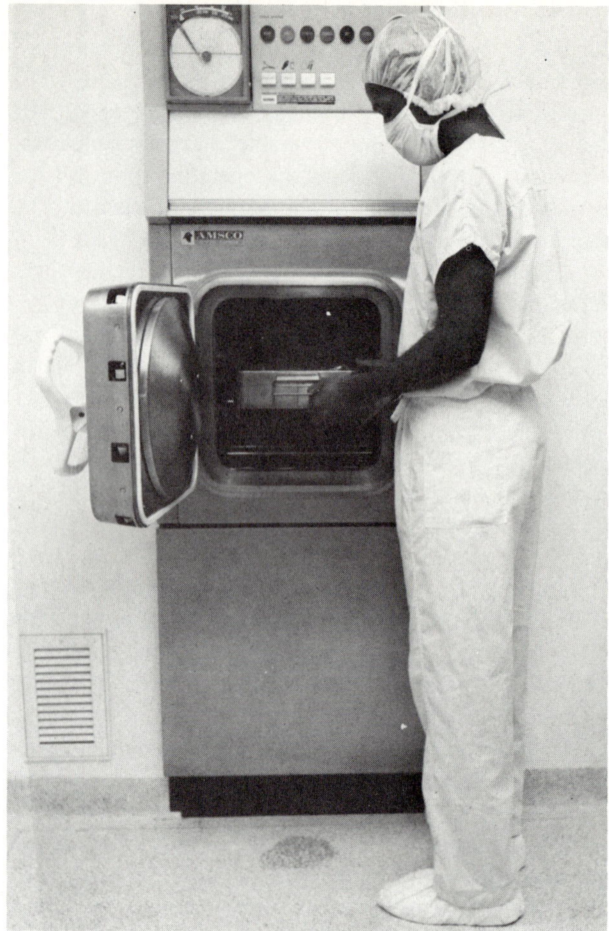

A

Fig. 5-10. General purpose, high-speed sterilizer can sterilize instruments, wrapped and unwrapped packs, utensils, and flasked solutions. **A,** Productivity of this high-speed cycle falls approximately halfway between standard gravity units and mechanical air removal (vacuum) high-temperature sterilizers. All human-engineered aspects of control panel have been zoned and color-coded for simplified selection of time, temperature, and cycle. Mechanism protects cycle from being changed while in progress. Mechanical timer permits timing from 0 to 60 minutes. **B,** Adjustable racks with four shelf positions are designed to permit maximum loading efficiency. **C,** Instrument trays featuring wire mesh bottoms and foldover, hinged handles are available in full-tray and half-tray lengths.

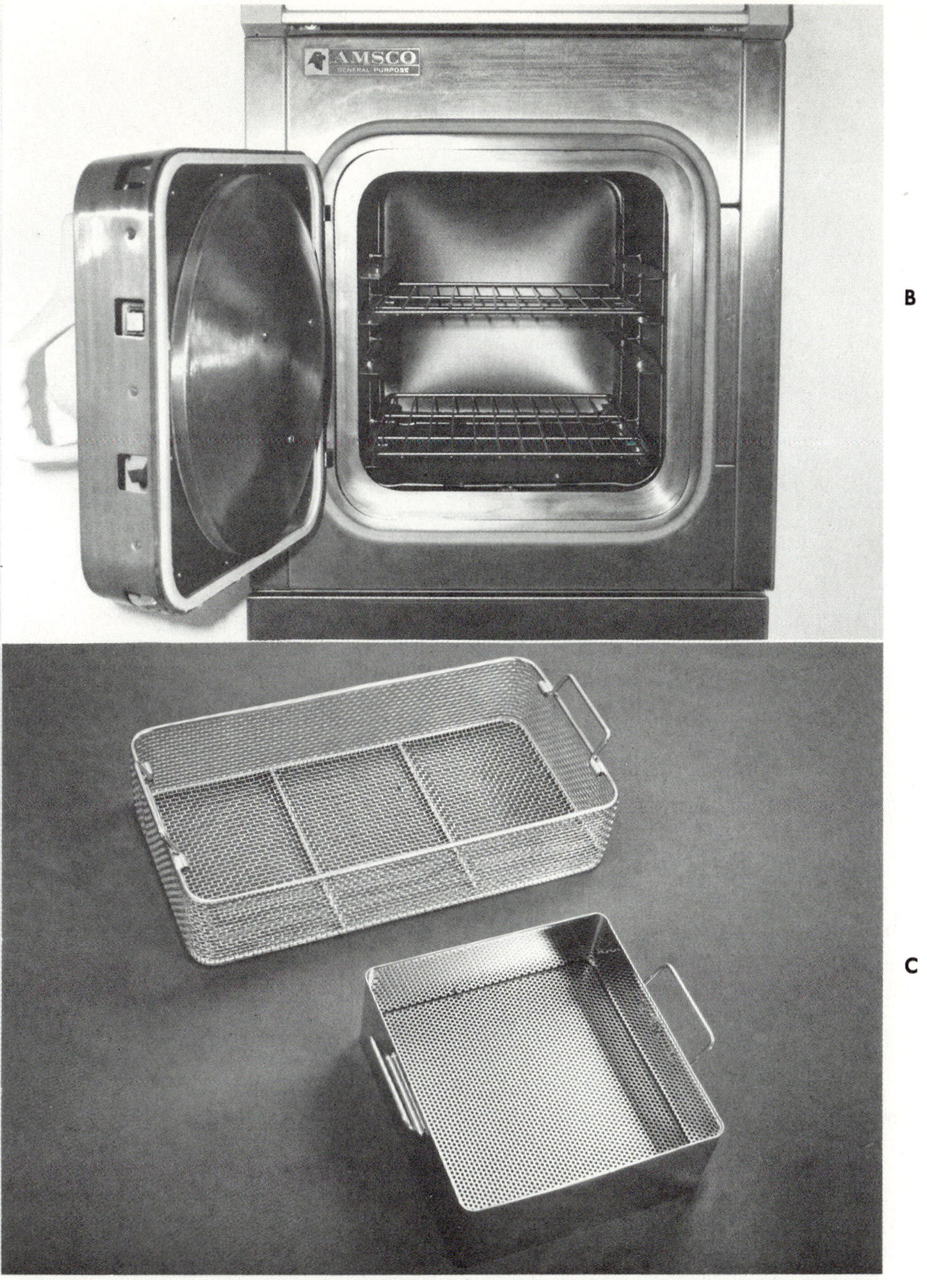

Fig. 5-10, cont'd. For legend see opposite page.

(canisters) that operate under manual control at room temperature to large chambers equipped with automatic controls. The automatic control cycle of the sterilizing process consists of air evacuation, humidification, sterilization, gas evacuation, and admission of filtered air to relieve the vacuum.

In general, ethylene oxide sterilization should be used only if the materials are heat sensitive and will not withstand sterilization by saturated steam under pressure. Any item that can be steam sterilized should never be gas sterilized.

As a sterilizing agent, ethylene oxide has the advantages that it is easily available; is effective against all types of microorganisms; penetrates through masses of dry material easily; does not require high temperatures, humidity, or pressure; and is noncorrosive and nondamaging to items.

Sterilization with ethylene oxide also has numerous disadvantages. The long exposure and aeration periods make it a lengthy process. When compared with steam sterilization, ethylene oxide sterilization is expensive. Liquid ethylene oxide may produce serious burns on ex-

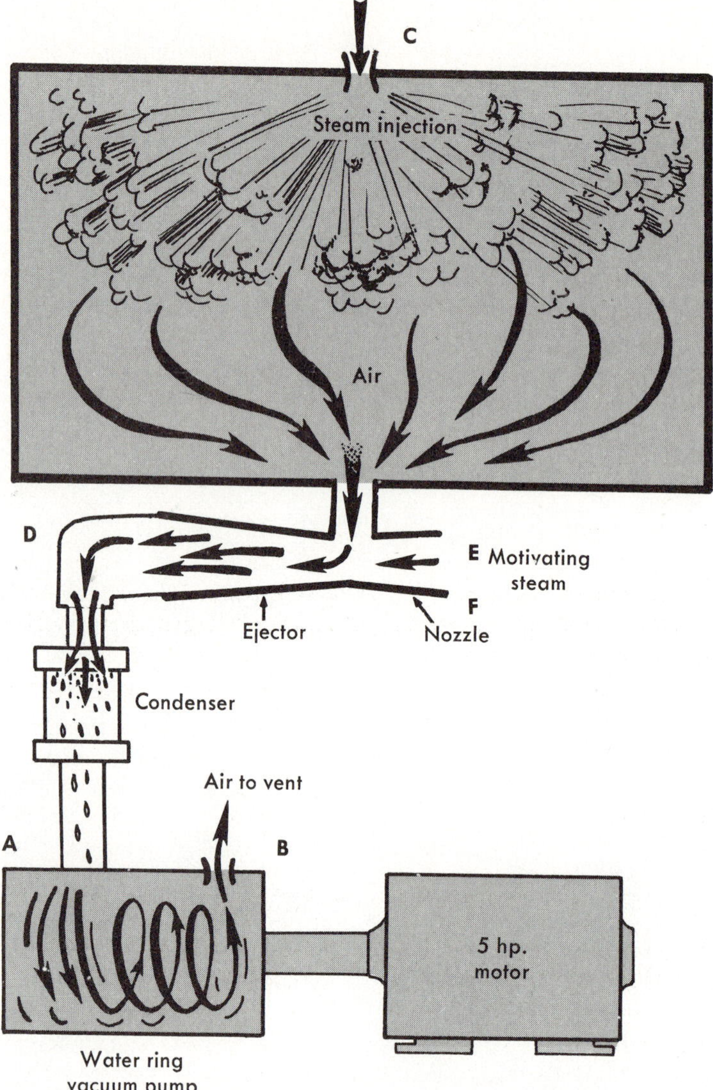

Fig. 5-11. Vacamatic sterilizer system. This type of sterilizer features simultaneous vacuum and steam injection. Air evacuation from chamber and load before sterilization is accomplished by means of high vacuum, coupled with simultaneous steam injection. This conditioning of load eliminates possibility of temperature lag when exposure period starts. Saturated steam enters chamber and penetrates densest packs in load, heating them rapidly to 133° to 136° C (272° to 276° F). Water-ring vacuum pump, together with steam ejector, forms direct, balanced, quiet element. Air to be evacuated from chamber is drawn into pump through an opening, **A,** and is exhausted through opening **B.** As air is being evacuated, "conditioning steam" is injected into chamber through **C,** thus diffusing air in space surrounding fabrics. Conditioning steam assisted by partial vacuum diffuses rapidly through fibers, thereby completely releasing absorbed air by displacement. Conditioning the load ensures fast heating to sterilizing temperature. Water-ring pump creates vacuum of about 50 mm Hg absolute at base of steam ejector. **D,** Steam from sterilizer jacket enters ejector through **E.** Incoming steam expanding through nozzle, **F,** creates tremendous velocity, which draws with it air from sterilizer chamber out to condenser and through pump. (Courtesy American Sterilizer Co., Erie, Pa.)

posed skin if not immediately removed; insufficiently aerated materials can cause skin irritation, burns of body tissue, and hemolysis of blood; and diluents used with ethylene oxide cause damage to some plastics. Human error and mechanical breakdown are more likely to occur.

Factors affecting sterilization with ethylene oxide are time of exposure, gas concentration, temperature, humidity, and penetration. The time exposure that is required depends on temperature, humidity, gas concentration, the ease of penetrating the articles to be sterilized, and the type of microorganisms to be destroyed. Manufacturers of gas sterilizers have developed recommended exposure periods for various ethylene oxide concentrations in relation to the material to be sterilized. In general, an exposure period of 3 to 7 hours is necessary for complete sterilization. Exposure time is set for absolute destruction of the most resistant microorganisms, which is a very slow process.

Gas concentration is affected by the temperature and humidity inside the sterilizing chamber, which also affects the exposure period. Concentration is considered effective within the margin of 450 to 1000 mg per liter of chamber space. If the concentration of gas is doubled, the exposure time may be shortened. The concentration and pressure of the ethylene oxide gas varies with types of sterilizers used; therefore manufacturer's instructions should be followed.

Temperature has a marked influence on the destruction of microorganisms. It is important in gaseous sterilization with ethylene oxide gas because it affects the penetration of the ethylene oxide through bacterial cell walls, as well as through wrappings and packaging material. The temperature for sterilizing is 21° to 60° C (70° to 140° F), and automatically controlled ethylene oxide sterilizers are usually preheated to 54° C (130° F). The small canister type of ethylene oxide sterilizers can be operated at the temperature and relative humidity of the room for a standardized time cycle. A higher gas concentration is used to compensate for the lower temperature.

Humidity of 40% to 60% is recommended with ethylene oxide to ensure enough moisture to kill microorganisms. Dry spores are most difficult to kill, but, when moistened, their resistance to gas penetration is lowered. Dehydration makes some microorganisms nearly immune to ethylene oxide sterilization, whereas too much moisture can slow the action of the gas below the lethal point. Ethylene oxide sterilizers with automatic controls most often provide for moisture injection to raise the relative humidity within the chamber, but less automated sterilizers require vials of water or soaked sponges to provide the necessary moisture.

Items to be sterilized must be thoroughly cleaned and towel or air dried so that no visible droplets will remain. This will inhibit the formation of ethylene glycol during the sterilization cycle. Lumina of tubing, needles, and the like should be dry and open at both ends. Caps, plugs, valves, or stylettes should be removed from instruments or equipment to permit the gas to circulate through the items. The packaging material used should possess the characteristics described previously in this chapter.

An ethylene oxide–sensitive chemical indicator should be used with each package to indicate only that the package was exposed to the gas; it does not indicate achievement of sterilization.

Specific instructions from the manufacturer of items to be sterilized should be followed closely. Penetration of gas throughout the load is essential. Care must be taken to avoid overloading the sterilizer. Compression of packages will prevent penetration of the gas; if packages are wrapped in plastic, compression will hinder evacuation of air and cause packages to open during the decrease in chamber pressure when a vacuum is drawn.

After completion of the sterilization cycle and before unloading, the sterilizer door should be opened approximately 6 inches and left for 15 minutes to permit dissipation of residual ethylene oxide from the chamber. Personnel should not reach into the chamber or remain close to the sterilizer during this period. No smoking is permitted in this area. Since ethylene oxide is highly explosive and flammable, the sterilizer should be installed in a well-ventilated room and should be vented to the outside atmosphere as recommended by the manufacturer.

The adequacy of every ethylene oxide cycle should be verified by the use of biological monitors that contain *Bacillus subtilis*. Where feasible, implantable or intravascular items should not be used until the results of the test are known.

When the sterilized items are removed from the sterilizer, they should be transferred immediately to the aerator or aeration area. The length of aeration required depends on the composition and porosity of the items, the sterilization wrap, the concentration of the diluent used with ethylene oxide for the sterilization process, and the airflow rate and temperature during aeration. Materials aerated in a mechanical aerator that provides a minimum of four air changes per hour and elevates the temperature within the cabinet to 50° to 60° C (122° to 140° F) require 8 to 12 hours of aeration based on the composition of the sterilized items and the aerator manufacturer's instructions. If a mechanical aerator is not available, items should be aerated at ambient room temperature for 7 days. Ambient aeration should be carried out in a limited access, well-ventilated room with controlled temperature between 18° and 22° C (65° and 72° F) and vented to the outside. Intravenous or irrigation fluids packaged in plastic bags should not be stored in this area.

Adherence to these guidelines will help protect patients and hospital personnel from any problems associated with ethylene oxide sterilization.

Liquid chemical sterilization

When used properly, liquid chemosterilizers can destroy all forms of microbial life, including bacterial and fungal spores, tubercle bacilli, and viruses. Only two liquid chemosterilizers are capable of causing sterilization: aqueous glutaraldehyde and aqueous formaldehyde. Although formaldehyde is one of the oldest chemosterilizers known to destroy spores, it is not used frequently because it takes from 12 to 24 hours to be effective, and its pungent odor is objectionable. Glutaraldehyde is more effective and less irritating than formaldehyde solutions.

Activated aqueous glutaraldehyde 2% is recognized as an effective liquid chemosterilizer. It is most useful in the sterilization of lensed instruments such as cystoscopes and bronchoscopes because it has no deleterious effects on the lens cement and is noncorrosive. Its low surface tension permits easy penetration and rinsing. Glutaraldehyde is not inactivated by organic matter and will not coagulate blood or protein. The sharpness of delicate instruments is not affected by this agent.

Instruments must be immersed in activated aqueous glutaraldehyde solution for 10 hours to achieve sterilization. Any period of immersion less than 10 hours will not kill spores that may be present and must be considered as only a disinfection procedure. (Activated glutaraldehyde is capable of disinfecting instruments in 10 minutes.) During immersion, all surfaces of the instrument must be contacted by the liquid chemosterilizer. Following immersion, instruments must be rinsed *thoroughly* with sterile distilled water before being used.

DISINFECTION

Disinfection is the process of destroying or inhibiting disease-producing microorganisms outside the body. It is most frequently achieved by chemicals in solution. The disinfection process may destroy tubercle bacilli and inactivate hepatitis viruses and enteroviruses but usually will not kill resistant bacterial spores.

Hospital disinfection is divided into two segments. When chemicals are used to disinfect inanimate materials, the chemical is called a *disinfectant;* when used to disinfect body surfaces, the chemical is called an *antiseptic*. Some chemicals can be used for both purposes. The term *germicide* refers to any solution that will destroy germs, or microorganisms. Many germicides can be employed on living tissue as well as on inanimate objects.

Concurrent disinfection refers to the immediate disinfection process following discharge of infectious materials from the body of an infected person or after contamination of articles by an infectious agent. *Terminal disinfection* is the process of rendering all articles, materials, and their immediate physical environment incapable of conveying infectious agents to other persons after the patient has left the room.

In recent years, physicians and hospital personnel have been faced with a continuous array of new germicides, many of which are claimed to be ideal for diverse purposes. Research data, however, do not support these claims.

Process

Disinfection is brought about by various types of reactions or by combinations of them. These include denaturation and coagulation of proteins in the cell, halogenation, poisoning of vital enzymes, hydrolysis, oxidation, and combination with proteins to form salts. The microbial destruction depends on the concentration of the chemical and the effects on the microorganism.

Selection of a disinfectant

Selection of a disinfectant depends on the type and population of microorganisms to be killed and the nature of the application. For disinfection purposes, microorganisms may be grouped into three classes: nonsporulating, vegetative bacteria, which possess the least resistance; tubercle bacilli, which have more resistance than the vegetative microorganisms; and spores, which are extremely resistant to any disinfectant.

Most disinfectants are capable of destroying vegetative bacteria and tubercle bacilli but not spores. The vegetative forms of molds and yeast, as well as animal parasites, are susceptible to disinfectants. Some fungi and antibiotic-resistant staphylococci have been shown to be as resistant as bacterial spores. Viruses vary in their resistance to disinfectants. At present no disinfectant will destroy with certainty the hepatitis virus.

A strong concentration kills more rapidly than a weak one. A disinfectant is primarily bacteriostatic when the range of concentration over which inhibition of growth occurs is a relatively wide one and is primarily bactericidal when the range is narrow. When the microorganisms are killed within a short period of time, the antimicrobial activity is termed lethal. When the rate of microbial death is slow, some microorganisms survive for a considerable time without multiplication. For those surviving, the antimicrobial activity is termed growth-inhibiting or bacteriostatic.

A disinfectant should be used at the lowest effective bactericidal concentration. A rapidly lethal concentration for microorganisms may cause corrosion and dullness of blades of delicate instruments. On the other hand, in a weak concentration, its disinfecting power is ineffective.

The larger the number of microorganisms present, the longer the disinfection time required to kill the resistant cells present. According to genetic principles, when the population is large, the proportion of higly resistant bacteria is correspondingly greater than when the population is small. However, when the size of the population is *extremely* large, there may be fewer highly resistant cells.

Temperature and surface tension of disinfectants

Increased temperature accelerates the rate of disinfection. The only practical value of this fact is in disinfection of inanimate objects. With some disinfectants, antimicrobial activity is increased when the chemical agent is added to warm or boiling water. The surface tension (wetness) of a disinfectant or antiseptic promotes contact between the agent and the microorganisms. A tension-reducing disinfectant, when combined with other chemicals, enhances the disinfecting power of that solution, thus decreasing the time-exposure rate.

Construction and condition of objects

An object must be thoroughly clean to provide for effective disinfection. Construction and composition of the object influence the disinfection time. A hard, flat, smooth-surfaced object requires less disinfection time than an uneven-surfaced object or a material of porous composition. The disinfectant coagulates the proteins in blood and other organic debris present on the object. Thus organic material creates a barrier on the object against the disinfecting solution. At present no ideal all-purpose disinfectant is available.

Types of disinfectants

The various disinfectants on the market may be divided into five major groups: halogens and halogen compounds, heavy metals, phenols and their derivatives, synthetic compounds, and alcohols.

Halogens and halogen compounds

Of the halogen compounds, the hypochlorites and iodines are widely used in hospitals. The hypochlorites are available as powders containing calcium hypochlorite and sodium hypochlorite, in combination with hydrated trisodium phosphate, and as liquids containing sodium hypochlorite. Preparations containing calcium hypochlorite (chlorinated lime) have been replaced by other detergents for cleaning purposes because of the former's unstable characteristics.

Chlorine acts primarily by oxidation, and its odor may therefore be objectionable. The many organic chlorine compounds that liberate their chlorine more slowly (such as chloride of lime) are effective as mild disinfecting agents. Inorganic chlorine is valuable in the disinfection of water.

Iodine acts directly by iodination and oxidation reactions. It is the most active antimicrobial of the halogens and combines readily with organic material. Because of its insolubility in water, it is prepared in various ways; the tinctures, or alcoholic solutions, are the most common forms.

Several syntheses of many organic iodine compounds in which iodine is held in dissociant complexes are available. The iodophors are iodine-detergent combinations capable of killing vegetative bacteria and tubercle bacilli if used in sufficient concentration (450 ppm of available iodine). Iodophors are not good sporicides.

Heavy metals

All metallic ions inhibit microorganisms if applied in sufficiently high concentrations.

The ions of the heavy metals have such a strong affinity for proteins that the bacterial cells absorb them out of the solution. However, the property that makes these ions appear lethal limits their usefulness because their activity is reduced in the presence of organic matter. The ions are also irritating to tissues and are poisonous.

Attempts have been made to decrease the toxic, corrosive, and irritating qualities of mercuric disinfectants by incorporating mercury in complex organic molecules in preparations such as merbromine (Mercurochrome), thimerosal (Merthiolate), and nitromersol (Metaphen). Data indicate that aqueous solutions of both inorganic and organic mercurials are ineffective in reducing cutaneous flora. Mercurials are poor disinfectants and have no place in modern surgical disinfection.

Phenols and their derivatives

Phenol in the pure state (carbolic acid) is not used as a disinfectant because many of its derivatives are more effective. Like phenol, its derivatives act mainly by coagulation and partly by lytic and toxic effects that are not clearly understood. Since phenols appear to have a greater affinity for nonaqueous than for aqueous media, it is believed that their action is dependent on their selective concentration at cell surfaces, resulting in the denaturation of proteins and an increase in permeability.

The aliphatic homologs of phenol have greater antimicrobial power than does phenol itself. Of this group, the methyl phenols—orthocresol, metacresol, and paracresol—and the halogenated phenols have phenol coefficients of three or more, but they are poorly soluble in water. The bisphenols have become the most useful of the phenolic disinfectants. The most important of these compounds are orthohydroxydiphenyl and chlorinated methylene and sulfur compounds. Of the chlorophenes, hexachlorophene is commonly used in soap. The bisphenols are relatively insoluble in water but are soluble in dilute alkali and in many organic solvents.

Synthetic detergent disinfectants

The quaternary ammonium compounds (often called *quats*) are among many surface-active detergents. These compounds are amines that contain pentavalent nitrogen and may be considered derivatives of ammonium chloride in which certain radicals are substituted for the hydrogen. There are three types of surface-active detergent substances: those in which the organic radical is a cation, those in which the organic group is the anion, and those which do not ionize (nonionic).

These compounds possess bacteriostatic power in high dilutions and are not highly irritating or toxic. They are effective surface-tension reductants. Their antimicrobial activity is affected by the kind of water (acid or alkaline, hard or soft) used and the material or substance involved. In the presence of hard, acid, or iron-rich waters, the antimicrobial activity is lowered, especially for the cationic compounds. Quaternary ammonium compounds may be mixed with nonionic detergents that have good solubilizing activity to provide effective cleansing agents.

Alcohols

Ethyl (grain) alcohol and isopropyl (rubbing) alcohol are much more useful as antiseptics than as disinfectants. Alcohol is an active germicide against tubercle bacilli in concentrations of 70% to 90%, but it is not sporicidal.

Frequently, alcoholic solutions are prepared by volume instead of by weight. The latter is the more accurate method of preparation. Alcohol is lighter than water and expands in the presence of heat.

Ethyl alcohol is nontoxic, colorless, tasteless, and nearly odorless and acts by denaturation of proteins. It may precipitate a protein covering around bacterial cells present in blood, pus, and mucus. Ethyl alcohol is less effective as a fat solvent than is isopropyl alcohol. A 70% solution of ethyl alcohol by weight is a satisfactory disinfectant for ordinary vegetative bacteria.

Formaldehyde

An aqueous solution of formaldehyde (formalin) is highly germicidal and sporicidal in a strong concentration. When a combination of 8% formaldehyde and 70% isopropyl alcohol is used, the action is even greater. Tubercle bacilli and viruses (except the hepatitis virus, whose destruction with certainty is not known) are promptly killed.

Irritating fumes limit formaldehyde's usefulness. It is also toxic to tissues; therefore materials treated with formaldehyde must be thoroughly rinsed before use.

Glutaraldehyde

Glutaraldehyde is related to formaldehyde but is more active. An aqueous solution of 2% is equivalent to an 8% solution of formaldehyde and alcohol. It is a high-level disinfectant that destroys tubercle bacilli in 10 minutes and is useful in disinfecting lensed instruments.

SKIN CLEANSING AND DISINFECTION

To prevent bacteria on the skin surfaces from entering the surgical wound, it is necessary to cleanse and disinfect the skin area of and around the proposed incision, as well as the hands and forearms of the members of the operating team. Proper skin cleansing and disinfection depend on knowledge of the physiology and bacteriology of the skin and on knowledge of the action of soaps, detergents, and antiseptic agents.

Objectives and influencing factors

Methods of skin preparation may vary; however, all are based on the same principles and share the same objectives: to remove dirt and transient microbes from the skin, to reduce the resident microbial count to as low as possible in the shortest time and with the least amount of tissue irritation, and to prevent rapid rebound growth of microbes.

The same general principles of skin cleansing apply whether the situation is preparation of the patient's skin at the operative site or preparation of the hands and arms of the members of the operating team. In either case, factors to be considered in skin disinfection are (1) the condition of the involved area, (2) the number and kinds of contaminants, (3) the characteristics of the skin to be disinfected, and (4) the general physical condition of the individual.

Structure and physiology of the skin

The skin consists of two distinct layers: the epidermis, which is a stratified squamous epithelium, and the true skin, or dermis. The outer layer, or epidermis, is the tissue to be treated by cleansing and disinfecting procedures (Fig. 5-12).

The *epidermis* constantly sheds the cells that form its horny outer layer, which are replaced by the multiplication and upward movement of cells from the lower levels. There are no blood vessels in the epidermis, although hair shafts, glandular ducts, and fine nerves reach through it. The *dermis* is a connective tissue containing blood and lymph vessels, sweat and sebaceous glands, nerves, and hair follicles.

Bacteria are found in all levels of the skin and comprise two groups, the transient and resident flora. *Transient* bacteria are usually limited to exposed areas of skin. They may be free on the skin or be loosely attached by grease or dirt, especially in the subungual areas. The transient flora are easily removed by mechanical cleansing of the skin.

Those which inhabit the deep structures of the dermis, the glands, and the hair follicles are considered the *resident* flora. They tend to move out and are shed with the old cells and skin secretions. The epidermal layers contain this debris from the dermis as well as soil and bacteria picked up by contact with various objects.

The resident flora of the skin are forced to the surface with perspiration and other secretions. This action is one way in which the skin disinfects and reconditions itself. The bacteria accompanying these secretions from the deep

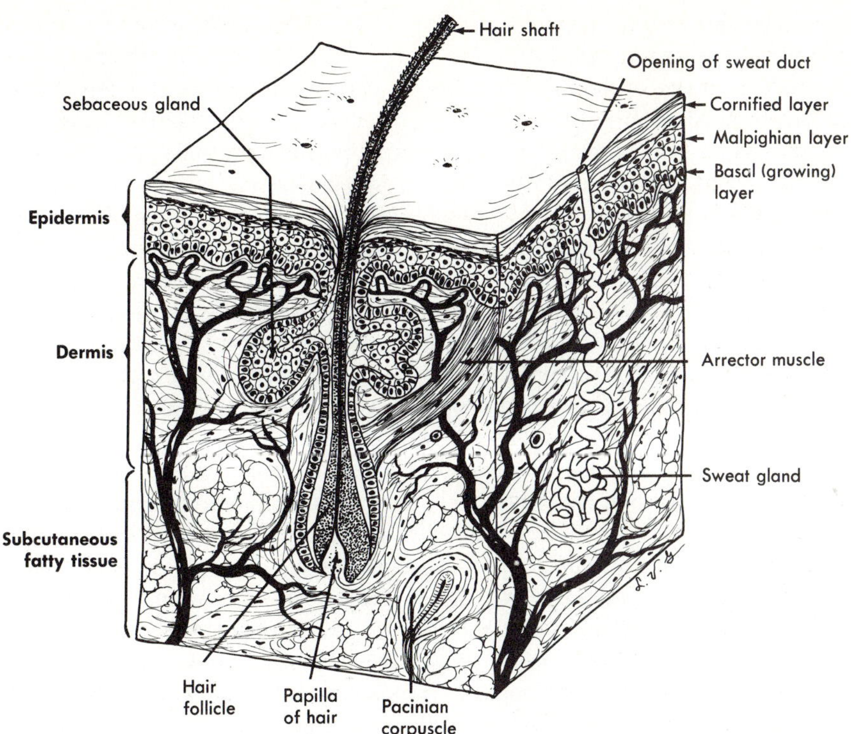

Fig. 5-12. Section of human skin showing several layers and many other structures appearing in skin. (From Schottelius, B.A., and Schottelius, D.D.: Textbook of physiology, ed. 18, St. Louis, 1978, The C.V. Mosby Co.)

layers may, however, become a source of infection. The activity of sweat glands is increased by external heat, emotional stress, and certain diaphoretic drugs.

Generally, the acidity of perspiration acts as a protective barrier against the growth of certain microorganisms. However, the perspiration in axillary and pubic regions has a higher pH and may permit more bacterial growth. Bacteria are also protected by the folds, ridges, and crevices of the skin from which detritus is not as readily shed as from smoother surfaces.

Agents for skin cleansing and disinfection

Many soaps and detergents are available for skin cleansing. Although most of them produce similar results in the immediate removal of soil and microorganisms, certain factors need further consideration in selecting a product for surgical use.

Action of soaps and detergents

Most soaps and detergents emulsify and peptize other waste products and oils that are absorbed in surface soil and permit the detritus to be rinsed off the skin with running water. The product selected should hydrolyze in the presence of water and yield a pH that corresponds to that of the average, normal skin. An odorless agent that produces a good lather for easy, comfortable use is usually preferred. It should not irritate the skin or in any way interfere with normal functioning. Careful rinsing and drying will help minimize skin irritation resulting from frequent scrubbing.

Hexachlorophene added to agents used for cleansing the skin has been found to suppress bacterial growth on the skin. Hexachlorophene retains its antibacterial power in the presence of soap and is combined with it in numerous liquid and solid forms.

It is impossible to sterilize the skin because chemicals that have the power to destroy bacteria are also injurious to the living tissues of the skin. Thus new bacterial populations are constantly being brought to the surface of normal skin.

Antiseptic agents

The antimicrobial agent employed for disinfection of the skin should be selected according to its ability to rapidly decrease the microbial count of the skin and its capability of being applied quickly and remaining effective throughout the operation. It should not cause irritation or sensitization and should not be incompatible with or inactivated by alcohol, organic matter, soap, or detergent.

Povidone-iodine, a complex of polyvinylpyrrolidone and iodine, is probably the newest antiseptic agent used for skin disinfection. It possesses the potent germicidal effect of iodine without many of its irritating properties. The activity of this agent is prolonged because it is released gradually from the binding polymer as the brownish iodine color fades from the skin. It is effective in the presence of pus, whereas the activity of the iodine complex is of somewhat shorter duration in the presence of blood or serum. It is nonstaining and can be safely used on mucous membranes. It should not be allowed to pool on the skin or in body cavities.

Many persons believe that tincture of iodine continues to be the most effective agent for skin disinfection. The modern iodine tincture (USP XVIII) contains 2% iodine, 2.4% potassium iodide, and 44% to 50% alcohol by volume. Iodine is a good bactericide but stains fabric and tissue. In combination with alcohol, iodine is tuberculocidal and appears to increase the efficiency of the alcohol as a skin antiseptic. Iodine has the disadvantage of potentially causing tissue irritation and sensitization.

The effectiveness of alcohol as an antiseptic is probably derived from the solution of lipoidal secretions of the skin and consequent mechanical removal of microorganisms. Absolute alcohol has little or no germicidal activity. For skin disinfection, 70% alcohol is the concentration usually used. The effectiveness of isopropyl alcohol as an antiseptic increases when the concentration is increased, in contrast to ethyl alcohol's effectiveness, which is not influenced by an increase in strength.

Hexachlorophene has been popular as a skin antiseptic. It is virtually insoluble in water, but it is soluble in alcohol. Hexachlorophene is a bacteriostatic agent that is active against gram-positive microorganisms but only minimally active against gram-negative microorganisms. With the increasing problem of *Pseudomonas* and other gram-negative microorganisms as sources of wound infections, the use of hexachlorophene should be carefully evaluated. If the skin surface is washed frequently each day with hexachlorophene, a relatively low flora population may gradually be achieved and maintained.

Hexachlorophene forms a long-lasting, imperceptible bacteriostatic film on the skin and develops a cumulative suppressive action with routine use. For this reason, no soap other than an agent with hexachlorophene added should be used daily by persons who scrub for surgery in order to obtain the best effect and to reduce the bacterial population of the skin significantly. In the preoperative preparation of a patient's skin, it is similarly useful to begin the regular use of a hexachlorophene compound for washing in the days immediately before surgery to take advantage of its suppressive bacteriostatic effect.

Benzalkonium chloride in a concentration of 1:1000 is bacteriostatic to vegetative bacteria but has no effect on tubercle bacilli or spores. It should not be considered a satisfactory disinfectant because it has marked incompatibility with anionic soaps, which causes the antibacterial activity to disappear, and it has very limited action against gram-negative microorganisms and fungi.

Preoperative skin preparation

Nursing considerations

The preoperative skin preparation of a surgical patient is the first step in the prevention of wound infection. Since the procedure may be alarming, embarrassing, or uncomfortable for the patient, every effort should be made to minimize these features by proceeding in a considerate, methodical, and professional manner.

If the preoperative skin preparation is done when the patient is awake, the nurse should explain the purpose and method of the procedure. Every effort should be made to allay any fears the patient may express and to answer questions in a reassuring manner. During the procedure, the nurse should observe the patient's general condition, particularly the condition of the skin under treatment. Any contraindication to the procedure because of an abnormal skin condition or an adverse reaction by or injury to the patient should be documented and reported to the physician.

In carrying out the procedure, the nurse should provide for the comfort, safety, and privacy of the patient. Good alignment of the patient's body should be maintained, and special supports for positioning should be used, as indicated.

Initial preparation of operative area

In the immediate preoperative period, the skin of the involved part of the body is prepared by special cleansing. Hair should be removed from the operative site only as necessary. Three alternatives for hair removal are clipping, use of depilatory, and wet shaving. Studies show that the wound infection rate is considerably higher for patients who are shaved preoperatively than for patients who have no preoperative shave preparation or for patients on whom a depilatory is used.[6] If a shave is ordered by the surgeon, the patient should be shaved immediately before surgery, preferably in a holding area within the operating room department that affords privacy and is equipped with good lighting facilities. The amount of time between the preoperative shave and the operation has a direct effect on the wound infection rate. In shaving the site, great care should be taken to avoid scratching, nicking, or cutting the skin because cutaneous bacteria will proliferate in these areas and increase the chances of infection. The decision of where and by whom the procedure is performed depends on when it is to be done, the facilities and personnel available, the patient's reactions, and the philosophy and policies that have been determined and established by the surgical committee.

Although specific orders for the skin preparation are written by the surgeon, a manual with diagrams and instructions concerning the preoperative skin shave is useful for the guidance and information of the personnel to whom the task is delegated (Figs. 5-13 to 5-22). The extent of the area to be shaved is determined by the site of the incision and the nature of the operation.

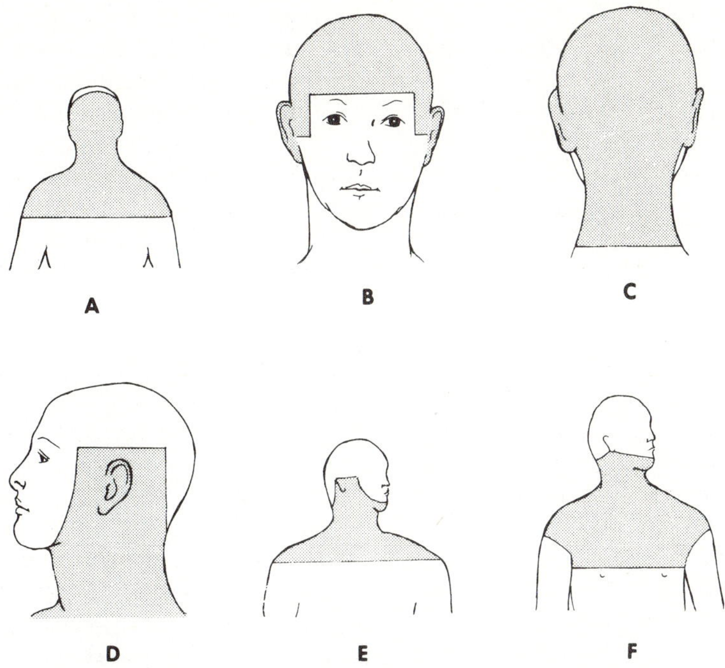

Fig. 5-13. Preparation for head, major neck, and upper thorax surgery. **A,** For posterior craniotomy. **B** and **C,** For craniotomy, frontal tumor excision. **D,** For major otological operations. **E,** For removal of lesions of neck and glands. **F,** For esophageal diverticulectomy, esophagotomy, scalenectomy, cervicothoracic anterior approach, thyroidectomy, and laryngectomy. (Adapted from Pate, M.O.: The preparation manual, Long Island City, N.Y., Edward Weck & Co., Inc.)

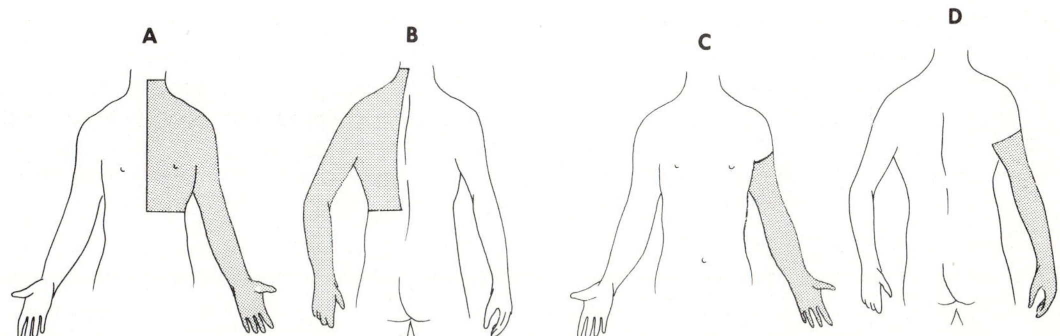

Fig. 5-14. Preparation for surgery of upper extremity. **A** and **B,** For major operations on shoulder and uppermost part of extremity, skin area is prepared from neckline to elbow line and axilla to midline anteriorly and posteriorly. **C** and **D,** For operations on forearm, preparation includes fingertips and axilla. (Adapted from Pate, M.O.: The preparation manual, Long Island City, N.Y., Edward Weck & Co., Inc.)

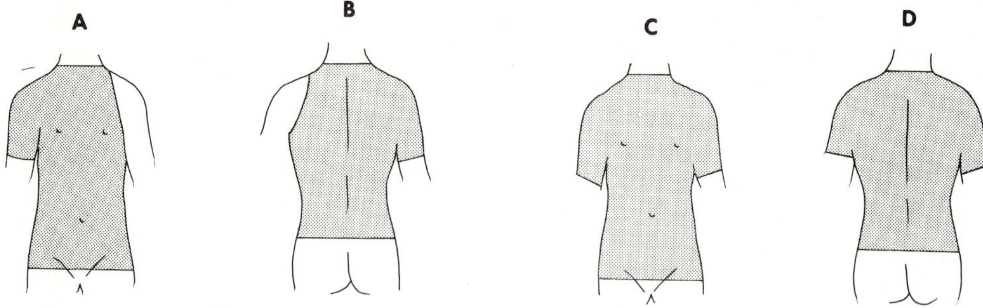

Fig. 5-15. A and **B,** For unilateral chest operations and radical mastectomies, affected chest, shoulder, and upper arm are prepared anteriorly and posteriorly. **C** and **D,** For combined thoracoabdominal operations, chest and shoulder are prepared bilaterally, anteriorly, and posteriorly. For cardiac surgery, this preparation may be extended to include legs. (Adapted from Pate, M.O.: The preparation manual, Long Island City, N.Y., Edward Weck & Co., Inc.)

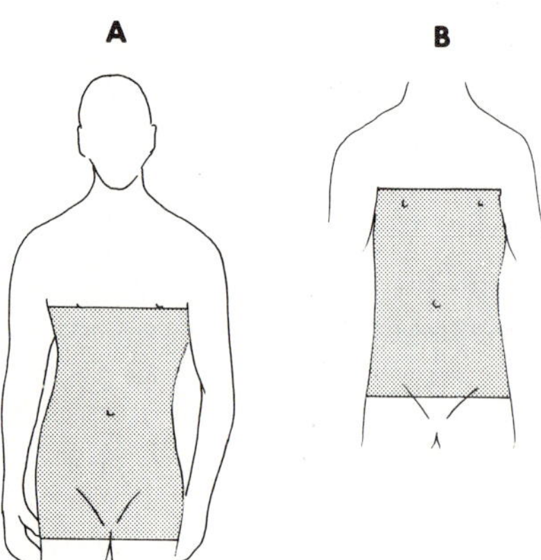

Fig. 5-16. Preparation for abdominal surgery. **A,** Skin area is cleansed and disinfected from nipple line to 3 inches below symphysis pubis, including external genitals, and from bedline to bedline. This preparation is done for gastrointestinal, biliary, and liver operations; splenectomy; herniorrhaphy; appendectomy; and surgery on great vessels of trunk. **B,** Skin prepared from above nipple line to above symphysis pubis. This preparation is done for gastrointestinal, biliary, and liver operations. (Adapted from Pate, M.O.: The preparation manual, Long Island City, N.Y., Edward Weck & Co., Inc.)

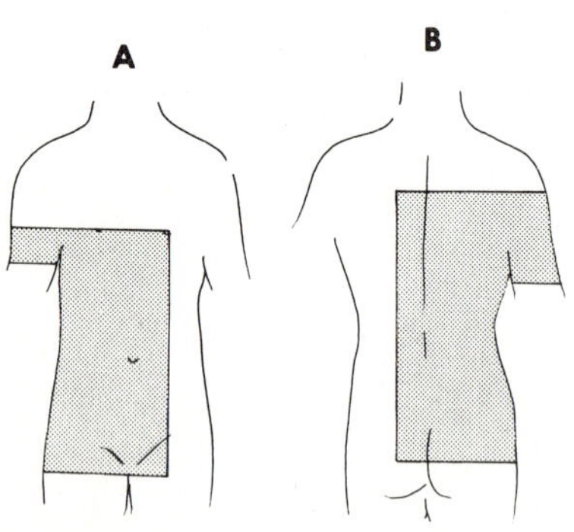

Fig. 5-17. Lateral preparation for operations on kidney and upper ureter. (Adapted from Pate, M.O.: The preparation manual, Long Island City, N.Y., Edward Weck & Co., Inc.)

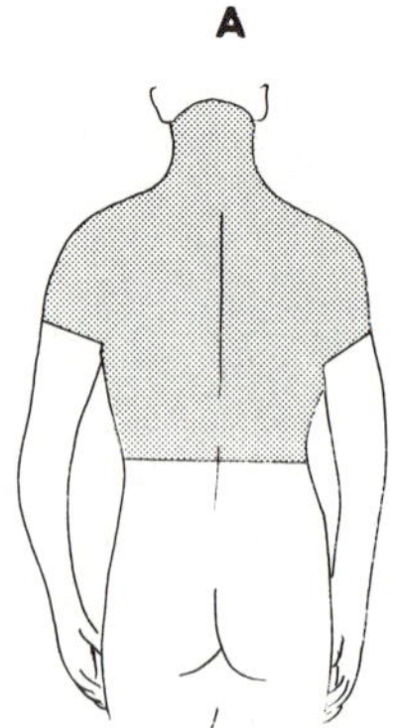

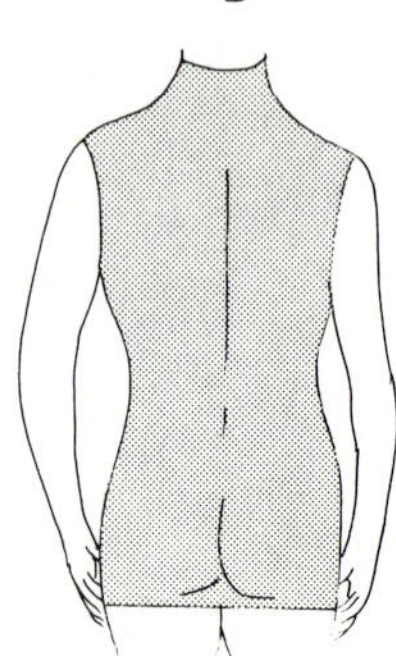

Fig. 5-18. A, Preparation for cervical laminectomy. **B,** Preparation for lumbar laminectomy. Preparation includes hairline to fold of buttocks and to bedline laterally. (Adapted from Pate, M.O.: The preparation manual, Long Island City, N.Y., Edward Weck & Co., Inc.)

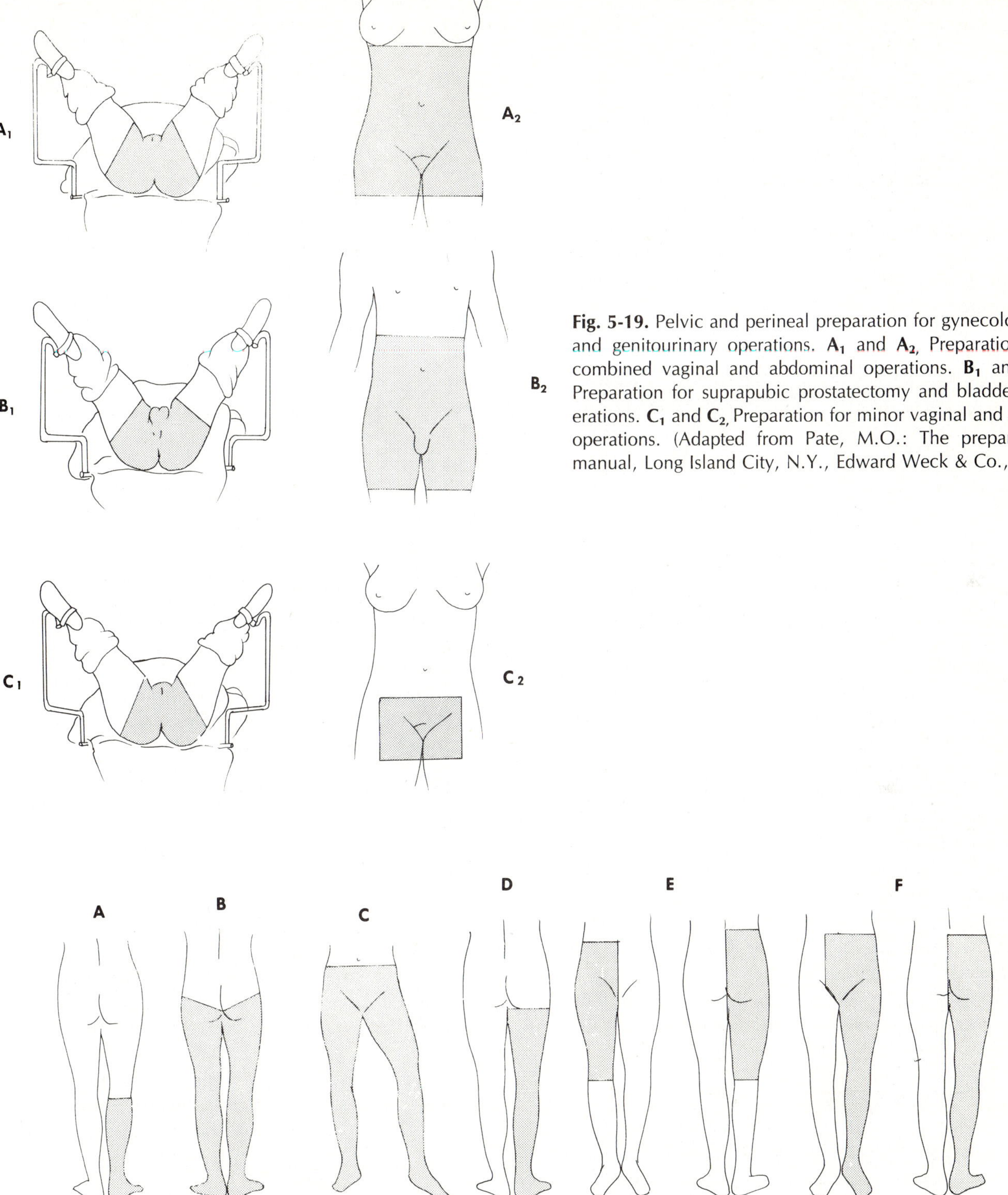

Fig. 5-19. Pelvic and perineal preparation for gynecological and genitourinary operations. $\mathbf{A_1}$ and $\mathbf{A_2}$, Preparation for combined vaginal and abdominal operations. $\mathbf{B_1}$ and $\mathbf{B_2}$, Preparation for suprapubic prostatectomy and bladder operations. $\mathbf{C_1}$ and $\mathbf{C_2}$, Preparation for minor vaginal and rectal operations. (Adapted from Pate, M.O.: The preparation manual, Long Island City, N.Y., Edward Weck & Co., Inc.)

Fig. 5-20. Preparation for surgery of lower extremity. **A,** For operations on ankle, foot, or toes, area is prepared anteriorly and posteriorly. **B** and **C,** For bilateral leg operations such as varicose vein ligation and skin and bone grafts. **D,** For operations of foot and lower leg. **E,** For unilateral hip operations. **F,** For unilateral operations involving hip and thigh. (Adapted from Pate, M.O.: The preparation manual, Long Island City, N.Y., Edward Weck & Co., Inc.)

It is rarely necessary to shave the face and neck of children or female patients. The eyebrows are never shaved, since hair will not grow back in scar tissue. The head and neck are not generally prone to wound infection because of the generous blood supply to this area. For cosmetic and psychological reasons, preparation for head and neck surgery may be done in the operating room after the induction of anesthesia.

For orthopedic surgery on the extremities, the shave preparation usually extends from one joint above to one joint below the area of incision. If a pneumatic tourniquet will be used during surgery, the entire extremity may be prepared to facilitate proper draping technique. Preparation and draping of the entire extremity also permit manipulation of the limb during surgery. Great care should be exercised in the preparation for surgery on bones, since wound infection resulting from improper cleansing may cause a stubborn condition leading to crippling, disfigurement and permanent dysfunction. The skin may be difficult to clean if it has been affected by casts, splints, or braces that interfere with normal skin care or cause skin damage. Daily soaking may help clean badly soiled feet in preparation for surgery, just as daily washing is advisable in preparation for general elective surgery.

Patients with traumatic injuries that may be excessively painful, such as fractures, burns, and soft tissue lacerations, may require anesthesia for skin preparation. Traumatic wounds usually require copious irrigation to flush out foreign matter. In cleansing the injured area, the surrounding skin is first carefully washed with an antimicrobial detergent. The open wound is irrigated with an isotonic solution, and the area is treated with an antimicrobial solution.

If a patient must be shaved in the operating room, a heavy lather should be used on the skin to control hair clippings and epithelium removed by the razor. Skin preparation in the operating room has the disadvantages that the patient's anesthesia time is prolonged, optimum use of the operating room is infringed on, loose hair remaining on the surrounding linen may get into the wound, and water used to wash the skin can result in sterile drapes becoming wet.

Procedure for preoperative shave

Individual sanitary supplies are used for each patient. Commercially prepared kits that contain the basic essentials for shaving the site of incision are available. The use of disposable preparation trays and razors can help ensure a safe, personal technique. The use of latex or plastic disposable gloves is an additional safeguard for the patient and for the worker and is often esthetically desirable.

Blankets and supports for the patient's position, as well as the necessary lighting and handwashing facilities, should be provided in the area where shaving is performed.

Basic equipment

Gloves
Basins with water and soap
Razor, as selected (straightedge, safety, or disposable) (Fig. 5-21)
Sponges for washing
Draping, as needed (towels and waterproof pads)

Accessory items

Brushes
Files or disposable nail cleaners for cleaning nails
Scissors and clippers for trimming long hair and nails
Applicators
Solvents for removal of adhesives and nail polish

Note: The use of volatile liquids such as alcohol, ether, benzine, and acetone should be strictly regulated in anesthetizing areas or where cautery or other electrosurgical equipment is in use because of the danger of fire, burns, and explosions.

Antimicrobial soap or detergent should be applied to the skin area using sponges moistened with water. A lather is created by using a circular motion and light friction, beginning with the proposed site of incision and working toward the periphery of the area. The principle is to progress from cleansed areas to uncleansed areas. Sponges are discarded as they become soiled, and the process is continued with fresh sponges.

Cotton-tipped applicators are needed to clean the umbilicus thoroughly, and a brush may be required for nails and calloused skin of the hands and feet.

Sensitive or denuded areas should be gently soaked with detergent and then rinsed or irrigated with sterile water.

A disposable or a terminally sterilized razor with a sharp blade is used to shave off the lathered hair. Holding the soft areas and loose skin taut with the free hand will raise the hair and permit easier accessibility to the area. A clean shave can be obtained without injury to the skin by gently stroking in the direction of the hair growth (Fig. 5-22). Nicks or cuts resulting from the shave should be reported as incidents, and the surgeon should be notified.

The surgeon may order a 5-minute scrub with an antimicrobial soap or detergent of the prepared area after it has been shaved. If so, the shaved area is scrubbed and rinsed carefully, and the skin is blotted dry to prevent chapping and irritation.

At the conclusion of the preparation, the patient should be made comfortable, the unit left in order, and the equipment disposed of or cleaned. Reusable items should be washed and sterilized. Expendable materials should be disposed of according to the prevailing regulations. The worker should follow the principles of aseptic technique for the removal of gloves and for terminal handwashing before proceeding to the care of other patients.

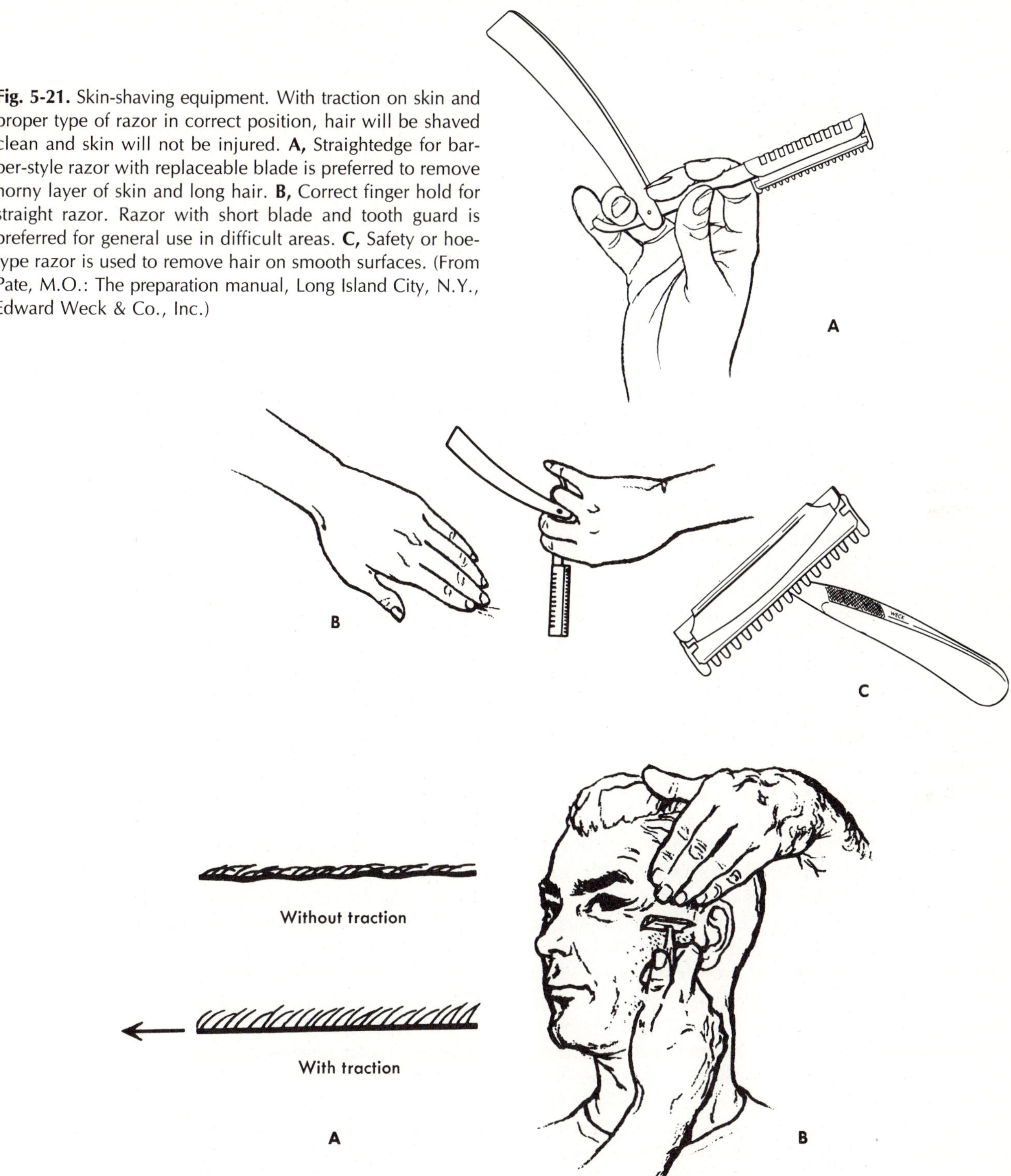

Fig. 5-21. Skin-shaving equipment. With traction on skin and proper type of razor in correct position, hair will be shaved clean and skin will not be injured. **A,** Straightedge for barber-style razor with replaceable blade is preferred to remove horny layer of skin and long hair. **B,** Correct finger hold for straight razor. Razor with short blade and tooth guard is preferred for general use in difficult areas. **C,** Safety or hoe-type razor is used to remove hair on smooth surfaces. (From Pate, M.O.: The preparation manual, Long Island City, N.Y., Edward Weck & Co., Inc.)

Fig. 5-22. Skin shaving. **A,** Skin traction is provided with free hand in direct opposition to slant of hair to tighten and smooth skin and raise hairs in more upright position. **B,** Hair and horny layer of skin are shaved off.

Continued.

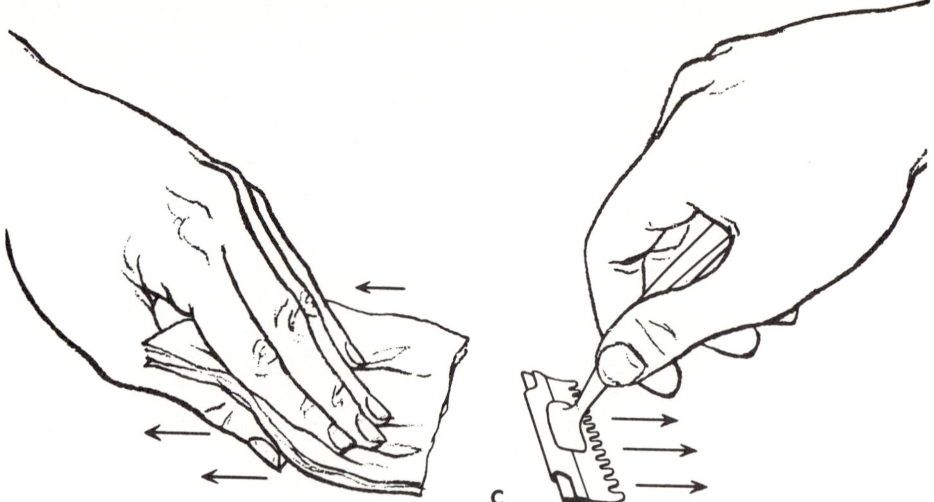

Fig. 5-22, cont'd. C, Traction is applied with sponge, and hoe-type razor head is held against skin, as shown in **A.** (From Pate, M.O.: The preparation manual, Long Island City, N.Y., Edward Weck & Co., Inc.)

Final skin disinfection of operative area

After the patient has been positioned on the operating table, final skin cleansing and disinfection are performed. If the patient has not showered with an antimicrobial detergent or soap immediately before leaving for the operating room, the operative area may be scrubbed with an antimicrobial scrub solution. While this is being carried out, the shave can be inspected and touched up or extended, as needed. Skin cleansing is followed by disinfection with an antimicrobial solution.

Procedure for final skin preparation

The supplies required for the final skin preparation may be arranged on a separate sterile preparation table. The items should include stainless steel cups for the cleansing agent and the selected antimicrobial agent, gauze sponges, and sponge-holding forceps if desired.

The scrub begins at the line of the proposed incision and proceeds to the periphery of the area. The sponges used in scrubbing are discarded as they become soiled, and fresh ones are taken. A soiled sponge is never brought back over a scrubbed surface. The lather is wiped off with dry sterile sponges. The antimicrobial agent is applied by sponges held in sponge-holding forceps or in the gloved hand.

In gynecology, the vulva and vagina are prepared by washing with a dilute detergent-germicide and applying an antimicrobial agent.

Open wounds and body orifices are potentially contaminated areas and as such are prepared after the surrounding unbroken skin is cleansed. This is in contrast to the principle of working from the line of the proposed incision into intact tissue to the periphery of the surgical field.

Sponges used to cleanse or disinfect a wound, sinus, ulcer, intestinal stoma, the vagina, or the anus are applied once to that area and are immediately discarded. After preparation of the area, intestinal fistulas may be walled off, using one of the plastic adhesive drapes.

The team member who has prepared the skin removes the gloves worn during preparation and dons sterile gown and gloves to join the scrubbed surgical team.

SURGICAL SCRUB

General considerations

The objectives of the surgical scrub are to remove dirt, skin oil, and microbes from hands and lower arms; to reduce the microbial count to as near zero as possible; and to leave an antimicrobial residue on the skin to prevent growth of microbes for several hours. The skin can never be rendered sterile, but it can be made *surgically clean* by reducing the number of microorganisms present. A lengthy mechanical scrub, even with strong antiseptics, will fail to remove all microorganisms. Friction and rinsing will significantly decrease the number of bacteria on the epidermis, but their numbers are constantly replenished by the continuous secretory activity of the skin glands.

Only persons who feel well and are free of upper respiratory infections and skin problems should scrub. Cuts, abrasions, pimples, and hangnails tend to ooze serum, which is a medium for prolific bacterial growth and can endanger the patient by increasing the hazards of infection.

Hospital regulations and physician preferences will govern the selection of materials and the methods used for the surgical scrub. The selection of a reusable or disposable brush for scrubbing should be based on realistic consideration of effectiveness and economy. Studies show that there is no significant difference in scrub effectiveness between reusable brushes and disposable brushes or sponges. A good reusable surgical hand brush with nylon bristles should be easy to clean and maintain and should be durable enough to withstand repeated heat sterilization without bristles becoming soft or brittle. Bristles should be rounded and firm, yet resilient, for effective friction without harshness. The backs of brushes should be of convenient size to fit the hand easily and may be grooved to permit nesting in containers. Wooden-backed brushes should not be used because wood is porous, absorbs foreign matter, and cannot be sterilized properly.

Brushes may be sterilized in metal dispensers that fit wall brackets or in covered metal boxes that fit on a shelf above the scrub sinks. The dispenser of metal box should permit the extraction of single brushes without contaminating the others. Brushes may be assembled with or without nail cleaners. They may also be packaged in individual wrappers, but this is a relatively expensive and time-consuming method. All containers and packages should be opened aseptically before the scrub is started.

The use of synthetic sponges in place of brushes has gained acceptance where long and repeated scrubbing may be traumatic to the skin. The antimicrobial soap or detergent used for the surgical scrub should act rapidly, have a broad spectrum, and not depend on cumulative action.

Two popular antimicrobial agents used for surgical hand scrubs are povidone-iodine and hexachlorophene. A third agent, chlorhexidene gluconate—used extensively in England for years—is also available for use as a surgical hand scrub. It is a rapid-acting, broad-spectrum antimicrobial agent that is effective against gram-positive and gram-negative microorganisms, possesses persistent residual activity, and has extremely low potential for causing skin reactions.

In scrubbing, light friction is effective in removing the detritus of the epithelium. The friction will produce heat, dilation of the blood vessels, and better circulation, which help recondition the skin (Fig. 5-12).

Hard scrubbing and harsh bristles tend to cause desquamation, leaving a bleeding or weeping dermis. This is painful and predisposes to infection. It also may massage bacteria into the deeper dermal layers.

An anatomical scrub using a prescribed amount of time or number of strokes plus friction is used to accomplish an effective cleansing of the skin.

A properly executed surgical scrub, using the anatomical counted brush stroke method, usually takes approximately 5 minutes. Studies indicate that there is no significant difference in microbial reduction between scrubs of 5 minutes' duration and those of 10 minutes' duration. Individual attention to detail is essential. The same scrub procedure should be used for every scrub, whether it is the first or last scrub of the day.

The prescribed number of strokes with a brush is usually thirty strokes to the nails and twenty strokes to each area of the skin. When scrubbing, the fingers, hands, and arms should be visualized as having four sides; *each* side must be scrubbed effectively.

The number of deep-resident flora is reduced by frequent scrubbing, but the number is increased when the surgical scrub is done only occasionally.

Procedure

Surgical scrub techniques that the staff must observe should be defined in writing.

Prior to beginning the surgical scrub, members of the operating team should inspect their hands to ascertain that their nails are short and free of polish, their cuticles are in good condition, and no cuts or skin problems exist. The cap or hood should be adjusted to cover and contain all hair. A fresh mask should be carefully placed over the nose and mouth and tied securely to prevent venting. Personnel should ascertain that the scrub shirt is fitted, tied, or tucked into the trousers or that the scrub dress is fitted or tied at the waist to prevent potential contamination of the scrubbed hands and arms from brushing against loose garments.

The basic steps of the procedure follow:

1. The faucet is turned on, and the water brought to a comfortable temperature. Most scrub sinks have automatic or knee controls for the faucets.

2. The hands and forearms are dampened.

3. By the foot control, a few drops of the antimicrobial soap or detergent are dispensed into the palms. Small amounts of water are added to make a lather.

4. The hands and forearms are washed to a level well above the elbows. The amount of time needed will vary with the amount of soil and the effectiveness of the cleansing agent.

5. If a prepackaged scrub brush is used, the package is opened, the brush and nail cleaner removed, and the package discarded. The brush is held in one hand while the nails are cleaned with the other hand (Fig. 5-23, *A*). All nails and subungual spaces are cleaned. If a disposable nail cleaner is not available, a metal nail file can be used. Orangewood sticks are prohibited because they cannot be sterilized properly after use.

6. The hands and arms are rinsed thoroughly; care is taken to hold the hands higher than the elbows. Splashing water onto the scrub suit or dress should be avoided because this moisture will cause contamination of the sterile gown.

7. If the brush is impregnated with antimicrobial soap, it should be moistened and scrubbing begun. If the brush is not impregnated with soap, antimicrobial soap or detergent solution is applied to hands. Starting at the fingertips, the nails are scrubbed vigorously while the brush is held perpendicular to them (Fig. 5-23, *B*). All

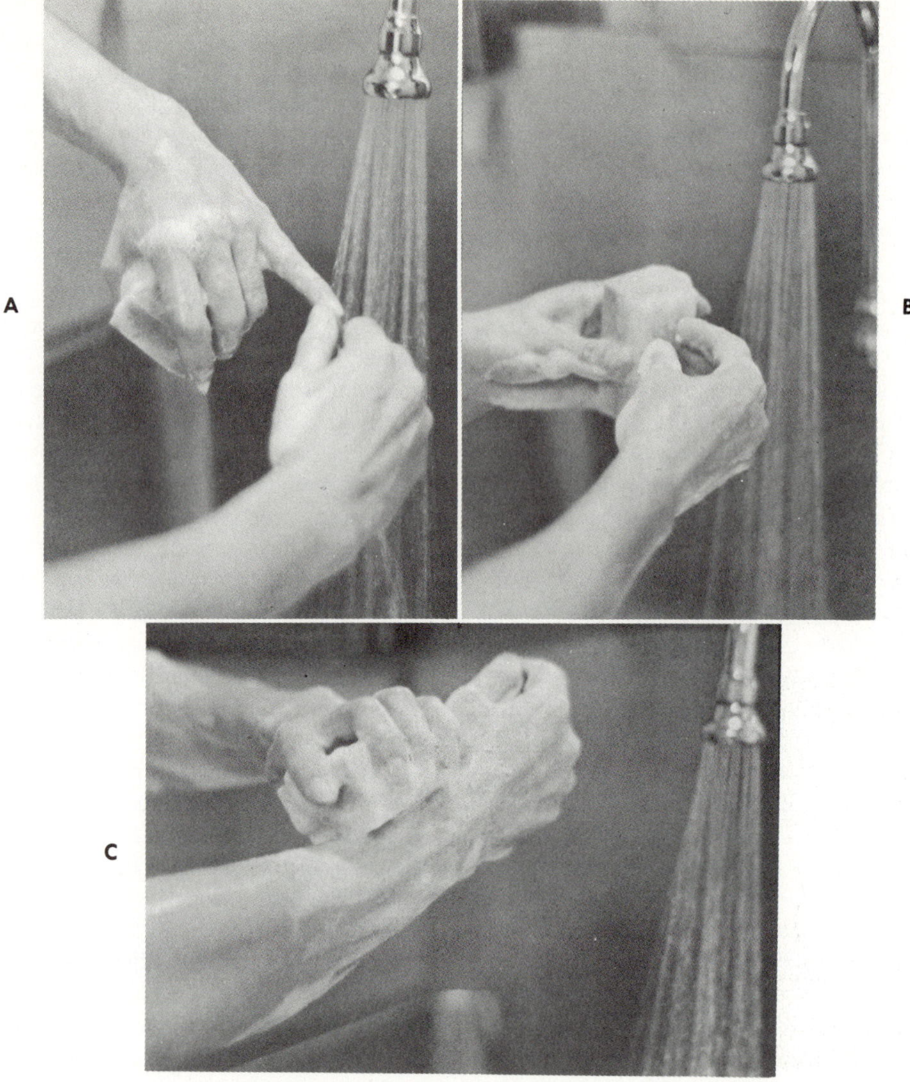

Fig. 5-23. Surgical scrub technique. **A,** Cleaning nails with plastic nail cleaner. **B,** Holding brush perpendicular to nails facilitates thorough scrubbing of undersides of nails. **C,** Holding brush lengthwise along arm covers maximum area with each stroke.

sides of each digit are scrubbed, including the web spaces between them. The palm and back of the hand are then scrubbed.

8. Each side of the arm, including the elbow and antecubital space, is scrubbed with a circular motion to 2 inches above the elbow (Fig. 5-23, *C*).

9. The hands are held above the level of the elbows while scrubbing to allow the water and detritus to flow away from the first-scrubbed and cleanest area. The hands and arms are also held away from the body. Small amounts of water are added during the scrub to develop suds and remove detritus.

10. The hands and arms are rinsed thoroughly. The brush is discarded in a proper receptacle.

11. If the sink is not automatically timed, the faucet is turned off by using the knee control or by using the edge of the brush on a hand control.

12. The hands and arms are held up in front of the body with elbows slightly flexed while entering the operating room.

Drying the cleansed area

Moisture remaining on the cleansed skin after the scrub procedure must be dried with a sterile towel before a sterile gown and gloves may be put on. The towel must be used with care to avoid contaminating the cleansed skin. The procedure for opening the sterile towel to dry the hands and forearms will vary, depending on the method used in folding the towel before sterilization. One method frequently used is to fold the towel to half its width, then to half its length, and then to half its length again.

The folded towel is grasped firmly near the open cor-

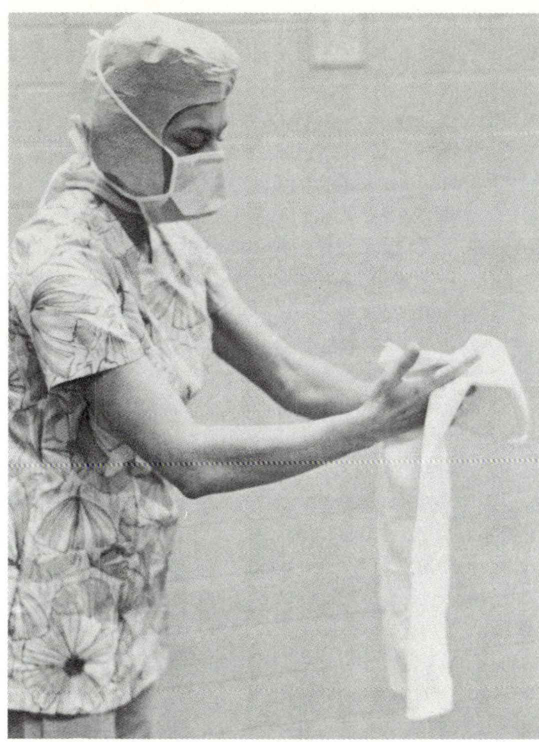

Fig. 5-24. Drying hands and forearms. Fingers and hand are dried thoroughly before forearm is dried. Extending arms reduces possibility of contaminating towel or hands.

ner and lifted straight up and away from the sterile field without dripping contaminated water from the skin onto the sterile field. The person steps away from the gown set and bends forward slightly from the waist, holding the hands and elbows above the waist and away from the body. The towel is allowed to unfold downward to its full length and width (Fig. 5-24).

The top half of the towel is held securely with one hand, and the opposite fingers and hand are blotted dry, making sure they are thoroughly dry before moving to the forearm. To avoid contamination, a rotating motion is used while moving up the arm to the elbow and an area is not retraced. The lower end of the towel is grasped with the dried hand, and the same procedure is used for drying the second hand and forearm. Care must be taken to prevent contamination of towel and hands. The towel is discarded.

GOWNING AND GLOVING PROCEDURES

Before scrubbed personnel can touch sterile equipment or the sterile field, they must put on sterile gowns and sterile surgical gloves to prevent microorganisms on their hands and clothing from being transferred to the patient's wound during surgery. The sterile gowns and gloves also protect the hands and clothing of personnel from microorganisms present in the patient or in the atmosphere.

Design and packaging of the gown

The gown should be made of a material that establishes an effective barrier, minimizing the passage of microorganisms between unsterile and sterile areas. Reusable fabrics must allow complete penetration of steam during the sterilization process and should withstand multiple in-house sterilization processes and multiple launderings. The material should be resistant to tearing and puncturing and as lint free as possible to reduce the dissemination of particles into the wound and the environment. It should facilitate aseptic technique and avoid excessive heat buildup. Regardless of the gown's material, the shape and size should fit the wearer and allow freedom of movement. To provide for extra protection, the gown's front from the waist upward and the forearms of the sleeves may be made of two thicknesses of material or a water-repellent material. Each sleeve should be finished with a tight-fitting wristlet, which prevents the inner side of the sleeve from slipping down onto the outer side of the sterile glove. Cotton tapes or Velcro fasteners are attached to the back of the gown to hold it closed. A wraparound gown should be used to achieve better coverage of the back.

Because the outer side of the front and sleeves of the gown will come in contact with the sterile field during surgery, the gown must be folded so that the scrub person can put it on without touching the outer side with bare hands. For in-house wrapping and sterilization, the gown is folded with the inner side out and the back edges together. The sleeves are not turned inside out; consequently, they remain within the folded gown. The side folds of the gown are folded lengthwise toward the center back opening, overlapping slightly at the center. With the open edges of the gown remaining on the inside, the bottom third of the gown is folded upward and the top third of the gown is folded over the bottom portion. The gown is then folded in half widthwise so that the inside front neckline of the gown is visible on top.

Gowns with wraparound backs are prepared in the same manner, with care taken to securely tie the tape on the wraparound back flap to the external side tie of the gown before initial folding. A folded hand towel with its free corners facing up is usually placed on top of the folded gown before the gown is wrapped and sterilized.

Preparation of gloves for surgical use

The use of prepackages sterile disposable surgical gloves has become common practice in hospitals throughout the United States. A few institutions, however, continue to reprocess reusable gloves for use in the operating room and for examining purposes. Reusable gloves must be washed, dried, tested, and sorted carefully to verify the integrity of the gloves.

Surgical gloves represent one of the most difficult items to be sterilized within hospital facilities. Ineffective air removal from the fingers of the gloves is a problem. To ensure sterilization of all surfaces, a wick of muslin or gauze should be inserted into the palms to separate the layers of the glove.

In the preparation of gloves, provision must be made for the scrub person to touch only the inner side of the glove when donning gloves. This is achieved by turning back a wide cuff on each glove. The cuffed gloves are placed right and left in the respective pockets of a wallet type of folder with the palms upward. Each glove folder is wrapped in an outer cover for sterilization. Although muslin is the traditional material for glove folders and wrappers, manufacturers of disposable products for operating rooms now offer nonwoven folders and wrappers.

Use of glove lubricants

The use of powder as a glove lubricant should be abolished because of two primary hazards: the postoperative complication of powder granulomata is an ever-present danger, and powder fallout from hands and gloves provides a convenient vehicle for dissemination of microorganisms throughout the hospital. If powder must be used, it should be distributed sparingly over the gloves before sterilization. The gloves must be washed thoroughly after they are put on and before the surgical team member approaches the sterile field.

Cream or liquid lubricants of various types have been developed. Some of these contain antiseptic or bacteriostatic agents that assist in keeping the gloved hands relatively free of bacterial growth. Manufacturers of surgical gloves have also used silicone films to eliminate stickiness. Little or no lubrication of the hands is needed to don these gloves easily. In assessing these new products and practices, it is necessary to determine their effectiveness for the purpose and their harmlessness to the skin and other body tissues of both patients and personnel.

Application of lubricant to hands

After scrubbed personnel have finished drying their hands, they may desire lubricant for their hands. Lubricants must be used before gowning if the closed method of gloving is employed. To lubricate the hands, each person grasps the end of the envelope containing the lubricant, stands near the waste receptacle, opens the envelope, pours or squeezes the lubricant carefully into the palms, discards the envelope in the waste receptacle, and applies the lubricant carefully over the surface of the hands.

Procedure for donning the sterile wraparound gown

Scrubbed personnel use the following procedure for donning the sterile wraparound gown:

1. The sterile gown is grasped at the neckline with both hands and lifted from the sterile gown wrapper; the person steps into an area where the gown may be opened without risk of contamination.
2. The gown is held away from the body and allowed to unfold with the inside of the gown toward the wearer.
3. The gown is completely unfolded while keeping the hands on the inside of the gown (Fig. 5-25, *A*).
4. Both hands are slipped into the open armholes at the same time, keeping the hands at shoulder level and away from the body.
5. The hands and forearms are pushed into the sleeves of the gown, advancing the hands only to the proximal edge of the cuff if closed gloving technique is used. If open gloving technique is employed, the hands are advanced completely through the cuffs of the gown.
6. The circulating nurse pulls the gown over the shoulders, touching only the inner shoulder and side seams (Fig. 5-25, *B*).
7. The circulating nurse ties or clasps the neckline and ties the inner waist ties of the gown, touching only the inner aspect of the gown (Fig. 5-25, *C* and *D*).
8. After gloving, the exterior gown ties (which were tied at the front of the gown before the gown was folded and sterilized) are untied, and both ties are held in the hands.
9. The tie attached to the back of the gown is handed to another gowned and gloved scrub person, the other tie is held securely, and the body is pivoted in the opposite direction from the other person, who extends the back tie to its full length (Fig. 5-26, *A*). This action effectively wraps the sterile back of the gown around the scrub person, who then retrieves the back tie from the assisting person and ties it securely with the other tie at the front or side of the gown (Fig. 5-26, *B*).
   a. If another gowned and gloved scrub person is not available, the end of the back tie is clamped with a sterile hemostat and handed to the circulating nurse. The scrub person then pivots in the opposite direction from the circulating nurse, who extends the back tie to its full length (Fig. 5-26, *C*). The back tie is retrieved as it is released from the hemostat by the circulating nurse (Fig. 5-26, *D*); care is taken to avoid touching the hemostat or the circulating nurse. Both ties are then tied.
   b. If closed gloving technique and commercially prepared disposable gloves are employed, an alternate method of tying the wraparound gown may be used by the scrub person. Most commercially prepared surgical gloves are double-wrapped. If the inner wrap is cardboard, it can be used as a protective covering for the gown tie when the circulating nurse assists with tying a wraparound gown. The end of the back tie in the center crease of the empty inner glove wrapper that is lying on the sterile gown wrapper is placed approximately two thirds of the way up to the edge of the opened wrapper (Fig. 5-26, *E*). The glove wrapper is then closed so that the tie is concealed. The closed

wrapper is handed to the circulating nurse, who grasps the folded edge of the wrapper securely, without touching the tie (Fig. 5-26, *F*). The scrub person then pivots in the opposite direction from the circulating nurse, who extends the back tie to its full length. The scrub person grasps the exposed portion of the back tie; pulls it out of the glove wrapper, taking care to avoid touching the glove wrapper or the circulating nurse (Fig. 5-26, *G*); and ties both ties. This method eliminates the need for removing a hemostat from the sterile field, which might potentially create a problem during the instrument count.

c. Most disposable gowns have a cardboard tab attached to the back tie and adhered to the front of the gown. When a disposable gown is worn, the scrub person releases the tab, hands it to the circulating nurse, and follows the same procedure as in step a.

Procedure for donning an open-back gown

If an open-back gown is used, the scrub person follows the preceding procedure from steps 1 through 6, then proceeds as follows: The circulating nurse ties or snaps the neckline and center back of the gown, touching only the ties or outer edges of the gown. When the circulating nurse is ready to tie the waist ties, the scrub person prevents potential contamination by bending slightly in the direction that will bring the ties away from the sterile gown. This allows the circulating nurse to grasp

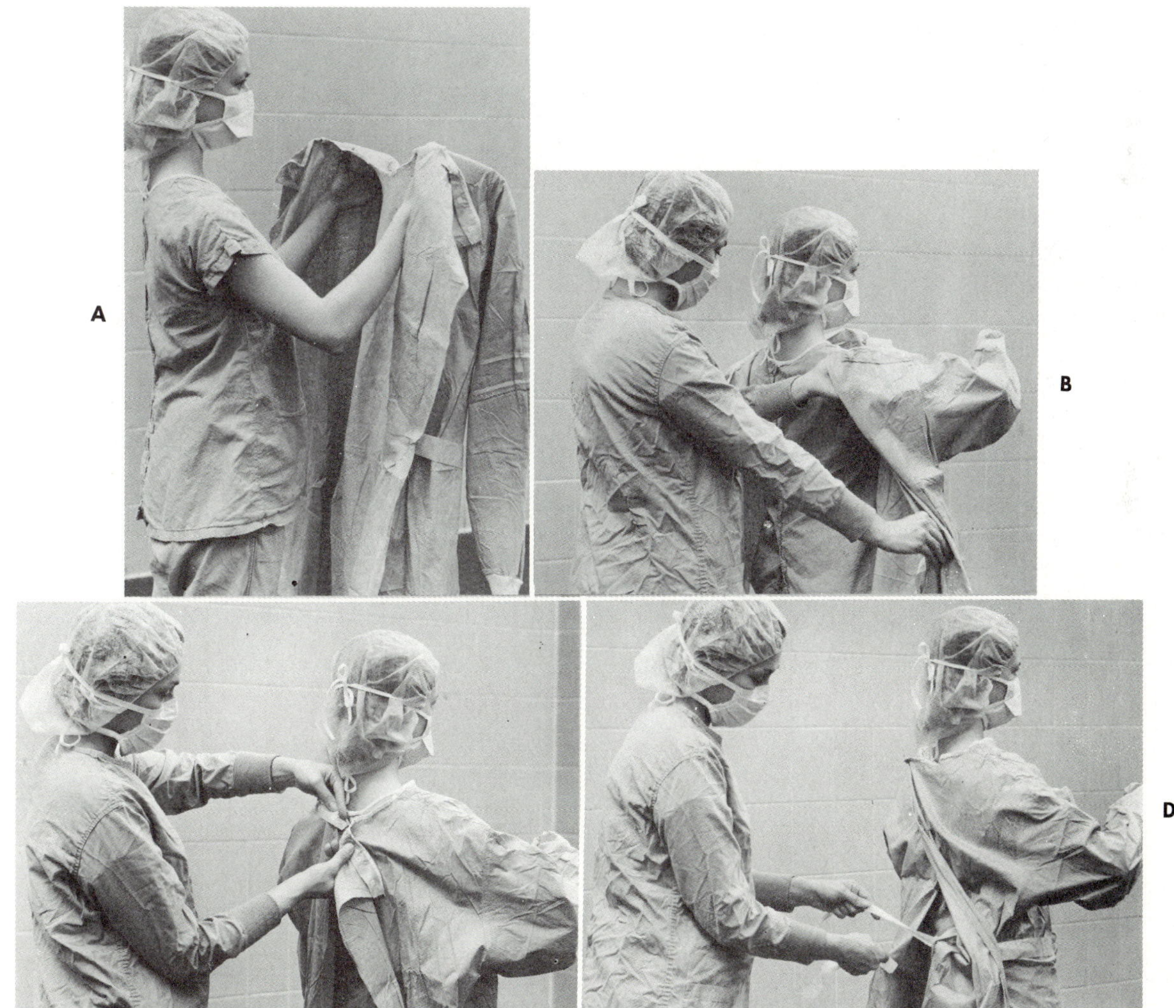

Fig. 5-25. Gowning procedure. **A,** Scrub person keeps hands on inside of gown while unfolding it at arm's length. **B,** Circulating nurse reaches under flap of gown to pull sleeves on scrubbed person. **C,** Circulating nurse snaps neckline of gown, touching only snap section of neckline. **D,** Circulating nurse ties inner waist ties of gown, maintaining margin of safety by touching only ties.

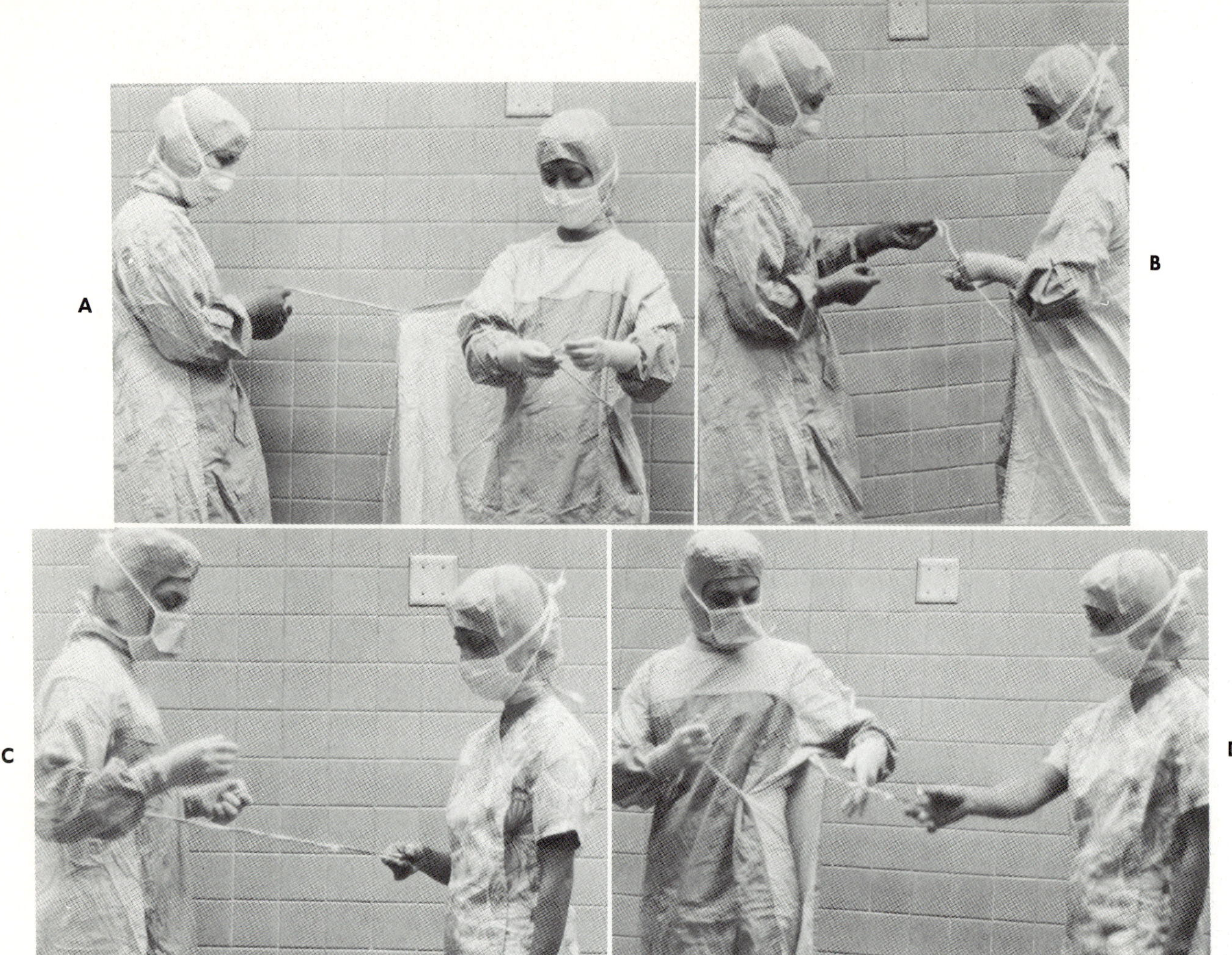

Fig. 5-26. Methods of tying wraparound gown. **A,** After handing back tie of gown to gowned and gloved person, scrub person turns toward left while holding other tie. **B,** Sterile back panel now covers previously tied unsterile ties; scrub person retrieves back tie and ties it securely with other tie. **C,** Circulating nurse accepts sterile hemostat clamped to end of back tie. **D,** After pivoting to left, scrub person retrieves back tie as circulating nurse releases it from hemostat.

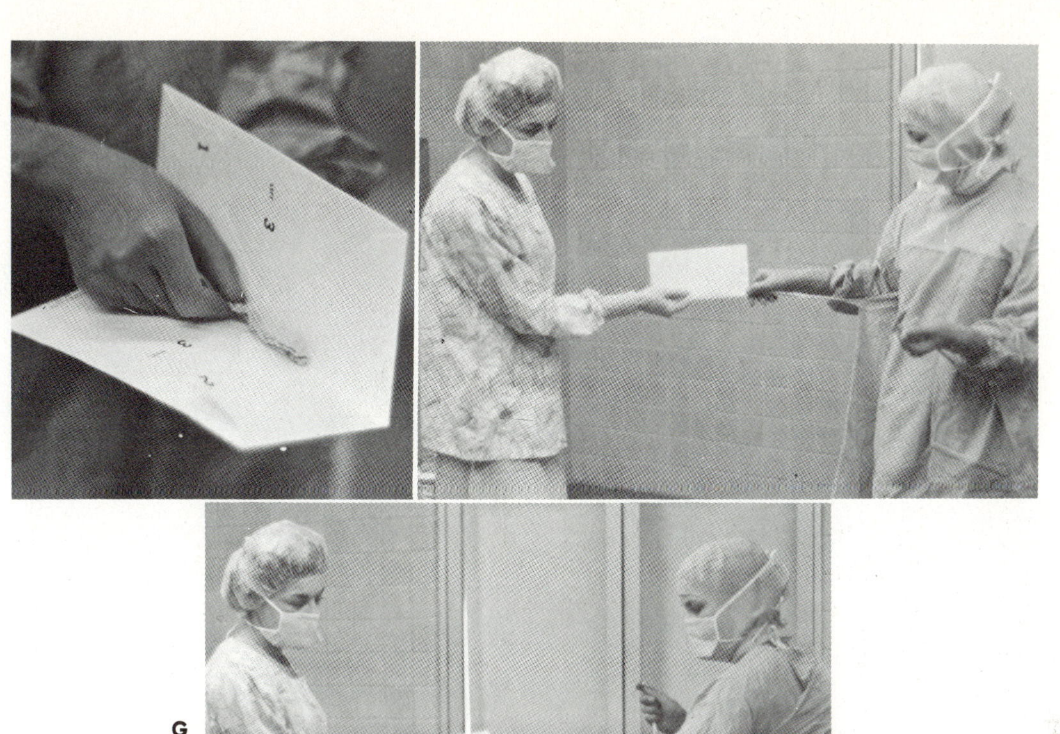

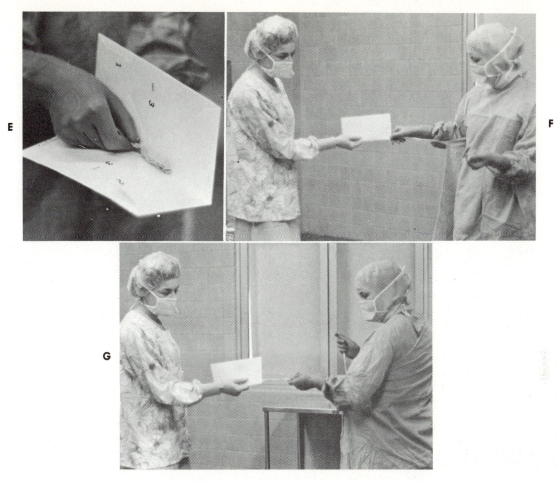

Fig. 5-26, cont'd. **E,** Using sterile inner glove wrapper, scrubbed person places end of back tie in crease of wrapper. **F,** After closing wrapper, scrub person hands it to circulating nurse, who grasps it carefully, touching neither tie nor gloved hand. **G,** After making three-quarter turn to left, scrub person carefully pulls back tie from wrapper.

the distal ends of the ties and draw them to the back to be tied. The circulating nurse grasps the bottom edges of the gown and pulls downward gently and firmly to remove any blousing effect on the gown.

Procedure for donning sterile gloves

Closed method (Fig. 5-27)

The closed method of gloving has the advantage of preventing the bare hands from coming in contact with the outside of the glove, which must remain sterile. The gloves are handled through the fabric of the gown sleeves. The hands are not extended from the sleeves and wristlets when the gown is put on. Instead, the hands are pushed through the cuff openings as the gloves are pulled in place.

Open method (Fig. 5-28)

The everted cuff of each glove permits a gowned person to touch the glove's inner side with ungloved fingers and to touch the glove's outer side with gloved fingers. Keeping the hands in direct view, no lower than waist level, the gowned person flexes the elbows. Exerting a light, even pull on the glove brings it over the hand, and using a rotating movement brings the cuff over the wristlet.

Assisting others with gowning (Fig. 5-29)

One gowned and gloved scrub person may assist another person in donning a sterile gown. The gown is opened in the manner previously described. The inner side with the open armholes is turned toward the individual

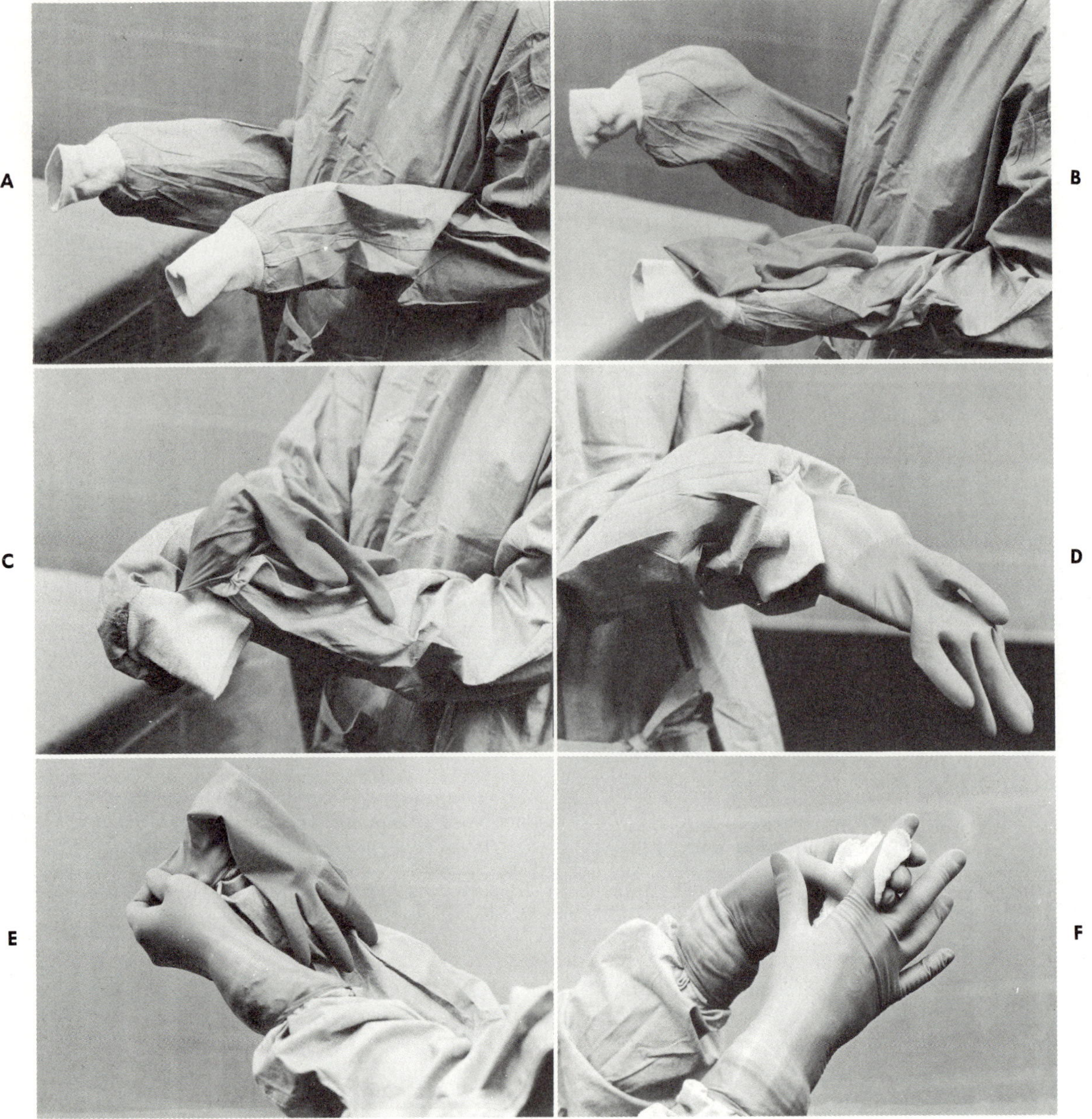

Fig. 5-27. Closed gloving procedure. **A,** When donning gown, scrub person does not slip hands through wristlets. Hands are not extended from sleeves. **B,** First glove is lifted by grasping it through fabric or sleeve. Cuff on glove facilitates easier handling of glove. Glove is placed palm down along forearm of matching hand, with thumb and fingers pointing toward elbow. Glove cuff lies over gown wristlet. **C,** Glove cuff is held securely by hand on which it is placed, and, with other hand, cuff is stretched over opening of sleeve to cover gown wristlet entirely. **D,** As cuff is drawn back onto wrist, fingers are directed into their cots in glove, and glove is adjusted to hand. **E,** Gloved hand is then used to position remaining glove on opposite sleeve in same fashion. Glove cuff is placed around gown cuff. Second glove is drawn onto hand, and cuff is pulled into place. **F,** Fingers of gloves are adjusted, and any powder that may be on gloves is removed by wet gauze sponge.

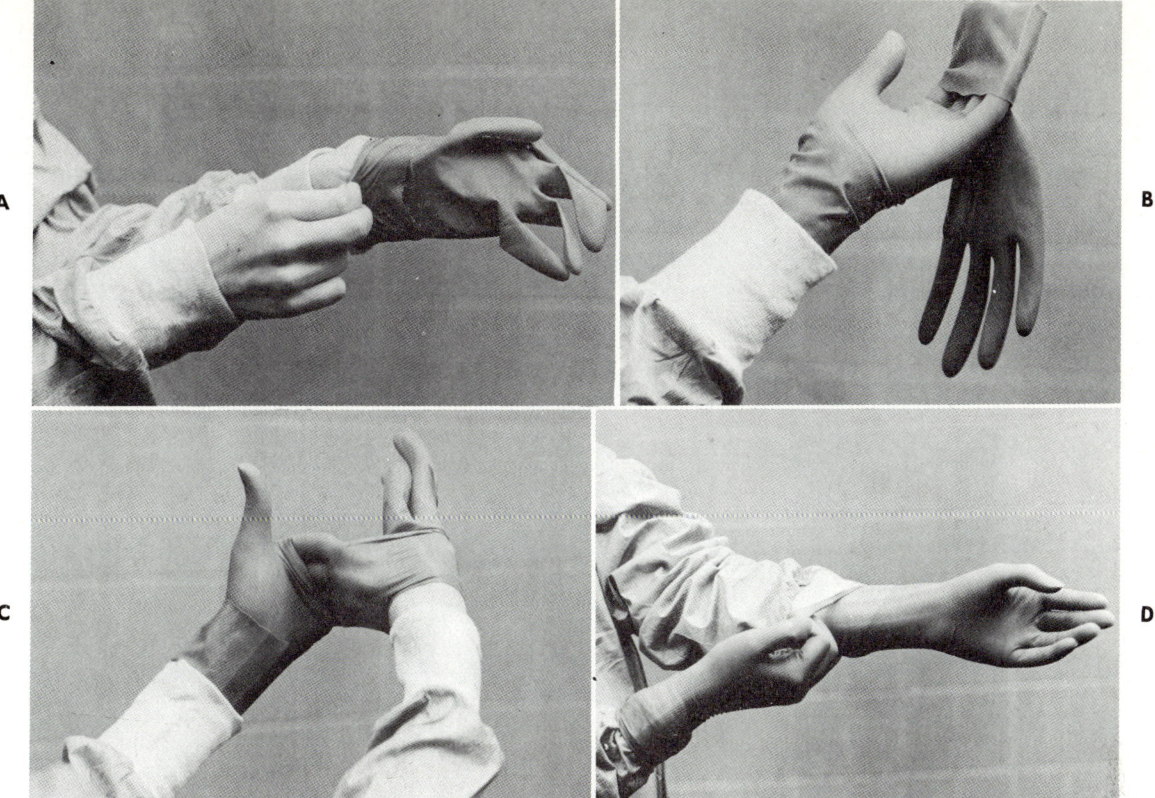

Fig. 5-28. Open gloving procedure. **A,** Gowned person takes one glove from inner glove wrapper by placing thumb and index finger of opposite hand on fold of everted cuff at a point in line with glove's palm and pulls glove over hand, leaving cuff turned back. **B,** Gowned person takes second glove from inner glove wrapper by placing gloved fingers under everted cuff. **C,** Gowned person, with arms extended and elbows slightly flexed, introduces free hand into glove and draws it over cuff of gown and upper part of wristlet by slightly rotating arm externally and internally. **D,** To bring turned-back cuff on other hand over wristlet of gown, scrub person repeats **C.**

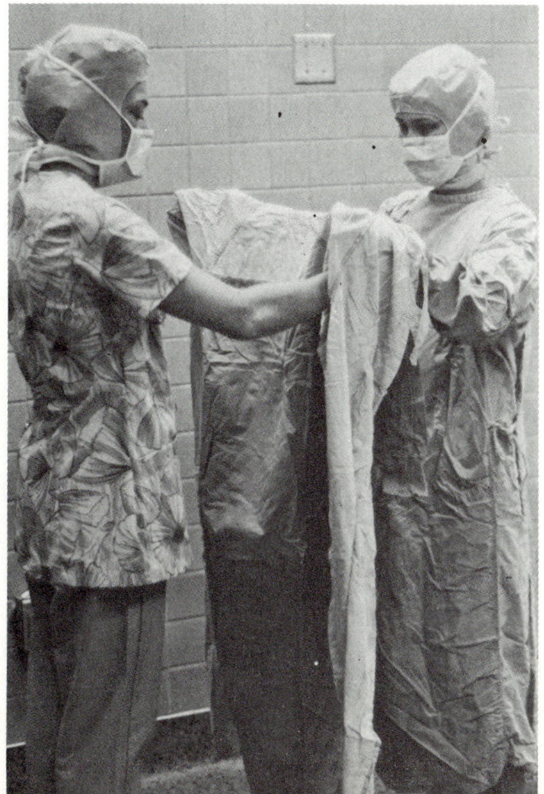

Fig. 5-29. Gowning another person. Gowned and gloved person cuffs neck and shoulder area of gown over gloved hands to prevent contamination as scrub person puts hands and forearms into sleeves.

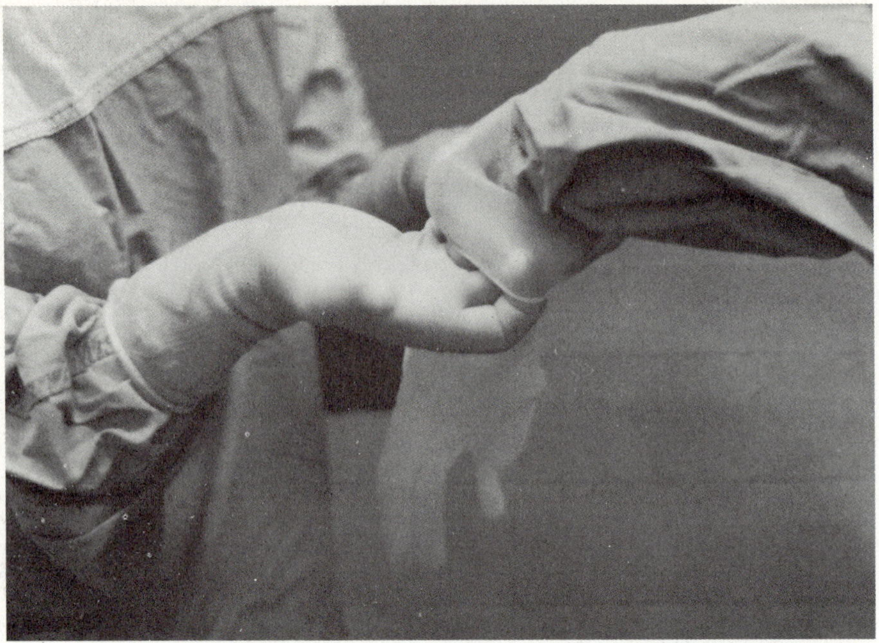

Fig. 5-30. Gloving another person. Gowned and gloved person places fingers of each hand beneath everted cuff, keeping thumbs turned outward and stretching cuff as gowned person slips hand into sterile glove, using firm downward thrust.

who is to be gowned. A cuff is made of the neck and shoulder area of the gown to protect the gloved hands. The gown is held until the person's hands and forearms are in the sleeves of the gown. The circulating nurse will assist in pulling the gown onto the shoulders, adjusting the back, and tying the tapes. The wraparound back on the gown is fixed into position by the scrub person after gloving is completed.

Assisting others with gloving (Fig. 5-30)

A gowned and gloved scrub person assists another gowned individual according to the following procedure:

1. The glove is grasped under the everted cuff.
2. The palm of the glove is turned toward the other individual's hand; the thumb of the other glove is opposed to the thumb of the person's hand.
3. The cuff is stretched to open the glove.
4. The gowned person exerts a slight upward pressure on the cuff while inserting the hand into the glove.
5. The gowned person brings the cuff over the wristlet of the gown while slipping the hand well into the glove.
6. The procedure is repeated to don the other glove.

Removing soiled gown, gloves, and mask (Fig. 5-31)

To protect the forearms, hands, and clothing from contacting bacteria on the outer side of the used gown and gloves, members of the scrubbed surgical team should follow steps 1 through 10:

1. The gloves are wiped with a clean wet sponge.
2. If a wraparound gown is worn, the front or side external waist tie is untied.
3. The circulating nurse unfastens the back closures of the gown.
4. The gown is grasped at one shoulder seam without touching the scrub clothes.
5. The neck of the gown and sleeve are brought forward and over and off the gloved hand, turning the gown inside out and everting the cuff of the glove.
6. Touching only the outside of the gown, step 5 is repeated for the other side, pulling the gown completely off.
7. The arms and soiled gown are kept away from the body while the gown is folded inside out and discarded carefully inside the linen hamper.
8. The gloved fingers of one hand are placed under the everted cuff of the other glove, and care is taken not to touch the skin with the soiled surface of either glove.
9. The glove is pulled off, inverting it in the process, and discarded in the appropriate receptacle.
10. The fold of the everted cuff on the remaining glove is grasped with the bare fingers of the ungloved hand; the glove is pulled off in the same way and discarded.

After leaving the operating area, the person removes the mask, touching only the strings, and discards it in the designated receptacle.

The hands and forearms are washed. If it is necessary to scrub for another operation immediately, the individual dons a fresh mask and repeats the prescribed scrub procedure.

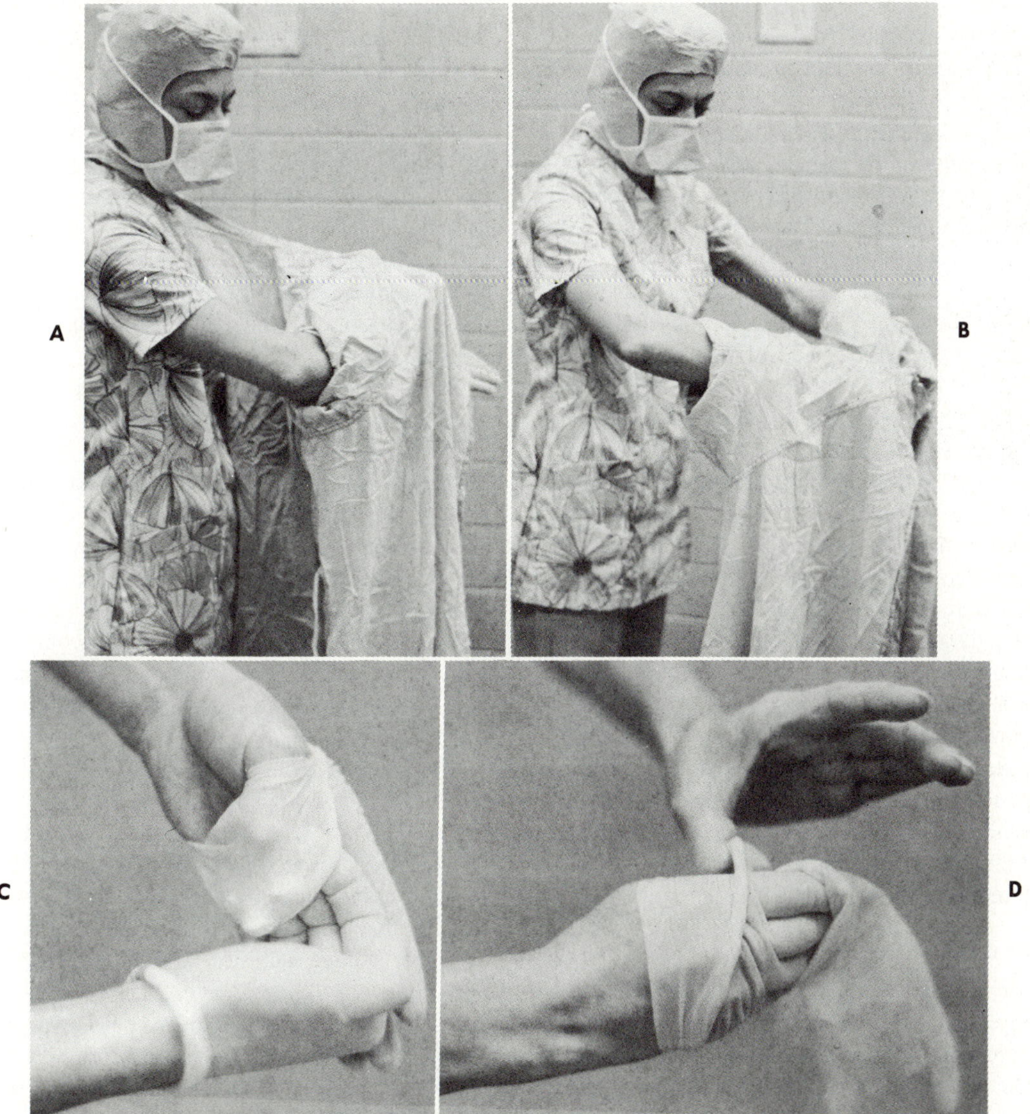

Fig. 5-31. Removing soiled gown and gloves. **A,** To protect scrub suit and arms from bacteria that are present on outer side of soiled gown, gowned and gloved person peels gown off one side of body, using opposite hand, and turns inner side of gown outward. **B,** Scrub nurse turns outer side of soiled gown away from body, keeping elbows flexed and arms away from body, so that soiled gown will not touch arms or scrub suit. **C,** To prevent outer side of soiled gloves from touching skin surfaces of hands, scrub nurse places gloved fingers of one hand under everted cuff of other glove and pulls it off hand and fingers. **D,** To prevent ungloved hand from touching outer side of soiled glove, scrub nurse hooks bare thumb on inner side of glove and pulls glove off.

SURGICAL DRAPING

Draping procedures create an area of asepsis called a *sterile field*. All sterile items that come in contact with the wound must be restricted within the defined area of safety to prevent transportation of microorganisms into the open wound.

The sterile field is created by placement of sterile sheets and towels in a specific position to maintain the sterility of surfaces on which sterile instruments and gloved hands may be placed. The patient and operating table are covered with sterile drapes in a manner that exposes the prepared site of incision and isolates the area of the surgical wound. Objects draped include instrument tables, basin and Mayo stands, and trays.

Draping materials

Draping materials are selected to create and maintain an effective barrier that will minimize the passage of microorganisms between nonsterile and sterile areas. To be effective, a barrier material should be resistant to blood, aqueous fluid, and abrasion; as lint free as possible, and drapable. It should maintain an isothermic environment that is appropriate to body temperature. It should meet or exceed the requirements of the current National Fire Protection Association standards so that there is no risk from a static charge. Draping materials must be penetrable by steam under pressure or by gas to achieve sterilization within hospital facilities.

Several reusable and numerous disposable materials currently available exhibit barrier qualities. All of them, however, do not remain equally impermeable to moist contaminants for given periods of time. Barrier properties vary, depending on the stresses applied to the draping materials during actual use.

Reusable drapes

Chemically treated cotton cloth and tightly woven 100% cotton cloth with an approximate thread count of 288 per square inch provide a barrier to liquids and are abrasion resistant. Manufacturers of these draping materials should be able to show that in-hospital sterilization can be achieved with practical sterilizer operating cycles.

Bleached and preshrunk muslin with a thread count of 140 to 160 per square inch has been used for years in the construction of surgical drapes. Although it conforms easily to body contours and remains in place when draped, muslin does not retard the passage of fluid effectively and therefore cannot be considered a barrier.

Heavy twill, denim, or canvas materials inhibit steam penetration, are difficult to handle, and retain heat on the patient. These factors prohibit the use of such materials as surgical drapes.

Care must be taken with reusable drapes to eliminate pinholes caused by towel clamps, needles, or other sharp objects. Special nonpenetrating towel clamps must be used.

Disposable drapes

Numerous synthetic disposable drapes prevent bacterial penetration and fluid breakthrough. These versatile materials can be manufactured to meet different specifications in both absorbent and nonabsorbent forms. The successful disposable drapes currently on the market are soft, lint free, lightweight, compact, flame and moisture resistant, nonirritating, and static free. These products are available prepackaged and presterilized from commercial sources. White or colored drapes are available. The use of colored drapes depends on the surgeon's preferences and convictions concerning glare, eyestrain, and morale factors.

Lightness and compactness of synthetic drapes prevent heat retention by patients, contribute to ease in handling and storage, and conserve storage space and personnel's time.

Disposable drapes reduce the hazards of contamination in the presence of known infectious microorganisms in body fluids and excretions and in situations in which laundering of grossly contaminated textiles is a problem.

The danger inherent in the use of synthetic drapes is that solvents, volatile liquids, and sharp instruments tend to penetrate the barrier. Loss of effectiveness may be caused by cracking at the folds or by pinholes from the use of regular towel clamps. Manufacturers are continually improving disposable flat sheets, fenestrated drapes, and towels to permit easy handling and adaptability to the body.

When considering the purchase of disposable drapes, the buyer must determine whether they will satisfy the needs of surgery, be acceptable to the users, and be cheaper than the cost of laundering reusable drapes. If the cost is not lower, other significant advantages may warrant the purchase of disposable drapes. Availability of items, storage facilities, and disposal method must be analyzed.

Compactors provide a relatively inexpensive method of discarding disposable drapes. They accept any material and reduce the volume by at least a 4:1 ratio. Collection, transportation, and storage of waste materials can be a problem. Hospital engineers must establish methods of controlling odor and maintaining sanitation in the compactor area. Since a portion of the compacted material may be grossly contaminated, certain city or county codes may prohibit transporting this potentially infectious material through city streets or dumping it at landfill operations.

Incineration is an alternate method for destroying waste disposables. If incinerators are used, they must be properly managed to prevent environmental contamination. Many hospital incinerators do not meet federal pollution standards; therefore their use is prohibited.

The ecological impact of disposable items can be only roughly estimated. Each hospital must carefully evaluate

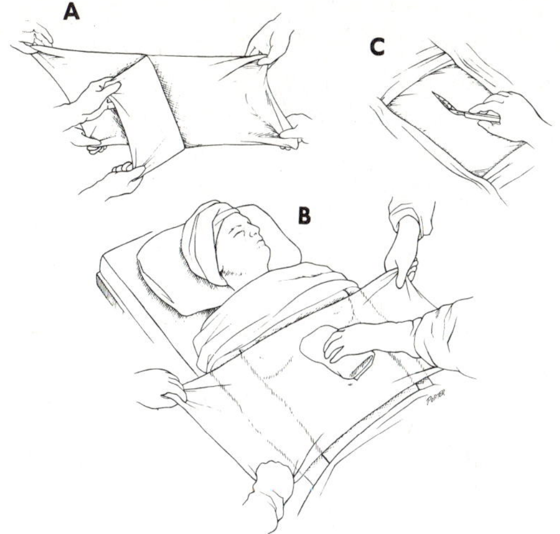

Fig. 5-32. Sterile plastic drape. For maximum sealing to prevent wound contamination, prepared area must be dry and drape applied carefully, preventing wrinkles and air bubbles. **A,** Surgeon and assistant hold plastic drape taut while another assistant peels off back paper. **B,** Surgeon and assistant apply plastic drape to operative site, and, using folded towel, apply slight pressure to eliminate air bubbles and wrinkles. **C,** Surgeon makes incision through plastic drape.

its capabilities and restrictions in the handling of disposable drapes before a conversion is implemented.

Plastic incisional drapes

Several types of plastic, impermeable polyvinyl sheeting are available in the form of sterile prepacked surgical drapes.

These plastic drapes are useful adjuncts to the conventional draping procedure. They can be applied after the fabric drape, alleviating the need for towel clamps.

Used alone they form a complete seal over the skin at the site of incision and prevent skin excretions and bacteria from coming in contact with the wound. They obviate the need for skin towels and sponges to separate the surgeon's gloves from contact with the patient's skin. Skin color and anatomical landmarks are readily visible, and the incision is made directly through the adherent plastic drape. These materials facilitate draping of irregular body surfaces, such as neck and ear regions, extremities, and joints. The draping procedure and surgical use of a commercial plastic drape are demonstrated in Fig. 5-32.

Standard drapes

Careful planning by nursing and surgical departments helps determine the desired types and sizes of sheets and towels required for surgery. The variety of drapes should be kept to a minimum. The most effective sheets and towels are simple and economical in terms of time, body motions, and materials. Standard methods provide management control that ensures the safety of patients, simplifies teaching of staff, and conserves human and material resources.

A *whole,* or *plain, sheet* is used to cover instrument tables, operating tables, and body regions. The sheet should be large enough to provide an adequate margin of safety between the surrounding physical environment and the prepared operative field. Usually two sizes of sheets suffice.

Surgical towels in one or two sizes should be available to drape the operative site. Four surgical towels of woven or nonwoven material are usually sufficient (Fig. 5-33).

Fenestrated, or *slit, sheets* are used for draping patients, leaving the operative site exposed.

A typical fenestrated (laparotomy) sheet is large enough to cover the patient and operating table in any position and to extend over the anesthetist screen at the head of the table and over the foot of the table (Figs. 5-34 to 5-36). In some cases, it may incorporate the Mayo stand that has been placed over the patient.

The typical fenestrated laparotomy sheet can be used for most procedures on the abdomen, chest, flank, and back. This type of sheet for adults should measure 9 to 10 feet long and 6 feet wide. A rectangular slit 10 inches long by 4 inches wide beginning 4 feet from the uppermost end of the sheet at a point in the center line of the sheet is usually suitable for a routine laparotomy sheet.

Other types of fenestrated sheets similar in length and width but with smaller or split fenestration may be used for the limbs, head, and neck with the patient in supine or prone position. The size of the fenestration is determined by the use for which the sheet is intended. The fenestrated sheet is fanfolded and handled as a typical laparotomy sheet.

A *perineal drape* is needed for operations on the perineum and genitalia with the patient in lithotomy position. A lithotomy drape consists of a fenestrated sheet and two triangularly shaped leggings. The leggings may be stitched to the sides of the sheet. The three-piece drape is less costly and is easier to handle and launder. A commercial, disposable lithotomy drape pack, including fenestration sheet, two leggings, absorbent and nonabsorbent towels, and a small sheet, is suitable for delivery, cystoscopy, hemorrhoidectomy, and vaginal procedures.

Folding drapes for use

Drapes should be folded so that the gowned and gloved members of the team can handle them with ease and safety. The larger, regular sheet is usually fanfolded from bottom to top. The bottom folds may be 4 inches wider than the upper ones. The small sheet is folded in half and then quartered, and the top corners of the sheet may be turned back or marked for easy identification and handling.

To provide for safe, easy handling and a wide margin

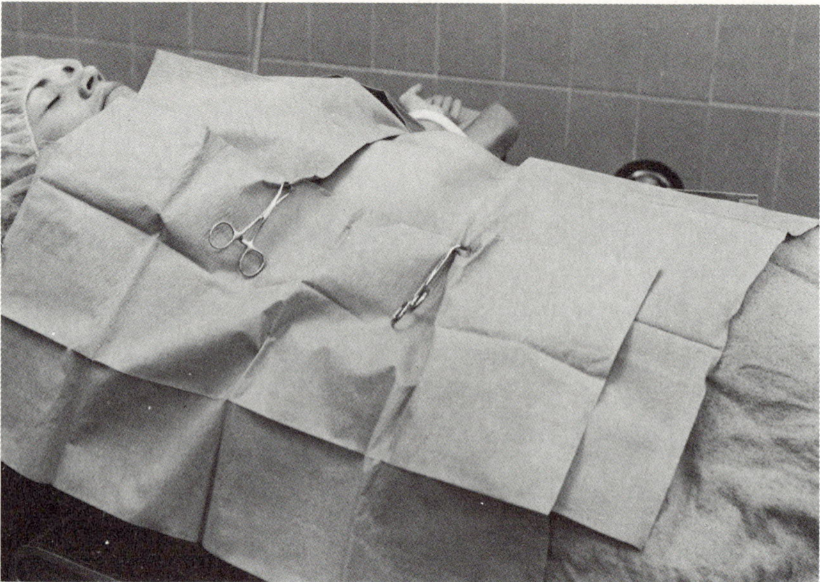

Fig. 5-33. Abdomen may be draped with four sterile towels, which are secured with non-perforating towel clamps. Standard method of placement of disposable towels is used.

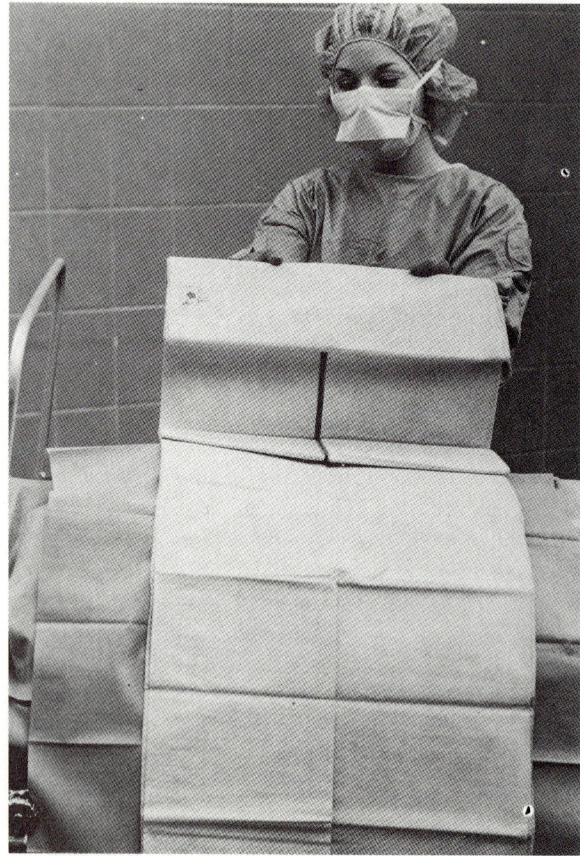

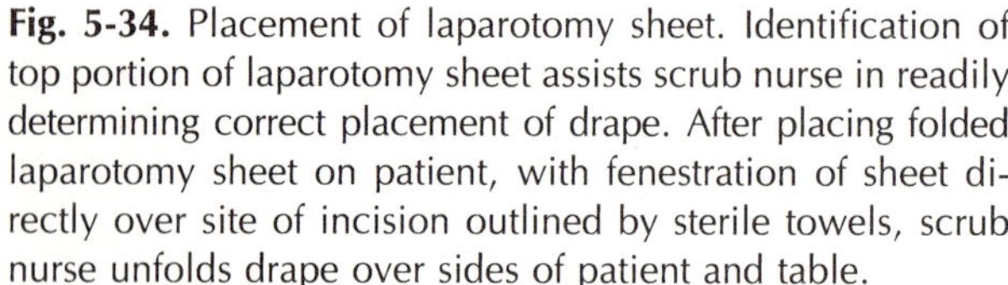

Fig. 5-34. Placement of laparotomy sheet. Identification of top portion of laparotomy sheet assists scrub nurse in readily determining correct placement of drape. After placing folded laparotomy sheet on patient, with fenestration of sheet directly over site of incision outlined by sterile towels, scrub nurse unfolds drape over sides of patient and table.

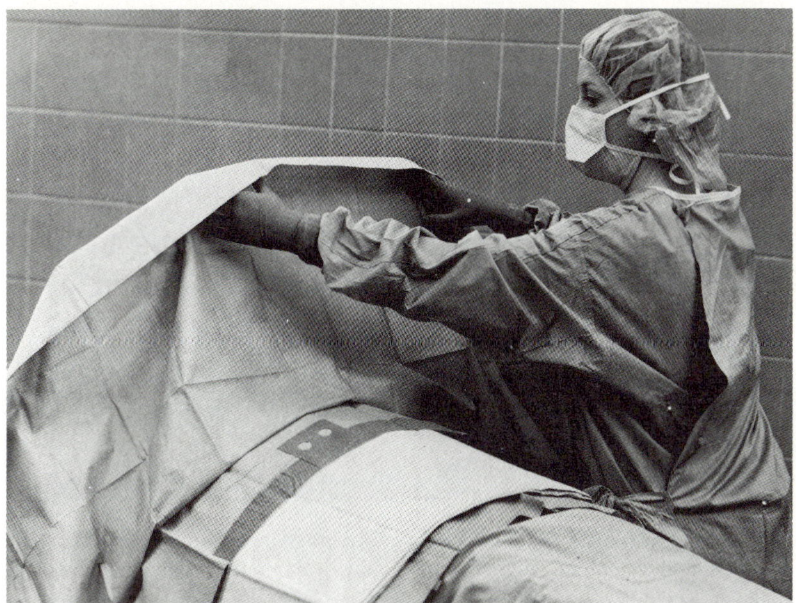

Fig. 5-35. Laparotomy draping continued. Scrub nurse protects gloved hands under cuff of fanfolded laparotomy sheet and draws upper section above fenestration toward head of table, draping it over anesthesia screen. Bottom portion of fanfolded sheet is then extended over foot of table in similar manner.

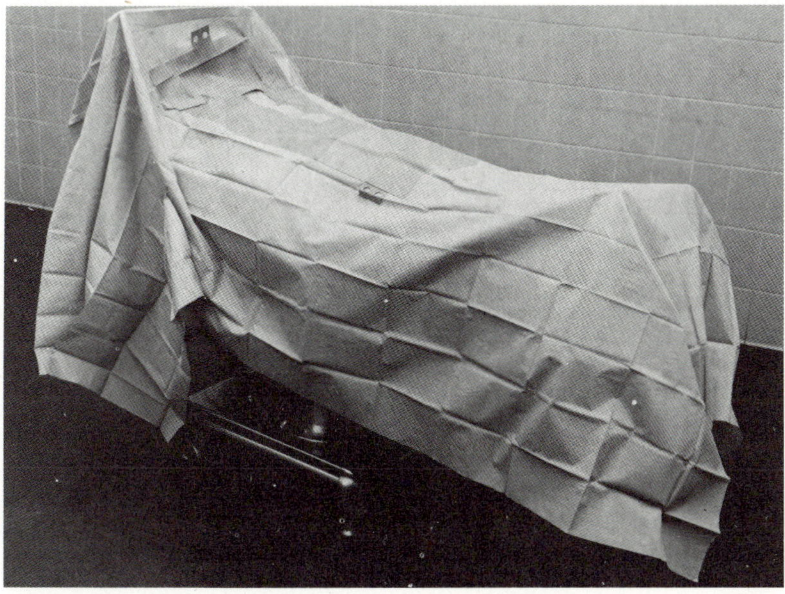

Fig. 5-36. Laparotomy draping completed. Fenestration provides exposure of prepared operative site. Special fabric surrounding fenestration is both absorbent and impermeable. Built-in instrument pad prevents instrument slippage. Perforated tabs provide means of controlling position of cords and suction tubes.

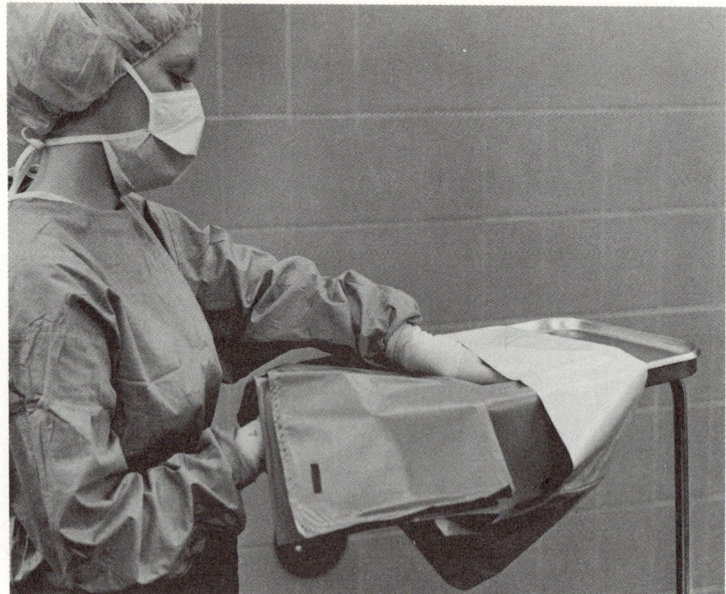

Fig. 5-37. Draping Mayo stand. Folded cover is slipped over frame. Scrub nurse's gloved hands are protected by cuff of drape. Wide margin is maintained between cover and lower portion of scrub nurse's gown. Cover is unfolded to extend over upright support of stand.

of safety between the unsterile item and the scrub nurse's gloved hands, the open end of the Mayo stand cover should be folded back on itself (Fig. 5-37).

Most fenestrated sheets are fanfolded to the opening from the top and the bottom, and then the folds are rolled or fanned toward the center of the opening. The edges of the top and bottom folds of the sheet are fanned so that they provide a cuff under which the worker may place gloved hands. The top and lower sections should be identified by a marking to facilitate easy handling (Fig. 5-34).

Draping procedure

If a sterile field is to be created and maintained, numerous important points must be remembered when draping for a surgical procedure:

1. The skin of the operative site must be dry before any sterile drapes are placed on it.

2. The surgical team should allow sufficient time and space to permit careful draping of the patient, employing proper aseptic technique.

3. Sterile drapes should be handled as little as possible.

4. The scrub person should carry the folded drape to the operative site, where the drape is carefully unfolded and placed in proper position. After a drape has been placed, it should not be moved.

5. Sterile drapes should be held above waist level until properly placed on the patient or object being draped. If the end of a drape falls below waist level, it should not be retrieved because the area below the waist is considered unsterile.

6. If a drape becomes contaminated during the draping procedure, it must be discarded immediately without contaminating the gloves or other sterile items.

7. While draping, the scrub person protects the gown by distance and the gloved hands by cuffing drapes over them (Fig. 5-38). The scrub person should have all parts of the drape under positive control at all times during placement and should use precise and direct motions. Draping is always done from a sterile area to an unsterile area, draping nearest first. The scrub person should never reach across an unsterile area to drape. When the opposite side of the operating table must be draped, the scrub person must go around the table to drape.

8. Drapes should not be flipped, fanned, or shaken. Rapid movement of drapes creates air currents on which dust, lint, and droplet nuclei may migrate. Shaking of a drape also causes uncontrolled motion of the drape, which may cause it to come in contact with an unsterile surface or object. A drape should be carefully unfolded and allowed to fall gently by gravity into position. The low portion of a sheet that falls below the safe working level should never be raised or lifted back onto the sterile area.

9. The incisional area should be draped first, followed by draping of the periphery.

10. If a towel clamp has been secured through a drape, it cannot be moved. If a drape must be removed during a procedure, the towel clamp must be considered contaminated and must be discarded at the same time as the

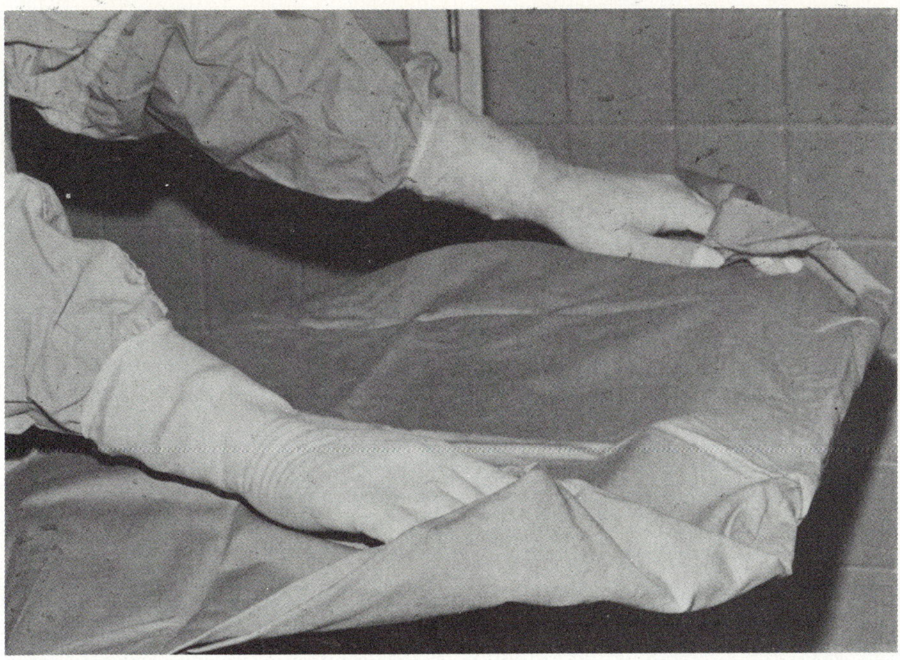

Fig. 5-38. When placing sterile drape on unsterile surface, scrub nurse rolls corners of drape over hands to avoid contamination.

drape. The use of nonperforating towel clips eliminates puncturing of the drape.

11. If sterility of a drape is questionable, it must be considered contaminated.

Arrangement of items on sterile tables

Standard arrangement of instruments, drapes, sutures, and other items on sterile tables for particular operations should be determined by nursing personnel. Factors to be considered include the surgeon's method of working; ease in handling, preparing, and transporting items; and reduction in human energy. Methods of work are based on work simplification and aseptic principles.

The arrangement of the various setups should be clearly defined and understood by operating room personnel. Visual aids are excellent tools for teaching personnel proper procedural methods.

DECONTAMINATION OF OPERATING ROOM, EQUIPMENT, AND SUPPLIES

Effective sanitation techniques should be established to control and reduce the possibility of cross-infection of patients in the operating room. Blood and tissue fluids from any patient may contain microorganisms that are pathogenic to other persons. Operating room practices should be developed to provide complete isolation for each patient. This is accomplished by considering every surgical wound to be potentially contaminated. Containment of contaminants is essential. Establishment of procedures concerning the terminal disinfection or sterilization of all equipment and supplies used in each operation prevents the transfer of microorganisms and protects patients and personnel.

During the surgical procedure, traffic within and through the room should be kept to a minimum to reduce air turbulence and to minimize human shedding. Sponges should be discarded in plastic-lined containers. As they are counted, they should be contained in an impervious receptacle. The circulating nurse must use gloves, instruments, or both when collecting and counting sponges or handling contaminated items. Spillage should be cleaned up immediately, using a broad-spectrum detergent-germicide. The exterior surfaces of all specimen containers should be cleaned before removal from the operating room.

Between surgical procedures personnel must remove their gowns and gloves and place them in the proper receptacles before leaving the operating room. All linens from open packs, whether soiled or not, should be discarded in linen hamper bags. Wet linen should be placed in the center of the bundle to prevent soaking through to the outside of the bag. The use of waterproof bags eliminates potential contamination. Used disposable and expendable items should be discarded in plastic bags and placed in containers for disposal.

The scrub nurse should place all instruments directly in wire mesh–bottom trays for processing in a washer-sterilizer. Basins, cups, and trays should also be washed and terminally sterilized. If a washer-sterilizer is not adjacent to the operating room, all these items should be covered for transportation to a central cleanup area, either in the surgical suite or in central service. Wall suction units should be disconnected by the circulating nurse to eliminate contamination of the wall outlet. Suction contents should be disposed of by the scrub nurse during the flushing of a hopper by the circulating nurse. If a flushing type of hopper is not available, the suction contents should be decontaminated with a detergent-germicide and disposed of in a toilet rather than in a conventional sink. Spillage during transport should be prevented. Glass suction containers should be rinsed and terminally sterilized with basins and trays. Disposable suction tubing should be discarded. If possible, reusable suction tubing should not be used because of difficulties in cleaning it properly.

The surgical spotlights and the horizontal surfaces of furniture and equipment that have been involved in the surgical procedure should be cleaned with a detergent-germicide. The floor should be cleaned with a detergent-germicide using the wet-vacuum method. If a wet vacuum is not available, a clean mophead should be used for each case. The wheels and casters of furniture used during the surgical procedure should be pushed through the solution used for floor cleaning.

At the end of the operative schedule, a complete housekeeping and maintenance program should be initiated.

REFERENCES

1. American Hospital Association: Infection control in the hospital, ed. 4, Chicago, 1979, The Association.
2. Association for the Advancement of Medical Instrumentation: Good hospital practice: steam sterilization and sterility assurance, Arlington, Va., 1980, The Association.
3. Association of Operating Room Nurses: AORN recommended practices for inhospital sterilization, AORN J. **32:**222, 1980.
4. Association of Operating Room Nurses: Standards for inhospital packaging material, Denver, 1978, The Association.
5. Buchanan, C.M.: Antisepsis and antiseptics, Newark, N.J., 1895, The Terhune Co.
6. Cruse, P.J., and Foord, R.: The epidemiology of wound infection: a ten-year prospective study of 62,939 wounds, Surg. Clin. North Am. **60:**27, 1980.
7. Youmans, G.P., Paterson, P.Y., and Sommers, H.M.: The biologic and clinical basis of infectious disease, ed. 2, Philadelphia, 1980, W.B. Saunders Co.

SUGGESTED READINGS

Association for the Advancement of Medical Instrumentation: EO sterilization: a guide for hospital personnel, Arlington, Va., 1976, The Association.

Association for the Advancement of Medical Instrumentation: Good hospital practice: ethylene oxide gas—ventilation recommendations and safe use, Arlington, Va., 1981, The Association.

Association of Operating Room Nurses: Standards for basic aseptic technique, Denver, 1978, The Association.

Association of Operating Room Nurses: Standards for O.R. wearing apparel, Denver, 1978, The Association.

Association of Operating Room Nurses: Standards for preoperative preparation of patients, Denver, 1978, The Association.

Association of Operating Room Nurses: Standards for surgical hand scrubs, Denver, 1978, The Association.

Association of Operating Room Nurses: Proposed recommended practices for O.R. sanitation, AORN J. **33:**1262, 1981.

Atkinson, L.J., and Kohn, M.L.: Berry and Kohn's introduction to operating room technique, ed. 5, New York, 1978, McGraw-Hill Book Co.

Board of Commissioners of Joint Commission on Accreditation of Hospitals: Accreditation manual for hospitals, Chicago, 1982, The Commission.

Brooks, S.M.: Fundamentals of operating room nursing, ed. 2, St. Louis, 1979, The C.V. Mosby Co.

Burrows, W.: Textbook of microbiology, ed. 21, Philadelphia, 1979, W.B. Saunders Co.

Grubb, R.D., and Ondov, G.: Operating room guidelines: an illustrated manual, St. Louis, 1979, The C.V. Mosby Co.

Gruendemann, B.J., and others: The surgical patient: behavioral concepts for the operating room nurse, ed. 2, St. Louis, 1977, The C.V. Mosby Co.

Harvey, C.K., and professional advisory committee: The experts research: questions and answers, AORN J. **34:**385, 1981.

Huth, M.E.: Rationale for O.R. attire standards, AORN J. **21:**1217, 1975.

Huth, M.E.: Principles of asepsis, AORN J. **24:**790, 1976.

Lawrence, C.A., and Block, S.S.: Disinfection, sterilization, and preservation, Philadelphia, 1977, Lea & Febiger.

Leichty, R.D., and Soper, R.T.: Synopsis of surgery, ed. 4, St. Louis, 1980, The C.V. Mosby Co.

LeMaitre, G., and Finnegan, J.: The patient in surgery: a guide for nurses, ed. 4, Philadelphia, 1980, W.B. Saunders Co.

McBride, M.E., Duncan, W.C., and Knox, J.M.: An evaluation of surgical scrub brushes, Surg. Gynecol. Obstet. **137:**934, 1973.

Moylan, J., and Kennedy, B.: The importance of gown and drape barriers in the prevention of wound infection, Surg. Gynecol. Obstet. **151:**465, 1980.

Perkins, J.J.: Principles and methods of sterilization in health sciences, ed. 2, Springfield Ill., 1978, Charles C Thomas, Publisher.

Rosenberg, A., Alatary, S.D., and Peterson, A.F.: Safety and efficacy of the skin antiseptic chlorhexidene gluconate, Surg. Gynecol. Obstet. **143:**789, 1976.

Ryan, P.: Inhospital packaging rationale, AORN J. **23:**980, 1976.

Smith, A.L.: Microbiology and pathology, ed. 12, St. Louis, 1980, The C.V. Mosby Co.

Tucci, V.J., and others: Studies of the surgical scrub, Surg. Gynecol. Obstet. **145:**415, 1977.

U.S. Department of Health, Education, and Welfare: A manual for hospital central services, Washington, D.C., April 1975, U.S. Government Printing Office.

Wells, P.: Fundamentals of aseptic technique, AORN Film Series, Denver, 1976, Association of Operating Room Nurses, Inc. (Film.)

6 Positioning the patient for surgery

Positioning of the operative patient is a key factor for the performance of a safe and efficient surgical procedure. All members of the surgical team have a duty to protect the patient from any deleterious effects of the surgical position. Although the choice of patient position is usually determined by the surgical approach, the responsibility for overall patient well-being rests with the surgeon, the anesthesiologist, and the nurse, who constantly monitor the physiological status of the patient. The circulating nurse may coordinate the details of restraints, support to the extremities, and safe transfers. The surgeon and the circulating nurse determine the position for patients who receive local anesthetics. The patient's position should provide optimum exposure and access to the operative site, should sustain circulatory and respiratory function, should not compromise neuromuscular structures, and should afford as much comfort to the patient as possible. Good positioning is that which promotes patient well-being and safety while meeting these needs.

ANATOMICAL AND PHYSIOLOGICAL FACTORS

The nurse must be cognizant of the anatomical and physiological changes that are associated with anesthesia, positioning of the patient, and operative procedure. These changes most frequently involve (1) the musculoskeletal system, (2) the nervous system, (3) the circulatory system, and (4) the respiratory system.

The **musculoskeletal system** of the patient may be subjected to unusual and exaggerated stress during operative positioning. The normal range of motion is maintained in the alert patient by pain and pressure receptors that warn against stretching and twisting of ligaments, tendons, and muscles. The tone of opposing muscle groups also acts to prevent strain and stress to the muscle bodies. When pharmacological agents such as anesthetics and muscle relaxants depress the pain and pressure receptors and loss of tone causes muscular relaxation, the normal defense mechanisms cannot guard against joint damage and muscle stretch and strain. Obvious resistance to unusual range of motion is often noted only in patients whose arthritic changes prevent even slight exaggeration of the position. The position chosen should provide physiological alignment while protecting the patient from pressure, abrasion, and other injuries.

Nervous system depression accompanies the administration of anesthetic agents and many other drugs. The degree of depression depends on the type of regional anesthesia or the level of general anesthesia. Pain and pressure receptors may be affected either regionally or systemically. The most important factor for the nurse to remember is that when nervous system depression occurs, the body's communication and command system is rendered totally or partially ineffective. Changes in physical status and compensatory actions are no longer possible. Lifesaving, physiological adaptive mechanisms do not function; the stresses of operative positioning are not automatically compensated. Pressure on superficial nerves should be prevented.

The **circulatory system** is most dramatically affected by the anesthesia causing a lack of nervous system control of vascular dilatation and constriction. It is also affected by direct peripheral pressure on the venous return; blood pools in veins to decrease circulating volume, and blood flow is distributed along variations of the horizontal body plane and follows laws of gravity in other manners than when it is upright. Blood pressure responds to redistribution of blood flow and the horizontal body plane in addition to inherent pathophysiological processes.

Poor positioning of the patient can adversely affect pulmonary function. Diaphragmatic movement may be impeded by the position or by shifting visceral pressure resulting from the position. The horizontal body plane changes the airflow and functional characteristics of the lungs. Not only airflow but also the flow of secretions is affected. The combination of circulatory changes and the compromised respiratory effort affects the oxygen saturation of the blood.

NURSING CONSIDERATIONS

Nursing assessment begins preoperatively with a review of the proposed schedule for the room to which the nurse is assigned. Based on the schedule and the operating surgeon's preferences, the basic patient position is anticipated. During the preoperative patient assessment, the nurse determines the patient's height and weight and reviews the record.

Specific nursing care is planned to encompass the surgeon's specification for the given basic position and to alleviate or prevent an individual patient problem. Planning may involve determining the appropriate mode of patient transport and transfer, determining equipment and positioning aids, or determining the need for ancillary personnel to accomplish the positioning.

Implementation of the plan begins when the nurse checks the operating table for proper functioning and gathers positioning aids. Implementation continues as the patient is assisted into the surgical position and culminates as the patient is returned to the stretcher for transport to the postanesthesia recovery room.

Details of the position should be recorded in the patient's records, including the type and placement of restraints, the position of the extremities, the site of the electrocautery plate, the positional changes made during the procedure (for example, supine to lithotomy to supine), and any abnormalities noted at the end of the procedure that could ultimately be attributed to the surgical position.

The nurse must be familiar with the normal functions, the maintenance, the various uses, and the potential hazards of the operating tables, their attachments, and other mechanical adjuncts to both patient position and the operative procedure (such as electrocautery, drills, and radiology). Mechanical malfunction must be recognized and repaired for the patient's safety.

Providing patient safety encompasses more than overseeing mechanical functions; it also includes direct patient care. The restraint strap should be snug but should not compromise venous circulation or exert pressure on bony prominences or nerves. It should never be placed directly on the patient's skin but rather over the blanket covering the patient. If possible, patient transfers should be made when the patient is awake. When the patient is anesthetized or unable to assist, a four-person lift or a Davis roller should be used to provide support to the torso and all extremities. Mayo tables should be positioned high enough to prevent pressure on the toes or the legs. The operative team should be reminded not to lean on the patient's trunk or extremities, since this pressure may compromise anatomical and physiological functions.

MODERN OPERATING TABLES

Modern operating tables are specifically designed to meet the peculiar and highly specialized requirements of surgical therapy. Modern manufacture and design have done much to facilitate safe and effective positioning of the patient while providing the surgeon with anatomical accessibility. Judicious manipulation of the table obviates untoward manipulation of the patient.

It is not feasible to describe here all types of operating tables available. It is the responsibility of the nursing personnel to be well versed in the use of the tables available in the institution. Nurses should keep abreast of new developments and should evaluate their usefulness in actual practice.

In common surgical use are the general operating table, the orthopedic (fracture) table, the urology table, and the eye table. The modern general operating table (Fig. 6-1) is so versatile that the need for specialty tables is declining. A table that is adapted to a wide range of uses is an economical investment and permits flexibility in the use of operating facilities. The orthopedic table with its multiple movable and removable parts and suspension frames remains one of few specialty tables required (Fig. 6-2).

The new urology table designed for cystoscopic procedures has radiological equipment attached, which facilitates operative filming of the genitourinary system.

Modern general operating tables can be adjusted for height and length and can be tilted laterally to either side and horizontally at the head and foot. Tables are divided into three or more sections that support the major body parts and permit their placement in flexion or extension. The head section is usually removable, and foot extensions may be added.

Controls and accessories may be employed to maintain the patient in standard or modified dorsal, lateral, or prone positions. Headrests of various designs enable the general table to be used for cranial and eye surgery. Electrically powered models make table movements swift and smooth.

Perineal cutouts and drainage trays fitted to the lumbar section adapt the general operating table to the perineal approaches used in gynecological, urological, and proctological surgery. Most tables are available with x-ray–penetrable tunnel tops that permit insertion of cassette holders at any position along the table.

Additional accessories for operating tables include pillows, pads, bolsters, and doughnut cushions of various sizes and shapes. These are made to fit the different anatomical structures of patients, thereby facilitating physiological functions and operative accessibility. Some accessories are soft and made of conductive foam rubber; others are firm, made of conductive rubber, and filled with kapok or fine sand. All of these accessories should be designed to permit terminal cleansing between patient usages.

STANDARD POSITIONS AND PHYSIOLOGICAL CONSIDERATIONS

Since operative procedures are performed with the patient resting on the back, abdomen, or side, three basic positions may be described: dorsal, prone, and lateral. These basic positions can then be modified in many ways. The following discussion of operative positioning is general; there is room for individuality to meet specific needs or preferences.

Dorsal position

In the *dorsal position,* the patient's spinal column is resting on the surface of the operating table mattress.

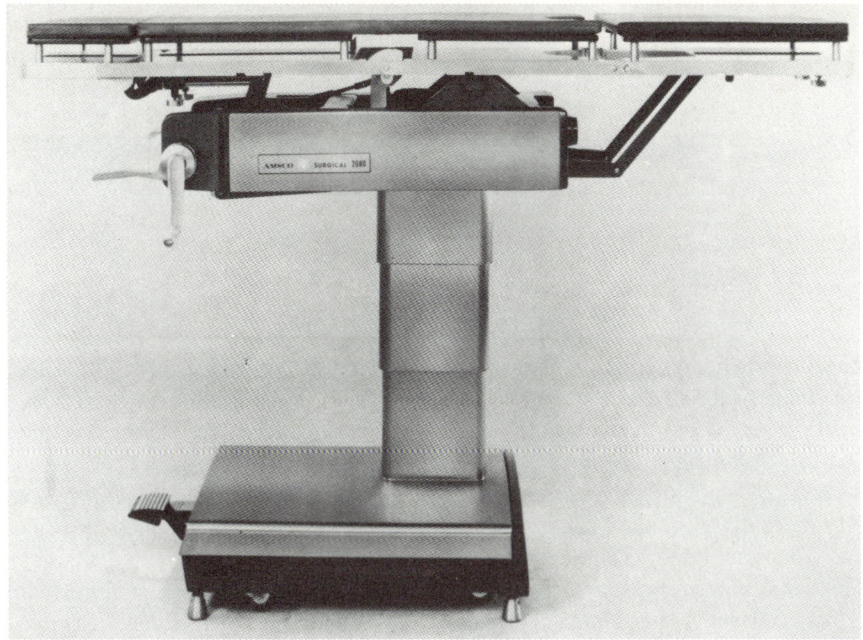

Fig. 6-1. Surgical operating table with x-ray–penetrable top. (Courtesy AMSCO—American Sterilizer Co., Erie, Pa.)

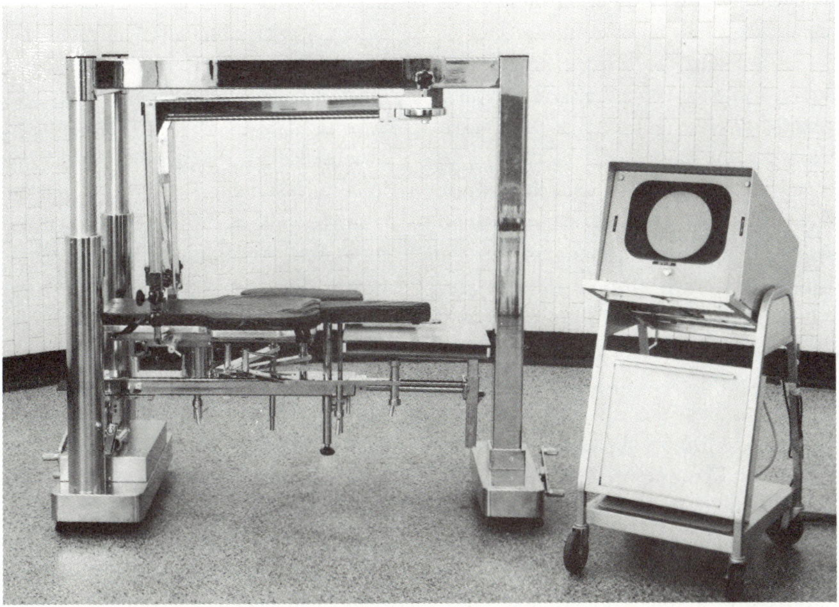

Fig. 6-2. Orthopedic and surgical table. (Courtesy Chick Orthopedic, Oakland, Calif.)

Modifications of the position allow approach to the major body cavities (cranial, thoracic, and peritoneal), the four extremities, and the perineum.

The *dorsal recumbent (supine) position* is the most common position. It is the most natural position of the body at rest. The patient is usually anesthetized in this position (Fig. 6-3), and modifications are made after induction of anesthesia.

The patient lies supine (face upward) with the arms at the sides and the legs extended. The position of the head should place the cervical, thoracic, and lumbar vertebrae in a straight, horizontal line. A small pad placed under the head allows the strap muscles to relax and prevents neck strain. Flexion or twisting may cause contractures in the neck and may interfere with a clear airway. A small soft pillow may be placed under the small of the

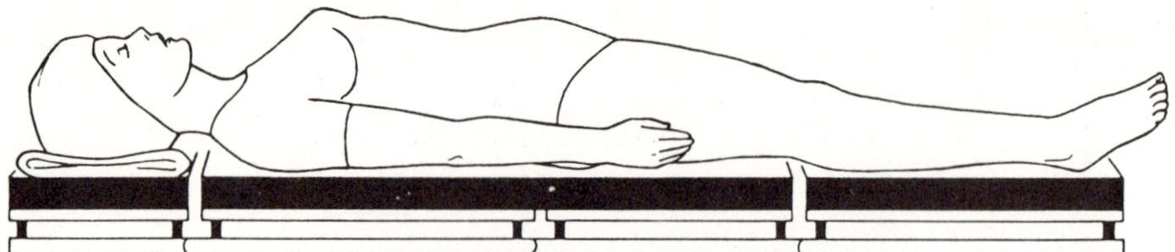

Fig. 6-3. Dorsal recumbent (supine) position.

back or under the knees to maintain normal lumbar concavity and to prevent strain on the relaxed back muscles and ligaments; such strain may occur if the muscles and ligaments are allowed to assume the configuration of the flat operating table surface. The hips are parallel. The legs are parallel and uncrossed to prevent peroneal and tibial nerve injury and compromised circulation. The legs are slightly separated so that skin surfaces are not in contact, since moisture from antiseptics, irrigating solutions, and body fluids contributes to irritation and maceration of the skin. The leg restraint (table strap) is placed across the thighs so that the patient is secured but superficial venous return is not impaired. Heel prominences also need protection from prolonged pressure. Doughnut cushions, ankle rolls, or foam heel protectors may be used.

The soles of the feet are supported on a firm foam rubber support or padded footboard that extends beyond the toes to prevent plantar flexion and to guard the toes from the weight and pressure of drapes.

The arms should rest easily at the sides with the palms against the padded body or with the hands pronated (palms down and fingers extended) on the mattress surface. A broad lift sheet can be used to tuck around the arms to support the full length of each arm. The elbows should neither be flexed nor rest on the metal edge of the table. An elbow resting on the table edge may cause pressure to the ulnar nerve as it passes over the epicondyle of the humerus. If the hands are placed under the buttocks, there is danger that the fingers will be compressed. Wristlets used to restrain the hands endanger the nerves and the blood supply to the hands. Leather restraints also may chafe and abrade the skin. When wrist restraints are necessary, the padded cloth clove hitch produces the least trauma.

Frequently one or both arms rest on armboards. Abduction, extension, and external rotation may stretch the brachial plexus. To prevent this, the arm should always be placed at less than a 90-degree angle to the body, with palms up to diminish the pressure on the brachial and ulnar nerves. The table mattress and armboard pad should be of the same height. The armboard should be the type that locks into position on the table to prevent inadvertent angle changes or sudden loss of support to the arm.

When the head is turned to one side or the other, it should be supported to keep the spine in alignment and secured in the desired position with a doughnut cushion, sandbag, or special headrest. Pressure on the ear and over bony prominences where nerves and blood vessels run superficially must be prevented. The eyes must be carefully guarded against pressure, and they must be protected as drapes are placed to prevent corneal irritation from textiles, solutions, and other foreign objects.

The circulatory system may be compromised in the dorsal recumbent position, not only by a tight leg restraint but also by the overall effect of the horizontal body posture and the changed effects of gravity. Depending on the degree of medullary and autonomic nervous system depression by general anesthesia, homeostatic compensatory mechanisms may not function to dilate and constrict blood vessels in response to cardiac or blood volume changes. The increased pressure of abdominal viscera or masses on the inferior vena cava may decrease blood return to the heart; blood pressure would then be lowered. Whenever possible, patient position should encourage venous drainage and avoid obstruction to the major veins. An example is tilting the supine cesarean section patient slightly to the left to prevent excessive pressure on the inferior vena cava before the baby is delivered, particularly with spinal anesthesia.

Respiratory function is also compromised in the dorsal recumbent position because the vital capacity is less than that in the erect posture, notwithstanding the effects of anesthesia. Although anterior and upward excursion of the chest during inspiration is not greatly impeded, diaphragmatic excursion may be lessened by the abdominal viscera. The dorsal recumbent position does allow a more even distribution of ventilation from apex to base of the lungs.

Trendelenburg's position is a variation of the dorsal recumbent position (Fig. 6-4). Occasionally in this position, the knees are flexed by "breaking" the lower portion of the table. Another modification is that of keeping the trunk level and elevating only the legs by raising the lower part of the table. This position is used either to provide better visualization of the pelvic organs or to improve circulation to the cerebral cortex and basal ganglia when blood pressure is suddenly lowered. In the latter instance, the position enhances arterial blood flow to the

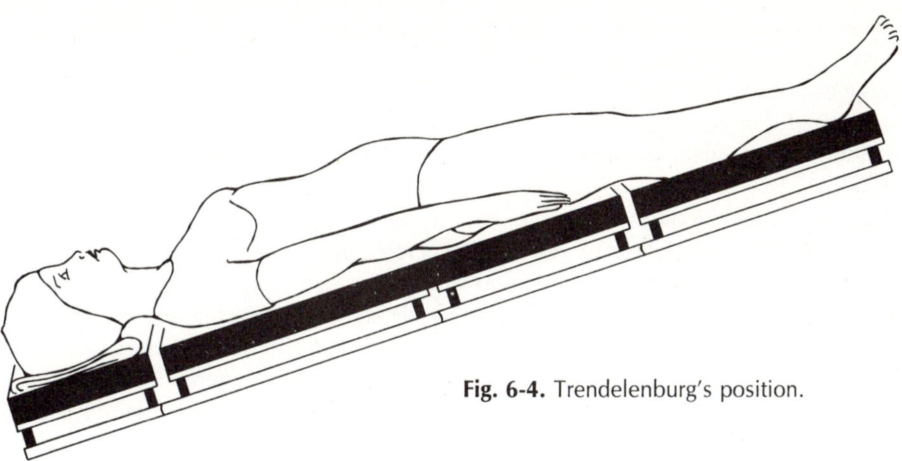

Fig. 6-4. Trendelenburg's position.

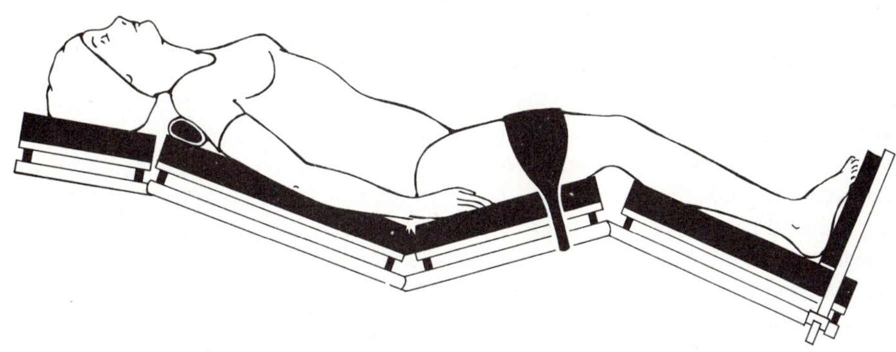

Fig. 6-5. Position for operations on thyroid and neck area.

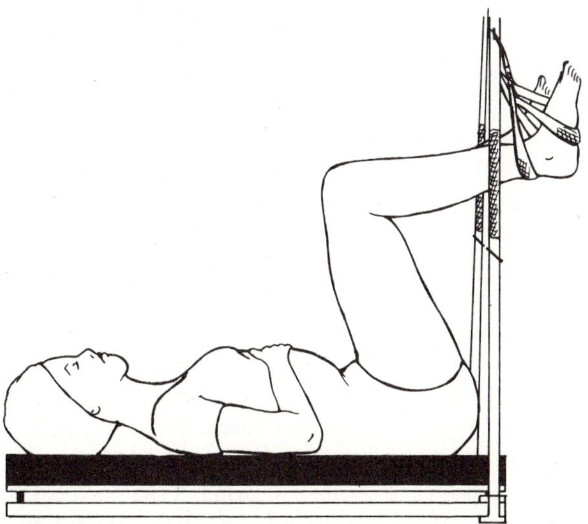

Fig. 6-6. Lithotomy position for vaginal and rectal operations. Stirrups or feet must be padded to prevent patient's skin from touching metal.

cranium, but the venous return pressure is also increased because of necessary venous antigravity flow. Both purposes for this position can be accomplished by modifying the standard, time-honored, "head down–toes up," tiltboard slant to a position more conducive to physiological homeostasis.

To reduce pooling of venous blood in the lower extremities, the legs and thighs may be elevated either by pillows or by adjusting the table. When it is desirable to place the entire trunk in Trendelenburg's position, the effects of gravitational pull can be improved. Flexion of the head on the headrest or a small pillow promotes cranial venous drainage. Although the head downward position facilitates drainage of secretions from the bases of the lungs and the oropharyngeal passages, the weight of the abdominal viscera further impedes diaphragmatic movement.

The less drastic slant of this modified Trendelenburg's position negates the need for wrist bracelets and shoulder braces that when improperly placed put pressure on the brachial plexus and blood vessels in the neck. This variation of Trendelenburg's position should be maintained only as long as necessary. The patient should be returned slowly to the dorsal recumbent position. Slow, smooth postural transitions allow sufficient time for the body to adjust to the imposed physiological changes.

Reverse Trendelenburg's position is frequently used to provide access to the head and neck and to facilitate gravitational pull on the viscera away from the diaphragm and toward the feet. When the foot of the table is tilted toward the floor, the patient's body must be supported by the padded footboard, by nonconstrictive body restraints, and by a lift sheet that supports the arms from elbows to fingers. Lumbar and popliteal pads also tend to prevent the body from slipping. In this position the tilted, head-up table is usually in a straight line, the opposite of Fig. 6-4.

When a modification of this position is used for thyroid or parathyroid surgery (Fig. 6-5), the neck may be hyperextended by raising the patient's shoulders (using inflatable pillow, bolster, or sandbag) and/or by lowering the table headpiece. There should be no gaps in the support of the neck in this position. When this position is used for biliary surgery, the right side of the patient may be elevated in the horizontal plane by a lengthwise bolster, inflatable gallbladder bag, or tapered foam pad (lemon slice). To prevent twisting of the spine, the full length of the trunk needs support. The hips and shoulders are kept in the same plane.

In reverse Trendelenburg's position, respiratory function is more like that in the erect position. Venous circulation may be compromised by an extended time in the legs downward position. When this is anticipated, the superficial venous return can be aided by the preoperative application of support hose. Return to the dorsal recumbent position from reverse Trendelenburg's position should also be accomplished slowly and smoothly.

Modified Fowler's (sitting) position causes most of the patient's weight to be on the dorsum of the body. The position of the body in relation to the table breaks must be carefully adjusted to prevent abnormal pressures. The backrest is elevated, the knees are flexed, and the footboard is set in place. The more erect the patient's posture, the greater the need to support the shoulders and torso. Such support requires adequate padding to protect the axilla and brachial plexus. Frequently, a special headrest is used for cranial ventricular procedures and for posterior fossa craniotomy (Chapter 24).

The sitting position requires special attention to positioning of the arms. Depending on the surgery, the arms may be flexed across the abdomen, resting on a large pillow in the lap, or may be placed in front of the patient on a padded stand. Hyperextension of the shoulder region must be prevented, and the arms must be secure from falling or pressing against hard surfaces. The vascular system of the arms and legs may require additional supportive measures.

The *lithotomy position* is the most extreme variation of the dorsal recumbent posture (Fig. 6-6). With the patient supine, the legs are raised and abducted to expose the perineal region to gain a surgical approach to the pelvic organs and genitals. This unnatural posture is fraught with danger and discomfort for the patient, and these hazards increase as the position is exaggerated for radical surgery of the groin, vulva, or prostate. Extreme flexion of the thighs impairs respiratory function by increasing intraabdominal pressure against the diaphragm and therefore decreasing the tidal volume. Gravity flow of blood from the elevated legs causes blood to pool in the splanchnic region during the operative procedure. Blood loss during surgery may not be immediately manifested because of this increased splanchnic volume. However, when the legs are lowered and 500 ml or more of blood is diverted to more total leg circulation, the circulating volume is depleted and the blood pressure may decrease. Normal compensatory mechanisms are depressed by the effect of anesthesia on the nervous system, and homeostasis may not be achieved easily.

Supports for the legs must be carefully chosen and applied. By placing the patient's anterior iliac spine on a line with the leg holder and the buttocks level and on a line with the edge of the table break, a good position can be achieved with a minimum of effort. A small lumbar pad will help maintain the physiological concavity of this area.

Modern leg holders provide secure support for the legs without the popliteal pressure of knee crutches and without undue external rotation and abduction, which stretch the abductor muscles and capsule of the hip joint.

The stirrups must be level. The height is adjusted to the length of the patient's legs. This prevents pressure at the knee and the lumbar spine. The patient's position must be symmetrical. The perineum is in line with the longitudinal axis of the table; the pelvis is level and the head and trunk are in a straight line. This aids the surgeon in identifying anatomical landmarks. Support is provided for the head and neck as previously described. If the table is to be tilted head downward to raise the operative area, padded shoulder braces may be applied over the acromioclavicular joint. All the cautions about the head downward position apply.

To place a patient in the lithotomy position, the patient's legs are raised simultaneously. Each leg is raised by grasping the sole of the foot in one hand and supporting the leg near the knee in the other. The leg is raised, and the knee is flexed slowly. The padded foot is secured in the holder by loops of canvas slings. One loop of the canvas sling is placed around the sole at the metatarsals, and the other loop around the ankle. The lower part of the leg should be free from pressure against the leg holders to prevent pressure on the common peroneal nerve. Some stirrups may require foam rubber padding between the calves of the legs and the metal posts. Pressure against the soft tissues of the leg may predispose to venous thrombosis. For high lithotomy position during extensive surgery or for patients with ankylosed hip joints, knee and footrest stirrups may be required.

Arms require special care in the lithotomy position. The hands should not extend along the table sides, since they will reach below the break of the foot section of the table and be in danger of injury from manipulation of the table parts. They may be folded loosely across the abdomen and supported by the folded gown or a cover sheet, or they may be extended on armboards. Arms must not impede chest movement and adequate respiration. The weight of the limbs on the chest, especially in infants and children, may tire the muscles used in respiration and induce respiratory failure.

Adequate assistance must be available for placing the patient in the lithotomy position and for releasing the patient from the position. Any change in body position affects hemodynamics. Movements must be slow and deliberate to allow gradual adjustment to the change. Muscles and joints must be protected from abnormal strain in their relaxed state. The legs should be raised simultaneously to place the feet in the loops of the canvas supports. They also must be lowered simultaneously, supporting the joints above and below to prevent strain on the lumbosacral musculature, which can stretch and tilt, thereby placing the pelvis and limbs in imbalance.

Prone position

In the *prone position,* the patient is lying with the abdomen on the surface of the operating table mattress. The surgical approach may be made to any dorsal surface. Modifications of the position allow approach to the cervical spine, back, rectal area, and lower extremities. After induction of anesthesia with the patient in the dorsal recumbent posture on a stretcher, the patient is turned to the abdomen when transferred to the operating table.

Turning can be accomplished safely, smoothly, and gently by four persons. The anesthesiologist supports the head and neck during the turn. One assistant stands at the side of the stretcher with hands at the patient's shoulders and buttocks to initiate the roll of the patient. A second assistant stands opposite, at the side of the operating table, with arms extended to support the chest and lower abdomen on outstretched arms as the patient is rolled forward and over. The third assistant stands at the foot of the stretcher to support and turn the legs. At the completion of the turn, the stretcher is removed.

An armboard is provided on each side of the table, and the patient's arms are brought down and forward to rest with elbows flexed and hands pronated at either side of the head. The head is positioned on a foam pillow or towels, keeping the neck in alignment with the spinal column. The eyes are carefully protected from pillow and drapes.

Body rolls extending lengthwise from the acromioclavicular joint to the iliac crests raise the chest and permit the diaphragm to move freely and the lungs to expand. Supports must not press against the female breasts. A bolster or pillow under the pelvis will decrease abdominal pressure on the inferior vena cava. A cushion or pillow is placed under the ankles to prevent pressure on the toes and plantar flexion of the feet. The table strap is again placed across the thighs and blanket so that the patient is secured but superficial venous return is not impaired.

The prone posture is initially hazardous as the anesthetized patient is turned from the dorsal recumbent position to the prone position. Normal compensatory mechanisms are depressed, and the patient cannot readily adjust to imposed hemodynamic change.

Neuromuscularly, the radial nerve may be compressed against the humerus if the forearm is allowed to hang over the side of the table. The shoulders may be overextended unless the elbows are flexed and the palms pronated. The venous return may be compromised by a tight leg restraint, dependent lower extremities, and visceral compression of the inferior vena cava.

The respiratory system is most vulnerable in the prone position because the normal anterolateral respiratory movement is restricted and the normal diaphragmatic movement is inhibited by the compressed abdominal wall.

For spinal operations the prone position may be modified to flex the affected part of spine, for example, the knee-chest position. The hips also may be flexed at one table break and the leg section raised to a "kneeling" position. The surgeon will specify the modifications preferred.

The *jackknife position* or *Kraske's position* is a modification of the prone position and is used for proctological procedures (Fig. 6-7). The patient's hips are placed

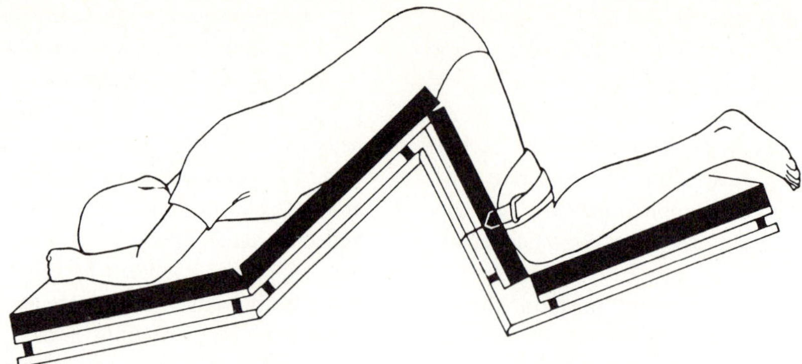

Fig. 6-7. Jackknife position for proctological operations.

on a bolster or pillow over the table break, and the table is flexed at a 90-degree angle, raising the hips and lowering the head and body. The patient's head, chest, and feet need the usual supports in this position. The leg restraint (strap) is across the thighs.

The buttocks may be separated with broad straps of adhesive tape secured firmly at the level of the anus a few inches from the midline on either side. These straps are pulled tight simultaneously and are fastened to the underside of the table surface. The straps are released at the end of the procedure to facilitate the approximation of the wound edges.

If the patient is to be placed on the recovery stretcher in the dorsal recumbent position, the turning is accomplished by reversing the four-person roll described earlier.

Lateral position

In the *lateral position,* the patient is lying on the unaffected side, and the surgical approach may be to the uppermost chest, the kidney, or the upper ureter (Figs. 6-8 and 6-9). Positioning of the extremities and trunk facilitates the desired approach.

After induction of anesthesia with the patient in the dorsal recumbent position on the operating table, the patient is turned to the side. The teamwork of four persons is necessary to accomplish a safe, smooth, gentle turn. The anesthesiologist supports the head and neck during the turn. One assistant stands at the shoulders of the operative side facing the patient's head; the assistant's arm and hand nearer the patient cross the chest and grasp the patient's shoulder; the other hand is placed under the nearer shoulder. The second assistant stands at the hips of the operative side, facing the patient's head; the assistant's arm and hand nearer the patient cross the hips and grasp the patient's opposite buttock; the other hand is placed under the nearer buttock. The third assistant stands at the foot of the table to support and turn the legs. A lifting sheet under the patient can be used by the team to facilitate the turn. At a signal from the anesthesiologist, the first and second assistants lift and bring the patient to his side at their edge of the operating table; the patient is then placed in the center of the table. A pillow is placed under the patient's head to maintain good alignment with the cervical spine and the thoracic vertebrae. Another pillow is placed between the patient's legs, the bottom leg flexed at the knee and hip, and the top leg straight or slightly flexed. The lateral aspect of the bottom knee must be padded to prevent pressure on the peroneal nerve, located superficially at the head of the fibula. One assistant should remain at the patient's back to steady and support the torso during positioning of the extremities.

The *lateral chest position* (Fig. 6-8) allows operative approach to the uppermost thoracic cavity. The upper arm is flexed slightly at the elbow and raised above the head to elevate the scapula and to provide access to the underlying ribs and to widen the intercostal spaces. This arm may be supported on a raised armboard. The lower shoulder is brought slightly forward to prevent pressure on the brachial plexus and is flexed at the elbow. The lower shoulder may rest on a thin foam pad to prevent tissue pressure from the bony prominence. In chest surgery, infusion needles may be placed in the upper or lower arm. Care must be taken to prevent compression of venous return in that arm.

The torso may be stabilized on the operating table by well-padded body braces or sandbags. Some surgeons prefer to secure the arms, hips, and legs and not use torso supports, which may impede respiratory expansion and decrease the surface area for the surgical approach. A roll may be placed at the apex of the scapula in the axillary space to relieve pressure on the arm and allow more chest movement with respirations. Slanting the upper section of the table downward places the trachea and mouth at a lower level than the lungs. This slanting of the table encourages bronchial secretions and fluids from the lung bases to drain into the mouth and not pass into the unaffected side of the chest.

For torso stabilization the legs may be positioned in several ways, according to the surgeon's preference: (1) both legs may be flexed at 90-degree angles at the hips and knees, a pillow placed between the legs, and adhe-

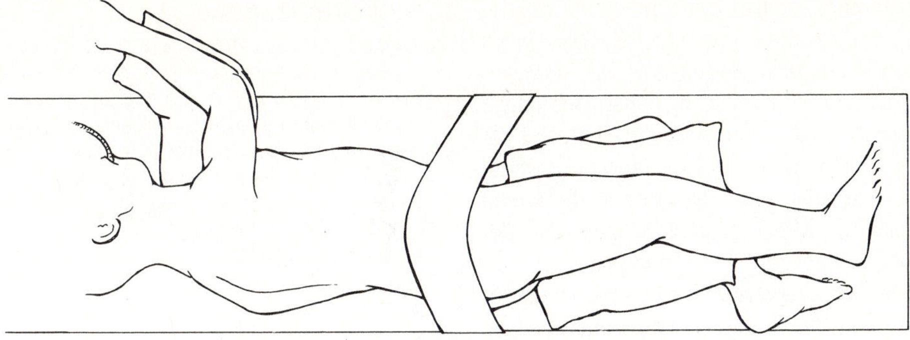

Fig. 6-8. Lateral position for chest operations.

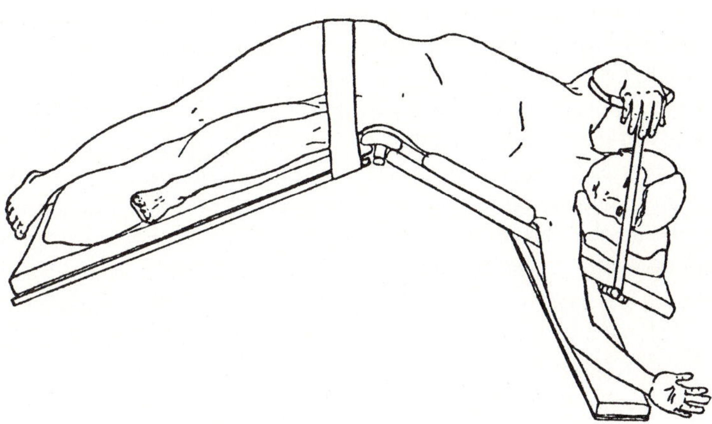

Fig. 6-9. Lateral position for kidney operations.

sive tape placed across the thigh to both sides of the tabletop; (2) the lower leg may be extended straight on the table, the upper hip and knee flexed at 90-degree angles with two pillows supporting this thigh and calf, the uppermost ankle secured in a padded restraint to the table top at the patient's back, and adhesive tape placed across the thigh to both sides of the tabletop; or (3) the lower hip and knee may be flexed at 90-degree angles, two or more pillows supporting the extended upper leg, the uppermost ankle secured in a padded restraint to the tabletop at the patient's back, and adhesive tape placed across the upper hip, between the iliac crest and greater trochanter, to both sides of the tabletop.

The *lateral kidney position* (Fig. 6-9) allows approach to the retroperitoneal space of the flank. After the anesthetized patient is turned from the dorsal position to the lateral position, the patient is moved so that the lower iliac crest is just below the kidney elevator of the table. To render the kidney region readily accessible, the bridge (kidney rest) of the table is raised and the table is flexed, so that the area between the twelfth rib and the iliac crest is elevated. A well-padded kidney brace may be placed against the iliac crest. Elevating is dependent on the cardiovascular response of the body to the increased pressure transmitted from this area. The kidney rest is slowly raised; blood pressure is measured frequently by the anesthesiologist. The table is then flexed to lower the patient's head and legs. In this position, the patient's affected side presents a straight horizontal line from shoulder to hip.

The upper arm is placed on a raised armboard. The lower shoulder is brought slightly forward, and the arm is flexed to rest near the face on the mattress. A small bolster is placed under the lower axilla to allow chest expansion. The lower extremity is flexed and supported by a sandbag or pillow. Two or more pillows support the extended upper leg. The feet should be protected against plantar flexion and the ankles or heels protected from undue pressure. In this position, the gravitational force on the head and torso opposes that on the extended limb to facilitate operative exposure. To stabilize the body, a restraining belt or adhesive strap is placed across the shoulder and hip areas and is secured to the tabletop. Before wound closure, the adhesive strap is released, the kidney rest lowered, and the table straightened to facilitate approximation of the suture line.

Physiological changes in the lateral position occur in the healthy alert person but may be more dramatic and stress producing in the anesthetized patient. Normally, there are systolic and diastolic pressure decreases when the lateral position is assumed. Because normal compensatory mechanisms are depressed by pharmacological agents and pathophysiological processes present, the patient may not readily compensate for abrupt postural changes. The acute angulation of the body in the lateral kidney posture and the effect of gravity may also decrease blood return to the right side of the heart.

Respiratory function is compromised by the weight of the body on the lower chest; chest movements are limited, and chest size may be decreased. Diaphragmatic movement is limited by the flexion of the lower limbs toward the abdomen. Another disadvantage of this position is that the weight of the body must rest on the unaffected side, which makes it more difficult to control the patient's aspiration of secretions from the lung on this side. In the lateral kidney position, pressure on the lower thorax and increased tension on the upper intercostal and lumbar musculature interfere with intercostal breathing.

The hazards of neuromuscular damage can largely be prevented through careful manipulation and adequate protective padding. Again, the brachial plexus and common peroneal nerve deserve thoughtful consideration.

SUGGESTED READINGS

Anthony, C.P., and Thibodeau, G.A.: Textbook of anatomy and physiology, ed. 10, St. Louis, 1979, The C.V. Mosby Co.

Eggers, G., DeGroot, W., and Tanner, C.: Hemodynamic changes associated with various surgical positions, J.A.M.A. **185:**105, 1963.

Foley, M.J.: Variations in blood pressure in the lateral recumbent position, Nurs. Res. **20:**64, Jan.-Feb. 1971.

Foster, C.G., and others: Effects of surgical positioning, AORN J. **30:**219, 1979.

Martin, J.T.: Positioning in anesthesia and surgery, Philadelphia, 1978, W.B. Saunders Co.

McCaig, C.: Review: positioning for neurosurgery, AORN J. **28:**1053, 1978.

Minckley, B.B.: Physiologic hazards of position changes in the anesthetized patient, Am. J. Nurs. **69:**2602, 1969.

Nelson, S.L.: Positioning the surgical patient, Danbury, Conn., 1982, Davis & Geck, American Cyanamid Co. (Film.)

Nicholson, M., and Eversole, U.: Nerve injuries incident to anesthesia and operation, AORN J. **2:**44, March-April 1964.

Schmidt, R.C.: Peripheral nerve injuries with anesthesia, Anesth. Analg. (Cleve.) **45:**748, 1966.

Souther, S., Carr, S., and Vistnes, L.: Pressure, tissue ischemia and operating table pads, Arch. Surg. **107:**544, 1973.

Sum, R.L.: Trendelenburg's position in hypovolemic shock, Am. J. Nurs. **71:**1758, 1971.

Works, R.F.: Hints on lifting and pulling, Am. J. Nurs. **72:**260, 1972.

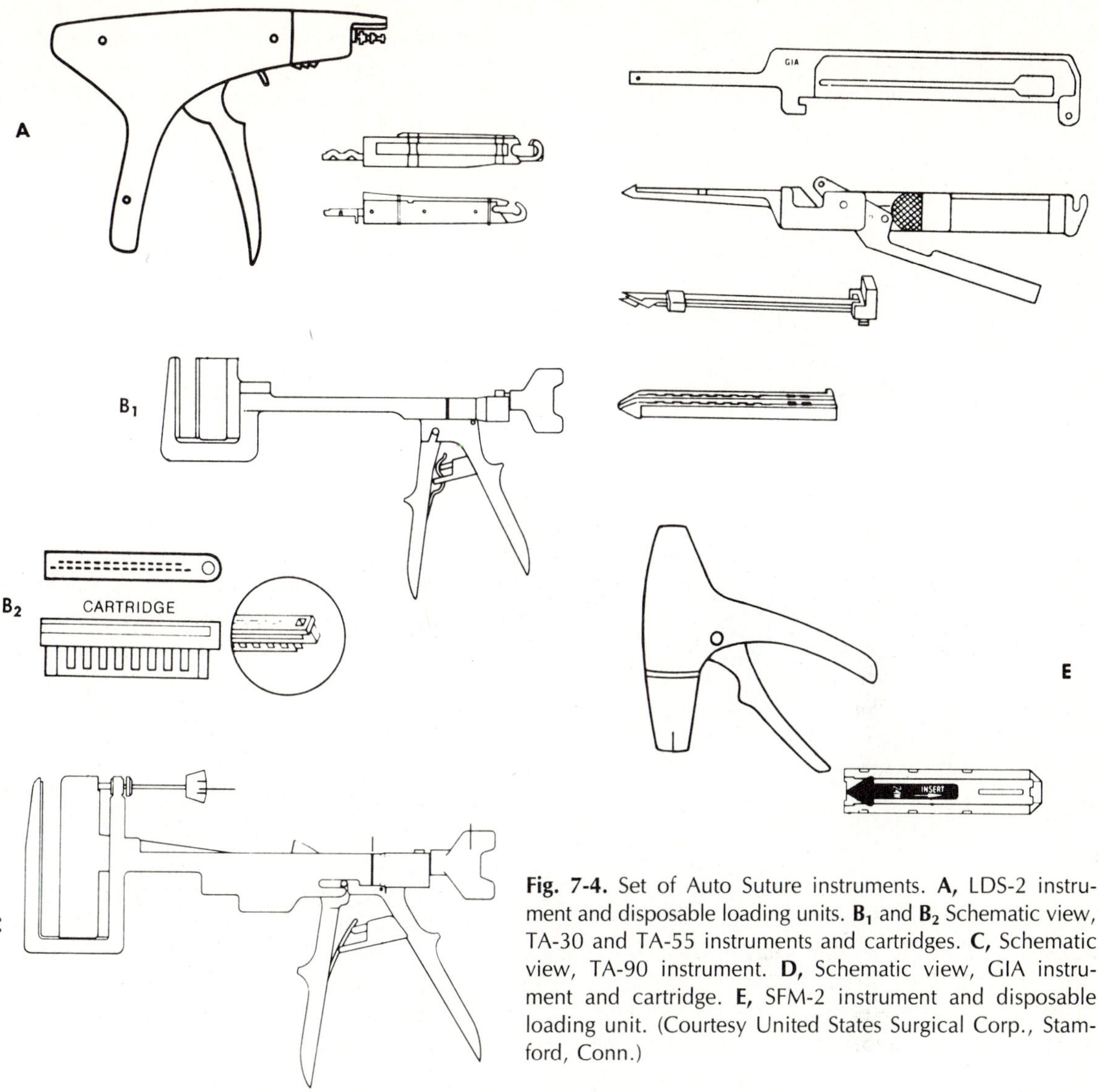

Fig. 7-4. Set of Auto Suture instruments. **A,** LDS-2 instrument and disposable loading units. **B_1** and **B_2** Schematic view, TA-30 and TA-55 instruments and cartridges. **C,** Schematic view, TA-90 instrument. **D,** Schematic view, GIA instrument and cartridge. **E,** SFM-2 instrument and disposable loading unit. (Courtesy United States Surgical Corp., Stamford, Conn.)

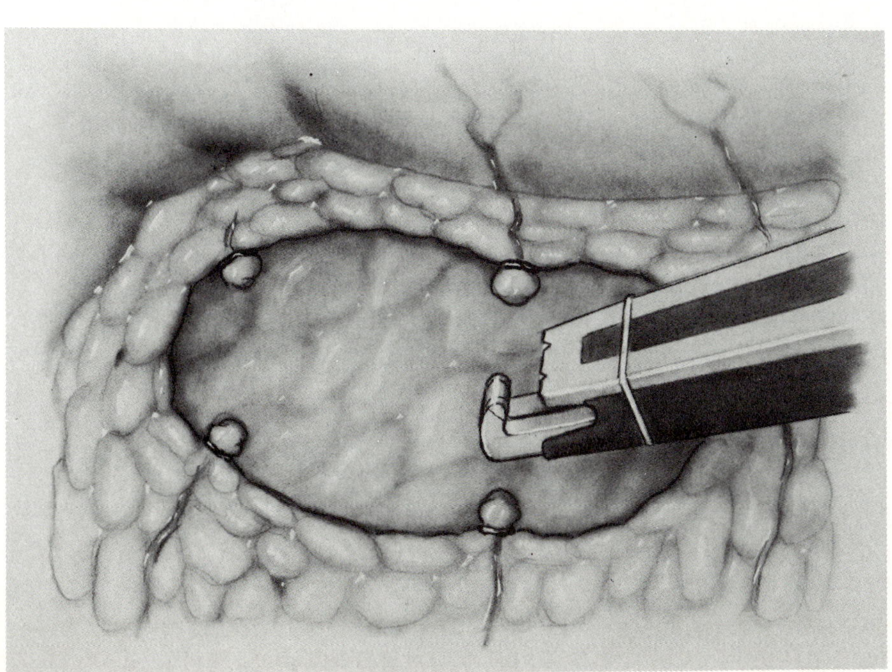

Fig. 7-5. Using LDS to ligate and divide omental vessels. (Courtesy United States Surgical Corp., Stamford, Conn.)

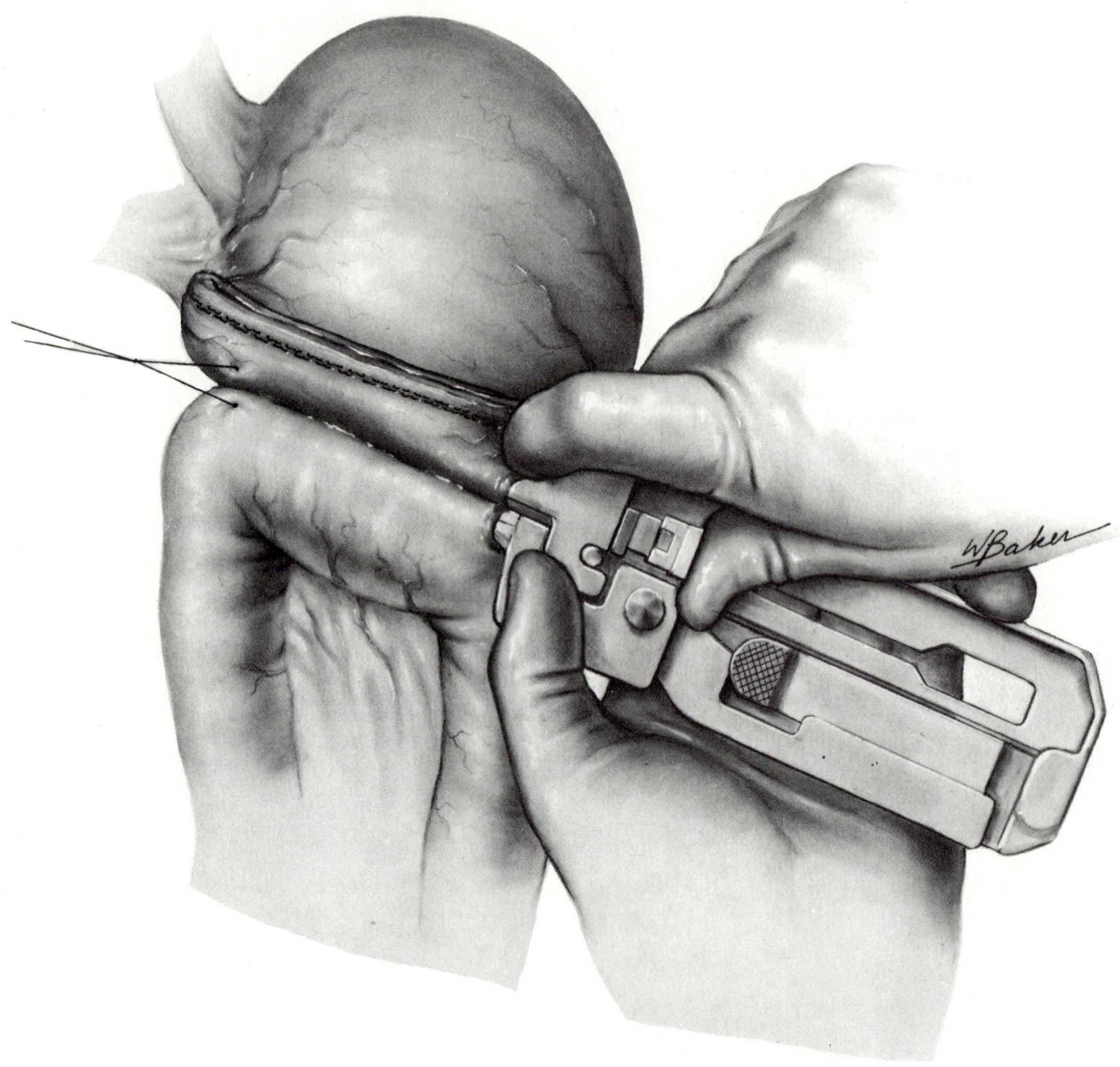

Fig. 7-6. Using GIA to staple and join stomach and jejunum. At same time, blade in GIA cuts between double staple lines, creating stoma for gastrojejunostomy. (Courtesy United States Surgical Corp., Stamford, Conn.)

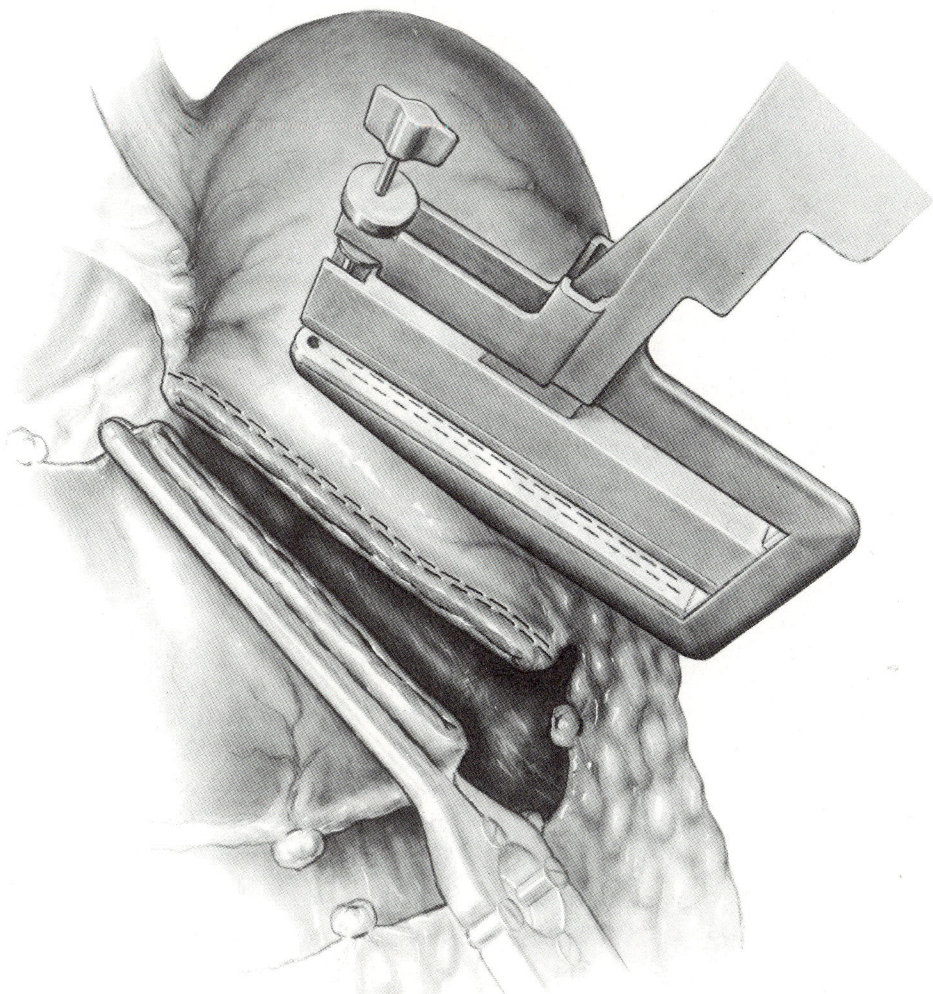

Fig. 7-7. Using TA-90 to close gastric pouch. Jaws of TA-90 are slipped around stomach at level of transection, pin is screwed into place, jaws are tightened, and staples are fired. (Courtesy United States Surgical Corp., Stamford, Conn.)

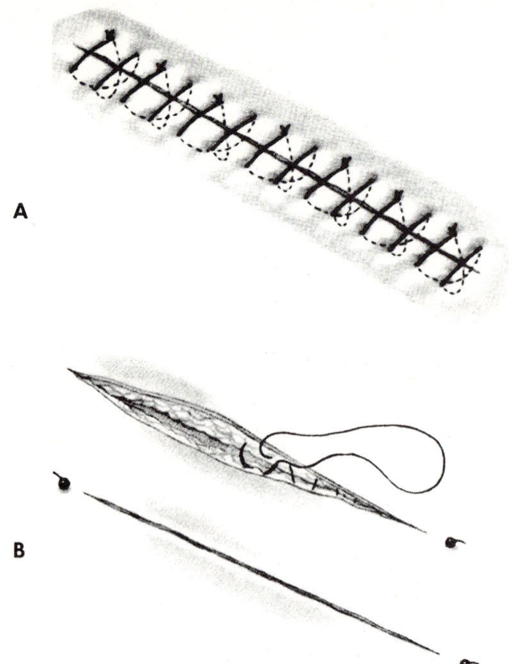

Fig. 7-8. Two types of skin closure. **A,** Interrupted figure-of-eight sutures. **B,** Continuous subcuticular closure anchored with lead shot. (Courtesy Ethicon, Inc., Somerville, N.J.)

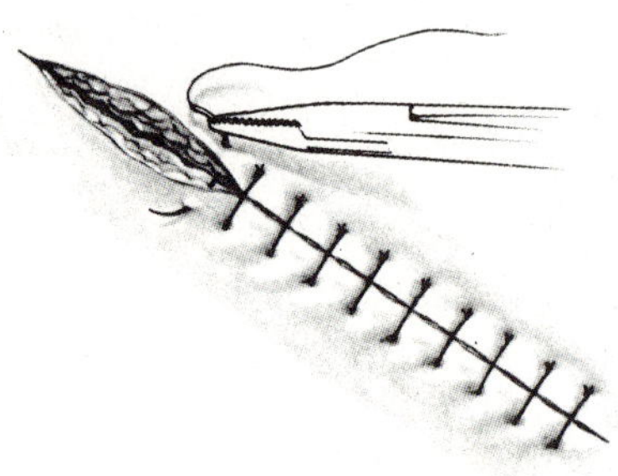

Fig. 7-9. Interrupted suture technique. (Courtesy Ethicon, Inc., Somerville, N.J.)

lationship of the wound's edges to each other. Such maneuvers cause the edges of the wound to either invert or evert; this, in turn, aids in wound healing, with fewer sutures used.

A *continuous suture* consists of a series of stitches, of which only the first and last ones are tied (Fig. 7-10). This type of suture is not widely used because a break at any point may mean a disruption of the entire suture line. It is used, however, to close a tissue layer such as the peritoneum, which does not have great strength but requires a tight closure to prevent the intestinal loops from protruding.

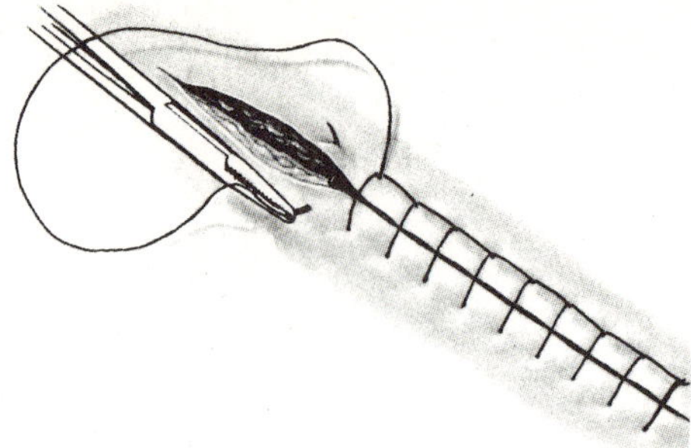

Fig. 7-10. Continuous suture technique. (Courtesy Ethicon, Inc., Somerville, N.J.)

A *purse-string suture* is a continuous suture that is placed in such a way that it surrounds an opening in a structure and causes it to close. This type of suture may be placed around the appendix before its removal or may be placed in an organ such as the cecum, gallbladder, or urinary bladder before opening it, so that a drainage tube can be inserted.

A *retention* or *stay suture* provides a secondary suture line (Fig. 7-11). These sutures, which are placed at a distance from the primary suture line, relieve undue strain and help obliterate dead space. They are placed in the wound in such a way that they include most, if not all, of the layers of the wound. A simple interrupted or figure-of-eight stitch is used. Usually heavy, nonabsorbable suture materials such as silk, nylon, polyester fiber, or wire are used to close long vertical abdominal wounds and lacerated or infected wounds. To prevent the suture from cutting into the skin surface, a small piece of rubber tubing or other type of "bumper" is passed over or through the exposed portion of the suture, or the suture is tied over a plastic bridge. The bridge device allows the surgeon to adjust tension over the wound postoperatively.

Holding a drain in place

If a drainage tube is inserted in the wound, the tube may be anchored to the skin with a nonabsorbable suture so that it will not slip in or out. If a tube is left in a hollow viscus, such as the gallbladder or common duct, it may be secured to the wall of that organ with an absorbable suture.

Knot-tying technique

The successful use of the many varieties of suture materials is, in the final analysis, dependent on the skill with which the surgeon ties the knot. The completed knot should be firm to prevent slipping and small, with ends cut short to minimize bulk of suture material in the wound. The suture may be weakened by excessive tension, sawing, friction between the strands, and inadvertent crushing with clamps or hemostats.

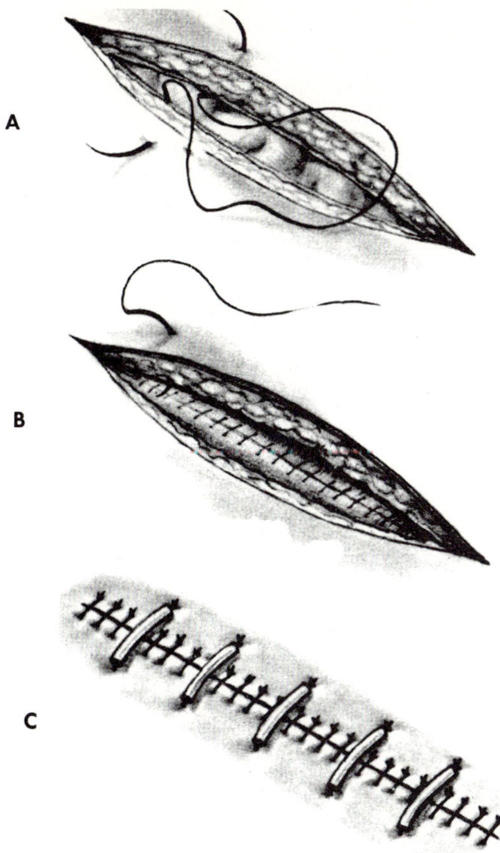

Fig. 7-11. Retention suture technique. A, Surgeons may place retention sutures from inside peritoneal cavity through to skin. B, Other surgeons prefer to close peritoneum first, then place retention sutures to penetrate only layers from fascia to skin. C, To prevent heavy materials from cutting into skin, "bolsters" or "bumpers" are used with retention sutures. (Courtesy Ethicon, Inc., Somerville, N.J.)

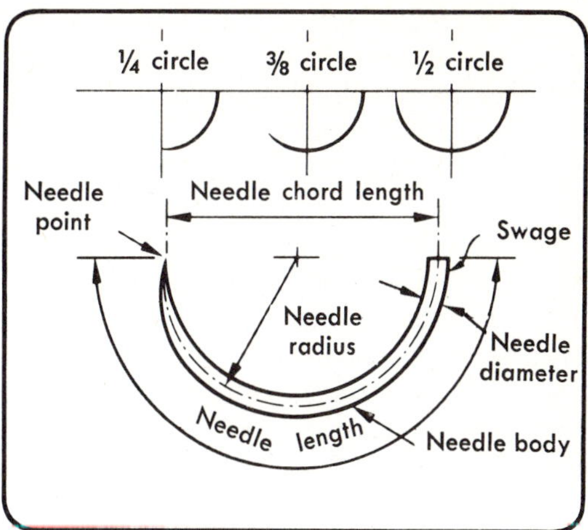

Fig. 7-12. Surgical needle differentiation by type, shape, and point. (Courtesy Ethicon, Inc., Somerville, N.J.)

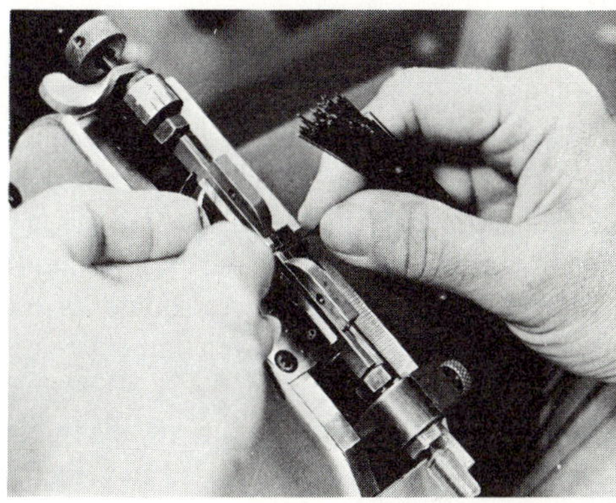

Fig. 7-13. Process of swaging needle to suture during manufacture. (Courtesy Ethicon, Inc., Somerville, N.J.)

SURGICAL NEEDLES

The surgical needles used vary considerably in shape, size, point design, and wire diameter, depending on the surgical procedure to be performed. Fig. 7-12 indicates the various types, shapes, and point designs available to the surgeon. The surgeon's selection of needle varies with the type of tissue to be sutured. Basically, cutting-edge needles are used on tough tissue (skin or eye tissues) and taper needles are used on soft tissue (bowel or subcutaneous tissues).

Surgical needles fall into three general categories: (1) eyed needles, in which the needle must be threaded with the suture strand, thus making it necessary to pull two strands of suture through the tissue; (2) spring or French eyed needles, in which the suture is forced through the spring; and (3) eyeless needles, a needle-suture combination in which a needle is swaged onto one or both ends of the suture material.

The most popular needle type is the swaged or atraumatic needle (Fig. 7-13). The surgeon draws a single strand of suture material through the tissue, thereby minimizing tissue damage, and uses a new, sharp needle with every suture strand. Swaged needles also eliminate threading eyed needles before and during surgery. Studies indicate that swaged needles provide greater safety to patients and economical use of materials and time. The swaged needle, permanently attached to the suture strand, must be cut off with scissors. A needle swaged for controlled release of the suture (semiswaged) facilitates interrupted suturing techniques. The needle remains attached until the surgeon releases it with a straight tug of the needle holder.

Surgical needles are made from either stainless steel or carbon steel. They must be strong, ductile, and able to withstand the stress imposed by tough tissue. Stainless steel is the most popular, not only because it provides these physical characteristics, but also because it is noncorrosive.

For use in certain types of delicate surgery, needles with exceptionally sharp points and cutting edges are produced. Microsurgery, ophthalmology, and plastic surgery require needles of this type; special honing wheels provide needles of precision-point quality for surgeons in these specialities.

In addition, recent developments include the application of a microthin layer of plastic to the needle surface, providing for easier penetration and a reduction in drag of the needle through the tissue.

Most operating rooms have instituted standardization programs to reduce the variety of needle-suture combinations available for different types of surgical procedures. A continuing program should be developed for keeping needle counts and for handling soiled needles. Such procedures should be described in the nursing procedure manual (Chapter 2).

SUTURING TECHNIQUES

In the preparation and use of sutures in surgery, every precaution must be taken to keep the sutures sterile, to prevent prolonged exposure and unnecessary handling, and to avoid waste. Before the nurses prepare the sutures, they should review the sutures listed in the card file for a particular procedure and surgeon. The scrub nurse should prepare only one of two sutures during the preliminary preparation, but the circulating nurse should have an adequate supply of sutures available for immediate dispensing to the sterile instrument table. Use of suture materials in dry packages provides sterile sutures ready for use, reduces length of time previously needed to prepare them, and decreases wasted motion (Fig. 7-14).

Opening primary packets

The scrub nurse tears the foil packet across the notch near the hermetically sealed edge and removes the suture. Plastic packets may be torn along designated lines or opened with suture scissors.

Handling suture materials

Surgical gut sutures should be removed from the packet immediately prior to use (Fig. 7-15).

To remove a suture that does not have a needle, the loose end is pulled out with one hand while the folder is grasped with the other hand. To straighten a long suture, the free end is grasped (using the thumb and forefinger of the free hand), and the kinks are removed by pulling gently. The free ends are secured in one hand and the center loop in the other, and then slowly the arms are abducted slightly to straighten the strands.

Kinks should never be removed by running gloved fingers over the strand, since this causes fraying. The tensile strength of a gut suture should not be tested before it is handed to the surgeon. Sudden pulls or jerks used to test the tensile strength of a suture may damage it so that it will break when in use.

To prepare individual ligatures and sutures, the strand is folded in equal parts and held between the fingers; then the strand is divided (Fig. 7-16). Sutures are also provided in 12- to 30-inch precut lengths.

In some hospitals, spiral wound sutures are used. Long sutures (surgical gut, silk, or cotton) are wound on cylindrical or circular reels supplied by suture manufacturers (Fig. 7-17). The surgeon holds the reel while ligating the bleeding vessels. This technique eliminates the need to rewind sutures on reels, saves nurses' time, and eliminates wasted motions.

To remove a suture-needle combination, the scrub nurse grasps the needle of the suture with fingertips or a needle holder and gently pulls the strand to remove and straighten it. The jaws of the needle holder are placed on the flattened surface of the needle to prevent breakage and bending (Fig. 7-18). The opening of a multiple sutures packet is shown in Fig. 7-19.

Cutting suture lengths

A suture or free ligature should not be too long or too short. A long suture is difficult to handle and increases the possibility of contamination because it may be dragged across the sterile field or fall below it. A short suture usually slips from the eye of the needle as it is being inserted and makes tying difficult.

The depth and distance to the site of tying or suturing, along with good judgment, will guide the scrub nurse in preparing ties or sutures of the correct length. In deep cavities, ties are often "mounted" on clamps to facilitate reaching the site where the use of hand, only, would be cumbersome.

For general surgery, a continuous suture is usually about 24 inches long after threading, and its short end is 3 to 4 inches long. An interrupted suture is 12 to 14 inches long, with 2 or 3 inches threaded through the needle. To ligate a vessel in the epidermal and subcutaneous layers, the ligature may be 12 to 15 inches long. However, vessels or structures deep in the wound are ligated with a suture 24 to 30 inches long.

Threading surgical needles

The scrub nurse pulls the suture about 4 inches through the eye of the needle to prevent the suture from being pulled out of the eye during suturing. A curved needle is threaded from within its curvature so that the short end falls away from the outside curvature. This helps prevent easy pullout. To keep the needle secure in the jaws of the needle holder and to prevent damage to the eye of the needle, the needle holder is placed on the flattened surface of the needle, at least ⅛ inch from its eye.

Different institutions vary in their policies regarding needle counts during operative procedures. Needles should be accounted for by the scrubbed personnel as they hand them to the surgeon on an exchange basis. Needles are counted in the operating room by the scrub nurse and the

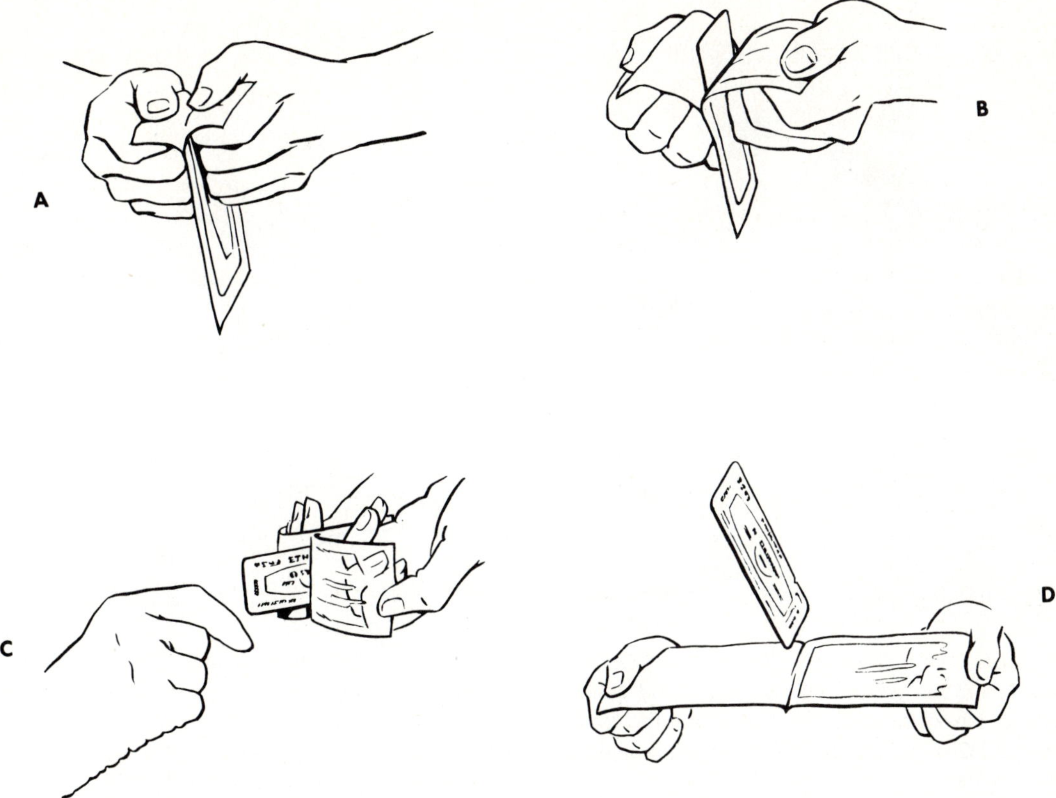

Fig. 7-14. Opening suture packet. **A,** Circulating nurse grasps two flaps between extended thumbs; **B,** rolls thumbs outward, peeling overwrap halfway down sealed edges; **C,** offers sterile inner pack to scrub nurse; **D,** or flips it onto sterile surface. (Courtesy Ethicon, Inc., Somerville, N.J.)

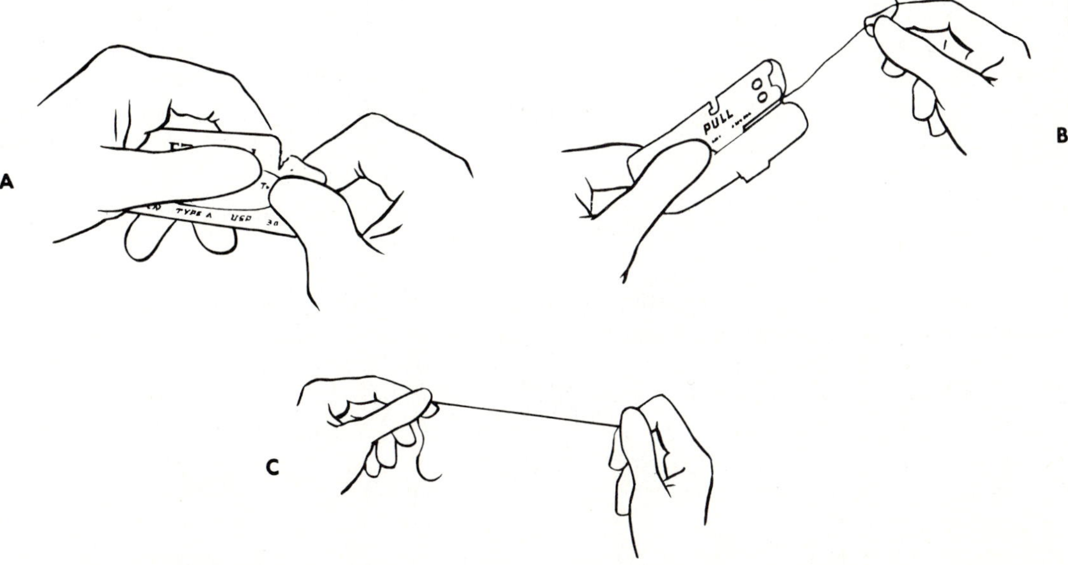

Fig. 7-15. Preparation of prepackaged individual suture. **A,** Sterile package. **B,** Suture strand is removed from package as unit. **C,** Strand is grasped at both ends. (Courtesy Ethicon, Inc., Somerville, N.J.)

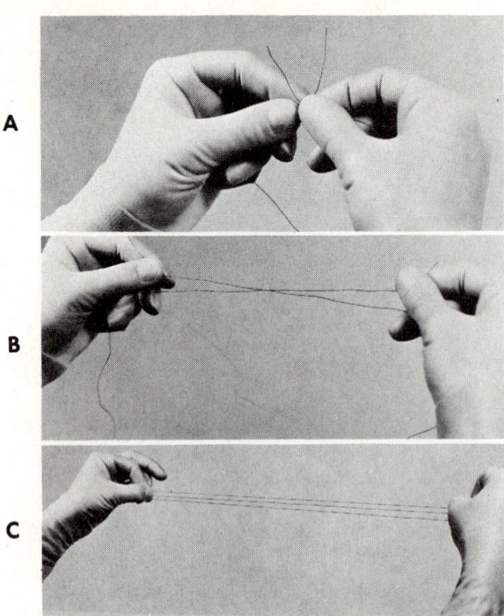

Fig. 7-16. Preparation of individual "freehand" ligatures. **A,** Free ends of ligature are grasped in each hand and gently pulled to remove kinks. **B,** Ligature is folded in equal parts of desired length. **C,** Ligatures are divided into individual strands. (Courtesy Ethicon, Inc., Somerville, N.J.)

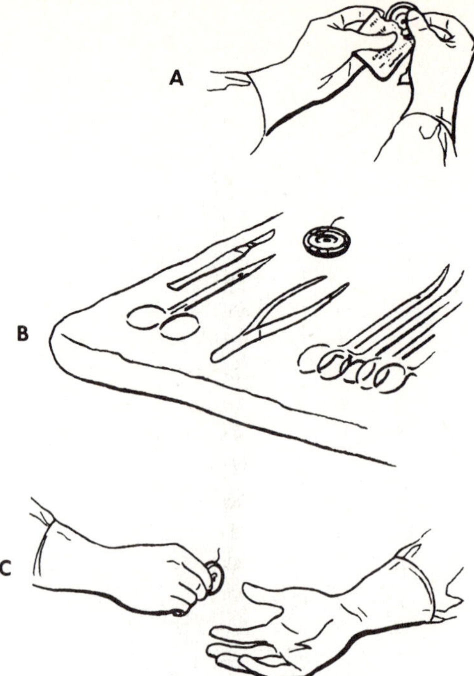

Fig. 7-17. Preparation of continuous ties on plastic disc type of reel. **A,** Foil packet containing appropriate material on reel is torn open. **B,** End of strand is extended slightly for easy grasping. Reel is placed conveniently on Mayo tray. **C,** It is passed to surgeon as needed, being certain end of ligating material is free to be grasped. (Courtesy Ethicon, Inc., Somerville, N.J.)

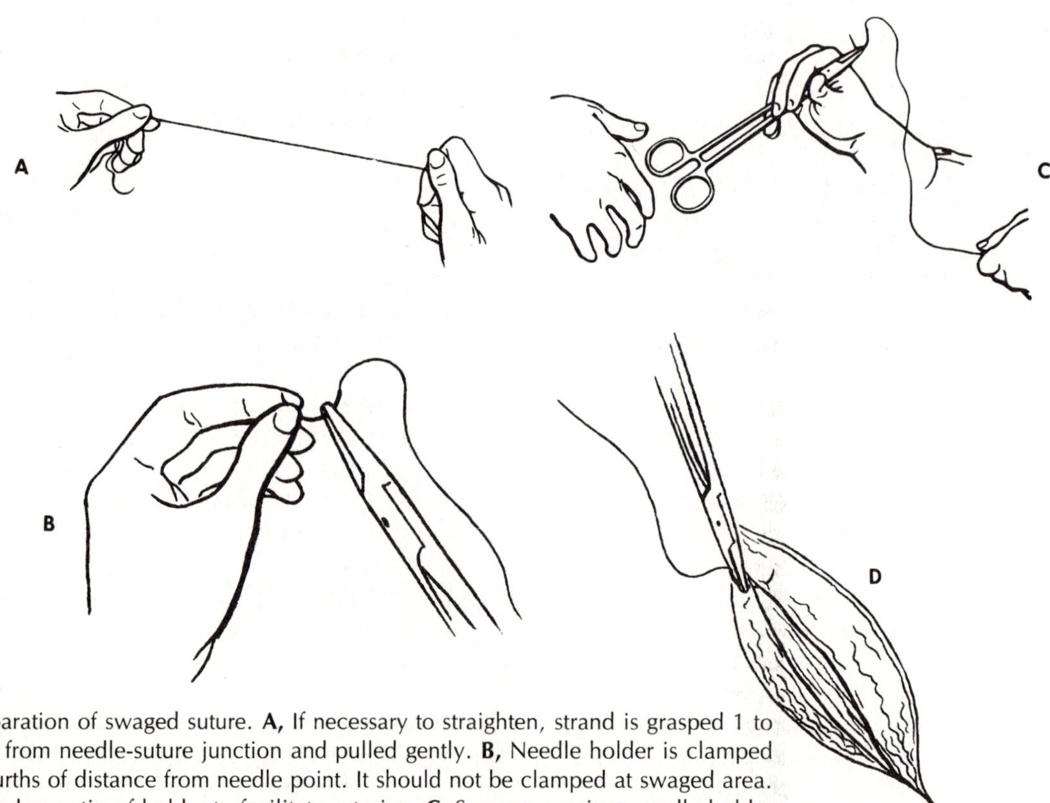

Fig. 7-18. Preparation of swaged suture. **A,** If necessary to straighten, strand is grasped 1 to 2 inches away from needle-suture junction and pulled gently. **B,** Needle holder is clamped about three fourths of distance from needle point. It should not be clamped at swaged area. Needle is placed near tip of holder to facilitate suturing. **C,** Surgeon receives needle holder with needle point toward thumb to prevent unnecessary wrist motion. Scrub nurse controls free end of suture. **D,** Surgeon begins closing with swaged needle. (Courtesy Ethicon, Inc., Somerville, N.J.)

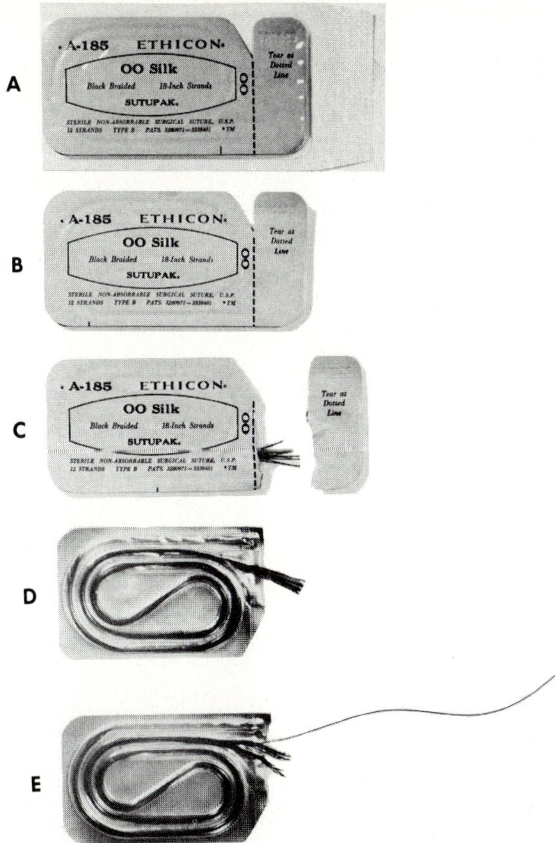

Fig. 7-19. Steps in opening multiple suture packet. **A,** Plastic packet enclosed in overwrap. **B,** Plastic packet as presented to scrub nurse. **C,** Packet torn open along dotted line. **D,** Reverse of packet showing strand packaging. **E,** Individual strand removed from packet. (Courtesy Ethicon, Inc., Somerville, N.J.)

circulating nurse before the operation, before wound closure begins, and when skin closure is started.

Used needles should be kept on a needle pad or in a container on the scrub nurse's table. Broken or missing needles must be reported to the surgeon and accounted for in their entirety.

INSTRUMENTS

The operating room nurse is responsible for use, handling, and care of hundreds of surgical instruments a day. A basic knowledge of how these instruments are manufactured and protected will help in their selection and maintenance. Surgical instruments are expensive and represent a major investment for every hospital.

Instruments used today are made predominantly in the United States, although some are also made in Germany and France. The United States does not have an agency that reviews or sets standards for surgical instruments. The quality is set by the individual manufacturer. If the instruments are inferior, they will not withstand normal usage, and the consumer will not receive full return for investment. A properly cared for instrument should last 10 years or more. A reputable company will stand behind its product.

Instruments today are manufactured from stainless steel. Stainless steel is a compound of iron, carbon, and chromium. This means that stainless steel can be of varying qualities. These qualities are designated by grading the steel into series. For example, the 400 series stainless steel has some noncorrosive characteristics and good tensile strength. It resists rust, takes a fine point, and retains a keen edge.

The raw steel is converted into instrument blanks by a machinist. These blanks, male and female halves, are then die forged into specific pieces. This process makes an impression of the piece in the stainless steel blank. The excess metal is trimmed away, and the instrument parts are ready for the final steps.

The two halves are then milled to prepare the box lock fittings, jaw serrations, and ratchets. After this is done, the halves are hand assembled. The pin is inserted through the box lock, and the jaws and shanks are properly aligned. Final grinding and hardening, accomplished by heat treating, bring the object to proper size, weight, spring temper, and balance. The final inspection tests for hardness, proper jaw closure, and smooth lock and ratchet action.

There are three types of instrument finishes. The first is the bright, highly polished mirror finish, which tends to reflect light and may restrict the vision of the surgeon. The second is the satin or dull finish, which tends to eliminate glare and lessen eye strain in the surgeon. The third finish is an ebonizing kind. This black finish is not widely used.

The last part of the process is called passivation. The instruments are put in nitric acid to remove any residue of carbon steel. Also the nitric acid produces a surface coating of chromium oxide. Chromium oxide is important because it produces in the stainless steel instrument a resistance to corrosion. Now the instrument is polished and ready for sale.

Instrument companies have brought highly skilled instrument makers to the United States, as well as bought instruments from overseas plants. There are now a limited number of 5-year apprentice programs to train instrument makers. They will design any instrument to a physician's specifications. The high cost of instruments is easily explained considering the small number of skilled artisans available and the amount of time necessary to make an instrument, as well as the cost of raw materials. Representatives of instrument companies often view surgery to observe a surgeon's needs. Manufacturers then conduct their own experiments and make suggestions that they hope will be beneficial to the surgeon.

The United States has made some contribution to the

history of instruments. The history of surgical instruments dates back to 2500 BC. These were sharpened flints and fine animal teeth. The ancient Greek, Egyptian, and Hindu instruments are amazing in their resemblance to present day instruments.

In the late 1700s, to be equipped for the practice of surgery, the surgeon had to employ various skilled artisans such as coppersmiths, steel workers, needle grinders, turners of wood, bone, and ivory, and silk and hemp spinners. The surgeon had to explain the mechanisms of the instruments and supervise their manufacture. This resulted in instruments that were crude and expensive and time consuming to make. Each artisan, using hand labor exclusively, devoted time to making only one type of instrument, thereby gaining proficiency. For example, a cutler would keep a small supply of surgical knives. Thus began the physician's supply houses and surgical instrument making in America.

In the mid-1800s, the physician's principal tools were their eyes and ears. Official records show that amputation, the trademark of the Civil War, was the result in three out of four operations. Surgeons were scarce, and medical instruments almost nonexistent. Kitchen knives and penknives, carpenter saws, and table forks did the job. After the Civil War the advent of the administration of ether and chloroform brought with it the demand for new ideas and methods in surgery and instruments. The division of general surgery into specialities took place in the late 1800s and early 1900s. Delicate instruments were seen as more useful than the force of crude and heavy instruments. So that instruments could withstand repeated sterilization, handles of wood, ivory, and rubber were discontinued.

During World War II, the development of stainless steel in Germany assured a better material for surgical instruments and other equipment. Today, surgeons have only to ask for what they need. Operating room nurses are involved in these needs through their care and sterilization of the surgical instruments.

Currently in operating rooms, it is the nursing personnel's responsibility to know the surgical instruments and their proper uses and care. Although there is no standard nomenclature for specific instruments, there are four main categories: sharps, clamps, holding instruments, and retractors.

Sharps, which include scissors and scalpels, are instruments with sharp or cutting edges as the usable parts.

Scalpels are probably the oldest of all surgical instruments (Fig. 7-20). Their purpose is to incise and dissect tissues. Most scalpels today are handles with one end suited to attaching disposable blades. During an operation, the blades may be conveniently changed by the scrub nurse as often as necessary. The blades come prepackaged and sterile and are passed onto the sterile field, as needed, by the circulating nurse. Careful disposal of blades at the end of a procedure is important so that no member of the operating room team, including housekeeping and central supply, is cut by a misplaced blade.

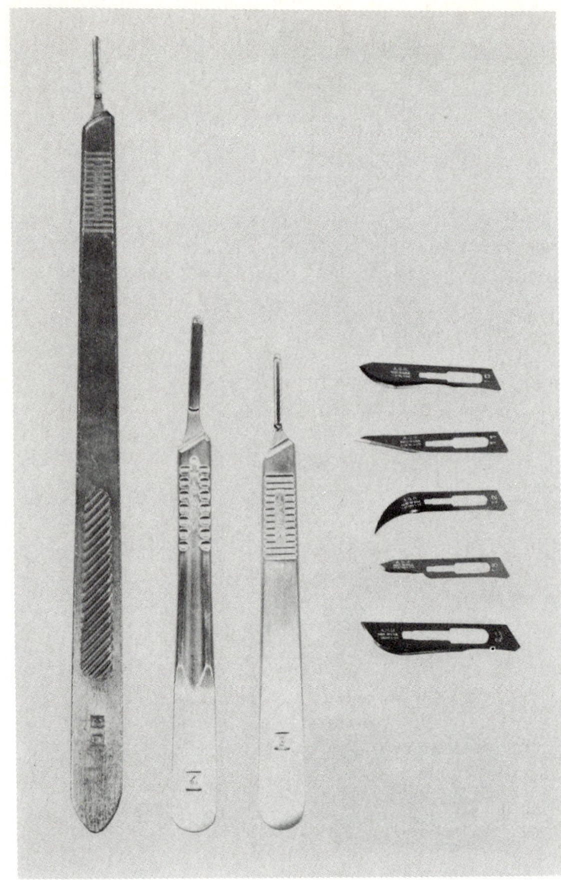

Fig. 7-20. Long and regular-length knife handles with assortment of blades. Blades, *top to bottom,* nos. 10, 11, 12, 15, and 20.

Scissors are designed in short, long, small, and large sizes and in various shapes for different purposes in cutting body tissues and surgical materials (Fig. 7-21). The basic design consists of two blades, each having a chisel-shaped edge, with the bevel consistent with the structure it has to cut. Scissors tips may be blunt or sharp, and the blades straight or curved. Conventional scissors require two movements to use—one to open and another to close the jaws. Other scissors may have a spring action in the body design that holds the jaws in an open position. A single movement pressing the spring together closes the jaws to cut. Scissors designed for delicate plastic and eye surgery are often of the latter type. A basic setup includes a Mayo scissors for dissection of heavy tissues, a Metzenbaum scissors for dissection of delicate tissues, and straight scissors for cutting the suture. For surgery in deep areas of the body, a scissors with long handles and short blades would be used for better control and easier use.

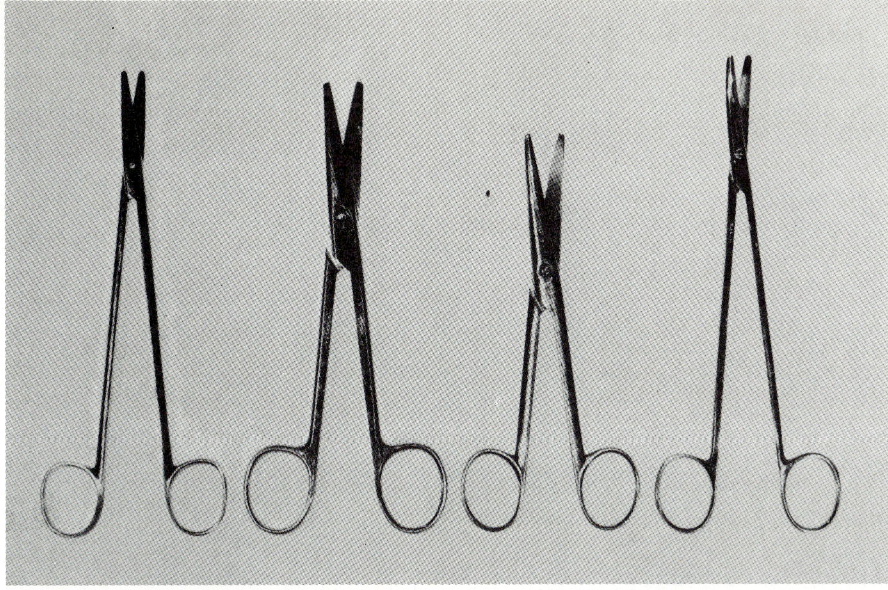

Fig. 7-21. Various regularly used scissors. *Left to right,* Straight, blunt dissecting scissors; heavy or suture scissors; Mayo scissors; Metzenbaum scissors.

Clamps are generally used as a method of hemostasis (Fig. 7-22). These are the instruments that make surgery possible by preventing excessive or fatal blood loss in the course of dissection. The well-designed modern instrument is styled for the lightness, balance, and security that yield maximum efficiency in closing the severed ends of each vessel with a minimum of tissue damage. The grasping ends have deep transverse cuts so that bleeding vessels may be compressed with sufficient force to stop the bleeding from smaller vessels if left for a couple of minutes. The serrations must be cleanly cut and perfectly meshed to prevent the clamps from slipping from the tissue to be held. Special jaws, having finely meshed, multiple rows of longitudinally arranged teeth, are made for vascular clamps to prevent leakage and to minimize trauma to the vessel walls when the severed vessels are anastomosed. The surgical service usually selects a hemostat or clamp design, according to surgeons' preferences.

The apposition of the clamp tips is necessary to its purpose and must be periodically checked. When the instrument is held up to the light and the handles are fully closed, no light should be visible between the jaws. These instruments, if used for purposes other than that for which they are intended, will be useless and need to be repaired.

There are three kinds of joints in instruments that are made up of two halves. The screw joint is the most popular. The two halves are only connected by a screw or pin. The joint must be checked and tightened periodically because the screw will work itself loose. Screw joint instruments are easy to make and comparatively inexpensive.

The second kind is the box lock joint instrument. One arm passes through a slot in the other arm. This is needed where accurate approximation of the tips is necessary, as in vascular forceps.

The final and less popular type is the semibox or aseptic joint. It has the advantage that the two halves can be separated for easy cleaning.

These joints must be cleaned regularly, and any dirt or rust collecting at the site must be removed to ensure proper functioning.

The *grasping* or *holding* instruments are used for tissue retraction or suturing. They must have a firm grip while inflicting a minimum of trauma to the tissues they hold. The most common kinds are the various simple two-armed spring forceps (Fig. 7-23). They vary in length and thickness and are available with teeth and without teeth. Nontoothed forceps create minimal damage and hold delicate, thin tissues. Toothed forceps are for holding thick or slippery tissues, where extra grip is needed.

Other holding forceps have handles like clamps with specialized tips or jaws (Fig. 7-24). These jaws may be triangular, straight, angular, or T shaped. The Allis forceps has multiple teeth that do not crush or damage tissue in its grasp. The Babcock forceps has curved, fenestrated blades with no teeth, and it grips or encloses delicate structures such as a ureter or fallopian tube. Sponge-holding forceps with ring-shaped jaws are available in 7- and 9-inch lengths. These can be used to handle tissue but are usually used as sponge holders. A gauze sponge is folded and placed in the jaws and is then used to retract tissue or to absorb blood in the field.

Needle holders are frequently used and are put through

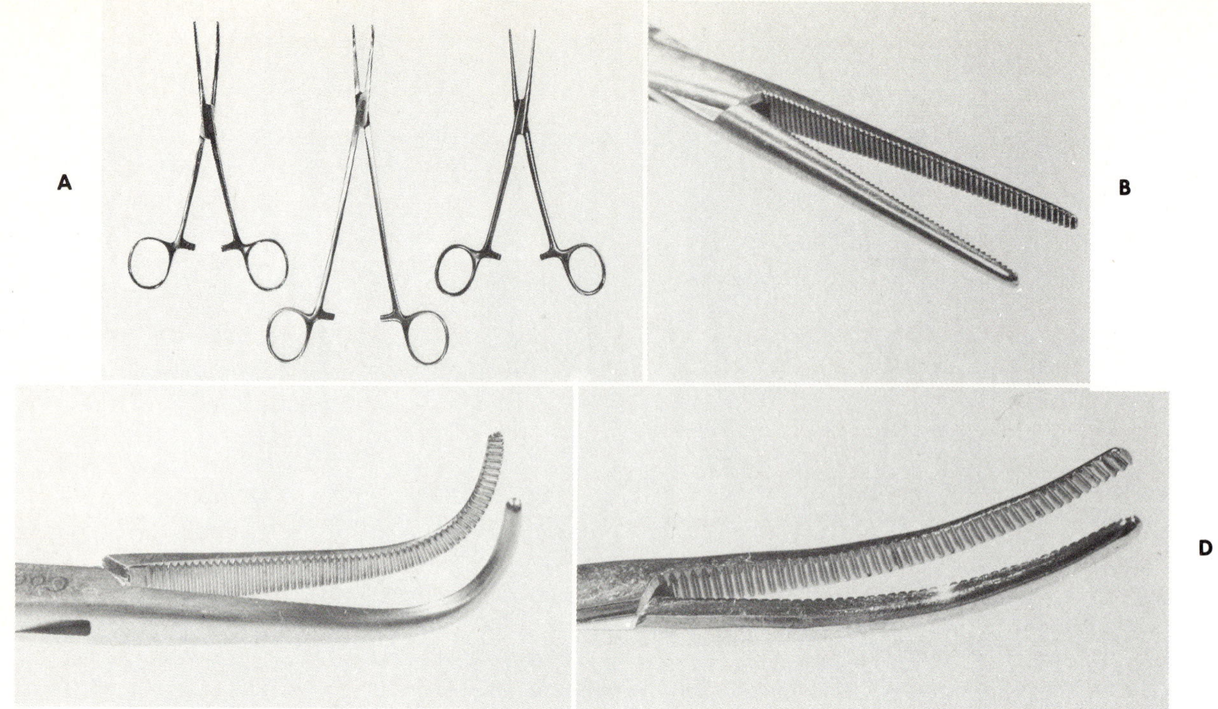

Fig. 7-22. A, Hemostatic clamps often used. **B,** Straight Kelly. **C,** Right-angle. **D,** Curved Kelly.

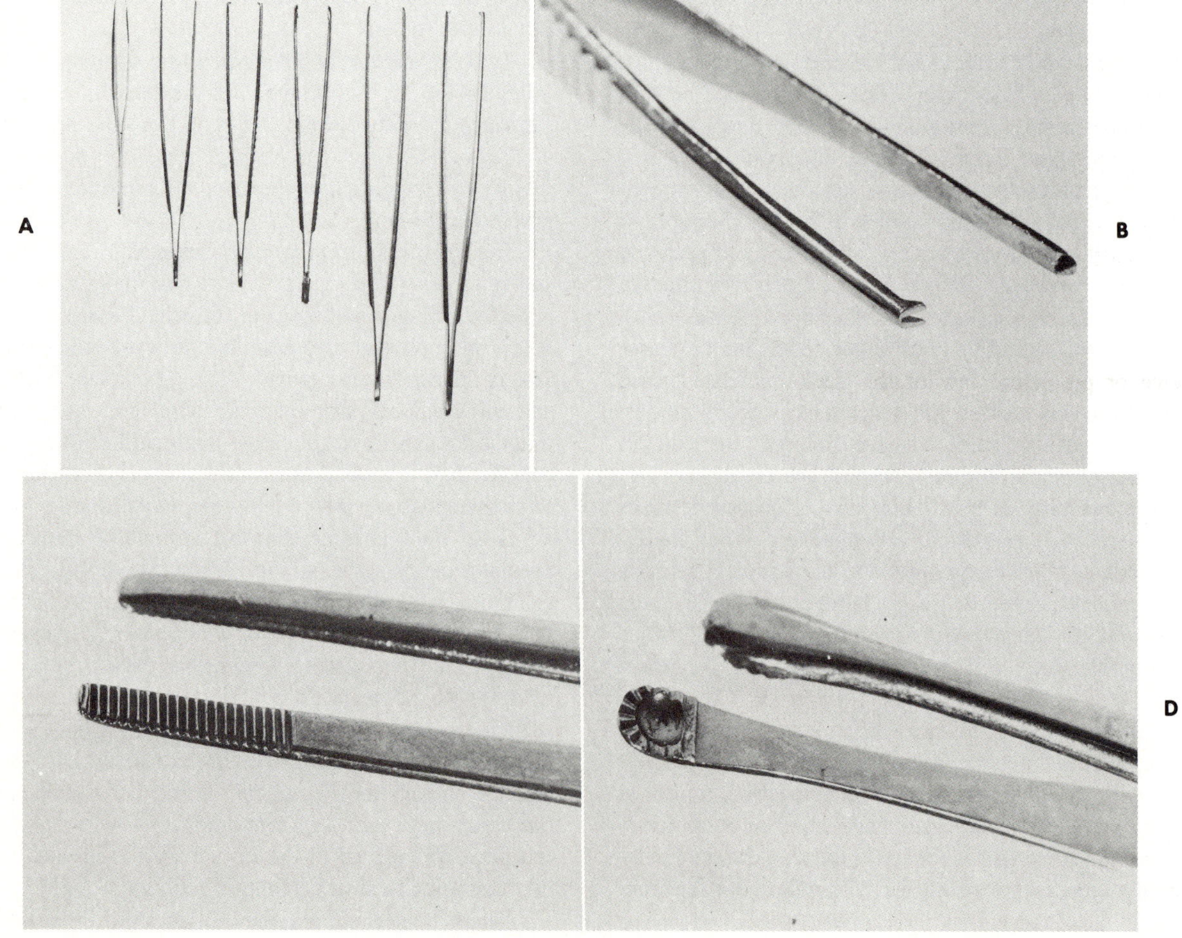

Fig. 7-23. A, Various forceps or pickups from those with very fine tips to heavy tips. **B,** Tips with teeth. **C,** Smooth tip. **D,** Tips of Russian forceps.

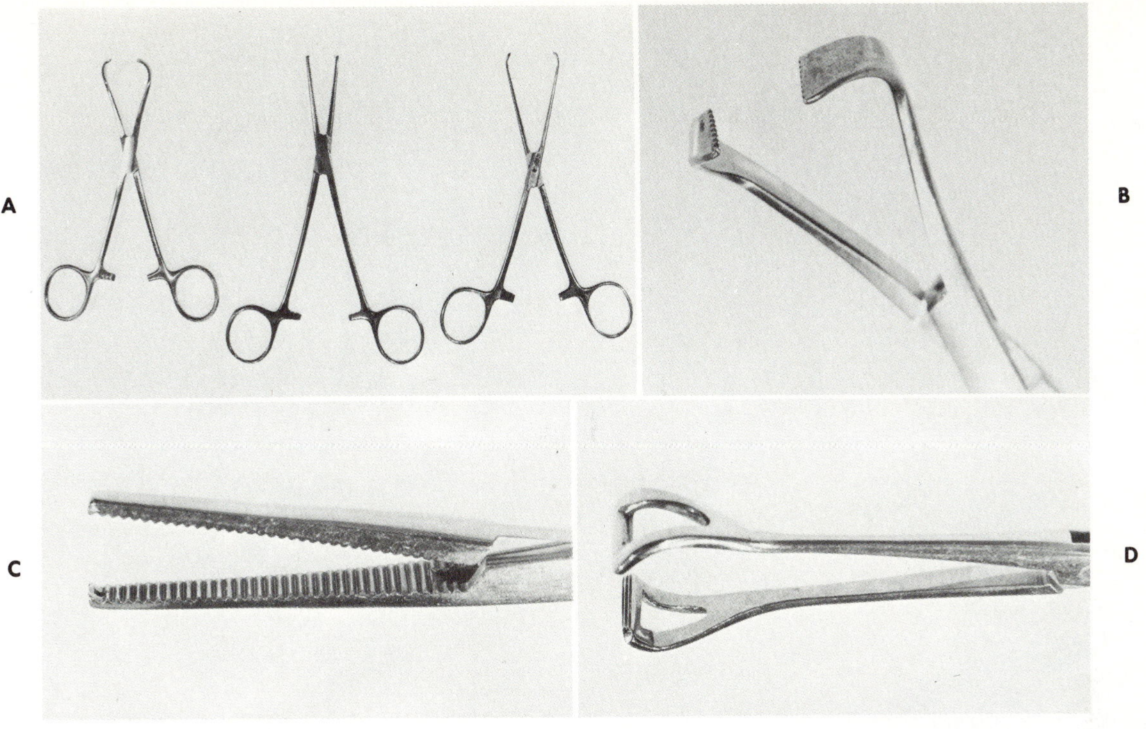

Fig. 7-24. A, Holding forceps with special jaws. **B,** Allis. **C,** Kocher or Ochsner. **D,** Babcock.

many different motions, even in a routine surgical operation. Since they must grasp metal rather than soft tissues, they are subject to greater damage. As a result, a fair number must be replaced regularly (Fig. 7-25).

To be of service, needle holders must retain a firm grip on the needle. Many types of jaws have been designed to meet this need, but all eventually become worn down and damaged beyond repair. The so-called diamond jaw needle holder has a tungsten carbide insert designed to prevent rotation of the needle. A longitudinal groove or pit in the jaw of the needle holder releases tension, prevents flattening of the needle, and holds the needle firmly in needle holders of standard design. Needle holders may work by a ratchet similar to that in a hemostat, or they may be of a spring action and lock type.

Towel clamps may be included here. There are two basic types. The first is a nonpiercing towel clamp used for holding in place barrier draping materials. The other type has sharp tips used to penetrate drapes and tissues but is damaging to both. The use of sharp towel clamps to penetrate drapes is highly discouraged.

Retractors determine the exposure of the operative field. A surgeon needs the best exposure possible while inflicting a minimum of trauma to the surrounding tissue. Retractors are either self-retaining (Fig. 7-26) or held in place by a member of the operative team. With the latter, the handles may be notched, hook shaped, or ring shaped to give the holder a firm grip without tiring (Fig. 7-27). The blade is usually at a right angle to the shaft and may be a smooth blade, rake, or hook. A malleable (ribbon) retractor is one which may be shaped by the surgeon at the field, with the original shape being a flat ribbon.

There are two types of self-retaining retractors: those with frames to which various blades may be attached and those with two blades held apart with a ratchet. An example of the latter is a Weitlaner retractor.

There are many miscellaneous instruments (Fig. 7-28) or specialty items particular to a certain service, such as mallets and screwdrivers in orthopedics. Microinstruments are extra fine for vascular and nerve repair. These are extremely delicate and should be handled separately from the other instruments. Power equipment driven by electric motors, nitrogen, or other means is discussed in Chapter 20.

When nursing team members can analyze the planned procedure and approach and are able to identify each instrument with its specific function, they can select instrument sets without omitting necessary items and without including items that will not be used. This intelligent, comprehending approach ensures economy of time and effort and protects instruments from abuse and unnecessary handling. During the operation, the informed nurse becomes a more valuable member of the surgical team.

Designated operating room or hospital supply personnel arrange the various instrument trays or sets. The trays

A

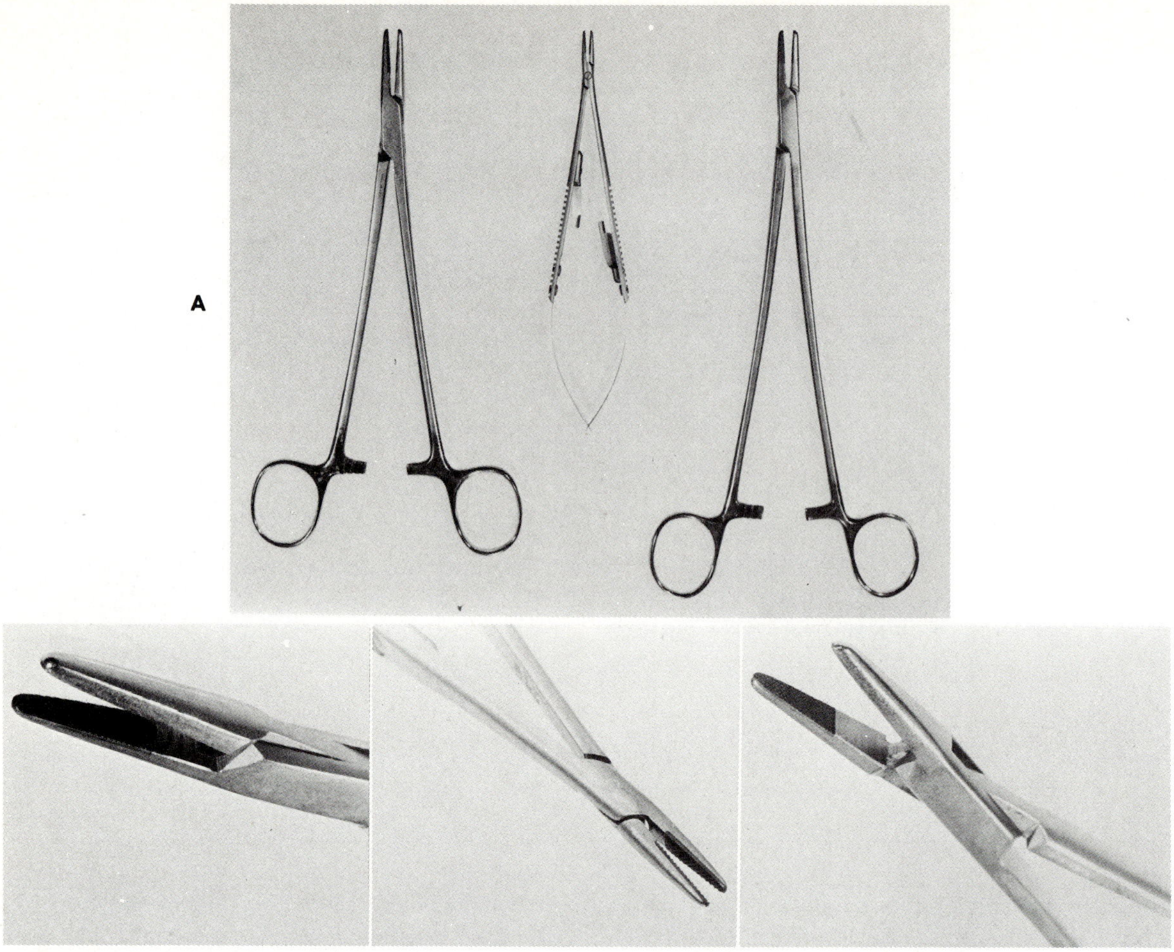

B C D

Fig. 7-25. A, Needle holders. **B,** Heavy. **C,** Fine. **D,** Regular.

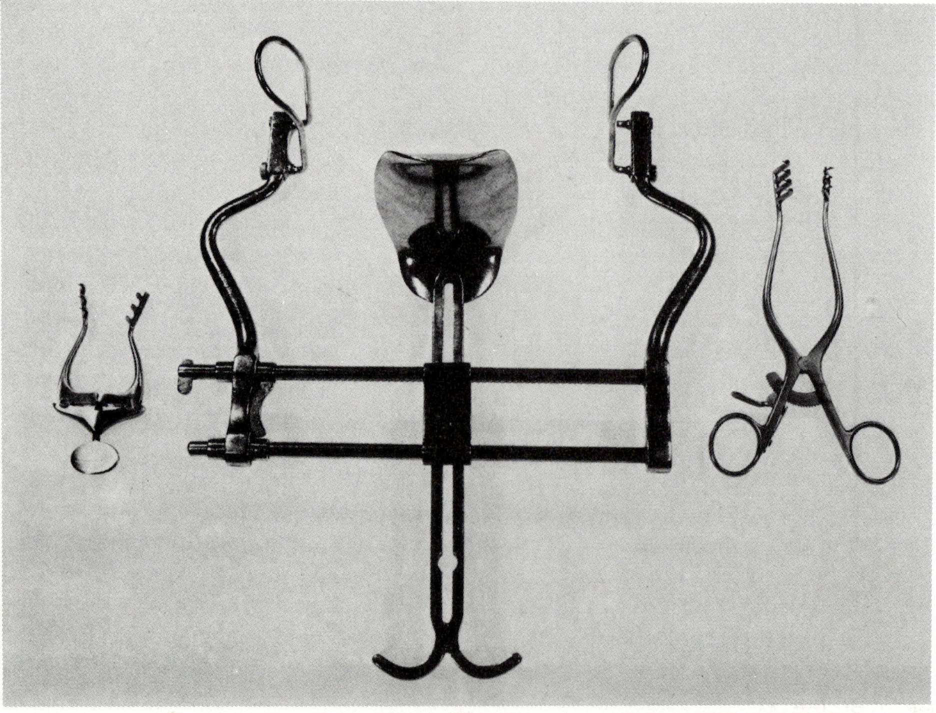

Fig. 7-26. Self-retaining retractors. *Left to right,* Mastoid, Balfour, and Weitlaner.

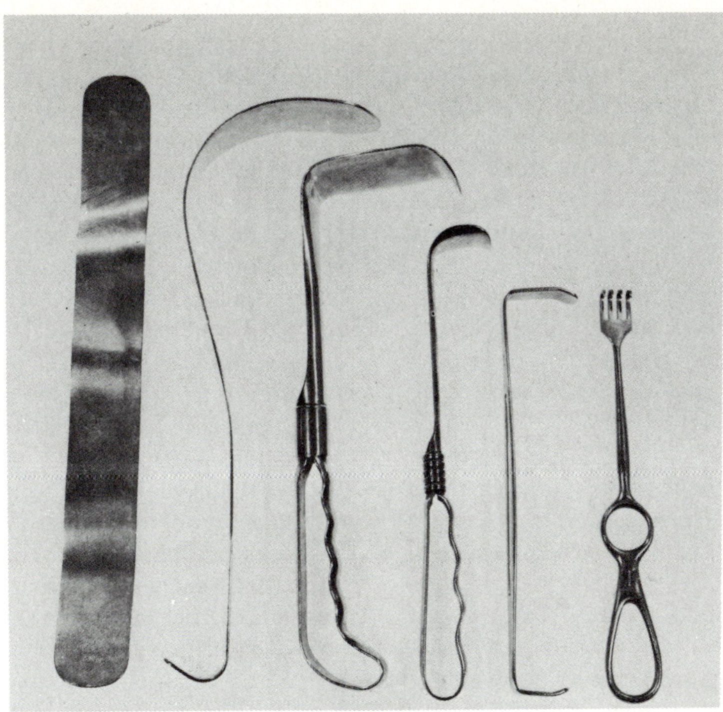

Fig. 7-27. Hand-held retractors. *Left to right,* Ribbon, or malleable; Deaver; two sizes of Richardsons; Army-Navy, or USA; and rake.

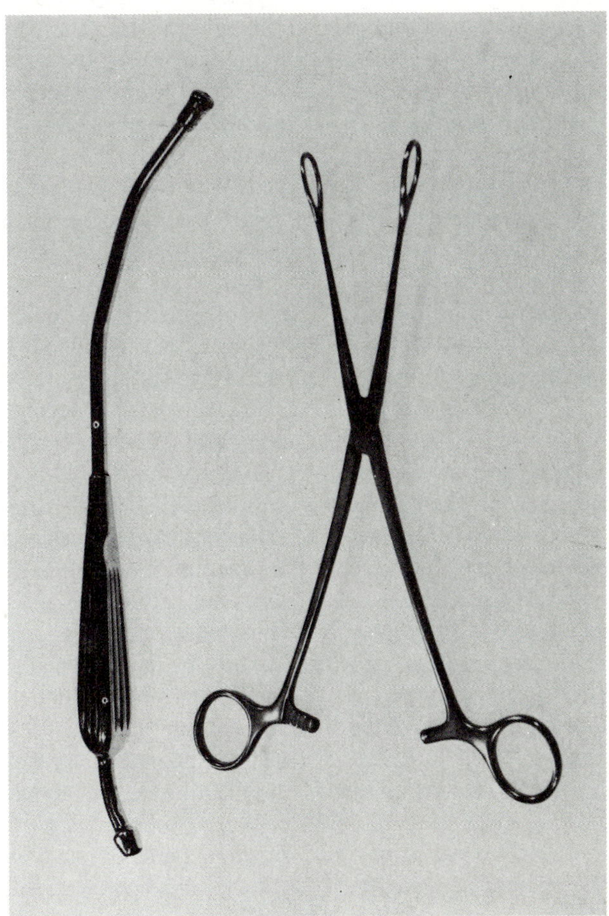

Fig. 7-28. *Left,* Metal suction tip to be attached to tubing; *right,* ring forceps used to hold sponges.

are named according to their functions. For example, a local (or plastic) set would include instruments needed for a simple superficial incision, excision, and suturing. A basic laparotomy set includes instruments to open and close the abdominal cavity and repair any gross defects in the major body musculature. An example of three *basic* operating room instrument sets would be major, minor, and plastic.

According to each patient's needs, more individualized instruments may be added, such as an intestinal set or a vascular set. In the same way, basic instrument sets may be selected for opening other cavities, such as the skull, chest, and pelvis.

Instruments are selected according to the size of the patient's body structures and the nature of the organs involved. Proper selection requires general understanding of surgical procedures and approaches and knowledge of anatomy, possible pathological conditions, and the design and purpose of instruments.

For example, the nurse needs to know that instruments for cutting and penetrating bones differ from those designed to cut soft tissues. Instruments designed for surgery on infants and for surgery of the eye, ear, blood vessels, nerves, brain, and facial structures are smaller, finer, and more delicate than those designed to handle thick, fibrous tissues such as cartilage and bone.

This knowledge is reinforced with the orientation of new personnel to the operating room. New personnel learn basic technique first in general surgery and then proceed to the speciality services where different instruments and devices are added but with the same basic principles.

In most operating rooms the instruments are set up on Mayo stands and back tables in a planned, standardized, organized, and functional manner to maintain continuity when the original scrub nurse is replaced by another. The teaching manual should have illustrations or diagrams to which all personnel may refer. Each item used by the scrub nurse should have its own position on the table to prevent the mass clutter that would occur if instruments and supplies were placed randomly.

A proficient and experienced scrub nurse must know the instrument inventory of the department, the routine instruments needed for each type of operation, the individual surgeon's preferences, and the correct use and handling, the method of preparation, and the aftercare of the instruments. A file of preference cards may be kept listing the procedures each physician performs, the physician's glove size, the preferred preparation solution, specific draping instructions, and instruments that will be desired for use during the procedure.

Before an operative procedure, the scrub nurse may assist the circulating nurse in gathering the needed supplies, equipment, and sutures. The scrub nurse scrubs, dons gown and gloves (Chapter 5), and begins to set up the sterile tables with drapes, instruments, supplies, and sutures. A Mayo stand is set up for use at the immediate operative site. Once the patient is on the operating table and is draped, the stand is brought across the patient. One or two back tables are also set up according to the number of instruments and supplies.

Instruments are arranged with those most frequently used on the Mayo stand (Fig. 7-29). The scrub nurse prepares the sutures and ligatures and places the knife blades on the handles. Other supplies needed are suction tubing and tips, cautery cord and tip, drains, basins, gowns, gloves, drapes, sponges, and needles. These are all sterile, given to the scrub nurse by the circulating nurse, and set up on a back table according to standardized hospital policy (Fig. 7-30).

The scrub nurse must be attentive to the operative field to anticipate the surgeon's needs. Instruments should be passed in a positive and decisive manner, with each instrument being slapped firmly into the surgeon's palm in such a manner that it is ready for immediate use with no wasted motion. For example, when a needle holder with a needle is passed to the surgeon, the needle should be pointing in the direction of the surgeon's thumb; there should be no need for readjustment. Because of this, it is important to know if a surgeon is left- or right-handed.

Often a surgeon will signal with hand motions for the type of instrument desired. This eliminates unnecessary talking and helps the scrub nurse pass the instruments more quickly.

Some institutions have now made instrument counts a standard practice. If done, they should be carried out by the circulating and scrub nurses before the procedure and again before wound closure begins. Instruments that break or are disassembled during surgery, like needles or certain retractors, must be accounted for in their entirety.

An instrument should be used only for the purpose for which it is designed. Proper use and reasonable care prolong its life and protect its quality. Scissors and clamps, which are most frequently abused, can be forced out of alignment, cracked, or broken when used improperly. Tissue scissors should not be used to cut suture or gauze dressings. Hemostatic clamps should not be used as towel clamps or to clamp suction tubing.

Instruments must be handled gently. Bouncing, dropping, and setting heavy equipment on top of them should be avoided. At the end of a procedure, the instruments should not be thrown together in a tangled heap. They should be handled individually or in small groups. Sharps and delicate instruments should be set aside for individual handling and cleaning.

Each instrument should be inspected before and after each use to detect imperfections. An instrument should function perfectly to prevent needlessly endangering a patient's life and increasing operative time because of the failure of an instrument. Before surgical use, instruments

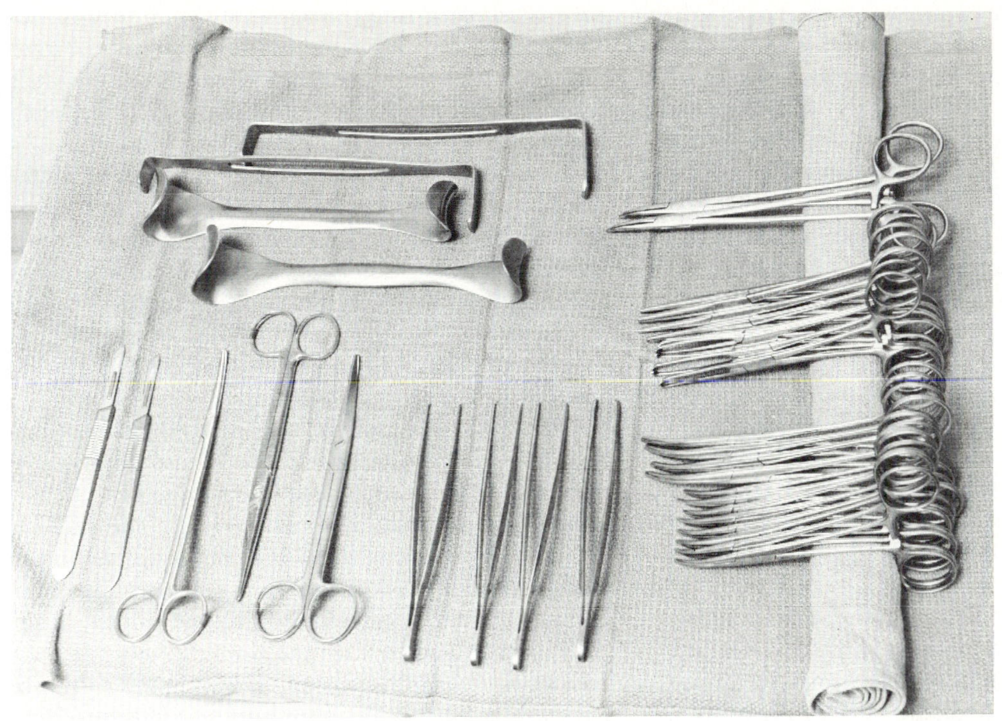

Fig. 7-29. Mayo stand setup.

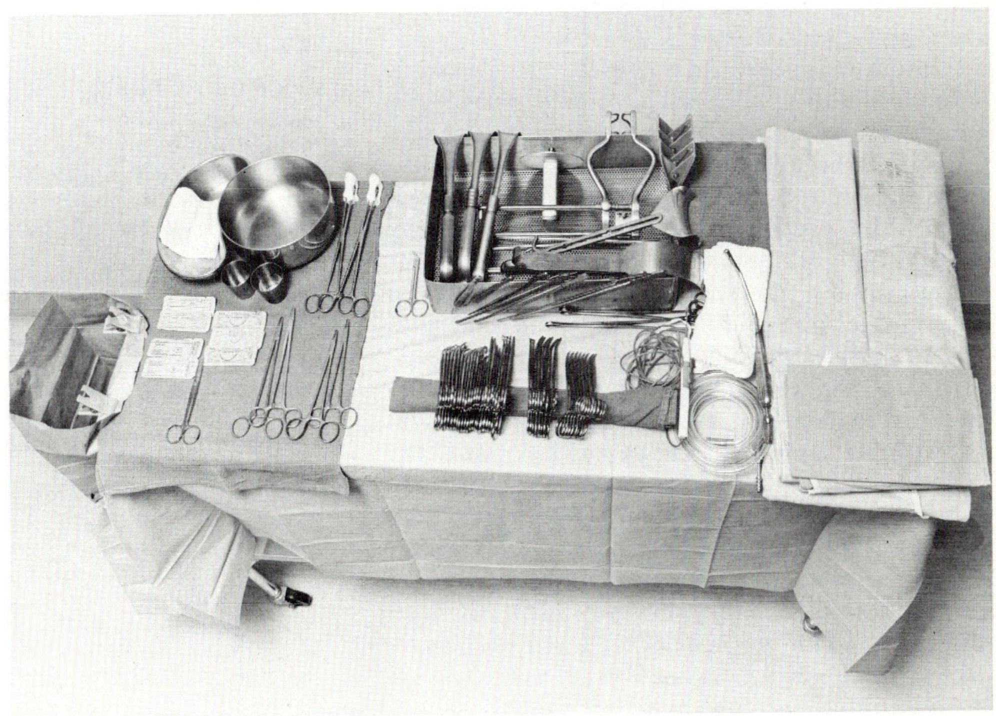

Fig. 7-30. Back table setup.

must be completely clean to ensure effective sterilization.

Forceps, clamps, and other hinged instruments must be inspected for alignment of jaws and teeth and for stiffness. Ratchets should hold firmly yet release easily when necessary. The tips of jaws and teeth should meet perfectly, and joints should work smoothly. The serrations on the ends of forceps must be perfectly fitted so that blood flow may be occluded but so as not to injure or cut the vein or artery.

The edges of scissors should be tested for sharpness. To cut, they must be beveled smoothly. All instruments should be checked for worn spots, chipping, dents, cracks, or sharp edges.

Cleaning should begin immediately after use to prevent blood and other substances from drying in the crevices or on the surfaces. The scrub nurse usually has a sterile basin to place the soiled instruments in after use or may wipe them clean with a damp sponge. The solution in the basin should be sterile, distilled water—never saline solution. The sodium chloride in saline solution is very corrosive.

There are two ways to clean instruments: manually and mechanically. Manual cleaning is difficult and time consuming. The instrument components must be cleaned thoroughly with a soft brush. Ideally, distilled water should be used for washing and rinsing. Different cities have varying qualities of tap water. Hard water will have many minerals and other corrosive particles. Soft water contains too much salt. Spotted or corroding instruments may be the result of either of these.

The pH of the detergent used is also very important. It should be as close to neutral as possible and no higher than 8. Too high a pH will be corrosive and promote stress. Household cleaners should not be used. The detergent used should meet all local, state, and federal regulations. The detergent should be a good wetting agent, low sudsing, and free rinsing, which means there is no detergent residue. The strength of a solution is increased when heated; therefore thorough rinsing with hot water is essential. Hot water also helps speed the drying time.

The washer-sterilizer is used by some institutions to wash and sterilize instruments after a procedure. Instruments should be arranged with the box locks open. The first cycle of the washer-sterilizer floods the chamber with cold detergent solution to dissolve blood and protein. This soil leaves by the overflow at the top of the chamber. The second cycle sends steam and air into the chamber to create a turbulence. This turbulence loosens and cleans the finer soil from the instruments, which will remove 60% of the soil from the instruments. Complete removal depends on the pH of the water, the efficiency of the detergent, the type of instrument, and the time of exposure. Steam then enters through the top of the chamber, forcing the water out through the bottom drain. Steam under pressure floods the chamber to achieve the sterilization phase. Ultrasonic cleaning, which is frequently used, is discussed further in Chapter 5.

Good cleaning is the only answer to proper instrument care. To temporarily ease stiffness, a water-soluble lubricant is recommended. Oil-based lubricants form a bacterial protecting film that is difficult and time consuming to remove. Also this film is not penetrated by steam during the sterilization process in sufficient quantity to be microbicidal. It is wise to periodically soak fine and delicate instruments in instrument milk.

Abrasive agents such as steel wool should never be used because the protective film of the instrument will be scratched or scoured off, predisposing it to rust.

Instruments should be stored safely. The use of locked cabinets or cupboards located in designated areas prevents theft and indiscriminate use. Cabinet shelving and hooks of cabinets should be adjustable and properly spaced for storage of various sizes and types of instruments. Attached labels and diagrams in cabinets assist personnel. An inventory should be taken at periodic intervals. Damaged instruments should be set aside and sent for repair or replacement. An instrument repair service should be selected carefully and used effectively for regular maintenance, such as sharpening and realignment of instruments.

SUGGESTED READINGS

Anderson, R.M., and Romfh, R.F.: Technique in the use of surgical tools, New York, 1980, Appleton-Century-Crofts.

Brooks, S.M.: Instrumentation for the operating room, ed. 2, St. Louis, 1983, The C.V. Mosby Co.

The care and handling of surgical instruments, Randolph, Mass., 1981, Codman & Shurtleff, Inc.

Crawford, M.L.: Surgical instruments in America, AORN J. **24:**150, 1976.

McElmurry, M., and Byrd, D.: Surgical instruments: manufacture and proper care, AORN J. **19:**1074, 1974.

Seawalt, S.: Eight steps to implementing a count system, AORN J. **28:**1098, 1978.

Standards for sponge, needle, and instrument procedures, AORN J. **23:**971, 1976.

Stapling techniques, general surgery, ed. 2, Norwalk, Conn., 1980, United States Surgical Corp.

Stroumtsos, O.: Perspectives on sutures, Pearl River, N.Y., 1978, Davis & Geck, American Cyanamid Co.

Suture use manual: use and handling of sutures and needles, Somerville, N.J., 1977, Ethicon, Inc.

Van Way, C.W., III, and Buerk, C.A.: Surgical skills in patient care, St. Louis, 1978, The C.V. Mosby Co.

8 Wound healing, dressings, and drains

WOUND HEALING

One of the most fundamental and marvelous defensive properties of living organisms is the power to heal wounds. This process is infallible in the absence of endogenous and exogenous infections, mechanical interferences, or certain disease processes. Apposition and maintenance of the edges of a cleanly incised wound almost always result in prompt healing.

The reaction of tissues to a surgical incision differs only in degree from that caused by a laceration (usually occurring in accidents). Bacteria on the skin are always carried into deeper tissues, even when the wound is a surgical incision.

Clean wound healing is an intricate, exact biological process that takes place in the following way. First, an exudate containing blood, lymph, and fibrin begins clotting and loosely binds the cut edges together. Blood supply to the area is increased, and the basic process of inflammation is set in motion. Leukocytes increase in number to fight bacteria in the wound area and by phagocytosis help remove damaged tissues. The incised tissue is quickly glued together by strands of fibrin and a thin layer of clotted blood, forming a scab. Plasma seeps to the surface, forming a dry protective crust. This seal prevents fluid loss and bacterial invasion. During the first few days of wound healing, however, there is little tensile strength.

After 3 to 4 days, connective tissue cells (fibroblasts) rapidly proliferate and give strength to the wound. At the same time, small blood vessels regenerate and build new blood channels. Granulation tissue (fibrous connective tissue) includes blood vessels and lymphatics that proliferate from the base of the wound. When wounds heal by primary union, granulation tissue is not visible.

As wound healing progresses, fibroblasts and capillaries greatly diminish in number. The resulting scar is composed chiefly of collagen connective tissue capped with epithelium. These rapidly growing and multiplying epithelial cells begin restoring the epithelial continuity of the skin. By the ninth or tenth day, the wound is moderately well healed and then becomes progressively stronger.

At this stage, the wound appears healed; however, healing is not complete until the granulation tissue organizes into scar tissue (the white protein called collagen). The whole process of repair takes 2 weeks or more, depending on factors such as physical condition of the patient, size and location of the wound, and stresses put on the incisional area. During this time, the scar (cicatrix) strengthens as the connective tissue shrinks.

The various types of wound healing are illustrated in Fig. 8-1.

Under favorable conditions primary union, or *healing by first intention,* takes place. This occurs in wounds made aseptically, with a minimum of tissue destruction and tissue reaction during the healing process. In first intention healing, there are no postoperative complications such as dehiscence, infection, excessive discharge or swelling, or abnormal scar formation.

Healing by first intention takes place under the following conditions:

1. Edges of an incised wound in a healthy person are promptly and accurately approximated.
2. Contamination is held to a minimum by impeccable aseptic technique.
3. Trauma to the wound is minimal.
4. After suturing, no dead space is left to become a potential site of infection.

Healing by granulation, or *healing by second intention,* involves the same fundamental repair process but involves a wound that is infected or one in which there is excessive loss of tissue and the skin edges cannot be adequately approximated. Generally, there is suppuration (pus formation), an abscess, or necrosis.

This type of wound is usually left open and allowed to heal from the inside toward the outer surface. In infected wounds, this process allows the proper cleansing and dressing of the wound as healthy tissue builds up from the inside. The gap gradually fills with granulation tissue (fiber cells and capillaries) that fills the area of the destroyed tissue.

Scar tissue is extensive because of the size of the tissue gap that must be closed. Contraction of surrounding tissue also takes place. Naturally, then, this healing process takes longer than first intention healing.

Healing by third intention implies that suturing is delayed for the purpose of walling off an area of gross infection, involving much tissue removal. An example is

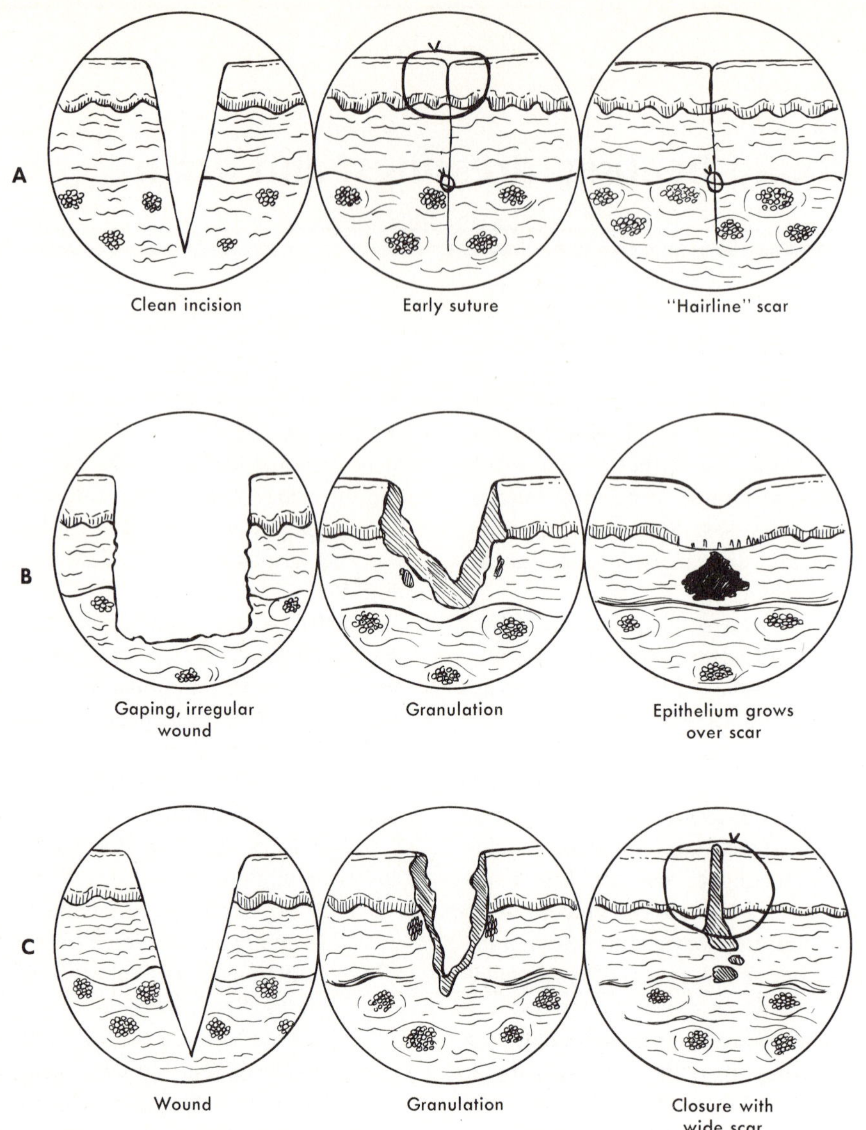

Fig. 8-1. Types of wound healing. **A,** First intention, primary union. **B,** Second intention, granulation. **C,** Third intention, secondary suture. (From Hardy, J.D., editor: Rhoads textbook of surgery: principles and practice, ed. 5, Philadelphia, 1977, J.B. Lippincott, p. 190.)

debridement of a third degree burn where actual suturing is done later, when conditions are more favorable for adequate healing.

Third intention healing means that two opposing granulation surfaces are brought together. Granulation tissue usually forms a wide fibrous scar.

Factors influencing wound healing

The patient's nutritional status, as well as overall recuperative power, is of utmost importance in tissue repair and healing. Especially significant is an adequate supply of protein, which is necessary for the growth of new tissues; the regulation of the osmotic pressure of blood and other body fluids; and the formation of prothrombin, enzymes, hormones, and antibodies. Also important is vitamin C, which aids connective tissue production and a strong scar formation.

Healthy tissues are able to tolerate and counteract a certain amount of contamination, but devitalized tissues have little resistive power. Large numbers or very virulent microorganisms can, however, overpower the body defenses of even a healthy person and interfere with wound healing. Therefore it is imperative that scrupulous aseptic technique be used to prevent any wound infection—the most common cause of delayed wound healing.

Many theories abound as to the genesis of wound infection. Cross-contamination from operating room, recovery room, and unit personnel is believed to be a pri-

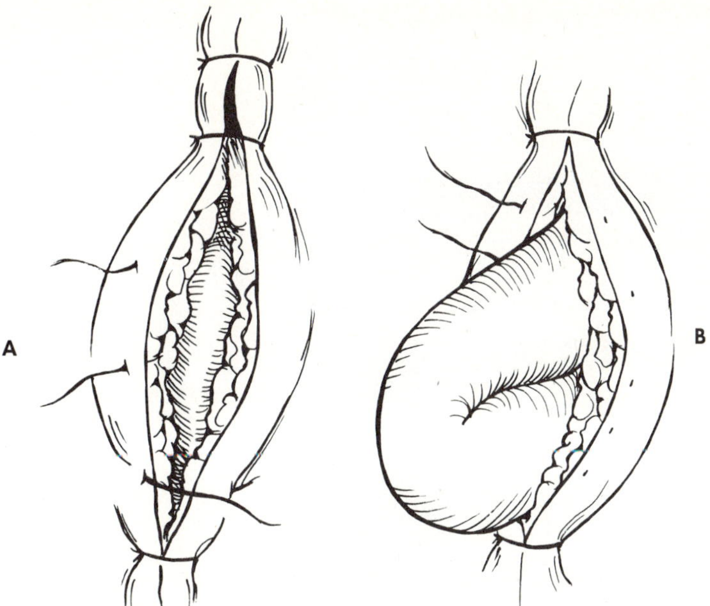

Fig. 8-2. A, Wound dehiscence. **B,** Evisceration. (From Barber, J.M., Stokes, L.G., and Billings, D.M.: Adult and child care: a client approach to nursing, ed. 2, St. Louis, 1977, The C.V. Mosby Co.)

mary source. Attention to aseptic principles and operating room environmental conditions are significant influencing factors. Length of time that the wound is open in the operating room has also been mentioned. Authorities are now suspecting, however, that the most common source of infection may be the patient himself, since many infections can be traced back to the patient's own endogenous flora. This points up the importance of meticulous preoperative antimicrobial preparation of the patient, thorough preparation of the surgical site, and careful observation of sterile technique, not only in the operating room but also during postoperative dressing changes.

Wound healing is impaired by poor surgical technique, believed by some to be the primary determinant of wound healing. Rough handling of tissue causes trauma that in turn can lead to dysfunction, bleeding, and other conditions conducive to infection. Other examples of surgical technique contributing to wound healing are inadequate hemostasis, poor cutting and suturing techniques, dead spaces, and excessive pressure from retractors and other instruments.

Other factors affecting wound healing are the patient's age, stress level, preexisting conditions such as diabetes, anemia, malnutrition, cancer, obesity, advanced age, or cardiovascular or respiratory impairments—in other words, overall physical and psychological conditions.

Following are terms used in connection with wound healing:

keloid Dense, unsightly connective tissue or excessive scar formation that is often removed surgically.

"proud flesh" Overgrowth of granulation tissue.

gangrene Process that may occur instead of healing; implies necrosis (death of tissue) and putrefaction (decomposition); usually caused by failure of nutriment or blood brought to a part.

adhesions Adherence of serous membranes to one another, causing fibrous tissue to form; sometimes occurring in healing and inflammatory processes; commonly occurring in or about gastrointestinal tract, where they may form bands and cause obstructions and subsequent surgical emergencies.

dehiscence Separation of layers of surgical wound (Fig. 8-2).

evisceration Extrusion of internal organs, or viscera, through gaping wound (Fig. 8-2).

DRESSINGS

After surgery, a dressing may be applied to the wound. Following are the purposes of a dressing:

1. To cushion and protect the wound from trauma and gross contamination
2. To absorb drainage
3. To support, splint, or immobilize the body part and incisional area
4. To aid in hemostasis and minimize edema, as in a pressure dressing
5. To enhance the patient's physical and esthetic (or psychological) comfort

Dressings are as varied as operations, but a standard dressing usually consists of gauze or nonadherent pads covered with a larger, bulkier absorbent (ABD) pad (Fig.

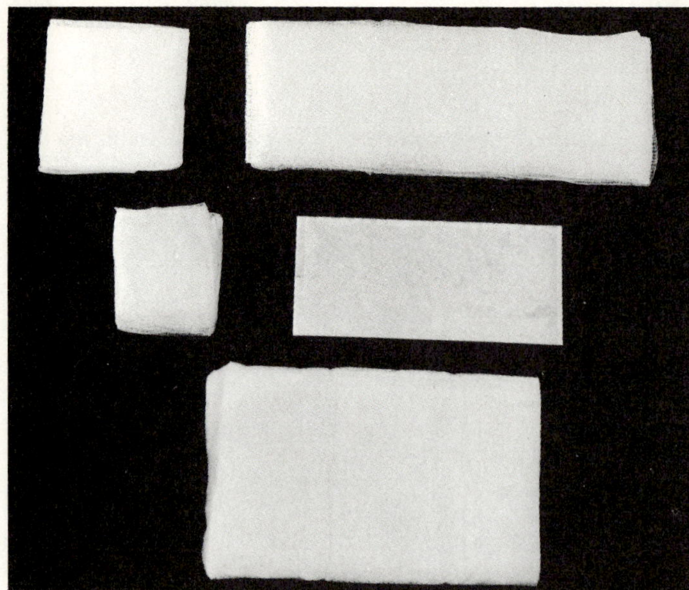

Fig. 8-3. Common dressing materials. *From left, top,* 4 × 4–inch gauze, 4 × 8–inch gauze, 2 × 2–inch gauze, Telfa-nonadherent pad, and ABD pad.

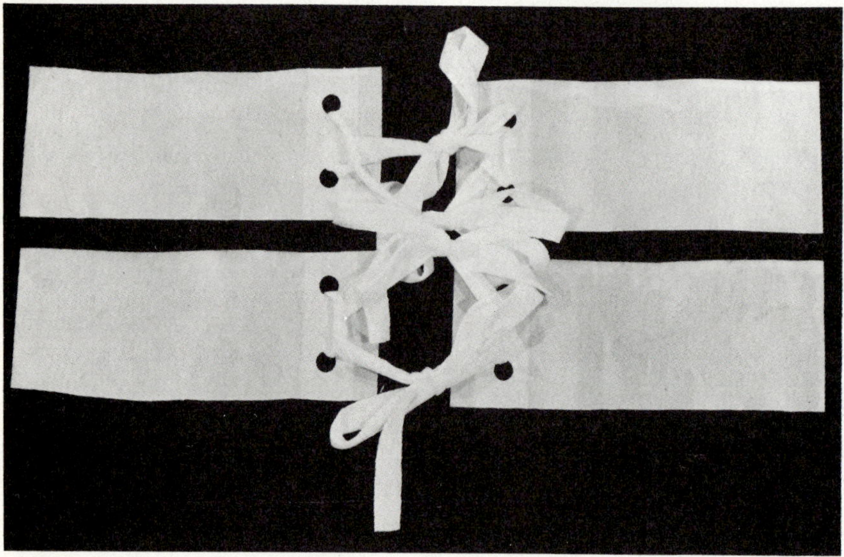

Fig. 8-4. Montgomery straps may be used when frequent dressing changes are anticipated.

8-3). Orthopedic patients may have splints or casts applied to their wounds (Chapter 20). Number and bulk of dressings depends on the area to be dressed, the pressure desired, and the drainage anticipated. Because many people have tape allergies, the dressings are secured with paper-like nonallergenic tape. Many varieties are available. If frequent dressing changes will be necessary, the dressings may be secured with Montgomery straps (Fig. 8-4).

In some instances, a clean wound may be covered with only a transparent protective spray dressing. This usually lasts from 3 to 6 days and either peels off or is removed with a solvent. This dressing is particularly advantageous for a small child who has an incision (for example, herniorrhaphy) in the diaper area, where standard gauze dressings would become contaminated immediately with urine or feces.

In some situations, the wound is not dressed at all. This allows a clean, dry incisional area to heal with the aid of air and light and eliminates the dark, moist, warm conditions conducive to microbial growth that frequently are present with a standard dressing. Other advantages are that having no dressing (1) allows for optimum observation of the incisional area, (2) aids bathing, (3) prevents possible adhesive tape reactions, (4) increases comfort and maneuverability for many patients, and (5) seems to minimize adverse responses to the operation by the patient.

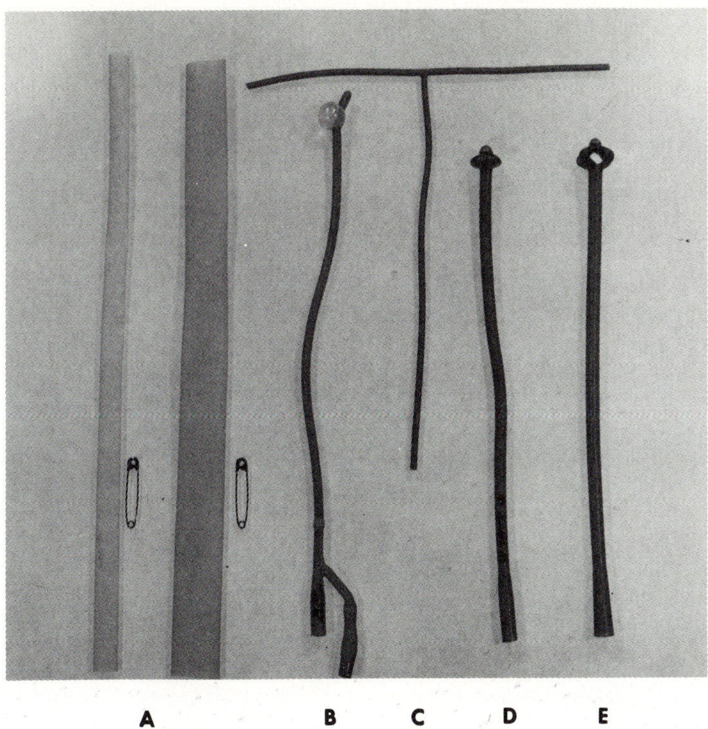

A B C D E

Fig. 8-5. Commonly used drains following surgery. **A,** Penrose drains. **B,** Foley catheter. **C,** T-tube. **D,** Mushroom, or Pezzer. **E,** Bat-wing, or Malecot.

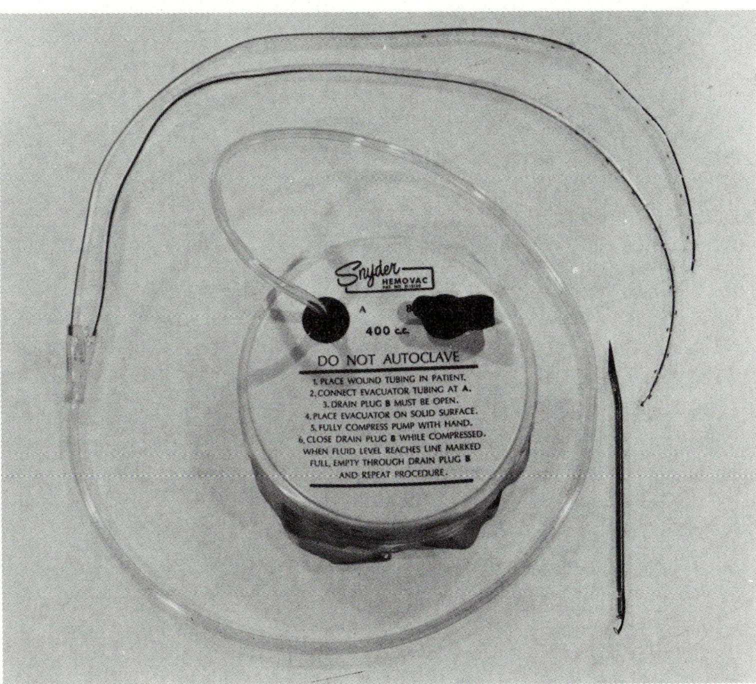

Fig. 8-6. Portable self-contained drainage system. (Courtesy Zimmer, Inc., Warsaw, Ind.; from Hoeller, M.L.: Surgical technology: basis for clinical practice, ed. 3, St. Louis, 1974, The C.V. Mosby Co.)

DRAINS

Drains provide exits through which air and fluids such as serum, blood, lymph, intestinal secretions, bile, and pus can be evacuated from the operative site. Drains may also be used to prevent the development of deep wound infections. They are usually inserted at the time of surgery, directly from the incision or through a separate small incision, known as a stab wound, close to the operative site.

In some instances (chest, common bile duct, bladder), drainage is directly through the tube. In other instances (peritoneal cavity), drainage of pus or blood is primarily along the outside surface of the drain (as with the Penrose drain). One specialized type of drain inserted into the bladder during many types of surgery is the Foley retention catheter, used to monitor urinary output and aid the healing process, especially in pelvic and genitourinary surgery.

Many types of drains are available, the most common of which are illustrated in Fig. 8-5. Some are self-retaining; others are taped or sutured into place or are secured in other ways that prevent slippage and excess movement. Other special drains are discussed in the chapters dealing with specific types of operations.

Some drains and drainage systems function by gravitational flow in areas in which body pressure is greater than atmospheric pressure or by capillary action (for example, the Penrose drain), drawing pus or fluid along their surfaces and through a wound outlet. Others are attached to or function by way of systems of continuous or intermittent vacuum and suction. Portable, self-contained suction units are available (Fig. 8-6), as well as those which are electrically powered and manually adjusted. The operating room nurse must know the exact location of drains to know the type and amount of drainage to expect and to be able to record and report this information.

SUGGESTED READINGS

Auld, M.E., Craven, R.F., and West, J.M.: What you can do to help and not hinder the miracle involved in wound healing, Nursing '72 **2**(10):36, 1972.

Bernhard, L.A., editor: Wound healing, AORN J. **35:**1067, 1982.

Bryant, W.M.: Wound healing, Clin. Symp. **3:**1, 1977.

Kildea, J.: The evolution of surgical wound drainage, Point of View **10:**2, 1973.

Laufman, H.: Surgical infection hazard control: the patient's defense, J. Surg. Prac. **7:**22, Sept.-Oct. 1978.

Marcinek, M.: Stress in the surgical patient, Am. J. Nurs. **77:**1809, 1977.

Myers, M.B.: Sutures and wound healing, Am. J. Nurs. **71:**1725, 1971.

Sanders, R.J., and DiCiementi, D.: Principles of abdominal wound closure, Arch. Surg. **112:**1188, 1977.

Schumann, D.: How to help wound healing in your abdominal surgery patient, Nursing '80 **10**(4):34, 1980.

Schumann, D., editor: Symposium on wound healing, Nurs. Clin. North Am. **14:**665, 1979.

Wilson, V.: Routine shaving and wound infections, AORN J. **28:**762, 1978.

9 Anesthesia

The first medical announcement of anesthesia occurred in the Bigelow paper of November 18, 1846. The article was in reference to the first "public" ether anesthesia performed in the amphitheater (now called Ether Dome) of the Massachusetts General Hospital. Here, Dr. William T.G. Morton, a dentist, anesthetized Gilbert Abbott. The surgeon, Dr. John Collins Warren, operated on an unconscious, still patient and at the conclusion of the operation announced, "Gentlemen, this is no humbug."

However, on December 10, 1844, another dentist, Dr. Riggs, had painlessly extracted a tooth from Horace Wells under the influence of nitrous oxide. A public demonstration by Horace Wells at Massachusetts General Hospital failed because of the magnitude of the surgery and the weakness as an anesthetic agent of nitrous oxide alone. Wells was ridiculed for this.

The first modern anesthetic actually was given in 1842 by Dr. Crawford W. Long in Jefferson, Georgia, who, using ether, painlessly removed a tumor from the neck of James Venable. However, the local populace threatened to lynch Dr. Long for this "heinous crime." He promptly gave up this practice and moved his office to Athens, Georgia.

The word *anesthesia* comes from the Greek word *anaisthesis,* meaning "negative sensation." The word appeared in Bailey's English Dictionary in 1721; later Dr. Oliver Wendell Holmes suggested the word anesthesia to William Morton in a letter in 1846 saying, "I think this state should be called anesthesia. This signifies insensibility more particularly to objects of touch."

Since these times, anesthesia has developed to an exact and sophisticated science, and an outline of modern concepts with its interrelationship to nursing is the subject of this chapter.

The choice of anesthesia for a surgical procedure, along with other considerations, is primarily decided on by the anesthesiologist. The additional considerations include the type of surgical procedure, the particular requirements of the surgeon, the position to be used, and the physical and mental state of the patient.

The two main forms of anesthesia used are general anesthesia and some type of block (local) anesthesia. Some forms of anesthesia are rarely used: hypnoanesthesia (using hypnosis) and, as commonly carried out in Oriental countries, acupuncture anesthesia. Other forms of anesthesia that are not used at present will not be considered here.

GENERAL ANESTHETICS

Action

Many theories as to the action of general anesthetics on the body have been proposed. None explains all the phenomena; a few explain many of the phenomena. Following are some theories of the action of anesthetic agents to provide a broader view of the subject:

1. In clinical concentration, transmission is not blocked in peripheral nerve fibers. Action is on specialized areas such as synapses and possibly on fine, unmyelinated nerve fibers.

2. It is possible that specialized areas on the membranes of cells are sensitive to anesthetic agents and other chemical agents.

3. Quastel in 1932 thought that anesthetics may interfere with intercellular oxidation, possibly by influencing enzyme action.

4. Overton and Meyer proposed that anesthetic agents are readily absorbed by lipids and that hence brain cells are especially susceptible to their action. The partition of a drug between lipid and water phases reflects its potency as a narcotic. This is true of volatile anesthetics but not for some of the parenteral anesthetics such as barbiturates or chloral hydrate.

5. Claude Bernard proposed a theory that anesthetics cause changes in cell metabolism of physiochemical nature, changes in surface tension or changes in permeability of the cell membrane.

6. Anesthetics may act by changing the electrical polarity of the cells of the nervous system.

7. Ferguson pointed out in 1939 that the potency of an anesthetic is inversely proportional to its vapor pressure provided that the agent was chemically reactive. This applies, of course, to volatile anesthetics.

In summary, these studies seem to indicate that a single theory of action that explains all anesthetic actions does not exist. Anesthetics can produce a spectrum of activity in the central nervous system, and different agents produce different patterns of activity. Differential effects at the cellular and membrane levels have been observed. Structurally dependent differences occur, and optical iso-

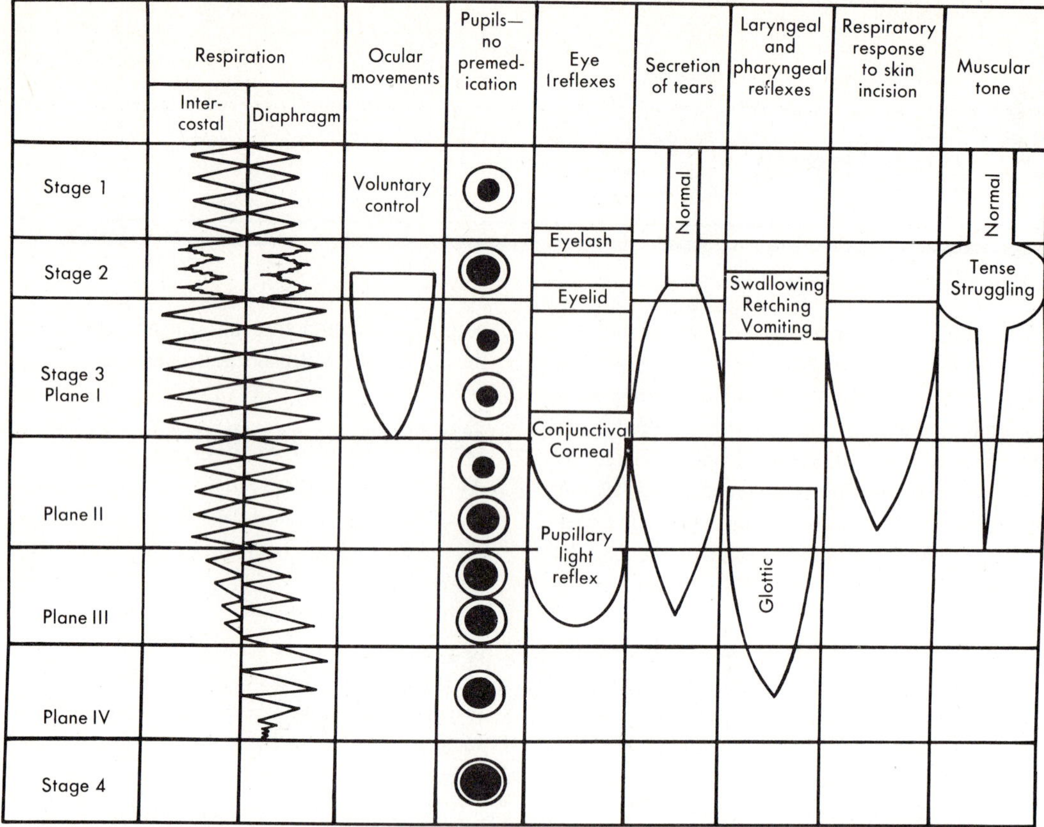

Fig. 9-1. Changes occurring during anesthesia as seen with ether anesthesia. The actions of different anesthetics vary slightly from this. (After Guedel; from Atkinson, R.S., Rushman, G.B., and Lee, J.A.: A synopsis of anaesthesia, London, 1982, John Wright & Sons, Ltd., Medical Publishers.)

mers display very different activities. Anesthetics are selective agents and produce their effects at multiple sites through a variety of mechanisms.

Four stages of anesthesia are classically described with ether anesthesia, but they are virtually the same for all anesthetic agents (Fig. 9-1). Stage 1 begins with the patient being awake and continues to the patient's loss of consciousness, during which analgesia occurs. Stage 2 is from loss of consciousness to the point at which the patient begins automatic breathing, during which excitement occurs with irregular breathing and limb movements. Stage 3 is heralded by regular respirations and is the stage of surgical anesthesia; it is divided into four planes. Stage 4 is apnea leading to death.

Usually, general anesthesia is begun with the intravenous injection of a rapidly acting agent that will take the patient immediately to stage 3, thereby eliminating the untoward responses of stages 1 and 2. Maintenance is usually accomplished with gaseous agents, sometimes supplemented with intravenous agents.

For pain-free surgery and a quiet patient, three different but interrelated events must occur: hypnosis (sleep), analgesia (freedom from pain), and amnesia (lack of recall of events). Different anesthetic agents possess different amounts of these properties; hence the use of drug combinations to produce a good anesthetic (for example, diazepam is a hypnotic and an amnesic, thiopental sodium is a hypnotic, and morphine is an analgesic). The correct combination provides the optimum depth of anesthesia that affects the body functions as little as possible.

To assist the surgeon, muscle relaxants, hypotensive agents, and other drugs may also be needed. Table 2 describes currently used agents.

Delivery

1. *Open drop* (reserved for ether, vinyl ether, and chloroform). The agent is dropped onto a gauze-covered mask placed over the face (rarely used now).

2. *Open circuit* (for example, Bain circuit, T piece circuit, and Magill circuit). This type of circuit uses a relatively high flow of fresh gas varying from approximately two thirds of the patient's minute volume for the Magill circuit to 100 cc or more per kilogram for the Bain and the T piece circuit. The majority of the exhaled gas is blown into the atmosphere with these circuits.

3. *Closed and semiclosed circuits.* These circuits incorporate soda lime, which is used to absorb carbon dioxide from the exhaled gas, which is then recycled.

Table 2. Anesthetic agents

Agent	Route	Use	Advantages	Disadvantages	Possible complications in operating room
Nitrous oxide	Inhalation	Maintenance; occasionally for induction	Rapid induction and recovery	No relaxation; usually needs other agents also	Patient becomes hypoxic if overdosed
Halothane (Fluothane)	Inhalation	Maintenance; occasionally for induction	Rapid induction and recovery; pleasant, nonirritating; fairly good relaxation	Narrow margin of safety; dangerous if used with epinephrine; may rarely cause liver damage postoperatively	May cause bradycardia and hypotension; premature ventricular contractions or ventricular fibrillation if epinephrine used
Enflurane (Ethrane)	Inhalation	Maintenance; occasionally for induction	Rapid induction and recovery; allows larger amounts of epinephrine to be used than with halothane; fairly good relaxation	May cause profound drops of blood pressure in older patients and convulsions in children	Hypotension; convulsions in children with high concentration
Isoflurane (Forane)	Inhalation	Maintenance; occasionally for induction	Good muscle relaxant; pleasant, nonirritating; cardiovascular stability	Expensive	
Ketamine (Ketaject, Ketalar)	Intravenous or intramuscular	Induction; occasionally for maintenance	Short acting; good for burned patients and small children; patient maintains airway	Large doses cause respiratory depression and hallucinations on emergence	Hallucinations on emergence; need perfectly quiet, dark room
Thiopental sodium (Pentothal)	Intravenous or rectal (children)	Induction	Fast, smooth induction; fast recovery	Large doses cause respiratory and circulatory depression and tendency to laryngospasm	Laryngospasm, particularly in smokers; hypotension
Sodium methohexital (Brevital sodium)	Intravenous	Induction; occasionally for maintenance	Fast acting, fast emergence	Hiccoughs	Few
Lidocaine (Xylocaine)	Spinal, epidural, block, or local infiltration	Block anesthesia	Low toxicity, well tried and tested; short acting; good relaxation	Accidental intravenous administration or overdosage can cause convulsions	Convulsions; may need resuscitation
Bupivacaine (Marcaine)	Epidural, block, or local infiltration	Block anesthesia	Low toxicity, long acting, good relaxation	Overdose can cause convulsions	Convulsions; may need resuscitation
Tetracaine (Pontocaine)	Intrathecal	Spinal anesthesia	Lasts 1 to 2 hours; very low toxicity		Block may get too high; may need resuscitation for hypotension

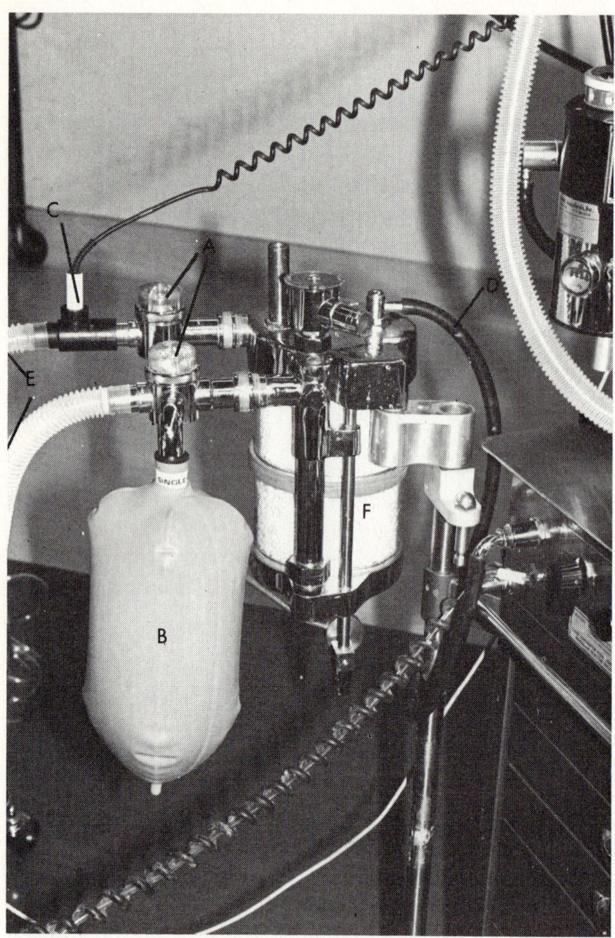

Fig. 9-2. Circle system of anesthesia administration. *A,* Unidirectional valves; *B,* rebreathing bag; *C,* oxygen analyzer sensor; *D,* fresh gas supply; *E,* anesthesia tubing; *F,* soda lime canister.

Closed circuit

With the circle system (Fig. 9-2) and a basal oxygen flow only (250 cc per minute), all the carbon dioxide is absorbed, and no gas is blown off from the circuit.

Semiclosed circuit

A higher fresh gas flow is used (1 to 6 liters per minute) with the circle system shown in Fig. 9-2. During exhalation some gas is eliminated, but some is recycled (hence semiclosed). This is the most common system used in the United States for anesthetizing adults.

Anesthesia can be delivered with these methods by way of a mask or an endotracheal tube. An endotracheal tube is inserted (intubation) to enable a clear airway to be maintained easily. For example, this would be done in facial or brain surgery, when maintenance with a mask is difficult (large tongue, small chin, etc.), or when the patient is paralyzed. The patient needs mechanical or manual artificial ventilation when this situation exists.

LOCAL ANESTHETICS

Local anesthetic agents (Table 2) primarily exert their action by inhibition of the excitatory process in nerve endings or nerve fibers. The normal nerve fiber has a negative electrical potential or resting potential of approximately −60 to −90 millivolts (mV). When the nerve is stimulated, the electrical potential inside approaches zero. When it reaches a threshold potential, which is often −30 or −20 mV, the rate of depolarization suddenly increases enormously and the electrical potential inside the cell changes from the original −60 to −90 mV to approximately 40 mV. After this depolarization process, a repolarization occurs until the resting potential is reestablished at −60 to −90 mV. The entire process normally occurs within 1 millisecond.

Although local anesthetics do not alter the resting potential of the nerves, they alter the rate of depolarization, which is depressed so that the threshold potential cannot be reached and therefore maximum depolarization cannot occur. Thus the nerve fails to transmit impulses. These drugs act by blocking the conductance of sodium across the cell membrane. At present, the following sequence of events is generally accepted as the mechanism of action of local anesthetic agents: (1) the agent binds to receptor sites on the nerve membrane; (2) sodium permeability is reduced; (3) there is a decrease in the rate of depolarization and then a failure to achieve threshold potential level; and (4) a lack of development of propagated action potential occurs, resulting in a conduction blockade. See also the section on administration of local anesthetics in Chapter 4.

GENERAL ANESTHESIA

Anesthesia machine

The anesthesia machine (Fig. 9-3) used for delivering general anesthesia looks more complicated than it is. However, the basic concepts on which any anesthesia machine functions remain the same and are actually very simple.

The machine is usually connected to a source of oxygen and nitrous oxide supplied to the machine at 50 to 60 psi by the hospital pipeline. In the event that this is not available or failure occurs, the machines are also equipped with cylinders that can supply the gas. The cylinders are attached to the side of the machine at yokes. The yokes are "pin indexed." The pin indexing system is a system in which the connection of the cylinder to the machine has two protruding pins. These two pins are at a particular sequence, meaning that cylinders cannot be connected to the wrong place on the machine.

Also of note is the fact that oxygen in cylinders is supplied at 2000 psi as a compressed gas. As the gas is used, the pressure on the gauge connected to the cylinder

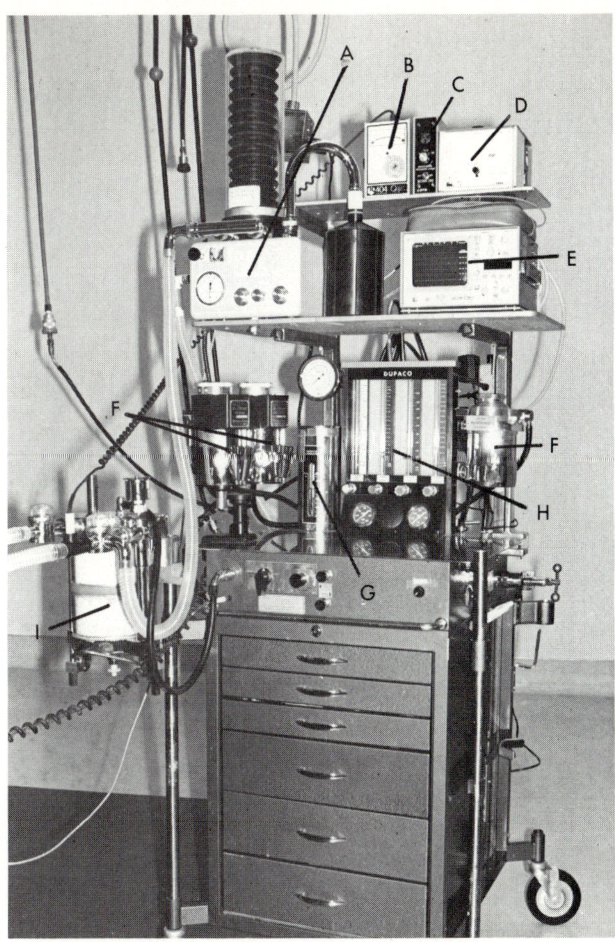

Fig. 9-3. Typical modern anesthesia machine. *A,* Ventilator; *B,* oxygen analyzer; *C,* disconnect alarm; *D,* temperature monitor; *E,* ECG monitor; *F,* flow-through vaporizers; *G,* Copper Kettle vaporizer; *H,* flowmeters; *I,* circle system.

progressively falls in a linear manner. Nitrous oxide is provided in liquid form in cylinders, and the pressure above the nitrous oxide is 750 psi. As the nitrous oxide is used, the pressure above the liquid stays constant; only when the liquid has gone does the pressure shown on the gauge fall. Therefore the nitrous oxide can be almost gone yet still show the same pressure on the gauge, whereas with oxygen the amount remaining can be readily determined.

Gases from these cylinders or the pipeline flow through flowmeters located on the front of the machine so that the concentration of nitrous oxide and oxygen and the total flow can be determined by the anesthesiologist. The mixed gases flow through a vaporizer in which the vaporized anesthetic of choice is added to the nitrous oxide oxygen mixture.

Vaporizers are of two types. The first is a "flow-through" vaporizer. *All* of the gas going to the patient flows through it. The second type of vaporizer is the Copper Kettle type, which is used in a different manner. A low flow of oxygen passes through this vaporizer from a separate special flowmeter and is totally saturated with the anesthetic vapor. This vapor is then mixed with the gases that have already been through the flowmeters, and the total amount flows out of the anesthetic machine to the patient. To determine the concentration of anesthetic agents going to the patient, the anesthesiologist must adjust the total flow of gases and the flow of gas going through the Copper Kettle vaporizer and must also note the temperature of the liquid in the Copper Kettle vaporizer, since this will affect the amount of vapor delivered to the patient.

In most situations in the United States, a *circle system* is used to deliver the anesthetic gases to the patient. The circle system is composed of a container in which a carbon dioxide–absorbing material (for example, soda lime or bara lime) is placed, two directional valves, and the two connections of this system to the patient through corrugated anesthetic hoses. As the patient breathes in, gases are drawn from the canister along one limb. As the patient breathes out, the gases leaving the patient flow back to the canister along the other limb, this flow being controlled by the two unidirectional valves found on the body of the canister. As the gases flow through the canister, the carbon dioxide is absorbed and any excess gas bleeds off from the blow-off valve. The advantage of this type of system is that much lower flows of anesthetic agents can be used, with accompanying financial savings. The substance used to absorb the carbon dioxide normally includes an indicator that will change in color as the substance becomes exhausted. As an example, soda lime may turn from white to blue. When the total canister contents are blue, the soda lime must be changed to stop carbon dioxide buildup in the patient.

Preparation of the patient

The patient is examined preoperatively by the anesthesiologist, the chart reviewed, and any premedication ordered.

The purpose of the premedication is to sedate the patient and, if necessary, dry secretions that may interfere with the smooth deliverance of an anesthetic. After the preoperative medication has been ordered, the patient may have nothing by mouth for at least 6 hours preoperatively. About an hour before surgery, the premedication, consisting often of a narcotic and possibly a drying agent such as atropine, hyoscine, or glycopyrrolate is given intramuscularly.

Next, the patient is taken to the operating room and placed on the operating room table, an intravenous infusion is started, the electrocardiogram is connected, and either general or block anesthesia is induced.

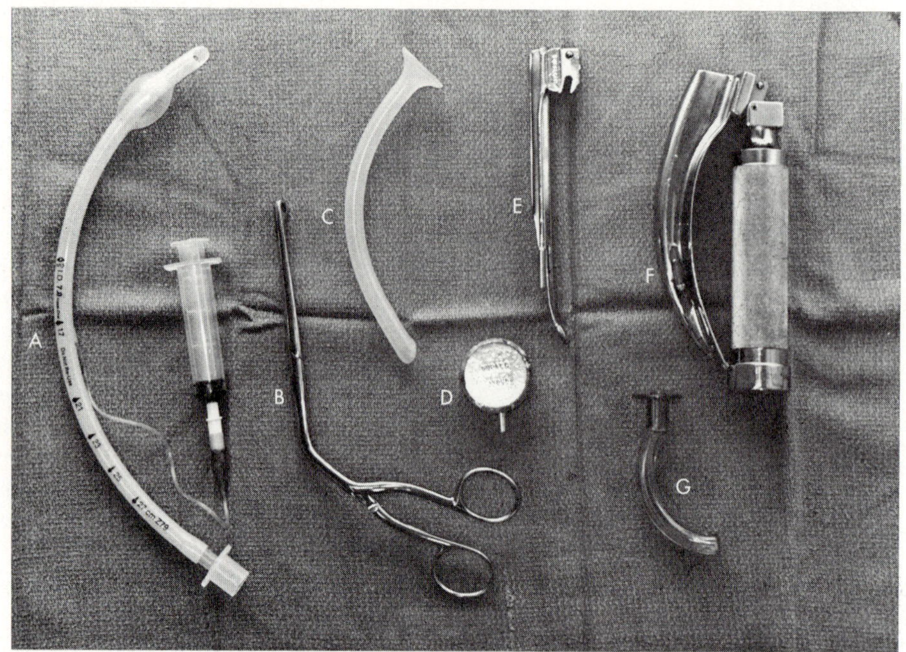

Fig. 9-4. Commonly used anesthesia equipment. *A,* Endotracheal tube; *B,* Magill forceps; *C,* nasal airway; *D,* precordial stethoscope; *E,* Magill blade; *F,* Macintosh blade on laryngoscope handle; *G,* oral airway.

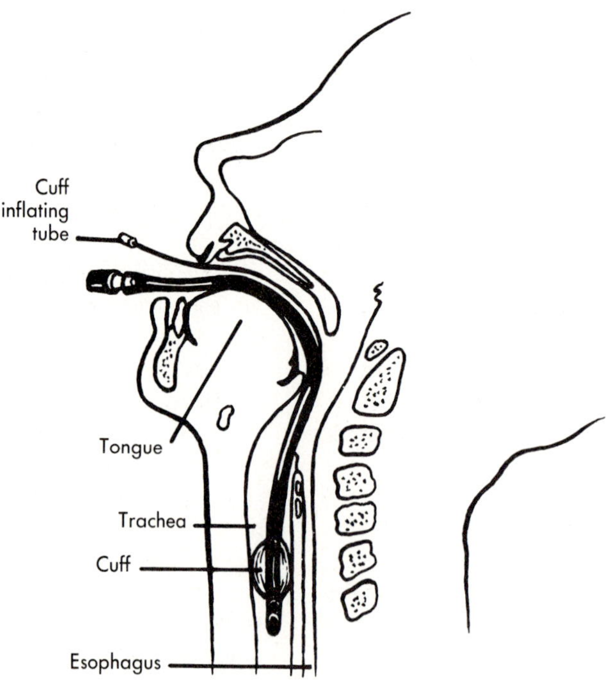

Fig. 9-5. Endotracheal tube in position.

Induction

To move the patient rapidly to stage 3 of general anesthesia (Fig. 9-1), induction is usually performed with an intravenous short-acting barbiturate such as thiopental sodium. Maintenance may be carried out with a mixture of nitrous oxide, oxygen, and a volatile anesthetic agent such as enflurane or halothane, with or without the addition of intravenous narcotics and with or without the addition of paralyzing drugs such as succinylcholine or pancuronium. Succinylcholine, which is short acting, is usually used during intubation.

A laryngoscope is used to visualize the vocal cords, and an endotracheal tube (Fig. 9-4) is placed in the trachea so that the cuff is just below the vocal cords. The cuff is then inflated to just seal (Fig. 9-5). (In children, it is usual for noncuffed tubes to be used because of a difference in the anatomy of small children's airways). After this, the paralyzed patient is either provided with artificial ventilation or allowed to breathe spontaneously when the dose of succinylcholine has worn off.

Alternatively, the anesthetic may be delivered with a mask, often held over the nose and mouth with a head strap and the patient breathing spontaneously. An oral or nasal airway may be placed to maintain an open airway for smooth breathing. Another variation is assisted ventilation, in which the patient breathes spontaneously but every so often the anesthesiologist assists respiration by squeezing the bag on the circle system.

At the end of the operation the anesthesiologist ensures that any nondepolarizing muscle relaxants (for example, curare or pancuronium) have completely worn off by reversing with a mixture of anticholinesterase such as neostigmine and an anticholinergic drug such as atropine. The patient is given oxygen to breathe to blow off as much nitrous oxide as possible before the endotracheal tube is removed. The patient is taken to the recovery room, soon to awake from the anesthetic experience.

BLOCK ANESTHESIA

If some form of block anesthesia is to be used, the patient arrives in the operating room and is prepared in a manner similar to that for general anesthesia. An intravenous cannula is put into place, a blood pressure cuff is placed on the arm, and an electrocardiogram is connected. A predetermined block is then carried out.

Block anesthesia can be induced by injecting a local anesthetic agent anywhere from the spinal cord (spinal anesthesia) to the tip of peripheral nerves (that is, surface application).

Spinal anesthesia

The local anesthetic agent (usually tetracaine) is injected into the subarachnoid space into the cerebrospinal fluid generally at the L2-3 or L3-4 interspace (Fig. 9-6). The drug is most often mixed with 10% dextrose solution and is injected (6 to 20 mg) in a total volume of 1 to 4 ml. This mixture is hyperbaric (heavier than the cerebrospinal fluid into which it is injected) and can therefore be made to "move" by positioning the patient's head up or down after the injection. For example, for prostate surgery the patient is usually left sitting for a minute or so after the injection, which may be done in the sitting position. A block of the S1 to S3 roots will result.

For gallbladder surgery the patient may be positioned in a 5-degree Trendelenburg position to allow the anesthetic to move toward the head while the anesthesiologist carefully checks the level; when the anesthetic is high enough, the table is leveled to stop the spread. After 10 minutes the block is usually "set"; that is, it will not extend further.

Problems

1. Rapid fall of blood pressure may occur. This is caused by vasodilatation as the sympathetic nerves governing vasomotor tone, as well as pain and motor fibers, are blocked. Treatment is rapid intravenous infusion of fluids and/or vasopressors.
2. Special care must be taken with these patients because burns and other trauma can occur on the anesthetized part of the body and the patient will obviously not feel them occurring. Personnel in the operating room have a false sense of security because the patient is awake.
3. Talking about the diagnosis or operation must be kept at an absolute minimum so as not to alarm the patient unless he has been *very* heavily sedated.
4. An inadvertently high anesthetic may cause problems with breathing, requiring "resuscitation" by the anesthetist. This is one instance in which the circulating nurse must be available to assist immediately.

Caudal and epidural anesthesia

Caudal and epidural anesthesia are the same in that the anesthetic agent is injected into the epidural space (Fig. 9-6). The epidural space is the area between the dura and the ligamentum flavum, a space occupied by fat and veins.

A caudal anesthetic is an epidural anesthetic. The only difference is that the site of injection of the caudal anesthetic is into the epidural space through the caudal canal in the sacrum. The site of injection of the epidural anesthetic is usually between the intervertebral spaces in the lumbar region, but thoracic and cervical epidural anesthetics have been given from time to time for specific operations. Single shot or continuous anesthesia is available with these techniques. In the continuous technique, either a malleable needle is used (for a caudal anesthetic) and left in position, or a catheter is inserted through the needle and the needle removed (for an epidural anesthetic).

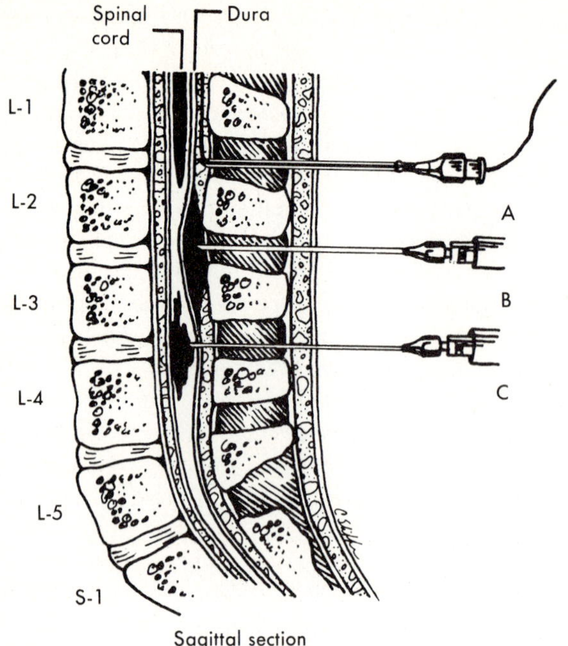

Fig. 9-6. Position of needles and injection sites. *A,* Epidural catheters; *B,* epidural anesthesia; *C,* spinal anesthesia.

The injected local anesthetic bathes the nerve roots as they leave the cord through the intervertebral foramina, blocking conduction of impulses through them. It is usual that only the nerve roots which are bathed by the anesthetic agent will be blocked by the anesthetic. It is, therefore, possible, particularly with the epidural anesthetic, to block only certain segments above and below the site of injection of the local anesthetic agent. As opposed to spinal anesthesia, much larger doses of the anesthetic are needed, usually 10 to 30 ml.

The most frequently used anesthetic agents are lidocaine, bupivacaine, and chloroprocaine. The position of the patient can affect the height of the anesthetic but to a much lesser extent than with spinal anesthesia. As with the spinal anesthetic, problems may occur: rapid falls of blood pressures, which will be somewhat slower with the epidural anesthetic because of the slower onset, and complications 2 through 4 as itemized previously. Two other specific complications related to epidural anesthesia may occur necessitating help from the nurses in attendance.

The first problem occurs when the local anesthetic is inadvertently injected into one of the epidural space veins. In this case, toxicity from the local anesthetic will occur and may result in a profound fall of blood pressure, a tachycardia if the local anesthetic contains epinephrine, and convulsions because of the effects of the anesthetic on the patient's brain. Under these circumstances, the anesthesiologist may do any of the following three things: (1) inject a paralyzing agent; (2) intubate the patient and keep the patient paralyzed until the convulsions end, usually within a few minutes; or (3) inject thiopental sodium or diazepam intravenously to counteract the effects of the local anesthetic on the patient's brain.

The second specific complication occurs if the needle or catheter is inadvertently placed in the subarachnoid space (that is, in the same place that the spinal needle is normally placed). Injection of a large volume of local anesthetic agent, used with epidural anesthesia, could cause what is known as total spinal anesthesia. In other words, the local anesthetic travels all the way to the brain. This will cause a fall of blood pressure due to vasodilatation, profound bradycardia as a result of blocking of the cardioaccelerator nerves, and a totally anesthetized and asleep patient. The treatment is usually intubation of the patient, maintenance of respiration, and support of the blood pressure until such time as the effects of the anesthetic agent have worn off. These two complications are not life threatening if they are treated correctly.

Nerve block anesthesia

In this form of anesthesia, local anesthetic agents are injected around peripheral nerves to block central specific areas of the body. Sometimes single nerves are blocked (intercostal nerve block), and sometimes many nerves are blocked by one injection (brachial plexus block).

Complications result from inadvertent intravascular injection or overdose leading to cerebral effects and convulsions.

ACUPUNCTURE ANESTHESIA

Acupuncture is commonly used for anesthesia in China but is frequently supplemented by narcotics. The original method is by inserting and twirling fine needles at specific points of the body. Recently, needles or surface electrodes have been placed in the same locations but connected to an electronic machine that creates current flow between these electrodes. Frequencies of 3 Hz to 250 Hz are used, with an average of 50 Hz.

The theory is that stimulation going to the brain from one source can effectively block painful stimuli from another source. This is known as the "gate control theory." The stimulation of acupuncture closes the gate on the pain stimuli, thereby eliminating the pain.

Interestingly enough, we all are aware of the effects of being hurt in two places. We usually feel only the more painful of the two injuries.

Endorphins can also be produced by acupuncture stimulation. Endorphins are naturally occurring morphine-like substances that are released in response to pain and that cause analgesia.

Acupuncture anesthesia can be used in the modern operating room. Its effects are produced by the "gate effect" and endorphin release. It is not satisfactory as an anesthetic in many persons and seems to work far better for Oriental than Occidental people.

HYPNOANESTHESIA

Hypnosis has been used for anesthesia during surgery. A sufficiently good subject, after appropriate training, may be able to make parts of the body go numb and insensible to pain. Hypnoanesthesia is rarely used.

POLLUTION OF THE OPERATING ROOM

All chemicals are potentially harmful until proved otherwise. Pollution of the operating room occurs with anesthetic gases, particularly nitrous oxide, but also with various halogenated agents such as enflurane and halothane.

Statistical surveys performed over the last 10 years have implicated pollution as causing complications such as an increased abortion rate, increased number of female children, and increased lymphoma rate in anesthesiologists who were receiving large doses of these agents. However, the interpretation of these figures is disputed.

All anesthesia machines should have a well-functioning scavenging system. According to the National Institute for Occupational Safety and Health (NIOSH), pollution levels should be less than 25 ppm for nitrous oxide and 0.5 ppm for halogenated agents. Often levels this low cannot be consistently obtained.

Although chronic occupational exposures to trace concentrations of anesthetic gases is a suspected cause of the previously mentioned complications, the evidence is equivocal. The question frequently raised is whether women who are pregnant or who are contemplating pregnancy should work in the operating room. The answer is that no "safe" exposure levels below which we can ensure that adverse effects will not occur exists. Persons with questions should consult a knowledgeable anesthesia or obstetrical department member for the latest information on this subject.

MALIGNANT HYPERPYREXIA

No chapter on anesthesia would be complete without mentioning malignant hyperpyrexia, a life-threatening complication of anesthesia. It is characterized by hyperpyrexia, tachycardia, acidosis, often rigidity, and ultimately death, which may occur at induction or at any time, even in the recovery room.

The mechanism is simply a generalized contraction of body muscles triggered by one of the anesthetic agents, most of which have been implicated in this disease. Succinylcholine and halothane in particular are possibly the most frequently implicated drugs.

Malignant hyperpyrexia is a rare occurrence, but when it appears, smooth functioning of the operating room team is needed to save the patient's life. Each operating room should have a procedure for dealing with this disease, which carries a 60% mortality. The important modalities of treatment include packing the patient in ice and administering iced intravenous solutions, steroids, diuretics, and dantrolene.

NURSING CONSIDERATIONS

1. The nurse checks the patient's chart to make sure all the laboratory work and pertinent studies are completed and reports available.

2. The nurse who assists in the positioning of the patient should remember never to move an unconscious patient without first obtaining the anesthesiologist's permission.

3. The nurse checks the position of the arms and legs to ensure that no pressure points exist.

4. The nurse assists the anesthesiologist during induction of anesthesia, making sure a functioning suction unit is close by. The nurse should be prepared to give cricoid pressure to stop regurgitation of stomach contents in patients with a full stomach and to help bring cords into better view during intubation.

5. The nurse assists with the insertion of arterial, intravenous, central venous pressure lines, and Swan-Ganz catheters.

6. Operating room personnel work as a team. Nurses may be asked to perform special duties for the anesthesiologist during the anesthetizing of a patient. It is important that this be done to the best of the nurse's ability.

SUGGESTED READINGS

Atkinson, R.S., Rushman, G.B., and Lee, J.A.: A synopsis of anaesthesia, London, 1982, John Wright & Sons, Ltd., Medical Publishers.

Birch, A.A., and Tolmie, J.D.: Anesthesia for the uninterested, Baltimore, 1976, University Park Press.

Cottrell, J.E., editor: Occupational hazards to OR and RR personnel, Int. Anesthesiol. Clin. **19**:1, Winter 1981.

Croushore, T.M.: Postoperative assessment: the key to avoiding the most common nursing mistakes, Nursing '79 **9**(4):47, 1979.

Hercules, P.R.: Nursing in the postoperative care unit: a review. 1. Respiratory complications, AORN J. **28**:1042, 1978.

Hercules, P.R.: Nursing in the postoperative care unit: a review. 2. Other complications, AORN J. **28**:1049, 1978.

Holley, H.S.: Anesthesia: methods to recovery, AORN J. **21**:822, 1975.

Lewis, K.P., and Cressey, I.: Nursing care for postanesthesia shivering, AORN J. **30**:357, 1979.

McConnell, E.A.: After surgery, Nursing '77 **7**(3):32, 1977.

Robertson, P.A.: Respiratory care in local anesthesia, AORN J. **21**:797, 1975.

Rosenberg, H.: Malignant hyperpyrexia, Am. J. Nurs. **81**:1484, 1981.

Smith, B.J.: Safeguarding your patient after anesthesia, Nursing '78 **8**(10):53, 1978.

Tobias, R.: Circulator, you can help your anesthetist, Point of View **17**:14, 1980.

Wilkinson, P.L., Ham, J., and Miller, R.D.: Clinical anesthesia: case selections from the University of California, San Francisco, St. Louis, 1980, The C.V. Mosby Co.

PART TWO

SURGICAL INTERVENTIONS

10 Laparotomy; abdominal incisions and closures; repair of hernias

Laparotomy

An opening made through the abdominal wall into the peritoneal cavity is called a laparotomy. Surgical procedures are performed for innumerable reasons, and the surgeon chooses the most suitable incision for the procedure to be performed.

Surgical intervention may be necessary to repair or remove traumatized tissue, to cure disease processes by organ removal, and to examine by biopsy or otherwise visualize internal organs for diagnosis. Surgery may be indicated for cosmetic, palliative, or prophylactic reasons.

ANATOMY AND PHYSIOLOGY

The abdominal wall consists of various tissue layers through which dissection must occur to enter the abdominal cavity (Fig. 10-1). The skin and subcutaneous tissue are incised, and blood vessels cauterized or ligated. The anterior fascia is incised, and subsequent muscle layers separated or divided. Fascia covers the muscles anteriorly and posteriorly (Fig. 10-2). The peritoneum is a serous membrane lining the interior abdominal cavity. Excision of this tissue layer exposes abdominal cavity contents.

NURSING CONSIDERATIONS

Nursing care for patients undergoing surgical intervention begins with assessment. A laparotomy may be indicated for any number of reasons, may occur at any age, and is frequently performed on an emergency basis. Individualized care is afforded each patient, integrating physiological preparation with psychological preparation. Explanations to dispel fear and offset the development of anxiety are paramount. Safe, efficient, and sound nursing care is rendered to alleviate the patient's problems, although preoperative contact may be brief.

The nurse should ensure that the patient understands the nature of the surgery and the site of the incision. Preoperative teaching of turning, coughing, and deep breathing is initiated and reinforced after surgery. Nursing considerations for specific surgical procedures are addressed in succeeding chapters.

Setup and preparation of the patient. After the patient is placed in the desired position (Chapter 6), the routine skin preparation is done and the patient is draped (Chapter 5). The basic instruments include the following:

Cutting instruments (Fig. 10-3)

6 Knife handles, no. 3 with blade no. 10, no. 4 with blade no. 20, and no. 7 with blade no. 15
1 Mayo scissors, straight, 6¼ inches
1 Mayo scissors, curved, 6¼ inches
1 Metzenbaum scissors, 7 inches
1 Suture scissors

Holding instruments (Fig. 10-4)

2 Tissue forceps without teeth, 5½ inches
2 Tissue forceps with teeth, 5½ inches
2 Tissue forceps without teeth, 7 and 10 inches
2 Tissue forceps with teeth, 7 and 10 inches
2 Russian tissue forceps, 7 and 10 inches
2 Adson-Brown forceps with teeth
6 Sponge-holding forceps, 10 inches
12 Towel clamps, 3½ or 5½ inches
12 Allis forceps, 6 and 9 inches
4 Babcock intestinal forceps, 6 inches

Clamping instruments (Fig. 10-5)

24 Crile forceps, straight or curved, 5½ inches
12 Rochester-Pean forceps, curved, 6¼ inches
8 Rochester-Pean forceps, curved, 10 inches
6 Rochester-Ochsner or Kocher forceps, straight, 6¼ inches
6 Rochester-Ochsner or Kocher forceps, straight, 9 inches

Exposing instruments (Fig. 10-6)

2 Malleable retractors, 1- to 1½-inch width
2 Vein retractors, small
2 Parker, Roux, Greene, or Army-Navy retractors
6 Richardson or Kelly retractors, small, medium, and large
4 Rake retractors, four- and six-pronged pairs, dull
3 Deaver retractors, small, medium, and large
1 Weitlaner retractor
1 Balfour retractor with blades (optional)

Suturing instruments (Fig. 10-7)

6 Needle holders, 6 and 8 inches
1 Needle set
2 Ligature carriers (optional)
2 Skin hooks (optional)

Accessory items (Fig. 10-8)

1 Frazier suction tip
1 Poole (sump) suction tube and tubing
2 Yankauer suction tubes and tubing
1 Silver probe
1 Grooved director

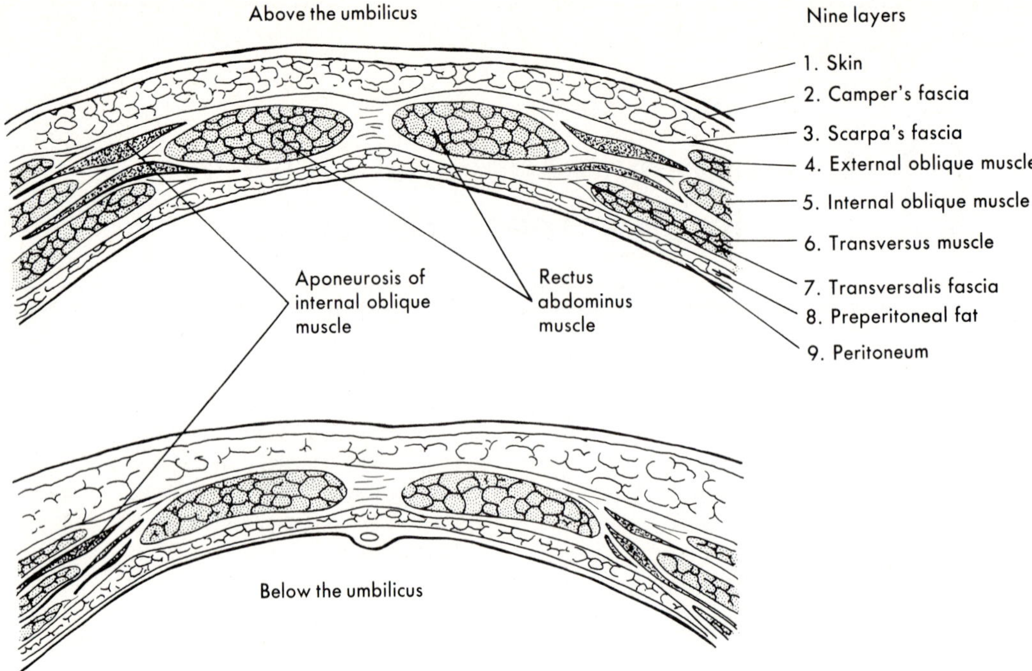

Fig. 10-1. Horizontal section of abdominal wall. Aponeurosis of internal oblique muscle splits into two sections, one lying anterior and other posterior to rectus abdominis muscle, thereby forming encasing sheath around muscle above umbilicus. Below umbilicus, aponeuroses of all muscles pass anterior to rectus. (Redrawn from Anthony, C.P., and Kolthoff, N.J.: Textbook of anatomy and physiology, ed. 9, St. Louis, 1975, The C.V. Mosby Co.)

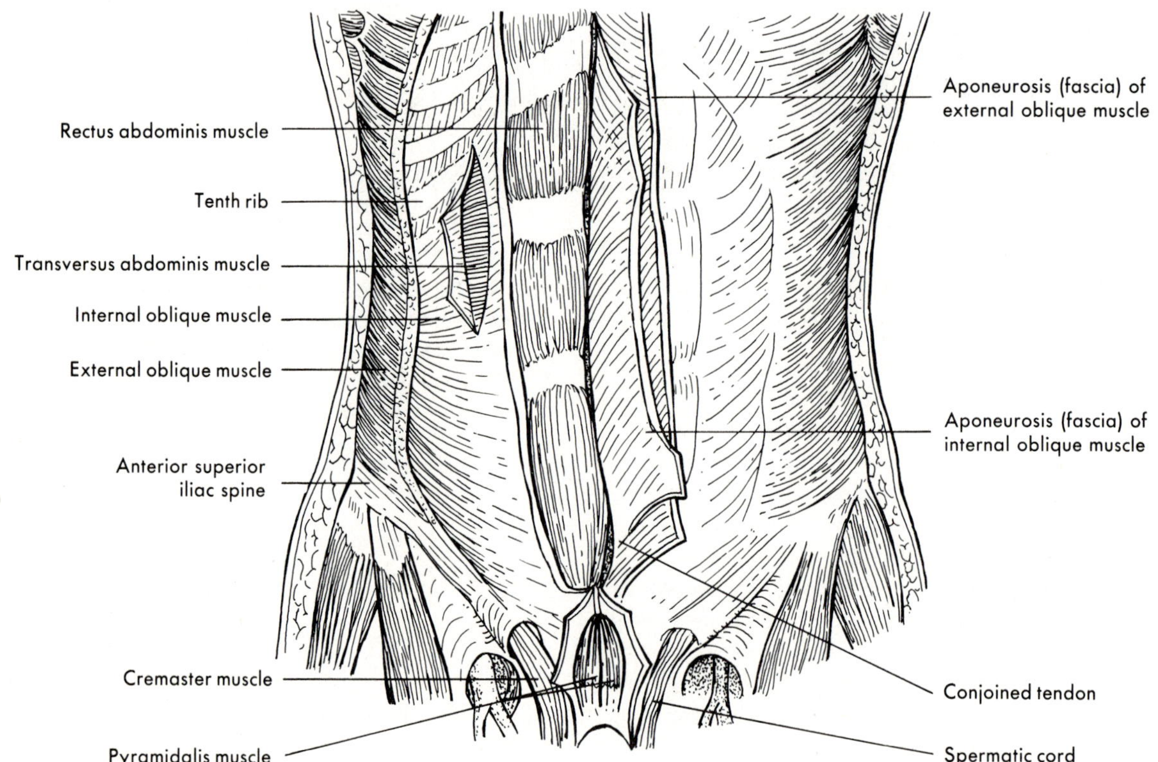

Fig. 10-2. Superior muscles of abdominal wall. (Redrawn from Anthony, C.P., and Kolthoff, N.J.: Textbook of anatomy and physiology, ed. 9, St. Louis, 1975, The C.V. Mosby Co.

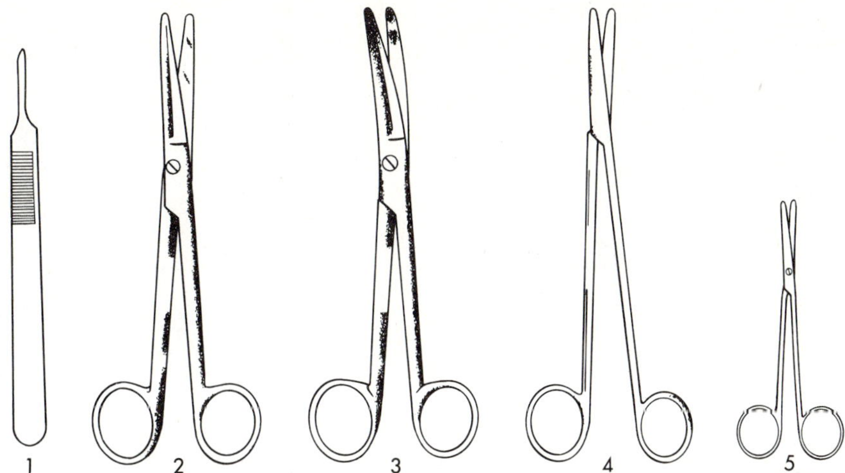

Fig. 10-3. Basic cutting instruments for laparotomy. *1,* Knife handle; *2,* Mayo scissors, straight; *3,* Mayo scissors, curved; *4,* Metzenbaum scissors, curved; *5,* suture scissors, straight. Specific cutting instruments for various procedures are illustrated in following chapters. (Courtesy Codman & Shurtleff, Inc., Randolph, Mass.)

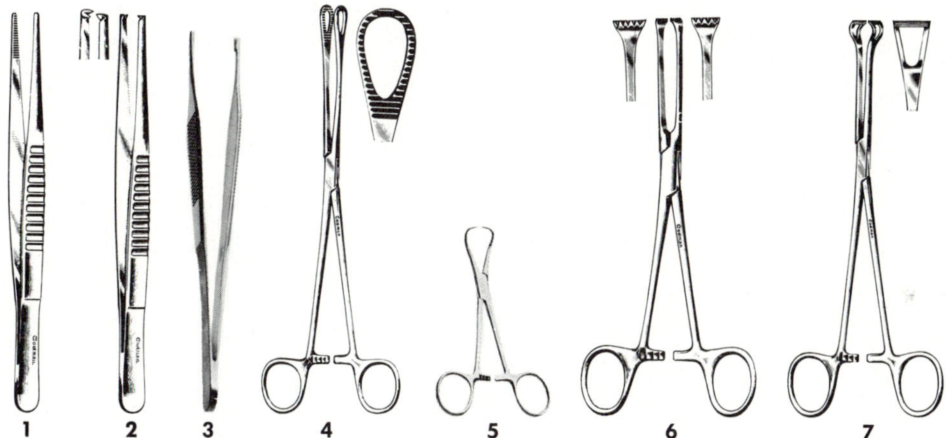

Fig. 10-4. Basic holding instruments for laparotomy. *1,* Tissue forceps, smooth; *2,* tissue forceps with teeth; *3,* Adson-Brown tissue forceps; *4,* sponge-holding forceps; *5,* towel clamps; *6,* Allis tissue forceps; *7,* Babcock intestinal forceps. Specific holding instruments for various procedures are illustrated in following chapters. (Courtesy Codman & Shurtleff, Inc., Randolph, Mass.)

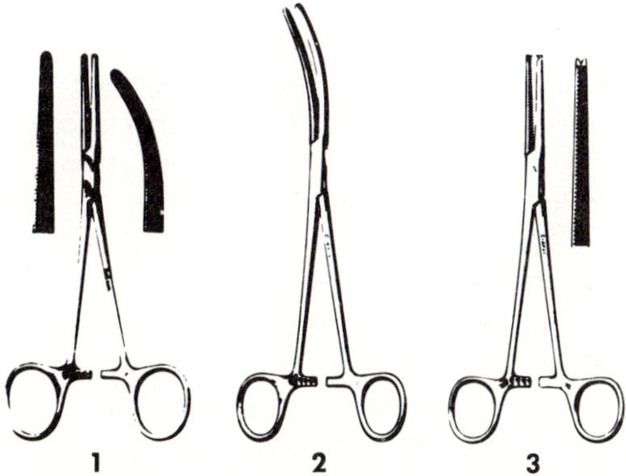

Fig. 10-5. Basic clamping instruments for laparotomy. *1,* Crile hemostatic forceps; *2,* Rochester-Pean hemostatic forceps; *3,* Ochsner or Kocher hemostatic forceps. Specific holding instruments for various procedures are illustrated in following chapters. (Courtesy Codman & Shurtleff, Inc., Randolph, Mass.)

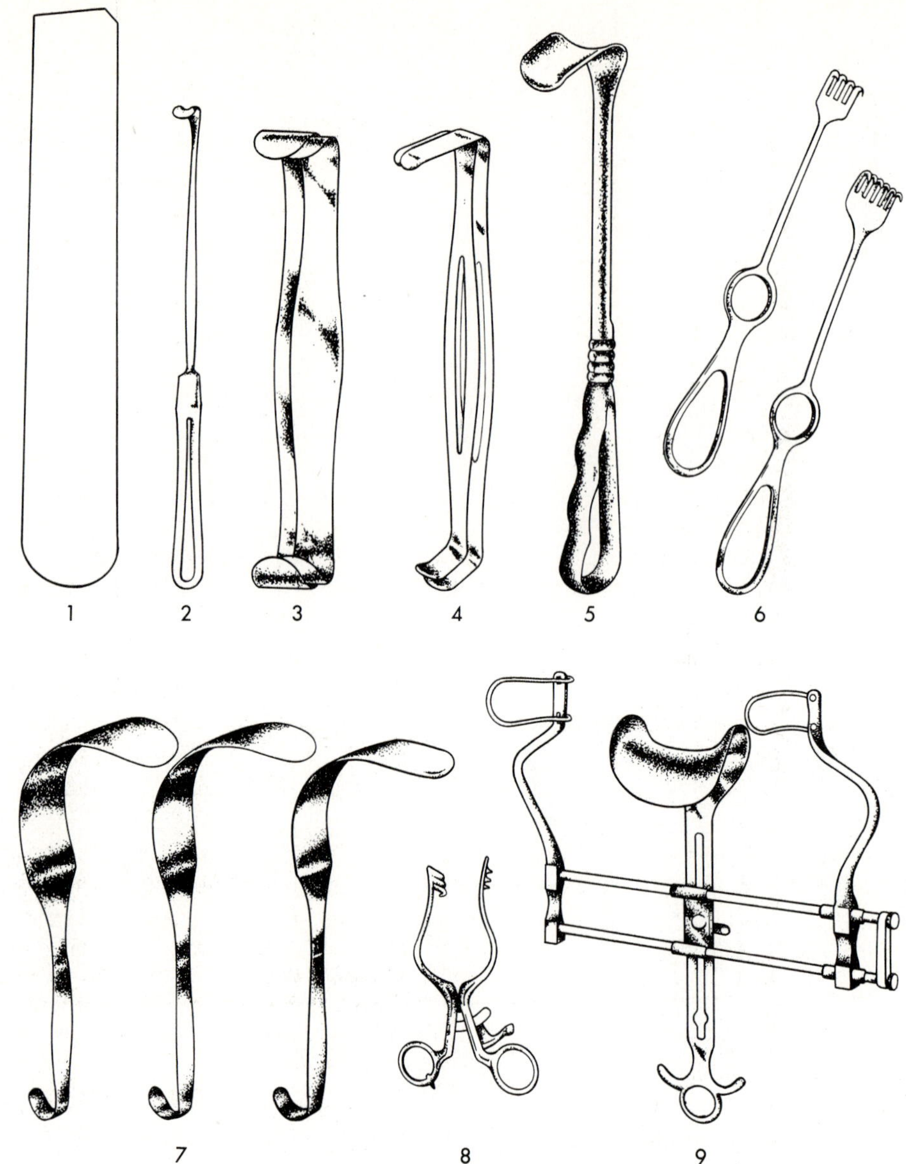

Fig. 10-6. Basic exposing instruments for laparotomy. *1,* Malleable copper retractor; *2,* vein retractor; *3,* Parker retractor; *4,* Army-Navy retractor; *5,* Richardson retractor; *6,* Volkmann rake retractor; *7,* Deaver retractor; *8,* Weitlaner retractor; *9,* Balfour self-retaining retractor with blades. Specific retractors for various procedures are illustrated in following chapters. (Courtesy Codman & Shurtleff, Inc., Randolph, Mass.)

OPERATIVE PROCEDURE

Laparotomy opening

1. Suction tube and tubing are connected, tested, and secured to the field.

2. Laparotomy packs are placed on each side of the proposed incision site to protect the surgeon's gloved hands from the patient's skin and to provide traction for making the skin incision.

3. With handle no. 4 and blade no. 20, the skin incision is made; then the scalpel is discarded.

4. With handle no. 3 and blade no. 10, the incision is continued down to the fascia.

5. Hemostats or ligating clips are used to control bleeding vessels. Clamped vessels are ligated with fine surgical gut, silk, or cotton or are cauterized.

6. If a plastic drape is not used, skin towels are placed to evert the skin edges and exclude them from the inside of the wound. Towel clamps or silk sutures no. 2-0 may be used to secure the skin towels.

   a. Two skin towels folded in half are placed together with folded edges parallel to the incision.
   b. The folded edge of the top towel is clipped or sutured to the skin edges at various points. The operator everts the skin edges with tissue forceps.

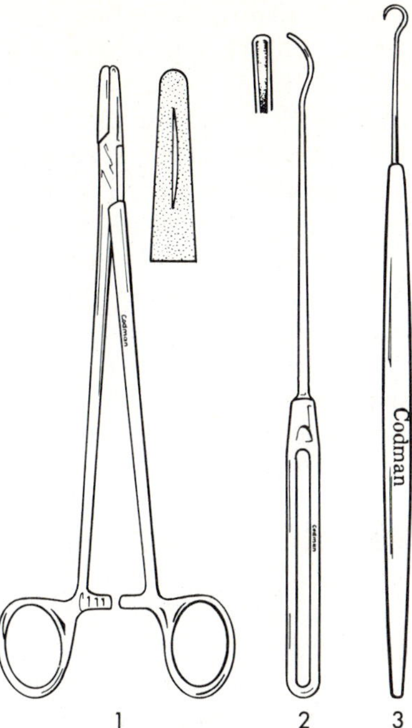

Fig. 10-7. Basic suturing instruments. *1,* Needle holder; *2,* ligature carrier; *3,* skin hook. Specific needle holders for various procedures are illustrated in the following chapters. (Courtesy Codman & Shurtleff, Inc., Randolph, Mass.)

c. The two towels are turned onto the other side of the wound and secured as in b.

d. The top towel is turned back, thereby exposing the wound.

e. The ends of the towels are overlapped at each end of the incision and secured with towel clamps.

7. The wound edges are retracted with small retractors.

8. With tissue forceps and scalpel, the external fascia is incised.

9. With Metzenbaum scissors, the external oblique muscle is split the length of the incision. Bleeding vessels are controlled with hemostats, ligating clips, and/or medium or fine ligatures.

10. The external oblique muscle is then retracted.

11. The internal oblique and transverse muscles are split, parallel to the fibers, up to the rectus sheath with a scalpel or a scissors. These muscles are then retracted. All free sponges are removed from the operative field.

12. The peritoneum is exposed, grasped with smooth tissue forceps, and nicked with scalpel no. 3 and blade no. 10.

13. Sponges and suction are used as needed. Cultures may be taken at this time.

14. The peritoneal incision is extended the length of the wound by Metzenbaum scissors.

15. The peritoneum is retracted with large Richardson retractors for exploration.

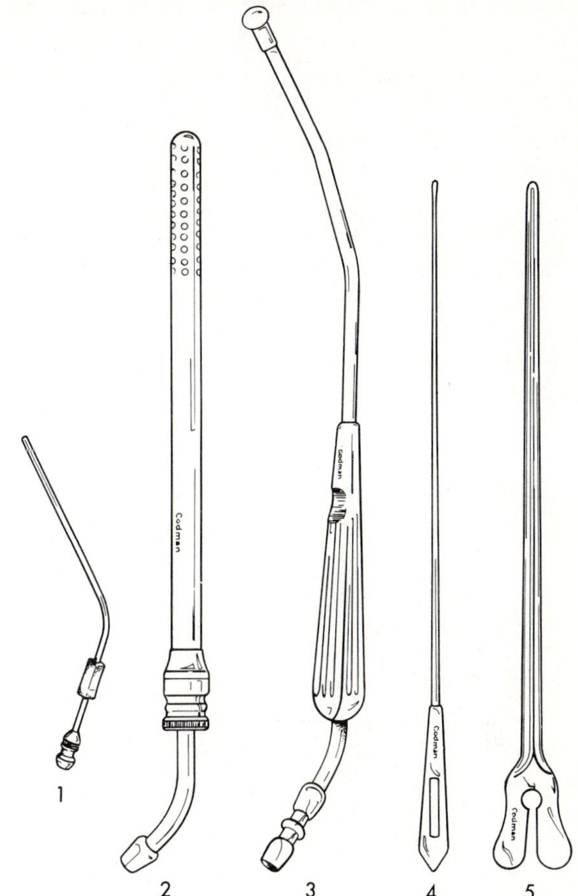

Fig. 10-8. Accessory items. *1,* Frazier suction tip; *2,* Poole suction tube; *3,* Yankauer suction tube; *4,* silver probe; *5,* grooved director. Special accessory items for various procedures are illustrated in following chapters. (Courtesy Codman & Shurtleff, Inc., Randolph, Mass.)

Laparotomy closure

1. Two tissue forceps or clamps are used to approximate the peritoneal edges, and the peritoneum is closed with a continuous chromic suture or interrupted nonabsorbable sutures.

2. The internal oblique and transverse muscles, the small opening at the outer border of the rectus sheath, and the external oblique fascia are closed in layers by interrupted sutures and/or staples. Retraction is necessary as the various layers are closed.

3. If towels and clamps are used, they are removed and discarded. Careful handling facilitates removal without contamination.

4. Clean towels are placed around skin edges.

5. Fine interrupted gut or absorbable synthetic or silk sutures may be used to close the subcutaneous tissue. Retraction is provided with sponges or small retractors.

6. Skin edges are approximated with Adson forceps, and interrupted fine silk or nylon sutures on a cutting needle are used for skin closure. Skin staples or dermaclips are often used to approximate skin edges.

■ Abdominal incisions and closures

The surgeon chooses an incision that will afford maximum exposure of the structures to be operated on, ensure minimal trauma and postoperative discomfort, and provide for primary wound healing with maximum wound strength.

VERTICAL INCISIONS

Vertical midline incision. The vertical midline incision is the simplest abdominal incision. It is an excellent primary incision and generally is preferred because it offers good exposure to any part of the abdominal cavity. It can be extended upward along the xiphoid process, diagonally across the costal border, downward around the umbilicus (avascular, tough connective tissue), back to the midline, and down to the symphysis pubis (Fig. 10-9). The peritoneum is incised, and the round ligament of the liver is divided.

To close the wound, the peritoneum and round ligament are approximated and sutured with surgical gut or nonabsorbable sutures. Sometimes the suture line is supported by using retention sutures, through-and-through sutures extending out through the subcutaneous tissue to the skin. Fascia, subcutaneous tissue, and skin are closed as layers. An alternative closure uses figure-of-eight sutures of stainless steel wire or Prolene; the peritoneum and posterior fascia may be closed in a single layer.

Paramedian rectus incision. When on the appropriate side, the paramedian rectus incision can be used in any intraabdominal surgery (Fig. 10-10). It is made parallel and about 4 cm lateral to the midline. The skin and subcutaneous tissue are incised, the anterior rectus sheath is divided, and the rectus muscle is retracted laterally, thus preserving the motor nerves. The posterior rectus sheath and peritoneum are opened vertically lateral to the midline.

The advantages of a paramedian incision are as follows: the abdominal cavity can be quickly entered; the incision avoids nerve injury, limits trauma to the rectus muscle, produces less bleeding, and permits anatomical layer closure; and the original incision can be extended upward to the costal margin or downward to the symphysis pubis.

The peritoneum can be approximated and closed with a continuous suture of chromic gut no. 2-0 or 0 or with interrupted natural or synthetic, nonabsorbable sutures no. 2-0 or 0. The posterior rectus sheath and fascial layers are approximated and closed with interrupted nonabsorbable sutures. Retention sutures may also be used. The superficial fascial layers are closed with finer interrupted sutures. The skin edges are approximated and closed with fine silk, nylon, staples, or dermaclips.

OBLIQUE INCISIONS

McBurney muscle-splitting incision. The McBurney muscle-splitting incision is used for the removal of the appendix. It is an 8-cm oblique incision that begins well

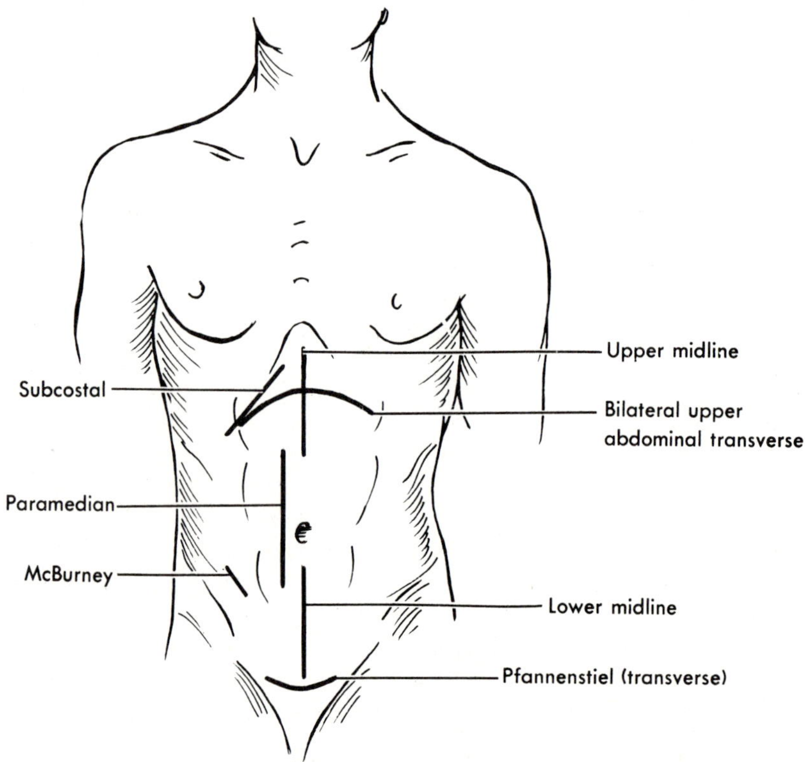

Fig. 10-9. Incisions made through abdominal wall.

below the umbilicus, goes through McBurney's point, and extends upward toward the right flank (Fig. 10-9). The external oblique muscle and fascia are split in the direction of their fibers and are retracted. The internal oblique muscle, transversalis muscle, and fascia are split and retracted. The peritoneum is incised transversely, and closure is as described for laparotomy. This incision is quick and easy to close and allows a firm wound closure. However, it does not permit good exposure and is difficult to extend. To extend the incision medially, the inferior epigastric vessels are ligated, and the rectus sheath is incised transversely.

Subcostal incision. The subcostal incision is made on the right side and preferred sometimes for operations on the gallbladder, common duct, or pancreas. When made on the left side, it may be used for splenectomy. This incision usually gives only limited exposure unless the patient is short with a wide abdomen and wide costal margins. The advantages of this type of incision are as follows: it provides good cosmetic results because it follows the skin lines, the nerve damage is limited because only one or two nerves are cut, tension on the incisional edges is less than in a vertical incision, it can readily be extended for wide exposure, and it causes less respiratory embarrassment.

This oblique incision begins in the epigastrium, extending laterally and obliquely downward to just below the lower costal margin (Fig. 10-11). Each muscle contains veins and arteries requiring ligation. If more exposure is needed, the incision is extended across the rectus muscle of the other side. The rectus muscle is either retracted or transversely divided. Vessels in the muscle must be ligated.

The closure of this incision includes approximation and closure of the falciform ligament, peritoneum, posterior rectus sheath, and anterior rectus sheath with interrupted, nonabsorbable sutures no. 2-0 or 0. The subcutaneous tissue and skin are closed as described for laparotomy. Absorbable sutures no. 2-0 or 0 may be used in conjunction with staples.

TRANSVERSE INCISIONS

Pfannenstiel incision. The Pfannenstiel incision is used frequently for gynecological surgery. It is a curved transverse incision across the lower abdomen through the skin, subcutaneous tissue, and rectus sheaths (Fig. 10-12). The rectus muscles are separated in midline, and the peritoneum is entered through a midline vertical incision. This incision provides for a strong closure; when the rectus muscles contract, there is less strain on the fascial sutures.

Midabdominal transverse incision. The midabdominal transverse incision is used on the left or right side or for a retroperitoneal approach. The incision begins slightly above or below the umbilicus on either side and is carried laterally to the lumbar region at an angle between the ribs and crest of the ilium. The skin and subcutaneous tissue are incised, the anterior rectus sheath is split, the rectus muscle is divided, and the vessels within the rectus are clamped and ligated. The posterior rectus sheath and

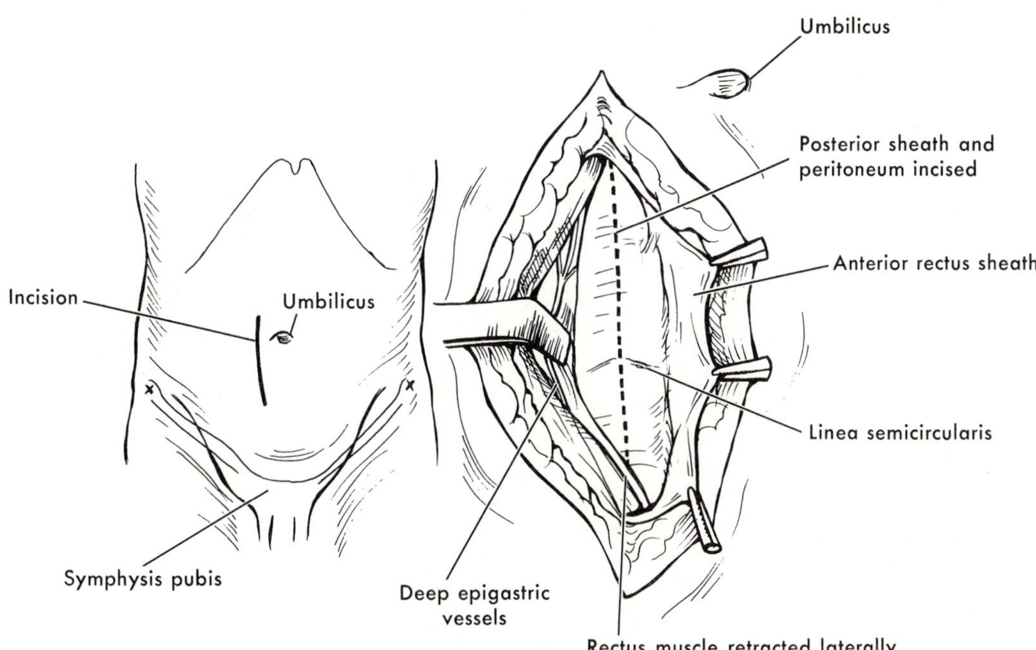

Fig. 10-10. *Left,* Location of right vertical paramedian rectus incision; *right,* anterior rectus sheath is divided, rectus muscle retracted, and posterior sheath and peritoneum exposed.

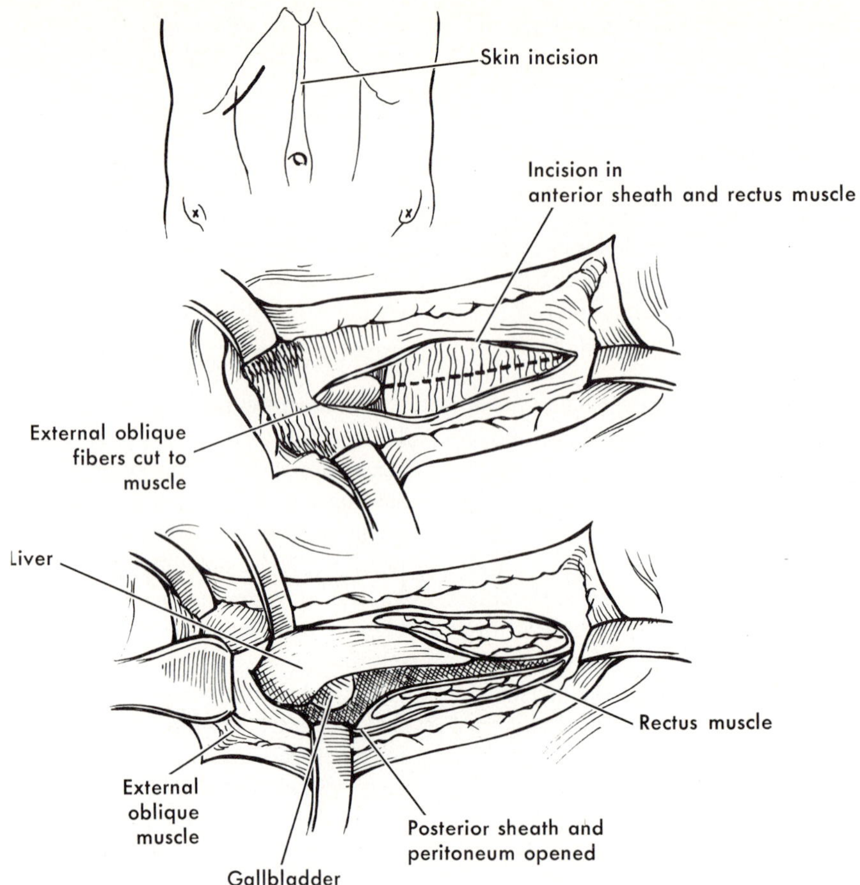

Fig. 10-11. Position of subcostal incision is shown in upper right quadrant. Anterior sheath has been divided transversely, and muscle is exposed. Posterior sheath and peritoneum have been opened transversely.

peritoneum are cut in the direction of the fibers, preserving the intercostal nerves. The peritoneum is incised near the midline, and the incision is extended laterally to the oblique muscle. The lateral muscles are incised to provide wide exposure. The closure is in layers with interrupted sutures; the subcutaneous tissue and skin are closed as for laparotomy.

Thoracoabdominal incision. The thoracoabdominal incision is used for operations on the proximal portion of the stomach and the distal section of the esophagus. Often the abdominal part of the incision is made first for exploration and then, if necessary, is extended across the costal margin into the chest.

The incision begins at a point midway between the xiphoid process and the umbilicus, extending across to the seventh or eighth interspace and to the midscapular line (Fig. 10-13). The rectus and oblique abdominal muscles are divided in the line of incision down to the peritoneum and pleura. Then the costal cartilage and the diaphragm are divided (Fig. 10-13).

The wound is closed in layers with interrupted sutures. Surgical gut may be used for the peritoneum and intercostal muscles. Nonabsorbable suture may be used for the muscle and fascial layers. Skin edges are approximated with silk or another nonabsorbable material.

Upper inverted-U abdominal incision. An upper inverted-U abdominal incision is not used frequently today; however, it can be used for gastrectomy, transverse colon resection, transverse colostomy, biliary, and pancreatic procedures. The incision extends from a point below the costal margin on one side in the anterior axillary line to the same point on the opposite side. It is curved, with the midpoint lying midway between the xiphoid process and the umbilicus. The intercostal nerves are preserved.

An upper abdominal transverse incision is closed by placing interrupted sutures in the peritoneum and anterior and posterior rectus sheaths. The muscle and fat need not be sutured. The skin edges are approximated and closed as described for laparotomy.

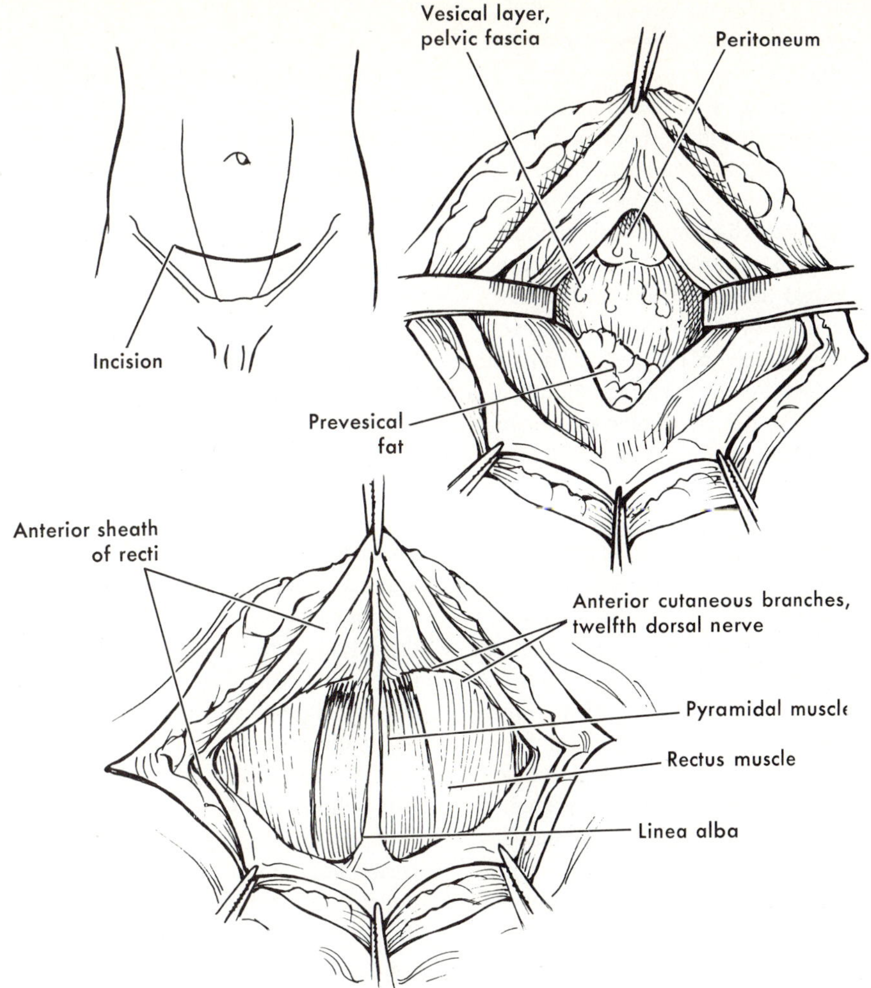

Fig. 10-12. Pfannenstiel incision (transverse).

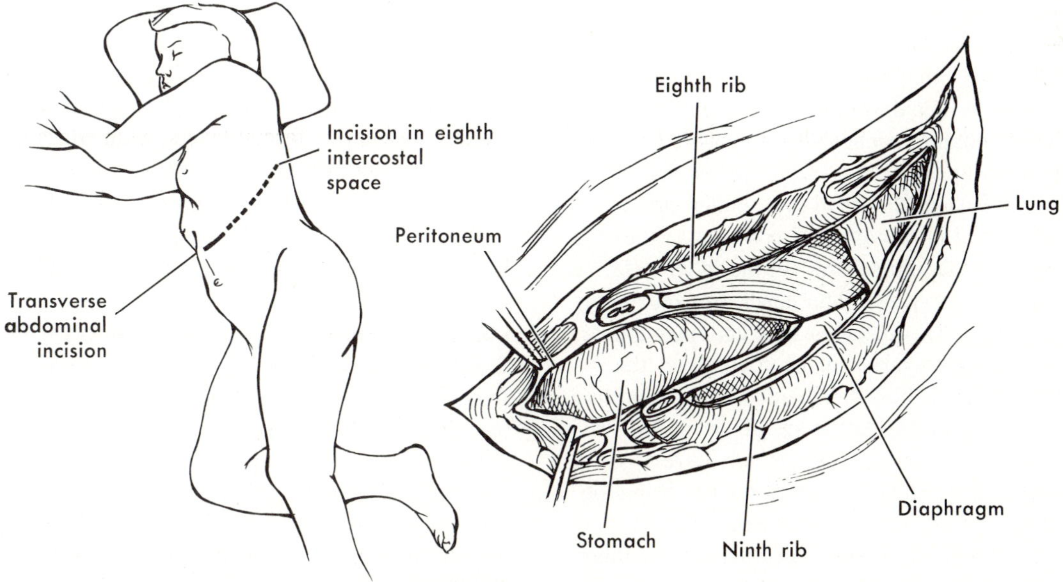

Fig. 10-13. Thoracoabdominal incision. Patient is placed on unaffected side. Incision is usually made from point midway between xiphoid process and umbilicus to costal margin at site of eighth costal cartilage. Dissection is carried down to peritoneum and pleura. Costal cartilage and diaphragm are divided, and stomach exposed.

■ Repair of hernias

A hernia is the displacement of intraabdominal tissue or viscus through a congenital or acquired opening or fascial defect in the abdominal wall. In general, hernias of the abdominal wall occur far less frequently in women than in men, with the greatest disparity in the incidence of indirect and direct inguinal hernias. Femoral hernias are more evenly distributed between males and females and account for more than 5% of all hernias in both sexes. About 75% of all hernias occur in the groin, with the remaining 25% distributed among ventral, umbilical, femoral, and other types. As the frequency and magnitude of abdominal surgery have increased in recent years, so has the incidence of incisional hernia. Herniorrhaphy is one of the most common operative procedures performed and is the preferred treatment for all population groups when a defect is detected. There are several places in the abdominal wall where rupture, with protrusion of a portion of the parietal peritoneum and often a part of the intestine, can occur.

The weak places or intervals in the abdominal aponeurosis are (1) the inguinal canals, (2) the femoral rings, and (3) the umbilicus. Any number of conditions causing increased pressure within the abdomen will contribute to the formation of a hernia in the patient. Contributing factors to hernia formation include age, sex, obesity, nutritional state, and pulmonary and cardiac disease. Loss of tissue turgor occurs with aging and in chronic debilitating disease.

ANATOMY AND PHYSIOLOGY

A *hernia* is a sac lined by peritoneum that is pushed through a defect in the layers of the abdominal wall. Generally, a hernial mass is composed of covering tissues, a peritoneal sac, and any contained viscera, which may be acquired or congenital. Depending on their location, hernias are classified as either direct inguinal, indirect inguinal, femoral, umbilical, or epigastric. Hernias in any of these groups are either *reducible* or *irreducible*. That is, the contents of the hernia sac either can be returned to the normal intraabdominal position, or they are trapped in the extraabdominal sac. In the latter case the hernia is called *incarcerated*. The conditions preventing the return of the hernial contents to the abdomen can result from (1) adhesions between the contents of the sac and the inner lining of the sac, (2) adhesions among the contents of the sac, or (3) narrowing of the neck of the sac. Patients with incarcerated hernias may have signs of intestinal obstruction, such as vomiting and distention. The great danger of an incarcerated hernia is that it may become *strangulated*. In a strangulated hernia, the blood supply of the trapped sac contents becomes compromised, and eventually the sac contents necrose. When bowel is trapped in such a hernia, resection of dead bowel, in addition to the repair of the hernia defect, becomes mandatory.

The anterolateral abdominal wall consists of an arrangement of muscles, fascial layers, and muscular aponeuroses lined interiorly by peritoneum and exteriorly by skin. The abdominal wall in the groin area seems to be composed of two groups of these structures: a superficial group—Scarpa's fascia, external and internal oblique muscles, and their aponeuroses—and a deep group—the internal oblique transverse fascia and peritoneum (Fig. 10-2).

Inguinal hernias

Essential to an understanding of inguinal hernia repair is an appreciation of the central role of the transversalis fascia as the major supporting structure of the posterior inguinal floor. The inguinal canal, which contains the spermatic cord and associated structures in the male and the round ligament in the female, is approximately 4 cm long and takes an oblique course parallel to the groin crease. The inguinal canal is covered by the aponeurosis of the external abdominal oblique muscle, which forms a roof (Fig. 10-14). A thickened lower border of the external oblique aponeurosis forms the inguinal ligament (Poupart's). This ligament stretches from the anterior superior iliac spine to the pubic tubercle. Structures that traverse the inguinal canal enter it from the abdomen by the internal ring, a natural opening in the transversalis fascia, and exit by the external ring, an opening in the external oblique aponeurosis to go to either the testis or the labium. If the external oblique aponeurosis is opened and the cord or round ligament mobilized, the floor of the inguinal canal is exposed. The posterior inguinal floor is the structure that becomes defective and gives rise to hernias, be they indirect, direct, or femoral.

The key component of this important posterior inguinal floor is the transversalis muscle of the abdomen and its associated aponeurosis and fascia. The posterior inguinal floor can be divided into two areas. The superior lateral area represents the internal ring, whereas the inferior medial area represents the attachment of the transversalis aponeurosis and fascia to Cooper's ligament (iliopectineal line). Cooper's ligament is the insertion of the transversalis aponeurosis along the superior ramus from the symphysis pubis laterally to the femoral sheath. It is important to appreciate that the inguinal portion of the transversalis fascia arises from the iliopsoas fascia and not from the inguinal ligament.

Medially and superiorly, the transversalis muscle becomes aponeurotic and fuses with the aponeurosis of the internal oblique muscle to form anterior and posterior rectus sheaths. As the symphysis pubis is approached, the contributions from the internal oblique muscle become less and less. At the pubic tubercle and behind the spermatic

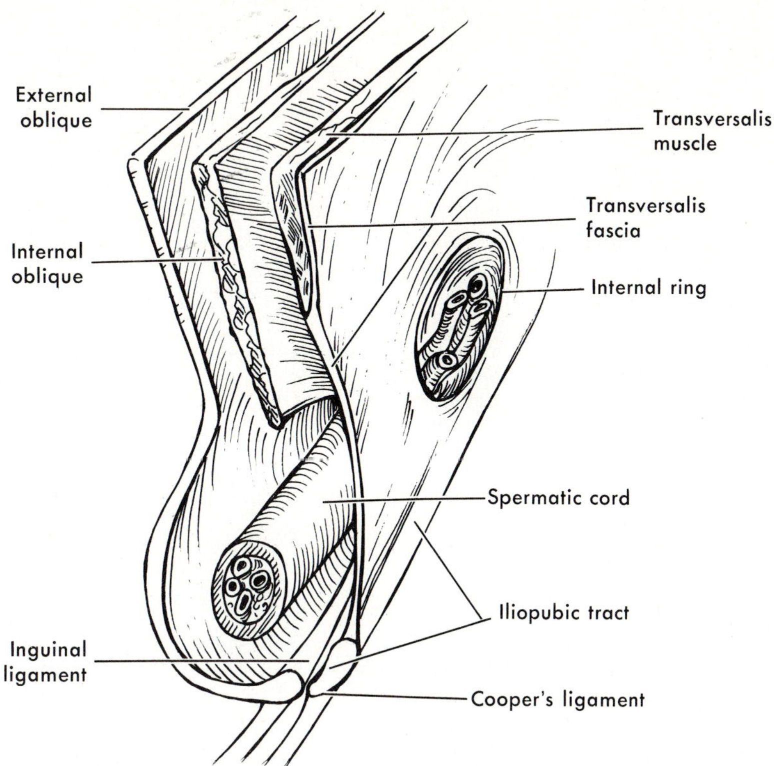

Fig. 10-14. Right inguinal region, parasagittal section. Roof of inguinal canal is formed by external oblique aponeurosis, while floor is formed by transversalis aponeurosis and fascia. (From Nyhus, L.M., and Harkins, H.N.: Hernia, Philadelphia, J.B. Lippincott Co.)

cord or round ligament, the internal oblique muscle makes no contribution, and the posterior inguinal wall (floor of the inguinal canal) is composed solely of aponeurosis and fascia of the transversalis muscle.

Direct versus indirect

The deep epigastric vessels (inferior epigastric) arise from the external iliac vessels and enter the inguinal canal just proximal to the internal ring. The triangle formed by the deep epigastric vessels laterally, the inguinal ligament inferiorly, and the rectus abdominis muscle medially is referred to as Hesselbach's triangle (Fig. 10-15). Hernias that occur within Hesselbach's triangle are called *direct hernias. Indirect hernias* occur lateral to the deep epigastric vessels (Fig. 10-16). Therefore both direct and indirect hernias represent attenuations or tears in the transversalis fascia.

Direct hernias protrude into the inguinal canal but not into the cord and therefore rarely into the scrotum. Direct inguinal hernias usually result from heavy lifting or other strenuous activities.

Indirect hernias leave the abdominal cavity at the internal inguinal ring and pass with the cord structures down the inguinal canal. Consequently, the indirect hernia sac may be found in the scrotum. Indirect hernias may be either congenital, representing a persistence of the processus vaginalis, or acquired. In the former case, the hernia sac has a small neck, is thin walled, and is closely bound to the cord structures. In an acquired indirect hernia, the neck is wide, and the sac is both short and thick walled. When both direct and indirect hernias are present, the defect is called a "pantaloon" hernia after the French word for pants, which this situation suggests. Clearly, with both direct and indirect hernias, the defect is in the transversalis fascia. The external oblique and the internal oblique muscles can only influence the direction that a hernia subsequently takes, but they are not responsible for the initial appearance of the hernia.

NURSING CONSIDERATIONS

Care of the patient encompasses the role of the scrub nurse. A review of anatomy will help the nurse anticipate instrumentation for the procedure. The scrub nurse's prime concern is to expedite the operation in an effective, efficient, and safe manner.

Instruments used for herniorrhaphies are those found in standard laparotomy sets. A self-retaining retractor facilitates the separation of tissue layers. A Penrose drain

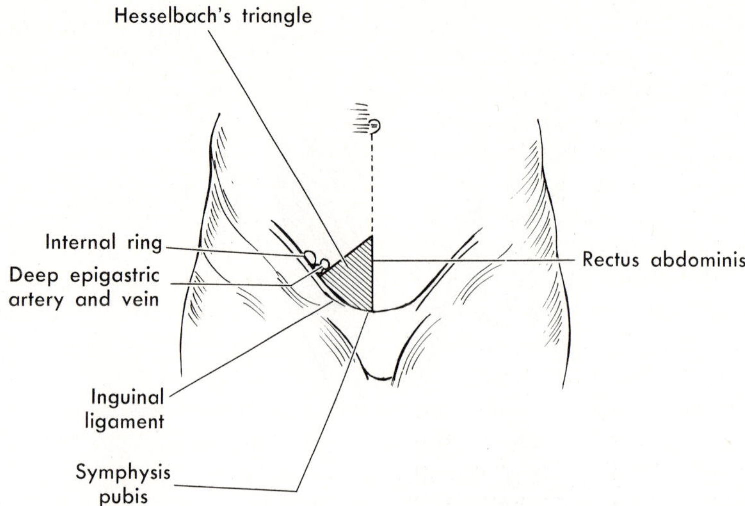

Fig. 10-15. Schematic representation of Hesselbach's triangle. Boundaries of Hesselbach's triangle are deep epigastric vessels laterally, inguinal ligament inferiorly, and rectus abdominus muscle medially.

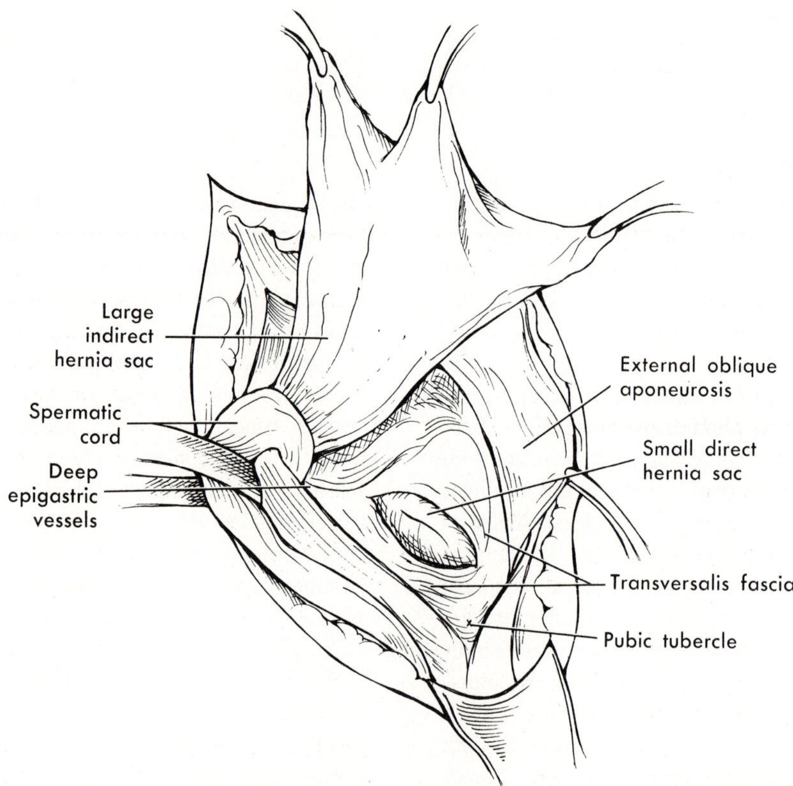

Fig. 10-16. Defect in transversalis fascia, medial to deep epigastric vessels, gives rise to direct hernia. Defect lateral to deep epigastric vessels results in indirect hernia. (From Maingot, R.: Abdominal operations, ed. 6, New York, 1974, Appleton-Century-Crofts.)

may be used to retract the spermatic cord structures for better exposure. Since the peritoneal cavity may be exposed in this procedure, accurate sponge and needle counts must be carried out.

In dealing with a sliding hernia or an incarcerated hernia, the possibility of having to enter the peritoneal cavity must be considered. If the hernia is strangulated, necrotic bowel must be resected, and instruments for making a bowel anastomosis must be ready.

Repair of the inguinal hernia includes approximation of the transversalis fascia with a heavy, nonabsorbable type of suture. With some indirect hernias, only two or three of these sutures may be necessary. In other cases, however, up to ten sutures in rapid succession may be requested. Numerous types of needles are used for hernia repair. Mayo and Ferguson needles are two of the most frequently requested. When actual repair of the hernia is completed, four additional layers of tissue are usually approximated. These layers add nothing to the strength of the repair and therefore are done with finer suture materials. The cremaster is approximated around the cord, and the external oblique aponeurosis is closed with a fine (4-0) nonabsorbable suture. Scarpa's fascia is approximated with an absorbable material, and the skin is closed by any number of methods. The scrub nurse should anticipate these multiple layers and have sufficient amounts of the different suture materials and an adequate supply of needles.

Routine nursing care is similar to that for any type of abdominal surgery. Preoperatively, the patient is assessed and protected from respiratory infections that may cause increased intraabdominal pressure postoperatively. Coughing and sneezing should be minimized to prevent tension on the newly repaired tissues. The patient is instructed to hold a hand firmly over the operative site if coughing occurs.

Urinary retention may occur after a herniorrhaphy, and measures must be taken to prevent overdistention of the bladder. Early ambulation is permitted to encourage the resumption of bladder and bowel function. If bowel has been resected because of strangulation, a nasogastric tube and suction may be required to reduce the incidence of postoperative vomiting and distention with subsequent strain on the suture line.

Postoperative inflammation or swelling of the scrotum from manipulation is reduced with the application of a suspensory and/or ice. The patient is reassured that ecchymosis and discomfort will diminish within a few days and that sexual functioning should not be affected.

The patient is discharged from 1 to 4 days after surgery. The patient who has had elective surgery for a hernia is restricted from strenuous activity for at least 3 weeks and needs to understand that good body alignment and/or possible modification in occupation is necessary. The potential for recurrence of a hernia always exists if old habits are continued.

OPERATIVE PROCEDURES

A number of operative procedures for repair of inguinal hernias exist. Approaches that reestablish the integrity of the transversalis layer and simultaneously reestablish the posterior inguinal floor are favored currently. An anatomical repair in which transversalis fascia is sewn to transversalis fascia accomplishes this goal. A McVay or Cooper's ligament repair approximates transversalis fascia superiorly to the inferior insertion of the transversalis fascia along Cooper's ligament. The following steps highlight the essentials of these repairs:

1. The patient is in the supine position. A 6-cm oblique incision is made parallel to the inguinal ligament, ending two finger breadths lateral to the pubic tubercle. Frequently, the skin is lightly crosshatched to facilitate later closure (Fig. 10-17).
2. The incision is carried through the superficial and deep (Scarpa's) fascia to the external oblique aponeurosis. Hemostasis is maintained with fine ties or electrocoagulation.
3. The external oblique aponeurosis is opened in the direction of its fibers to the external ring, and the aponeurotic flaps are reflected back along the iliohypogastric and ilioinguinal nerves, which are usually encountered at this point (Fig. 10-17).
4. The cremaster muscles that form an envelope around the cord and represent the continuation of the internal oblique muscles are opened and the cord exposed.
5. By gentle dissection, the spermatic vessels and the vas deferens are separated. While this is being done, the cord is examined for an indirect hernia, which arises from the internal ring and is initially adherent to the cord.
6. If an indirect sac is identified, it is carefully dissected away from the cord until the neck of the hernia is clearly delineated (Fig. 10-18).
7. The sac is opened, and any abdominal contents are returned to the abdominal cavity.
8. A suture ligature is placed high in the neck of the sac, and the excess peritoneum of the hernia is excised. The ligated stump quickly retracts into the peritoneal cavity. If only a direct sac is present, usually no resection of the hernia is done, since the sac easily returns to the abdominal cavity.
9. If transversalis fascia is present on either side of the hernia defect, it is sutured together (Fig. 10-19). Suturing begins at the symphysis pubis and continues laterally to the internal ring. If the transversalis fascia inferiorly is weak or not present, the superior portion of the transversalis fascia is sutured to Cooper's ligament, the site of insertion of the transversalis fascia. In this case, suturing again begins at the pubic tubercle and is continued laterally along Cooper's ligament to the medial border of the femoral sheath, where a transition stitch is placed. The repair is then carried laterally, approximating transversalis fascia to inguinal ligament (Fig. 10-20).

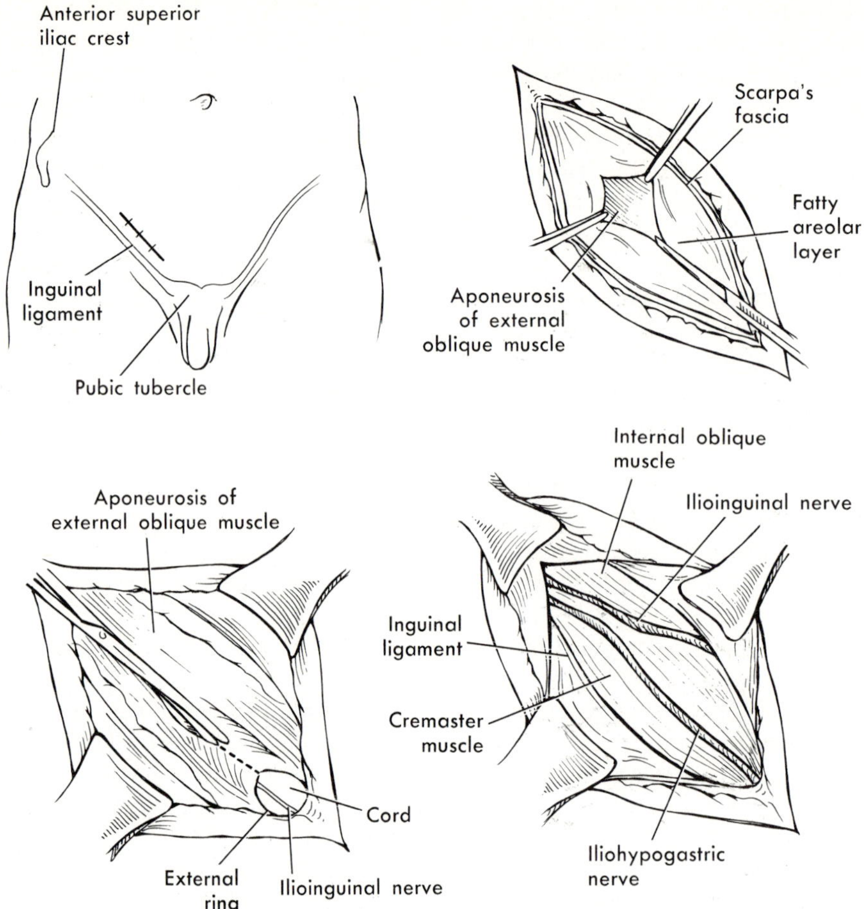

Fig. 10-17. Skin incision with division of superficial muscle and fascial layers. (From Madden, J.L.: Atlas of techniques in surgery, ed. 2, New York, Appleton-Century-Crofts.)

10. When the transversalis fascia is pulled down to Cooper's ligament, a relaxing incision in the rectus sheath is sometimes necessary to relieve excess tension. Essentially, this is an incision 5 to 7 cm long in the anterior rectus sheath. The incision begins immediately above the pubic crest, approximately 1 cm from the midline, and extends cephalad, following the line of fusion of the external oblique aponeurosis with the rectus sheath. The posterior rectus sheath and the rectus muscle itself guard against later herniation at the point where the relaxing incision is made. In some situations, a prosthetic patch, such as Marlex mesh, may be used to cover the hernia defect to allow repair without undue stress.

11. After the integrity of the posterior inguinal floor has been reestablished, the cremaster muscles are reapproximated around the cord. Repair is completed with the approximation of the external oblique aponeurosis, Scarpa's fascia, and the skin.

Bassini repair

The Bassini repair approach to the hernia and the treatment of the sac is identical to that previously described. The major difference with this repair is that the superior transversalis fascia is sutured to the inguinal ligament with no attempt made to approximate it to the inferior portion of the transversalis fascia or Cooper's ligament. Critics of this procedure claim that it is not anatomical, since layers that originally are not one (transversalis fascia and inguinal ligament) now are approximated. Nonetheless, this repair is extremely popular and is used successfully by many surgeons.

Shouldice repair

Again the approach to the hernia is the same as previously described, but in the Shouldice repair, a double layer of transversalis fascia is sutured to the inguinal ligament. This is reinforced by a layer of internal oblique muscle and conjoined tendon approximated to the undersurface of the fascia of the external oblique. At the Shouldice Clinic in Toronto, where this procedure was developed and now is used exclusively, the recurrence rate is about 1%.

Repair of hernias in females

Regardless of the specific technique used, the initial approach to the repair of a hernia in the female is the

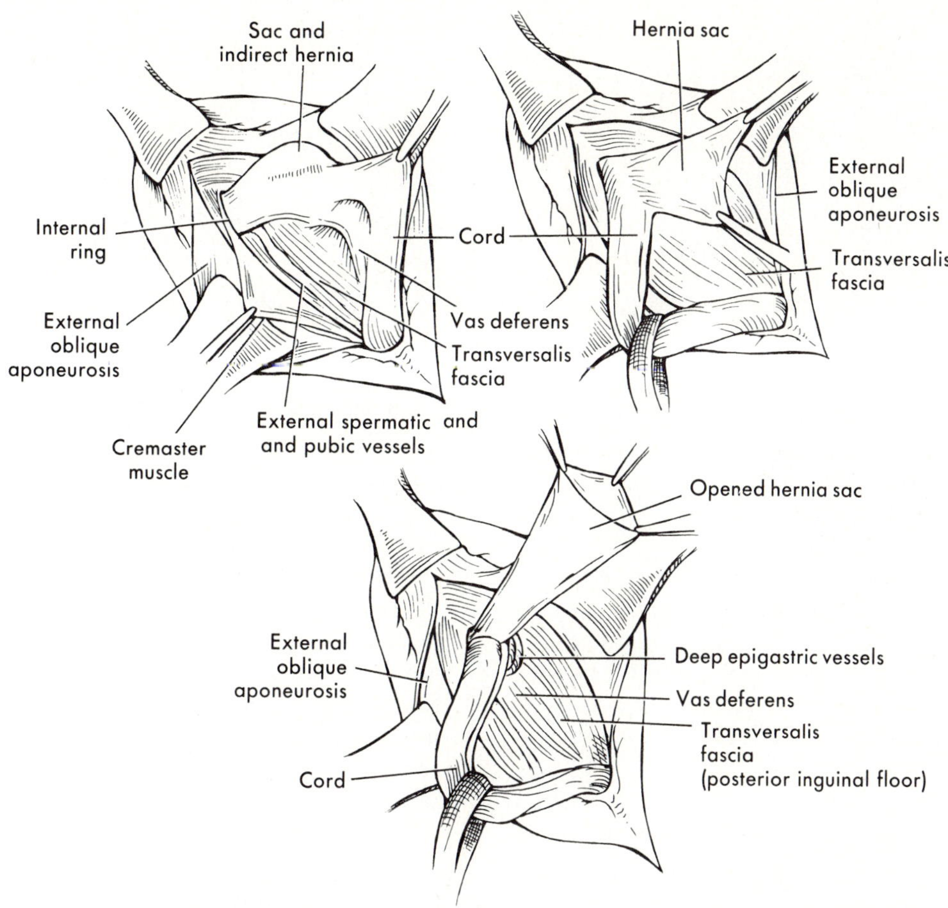

Fig. 10-18. Indirect hernia sac is identified along with cord structures and dissected away from cord. Neck of hernia sac is clearly delineated, and sac opened to check for abdominal contents. (From Madden, J.L.: Atlas of techniques in surgery, ed. 2, New York, Appleton-Century-Crofts.)

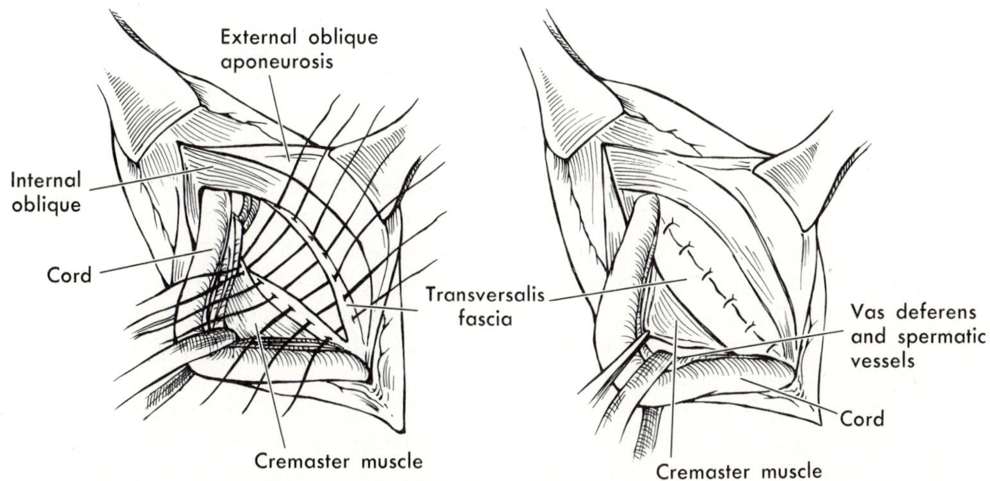

Fig. 10-19. Transversalis fascia on either side of large hernia defect is approximated. (From Madden, J.L.: Atlas of techniques in surgery, ed. 2, New York, Appleton-Century-Crofts.)

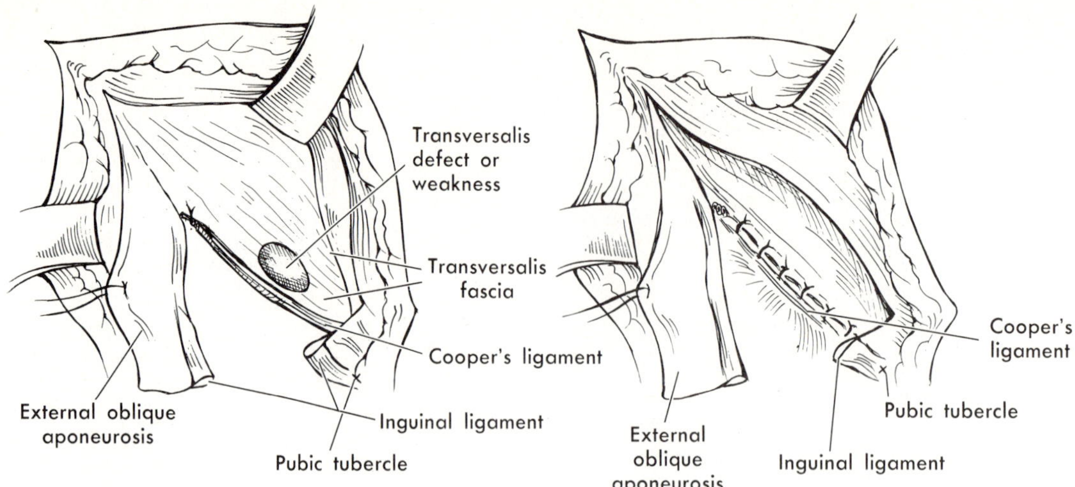

Fig. 10-20. Defect in transversalis fascia repaired by approximation of transversalis fascia to Cooper's ligament. (From Nyhus, L.M., and Harkins, H.N.: Hernia, Philadelphia, J.B. Lippincott Co.)

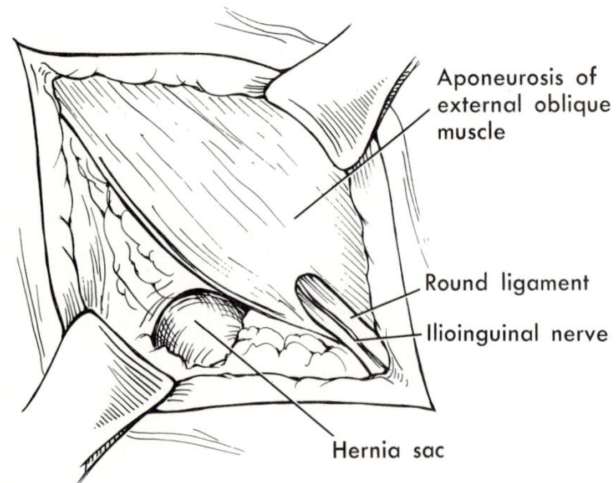

Fig. 10-21. Bulge from femoral hernia occurring below inguinal ligament. (From Madden, J.L.: Atlas of techniques in surgery, ed. 2, New York, Appleton-Century-Crofts.)

same as that used in the male. After the cremaster muscles are opened to expose the round ligament, variations that may be encountered include the following: (1) with the sac exposed and cleared from the round ligament, the round ligament and accompanying vessels are dissected free from the inguinal floor to the labium; (2) at the labium the round ligament is clamped, ligated, and divided; (3) the sac at the internal ring is opened, checked to be sure that no abdominal contents are present, and ligated at its neck, together with the round ligament and associated vessels; (4) the sac distal to the ligature is removed with the distal round ligament, while the ligated stump retracts promptly into the abdomen; (5) the remainder of the repair is the same as that previously described.

Repair of femoral hernias

A femoral hernia protrudes from the groin, below the inguinal ligament into the thigh (Fig. 10-21). In its most obvious form, a femoral hernia presents as an inflamed, tender mass with bowel sounds below the inguinal ligament. Unfortunately, the presentation is frequently more subtle, and the diagnosis is completely missed or confused with enlarged inguinal lymph nodes, a psoas abscess, a saphenous varix, or a lipoma. Usually the defect is small and, frequently, irreducible. The general approach is surgical treatment to free the tightly bound hernia, closely examine the contents of the hernia for ischemic change, and repair the hernia defect. The principles for repair of this type of hernia are the same as those which are the basis for other inguinal herniorrhaphies. Ultimately, repair of the transversalis fascia must be accomplished.

Preperitoneal (properitoneal) repair

Preperitoneal (properitoneal) repair also is based on the essential role of the transversalis fascia in the cause and subsequent correction of a hernia. This repair is suitable for direct, indirect, and femoral hernias. It is particularly applicable in dealing with recurrent hernias, since exposure is obtained by operating through virgin surgical fields rather than through previous scars. Steps for this procedure are as follows:

1. A transverse incision is made 2 cm above the symphysis pubis, over the rectus on the affected side (Fig. 10-22, *A*).
2. The wound is deepened by cutting the external oblique, internal oblique, and transversalis muscles.
3. The transversalis fascia is then cut, and the preperitoneal space is entered. This is the proper plane of dissection for the remainder of the operation.

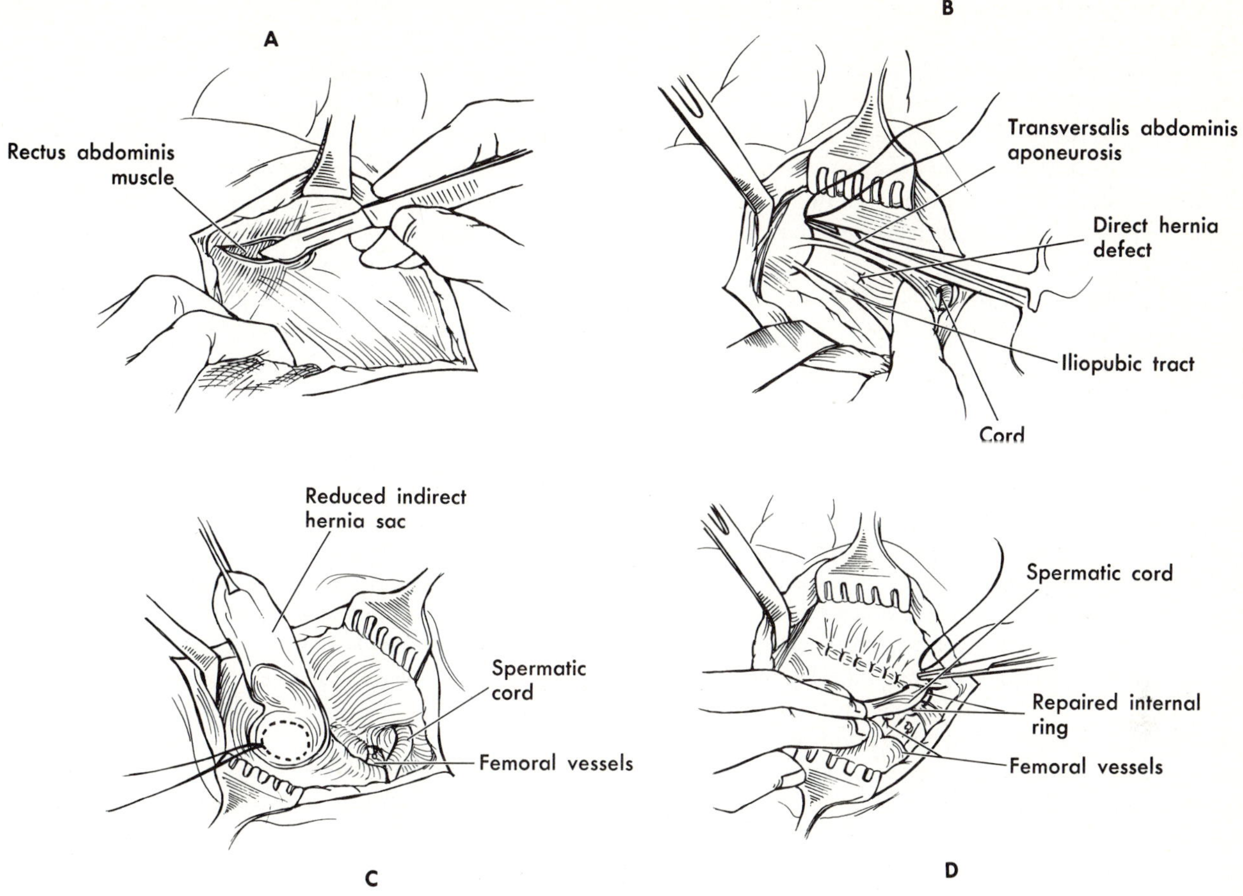

Fig. 10-22. Preperitoneal repair. **A,** Skin incision starts 2 cm above symphysis pubis and is extended through external oblique, internal oblique, and transversalis muscles. **B,** With finger in direct hernia defect surgeon sutures transversalis abdominis aponeurosis to iliopubic tract. **C,** In case of indirect defect, sac is reduced and then excised, with high ligation being achieved by use of a purse-string suture. **D,** Internal ring is tightened after transversus abdominis aponeurosis has been approximated to iliopubic tract. (From Nyhus, L.M., and Harkins, H.N.: Hernia, Philadelphia, J.B. Lippincott Co.)

4. Retraction on the lower side of the incision will reveal the posterior inguinal wall and the hernia defect.

Variations in the procedure are performed for different types of hernias.

1. If the hernia is direct, it can be reduced easily (Fig. 10-22), *B*), and the superior edge of the hernia defect (the transversalis fascia) is sutured to the iliopubic tract (origin of the transversalis fascia).

2. In an indirect hernia, the sac is gently retracted from the inguinal canal. A purse-string suture is placed around the peritoneal defect as the sac is excised (Fig. 10-22, *C*). The lateral aspect of the internal abdominal ring is closed, and the posterior wall is reinforced as with the direct hernia.

3. In repairing a femoral hernia, the sac is again reduced by traction. After inspection of the sac for contents, a high ligation is performed. As it approaches Cooper's ligament, the defect in the posterior inguinal floor, the transversalis fascia, is clearly identified and is repaired by direct approximation (Fig. 10-22, *D*).

After repair of any of the foregoing hernias, the preperitoneal space is irrigated with saline, and the appropriate layers are approximated.

Sliding hernias

Direct or indirect hernias may occur as sliding hernias. A sliding inguinal hernia is one in which the wall of a viscus forms a portion of the wall of the hernia. The most common sliding hernias involve the bladder in direct hernias, the sigmoid colon in left indirect hernia, and the cecum in right indirect inguinal hernias (Fig. 10-23). It is essential to recognize this hernia early in the repair, since attempts at surgical removal of the entire sac will injure the sliding viscus.

All operations designed to repair sliding hernias adhere to the basic principle of repairing the defect in the transversalis fascia. To free the bowel from the sac, the following steps must be taken:

1. The sac is opened in an area in which no bowel is present and is excised medially and laterally to a point at which the bowel can be reduced (Fig. 10-24).
2. The lateral and medial peritoneal margins are approximated.
3. High ligation of the sac is performed.
4. Repair of the transversalis fascia is done by one of the methods previously described.

Ventral hernias

Ventral hernias can appear either spontaneously or after previous operations. Spontaneously occurring ventral hernias include epigastric and umbilical hernias. Postoperative ventral hernias are called *incisional hernias*. Incisional hernias appear more frequently when the original incision was a T-shaped incision or a vertical midline incision. Operations that involve a potential for contamination, such as for acute perforated ulcer or other perforated abdominal viscus, are more prone to developing subsequent ventral hernias. Poor nutritional state with resulting hypoproteinemia predisposes to ventral hernia formation. Finally, faulty surgical technique, such as the wrong choice of suture materials, may result in the ultimate appearance of a ventral hernia.

Several methods have been developed for repairing ventral hernias. If all layers of the abdominal wall are easily identified, anatomical layer-by-layer repair may be done. Frequently, a type of overlap method for repair is employed. Vertical and transverse overlap procedures are referred to as "vest-over-pants" repairs. For large defects, in which approximation of tissue would result in closure under stress or would cause either circulatory or respiratory compromise, synthetic materials such as Marlex are employed.

Umbilical hernias

Umbilical hernias are extraabdominal hernias that occur as small fascial defects under the umbilicus. They are common in children and frequently disappear spontaneously by the time a child is 2 years old. If the defect is persistent, a simple approximation of the overlying fascia is all that is necessary for repair. In adults, umbilical hernias represent a defect in the linea alba just above the umbilicus. These hernias tend to occur more frequently in obese people, thus making diagnosis more difficult. These hernias are potentially very dangerous, since they have small necks and frequently incarcerate. Surgical repair is indicated in all adults with asymptomatic umbilical hernias.

Epigastric hernias

Epigastric hernias are protrusions of fat through defects in the abdominal wall between the xiphoid process and the umbilicus. Patients with these hernias can have nausea, vague abdominal pain, or epigastric pain similar to that observed with cholecystitis or duodenal ulcers. Surgical repair of these hernias is simple and very successful.

Synthetic mesh repairs

Synthetic meshes, such as Mersilene or Marlex, have been particularly helpful in repairing recurrent hernias or large ventral hernias. These synthetic materials are strong and durable. Mersilene and Marlex promote fibrovascular growth within their pores, which lends extra strength to the repair. A major criticism of synthetic meshes is that, as with any foreign body implant, the risk of infection is increased.

Essential to the use of Mersilene or Marlex in a repair is the identification and cleaning of tissue planes to which the mesh will be attached (Fig. 10-25, *A*). In a ventral hernia, the peritoneum is dissected from the undersurface

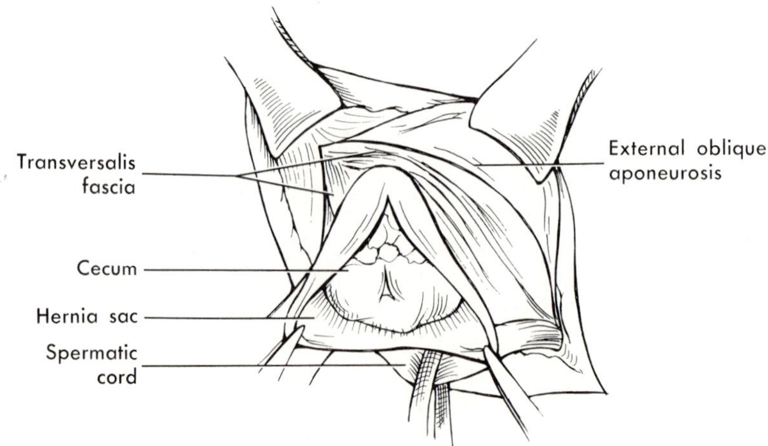

Fig. 10-23. Sliding hernia with cecum forming portion of posterior hernia sac wall. (From Madden, J.L.: Atlas of techniques in surgery, ed. 2, New York, Appleton-Century-Crofts.)

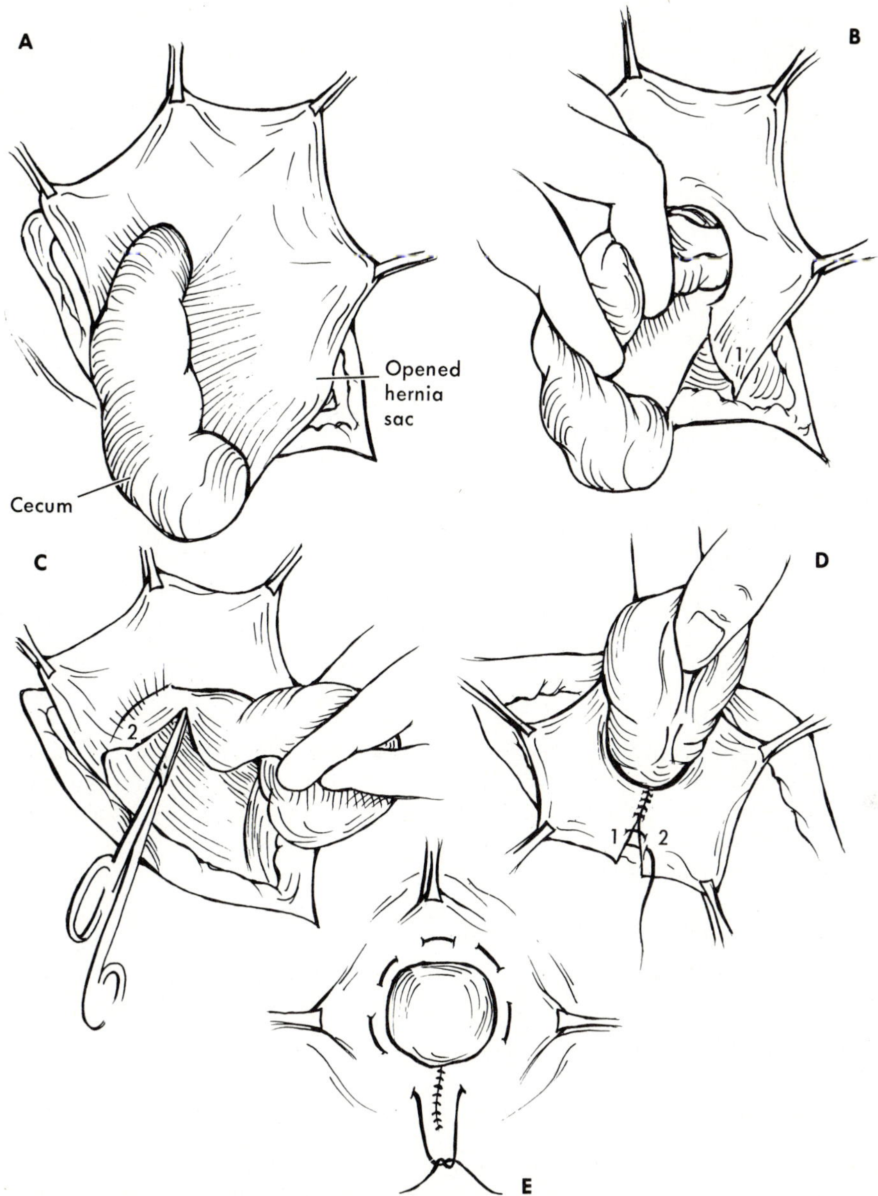

Fig. 10-24. Right sliding hernia. **A,** Cecum forms posterior wall of hernia sac. **B,** Peritoneum is excised medially, **C,** and laterally, **D,** allowing mobilization of cecum and subsequent reduction to abdomen. **E,** After reduction, high ligation is accomplished by using purse-string suture. (Redrawn from Ponka, J.L.: Surgical management of large bilateral indirect sliding inguinal hernias, Am. J. Surg. **112**[7]:52, 1966.)

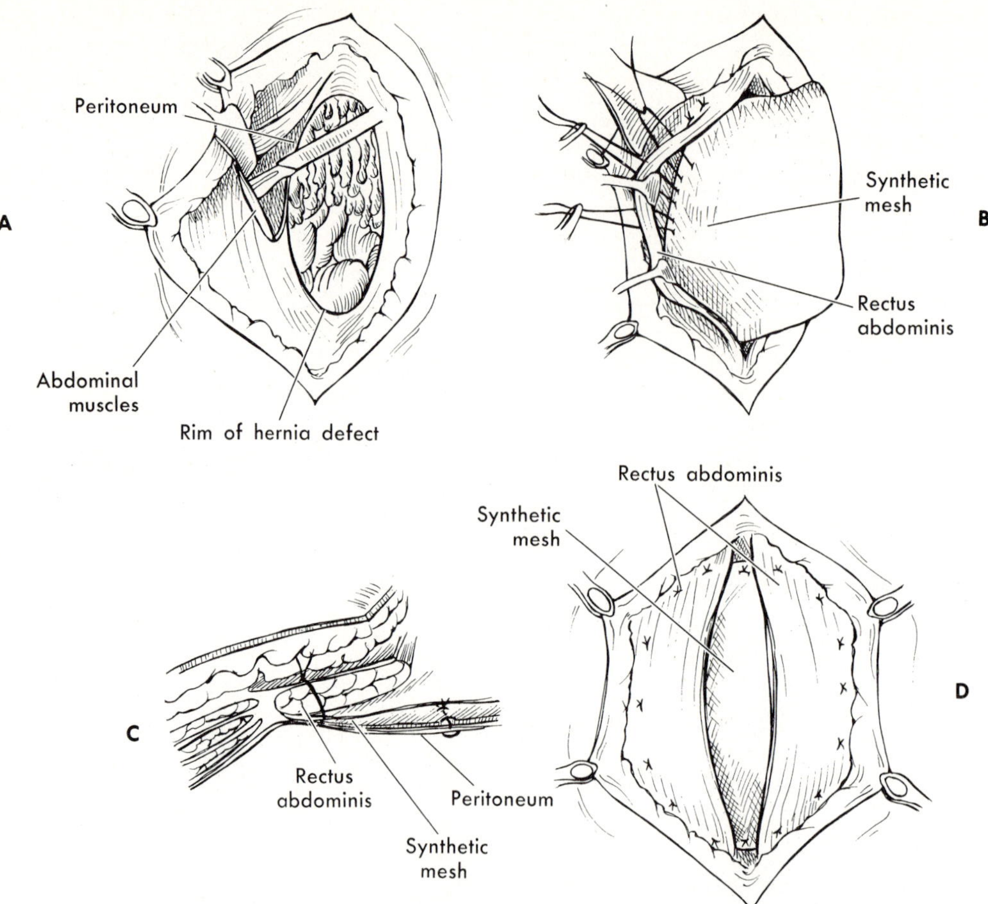

Fig. 10-25. Use of mesh in hernia repair. **A,** After layers of abdominal wall surrounding ventral hernia are identified, **B** and **C,** mesh is inserted between rectus and peritoneum. **D,** With moderate tension on mesh, it is inserted between appropriate layers on opposite side and is sutured into place. (From Maingot, R.: Abdominal operations, ed. 6, New York, 1974, Appleton-Century-Crofts.)

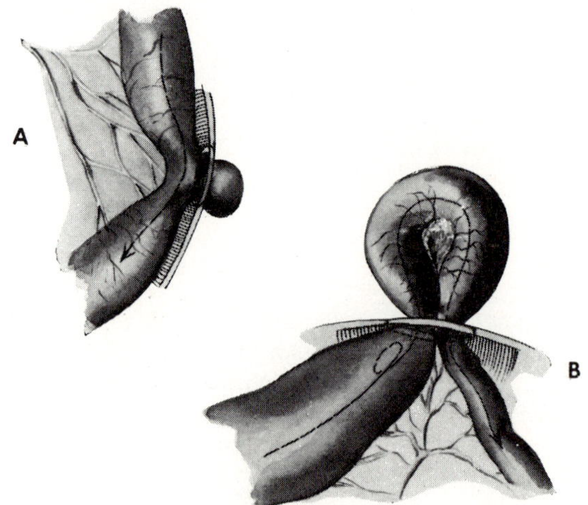

Fig. 10-26. A, Richter's hernia. Only a portion of bowel passes through hernial ring; arrow indicates that bowel need not be obstructed mechanically even with strangulation. **B,** Incarcerated hernia. Distended bowel in hernia cannot return to abdomen through narrow fascial defect. (From Liechty, R., and Soper, R.: Synopsis of surgery, ed. 4, St. Louis, 1980, The C.V. Mosby Co.)

of the rectus, and the mesh is placed between the peritoneum and the rectus (Fig. 10-25, *B*). After the mesh is positioned, it is sutured in place on one side, using the synthetic suture material compatible with the type of mesh employed (Fig. 10-25, *C*). At this point, the peritoneum can be closed, if possible. If the peritoneum cannot be closed, mesh can be placed directly over the omentum. The mesh is then placed and sutured to the other side of the defect, with moderate tension maintained (Fig. 10-25, *D*). If possible, the mesh is then covered with a fascial or muscular layer before the subcutaneous fat and skin are closed. Suction catheters are usually placed in the wound, and antibiotics are frequently used prophylactically. Using mesh to repair inguinal hernias is based on the same principles used for closing ventral hernias. With inguinal hernias, the mesh is sutured to transversalis fascia on either side of the defect.

Miscellaneous hernias

Spigelian hernias are uncommon and occur between the walls of the abdominal musculature. Lumbar hernias (Petit's hernias) occur anywhere in the back between the twelfth rib, superiorly; the ilium, inferiorly; the vertebral column, medially; and a line between the tip of the twelfth rib and ilium, laterally. Hernias may occur through the obturator canal or the greater or lesser sciatic foramen. An inguinal hernia containing a Meckel diverticulum is called Littre's hernia, whereas one containing two loops of bowel is called Maydl's hernia. A special type of strangulated hernia is Richter's hernia (Fig. 10-26). In this case, only a part of the circumference of the bowel is incarcerated or strangulated in the hernia. Frequently, this is described as a knuckle of bowel that becomes trapped and ischemic. Since initially a very small area is necrotic, diagnosis may be delayed and the probability of mortality becomes significant. It is most frequently found in femoral hernias because of the small size and sharp, relatively inflexible nature of the fascial ring in this area. A strangulated Richter hernia may spontaneously reduce and the gangrenous piece of intestine be overlooked at operation.

Esophageal hiatal hernia is discussed in Chapter 14.

SUGGESTED READINGS

Anthony, C.P., and Thibodeau, G.A.: Textbook of anatomy and physiology, ed. 10, St. Louis, 1979, The C.V. Mosby Co.

Beyers, M., and Dudas, S.: The clinical practice of medical-surgical nursing, Boston, 1977, Little, Brown, & Co.

Dunphy, J.E., and Way, L.: Current surgical diagnosis and treatment, ed. 4, Los Altos, Calif., 1979, Lange Medical Publications.

Grew, H.E., and Kremer, K.: Atlas of surgical operations, vol. 2, Philadelphia, 1980, W.B. Saunders Co.

Gruendemann, B.J., and others: The surgical patient: behavioral concepts for the operating room nurse, ed. 2, St. Louis, 1977, The C.V. Mosby Co.

Liechty, R. and Soper, R.: Synopsis of surgery, ed. 4, St. Louis, 1980, The C.V. Mosby Co.

Netter, F.: The Ciba collection of medical illustrations, vol. 3, Digestive system, pt. 2, Lower digestive tract, Summit, N.J., 1973, Ciba Pharmaceutical Co.

Nyhus, L.M., and Condon, R.: Hernia, ed. 2, Philadelphia, 1978, J.B. Lippincott Co.

Ponka, J.L.: Hernias of the abdominal wall, Philadelphia, 1980, W.B. Saunders Co.

Schumann, D.: How to help wound healing in your abdominal surgery patient, Nursing '80 **10**(4):34, 1980.

Tinckler, L.: The surgery of groin hernia, Nurs. Times **74:**1519, 1978.

Usher, F.C.: The repair of incisional and inguinal hernias, RN **34:**1, April 1971.

11 Breast surgery

Pathologic breast conditions, indicated by benign or malignant tumors and infections, are currently one of the most common and emotionally upsetting health problems confronting women and occasionally men. In women particularly, changing hormone levels from puberty throughout the remainder of life affect breast tissue in its physical and microscopic characteristics. In association with these changes, numerous dysfunctions, malformations, and tumors may occur.

Operative procedures on the mammary glands may be indicated in the presence of disease or as a result of other physical or psychological patient considerations (reconstructive surgery of the breast is discussed in Chapter 21).

ANATOMY AND PHYSIOLOGY

The breasts are bilateral mammary glands that lie on the pectoralis major fascia of the anterior chest wall. The breasts are surrounded by a layer of fat and are encased in an envelope of skin. The breasts extend from the second to the sixth rib and horizontally from the lateral edge of the sternum to the anterior axillary line. The largest part of the mammary gland rests on the connective tissue of the greater pectoral muscle and laterally on the serratus anterior, with a normal global contour occurring as a result of the fascial support (Cooper's ligaments). An elongation of mammary tissue normally extends on the pectoralis major toward the axilla and is known as the tail of Spence (Fig. 11-1).

Each breast is made up of twelve to twenty glandular lobes that are separated by connective tissue and adipose tissue deposits. Each lobe is subdivided into lobules in which are embedded the secreting cells (alveoli) arranged in grape-like clusters around minute ducts. The lobes are positioned in a spiral fashion around the nipple. Each lobe is drained by a single lactiferous duct that opens on the nipple (Fig. 11-2). The nipple, located in the fourth intercostal space, forms a conical projection into which the ducts open independently of each other on the surface. A pigmented circular area called the areola surrounds the nipple. Smooth contractile muscle fibers of the areola allow for nipple contraction.

Three major arterial systems generously supply the mammary glands with blood. Branches of the internal mammary and the lateral branches of the anterior aortic intercostal arteries are the two main sources, all which form an extensive network of anastomoses over the breast. A third source is the pectoral branch deriving from a branch of the axillary artery.

The main veins follow the courses of the arteries. The superficial veins frequently become dilated during pregnancy. They are also often dilated over an area that contains disease. One route of venous drainage from the breast is significant in that it forms an anastomosis with the intercostal veins that in turn joins with the vertebral veins.

The lymph drainage system generally follows the course of the vessels. These drain into two main areas represented by the axillary nodes and the internal mammary chain of nodes (Fig. 11-3). An average of fifty-three lymph nodes occur in the axillary area. The internal mammary nodes are fewer in number but are responsible for most of the lymph drainage from the upper and lower inner quadrants of the breast. Thus one can see how the lymph system may act as channels for the spread of malignant disease from the breast to associated areas of the chest wall or to the axilla.

The nerve supply is mainly from the anterior cutaneous branches of the upper intercostal nerves, the third and fourth branches of the cervical plexus, and the lateral cutaneous branches of the intercostal nerves.

The mammary glands are affected by three types of physiological changes: (1) those related to growth and development, (2) those related to the menstrual cycle, and (3) those related to pregnancy and lactation. The mammary glands are present at birth in both the male and female. Hormonal stimulation, however, produces the development and function of these glands in the female. Estrogen promotes growth of the ductal structures, while progesterone promotes development of the alveoli. Both of these hormones act synergistically with the pituitary growth hormones, prolactin and corticotropin, to produce the structure and function of the glands.

Occasionally, developmental errors of the breast may occur. Additional nipples may be present as well as extra mammary tissue in the axilla or over the upper abdomen. The preferred treatment of these supernumerary structures often is excision. Absence of one or both nipples also may occur and may be associated with the absence of the underlying pectoral muscle and chest wall.

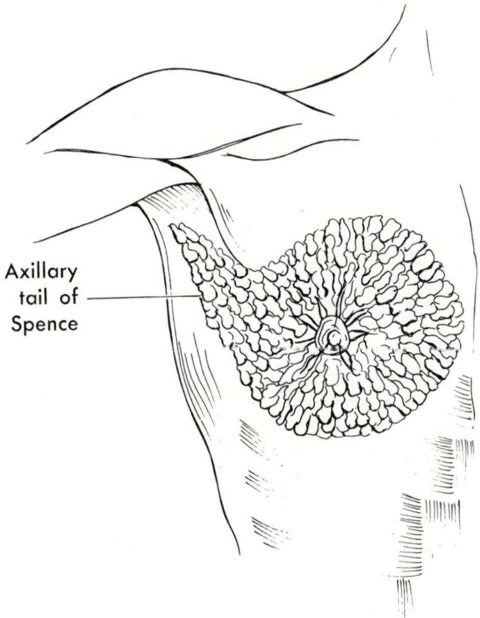

Fig. 11-1. Normal distribution of mammary tissue of adult female breast. Note long tail of Spence extending into axilla. (Adapted from Schwartz, S.I., and others: Principles of surgery, New York, 1974, McGraw-Hill Book Co.)

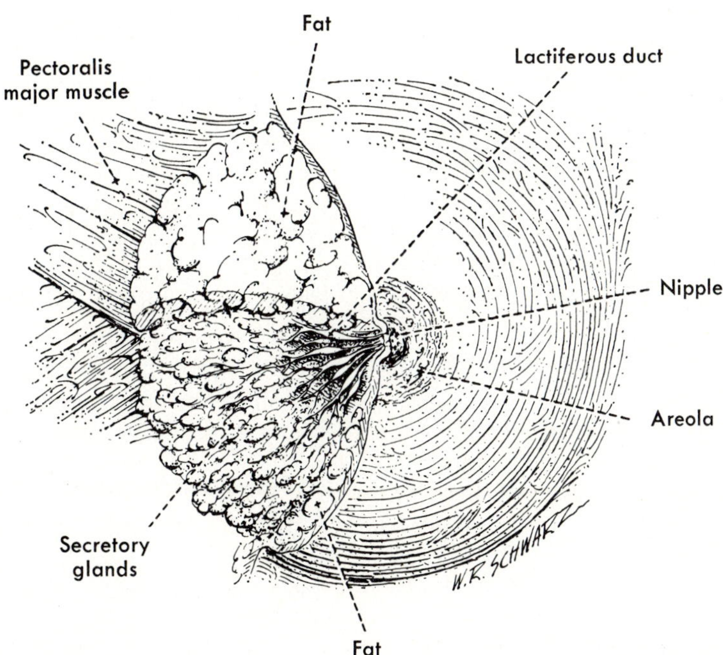

Fig. 11-2. Diagrammatic cross section of mammary gland showing relationship of various anatomical structures. (From Jorstad, L.H.: Surgery of the breast, St. Louis, The C.V. Mosby Co.; drawing by W.R. Schwarz.)

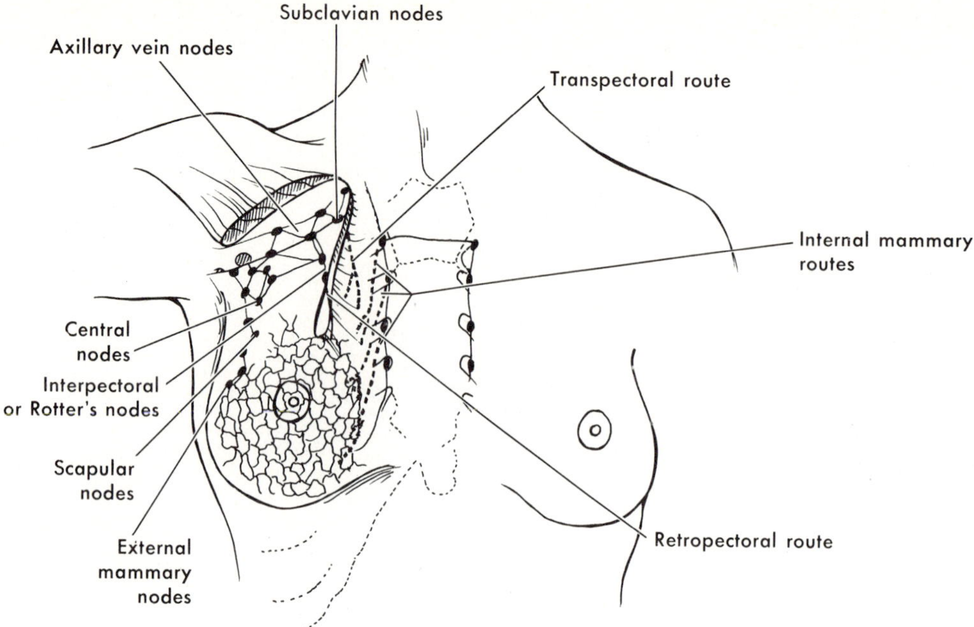

Fig. 11-3. Normal distribution of mammary tissue and lymphatic system of adult female breast. (Adapted from Southwick, H.W., Slaughter, D.P., and Humphrey, L.J.: Surgery of the breast. Copyright by Year Book Medical Publishers, Inc., Chicago. Used by permission.)

NURSING CONSIDERATIONS

Preoperative considerations

Each patient requiring breast surgery has a special need for understanding and acceptance. Before hospitalization for biopsy, it is the surgeon's responsibility to discuss with the patient the preliminary findings, including mammography, what should be done, how it is to be done, and expected results. It is vital that the patient's questions be answered.

During a preoperative interview, the operating room nurse is in a unique position to assist the patient in understanding routine occurrences in the operating room and at the same time assess and plan for individualized instrumentation, equipment, and physiological needs. Preoperative anxiety is an emotional reality, and the breast patient is apprehensive about the possibility of losing a body part, a negative reaction by the family, and a change in self-image. The operating room nurse can help allay the patient's fears by answering questions, giving information relating to early activity and recommended exercises, and discussing prosthetic reconstruction if appropriate. Early preoperative teaching and reassurance allow for a smoother postoperative course.

Intraoperative considerations

Special considerations must be given to the positioning process. Nursing care must provide for physiological safety of the patient, best access to the airway for the anesthesiologist, and optimum exposure of the incision site for the surgeon.

The patient is placed on the operating table in the supine position. The operative side is placed nearest the edge of the table with the arm on the involved side extended on a padded armboard. Unnecessary breast exposure is avoided.

Skin preparation technique differs among surgeons, but generally the site is shaved and cleansed with an antimicrobial solution. The margin of the operative area varies depending on the type of procedure to be performed. Skin preparation usually includes the area from above the clavicle to the umbilicus and from the opposite nipple to and including the upper arm on the involved side. Gentle handling of the breast is encouraged to avoid dislodging tumor cells.

If a skin graft is to be used, the donor site is separately prepared. Usually the anterior thigh on the same side as the operative breast is preferred.

Postoperative considerations

Evaluation immediately after surgery includes checking the status of patient's skin and neuromuscular skeletal system. Special attention should be given to intactness of dressing, wound suction, and proper drainage. Protection of the arm on the involved side is essential.

When the patient awakens, the nurse or surgeon should be available to answer the patient's questions regarding the extent of surgery. If a breast has been removed, the response and support, or lack of it, by the nurse will have an effect on the patient's attitude and should be based on individual patient needs.

Discharge planning may begin as soon as the patient

is ready. This may include information about exercises, activities, prosthetic devices, and available support organizations.

OPERATIONS

Incision and drainage for abscess

Definition. Surgical opening and drainage of an inflamed and suppurative area of the breast.

Considerations. Abscesses occur most frequently as a result of infections in the lactating breast. Staphylococcal or streptococcal organisms enter the breast either through abraded or lacerated nipple surfaces or through the lactiferous ducts. Chronic abscesses are rare. Free drainage is required with the association of an abscess around the nipple or in the breast tissue.

Setup and preparation of the patient. The patient is placed on the operating table in a supine position, and the operative area cleansed. General anesthesia is used. Instruments include the following:

1 Knife handle with no. 10 blade
2 Mayo scissors, 1 curved and 1 straight
1 Tissue forceps with teeth
2 Hemostats, straight
2 Hemostats, curved
2 Kelly clamps
2 Allis forceps
1 Probe
Culture tube
Gauze packing
Tissue drain

Operative procedure

1. Generally, a radial incision extending outward from the nipple or a circumareolar incision is preferred. A short thoracomammary fold may be used for deep breast abscesses in the lower or outer quadrant.

2. After skin incision, the wound is deepened until pus is encountered.

3. A curved hemostat is directed into the cavity to determine the extent of the abscess cavity, and a culture is taken.

4. Loculations are broken up by exploring the cavity with the index finger.

5. The opening is enlarged to ensure adequate drainage, the cavity is irrigated with warm saline solution, and bleeding vessels are ligated with absorbable sutures.

6. The wound is drained or loosely packed with gauze. Healing occurs by granulation.

Biopsy

Definition. Removal of tissue for pathologic examination.

Needle biopsy. A Vim Silverman or a disposable cutting type of needle is introduced and advanced into the breast mass and entraps a core or plug of tissue specimen. The needle is withdrawn, and the tissue sent for diagnostic examination (Fig. 11-4).

Incisional biopsy. Using a curved incision line, a portion of the mass is surgically excised and sent for pathologic examination and estrogen-progesterone receptor assay.

Excisional biopsy. The entire tumor mass is excised from adjacent tissue for examination as with incisional biopsy.

Considerations. Biopsy is indicated in the presence of a tumor mass detected by palpation, mammography, thermography, nipple discharge, or skin changes. Fibroadenoma, an isolated cyst, and intraductal papilloma may be encountered. Definitive surgical treatment should never be performed without a formal biopsy. The biopsy procedure has little risk and can be done under local anesthesia. The short delay between biopsy and further treatment does not adversely affect survival. However, when an extensive procedure is anticipated, general anesthesia is preferred.

Setup and preparation of the patient. The patient is placed in the supine position with the operative side nearest the edge of the table and arm abducted on a padded armboard. The prep solution and draping manner vary with the surgeon's preference. The arm on the involved side may be draped to allow movement. A separate biopsy instrument set is used:

Cutting instruments

2 Knife handles with no. 10 blades
2 Mayo scissors, 1 straight and 1 curved
2 Tissue forceps with teeth
1 Dura scissors

Holding instruments

6 Allis forceps
6 Kelly clamps
12 Hemostats
6 Towel clamps

Exposing instruments

2 Muscle retractors, small
2 Rake retractors, small
1 Set of intraductal probes
4 Skin hooks

Suturing items

1 Needle holder
2 Packages of sutures, 1 absorbable and 1 nonabsorbable, usually on atraumatic cutting needles
Collodion sealer

Operative procedure

1. An incision in the direction of the skin lines or along the border of the areola is made over the tumor mass. The circumareolar incision gives the best cosmetic effect.

2. Gentle traction is applied to the mass with holding forceps. If the lesion is small, the entire mass and an edge of normal tissue are removed by sharp dissection.

If a large lesion is present, a small incisional biopsy of the main mass is done. The tissue specimen is examined by a frozen section to determine immediate diagnosis while the patient is still anesthetized. If a 48-hour permanent section is required, the patient will be rescheduled for any further surgery that may be necessary.

3. Wound closure
   a. Benign lesion. Breast tissue is approximated with plain or chromic gut, the skin is closed with fine sutures, and a firm pressure dressing is applied.
   b. Malignant lesion. The incision is tightly closed with continuous locking sutures on a cutting needle, and the wound is sealed with collodion to prevent the spread of tumor cells through leakage.

After the biopsy, the instruments used are removed for cleaning and terminal sterilization. If a more extensive operation becomes necessary, the team members rescrub, gown, and glove; the operative site is again prepared and draped. A set of instruments for a radical procedure is now used.

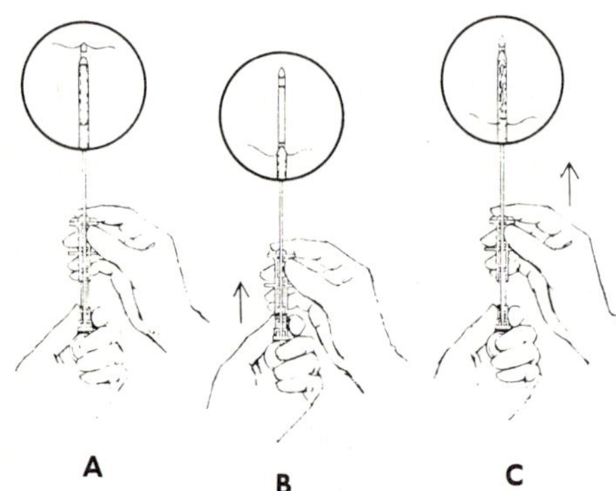

Fig. 11-4. Technique for needle biopsy of breast:

1. Site is prepared as required. For percutaneous procedures, adequate anesthesia is ensured and skin incised with scalpel. If distance measurement is desired, tissue depth spacer is slipped on needle before procedure.

2. With obturator fully retracted to cover specimen notch, cannula hub is held and needle assembly inserted *up* to tissue from which specimen is to be secured as shown in **A.**

3. Larger H-shaped cannula handle is held firmly to stabilize assembly, and obturator hub is quickly advanced as far as permitted, which will position specimen notch in tissue to be biopsied as shown in **B.**

4. To cut tissue that has prolapsed into specimen notch, H-shaped cannula handle is quickly advanced as shown in **C.**

5. Needle assembly is withdrawn with cannula still advanced over obturator.

6. Obturator is advanced to remove biopsy specimen from specimen notch. (Courtesy Travenol Laboratories, Inc., Deerfield, Ill.)

Mastectomy

Definition. Excision of the total breast.

Considerations. The various methods of breast cancer treatment are surrounded by controversy and still under study. Physicians and researchers are comparing and evaluating treatment methods and survival rates, but it is ultimately the patient's decision as to which type of treatment will be used.

Breast cancer primarily affects women, and, until it can be prevented, early detection is the greatest hope for its control. All women should practice self-examination monthly, and any changes or abnormalities should be immediately reported to a physician. Periodic palpation by a trained person is also an effective and simple method of detecting breast cancer.

Diagnostic study techniques used to detect early disease are continually improving. Good results have been obtained with x-ray mammography. This technique visualizes the entire breast by directing the x-ray beam vertically through the breast and by using a mediolateral exposure. Such mammograms are best analyzed by a trained radiologist, who sends the reports to the referring physician. In some instances mammograms are done immediately before surgery, and the detected lesions (Figs. 11-5 and 11-6) are localized by insertion of a needle or needles or a barbed-wire stylet, which is inserted through the needle. The needle or needles may be left in place or removed after insertion of the barbed wire (Fig. 11-7). Once the suspicious area is identified, the needle or needles or barbed wire is taped in place and the patient is sent directly to the operating room for surgical biopsy.

Mammography is a widely used screening device for early breast cancer detection. Its accuracy depends on careful x-ray techniques and on breast size, structure, and density. Radiation dosage varies with individual women and techniques. Research continues to lead to improved equipment and techniques to lower doses of radiation in mammographic studies.

Other detection techniques available include thermography and ultrasound. Thermography (measuring heat emissions from the breast by an infrared scanner) and ultrasound (projection of high-frequency sound waves into the breast to produce an interior image of the breast) have the greatest appeal but are of limited use and should be used as an adjunct to mammography and physical examinations.

Surgical treatment ranges from removal of only the tumor to the extended radical mastectomy, which includes the pectoral muscles, the axillary and internal mammary lymph nodes, and a section of the ribs. The choice of operation depends on the size, site, and stage of disease advancement. Treatment methods of radiation therapy, chemotherapy, endocrine manipulation, and immunotherapy may be used in conjunction with surgery or as alternative treatment methods.

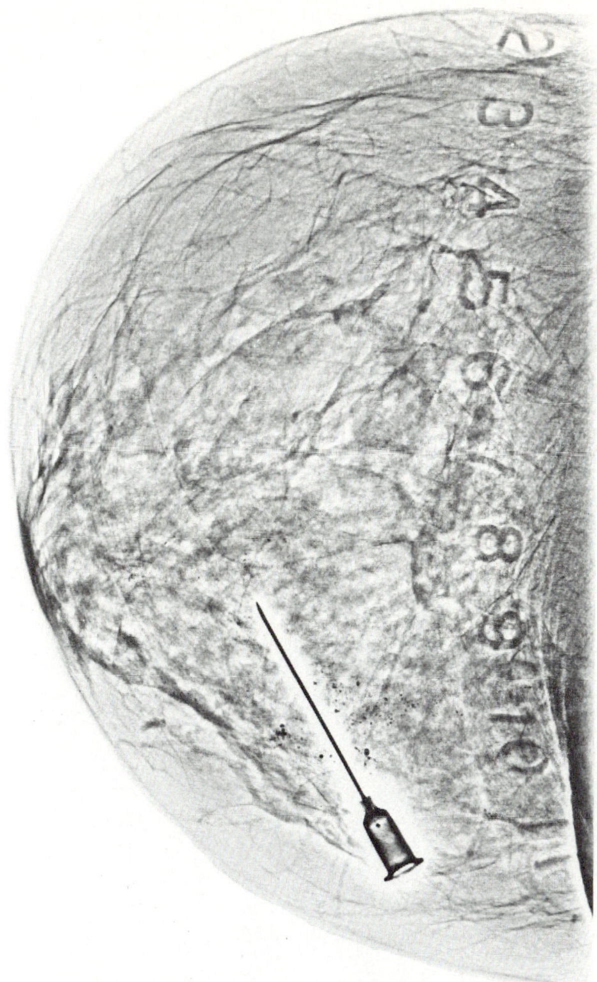

Fig. 11-5. Xeromammogram: craniocaudal view of breast. Needle has been placed from lateral surface of breast through area of calcification before biopsy, which showed intraductal carcinoma. (Courtesy Dr. Renate Duchesneau, Department of Radiology, University Hospitals of Cleveland, Cleveland, Ohio.)

Partial mastectomy (lumpectomy, tylectomy, quadrant resection, wedge resection)

Definition. Removal of the tumor mass with at least 1 inch of surrounding normal tissue.

Considerations. This procedure has been the subject of much controversy and is currently recommended only for patients with small, peripherally located lesions. Data reported by opponents of this procedure indicate that the 10-year survival rate for patients having partial mastectomy is half that of women receiving conventional treatment; however, the number of patients is so limited that statistically valid conclusions cannot be made at this time. Some physicians recommend that all such patients receive radiation therapy to the breast and usually to the surrounding nodes as well. In addition, many patients who have had a partial mastectomy subsequently need additional procedures because of the multicentric origin of cancers.

Setup and preparation of the patient. As described for radical mastectomy, particularly in patients with large breasts, in which increased bleeding may occur.

Operative procedure. As described for excisional biopsy.

Subcutaneous mastectomy (adenomammectomy)

Definition. Removal of all breast tissue with the overlying skin and nipple left intact.

Considerations. Subcutaneous mastectomy is recommended for patients with central tumors of noninvasive origin, with chronic cystic mastitis, when a number of previous biopsies have been carried out, or with hyperplastic duct changes or multiple fibroadenomas. A prosthesis may be inserted at the time of mastectomy or at a later date. Marked bleeding at the time of surgery is a contraindication for the insertion of a prosthesis.

Setup and preparation of the patient. As described for radical mastectomy. If a prosthesis is to be inserted, equipment listed for augmentation mammoplasty (Chapter 21) is also required.

Operative procedure

1. An incision is usually begun in the inframammary crease and may be made on the medial or the lateral aspect of the breast. Some surgeons may choose to initially remove and preserve the nipple areola complex by employing lateral extensions of wide periareolar incisions.

2. Blunt dissection is performed to elevate the breast from the pectoral fascia.

3. The breast tissue is removed from the skin with an attempt made to remain in a plane between the subcutaneous tissue and the breast. Dissection is carried out toward the axilla; with care, 90% or more of the breast tissue can be removed, including the tail of Spence. Some lymph nodes in the axillary area also may be removed. Bleeding vessels are clamped and ligated.

4. A decision is made at this time as to whether it is possible to insert a prosthesis (augmentation mammoplasty). If the subareolar tissue shows no signs of tumor, as verified by a pathologist, the areolar complex is placed on a deepithelialized dermal bed.

5. A small tissue drain may be inserted. The wound is closed, and a light pressure dressing is applied.

Simple mastectomy (total mastectomy)

Definition. Removal of the entire involved breast without lymph node dissection.

Considerations. A simple mastectomy is performed to remove extensive benign disease, if malignancy is believed to be confined only to the breast tissue, or as a

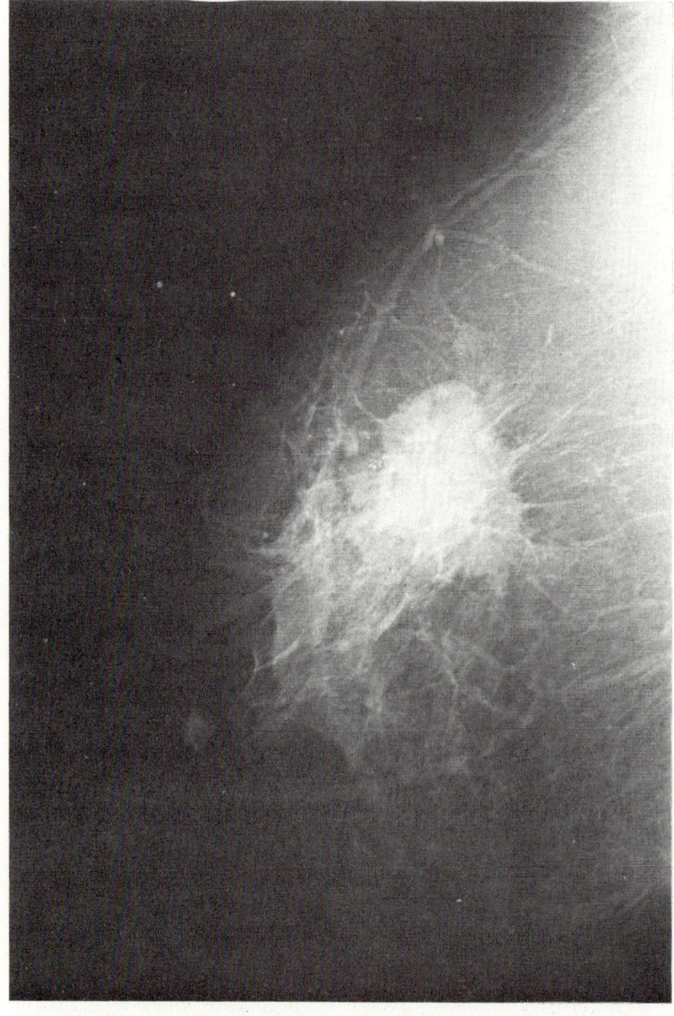

Fig. 11-6. Xonics mammogram. Lateral view of breast showing typical infiltrating carcinoma occurring as 4-cm speculated mass containing fine tumor calcifications. (Courtesy Dr. Renate Duchesneau, Department of Radiology, University Hospitals of Cleveland, Cleveland, Ohio.)

palliative measure to remove an ulcerated advanced malignancy.

Setup and preparation of the patient. As described for radical mastectomy.

Operative procedure

1. Through a transverse elliptical incision, using a knife and curved scissors, the skin edges are freed from the fascia (Fig. 11-8, *A*). Bleeding vessels are clamped with hemostats and ligated with fine silk or chromic sutures.

2. The skin edges of the wound are protected by warm laparotomy packs; the breast tissue is grasped with Allis forceps and is dissected free from the underlying pectoral fascia with curved scissors and knife.

3. The tumor and all breast tissue are removed. Bleeding vessels are clamped and ligated.

4. A tissue drain or closed wound drainage system catheters may be inserted and anchored to the skin with a fine suture. The wound is closed with skin sutures, and a moderate pressure dressing is applied.

Radical mastectomy

Definition. Following a tissue biopsy with positive diagnosis of malignancy, en bloc removal of the entire involved breast, the pectoral muscles, the axillary lymph nodes, and all fat, fascia, and adjacent tissues.

Considerations. A radical mastectomy is done to remove the involved area with the hope of decreasing the spread of malignancy. Preoperatively, the surgeon may also prepare skin of the anterior surface of the thigh in the event a skin graft may be needed.

Setup and preparation of the patient. As described for breast biopsy. The following radical set supplies and instruments should be available:

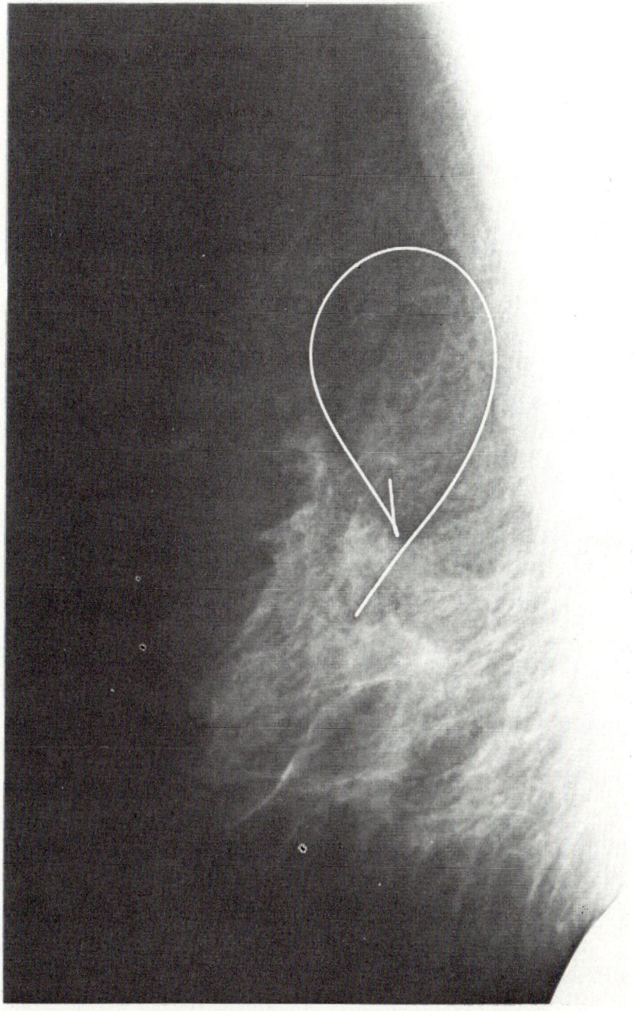

Fig. 11-7. Lateral xonics film after removing localizing needle with barbed wire hooked posterior to 1-cm carcinoma. (Courtesy Dr. Renate Duchesneau, Department of Radiology, University Hospitals of Cleveland, Cleveland, Ohio.)

Cutting instruments

2 Knife handles with no. 10 blades
2 Mayo scissors, 1 straight and 1 curved
1 Tissue scissors
2 Tissue forceps with teeth
2 Tissue forceps without teeth
2 Adson forceps with teeth

Holding instruments

12 Allis forceps
6 Kocher clamps
12 Kelly clamps
24-48 Hemostats (will vary with size of breast)
12 Towel clamps

Exposing instruments

2 U.S. Army retractors
4 Richardson retractors, 2 small and 2 medium
4 Rakes, four-prong, 2 small and 2 medium
4 Skin hooks
3 Berens skin-flap retractors

Suturing items

4 Needle holders
Applicators with skin clips (optional)
Suture material, usually atraumatic on cutting needles

Accessory items

1 Tissue drain or closed wound drainage system
Electrocautery unit
Marking pen
Suction tip and tubing

When a skin-grafting procedure is to be performed, a separate setup will be needed for taking the graft from the donor site and should include the following:

6 Hemostats
6 Allis forceps
2 Adson forceps with teeth
1 Dermatome with supplies
2 Vein retractors
4 Mosquito hemostats, curved
Suture material: plain and chromic gut and silk, as desired, for ligatures and closure

Operative procedure

1. The elliptical skin incision is made through the fat to the fascia with a knife (Fig. 11-8, *A*). The bleeding points are controlled with hemostats; warm, moist pressure packs; and ligatures or electrocautery.

2. The skin is undercut in all directions to the limits of the dissection by means of a fresh knife, curved scissors, and retractors. (Knife blades may need to be changed frequently.)

3. The margins of the skin flaps are covered with warm, moist pressure packs and are held away with retractors; the greater pectoral muscle at the point of insertion into the humerus is freed and divided by means of a knife, hemostats, and ligatures.

4. The vessels and nerves of the greater and smaller pectoral muscles are dissected free, clamped with hemostats, divided, and ligated with fine silk or chromic gut ligatures swaged on a needle.

5. The cut end of the greater pectoral muscle is grasped with holding forceps and is held medially by a right-angle retractor. The attachments of this muscle to the clavicle are clamped with a hemostat and are cut (Fig. 11-8, *B*).

6. The smaller pectoral muscle is cut and ligated close to its insertion into the coracoid process of the scapula with hemostats, a knife, and ligatures (Fig. 11-8, *C*).

7. The axillary node dissection is completed, and the axillary vein is stripped of its lymphatic tissues; preservation of the cephalic vein is imperative (Fig. 11-8, *D*). Bleeding venous and arterial vessels are clamped and ligated with silk or fine chromic gut ligatures. Electrocautery hemostasis is also used.

8. The fascia overlying the anterior sheath of the rectus abdominis muscle is freed from the chest wall; bleeding vessels are clamped and ligated. The sternal and costal origins of the pectoral muscles are severed by sharp dissection. The breast and tumor are removed. The wound is cleansed by irrigation or with laparotomy packs saturated in warm saline solution.

9. The skin edges are carefully approximated with skin hooks. If drainage is desired, a knife is used to make an opening through the skin flap in the axillary region. A tissue drain, soft multieyed tube, or closed wound drainage catheter is introduced with tissue forceps. The free end of the drain is secured to the skin with a suture.

10. The wound is closed with interrupted silk sutures; a skin graft is often used (Fig. 11-8, *E*). A moderate pressure dressing is applied and held in place with Ace bandages; suction may be applied to the drainage tube. A Surgi-Bra may also be applied over the dressing.

Modified radical mastectomy

Definition. Removal of the involved breast and all axillary contents (all three levels of nodes—axillary, pectoral, and superior apical). The underlying pectoral muscles generally are not removed before or after removal of the axillary nodes. There are several variations of this procedure.

Considerations. A modified radical mastectomy is often performed for early malignant lesions of the breast. Consideration must be given to the high incidence of multicentricity of these malignant lesions and there is much controversy as to the appropriate operation for patients with operable breast cancer. Because of the variance in this procedure, the surgeon must weigh all factors before selecting an operation.

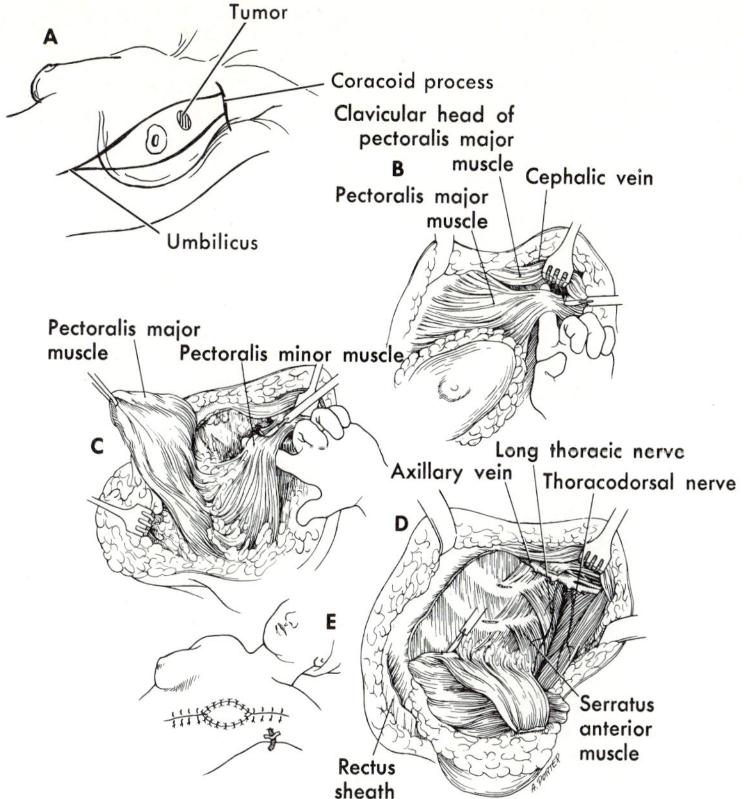

Fig. 11-8. Radical mastectomy. **A,** Lines of incision. **B,** Resection of pectoralis major muscle at clavicular attachment. **C,** Resection of pectoralis minor muscle at coracoid attachment. **D,** Axillary contents are dissected free and resected. **E,** Incision is closed (skin graft may be necessary), and drain is placed. (Redrawn from Moseley, H.F., editor: Textbook of surgery, ed. 3, St. Louis, The C.V. Mosby Co.)

Setup and preparation of the patient. As described for radical procedure.

Operative procedure. As described for radical mastectomy with the possible variations mentioned.

Extended radical mastectomy (supraradical mastectomy)

Definition. En bloc removal of the involved breast, axillary contents, underlying pectoral muscles, and internal mammary chain of lymph nodes.

Considerations. An extended radical mastectomy is indicated when the malignant lesion is located in the medial quadrant or subareolar tissue, since it tends to metastasize to the internal mammary lymph nodes. The literature suggests that this procedure be done only by surgeons well trained in this field because it carries an increased morbidity and mortality rate. Whether extended survival is obtained has not been proved.

Setup and preparation of the patient. As described for radical mastectomy. In addition, periosteal elevators and rib shears are needed. Pleural drainage tubes and collection bottles also should be available.

Operative procedure

1. After the skin incision is made and the skin flaps freed, as described for radical mastectomy, the greater pectoral muscle at the point of insertion into the humerus is freed and divided by means of a knife, hemostats, and silk ligatures.

2. The sternal origin of the greater pectoral muscle is divided with a scalpel. As the first interspace is exposed, a thoracotomy is established: through this opening, the internal mammary vessels are isolated and divided lateral to the sternum.

3. With rib shears, a segment of chest wall between 3 and 4 cm wide is resected, including portions of the second through the fifth ribs and possibly part of the sternum. As they are encountered, the intercostal vessels are clamped and ligated with silk ligatures.

4. The bone flap and lymphatic tissues are resected in continuity with the breast specimen. Resection is then continued on to the pectoral muscles and the axillary contents.

5. On excision of the en bloc specimen, closure of the wound is begun. The chest wall defect may be grafted

with a piece of rectus fascia sheath sewn to the intercostal muscles and sternal sheath, chest catheters are inserted into the eighth or ninth intercostal space, multieyed suction catheters are placed in the wound, the skin edges are approximated with interrupted silk sutures, and light pressure is applied.

6. A chest x-ray film may be taken while the patient is in the operating or recovery room.

SUGGESTED READINGS

Anthony C.P., and Thibodeau, G.A.: Textbook of anatomy and physiology, ed. 10, St. Louis, 1979, The C.V. Mosby Co.

Barth, V.: Atlas of diseases of the breast, Chicago, 1979, Year Book Medical Publishers, Inc.

Bassett, L.W.: Detecting early breast cancer, AORN J. **27:**850, 1978.

Dadd, G.D.: Present status of thermography, ultrasound, and mammography in breast cancer detection, Cancer **39:**2796, 1977.

del Regato, J.A., and Spjut, H.J.: Ackerman and del Regato's cancer diagnosis, treatment and prognosis, ed. 5, St. Louis, 1977, The C.V. Mosby Co.

Donnegan, W.L.: General considerations. In Nora, P.F.: Operative surgery, ed. 2, Philadelphia, 1980, Lea & Febiger.

Foster, C.G., and others: Effects of surgical positioning, AORN J. **30:**219, 1979.

Gallagher, H.S., and others, editors: The breast, St. Louis, 1978, The C.V. Mosby Co.

Handley, R.S., and Scanlon, E.F.,: Modified radical mastectomy. In Nora, P.F.: Operative surgery, ed. 2, Philadelphia, 1980, Lea & Febiger.

Holt, J.A., and others: Hormone receptors and breast cancer, AORN J. **27:**841, 1978.

Kneedler, J.A.: Perioperative role in three dimensions, AORN J. **30:**859, 1979.

Leis, H.P., Jr.: Risk factors for breast cancer: an update, Breast **6:**4, Oct.-Dec., 1980.

Levinger, G.E.: Working through recovery after mastectomy, Am. J. Nurs. **80:**1119, 1980.

Libshitz, H.I., Feig, S.A., and Fetouh, S.: Needle localization of nonpalpable breast lesions, Radiology **121:**557, 1976.

Marchant, D.J., and Nyerjesy, I.: Breast disease, New York, 1978, Grune & Stratton, Inc.

Mauldin, B.: Breast reconstruction after mastectomy, AORN J. **31:**612, 1980.

Phippin, M.L.: Nursing assessment of preoperative anxiety, AORN J. **31:**1019, 1980.

Rhoads, J.E., and others: Surgery: principles and practice, ed. 5, Philadelphia, 1977, J.B. Lippincott Co.

Rush, B.: Breast. In Schwartz, S.: Principles of surgery, ed. 3, New York, 1979, McGraw-Hill Book Co.

Sabiston, D.C., Jr., editor: Davis-Christopher textbook of surgery: the biological basis of modern surgical practice, ed. 11, Philadelphia, 1977, W.B. Saunders Co.

Spratt, J.S., Jr.: Radical mastectomy. In Nora, P.F.: Operative surgery, ed. 2, Philadelphia, 1980, Lea & Febiger.

Sugarbaker, E.D.: Extended radical mastectomy. In Nora, P.F.: Operative surgery, ed. 2, Philadelphia, 1980, Lea & Febiger.

Townsend, C.M., Jr.: Clin. Symp. **32**(2):3, 1980.

Tully, J.P., and Wagner, B.: Breast cancer: helping the mastectomy patient live life fully, Nursing '78 **8**(1):18, 1978.

U.S. Department of Health and Human Services: the breast cancer digest, Washington, D.C., May 1980, National Institute of Health.

Williams, P.L., and Warwick, R.: Gray's anatomy, Philadelphia, 1980, W.B. Saunders Co.

Zollinger, R.M., and Zollinger, R.M., Jr.: Atlas of surgical operations, ed. 4, New York, 1975, Macmillian Publishing Co.

12 Thyroid and parathyroid surgery

■ Thyroid gland

Surgery of goiter has long been a part of modern surgery. The introduction of iodine therapy in 1923 greatly reduced the incidence of endemic goiter and consequently the need for goiter surgery. Since 1941, indications for operations on the thyroid gland have changed because of the use of radioactive iodine and antithyroid drugs that decrease the size and vascularity of the gland.

ANATOMY AND PHYSIOLOGY

The thyroid gland is a very vascular organ situated at the front of the neck. It consists of right and left lobes united by a middle portion, known as the isthmus. The isthmus is situated near the base of the neck, and the lobes lie below the larynx and beside the trachea. The upper pole of the gland is hidden beneath the upper end of the sternothyroid muscle. The lower pole extends to the sixth tracheal ring. The posterior surface of the isthmus is adherent to the anterior surface of the tracheal rings, and the gland is enclosed by the pretracheal fascia (Fig. 12-1).

Blood supply to the thyroid is from the external carotid arteries, via the superior thyroid arteries, and from the subclavian arteries, via the inferior thyroid arteries. The thyroid gland is drained by three pairs of veins that extend from a plexus formed on the surface of the gland and on the front of the trachea. The capillaries form a dense plexus in the connective tissue around the follicles.

On each side, the superior laryngeal nerve lies in proximity to the superior thyroid artery. The recurrent laryngeal nerve that supplies the vocal cord ascends from the mediastinum and is in close association with the tracheoesophageal sulcus and the inferior thyroid artery. Sympathetic and parasympathetic nerves enter the gland, probably exerting their influence primarily on blood flow.

Numerous lymphatics of the pretracheal fascia and carotid sheath drain the gland.

The thyroid gland is important in maintaining the metabolic rate at a level compatible with health and efficiency. It is not, however, essential to life. Removal of the thyroid results in reduction of the oxidative processes of the body. Supplemental drugs help maintain a more normal metabolic rate for body processes.

The primary function of the thyroid gland is iodine metabolism. Ingested iodides are absorbed from the gastrointestinal tract into the circulatory system, from which they are sequestered by the thyroid gland. Iodides are converted into thyroid hormones, some of which are stored in the gland as thyroglobulin or are secreted into the blood as thyroid hormone.

NURSING CONSIDERATIONS

The preoperative nursing care includes assessing if the patient has been treated with drugs, if thyroid function tests have been completed, and if the ECG shows a normal rhythm. Of great importance is assessing the patient's emotional status. Many people have high anxiety levels concerning head or neck surgery. The neck is a highly visible area. Many patients, especially females, fear the cosmetic results of such surgery. The patient's own body image should be ascertained and reassurance given. Specific goals are then set to meet identified patient needs and to expedite the surgical intervention.

Implementation of nursing care begins preoperatively as the nurse answers patient questions. The successful surgical outcome is reinforced by teaching the patient postoperative comfort measures, such as turning and moving the head and shoulders as one unit to decrease tension on the muscles and suture lines of the neck.

A standard instrument setup for thyroid surgery should include the following:

- Basic instrument set (Chapter 10)
- 2 Tissue forceps, fine with several teeth
- 12 Hemostats, straight, fine
- 12 Hemostats, curved, fine
- 2 Plastic scissors, fine
- 4 Lahey vulsellum clamps
- 2 Greene retractors
- 2 Spring retractors or self-retaining retractors (Fig. 12-2)

The nurse further implements nursing care by assisting in situating the patient in the dorsal recumbent position. This is modified (Chapter 6) by placing an inflatable pillow or rolled sheet between the scapulae to extend the neck and raise the shoulders. The table is slanted feet downward to elevate the upper part of the body for the convenience of the surgeon. A padded footboard is used to keep the feet in proper alignment, and to prevent the patient's body from sliding down on the operating room bed. The arms are restrained at the side by the lift sheet, with the elbows adequately protected. A functioning suction apparatus is essential, especially during the induction and intubation phases of anesthesia. The proposed operative site, including the anterior neck region, lateral surfaces of the neck down to the outer aspects of the shoulders, and the upper anterior chest region, is cleansed in the usual manner (Chapter 5). The patient is draped with sterile towels and a fenestrated sheet, as described in Chapter 5. The surgeon may wish to mark the incision site with a silk suture strand or a "scratch" of a scalpel. This ascertains the normal neck creases and skin lines, which helps ensure a wound line that blends with the patient's neck anatomy.

As with other procedures, the instrument table is kept sterile until the dressing is applied, the patient extubated, and adequate respiratory exchange ensured.

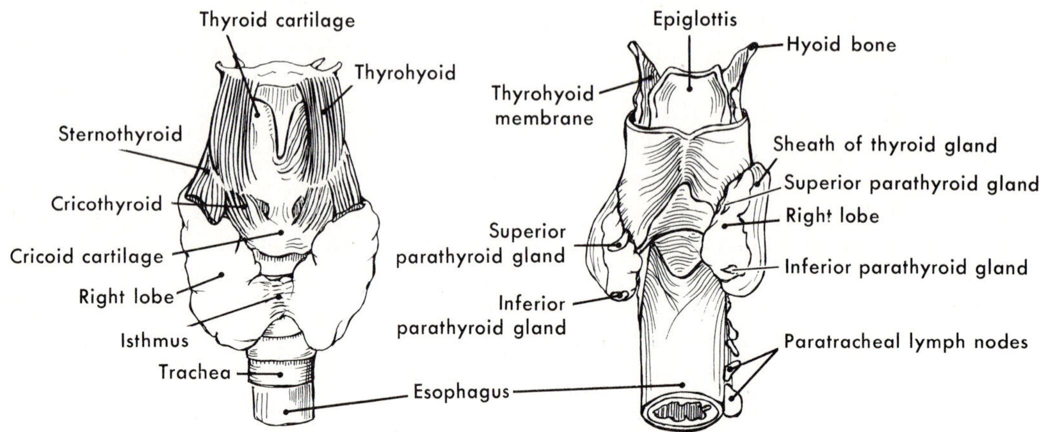

Fig. 12-1. Thyroid and parathyroid glands. Note their relation to each other and to trachea.

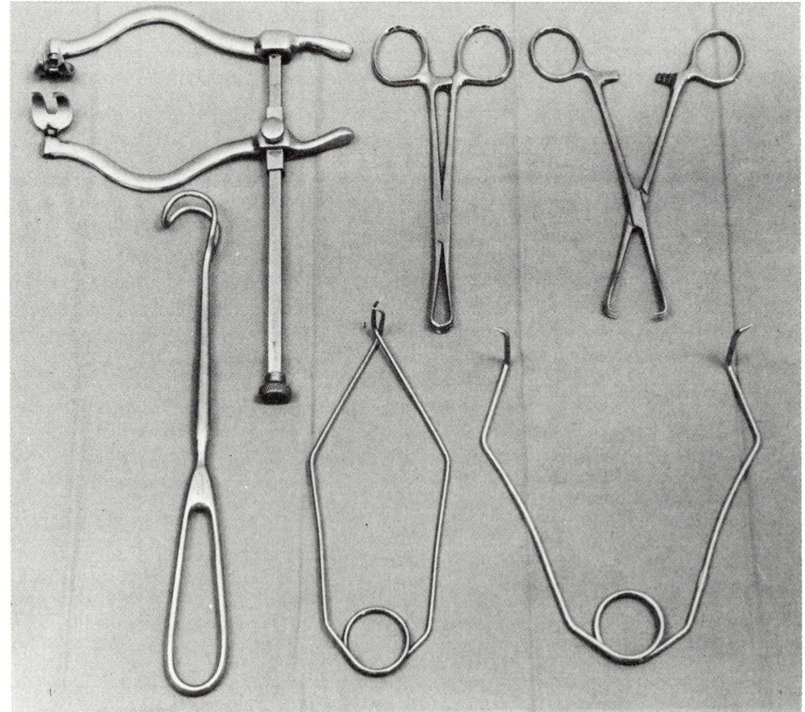

Fig. 12-2. Special instruments for thyroidectomy. *Top row, left to right,* Self-retaining thyroid retractor and Lahey vulsellum clamps; *bottom row, left to right,* Greene thyroid retractor and wire or spring retractors (set).

OPERATIONS

Thyroidectomy

Definition. Removal of the thyroid gland.

Considerations. Hyperthyroidism (Graves' disease) is associated with diffuse, bilateral enlargement of the thyroid gland. In surgical treatment of hyperthyroidism, the objective is to resect enough of the gland to reduce the level of circulating hormones to normal, yet leave a sufficient amount of the gland to secrete a supply of the hormone.

In Hashimoto's thyroiditis, thought to be an autoimmune disease, there is nontender enlargement of the gland. Surgery is done to relieve tracheal obstruction.

Nontoxic nodular goiter does not produce an excess of hormones and is not inflammatory in character. This condition is a proliferation of the thyroid tissue in an attempt to produce the minimal hormonal requirement. Surgery may be indicated to relieve tracheal or esophageal obstruction, to forestall or rule out a malignant nodule of the thyroid gland, or to relieve cosmetic disfigurement.

In the presence of papillary carcinoma and some thyroid nodules in children, a total or near total thyroidectomy is usually done. In the presence of a primary tumor of one lobe, total thyroid lobectomy and some form of neck dissection of the involved side may be performed, since the primary route of metastasis is through the regional lymph nodes.

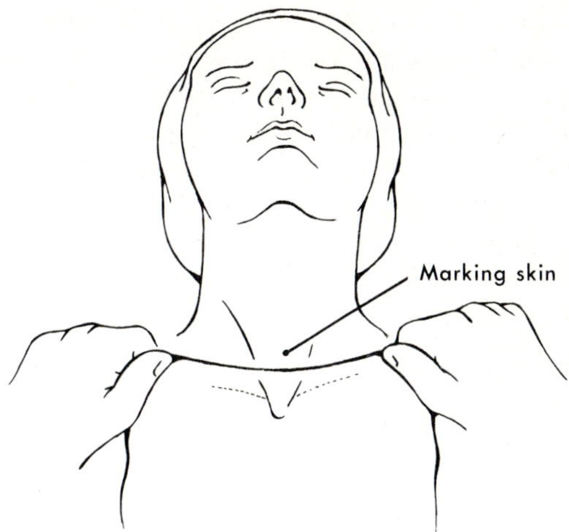

Fig. 12-3. Thyroidectomy. Proposed area of skin incision is outlined by pressure with fine silk suture strand to ensure even cosmetic incision.

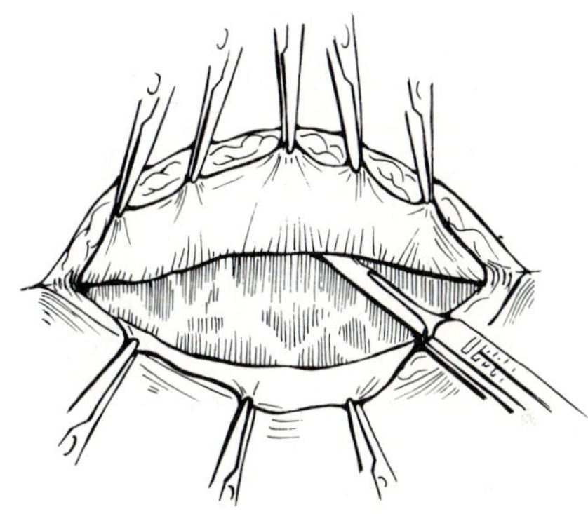

Fig. 12-4. Thyroidectomy, continued. Skin flaps are created by dissection deep to platysma and cervical fascia.

Thyroid lobectomy

Definition. Removal of a lobe of the thyroid gland.

Operative procedure

1. A transverse incision is made through the skin and first layer of the cervical fascia and platysma muscle, approximately 2 cm above the sternoclavicular junction or in the normal skin crease marked by pressing the crease with a length of silk suture strand for marking skin (Fig. 12-3).

2. Flaps may be held away from the wound with stay sutures inserted through the cervical fascia and platysma muscle, or the skin edges of flaps may be inverted and covered with skin towels by means of heavy sutures or small towel clamps.

3. The upper skin flap is undermined to the level of the cricoid cartilage; then the lower flap is undermined to the sternoclavicular joint with a knife, curved scissors, tissue forceps, and moist gauze compresses (Fig. 12-4). Bleeding vessels are clamped with hemostats and ligated with fine, nonabsorbable sutures.

4. The fascia in the midline is incised between the strap (sternohyoid) muscles with a knife (Fig. 12-5, *A*); the sternocleidomastoid muscle may be retracted with a loop retractor; the strap muscles may be divided between clamps, using Ochsner or Crile hemostats and a knife. The divided muscles are retracted from the operative site with Lahey vulsellum clamps, thereby exposing the diseased lobe. This maneuver is necessary only for markedly enlarged lobes. Usually, the strap muscles may be retracted to provide adequate exposure.

5. The inferior and middle thyroid veins are clamped, divided with Metzenbaum scissors, and ligated with no. 3-0 fine silk or other nonabsorbable sutures of choice (Fig. 12-5, *B* and *C*).

6. The lobe is rotated medially, and the loose areolar tissue is divided posteriorly and medially toward the tracheoesophageal sulcus with hemostats and Metzenbaum scissors. Small sponges are useful for blunt dissection here. Bleeding is controlled by hemostats and ligatures as well as by electrocautery. The recurrent laryngeal nerve is identified and carefully preserved.

7. The thyroid lobe is pulled downward, and the avascular tissue between the trachea and upper pole of

the thyroid is dissected by means of Metzenbaum scissors.

8. The superior thyroid artery is secured with two or three curved hemostats; the artery is ligated and divided and then is transfixed with chromic gut or silk sutures.

9. The inferior thyroid artery is identified and ligated by means of fine forceps, sutures, and scissors (Fig. 12-6, *A*). The thyroid lobe is then dissected away from the recurrent nerve with Metzenbaum scissors, hemostats, and retractors. Bleeding vessels are clamped with hemostats and ligated with fine silk sutures.

10. The lobe is elevated with Lahey vulsellum clamps; it is freed from the trachea with fine scissors, forceps, knife, and hemostats. The fibrous bands attached to the trachea and cricoid cartilage are divided.

11. The isthmus of the gland is elevated with fine forceps and divided between Crile hemostats with scissors (Fig. 12-6, *B*). The resection of the lobe is completed, and the lobe is removed. Care is taken throughout the procedure to carefully identify and preserve the parathyroid glands.

12. The cut surface of the opposite lobe requires careful hemostasis (Fig. 12-6, *C*).

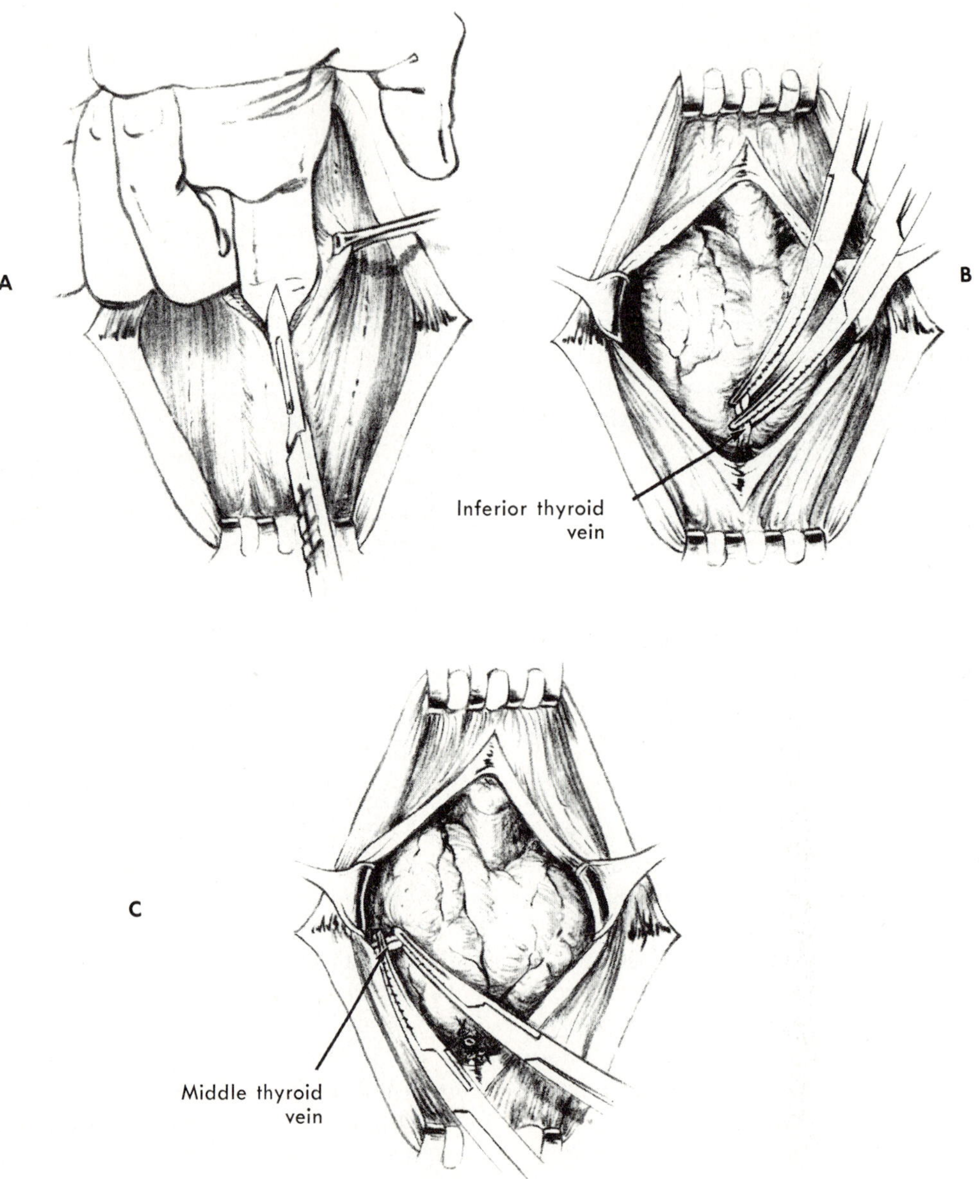

Fig. 12-5. Thyroidectomy, continued. **A,** Strap muscles reflected. **B,** Ligation of inferior thyroid vein. **C,** Ligation of middle thyroid vein. (From Wilder, J.R.: Atlas of general surgery, ed. 2, St. Louis, The C.V. Mosby Co.)

13. The strap muscles, if severed, are approximated with interrupted, absorbable or nonabsorbable sutures. A Penrose drain may be inserted in the thyroid bed and brought out between the strap muscles and sternocleidomastoid muscle. Many surgeons prefer to drain laterally through the sternocleidomastoid muscle and the lateral extremity of the incision, believing this to produce a better cosmetic result. Drainage is usually not necessary.

14. The edges of the platysma muscle are approximated; then the skin edges are approximated with interrupted, fine silk sutures.

15. Gauze dressings are applied to the wound; a thyroid collar type of dressing is applied. This dressing consists of a strip of adhesive tape or Elastoplast 2 inches wide and 28 inches long, with a folded gauze compress covering its center portion (Fig. 12-7). The gauze prevents the hair from coming in contact with the tape. The dressing is brought from the back of the neck to the front, and the free ends of the collar are crossed and secured over the chest region. The dressing is further secured by additional strips of tape.

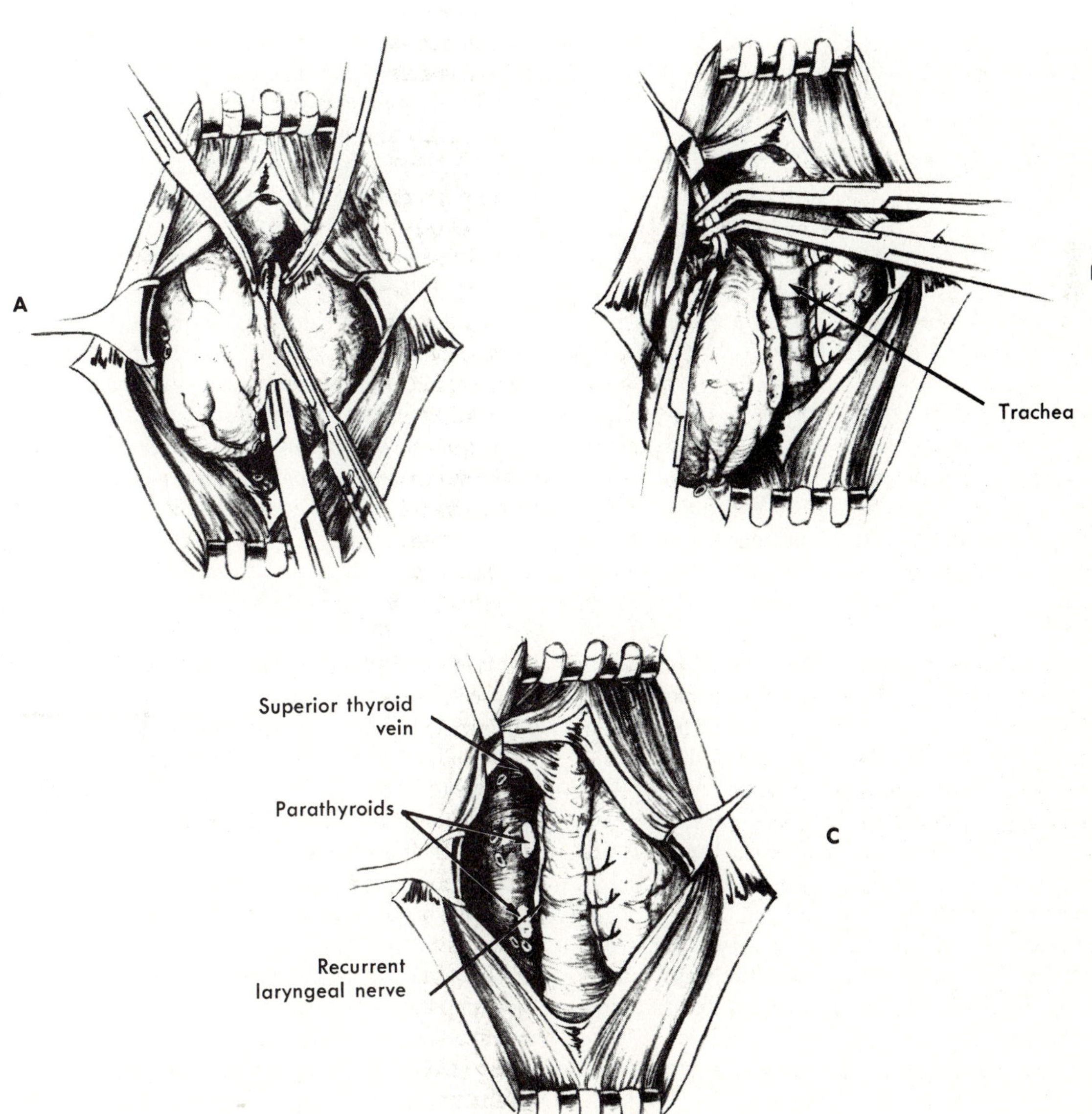

Fig. 12-6. Thyroidectomy, continued. **A,** Ligation of pole vessels. **B,** Isthmus divided. **C,** Anatomical structures identified, and wound examined for bleeding. (From Wilder, J.R.: Atlas of general surgery, ed. 2, St. Louis, The C.V. Mosby Co.)

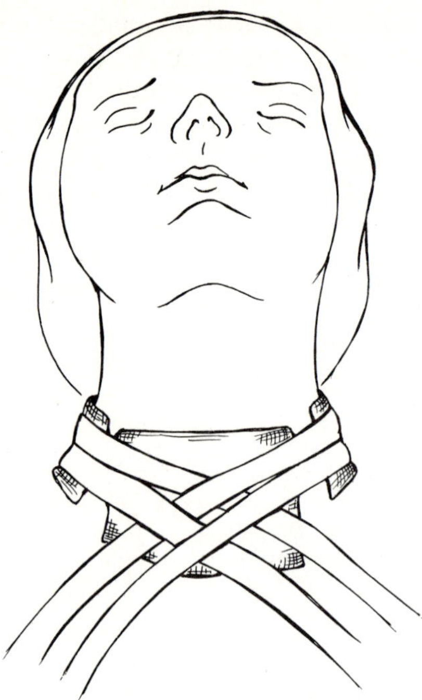

Fig. 12-7. Thyroid collar type of dressing.

Nerve damage is more likely to occur in patients undergoing a bilateral total thyroidectomy.

Substernal or intrathoracic thyroid

Extensions of enlarging goiters into the substernal and intrathoracic regions are frequently seen. They may cause tracheal and esophageal obstruction, in which case they may be surgically excised. Longer instruments are usually required. Splitting of the sternum is rarely necessary.

Thyroglossal duct cystectomy

Definition. Complete excision of all portions of the cyst and duct, as well as a portion of the hyoid bone, which contains the duct, to avoid recurrent cystic formation and prevent infections. The thyroglossal duct is an embryological structure present during the descent of the thyroid gland into the anterior neck. When present in the adult, it exists as a pretracheal cystic pouch attached to the hyoid bone, with or without a sinus tract to the base of the tongue at the foramen cecum.

Considerations. The preoperative nursing assessment should be conducted appropriate to the patient's age, since the patient is frequently a child or teenager. Reassurance regarding the procedure should be given.

A thyroidectomy setup plus the following instruments is used:

1 Periosteal elevator, small
1 Duckbill rongeur, small
1 Bone cutter, small
1 Syringe, 5 ml, with appropriate needle
Methylene blue dye for injection

Operative procedure

1. After the head is extended and the chin is elevated, an incision is made between the hyoid bone and the thyroid cartilage through the subcutaneous tissue.
2. The platysma muscle is incised and the flaps raised as described previously.
3. The strap (sternohyoid) muscles are separated in the midline.
4. Sharp and blunt dissections are used to mobilize the cyst and duct up to the attachment to the hyoid bone. The hyoid bone is transected twice with bone-cutting forceps, and the segment of bone and cyst is freed from adjacent structures.
5. The cephalic part of the duct is identified; a transfixion suture no. 3-0 is passed through it, and the duct transsected. (Methylene blue dye injection is used rarely to visualize the whole tract.)
6. The cyst is removed. The strap muscles are closed with interrupted, nonabsorbable, fine silk sutures. A drain may be placed if necessary. The skin is closed with interrupted, fine no. 5-0 nylon sutures.

■ Parathyroid glands

Interest in the parathyroid glands began in 1880, when they were discovered by the Swedish anatomist Sandström. Through the years, subsequent discoveries have been made linking disturbances of these endocrine glands with tetany, bone diseases, renal calculi, and many other systemic abnormalities. Current surgical interest is focused on definitive treatment of hyperparathyroidism.

ANATOMY AND PHYSIOLOGY

The parathyroid glands are four small masses of tissue lying behind or, rarely, within the thyroid gland, inside the pretracheal fascia. The upper pair lie behind the superior pole of the thyroid; the lower pair lie near the lower pole of the thyroid. Aberrant nodules of the parathyroid tissue may be found outside the pretracheal fascia as low as the superior mediastinum, especially within the thymus. The glands are brownish and normally measure 3 to 4 mm in diameter. Their blood supply is derived from the superior and inferior thyroid arteries (Figs. 12-5 and 12-6).

The function of these glands in body metabolism is most important. The endocrine secretion of parathormone regulates and maintains the metabolism and hemostasis of blood calcium concentration. Removal of all parathyroid tissue results in severe tetany or death. The diseases attributed to the parathyroid glands are hyperparathyroidism, which results in elevation of calcium in the blood, and hypoparathyroidism, resulting in decreased calcium in the blood.

OPERATIONS

Parathyroidectomy

Definition. Excision of one or more diseased parathyroid glands. Normal or atrophic glands are not to be damaged or resected.

Considerations. The presence of adenomas (hypersecreting neoplasms), hyperplasia, or carcinomas requires surgical excision. In the last case, resection of lymphatics is essential, although metastasis may also occur by way of the bloodstream. After local excision, a metastasis may continue the hypersecretion of parathormone.

The instrument setup is identical to that for thyroid operations, with the addition of numerous specimen containers that are necessary for the multiple biopsies to determine the presence or absence of parathyroid tissue.

Operative procedure

1. See approach to the thyroid gland, described previously.

2. The thyroid gland is now visible. A thorough exploration of the "normal" locations of the four parathyroid glands is conducted to find them. Meticulous hemostasis by means of mosquito hemostats and fine ligatures is a prerequisite to location and identification of these small glands.

3. The thyroid gland is gently rotated anteriorly to provide access to the posterior thyroid sulcus, where the parathyroid glands are almost always found. Identification of the parathyroid vascular pedicle as it leaves the superior thyroid artery is an excellent means of finding the upper gland. Metzenbaum scissors, mosquito hemostats, and Kitner sponges are used in the dissection.

4. Attention is then directed toward the posterior lateral surface of the thyroid lobe or just beneath the lower thyroid pole, where the lower parathyroid gland is frequently found. Again, finding the vascular pedicle from the inferior thyroid artery may aid in identification. Occasionally the lower pair may be found in the thymic capsule or tissue, in which case a portion of the thymus is resected.

5. Should one of the parathyroid glands evidence disease, it is resected by clamping the vascular pedicle with mosquito forceps, dividing with small scissors or knife, and ligating with a fine nonabsorbable suture. The question of how much parathyroid tissue to remove is controversial and relates to whether a single or multiple glands are involved, regardless of their size and/or appearance. A portion of one gland must remain to prevent complications.

6. The neck region is explored for aberrant parathyroid tissue, which is also resected.

7. The remainder of the operation is the same as that described for the thyroid gland.

8. A dressing is applied as described for thyroid surgery.

SUGGESTED READINGS

Anthony, C.P., and Thibodeau, G.A.: Textbook of anatomy and physiology, ed. 10, St. Louis, 1979, The C.V. Mosby Co.

Ballinger, W.F., and Haff, R.C.: Hyperparathyroidism: increased frequency of diagnosis, South. Med. J. **63**:571, 1970.

Beland I.L., and Passos, J.Y.: Clinical nursing, ed. 3, New York, 1975, Macmillan Publishing Co.

Bondy, P.K., and Rosenberg, L.E.: Duncan's diseases of metabolism, ed. 7, Philadelphia, 1974, W.B. Saunders Co.

Bradley, E.L., DiGirolamo, M., and Tarcan, Y.: Modified subtotal thyroidectomy in the management of Graves' disease, Surgery **87**:623, 1980.

Gruendemann, B.J., and others: The surgical patient: Behavioral concepts for the operating room nurse, ed. 2, St. Louis, 1977, The C.V. Mosby Co.

Haff, R.C., Black, W.C., and Ballinger, W.F.: Primary hyperparathyroidism: changing clinical, surgical, and pathologic aspects, Ann. Surg. **171**:85, 1970.

LeMaitre, G.D., and Finnegan, J.A.: The patient in surgery: a guide for nurses, ed. 4, Philadelphia, 1980, W.B. Saunders Co.

Luckmann, J., and Sorenson, K.C.: Medical surgical nursing, Philadelphia, 1974, W.B. Saunders Co.

Madden, J.L.: Atlas of techniques in surgery, ed. 2, New York, 1964, Appleton-Century-Crofts.

Martis, C., and Athanassiades, S.: Post-thyroidectomy laryngeal edema, Am. J. Surg. **122**:58, 1971.

Norton, J.A., Doppman, J.L., and Brenan, M.F.: Localization and resection of clinically inapparent medullary carcinoma of the thyroid, Surgery **87**:616, 1980.

Paparella, M.M., and Shumrick, D.A.: Otolaryngology, vol. 3, Philadelphia, 1973, W.B. Saunders Co.

Rhoads, J.E., and others: Surgery: principles and practice, ed. 4, Philadelphia, 1970, J.B. Lippincott Co.

Rosoff, L., and Bethune, J.E.: Surgical management of primary hyperparathyroidism, Hosp. Prac. **9**:70, April 1974.

Stone, D.B.: Hyperparathyroidism, Curr. Med. Dialogue, **41**:377, 1974.

13 Gallbladder, ducts, liver, pancreas, and spleen surgery

ANATOMY AND PHYSIOLOGY

The *liver* is situated in the right upper quadrant of the abdominal cavity, beneath the dome of the diaphragm and directly above the stomach, duodenum, and hepatic flexure of the colon (Fig. 13-1). The external covering, known as *Glisson's capsule,* is composed of dense connective tissue. The peritoneum extends over the entire surface of the liver, except at the point of posterior attachment to the diaphragm. The arterial blood supply is maintained by the hepatic artery, and venous blood from the stomach, intestines, spleen, and pancreas is carried to the liver by the portal vein and its branches. The hepatic venous system returns blood to the heart by way of the inferior vena cava.

The *bile,* manufactured by the liver cells, is secreted into the fine biliary radicles and, in turn, flows into the large ducts. It ultimately leaves the liver through the right and left hepatic ducts. These ducts join immediately after leaving the liver to form one common hepatic duct that merges with the cystic duct from the gallbladder to form the common bile duct. The common bile duct opens into the duodenum in an area called the *ampulla* or *papilla* of Vater, located about 7.5 cm below the pyloric opening from the stomach.

The bile contains bile salts, which facilitate digestion and absorption, and various waste products. The liver is essential in the metabolism of carbohydrates, proteins, and fats.

The *gallbladder,* which lies in a sulcus on the undersurface of the right lobe of the liver, terminates in the cystic duct. This ductal system provides a channel for the flow of bile to the gallbladder, where it becomes highly concentrated during the storage period. However, as food is ingested, especially fats, the musculature of the gallbladder contracts, forcing bile into the cystic duct and through the common duct. As the sphincter of Oddi in the ampulla of Vater relaxes, bile pours forth, flowing into the duodenum to aid in digestion. The gallbladder receives its blood supply from the cystic artery, a branch of the hepatic artery (Fig. 13-1).

The *pancreas* (Fig. 13-1) is a fixed structure lying transversely behind the stomach in the upper abdomen. The head of the pancreas is fixed to the curve of the duodenum and shares the same blood supply with the duodenum. The body of the pancreas lies across the vertebrae and over the superior mesenteric artery and vein. The tail of the pancreas extends to the hilus of the spleen. The pancreatic juice, containing digestive enzymes, is collected in the pancreatic duct, or duct of Wirsung, which unites with the common bile duct to enter the duodenum about 7.5 cm below the pylorus. The ampulla of Vater is formed by the dilated junction of the two ducts at the point of entry.

The pancreas also contains groups of cells, called *islets* or *islands of Langerhans,* which secrete hormones into the blood capillaries instead of into the duct. These hormones are insulin and glucagon, and both are involved in carbohydrate metabolism.

The *spleen* (Fig. 13-2) is situated in the upper left abdominal cavity, with full protection provided by the tenth, eleventh, and twelfth ribs; the lateral surface is directly beneath the dome of the diaphragm. The anterior medial surface is in proximity to the cardiac end of the stomach and the splenic flexure of the colon. The spleen is covered with peritoneum that forms supporting ligaments. The arterial blood supply is furnished by the splenic artery, a branch of the celiac axis. The splenic vein drains into the portal system (Fig. 13-2).

The spleen has many functions. Among them are the defense of the body by phagocytosis of microorganisms, formation of nongranular leukocytes and plasma cells, and phagocytosis of damaged red blood cells. It also acts as a blood reservoir.

NURSING CONSIDERATIONS

General procedures of skin preparation and draping are discussed in Chapter 5. The following pertinent factors are to be considered in caring for the patient undergoing biliary surgery.

Positioning the patient. The patient is placed in a supine position with the patient's right upper quadrant elevated with an inflatable "gallbladder bag," folded sheet, or other device. Some surgeons do not use elevation because they do not believe that it aids in exposure, and it may cause backaches postoperatively.

When an operative cholangiogram is anticipated, the operating table is prepared with an x-ray cassette holder before the patient is positioned. A preliminary x-ray film may be taken to ensure correct placement of the cassette. The holder must be directly beneath the patient's right

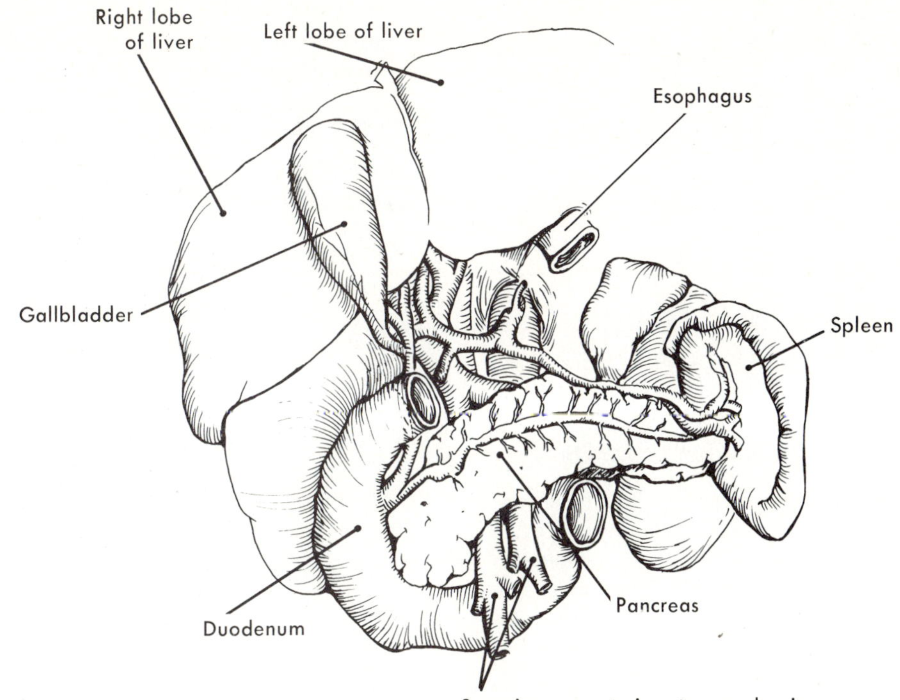

Fig. 13-1. Gallbladder and surrounding anatomy.

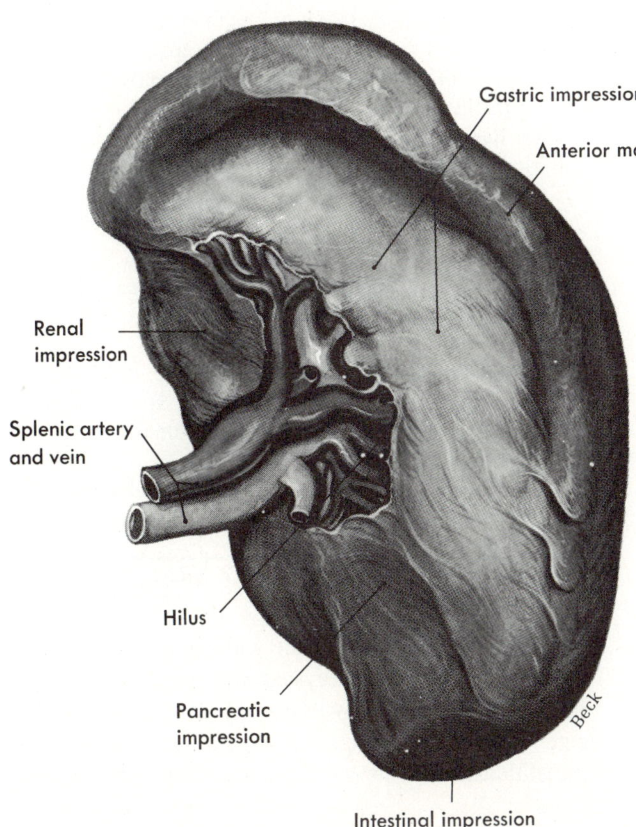

Fig. 13-2. Spleen, medial aspect. Arrangement of vessels at hilus is highly variable. (From Anthony, C.P., and Kolthoff, N.J.: Textbook of anatomy and physiology, ed. 9, St. Louis, 1975, The C.V. Mosby Co.)

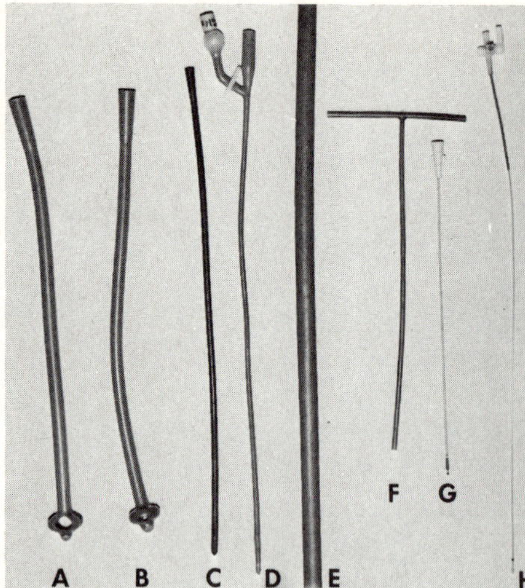

Fig. 13-3. Drainage tubes and catheters for biliary surgery. *A*, Malecot or batwing catheter; *B*, mushroom or Pezzer catheter; *C*, red Robinson catheter; *D*, Foley catheter; *E*, Penrose soft latex tubing; *F*, T tube (latex); *G*, biliary balloon probe; *H*, cholangiography catheter.

upper quadrant, since correct positioning is imperative to ensure accurate visualization of the biliary tract.

Drainage materials. Tubes and catheters must be in perfect condition and suitable for the areas to be drained. If a defective drain is used, a free fragment may remain in the wound on removal of the tube (Fig. 13-3).

The scrub nurse should note the condition of all drainage materials and should test them for patency before giving them to the surgeon.

Soft rubber or latex tissue drains (Penrose) are used after a cholecystectomy or a choledochotomy. The Penrose or capillary drain may be used the way it comes from the package, or it may be made into a cigarette drain. The latter can be made by passing folded gauze packing of suitable width and length through the lumen of the drain. The packing will serve as a wick.

A T tube drain of latex rubber (Fig. 13-3) and of suitable size is prepared by the surgeon after the duct has been explored. The center of the crossbar is notched opposite the junction of the vertical limb so that its ends will bend more readily during removal. The ends are beveled and tailored to fit the duct. In operations involving the ampulla of Vater, a Cattell-type T tube may be passed through this sphincter and into the duodenum, although this is rarely used today.

Drains are usually exteriorized through separate stab wounds and anchored to skin edges to prevent retraction of the drain.

Aseptic measures. When the common duct is opened or an anastomosis is established between a duct and other parts of the tract, care should be exercised to isolate contaminated instruments and materials from the remainder of the operative field, as described for gastrointestinal surgery (Chapter 14).

Instruments and materials used for the exteriorization of a drain should be treated as contaminated.

INSTRUMENTATION

The setup includes the basic laparotomy set (Chapter 10), plus the following:

Cutting instruments

1 Metzenbaum or Nelson scissors, 9¼ inches

Clamping and exposing instruments (Fig. 13-4)

1 Wolfson gallbladder retractor
2 Harrington retractors
2 Mixter gallbladder forceps, 7¼ inches
2 Johns Hopkins gallbladder forceps, 8 inches
2 Lahey gall duct forceps, 7¼ inches
6 Schnidt gall duct forceps

Duct instruments (Fig. 13-5)

1 Mayo common duct scoop, malleable shaft, 10½ inches
1 Mayo cystic duct scoop, malleable shaft, 10 inches
1 Moore gallstone scoop
1 Set gall duct spoons, malleable copper, sizes 1 to 5
1 Ochsner gallbladder aspirating trocar
2 Potts-Smith forceps

Stone instruments (Fig. 13-6)

1 Set Randall kidney stone forceps (may be used instead of Blake and Desjardin gallstone forceps)
2 Blake gallstone forceps, 1 straight and 1 curved, 8¼ inches
1 Desjardin gallstone forceps, 9¼ inches
1 Set Bakes common duct dilators
1 Moynihan bile duct probe and scoop

Accessory items

Hemostatic clips and applicators
2 Penrose drains, ⅝- or ½-inch diameter, each 12 inches long
2 Safety pins
1 Yard plain gauze packing, 2 inches wide, if desired
Drainage catheters, as desired (Fig. 13-3)
Sutures, as listed for surgeon in card file (Chapter 7)
Fogarty biliary catheters (Fig. 13-3)
Contrast media (Hypaque, Conray, or Reno-M)
Culture tubes

OPERATIONS ON THE BILIARY TRACT

Cholecystectomy

Definition. Removal of the gallbladder.

Considerations. Cholecystectomy is performed for the treatment of diseases involving the gallbladder, such as acute or chronic inflammation with or without stones (cholelithiasis), or in the presence of polyps or carcinoma.

Setup and preparation of the patient. As described for laparotomy and biliary surgery.

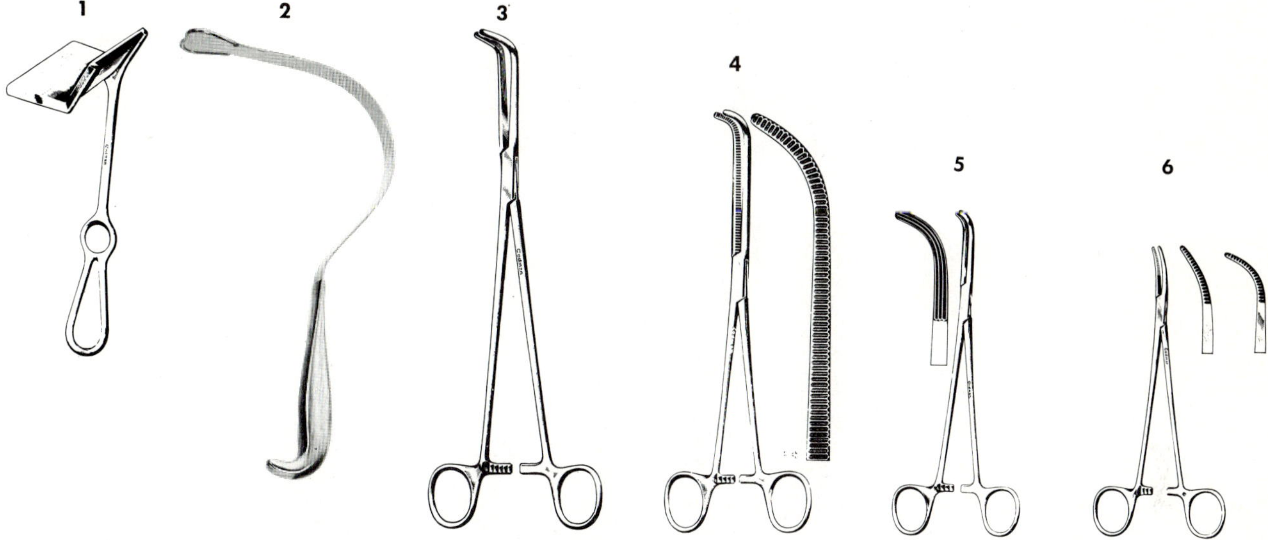

Fig. 13-4. Clamping and exposing instruments for gallbladder surgery. *1,* Wolfson gallbladder retractor; *2,* Harrington retractor; *3,* Mixter (right-angle) gallbladder forceps; *4,* Johns Hopkins gallbladder forceps; *5,* Lahey gall duct forceps; *6,* Schnidt gall duct forceps. (Courtesy Codman & Shurtleff, Inc., Randolph, Mass.)

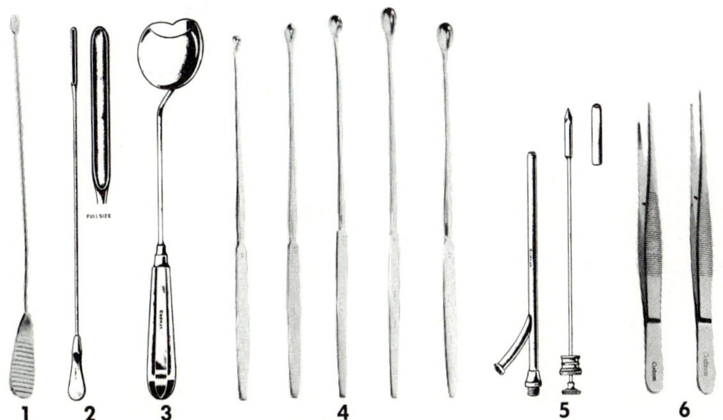

Fig. 13-5. Duct instruments: *1,* Mayo common duct scoop; *2,* Mayo cystic duct scoop; *3,* Moore gallstone scoop; *4,* gall duct spoons; *5,* Ochsner gallbladder trocar; *6,* Potts-Smith forceps. (Courtesy Codman & Shurtleff, Inc., Randolph, Mass.)

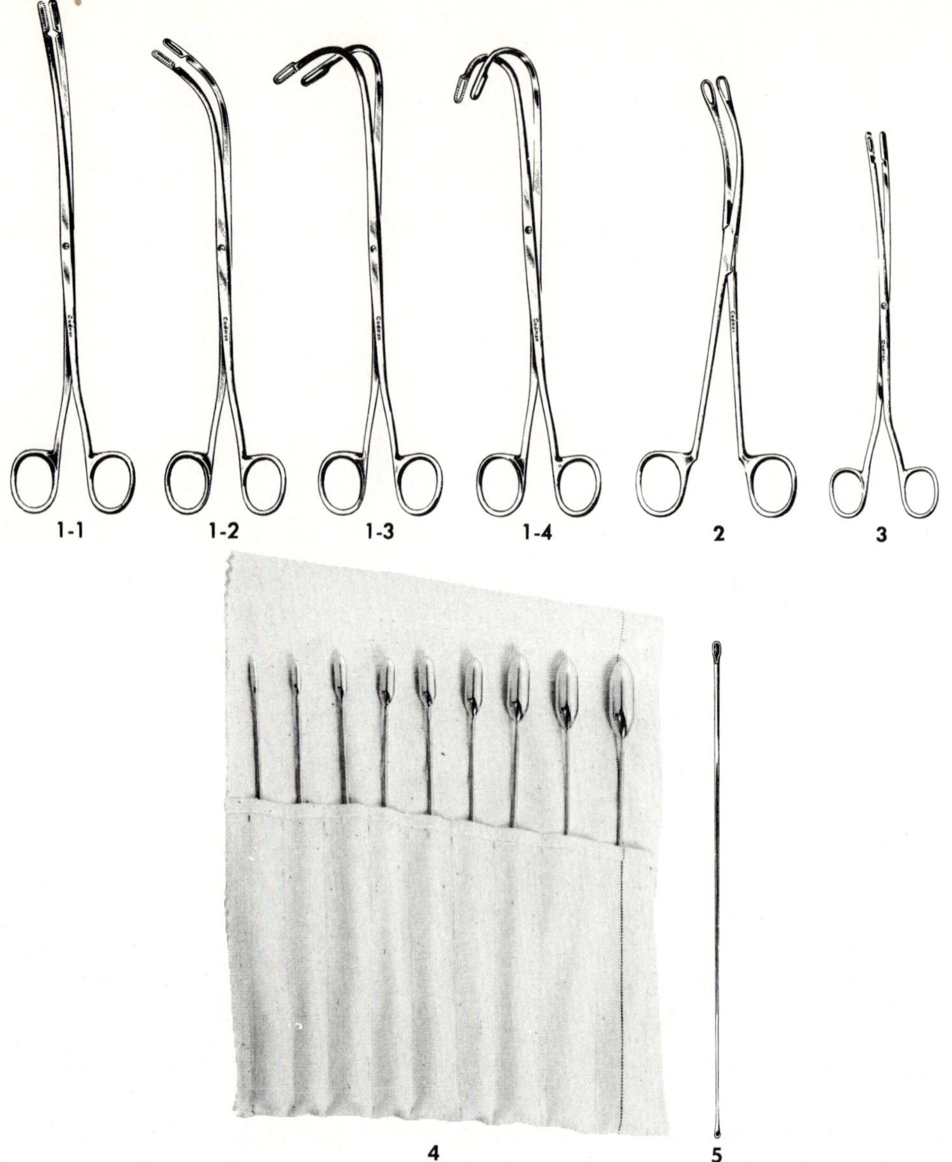

Fig. 13-6. Stone instruments. *1-1* to *1-4,* Randall kidney stone forceps (four sizes and shapes); *2,* Blake gallstone forceps; *3,* Desjardin gallstone forceps; *4,* Bakes common duct dilators; *5,* Moynihan gall duct probe and scoop. (Courtesy Codman & Shurtleff, Inc., Randolph, Mass.)

Operative procedure (Fig. 13-7)

1. Through a right subcostal, right paramedian, or midline incision, the abdominal cavity is opened, as described for laparotomy (Chapter 10). Retractors and laparotomy packs are employed as the abdominal cavity is carefully examined.

2. The common duct is palpated for evidence of stones, and the pathological condition determined. Harrington retractors, moist or dry laparotomy packs, long tissue forceps, and suction are used.

3. The surrounding organs are walled off from the gallbladder region by laparotomy packs and deep retractors.

4. To facilitate gentle traction, Peans are usually placed on the body of the gallbladder (Fig. 13-7, *A*).

5. The peritoneal fold overlying the junction of the cystic and common duct is incised with a long no. 7 knife handle and a no. 15 blade, long Metzenbaum scissors, and forceps. Suction is available, and bleeding points are clamped and ligated or electrocoagulated.

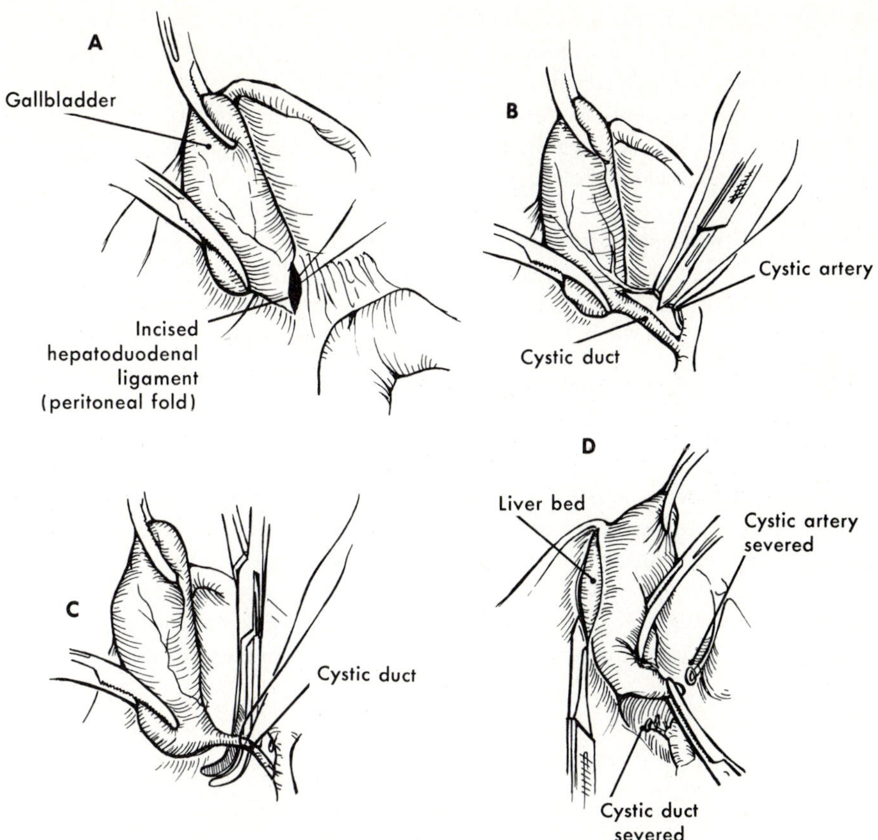

Fig. 13-7. Cholecystectomy. **A,** With Pean clamps in place, gentle traction is maintained as peritoneum over Calot's triangle is incised. **B,** Cystic artery is clearly visualized, doubly ligated, and divided. **C,** Cystic duct is carefully dissected and identified before clamps and ligatures are applied. **D,** Dissection of gallbladder from liver bed is completed.

6. Adhesions are separated by blunt dissection with small, round, dry dissector sponges; sponges on holders; and blunt right-angled clamps. Dissection is continued to expose the neck of the gallbladder, the cystic artery, and the cystic duct (Fig. 13-7, *B* and *C*).

7. Dissection is continued to expose the cystic artery as it enters the wall of the gallbladder. On complete exposure and visualization of the branches, the cystic artery is doubly ligated with silk or clamped with hemostatic clips and divided (Fig. 13-7, *B*). Occasionally, a third ligature or clip may be used. If there is more than one branch of the cystic artery, each will be ligated and divided separately. Abnormalities of the arterial and ductal anatomy are common, and the surgeon works with meticulous care to identify these structures.

8. The true junction of the cystic duct with the common bile duct is visualized. The cystic duct is identified and carefully dissected from the common bile duct to the gallbladder neck. It is then doubly ligated and divided (Fig. 13-7, *C*). A transfixion suture of fine chromic gut may be used on the stump of the cystic duct near the common bile duct. The gallbladder is freed from the liver, working upward to the fundus, and the specimen is removed (Fig. 13-7, *D*). In some cases it may be necessary to work from the fundus downward to the neck of the gallbladder.

9. All bleeding is controlled; reperitonealization of the liver bed, if indicated, is accomplished with interrupted or continuous fine chromic intestinal sutures.

10. A Penrose, Jackson-Pratt, or cigarette drain is inserted near the cystic duct stump. The free end of the drain is exteriorized through a stab wound in the lateral abdominal wall.

11. The wound is closed in layers, as described for laparotomy (Chapter 10). A safety pin may be attached to the protruding Penrose drain, and a dressing applied.

Cholecystostomy

Definition. Establishment of an opening into the gallbladder to permit drainage of the organ and removal of stones.

Considerations. Cholecystostomy is usually selected

for patients with acute gallbladder disease and a general physical condition that will not permit more extensive surgery. A local anesthetic may be administered.

Setup and preparation of the patient. As described for laparotomy and biliary surgery, plus selected drainage tubes or catheters of suitable sizes, such as Foley, Malecot, mushroom, or Robinson.

A large syringe (50 ml) or an Asepto syringe may be needed for irrigation purposes. If a local anesthetic is used, the agent and a selection of syringes and needles are necessary.

Operative procedure

1. Although many surgeons prefer the right subcostal incision, cholecystostomy procedures are often done as emergencies, so a quicker vertical incision may be used.

2. The fundus of the gallbladder is grasped with an Allis or Babcock clamp, and the proposed opening is encircled by means of a chromic purse-string suture, leaving the ends long (Fig. 13-8, *A*).

3. To protect the abdominal cavity from infection, the gallbladder is isolated by means of laparotomy packs, and suction is available.

4. Within the purse-string suture, the gallbladder is aspirated by means of a trocar with tubing and suction attached (Fig. 13-8, *A*).

5. As the contents are aspirated, cultures should be taken. The contaminated trocar is removed and discarded.

6. The opening can be enlarged with Metzenbaum scissors; gallstones are removed with malleable scoops and stone forceps (Fig. 13-8), *B*). It is necessary to irrigate the gallbladder with isotonic saline solution to remove small stones, grit, or paste-like material. A syringe with a catheter or an Asepto syringe may be used for irrigation. Contaminated instruments are placed in a basin on the operative field.

7. A drainage tube is inserted in the gallbladder opening (Fig. 13-8, *C*). The purse-string suture is tightened around the catheter, care being taken not to occlude it. A second purse-string suture or separate mattress sutures may be used to secure the gallbladder to the peritoneum and the posterior rectus fascia.

8. The free end of the catheter or tube is exteriorized

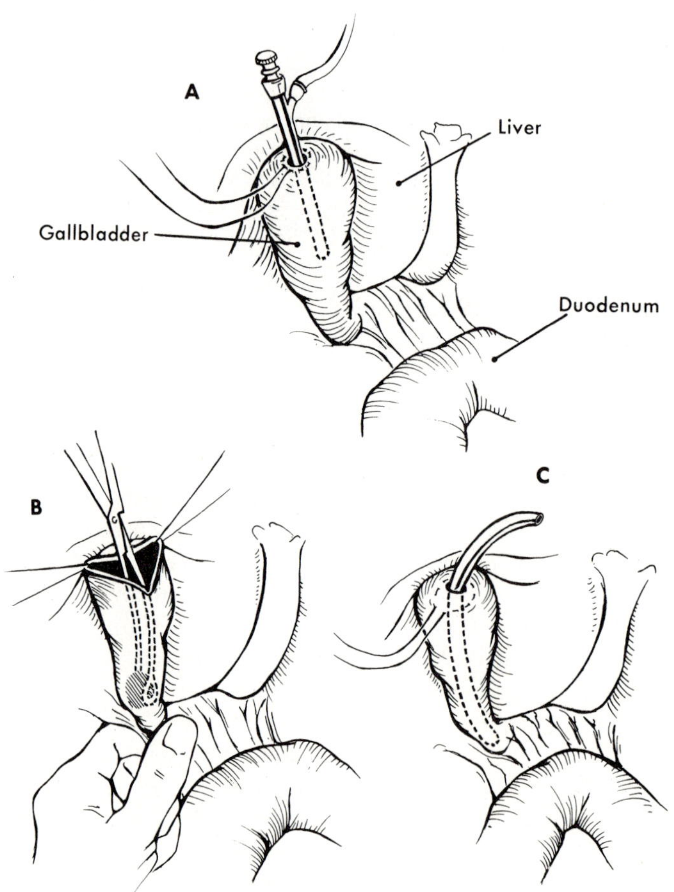

Fig. 13-8. Cholecystostomy. **A,** Purse-string suture and trocar are in place. **B,** Calculus is removed through opening in fundus. **C,** Drainage catheter is in place.

through a stab wound and then anchored to the skin edges, as described for cholecystectomy.

9. Drainage of the abdominal cavity is established by means of a Penrose or cigarette drain. The exterior end of each drain is secured by a safety pin or suture.

10. The wound is closed in layers, as described for laparotomy, and dressings are applied without disturbing the drains.

Choledochostomy and choledochotomy

Definitions

choledochostomy Establishment of an opening into the common bile duct by means of a drainage T tube.

choledochotomy Incision into the common bile duct for removal of stones.

Considerations. Choledochotomy is performed to treat choledocholithiasis or to relieve an obstruction in the common bile duct.

Before exploration is begun, open cholangiography may be performed to locate all stones within the ductal system. X-ray films are repeated after the T tube drain is in place to confirm the successful evacuation and patency of the ducts.

A subcostal or upper right rectus incision may be made.

Setup and preparation of the patient. As described for biliary surgery, plus the following additional instruments:

1 Set Bakes common duct dilators, malleable shafts, sizes 3 to 11 mm (Fig. 13-6)
1 Ochsner flexible spiral gallstone probe, 14 inches
1 Malleable silver probe, 8 inches
1 Asepto syringe, 2 ounces
4 Syringes, 2, 20, 30, and 50 ml
3 Aspirating needles: 24 gauge, ¾ inch; 19 gauge, 3½ inches; and 16 gauge, 2 inches
1 Catheter adapter for saline solution irrigation
2 Ampules contrast media
3 Robinson catheters, 8, 12, and 16 Fr
3 T tubes, Cattell-type, 8 to 26 Fr, as desired
Fogarty biliary catheters (Fig. 13-3)

Operative procedure

1. The abdomen is opened as for cholecystectomy. If the gallbladder has not been previously removed, it is now exposed and removed or retracted by means of laparotomy packs and retractors.

2. The common duct (Fig. 13-9, *A*), may be identified by means of an aspirating syringe and fine-gauged needle to make certain that the suspected duct is not a blood vessel. A specimen for cultures may be obtained.

3. Two fine traction sutures are placed in the wall of the duct, below the entrance of the cystic duct (Fig. 13-9, *B*).

4. The common duct region is walled off with laparotomy packs and narrow blade retractors. A discard basin for contaminated instruments is placed at the lower end of the operative field; a suction apparatus is made ready for immediate use.

5. A longitudinal incision is made in the common duct (Fig. 13-9, *A*), between the traction sutures, with a long no. 3 handle and a no. 15 or no. 11 blade. Constant suction is maintained with a Yankauer suction tube to keep the field free of oozing bile as the incision is enlarged with a Potts angled or Metzenbaum scissors. Additional stay sutures may be applied to the ductal opening.

6. Visible stones are removed with gallstone forceps, after which exploration of the duct is begun with small malleable scoops proximally and then distally to the opening. Probing is continued as stones are removed from both the common and hepatic ducts. Isotonic saline solution in a bulb syringe and a small-lumen catheter or a Fogarty-type, balloon-tipped catheter is used to facilitate the removal of small stones and debris, as well as to demonstrate patency through to the duodenum (Fig. 13-9, *B* to *D*).

7. A duodenotomy may be performed if patency of the sphincter of Oddi and ampulla of Vater cannot be demonstrated.

a. An area of the duodenum is walled off with laparotomy packs. The incision is made longitudinally with a scalpel, using blade no. 15 and Metzenbaum scissors.
b. Bleeding vessels are clamped with mosquito hemostats and ligated with fine silk or chromic sutures or electrocoagulated.
c. Fine silk traction sutures are inserted, and exploration is carried out.
d. The duodenal opening is usually closed transversely in two layers with fine chromic and silk intestinal sutures.

8. The T tube is prepared by the surgeon (Fig. 13-9, *E*), irrigated for patency, and introduced into the common duct with fine vascular forceps.

9. The common duct incision is closed with fine chromic intestinal sutures. Contaminated instruments are placed in the discard basin.

10. The T tube is irrigated to demonstrate patency (Fig. 13-9, *E*), and a cholangiogram is done.

11. The gallbladder may be removed, as described for cholecystectomy.

12. A Penrose, Jackson-Pratt, or cigarette drain is introduced into the foramen of Winslow. Both drain and tube are exteriorized through a stab wound.

13. The wound is closed in layers; the tube and drain are carefully anchored to the skin, and each wound is dressed individually to prevent undue tension that could result in displacement of tube and drain.

14. Sterile tubing is used to connect the T tube to the small drainage container.

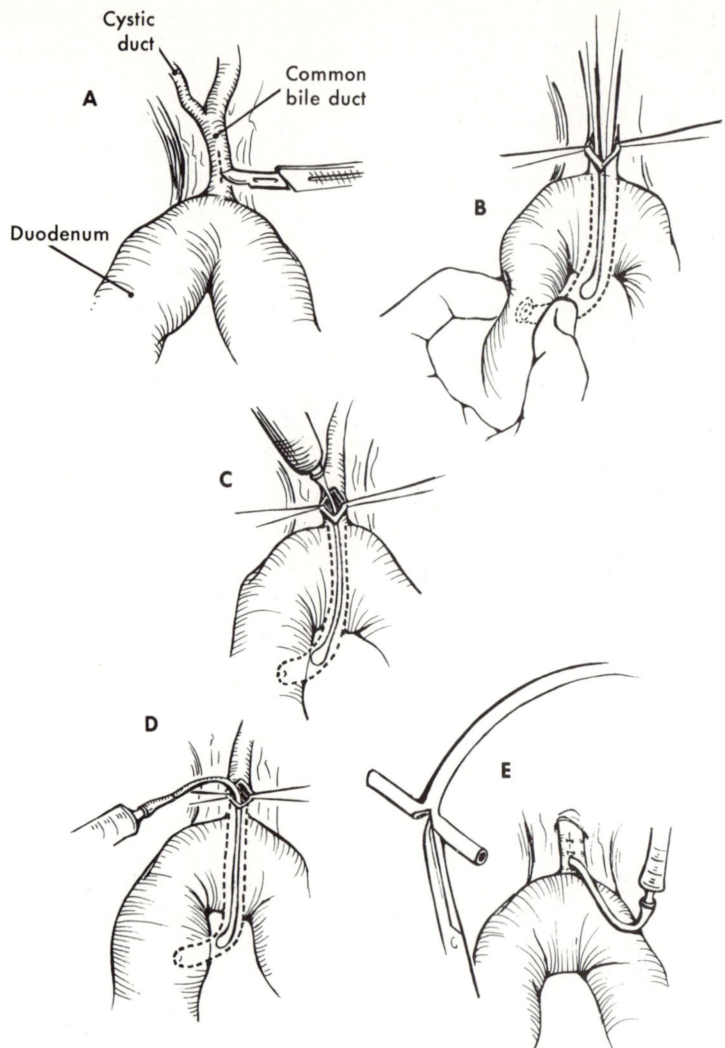

Fig. 13-9. Choledochotomy. **A,** Opening common duct. **B,** Introducing stone forceps. **C,** Probing common duct. **D,** Irrigating duct. **E,** Preparing and irrigating T tube.

Choledochoscopy

Definition. Direct visualization of the common bile duct by means of an instrument (choledochoscope) introduced into the common bile duct.

Considerations. Choledochoscopy may take the place of operative cholangiography. It provides a means for extraction of stones that are difficult to remove from the common bile duct. To visualize the common duct, it is necessary to distend it while viewing. This is done by irrigating the duct with copious amounts of sterile saline. To accomplish this, a pressure bag must be used on the saline and pressure applied to 300 mm Hg. Sterile cystoscopy tubing is then attached to the saline and directly to the irrigating stopcock on the scope (Fig. 13-10).

Setup and preparation of the patient. As described for biliary surgery, plus the following additional instruments:

Choledochoscope with accessories: biopsy forceps, stone grasping forceps and a sheath that can be used to direct other instruments into various portions of the biliary tract
Eyepiece protector disc
Light cord
Normal saline, 1000-ml bag
IV pole
Pressure bag
Light source

Operative procedure

1 to 5. As described for choledochotomy.

6. The choledochoscope is inserted into the duct, and the common duct is flushed with saline. Stones are grasped with the stone forceps and removed. The choledochoscope allows visualization of the entire duct so that no stones will remain. After all stones are removed, the

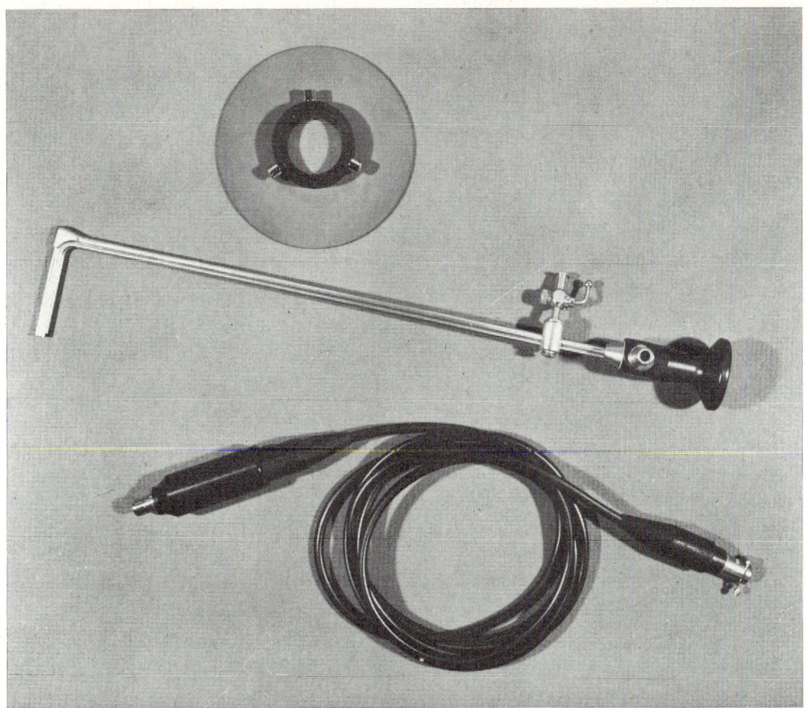

Fig. 13-10. Choledochoscopy set. *Top to bottom,* Eyepiece protector disc, choledochoscope, light cord.

common duct is again thoroughly flushed with saline. Closure of the duct and wound is completed.

Cholecystoduodenostomy or cholecystojejunostomy

Definition. Establishment of continuity by an anastomosis between the gallbladder and duodenum or jejunum to relieve an obstruction in the distal end of the common duct.

Considerations. An obstruction in the biliary system may be caused by a tumor of the ducts involving the head of the pancreas or the ampulla of Vater, the presence of an inflammatory lesion, a stricture of the common duct, or the presence of stones.

Setup and preparation of the patient. As described for cholecystostomy, plus two Doyen intestinal forceps, curved with guards, or similar nontraumatic holding forceps.

Operative procedure

1. The abdomen is opened, the gallbladder is exposed and aspirated, and the pathological condition is confirmed, as described for cholecystostomy.
2. The anastomosis site is prepared, posterior serosal silk sutures are placed, and open anastomosis is performed. The technique as described for gastrointestinal anastomosis is followed (Chapter 14).
3. Contaminated instruments are placed in the discard basin, and the operative field is prepared for closure.
4. A Penrose, Jackson-Pratt, or cigarette drain may be introduced; the wound is closed in layers, and dressings are applied.

Choledochoduodenostomy and choledochojejunostomy

Definitions. Anastomosis between the common duct and the duodenum or between the common duct and the jejunum.

Considerations. These procedures are usually necessary in postcholecystectomy patients to circumvent an obstructive lesion and reestablish the flow of bile into the intestinal tract.

Setup and preparation of the patient. As described for choledochostomy and cholecystojejunostomy.

Operative procedures

Choledochoduodenostomy

1. The abdomen is opened, and the common duct and duodenum are exposed.
2. The common duct is identified and dissected free.
3. The common duct and duodenum are approximated, either side to side or end of common duct to side of duodenum, and an anastomosis is established (Fig. 13-11).
4. The wound is closed in layers, and dressings are applied.

Choledochojejunostomy

1. The abdomen is opened, the jejunum is mobilized, and the common duct is identified.

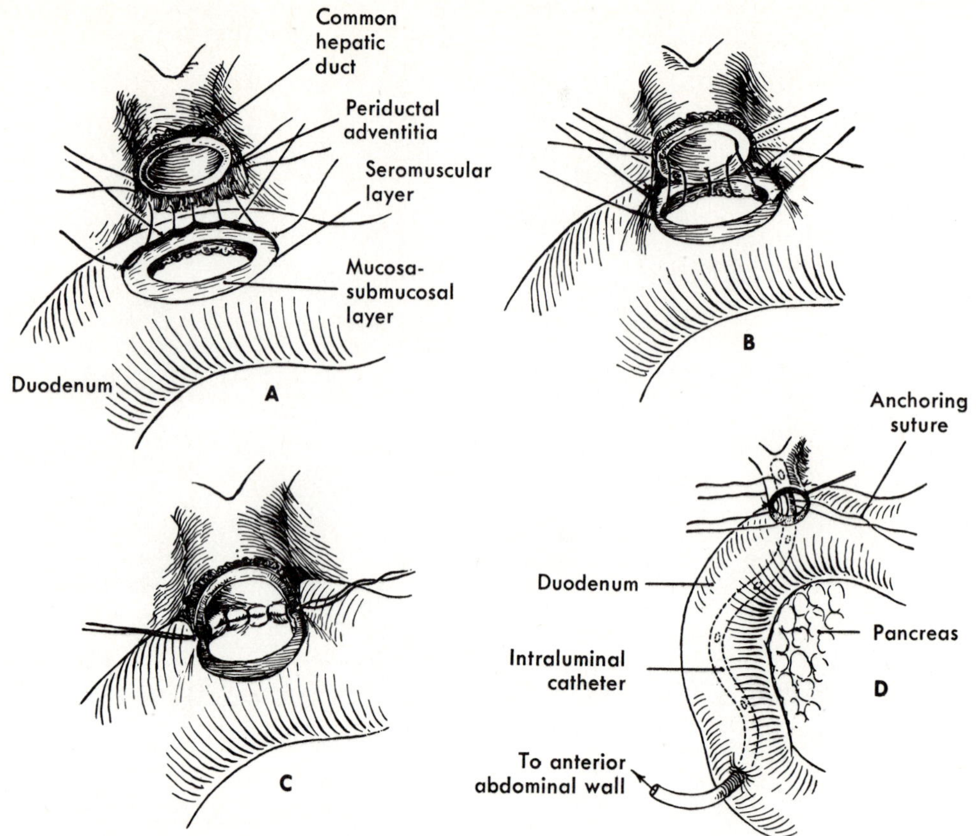

Fig. 13-11. Technique for choledochoduodenostomy. **A,** First posterior row of interrupted, silk sutures approximates adventitia around proximal biliary segment and seromuscular layer of anterior aspect of duodenum. **B,** Second posterior row approximates full thickness of duct and mucosa-submucosal layer of bowel. Knots are on outside of lumen. **C,** Two posterior rows are completed. **D,** Intraluminal catheter is in place, secured by gut suture at line of anastomosis. Extra holes in catheter provide egress of bile to bowel. (From Longmire, W.P., Jr., and Lippman, H.N. In Allen, A.W., and Barrow, D.W., editors: Abdominal surgery, New York, Harper & Row, Publishers.)

2. Anastomosis is established between the common duct and the transected jejunum (Fig. 13-12, *A*). A catheter is introduced, as described for cholecystoduodenostomy.

3. Jejunal continuity is reestablished by Roux-en-Y anastomosis (Fig. 13-12, *B*).

4. As an alternative, anastomosis may be fashioned between the end of the severed duct to the side of a loop of jejunum, with a side to side jejunal anastomosis below (Fig. 13-12).

5. Contaminated instruments are removed from the operative field.

6. The drain is exteriorized, the wound is closed in layers, and dressings are applied.

Repair of strictures of the common and hepatic ducts

Definition. Relief of biliary obstruction either by resection of a stricture of the duct and an end-to-end anastomosis over a T tube splint (Fig. 13-13) or by means of an anastomosis between the duct or ducts and the intestinal tract. These are usually very difficult operations, since they practically always follow previous unsuccessful operations on the biliary tract with resultant scarring, stricture, and fistulas.

Setup and preparation of the patient. As described for choledochostomy and gastroenterostomy (Chapter 14), with a complete selection of drainage tubes and fine intestinal chromic and silk sutures.

Operative procedure

1. The abdomen is opened, and the anastomotic procedure to be performed is selected after careful exploration and evaluation of the existing pathological condition (Fig. 13-13).

2. After anastomosis, the selected T tube and drain are inserted. Extreme caution is exercised to prevent displacement of the vital drainage tubes (Fig. 13-13).

3. The wound is closed, as described in Chapter 10.

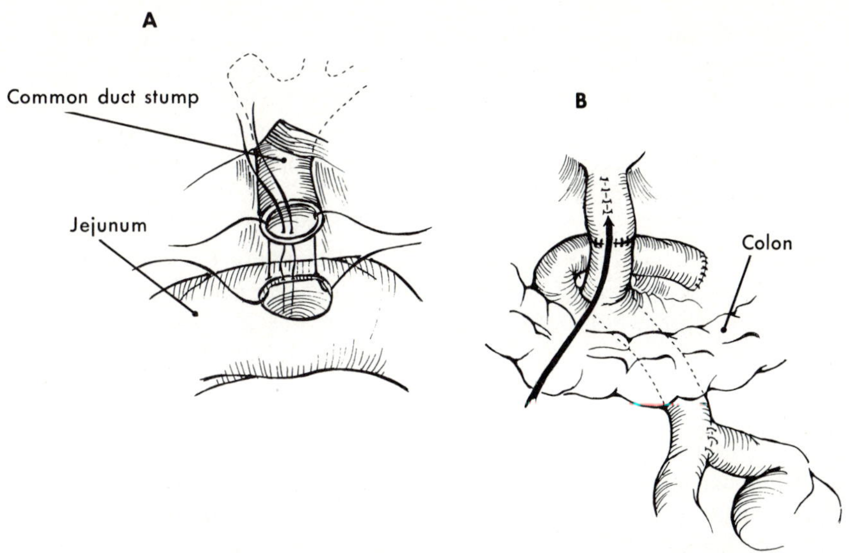

Fig. 13-12. Technique for choledochojejunostomy. **A,** Stay sutures are placed in lumen of prepared jejunum and common duct stump prior to anastomosis. **B,** Completed Roux-en-Y anastomosis with intraluminal catheter in place. (Adapted from Wilder, J.R.: Atlas of general surgery, ed. 2, St. Louis, The C.V. Mosby Co.)

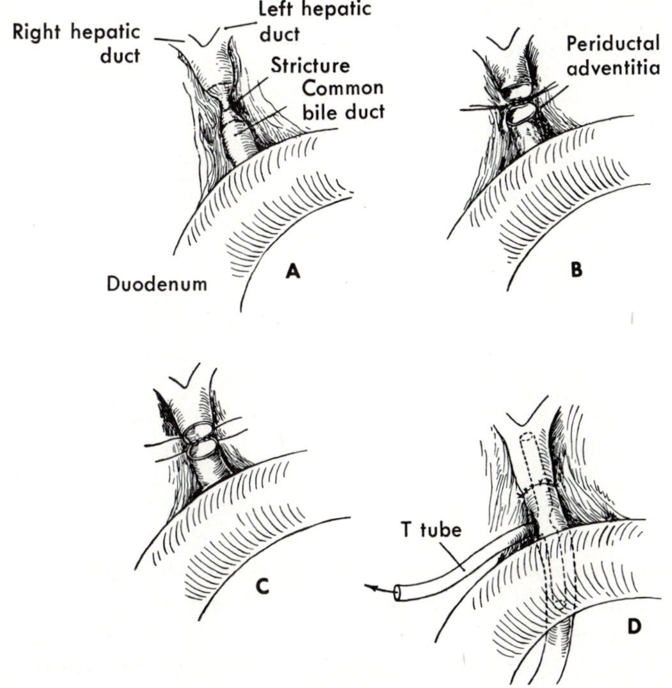

Fig. 13-13. Technique for duct-to-duct anastomosis with T tube in place. **A,** Strictured area is defined; dotted lines indicate area to be excised. **B,** First posterior row of sutures has been placed in adventitia around duct. **C,** Posterior inner row of interrupted, catgut sutures has been completed. **D,** Completed anastomosis with T tube in place, brought out below line of anastomosis. (From Longmire, W.P., Jr., and Lippman, H.N. In Allen, A.W., and Barrow, D.W., editors: Abdominal surgery, New York, Harper & Row, Publishers.)

Transduodenal sphincterotomy

Definition. Partial division of the sphincter of Oddi and exploration of the common duct to treat recurrent attacks of acute pancreatitis as a result of formation of calculi in the pancreatic duct or blockage of the sphincter of Oddi.

Setup and preparation of the patient. As described for choledochotomy, plus a ureteral knife or sphincterotome.

Operative procedure

1. The gallbladder may have been removed; the common duct is opened and explored for stones, as described for choledochotomy.

2. For the Doubilet and Mulholland techniques, a sphincterotome is inserted through the common duct into the duodenum, and the sphincter is severed; or the ampulla of Vater is exposed through an incision made in the duodenum, and a probe is passed through the common duct into the duodenum. The sphincter is incised over the probe.

3. The duodenum is closed usually transversely in two layers, with interrupted silk sutures. A T tube usually is introduced into the common duct and held in place with sutures. The abdominal cavity is drained, and the wound is closed.

OPERATIONS ON THE PANCREAS

Drainage or excision of pancreatic cysts

Definition. Usually, internal drainage of the cyst into the small intestine or stomach; less frequently, excision or external drainage (marsupialization).

Considerations. Cysts of the pancreas have been classified according to etiological factors as follows: developmental or congenital, inflammatory, traumatic, neoplastic, and parasitic. Their cause and size, location, and anatomical relationships are important deciding factors in selection of the surgical procedure.

Pancreatic pseudocysts arise from within the substance of the pancreas, enlarging and displacing the stomach anteriorly. Complete excision of retention cysts is usually considered the preferred method; however, this may not be possible in the presence of an acute or secondary inflammatory reaction. In the latter, internal or external drainage of the cyst may be established.

Setup and preparation of the patient. As described for common duct and gastrointestinal procedures, plus appropriate drains.

Operative procedure

1. Simple external drainage is established by direct introduction of a retention type of catheter into the cyst, following decompression and inspection (Fig. 13-14).

2. Internal drainage may be accomplished by an incision into the anterior wall of the stomach, directly opposite the cyst as it adheres to the posterior wall (Fig. 13-15). A fistula is established between the anterior wall of the cyst and the posterior wall of the stomach, thereby providing drainage through the gastrointestinal canal.

3. The anterior gastrotomy is closed, and the wound closure is completed in the usual manner.

4. Many surgeons prefer an anastomosis between the cyst and a Roux-en-Y loop of jejunum or into the duodenum directly, depending on the location of the cyst.

Pancreaticoduodenectomy (Whipple operation)

Definition. Removal of the head of the pancreas, the entire duodenum, a portion of the jejunum, the distal third of the stomach, and the lower half of the common bile duct, with the reestablishment of continuity of the biliary, pancreatic, and gastrointestinal tract systems.

Considerations. Radical excision of the head of the pancreas for carcinoma is a technically hazardous procedure because it involves many vital structures and organs. Resectability of the tumor in the presence or absence of metastasis and the general overall condition of the patient are evaluated carefully before resection.

Once the surgeon opens and explores the abdomen, including the liver, pancreas, and biliary tree, and feels the patient will benefit from extensive surgery, the supervisor, along with the blood bank, should be advised. Surgery of this type may require 5 to 6 hours and the transfusion of many units of blood. This procedure is one of the most extensive of all abdominal procedures.

After surgery, it is important to reevaluate the insulin requirements, as well as those of supplementary pancreatin.

Setup and preparation of the patient. As described for gastrointestinal surgery, plus drainage tubes and drains, as in cholecystoduodenostomy.

Operative procedure

1. The abdomen is entered through an upper transverse, bilateral subcostal, or long paramedian incision. Laparotomy packs and retractors are used to expose the operative site and protect structures.

2. Mobilization of the duodenum is achieved with an adequate Kocher maneuver, which consists of incision of peritoneal reflection, lateral to the second portion of the duodenum, with Metzenbaum scissors and subsequent blunt dissection of loose areolar tissue.

3. Mobilization is continued; bleeding vessels are ligated with silk.

4. The gastrocolic ligament and the gastrohepatic omentum are divided between curved forceps and are ligated or transfixed.

5. The gastroduodenal and right gastric arteries are clamped, divided, and ligated.

6. The prepyloric area of the stomach is mobilized. The operative field is prepared for open anastomosis. By placing two long Allen or Payr clamps near the midportion of the stomach, the transection is completed (Fig. 13-16, *A*).

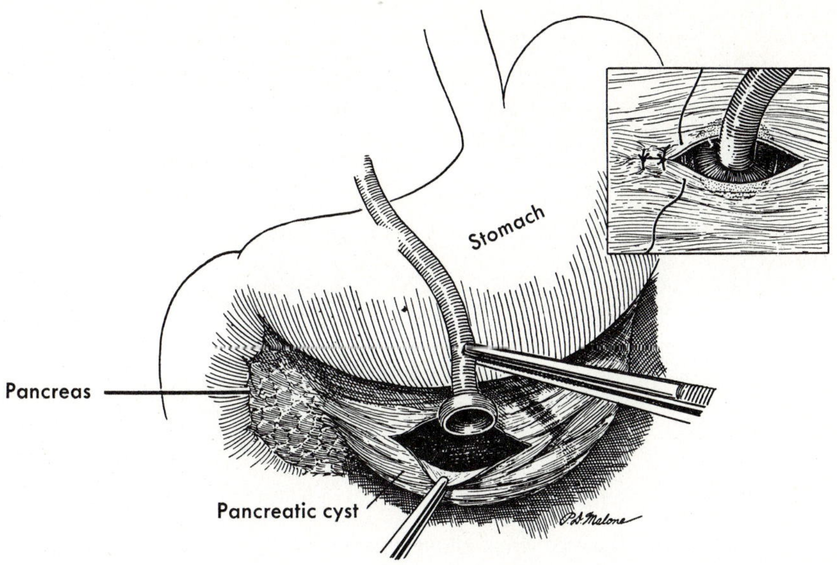

Fig. 13-14. Simple drainage of pancreatic cyst. Cyst is incised sufficiently to permit complete evacuation of contents and inspection of lining of cavity. Flanged end of Pezzer catheter is sutured into cyst, and other end is brought out through stab wound. (From Warren, K.W., and Baker, A.L., Jr. In Lahey Clinic: Surgical practice of the clinic, Philadelphia, W.B. Saunders Co.)

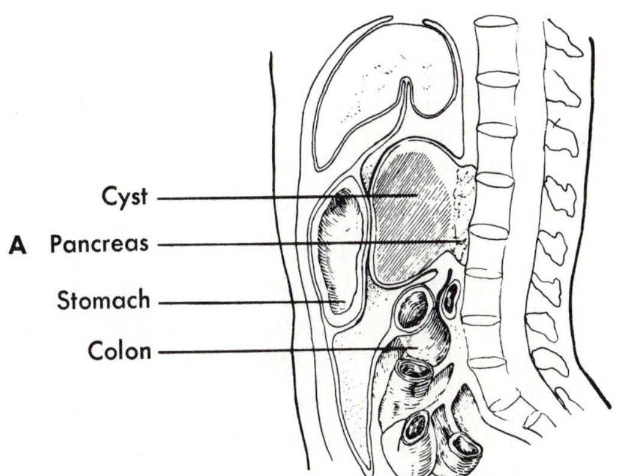

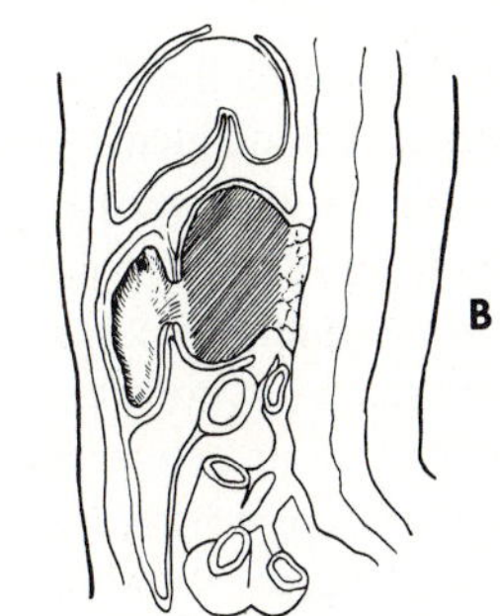

Fig. 13-15. Treatment of pancreatic pseudocyst by internal drainage by means of anastomosis of cyst to stomach. **A,** Sagittal section showing relationship of cyst of body of pancreas to posterior wall of stomach. **B,** Cystogastrostomy, sagittal view. **C,** Cystogastrostomy, anterior view. Stomach has been lifted cephalad to demonstrate anastomosis between pseudocyst and posterior wall of stomach. (From Dreiling, D.A., Janowitz, H.D., and Perrier, C.V.: Pancreatic inflammatory disease, New York, Harper & Row, Publishers.)

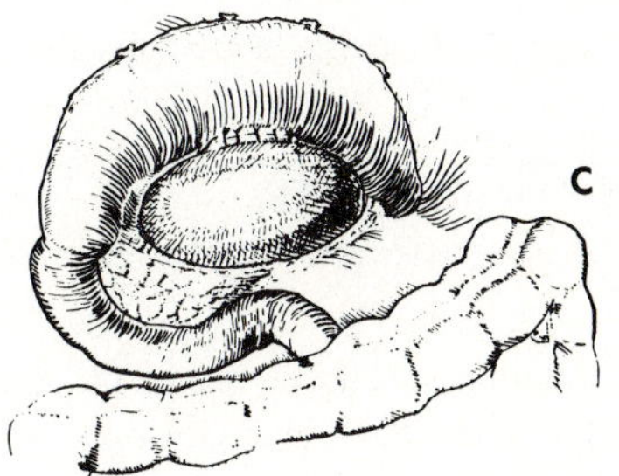

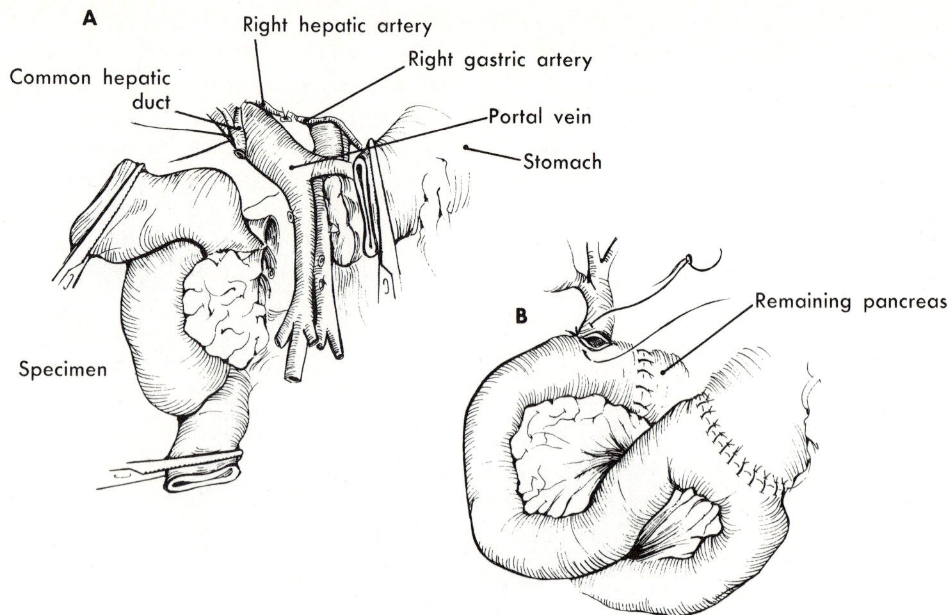

Fig. 13-16. Radical one-stage pancreatoduodenectomy. **A,** Operative field prepared for anastomosis and transection completed. **B,** Reconstruction of gastrointestinal canal completed by means of three anastomoses—establishment of continuity with pancreas and jejunum or duodenum, with gallbladder and jejunum, and with stomach and jejunum.

7. The duodenum is reflected, the common duct is divided, and the hepatic end is marked or tagged for later anastomosis.

8. The jejunum is clamped with two Allen forceps, and the duodenojejunal flexure is divided.

9. The pancreas is divided, and the duct is carefully identified.

10. Further mobilization of the duodenum and division of the inferior pancreatoduodenal artery is done to permit complete removal of the specimen.

11. Reconstruction of the gastrointestinal tract is completed by the following anastomoses: retrocolic end-to-end pancreatojejunostomy, retrocolic end-to-side choledochojejunostomy, and an antecolic long-loop isoperistaltic gastrojejunostomy (Fig. 13-16, *B*).

12. Drains are introduced, as for cholecystostomy. Some surgeons prefer to place a sump drain near the pancreatic anastomosis.

13. The wound is closed in layers, usually with wire sutures.

OPERATIONS ON THE LIVER

Drainage of intrahepatic, subhepatic, or subphrenic abscess

Definition. Drainage of abscesses of the liver.

Considerations. Hepatic abscesses may be pyogenic or parasitic and single or multiple.

Extreme care is used in removal of an *Echinococcus* (hydatid) cyst, since the fluid is under high tension and any spillage into the peritoneal cavity may result in anaphylactic reaction. Even more important is the possible escape of ''daughter'' cysts that will spread through the abdomen producing multiple cysts, an extremely difficult situation to treat. Hydatid cysts are rare in the United States.

Setup and preparation of the patient. As described for biliary surgery, plus drainage materials such as several Penrose or sump drains. Aerobic and anaerobic culture tubes should be available.

Operative procedure

1. The incision and type of procedure selected depend on the cause and location of the abscess. For the anterior approach, a right transperitoneal incision is made. For the posterior approach, the patient is prepared and the incision selected, as described for a posterior thoracotomy.

2. Drainage of an abscess may be treated in one or two stages. In the one-stage procedure, the approach is through the outer third of the right twelfth rib, reaching the liver abscess retroperitoneally and extrapleurally.

A two-stage operation is selected rarely to obliterate the right pleural cavity. The objective of the first stage is to seal off the pleural cavity by stimulating adhesions with the insertion of iodoform packing. When the second stage, which is done at a higher level, is performed, the chest cavity will not become contaminated.

Hepatic resection

Definition. Resection of the liver that may involve a small wedge biopsy, excision of simple tumors, or a major lobectomy. Increased knowledge of liver function and circulatory physiology and improved methods of hemostasis now permit the surgeon to offer safer, more definitive treatment to the patient with liver disease or trauma.

Considerations. Facilities should be available for hypothermia, electrocoagulation, measuring portal pressure, thoractomy drainage, and accurate replacement of blood loss; special needles for suturing liver tissue are available.

Setup and preparation of the patient. The patient is placed in the supine position. Some surgeons elevate the hepatic area with an inflatable "gallbladder bag," folded sheet, or other device. An abdominal incision through the midline, occasionally with division of the lower sternum, provides access to the left lobe, whereas a combined right thoracoabdominal incision is needed to expose the right hepatic region for major resection. Vertical abdominal incisions are also advantageous, since they can be made and closed more rapidly and permit better exposure of all abdominal organs.

Instrument setup includes those for portacaval shunt and common duct procedures, plus additional items as follows:

- Manometer
- 2 Chest drainage catheters
- 12-18 Liver sutures, silk or chromic, according to surgeon's preference
- Hemostatic material: Gelfoam, Surgicel, Avitene

Operative procedure for right hepatic lobectomy

1. Through a right subcostal or upper midline incision, the abdominal cavity is opened; examination is carried out, using items as described for biliary surgery. Pathological condition is determined, and resectability evaluated.

2. Thoracoabdominal incision is completed through the seventh or eighth interspace (Fig. 13-17, *A*). Moist laparotomy packs are inserted, and a chest retractor is placed.

3. Exposure of the hilar structures is obtained by upward displacement of the right lobe toward the right chest cavity, application of a clamp to the falciform ligament to facilitate traction, and inferior displacement of intestines with moist packs and retractors.

4. The cystic duct is carefully exposed, using Metzenbaum scissors, vascular forceps, small dry dissectors on curved holders, and fine right-angled forceps. It is clamped, transected, and doubly ligated with chromic or silk ligatures and transfixion sutures (Fig. 13-17, *B*).

5. The right hepatic duct, right hepatic artery, and right branch of the portal vein are also transected and doubly ligated with silk ligatures and transfixion sutures.

6. The liver is rotated forward, and the multiple right hepatic veins entering the inferior vena cava are carefully identified, clamped, divided, and ligated.

7. A double row of interlocking liver sutures are placed (Fig. 13-17, *C*). Blunt needles are used to prevent undue trauma or tearing of the liver. A scalpel is used to excise the specimen through the devascularized section. Fine suture ligatures may be needed to ligate bile ducts and small blood vessels (Fig. 13-17, *D*). As additional sutures are placed, care should be exercised to avoid injury to the left hepatic veins.

8. The omentum may be sutured to the raw liver surface to decrease bile and serum loss (Fig. 13-17, *E*).

9. Chest and abdominal drainage tubes are inserted, and layer closure is completed (Fig. 13-17, *F*).

TRAUMA

Nothing else requires an operating room nurse's expertise as does a trauma patient. Often the demand occurs during the night when the nurse is on call. The nurse is awakened from a sound sleep to be told by an excited voice that there has been a terrible accident—"Come quickly!" Information is often sketchy: "It's an exploratory something."

Trauma is the third leading cause of death in the United States, following coronary artery disease and cancer. For people under the age of 40, it is the number one cause of death. Traumatic emergencies include serious injury to the head, chest, or abdomen and the loss of a limb. A trauma patient may also require immediate surgery to stop internal bleeding. Gunshots, knife stabbings, and automobile accidents cause many of these life-threatening injuries. Trauma centers are being established, and hospital operating rooms, with specialized equipment and trained staff, are increasingly being called on to handle the severely injured patient.

Trauma is fast becoming a speciality that involves a combination of emergency room, operating room, and intensive care nursing expertise. Many times the operating room nurse is put in a situation in which she is required to have many skills that before were credited to intensive care nurses, for example, setting up central venous pressure (CVP) and arterial lines, administering emergency drugs, and performing a nursing assessment of the traumatized patient. While acting on this assessment, the anesthesiologist and other team members are supplied with needed equipment; direct nursing care of the patient is a priority. Perhaps in the future, some operating room nurses will specialize in trauma only.

Setup and preparation of the patient. When arriving at the hospital, the operating room nurse should check with the emergency room personnel or the surgeon to determine exactly what is to be done. If possible, the patient should be examined and a nursing assessment that focuses on immediate priorities performed. A report should be obtained from the emergency room nurse on the patient regarding allergies, oral intake status, fluid replacement, other traumatized parts of the body, and any other

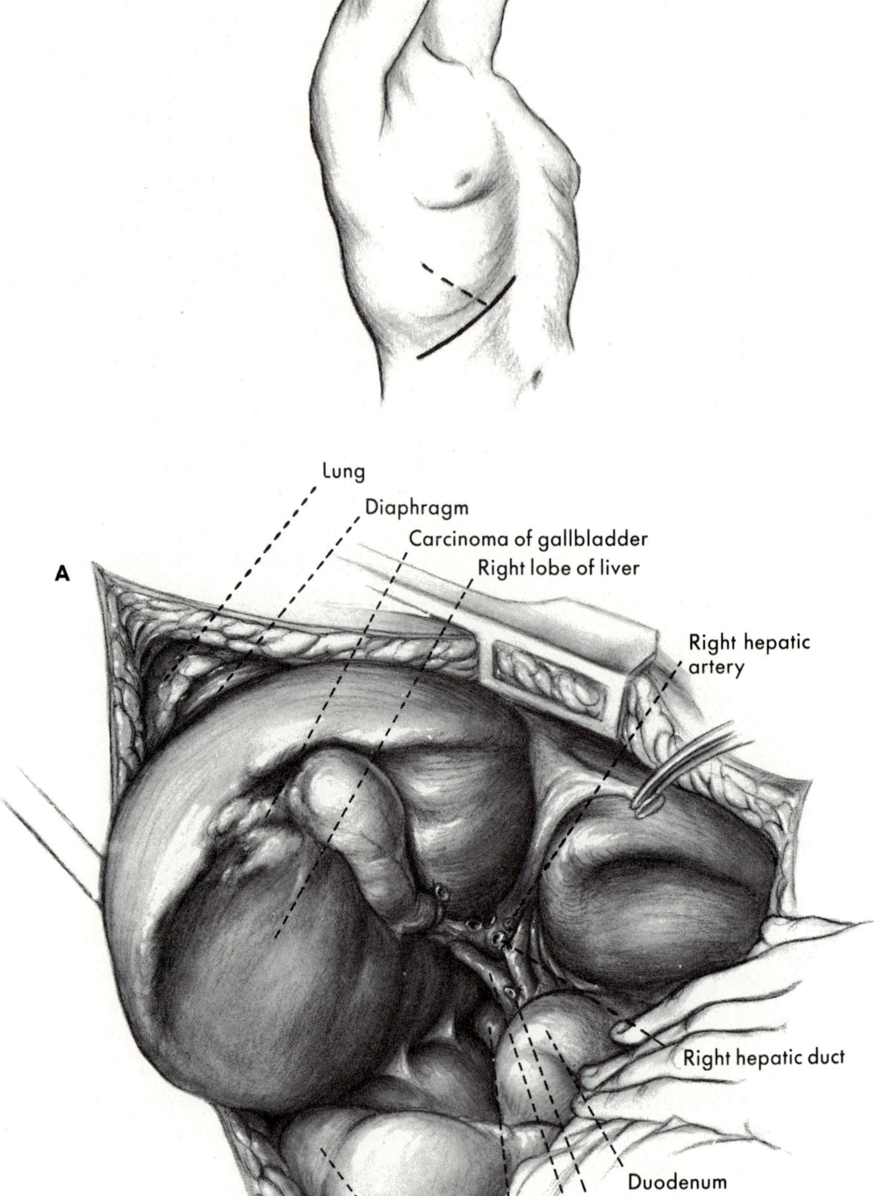

Fig. 13-17. Right hepatic lobectomy. **A,** Extension of subcostal incision through seventh or eighth interspace.

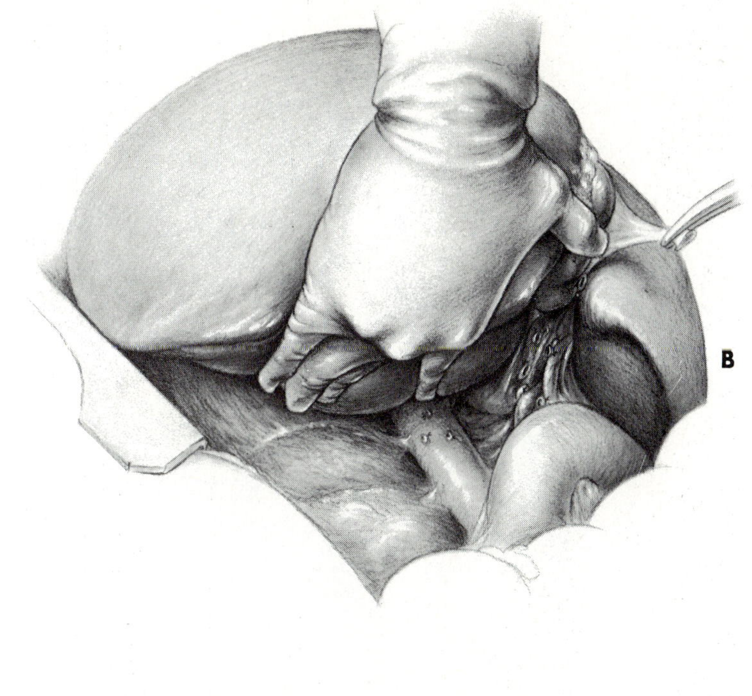

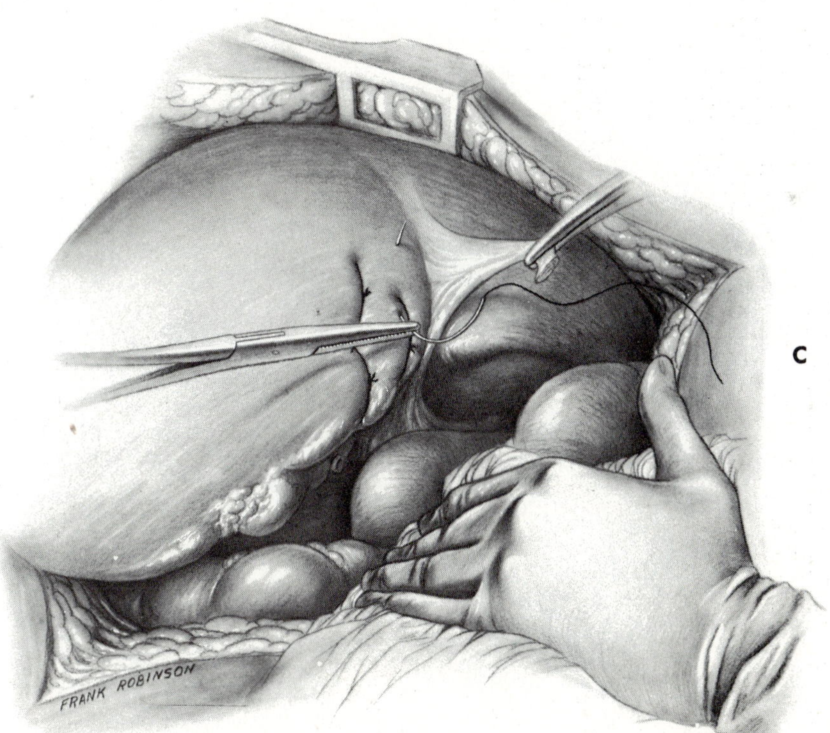

Fig. 13-17, cont'd. B, Hilar structures ligated preparatory to transection of right lobe. **C,** Preparation of devascularized channel for transection by placement of interlocking sutures.

Continued.

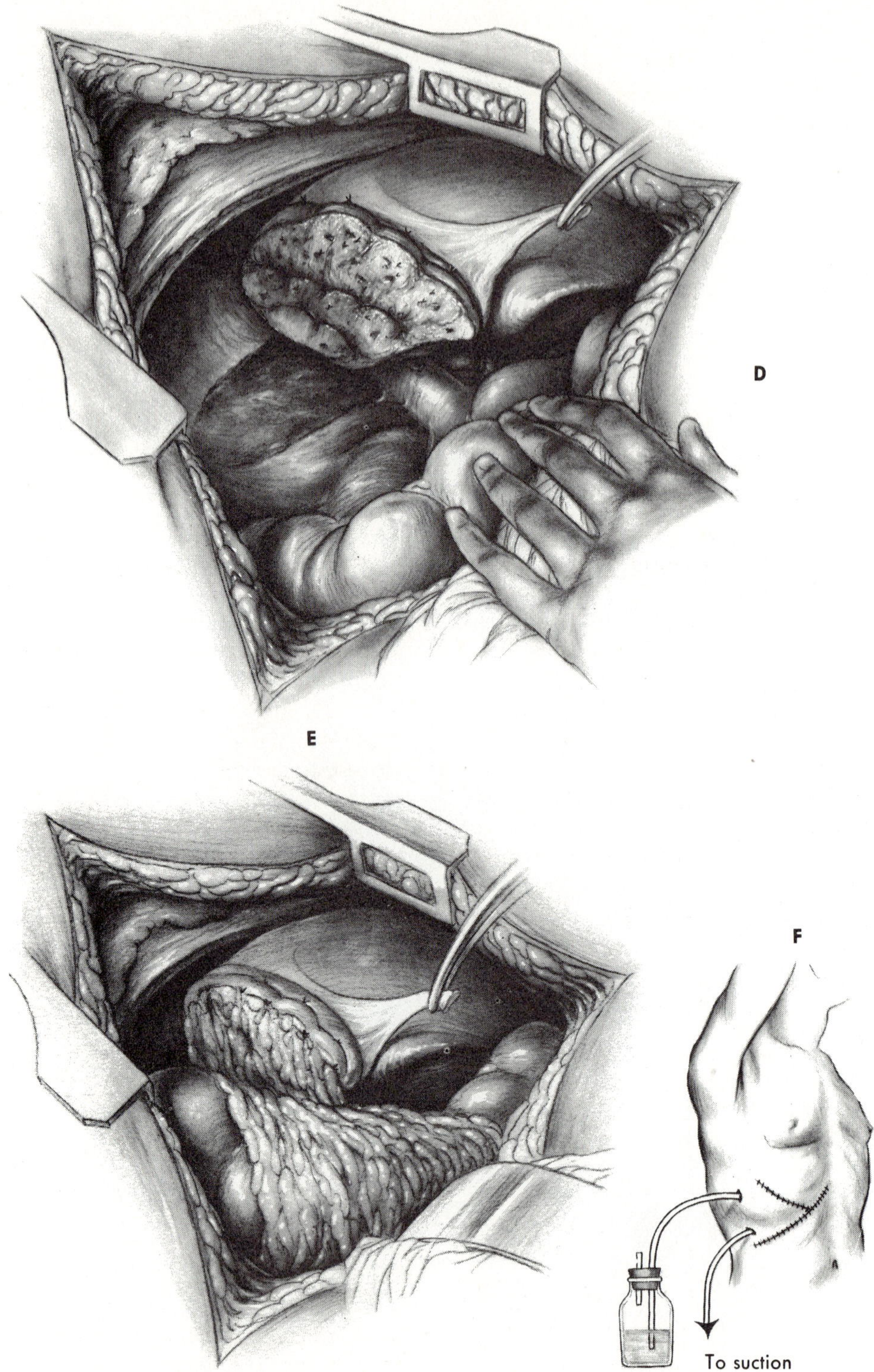

Fig. 13-17, cont'd. D, Pattern of hemostatic sutures following removal of specimen. **E,** Omentum sutured over raw liver surface to decrease bile and serum loss. **F,** Position of drainage catheters. (From Indications and technique of right hepatic lobectomy, Somerville, N.J., Ethicon, Inc.)

pertinent information. An exploratory laparotomy may be scheduled first. The patient will usually come to the operating room, intubated and on a respirator, with peripheral intravenous lines and/or a CVP line, a Foley catheter (which should be attached to a urinometer), a nasogastric tube, and sometimes an arterial line.

On the patient's arrival in the operating room, it is important to remember that this is a person and not a "trauma case." It is easy to get caught up in the excitement and forget about the human, interpersonal aspects. The nurse should talk with the patient even if he is unconscious. What is being done should be explained.

If the hospital has a helicopter base station, the patient will often be received in the helicopter basket. This presents a problem of transferring the patient to the operating room bed. In this case, sterile technique often becomes secondary in importance to the emergency of the situation. Emergency room personnel who are to help transport the patient will have to enter the operating room suite wearing their uniforms or street clothes.

The patient will sometimes be wearing a military antishock trouser (MAST) suit. The suit is usually applied in the field or in the emergency room. It is used in cases of hemorrhagic injury. The MAST suit is said to increase central venous pressure and improve cardiac filling. The suit is in one piece, similar to a pair of wraparound trousers. The trousers enclose the body from the rib cage margin down to the ankles. The suit is inflated by a foot pump until it is smooth. The MAST suit is not to be removed by anyone but the surgeon or by the surgeon's specific order. When the suit is deflated, the patient's blood pressure will usually drop, sometimes drastically. In removing the suit, the abdominal compartment is deflated first, then each leg. If, after the abdominal compartment is deflated, the blood pressure drops too low, the leg trousers may be kept inflated during the surgery. If the patient's pressure is too low, either preparation is not done or some preparatory solution can be poured onto the operative site.

The packs, instruments, and needed supplies should be opened before the patient arrives. If possible, the patient's x-ray studies should be placed in the room. It is a good idea to have a thermia blanket on the operating room bed and to have the autotransfuser set up and available.

Autotransfusion. The purpose of the autotransfuser is to retrieve blood from and return it to a traumatically injured patient. Autotransfusion is contraindicated if the wounds are more than 4 hours old, if the patient has cancer, or if gross contamination from bowel or stomach contents has occurred. The blood is immediately available, it is fresh, and it is type specific for that patient. Although hemothorax is the most frequent indication for autotransfusion, others include injury to the liver, spleen, chest wall, heart, pulmonary vessels, kidney, iliac vein, portal vein, and inferior vena cava. Using a patient as a self-donor was first reported in 1818. Since that time, autotransfusers that are safe and relatively simple to use have been manufactured (Fig. 13-18).

Sterile equipment

Trauma blood liner, 1900-ml, disposable, flexible
Trauma drainage tubing set: 28 Fr thoracic catheter, male-male adaptor, drainage tubing, and anticoagulant connector
Volume control device, 150-ml–capacity burette with intravenous administration set
Citrate-phosphate-dextrose (CPD) anticoagulant set, obtained from hospital pharmacy
Sodium chloride, 1000 ml, with blood administration set
Microemboli filter

Nonsterile equipment (Fig. 13-18, *A*)

The following nonsterile items are mounted on an IV pole:
Vacuum regulator with gauge and mounting clamp
Receptal ATS canister, 2000-cc, graduated every 25 cm, numbered every 100 cc
Room vacuum line, able to hook up to wall suction

Procedure

1. The vacuum is connected to the regulator, and the suction is connected.
2. The sterile liner (Fig. 13-18, *B*) is removed from its package and extended to its full length. Care should be taken not to contaminate the sterile spacer.
3. The liner is inserted in the canister, and the lid snapped in place by placing the thumb tab directly over the canister tee (Fig. 13-18, *C*).
4. The liner lid tubing is connected to the canister tee by way of the sterile spacer.
5. The vacuum is turned on; the regulator is set at between 10 and 30 mm Hg.
6. The thoracic catheter and the suction tubing are placed on the sterile field.
7. The anticoagulant is hung from the IV pole. (CPD, 25 to 60 ml, is used for every 500 ml of blood collected.) The anticoagulant is connected to the volume control administration set. The line is flushed and attached to the anticoagulant connector after the cap is removed (Fig. 13-18, *D* and *E*).
8. If used thoracically, the patient line must be clamped whenever the vacuum is turned off. If clamping is not done, pneumothorax may occur.

Removal of liner

1. The patient line is clamped near the distal end of the tubing (only if used thoracically).
2. The patient line and anticoagulant are disconnected from the patient port of the inner lid.
3. The sterile spacer is removed and discarded (Fig. 13-18, *F*).
4. The patient port is securely capped with the liner lid tubing connector.
5. The blood bag is removed from the canister by pushing up on the thumb tab.
6. A new liner is inserted.

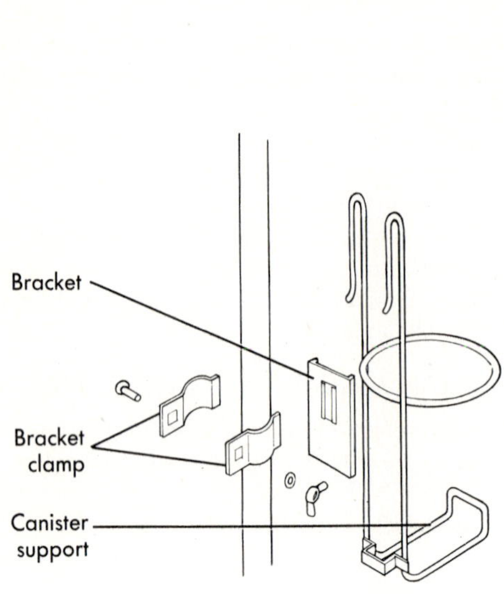

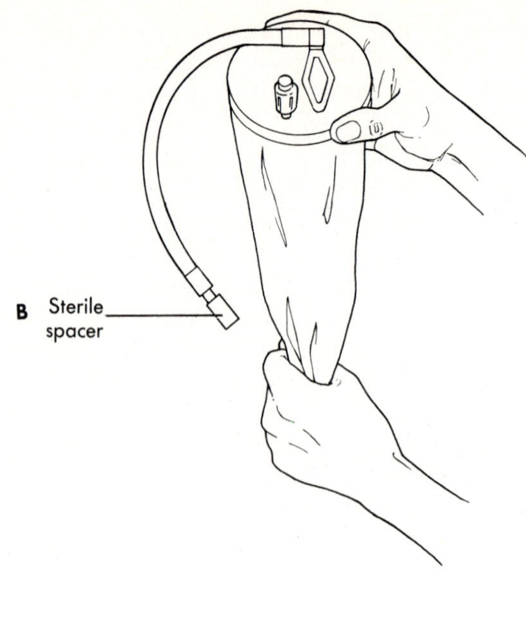

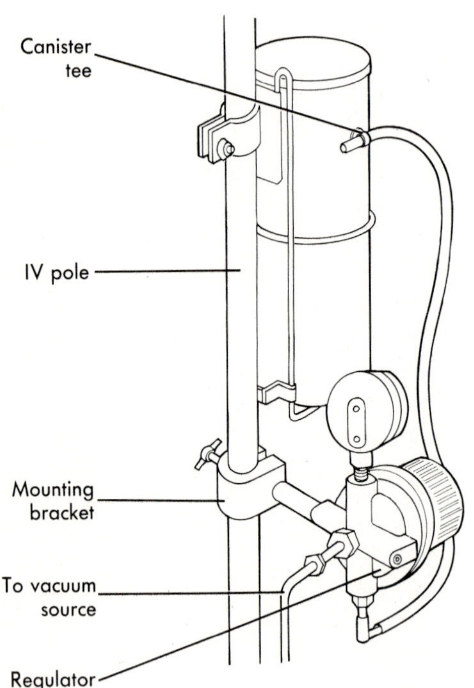

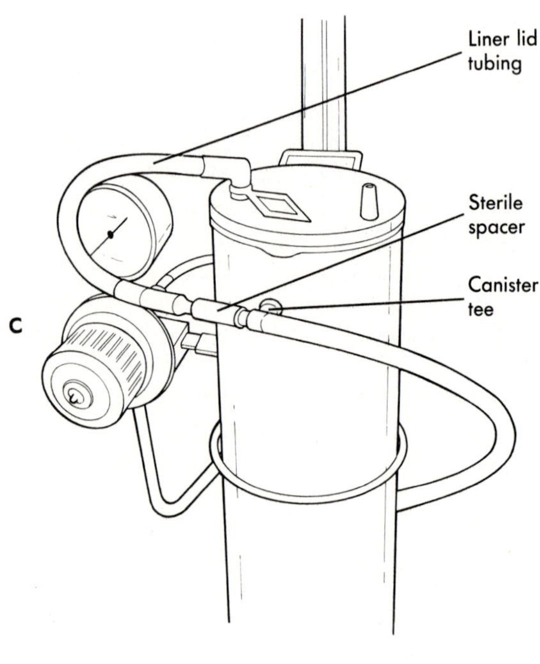

Fig. 13-18. Autotransfuser. **A,** Equipment mounted on intravenous pole. **B,** Suction liner. **C,** Liner inserted in canister. **D** and **E,** Unit assembled and ready to use. **F,** Liner filled with patient's blood; removal of sterile spacer.

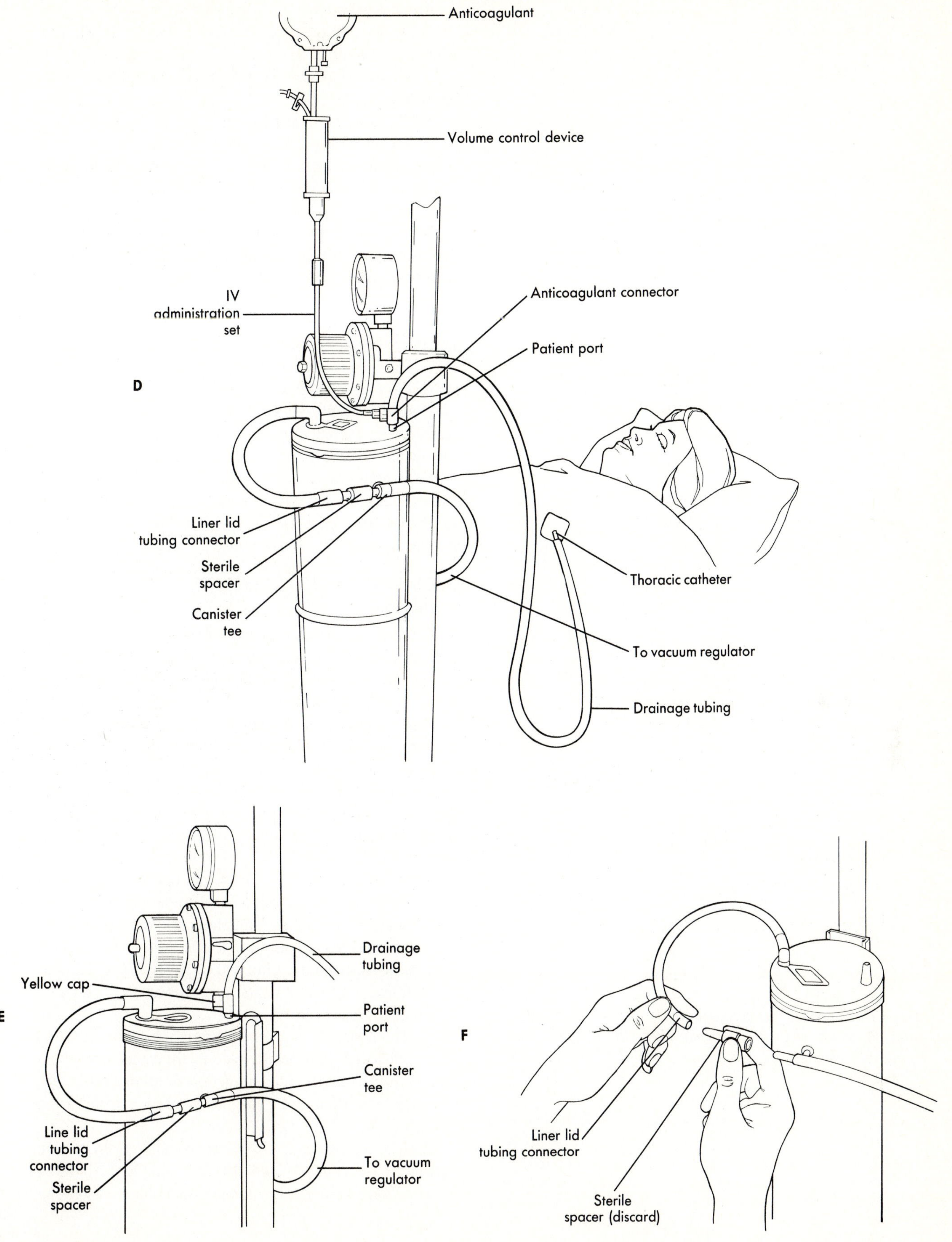
Anticoagulant
Volume control device
IV administration set
Anticoagulant connector
Patient port
D
Liner lid tubing connector
Sterile spacer
Canister tee
Thoracic catheter
To vacuum regulator
Drainage tubing
Drainage tubing
Yellow cap
E
Patient port
Canister tee
Line lid tubing connector
Sterile spacer
To vacuum regulator
F
Liner lid tubing connector
Sterile spacer (discard)

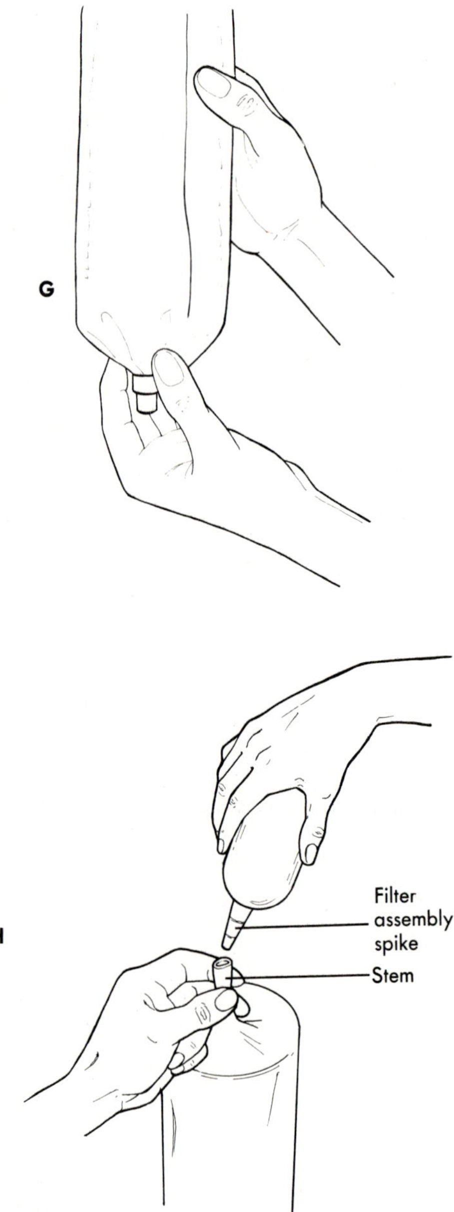

Fig. 13-18, cont'd. G, Preparation of liner for autotransfusion. **H,** Insertion of microemboli filter into inverted liner. (Original design courtesy Sorenson Research Co., Salt Lake City, Utah.)

Autotransfusion

1. A blood administration set should be ready and primed with sodium chloride.

2. The recessed stem of the liner is grasped and pulled down (Fig. 13-18, *G*).

3. The liner is inverted so that the stem points up.

4. The protective cap is removed from the stem, and the microemboli filter is inserted. The wall of the liner should not be punctured with the filter spike (Fig. 13-18, *H*).

5. The bag should be held with the filter and drip chamber upright. The clamp is opened, and any air is gently squeezed from the bag until the drip chamber is partially filled. The clamp is then closed.

6. The bag is inverted and hung from the IV pole. (A new microemboli filter is used every time a liner is hung.)

7. The clamp is opened, and blood is infused according to hospital procedure.

Considerations. Autotransfusion is indicated whenever enough uncontaminated blood is recovered to make transfusion worthwhile, that is, 2 or 3 units. The blood is warm and immediately available. This is especially useful if there is a blood shortage or if the patient has a rare blood type. Because the blood is the patient's own, transfusion reactions are decreased.

OPERATIONS ON THE SPLEEN

Splenectomy

Definition. Removal of the spleen.

Considerations. A splenectomy is usually performed for trauma to the spleen or for specific conditions of the blood, such as hemolytic jaundice or splenic anemia, or for tumors, cysts, or splenomegaly. Actually, the most common indication for splenectomy is accidental injury to the spleen during vagotomy or other gastric procedures or operations involving mobilization of the splenic flexure of the colon. If accessory spleens are present, they are also removed, since they are capable of perpetuating hypersplenic function.

Massive splenomegaly may on occasion require a thoracoabdominal approach. Abdominal suction apparatus should be available throughout all splenectomies.

Setup and preparation of the patient. As described for a basic laparotomy, plus two large, right-angled pedicle clamps, long instruments, and hemostatic material.

Operative procedure

1. The abdomen is opened through an upper midline or left subcostal incision. Retractors are placed over laparotomy packs, and gentle retraction is employed as exploration is carried out. The costal margin is retracted upward.

2. The splenorenal, splenocolic, and gastrosplenic ligaments are clamped and divided with long dressing forceps, long hemostats, sponges on holders, and long

Metzenbaum or Nelson scissors. Adhesions posterior to the spleen are freed.

3. The spleen is delivered into the wound after these attachments are freed. The short gastric vessels are now easily identified, clamped, divided, and ligated.

4. The cavity formerly occupied by the spleen is packed with laparotomy packs, if necessary.

5. The splenic artery and vein are dissected free with fine dissecting scissors and forceps.

6. The artery is clamped and doubly ligated with silk. The artery is ligated first, and then the vein, thus permitting disengorgement of blood from the spleen and facilitating the return of venous blood to the circulatory system.

7. The splenic vein is then clamped, divided, and ligated.

8. The specimen is removed; all bleeding vessels are controlled.

9. The wound is closed in layers, as described for routine laparotomy, and dressings are applied. Drainage is usually required only if many adhesions to the diaphragm were divided or if significant clotting abnormalities exist.

SUGGESTED READINGS

Aronsen, K.F., and others: Liver resection in the treatment of blunt injuries to the liver, Surgery **63:**236, 1968.

Balasegaram, M.: Hepatic resection for malignant tumors, Surg. Rounds, p. 14, Sept. 1979.

Ballinger, W.F., II, and Erslev, A.J.: Splenectomy: indications, technic, and complications, Curr. Probl. Surg., p. 1, Feb. 1965.

Barber, J.M.: Blunt abdominal trauma, Nurs. Clin. North Am. **13:**211, 1978.

Barber, J.M., and Budassi S.A.: Mosby's manual of emergency care: practices and procedures, St. Louis, 1979, The C.V. Mosby Co.

Bell, J.: Just another patient with gallstones? Don't you believe it, Nursing '79 **9**(10):26, 1979.

Bell W.: The hematology of autotransfusion, Surgery **84:**695, 1978.

Bergin, J., Zuck, T, and Miller, R.: Compelling splenectomy in medically compromised patients, Ann. Surg. **178:**761, 1973.

Budassi, S.A.: Giving an autotransfusion with MAST, Nursing '81 **11**(10):50, 1981.

Budassi, S.A., and Barber, J.M.: Emergency nursing: principles and practice, St. Louis, 1981, The C.V. Mosby Co.

Caldwell, E.: The psychological impact of trauma, Nurs. Clin. North Am. **13:**247, 1978.

Cooperman, A.M., and Hoerr, S.O., editors: Surgery of the pancreas: a text and atlas, St. Louis, 1978, The C.V. Mosby Co.

Davidson, S.J.: Emergency unit autotransfusion, Surgery **84:**703, 1978.

Davis, J.W., McKone, T.K., and Cram, A.: Hemodynamic effects of military anti-shock trousers (MAST) in experimental cardiac tamponade, Ann. Emerg. Med. **10:**185, 1981.

Ellis H., and Wastell, C.: General surgery for nurses, ed. 2, London, 1980, Blackwell Scientific Publications, Ltd.

Gilroy, A., and Caldwell, E.: Initial assessment of the multiply injured patient, Nurs. Clin. North Am. **13:**177, 1978.

Liechty, F.D., and Soper, R.T.: Synopsis of surgery, ed. 4, St. Louis, 1980, The C.V. Mosby Co.

Lockhart, C., and Mattox, K.L.: Autotransfusion: a technique for the trauma patient, Nurs. Clin. North Am. **13:**235, 1978.

Madding, G., and Kennedy, P.: Major problems in clinical surgery, vol. 3, Philadelphia, 1965, W.B. Saunders Co.

Noon, G.: Intraoperative autotransfusion, Surgery **84:**719, 1978.

Perdue, P.: Abdominal injuries and dangerous fractures, RN **44:**34, July 1981.

Phipps, W.J., Long, B.C., and Woods, N.F.: Shafer's medical-surgical nursing, ed. 7, St. Louis, 1980, The C.V. Mosby Co.

Pliam, M., and ReMine, W.: Further evaluation of total pancreatectomy, Arch. Surg. **10:**506, 1975.

Puestow, C.B.: The biliary tract, Philadelphia, 1969, Lea & Febiger.

Ranson, J.H., and others: New diagnostic and therapeutic techniques in the management of pyrogenic liver abscesses, Ann. Surg. **181:**508, 1975.

Sabiston, D.C., Jr., editor: Davis-Christopher textbook of surgery: the biological basis of modern surgical practice, ed. 12, Philadelphia, 1981, W.B. Saunders Co.

Stephenson, H.E., Jr., editor: Immediate care of the acutely ill and injured, ed. 2, St. Louis, 1978, The C.V. Mosby Co.

Zimmerman, L., and Levine, R.: Physiologic principles of surgery, ed. 2, Philadelphia, 1965, W.B. Saunders Co.

14 Gastrointestinal surgery

The alimentary canal comprises a series of organs joined to form a tube-like structure that extends the entire length of the trunk (Fig. 14-1). The alimentary tract includes the mouth, pharynx, esophagus, stomach, small intestine (duodenum, jejunum, and ileum), large intestine, colon, rectum, and anus. These organs are responsible for the supply of nourishment to the body and the elimination of solid wastes.

ANATOMY

The *esophagus* extends from the pharynx, at the level of the sixth cervical vertebra, and passes through the neck, posterior to the trachea and heart and anterior to the vertebral column. The lower portion of the esophagus passes in front of the aorta and through the diaphragm, slightly to the left of the midline, to join the cardia of the stomach.

Blood is supplied to the esophagus from branches of the inferior thyroid, thoracic aorta, and celiac arteries. The nerve supply comes from branches of the vagi and sympathetic chain. The esophagus of an adult is about 10 inches in length and is a collapsible musculomembranous tube.

The *stomach* is situated between the esophagus and the duodenum and lies in the upper left abdominal cavity, slightly to the left of the midline and beneath the diaphragm. The stomach is divided into three parts: the fundus, the body, and the pyloric antrum (Fig. 14-2). The *fundus* lies beneath the left dome of the diaphragm, behind the apex of the heart, while the *body* and *antrum* lie in an oblique direction within the abdominal cavity. The stomach is stabilized indirectly by the lower portion of the esophagus and directly by its attachment to the duodenum, which is anchored to the posterior parietal peritoneum. The stomach is associated with branches of the celiac vessel, with the peritoneal ligaments and the omentum providing additional support.

The convex, or lower, margin of the stomach is known as the *greater curvature,* and the concave margin, the *lesser curvature*. Attached to the greater curvature is the *greater omentum,* which is a double fold of peritoneum, containing fat. It covers the intestines loosely and is not to be confused with the mesentery, which connects the intestines with the posterior abdominal wall. The left gastroepiploic branch of the splenic artery and the right gastroepiploic branch of the hepatic artery run through the greater omentum. The *lesser omentum,* which is attached to the lesser curvature of the stomach, contains the left gastric artery, a branch of the celiac axis, and the right gastric branch of the hepatic artery. During a gastrectomy, these vessels are clamped and ligated (Fig. 14-3).

The *small intestine* begins at the pylorus and ends at the ileocecal valve (Fig. 14-1) and is also divided into three parts: the duodenum, which is about 11 inches long; the jejunum, which is about 7½ feet long; and ileum, which is about 11½ feet long. The small intestine varies in size with the degree of contraction but is usually about 20 feet in length and 1 inch in diameter (Fig. 14-1). The *duodenum,* the proximal portion of the small intestine, begins at the pylorus, is continuous with the jejunum, and is stabilized by a fusion between the pancreas and the posterior parietal peritoneum. The duodenum also communicates with the common bile duct, and the duodenojejunal angle is stabilized by the ligament of Treitz that suspends the duodenum. The ligament of Treitz serves as an important landmark during any abdominal operation.

The middle portion of the duodenum forms an acute angle in its descent. It passes along the right side, then its inferior portion traverses to the left, so that it lies in front of the right ureter, the inferior vena cava, and the aorta. It then turns upward and forward to become a part of the duodenojejunal flexure that in turn joins the jejunum. The bile and pancreatic ducts enter the descending portion of the duodenum; the blood supply of the duodenum comes from the arterial branches of the celiac axis.

The *jejunum,* which is situated in the upper portion of the abdomen, joins the *ileum,* which is situated in the lower portion of the cavity. The ileum empties into the large intestine through the ileocecal valve. The jejunum and ileum are suspended by the mesentery, which is attached to the posterior abdominal wall. The free border of the mesentery (Fig. 14-4), which is about 18 feet long, contains branches of the superior mesenteric artery, many veins, lymph nodes, and nerve fibers.

The *large intestine* begins at the ileocecal valve and terminates at the anus. It is divided into the cecum and the colon.

The *cecum* is attached to the ileum and extends about

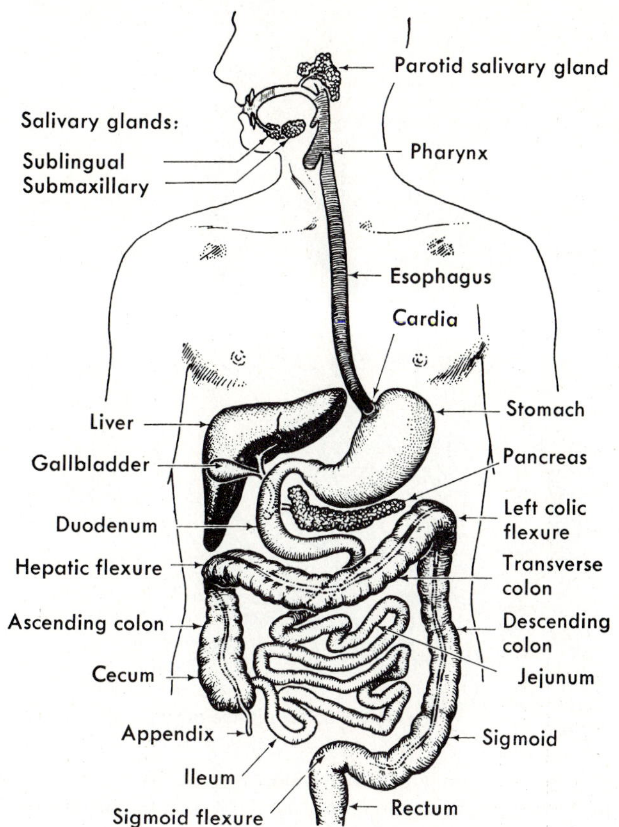

Fig. 14-1. Alimentary canal and its appendages. (From Schottelius, B.A., and Schottelius, D.D.: Textbook of physiology, ed. 18, St. Louis, 1979, The C.V. Mosby Co.)

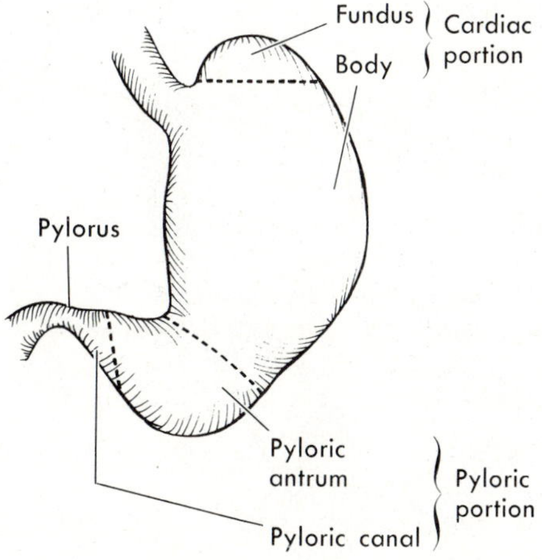

Fig. 14-2. Regional anatomy of stomach.

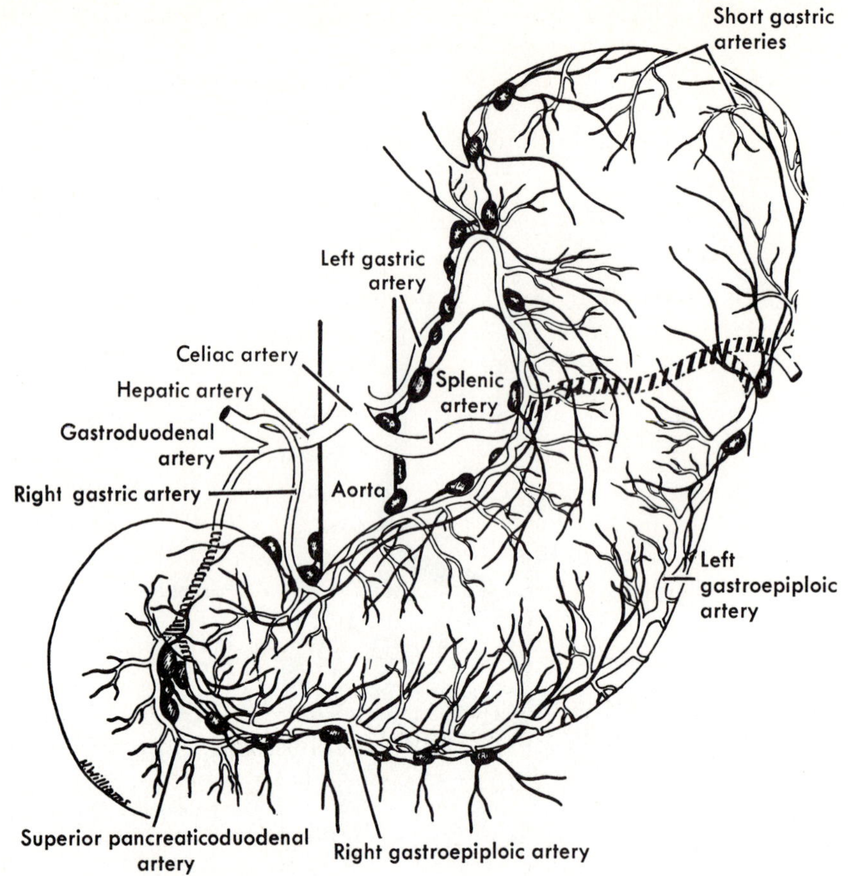

Fig. 14-3. Arterial supply of stomach. (After Cutler and Zollinger; from Francis, C.C., and Martin, A.H.: Introduction to human anatomy, ed. 7, St. Louis, 1975, The C.V. Mosby Co.)

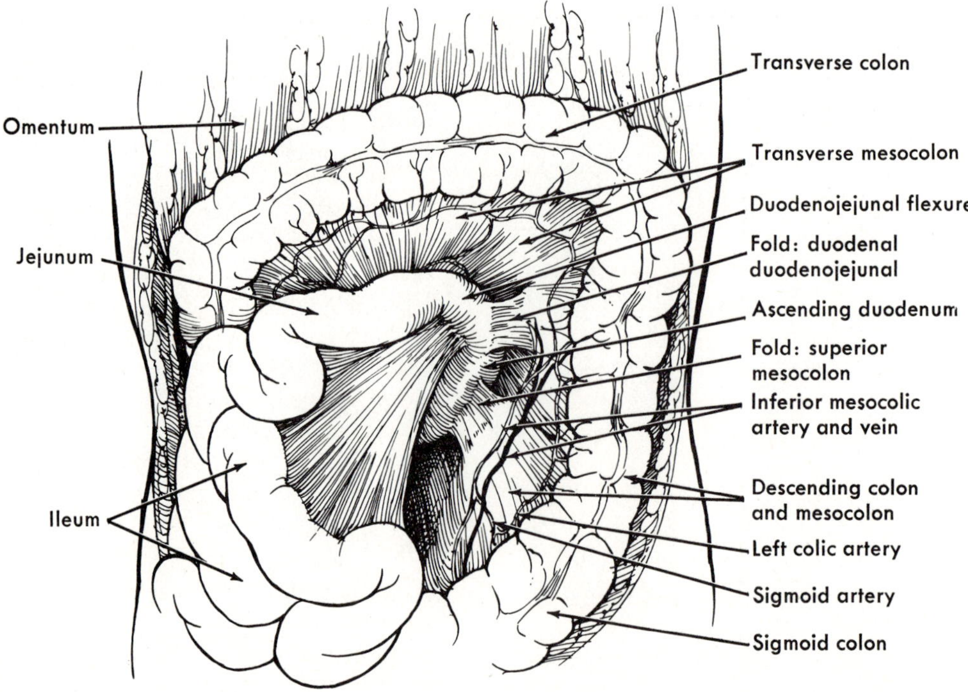

Fig. 14-4. Mesentery, as seen when intestine is pulled aside.

2½ inches below it (Fig. 14-1). The cecum in an adult is usually adherent to the posterior wall of the peritoneal cavity and has a serosal covering on its anterior wall only. The cecum forms a blind pouch from which the appendix projects.

The *colon* is divided into five parts: the ascending colon, the transverse colon, the descending colon, the sigmoid colon, and the rectum (Fig 14-5).

The ascending colon is about 6 inches long and extends upward from the ileocecal valve to the hepatic flexture. The upper portion of the ascending colon lies behind the right lobe of the liver and in front of the anterior surface of the right kidney.

The transverse colon, which is about 20 inches long, begins at the hepatic flexture and ends at the splenic flexture. It lies below the stomach and is attached to the transverse mesocolon.

The descending colon extends downward from the splenic flexure to the area just below the iliac crest and is about 7 inches long. The iliac portion of the sigmoid colon, which is about 6 inches long, lies on the inner surface of the left iliac muscle. The remaining portion of the colon passes over the pelvic brim into the pelvic cavity and lies partly in the abdomen and partly in the pelvis. It then forms an S curve in the pelvis and terminates in the rectum at the level of the third segment of the sacral vertebrae.

The blood supply to the ascending colon, hepatic flexure, and transverse colon comes from the superior mesenteric artery, whereas the blood supply to the descending colon and rectum comes from the inferior mesenteric artery.

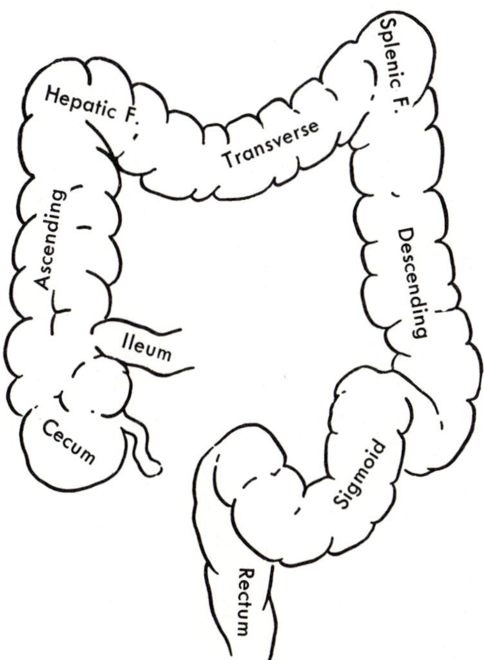

Fig. 14-5. Anatomical division of large intestine (colon), showing placement of ileocecal valve, hepatic flexure, and splenic flexure.

The wall of the colon is made up of teniae coli, epiploic appendices, and haustra. The teniae coli are three longitudinal, or axial, strips of muscles distributed around the circumference of the colon. They represent the longitudinal muscle layer, which is not complete in the colon. The small intestine and rectum have both circular and complete longitudinal muscle layers. The epiploic appendices are fatty appendages along the bowel that have no particular function; the haustra are sacculations that are the outpouchings of bowel wall between the teniae coli.

The diameter of the colon varies in size from about 3½ inches in the cecum to an average of about 1½ inches in the sigmoid colon (Fig. 14-5).

The rectum, which is a continuation of the sigmoid colon, terminates in the anus. The rectum, a slightly curved passage about 6 inches long, is surrounded by pelvic fascia as it lies on the anterior surface of the sacrum and coccyx. In the male, the rectum lies behind the prostate gland and the bladder. In the female, the rectum lies behind the uterus and the vagina. The rectum dilates just before it becomes the anal canal, and this dilatation or ampulla presents folds called Houston's valves. The wall of the rectum consists of four layers, similar to those of the small intestine.

The anal canal is a narrow passage about 1 inch long, which passes downward and backward. It is surrounded and controlled by two circular muscle groups, which form the external and internal anal sphincters. The internal sphincter is a continuation of the longitudinal muscle layer.

PHYSIOLOGY

The esophagus serves as the route from which food enters the stomach from the mouth. When food enters the stomach, it undergoes chemical and mechanical changes and then enters the duodenum, where it is mixed with bile and pancreatic juices. The stomach is never entirely empty because it always contains some gastric juice, which is acid in nature and is produced by numerous tubular glands in the wall of the stomach.

When food is in the stomach, the stomach becomes distended and flattens out the *rugae,* or folds of the stomach. Little absorption takes place in the stomach, and liquid enters the duodenum within half an hour after its ingestion. Food enters the stomach by passing through the cardiac sphincter and leaves the stomach by passing through the pyloric sphincter. Peristalsis, which causes the food to move, consists of waves of motion in the stomach and intestines by successive contractions of the muscles in the walls.

Absorption of food is a function of the small intestines. The large intestine absorbs water from the contents and acts in expelling the indigestible residue from the body. The residue is composed primarily of cellulose from carbohydrates, connective tissue, and undigested fats. The act of defecation is accomplished by contraction of the rectal and abdominal muscles, the descent of the diaphragm, and the relaxation of the anal sphincter muscles.

The gastrointestinal tract is probably affected by psychological factors at least as much as are other body systems. In our high-pressured society, people tend to overeat or undereat, and the pressures of everyday living frequently show their effects on the gastrointestinal tract. Although there is no conclusive evidence, some disease entities seem to be exacerbated by psychological factors, for example, pylorospasm, peptic and duodenal ulcers, colitis, and obesity. Some of these diseases can be treated medically; others require adjunctive psychotherapy. All of them necessitate diagnostic studies, and many require surgery.

NURSING CONSIDERATIONS

Patients undergoing gastrointestinal surgery should understand why they need preoperative preparation, what the intended surgical intervention will be, and how it will affect them postoperatively. Many patients require nasogastric tubes. Fluid and electrolyte balance must be maintained before, during, and after surgery. Preoperative mechanical preparation of the gastrointestinal tract must be employed for elective surgery, and often bactericidal and bacteriostatic agents will be used to attempt to eliminate pathogenic organisms, especially in the lower gastrointestinal tract. Often, Foley catheters are inserted preoperatively, or immediately after induction, to maintain fluid balance during surgery and to keep the bladder empty, allowing more space for the surgeon to work.

Skin preparation should be done immediately before the patient comes to the operating room. Hair should be shaved according to the protocol for the type of surgery the patient is to have, as well as the surgeon's preference.

If the surgeon anticipates the need to replace blood loss, the patient's blood is typed and cross-matched before the operation.

Preoperative assessment enables the nurse to plan for the specific needs of the individual patient. An example is patient size, which has a definite bearing on positioning and which may necessitate additional instrumentation such as retractors and longer forceps and scissors.

As in all surgery, careful consideration should be given to the positioning of the patient, so that the surgeon will gain optimum exposure without compromising the respiratory, circulatory, and nervous systems and without producing undue pressure on any body part (Chapter 6).

The circulating nurse should be well informed as to what the procedure will be and should ensure that all necessary equipment is on hand and that the integrity of the equipment is without question.

Suture materials used on gastrointestinal tissue have traditionally been silk and chromic gut. With the increased number of synthetic absorbable and nonabsorbable suture materials available, surgeons have a variety of materials from which to choose. Polyester fiber sutures and polyglycolic acid sutures are frequently employed on gastrointestinal tissue. It is important to check the surgeon's preference card for appropriate suture materials. This not only ensures the availability of necessary supplies but also is a cost-effective measure.

Irrigating solution is frequently used during gastrointestinal procedures. The surgeon specifies the solution of choice. Normal saline, an isotonic solution, may be used to moisten laparotomy sponges and for irrigation. Moist packs are used to isolate open and diseased portions of the stomach and bowel from the abdominal cavity and to protect other viscera. During procedures involving a suspected malignancy, sterile distilled water may be the solution of choice because of the hypotonic properties. Solutions should be warm when used for these purposes.

As in all operations, the excised specimen is handled carefully and prepared for examination by the surgical pathologist. The surgeon determines how the specimen will be handled before examination. It may be sent to the pathology department fresh, in saline, or in a preservative solution. Tissue also may be sent for frozen section examination to verify the pathological condition and determine if tissue margins are free of malignant cells.

To reduce tissue trauma, the jaws of heavy intestinal forceps may be protected by pieces of soft rubber tubing. These guards (shods) should fit the jaws firmly but not tightly and should extend slightly beyond the tip of forceps. Before sterilization, the rubber shods should be separated from the forceps to facilitate steam penetration.

The advent of surgical stapling instruments has had a great impact on the technical aspects of gastrointestinal surgery. For some surgeons, the use of these devices has, to a certain extent, replaced conventional suturing techniques. The stapling instruments can be employed to divide and ligate, resect and anastomose. The "B" design of the staple does not compromise the vascularity of the resected tissue edges. These devices are available in reusable as well as disposable models. Personnel must be familiar with the stapling equipment, application, and proper loading.

Whenever a portion of the gastrointestinal tract is entered, bowel technique must be performed. Bowel technique means that any instrument coming in contact with the gastrointestinal mucosa is not used after the lumen of the gastrointestinal tract has been restored. These instruments are discarded in a separate basin and do not come in contact with other instruments. Some surgeons may desire a new set of instruments for closure, additional draping materials, as well as a change of gown and gloves.

BASIC INSTRUMENT SETUP

Since many varieties of resection instruments are available, the basic set should be standardized with the approval of the attending physicians. Frequently it is impossible for the surgeon to determine in advance the specific type of operation to be performed until examining the involved organs. The gastrointestinal instrument set comprises the basic major laparotomy setup.

Cutting instruments

1 Metzenbaum scissors, 9 inches
2 Metzenbaum scissors, 5¾ inches, 1 straight and 1 curved
2 Mayo scissors, 9 inches, 1 straight and 1 curved

Clamping instruments (Fig. 14-6)

1 DeMartel clamp
1 Best colon clamp
4 Allen intestinal anastomosis clamps
4 Rochester-Carmalt forceps, straight, 8 inches
4 Doyen intestinal forceps, longitudinal serrations, 9 inches, 2 straight and 2 curved
2 Mayo vessel clamps, angled, 9 inches
2 Mayo-Robson intestinal forceps, straight
2 Dennis intestinal clamps
4 Payr pylorus clamps, 8 inches
2 Payr pylorus clamps, 11 inches
1 Payr pylorus clamp, 13¾ inches
4 Gallbladder forceps, right-angled, assorted sizes
4 Rochester-Pean forceps, curved, 8 inches
12 Rochester-Pean forceps, curved, 6¼ inches
12 Crile forceps, curved, 5½ inches
36 Halsted mosquito forceps, 5 inches, 24 curved and 12 straight

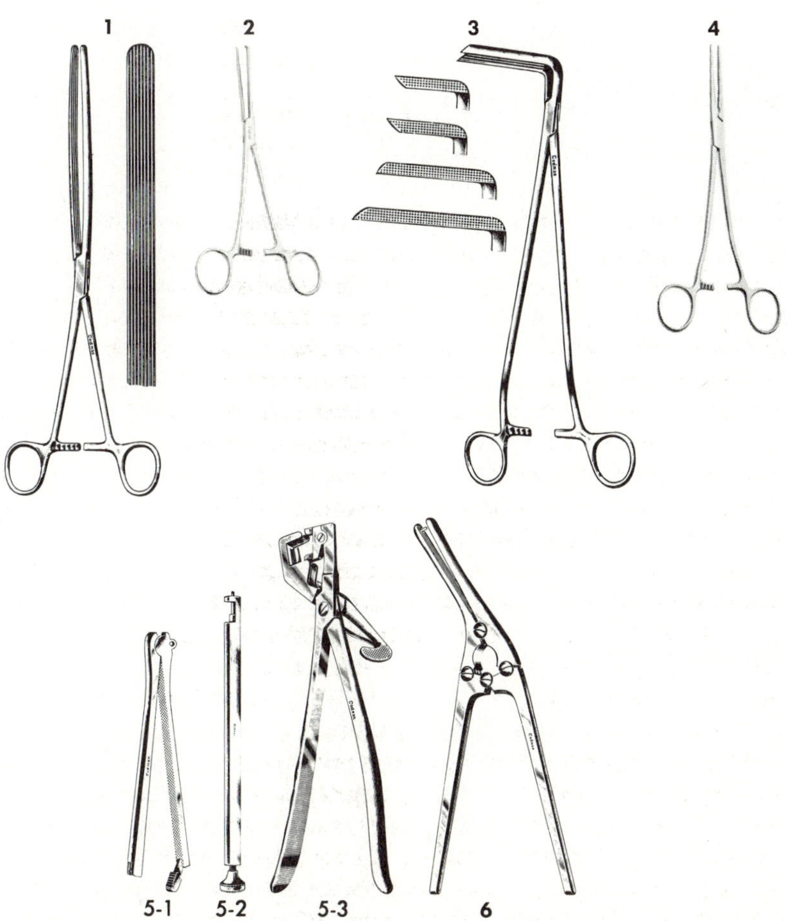

Fig. 14-6. Instruments for stomach and intestinal operations. *1,* Doyen intestinal forceps; *2,* Allen intestinal anastomosis clamp; *3,* Best colon clamps; *4,* Dennis intestinal forceps; *5-1* to *5-3,* DeMartel anastomosis clamp set; *6,* Payr pylorus clamp. (Courtesy Codman & Shurtleff, Inc., Randolph, Mass.)

Holding instruments

2 Tissue forceps without teeth, 5½ inches
2 Fixation or Adson forceps, 5 inches
2 Potts-Smith dressing forceps, 8 inches
6 Babcock intestinal forceps, 6¼ inches

Exposing instruments

1 Doyen retractor, large blade, 2¼ inches wide × 3½ inches deep
2 Kelly retractors, large blade, 2½ inches wide × 3 inches deep
Self-retaining retractor and blades

Suturing items

2 Fine needle holders, 6 inches
2 Medium ligating clip applicators with clips
2 Long ligating clip applicators with clips
Suture materials for gastrointestinal operations:
Ligatures for small blood vessels: chromic no. 4-0 and silk no. 5-0, 4-0, or 3-0
Ligatures for larger blood vessels: chromic no. 0 or silk no. 2-0 or 0
Closure of gastrointestinal layers:
Mucosal—chromic no. 4-0 or 3-0 with curved atraumatic intestinal needle; usually continuous
Seromuscular—chromic no. 3-0 or 2-0 and silk no. 4-0 or 3-0 with curved or straight atraumatic intestinal needles; interrupted silk sutures on intestinal needles may be used
Abdominal closure and retention sutures, as previously described (Chapter 7)

Accessory items

3 Penrose drains, 12 inches long, narrow and medium diameters
2 Malecot, Pezzer, or Foley catheters, desired size
1 Robinson catheter, desired size
1 Rectal tube (optional)
1 Baker jejunostomy tube
Sump drain
Suction drain

OPERATIONS

Esophagectomy and intrathoracic esophagogastrostomy

Definition. Removal of the diseased portions of the stomach and esophagus through a left thoracoabdominal incision in the left chest—including a resection of the seventh, eighth, or ninth rib or separation of the two appropriate ribs—and establishment of an anastomosis (Fig. 14-7).

Considerations. Esophagectomy and intrathoracic esophagogastrostomy are performed to remove strictures in the lower esophagus that may develop after trauma, infection, or corrosion or to remove tumors that are situated in the cardia of the stomach or in the distal esophagus.

Setup and preparation of the patient. The basic thoracotomy set (Chapter 17), laparotomy set, and intestinal set are required.

Operative procedure

1. The skin incision is carried downward midway between the vertebral border of the scapula and the spinous processes to the eighth rib and then forward along this rib to the costochondral junction. The extent of the vertical portion of the incision depends on the location of the tumor. The wound is retracted, and bleeding vessels are ligated.
2. The chest cavity is opened, and the rib spreader is placed. Moist packs are placed, and with a Deaver or Harrington retractor, the lung is retracted.
3. The mediastinal pleura is incised in line with the esophagus and the lesion with long plain forceps and long Metzenbaum scissors. The esophagus is dissected free from the aorta with dry dissectors. Suture ligatures of silk nos. 2-0 and 3-0 are used for controlling bleeding vessels.
4. The diaphragm is opened, and a series of traction sutures are attached. The stomach is mobilized by dissection of its ligamental attachment with long scissors and curved thoracic clamps.
5. The left gastric artery is clamped, cut, and doubly ligated with silk no. 2-0 and a suture ligature of silk no. 3-0.
6. The sterile field is prepared for the open method of anastomosis. The stomach is transected well below the lesion with the selected resection instruments. Closure of the stomach is completed with two rows of intestinal sutures of chromic gut no. 2-0 and sometimes with an additional row of silk no. 3-0 sutures for reinforcement. A separate circular opening is usually made in the upper portion of the stomach for anastomosis to the esophagus.
7. Two Allen clamps or a stapler type of clamp is applied above the stricture, and the freed esophagus is divided.
8. The circular opening in the stomach and the severed end of the esophagus are sutured together by the open method of anastomosis. The mucosal layers are approximated; then the muscular layers of the esophagus and stomach are closed by two rows of interrupted sutures.
9. The stomach is anchored to the pleura, and the edges of the diaphragm are sutured to the wall of the stomach with interrupted sutures of silk no. 3-0 or 2-0.
10. The pleura is cleansed with normal saline solution that is suctioned off. A catheter is inserted for closed drainage. The chest wall is closed as described for thoracotomy (Chapter 17).

Excision of esophageal diverticulum

Definition. Excision of a weakening in the wall of the esophagus that collects small amounts of food and

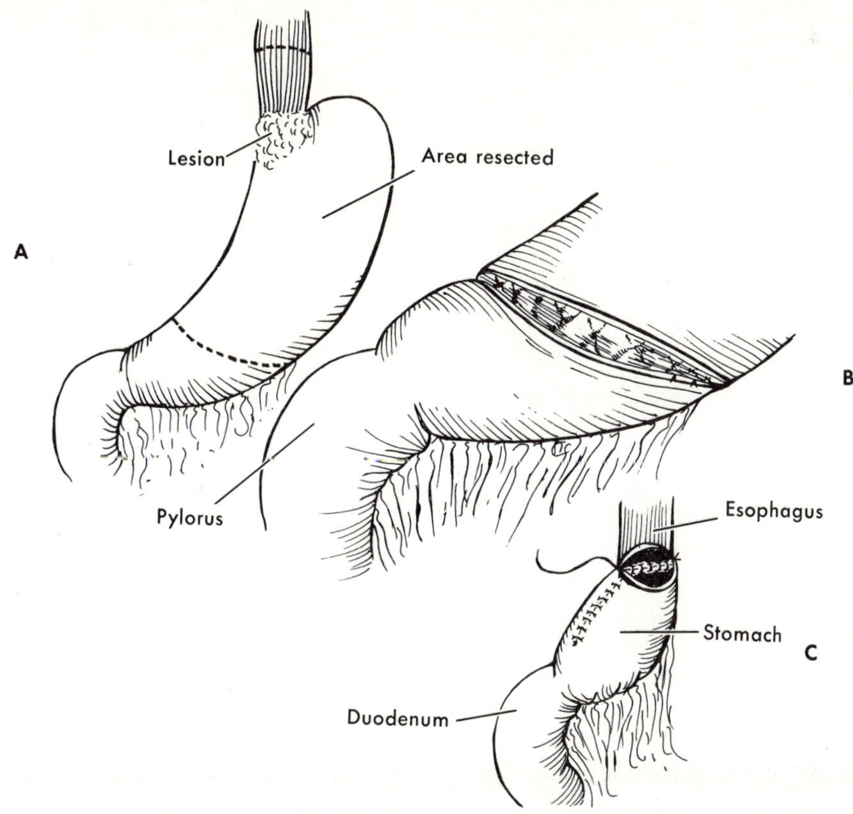

Fig. 14-7. A and **B,** Resection of cardia and distal esophagus for carcinoma. **C,** Tailoring of antrum for esophagogastric anastomosis.

causes a sensation of fullness in the neck. Since this usually occurs in the cervical portion of the esophagus, excision of the diverticulum gives complete relief of symptoms.

Setup and preparation of the patient. A thyroid set (Chapter 12), plus two Pennington clamps, six Halsted curved mosquito clamps, two 5-inch Adson forceps, and two lateral retractors are required.

Operative procedure (Fig. 14-8). An incision is made over the inner border of the sternocleidomastoid muscle and is extended from the level of the hyoid bone to a point 2 cm above the clavicle. The sac of the diverticulum is freed and ligated, and the pharyngeal muscle and surrounding tissues are closed. In conjunction with this procedure, an esophageal myotomy is often performed distal to the diverticulum. A myotomy seems to lessen the likelihood of recurrence.

Esophageal hiatal hernia repair

Definition. Hiatal herniorrhaphy to restore the cardioesophageal junction to its correct anatomical position in the abdomen and to secure it firmly in place.

Considerations. A hiatal hernia is a special type of hernia in which a defect, either congenital or accidental, in the diaphragm permits a portion of the stomach to enter the thoracic cavity (Fig. 14-9).

Hiatal hernias are usually of two distinct types, paraesophageal hiatal hernias and sliding hiatal hernias. Symptoms vary from none to severe heartburn, reflux, regurgitation, and dysphagia. When symptoms are severe enough, a repair of the hernia is done, usually through a transabdominal approach. An antireflux procedure, which prevents reflux of gastric juices into the esophagus, is also done when the hernia is repaired. The three most frequently performed antireflux procedures are the Nissen, Hill, and Belsey Mark IV procedures. A transthoracic approach is used in patients who previously have had left upper quadrant surgery or are extremely obese, or if a Belsey Mark IV procedure is selected.

Setup and preparation of the patient. Instrumentation is as follows:

Laparotomy short and long sets
Thoracic set (Chapter 17), if requested
2 Forceps, smooth, extra long
1 Semb ligature carrier
2 Crile nerve hooks
2 Schnidt thoracic forceps, long
2 Vessel clip applicators, long, with clips

Operative procedure

1. Through a transabdominal incision, the hernia is located, and a crural repair is done.

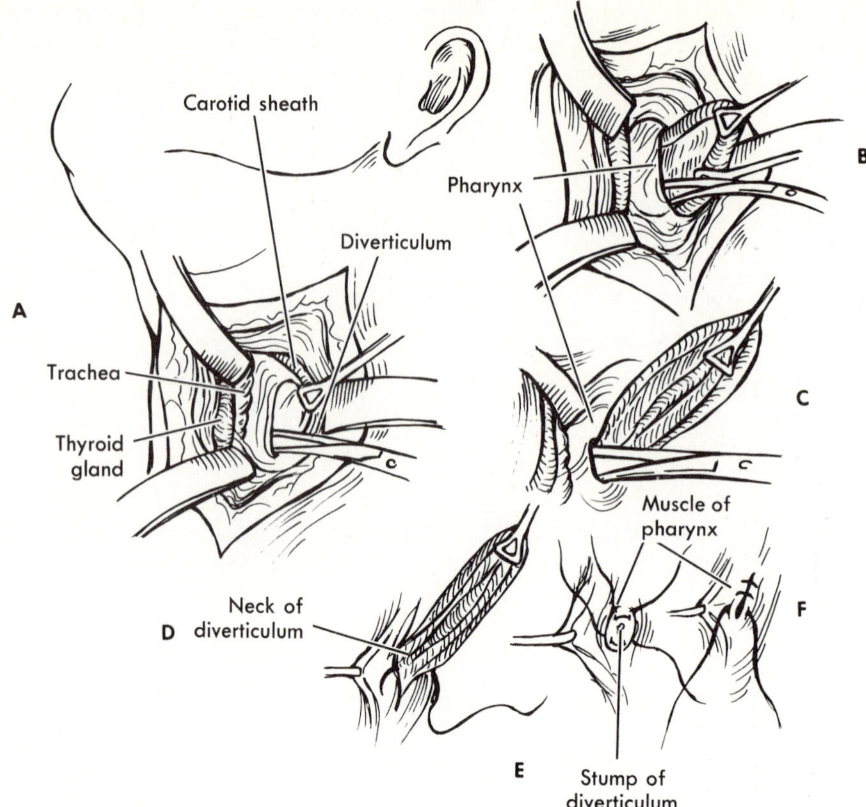

Fig. 14-8. Harrington technique for one-stage esophageal diverticulectomy. **A,** Wound is opened, thyroid is retracted medially, and carotid sheath with sternocleidomastoid muscle is retracted laterally, exposing diverticulum. **B,** Diverticulum is dissected free from surrounding structures down to neck. **C,** True neck of sac is dissected from surrounding muscles of posterior wall of pharynx. **D,** Neck of sac is ligated with chromic gut sutures. **E,** Stump of sac invaginated into wall of pharynx. **F,** Opening in pharyngeal muscles is closed.

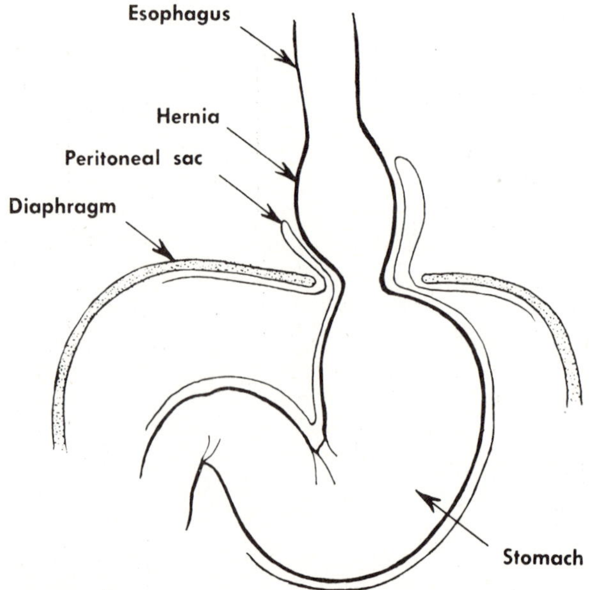

Fig. 14-9. Schematic drawing showing displacement of portion of cardia of stomach through normal hiatus into thoracic cavity in sliding hiatus hernia. (From Anderson, H.C.: Newton's geriatric nursing, ed. 5, St. Louis, 1971, The C.V. Mosby Co.)

2. The fundus of the stomach is wrapped around the lower 4 to 6 cm of the esophagus and is sutured in place (Nissen procedure), or the upper part of the lesser curvature of the stomach and the cardioesophageal junction are sutured to the median arcuate ligament (Hill procedure).

3. Vagotomy and/or pyloroplasty may be performed at the same time.

4. The wound is closed.

An alternative to traditional surgical repair of gastroesophageal reflux and sliding hiatal hernia is the use of a silicone prosthesis (Fig. 14-10). Through an upper abdominal vertical incision, the prosthesis is placed around the esophagus under the diaphragm and above the stomach. A radiopaque marker on the device facilitates x-ray location after surgery. Proper placement of the prosthesis allows passage of food into the stomach yet prevents the stomach from sliding into the chest cavity. Although this procedure seems to be effective, long-term results are not available.

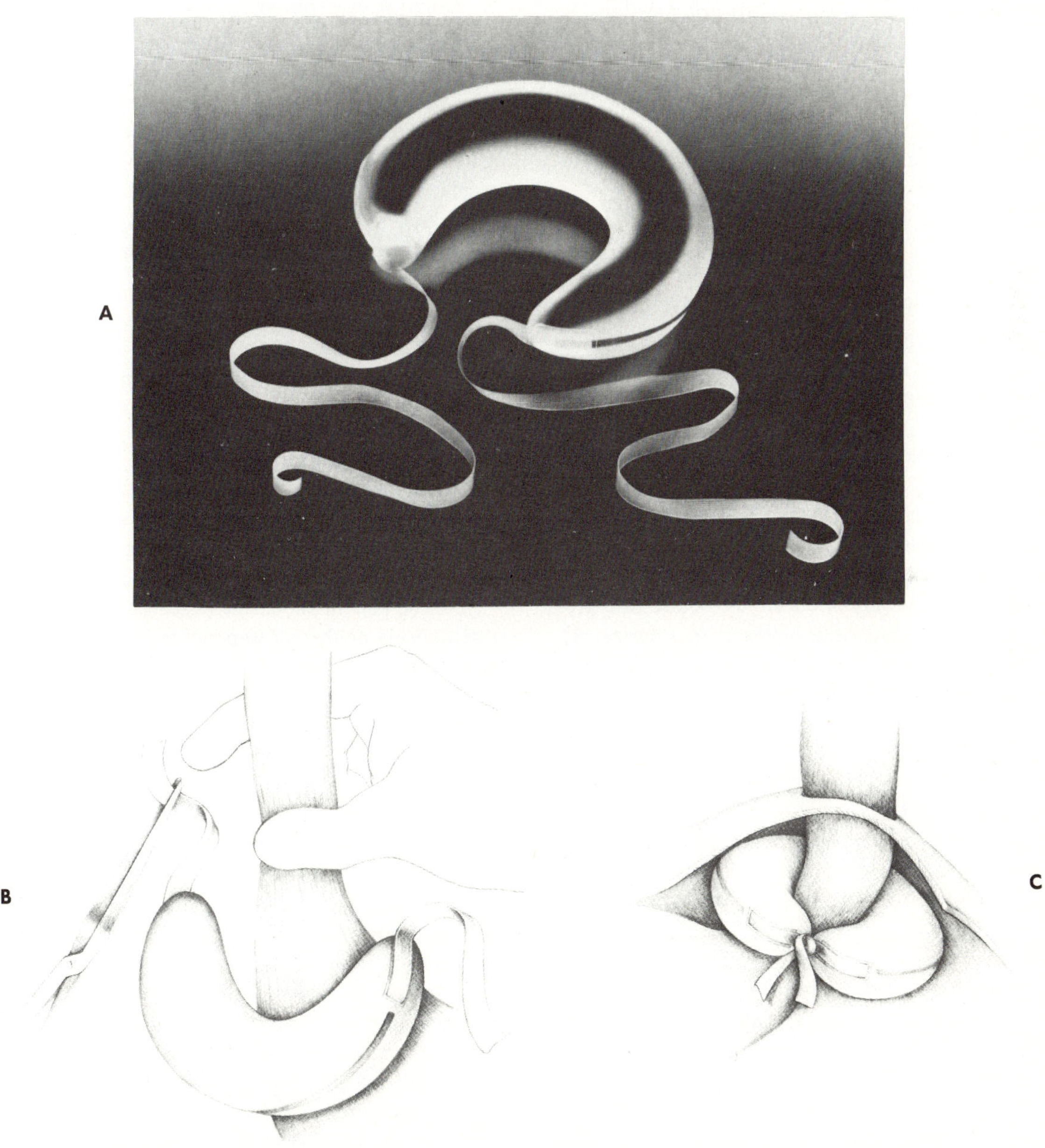

Fig. 14-10. A, Angelchik antireflux prosthesis is C-shaped, soft silicone elastomer collar with radiopaque markings. **B,** Prosthesis is held in place by anteriorly tied Dacron straps, not sutures. **C,** Prosthesis wraps around esophagus below diaphragm and above stomach. (Courtesy American Heyer-Schulte Corp., Goleta, Calif.)

Esophagomyotomy (Heller cardiomyotomy)

Definition. Myotomy of the esophagogastric junction.

Considerations. Esophagomyotomy is done to correct esophageal obstruction resulting from cardiospasm. Selection of transthoracic or transabdominal incision depends on the patient's general condition and other existing pathological factors. The surgeon may elect to perform a pyloroplasty to prevent reflux (backward flow).

Operative procedure

1. The surgeon uses a transthoracic or a transabdominal incision.

2. After exposure of the esophagogastric junction, the anesthesiologist inserts a nasogastric tube to serve as a splint.

3. With a scalpel and a no. 15 blade, a longitudinal incision is made through the muscular wall of the distal esophagus and proximal stomach, leaving the mucosa intact.

4. The wound is closed.

Endoscopic procedures

Endoscopic procedures that permit direct visual inspection of the contents and walls of the esophagus, stomach, and colon may be pertinent to establishing diagnosis or determining preferred treatment of the disease process.

Care must be taken in handling fiberoptic equipment. Flexible scopes can be easily damaged if handled improperly. The endoscopic equipment is terminally cleaned according to the manufacturer's instructions (Chapter 17).

Endoscopic procedures may be performed with local anesthesia or sedation only or during the course of a procedure being performed with general anesthesia. Although medications may be used for sedation, the nurse must be immediately available to provide emotional support to the patient.

Gastroscopy

Definition. Visual inspection of the stomach, with aspiration of contents and biopsy, if necessary, by an instrument known as a gastroscope.

Considerations. When gastroscopy is performed with local anesthesia or sedation, the patient is usually not allowed to eat solid food 4 to 6 hours before the procedure but may take liquids up to 2 hours before it. The position selected for gastroscopy depends on the areas of the stomach to be visualized. For inspection of lesions in the gastric fundus and cardia, an upright sitting position may be used.

Setup and preparation of the patient. Instrumentation is as follows:

Local anesthesia set	Suction set
Gastroscope	Lubricating jelly
Light source	Aspiration tubes
Biopsy forceps	

Operative procedure

1. The gastroscope is thinly but completely covered with water-soluble lubricating jelly.

2. During introduction of the gastroscope, the patient's head and neck must remain in the sagittal plane of the spine so that the axis of the mouth is in line with the esophagus.

3. The gastroscope is slowly passed into the stomach.

4. The stomach is inspected, and stomach contents may be aspirated for cytologic analysis. A biopsy can be performed.

Colonoscopy/sigmoidoscopy

Definition. Visualization of the entire large intestine by means of a colonoscope (160 cm). The colonoscope is an important diagnostic tool and may be used for biopsy and the removal of polyps. The patient must receive a liquid diet for 2 days before the colonoscopy and may receive laxatives. Enemas are given until clear before the procedure.

Setup and preparation of the patient. The following instruments are required:

Colonoscope	Snares
Light source	Cautery
Carbon dioxide tank	Lubricating jelly
Biopsy forceps	Suction

Operative procedure

1. Analgesia is induced intramuscularly or intravenously.

2. The well-lubricated colonoscope is passed slowly and continuously until it reaches the cecum.

3. The patient should be observed carefully to ensure that there is neither postoperative bleeding nor signs of perforation.

Pyloroplasty

Definition. Formation of a larger passageway between the prepyloric region of the stomach and the first or second portion of the duodenum with excision of peptic ulcer, if present.

Considerations. A pyloroplasty may be done to treat a peptic ulcer under selected conditions but is more frequently employed to remove cicatricial bands in the pyloric ring to relieve spasm and permit rapid emptying of the stomach. In adults, a vagotomy is usually performed in conjunction with a pyloroplasty.

Setup and preparation of the patient. Laparotomy short and long sets and an intestinal set are required.

Operative procedure

1. The abdominal cavity is opened through a midline incision.

2. The field is prepared for gastric technique.

3. An incision is made through the stomach and the duodenum (Fig. 14-11).

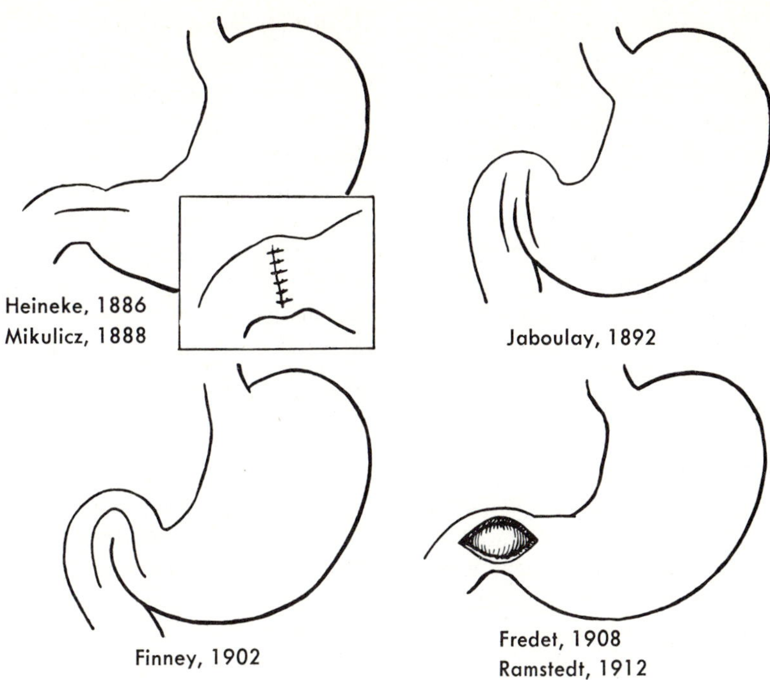

Fig. 14-11. Different types of pyloroplastic procedures: Heineke-Mikulicz longitudinal incision with transverse closure to enlarge lumen; Jaboulay anastomosis of two longitudinal incisions; Finney closure of inverted U incision; Ramstedt longitudinal incision down to muscle layer, with mucosa pouching out to level even with adjoining serosa. (After Waugh and Hood; from Moyer, C.A., and others: Surgery: principles and practices, ed. 3, Philadelphia, J.B. Lippincott Co.)

4. The pyloroplasty is closed with silk or chromic intestinal sutures.

5. The abdominal wound is closed in layers, and a dressing is applied.

Gastrostomy

Definition. Through a high left rectus abdominal or midline incision, establishment of a temporary or permanent channel from the gastric lumen to the skin to permit liquid feeding or retrograde dilatation of an esophageal stricture.

Considerations. This palliative procedure is performed to prevent starvation, which may be caused by a lesion or stricture situated in the esophagus or in the cardia of the stomach. A temporary procedure is done when the obstruction is capable of being corrected. A permanent gastrostomy, in which a stomach flap is formed around the catheter, is advised by some surgeons in an extensive lesion of the esophagus. The catheter is brought out of the abdomen through a separate stab wound. By avoiding the incisional area, improved tissue healing occurs and there is a decreased incidence of postoperative wound healing problems.

Operative procedure

1. The abdominal cavity is opened through an upper midline or transverse incision.

2. The stomach is held with Allis or Babcock forceps, and a purse-string suture is placed at the proposed site for the catheter.

3. A scalpel with a no. 15 blade is used to make an incision within the purse-string suture, and the contents of the stomach are suctioned.

4. Bleeding points are controlled. The catheter is inserted, and the purse-string suture is tied around it.

5. The catheter is brought through a stab wound in the area of the left rectus muscle.

6. The stomach may be sutured to the peritoneal layer, and the abdominal wound is closed in layers (Fig. 14-12).

Gastrotomy

Definition. Opening of the anterior stomach wall through a left paramedian abdominal incision and exploration of the interior.

Considerations. Gastrotomy is usually done to explore for upper gastrointestinal tract bleeding, perform a tissue biopsy, or remove a gastric lesion or foreign body.

Setup and preparation of the patient. A laparotomy short set and an intestinal set are required.

Operative procedure

1. A longitudinal incision is made through the anterior wall of the stomach, halfway between the curvatures.

2. The stomach wall is grasped and elevated by Allis or Babcock forceps.

3. An incision is made, and a suction tube is inserted into the stomach to remove gastric contents.

4. The lesion or foreign body is removed, and the stomach wall and abdominal wall are closed.

Closure of perforated gastric or duodenal ulcer

Definition. Closure of a perforation in the stomach or duodenum through a high right rectus or midline abdominal incision.

Considerations. A perforated gastric or duodenal ulcer is treated as a surgical emergency, and the operation is performed as soon as the diagnosis is made. The patient's blood should be typed and crossmatched so blood will be available for emergency replacement. A gastric lavage is not performed, but continuous suction is used.

Setup and preparation of the patient. Laparotomy short and long sets and an intestinal set are required.

Operative procedure

1. Through a right rectus or midline abdominal incision, the perforation is located.

2. Suction is used to remove exudate in the peritoneal cavity.

3. The perforation is closed with a purse-string suture by inverting the raw edges and suturing a piece of omentum over the closure.

Gastrojejunostomy

Definition. Establishment of a permanent communication through a midline or a paramedian abdominal incision, either between the proximal jejunum and the anterior wall of the stomach or between the proximal jejunum and the posterior wall of the stomach, without removing a segment of the gastrointestinal tract.

Considerations. Gastrojejunostomy may be performed to treat a benign obstruction at the pyloric end of the stomach or an inoperable lesion of the pylorus when a partial gastrectomy would not be feasible and also to provide a large opening without sphincter obstruction.

Setup and preparation of the patient. As described for gastrointestinal surgery.

Operative procedure

1. Through an upper midline or paramedian abdominal incision, exploration of the peritoneal cavity is completed, as described for routine laparotomy. The pathological condition is confirmed.

2. Moist packs are placed, and a loop of proximal jejunum is grasped with Babcock forceps and freed from the mesentery. It is approximated to either the anterior or posterior stomach wall several centimeters from the greater curvature. Silk no. 2-0 traction sutures are placed through the serosal layers at each end of the selected portion of

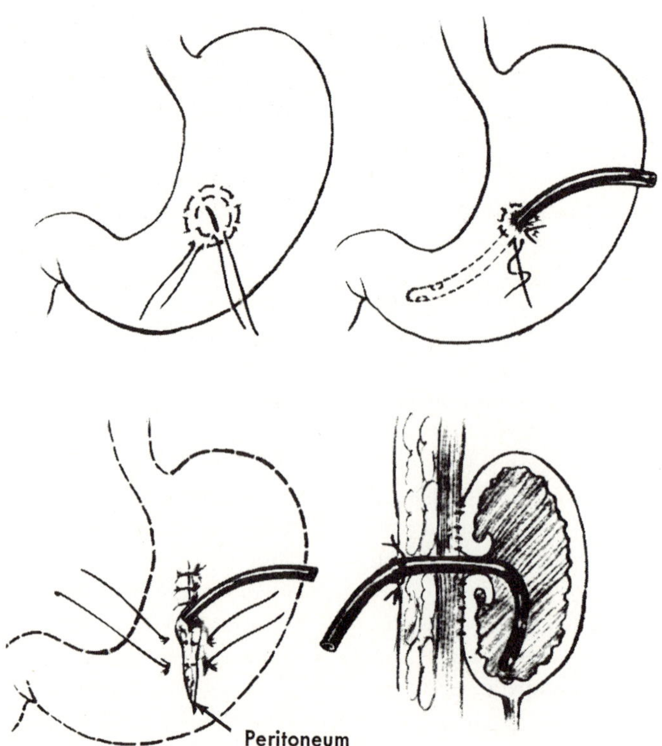

Fig. 14-12. Stamm technique of simple gastrostomy. (From Wilder, J.R.: Atlas of general surgery, ed. 2, St. Louis, The C.V. Mosby Co.)

the jejunum and stomach. Rubber-shod or gastroenterostomy clamps may be placed before insertion of the posterior interrupted silk no. 3-0 or 2-0 serosal sutures.

3. The field is draped for open anastomosis. The jejunum and stomach are opened. Bleeding points are clamped with mosquito forceps and ligated with chromic no. 3-0 sutures. The inner posterior row of sutures is placed, using continuous chromic no. 2-0 or 3-0 with ½-circle intestinal needles, and continued for the first anterior row. The anastomosis is completed with anterior serosal sutures of silk no. 3-0 or 2-0. Traction sutures are removed. Interrupted silk no. 4-0 sutures may be used for reinforcement.

4. The contaminated instruments are discarded. The abdominal wound is closed in layers and a dressing applied.

Partial gastrectomy

Billroth I

Definition. Resection of the diseased portion of the stomach through a right paramedian or midline abdominal incision and establishment of an anastomosis between the stomach and duodenum.

Considerations. The Billroth I procedure is performed to remove a benign or malignant lesion located in the pyloric half of the stomach.

One of several techniques may be followed to establish gastrointestinal continuity, including the Schoemaker, the von Haberer-Finney, and other modifications of the Billroth I procedure (Fig. 14-13).

Operative procedure

1. The abdominal wall is incised, and the peritoneal cavity opened and explored. Bleeding vessels are clamped and ligated.

2. The abdominal wound is retracted, and the surrounding organs protected with moist packs.

3. The gastrocolic omentum is freed from the colon mesentery to prevent injury to the middle colic artery. With hemostats and Metzenbaum scissors, the right and left gastroepiploic arteries and veins are clamped, divided, and ligated with silk no. 2-0 and suture ligatures of silk nos. 2-0 and 3-0, thereby freeing the greater curvature of the stomach. The gastrohepatic vessels are also clamped, divided, and ligated to completely free the diseased portion of the stomach (Fig. 14-14).

4. The operative field is prepared for open anastomosis. Two Payr, Allen, or other suitable clamps are placed on the upper portion of the duodenum just distal to the pylorus. Division is accomplished by scalpel or cautery, as preferred. Additional moist packs are placed for protection, and two sets of anastomosis clamps are placed across the stomach. Division is completed by the surgeon's preferred method.

5. At the lower margin the opened stomach is approximated to the duodenum by a series of interrupted sutures placed in the serosal layers. Silk no. 3-0 threaded on intestinal or atraumatic needles is used. Suture ends are held with hemostats, and the intestinal clamps are removed. Stumps of the stomach and duodenum are cleansed with moist sponges, and bleeding vessels are ligated with fine suture. During the anastomosis, the involved segments may be held with rubbershod clamps.

6. The excess of the lesser curvature in the stomach is closed on completion of the anastomosis (Fig. 14-14). Soiled instruments are discarded.

7. Routine laparotomy closure is completed.

Billroth II

Definition. Resection of the distal portion of the stomach through an abdominal incision and establishment of an anastomosis between the stomach and jejunum.

Considerations. The Billroth II procedure is performed to remove a benign or malignant lesion in the stomach or duodenum. This technique and modifications may be selected because the volume of acidic gastric juice will be reduced, and the anastomosis can be made along the greater curvature or at any point along the stump of the stomach. Modifications of the Billroth II procedure include the Polya and Hofmeister operations, which also establish gastrointestinal continuity through bypassing the duodenum.

After surgery, duodenal and jejunal secretions empty into the remaining gastric pouch. The stomach empties more rapidly because of the larger opening, and a limited amount of gastric juice remains.

Setup and preparation of the patient. Laparotomy short and long sets and an intestinal set are required.

Operative procedure

1. Through an abdominal incision the distal portion of the stomach is resected, and an anastomosis is established between the stomach and jejunum (Fig. 14-15).

2. The abdomen is closed.

Total gastrectomy

Definition. Complete removal of the stomach and establishment of an anastomosis between the jejunum and the esophagus. It may include an enteroenterostomy, if indicated.

Considerations. Total gastrectomy is done as a potentially curative or palliative procedure to remove a malignant lesion of the stomach and metastases in the adjacent lymph nodes. The incision may be bilateral subcostal, long transrectus, long midline, or thoracoabdominal.

Setup and preparation of the patient. Laparotomy short and long sets, a basic thoracic set (if a thoracoabdominal incision is to be used), and an intestinal set are required, plus two long, blunt nerve hooks and two 10-inch needle holders.

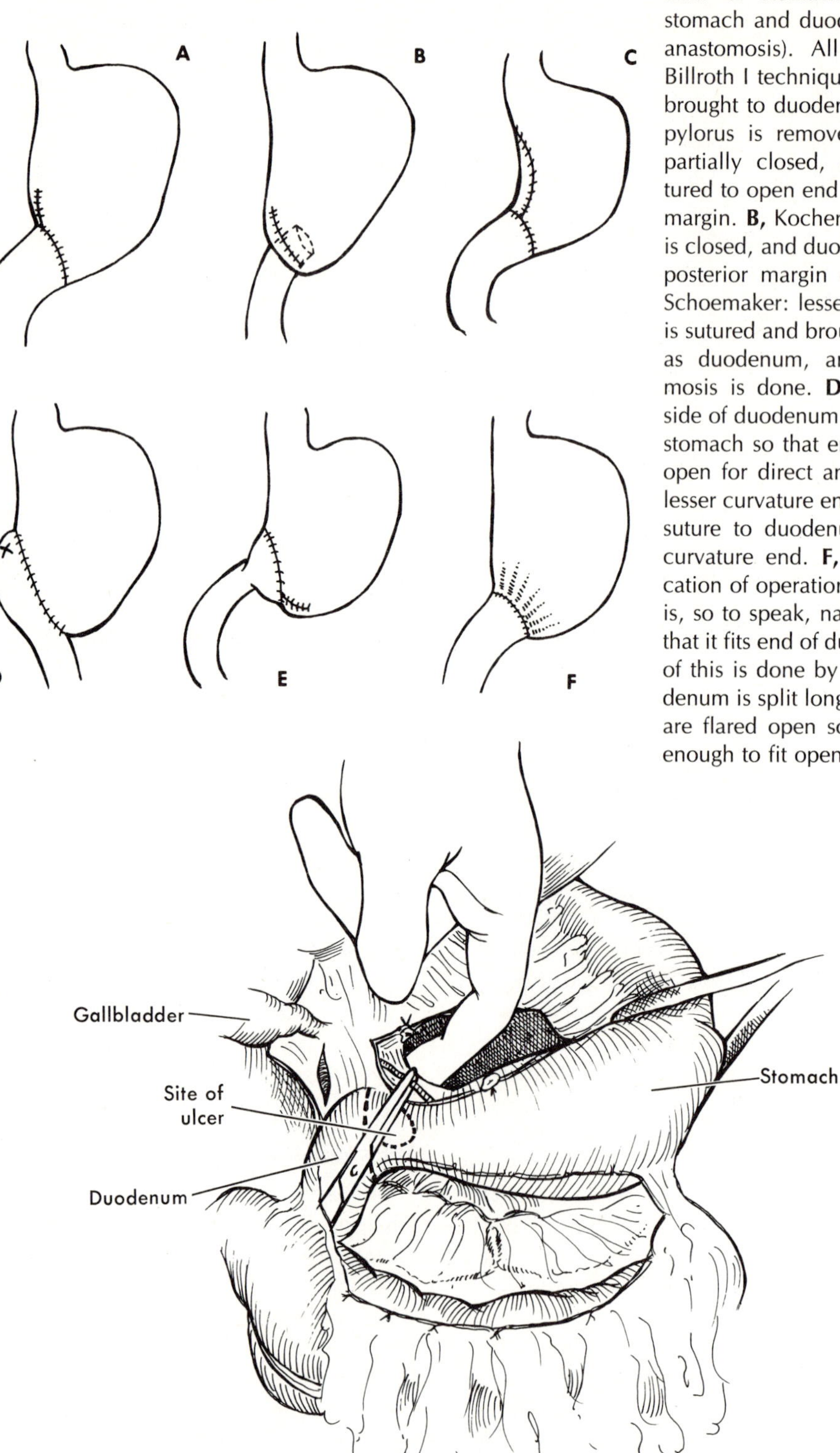

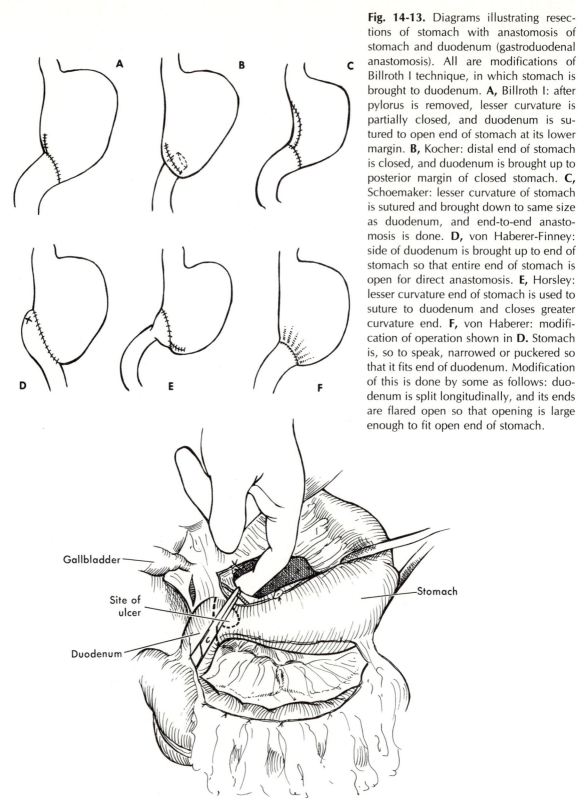

Fig. 14-13. Diagrams illustrating resections of stomach with anastomosis of stomach and duodenum (gastroduodenal anastomosis). All are modifications of Billroth I technique, in which stomach is brought to duodenum. **A,** Billroth I: after pylorus is removed, lesser curvature is partially closed, and duodenum is sutured to open end of stomach at its lower margin. **B,** Kocher: distal end of stomach is closed, and duodenum is brought up to posterior margin of closed stomach. **C,** Schoemaker: lesser curvature of stomach is sutured and brought down to same size as duodenum, and end-to-end anastomosis is done. **D,** von Haberer-Finney: side of duodenum is brought up to end of stomach so that entire end of stomach is open for direct anastomosis. **E,** Horsley: lesser curvature end of stomach is used to suture to duodenum and closes greater curvature end. **F,** von Haberer: modification of operation shown in **D.** Stomach is, so to speak, narrowed or puckered so that it fits end of duodenum. Modification of this is done by some as follows: duodenum is split longitudinally, and its ends are flared open so that opening is large enough to fit open end of stomach.

Fig. 14-14. Partial gastrectomy for peptic ulcer. Stomach is mobilized and elevated by traction tape. Omentum is preserved in this instance but frequently is excised with stomach. Right gastroepiploic vessels are ligated; right gastric artery is isolated and clamped. Incision into hepatoduodenal ligament is made to expose common bile duct. (Courtesy Lahey Clinic, Boston, Mass.; from Marshall, S.F.: Surg. Clin. North Am. **6:**665, 1955.)

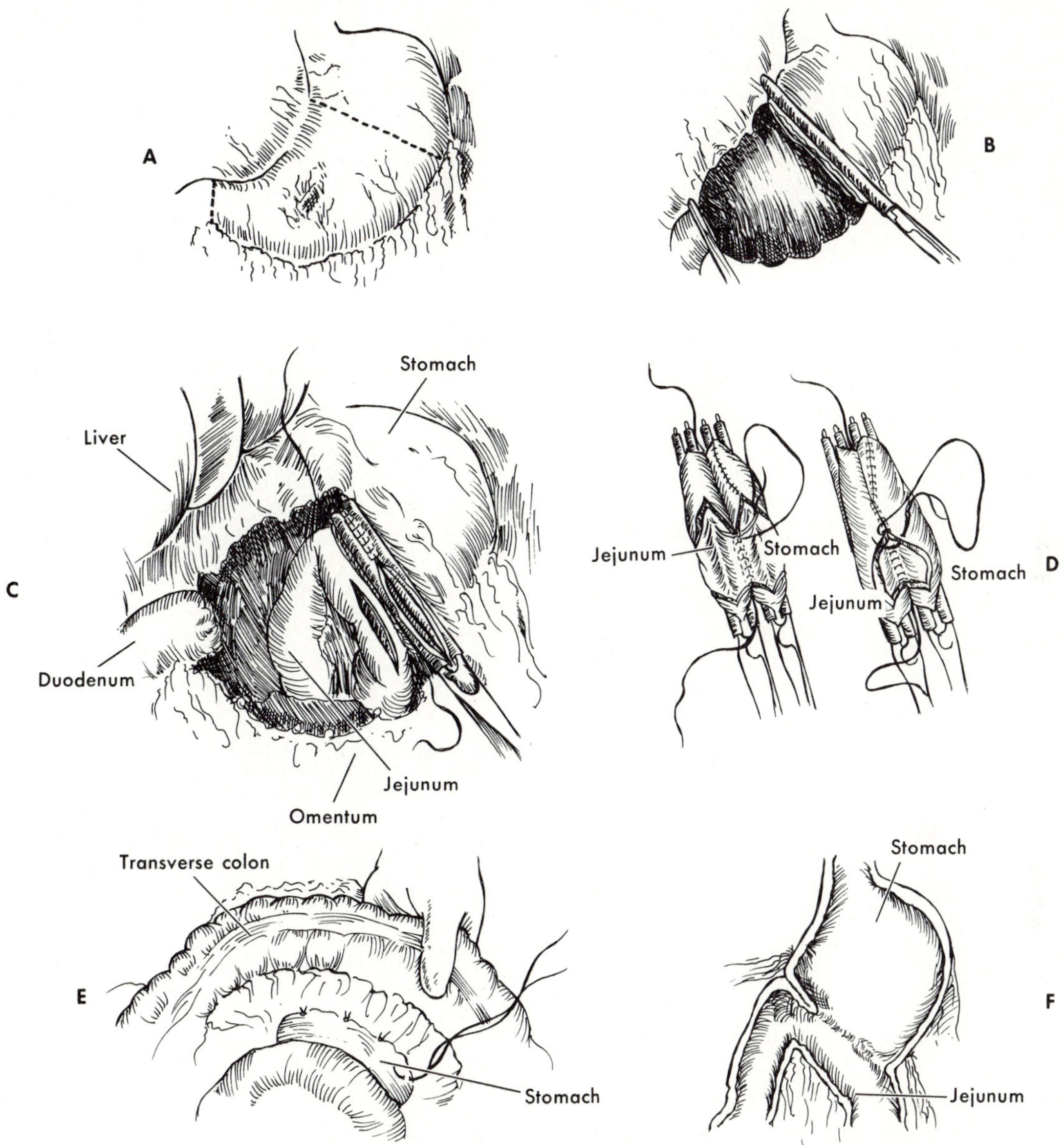

Fig. 14-15. Subtotal gastric resection. **A,** Diagram of stomach showing lesion. *Dotted lines,* Section of stomach to be removed. **B,** Portion of stomach has been clamped and resected: Duodenal stump is now prepared for inversion. **C,** Duodenal invagination is completed. Upper third of stomach is closed. Jejunum is brought through mesocolon. **D,** Anastomosis is established between jejunal loop and lower two thirds of incompleted stomach opening. **E,** Gastrojejunal anastomosis is completed. Stomach is now fixed to edges of slit in mesocolon. **F,** Cross section demonstrating completed operation, showing anastomosis between stomach and jejunum. (From Manual of operative procedures, Somerville, N.J., 1977, Ethicon, Inc.)

Operative procedure

1. The abdomen is opened, and the wound edges are protected and retracted, as previously described.

2. Careful and complete exploration for the extent of metastasis is carried out.

3. The omentum is freed from the colon, using sharp dissection; vessels are ligated with silk no. 2-0.

4. The splenic vessels are ligated and transfixed with silk nos. 2-0 and 3-0 at the tail of the pancreas, leaving the spleen attached to the omentum.

5. The duodenum is mobilized, intestinal clamps are applied, and the operative field is protected for transection and closure of the distal duodenum.

6. The right gastric artery is ligated and transfixed with silk nos. 2-0 and 3-0, and the gastrohepatic omentum is separated from the liver. Following ligation of the left gastric artery, the mobilized stomach, spleen, omentum, and lesser and greater curvature ligamentous attachments are delivered into the wound.

7. Division of the coronary ligament of the left lobe of the liver permits exposure of the diaphragmatic peritoneum over the esophagogastric junction. The liver is protected by moist packs, and gentle retraction is maintained with a Harrington, Deaver, or malleable retractor.

8. A flap of peritoneum is freed from the diaphragm, and branches of the vagus nerves are divided, as seen in Fig. 14-16.

9. A loop of jejunum is selected and delivered antecolic to the esophagogastric junction for anastomosis. With the specimen for traction, the posterior layer of interrupted silk no. 3-0 sutures is inserted.

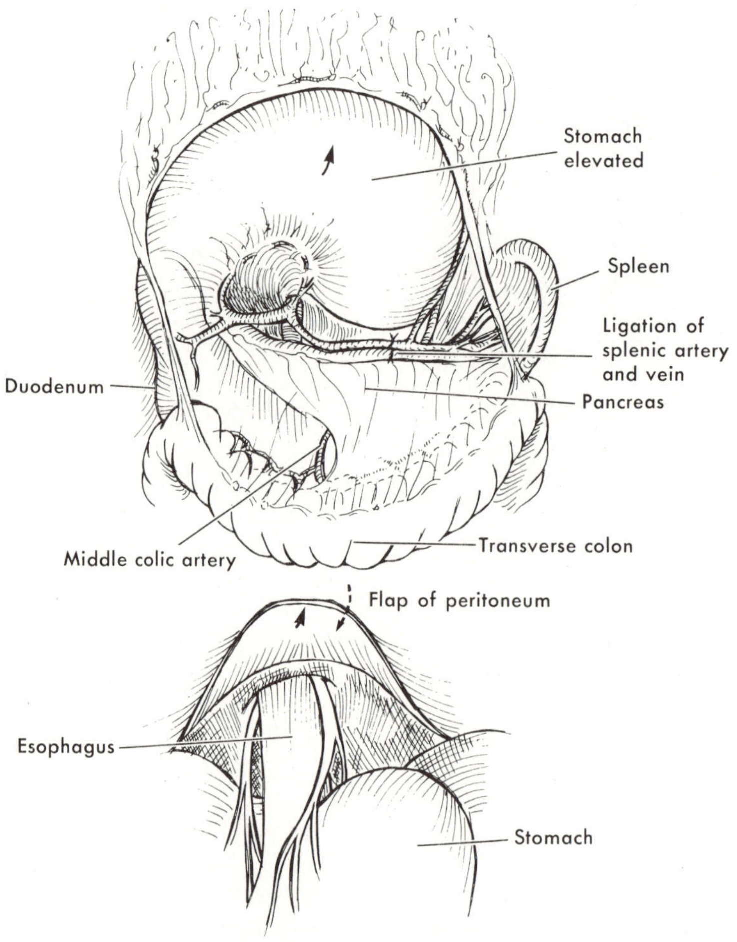

Fig. 14-16. Total gastrectomy. *Top,* Method of detaching greater omentum from transverse colon so that entire lesser peritoneal cavity is exposed. Spleen left attached to omentum and stomach and gastrohepatic omentum are removed in one block. *Bottom,* Flap of peritoneum cut from front surface of esophagus and reflected over diaphragm is diagrammatically shown. This flap will be used to suture to jejunum, reinforce anterior suture line, and take up weight of jejunum anastomosed to esophagus. Vagi also are shown diagrammatically. It is necessary to sever nerves before free delivery of esophagus can be obtained.

10. As the jejunum and esophagus are incised, bleeding is controlled by mosquito hemostats and ligatures of chromic no. 3-0. The posterior layer is reinforced with chromic no. 3-0, intestinal, interrupted sutures.

11. Division of the esophagus is completed, and the entire specimen is removed. Interrupted, chromic no. 4-0 sutures also are used to approximate the mucosal anterior wall of the anastomosis. A second layer of sutures, silk or chromic no. 3-0, is placed anteriorly in the seromuscular and muscular coat of the intestine. A flap of the peritoneum is attached to the jejunum with interrupted, silk no. 3-0 sutures to relieve traction on the anastomosis. A lateral jejunojejunal anastomosis is completed to permit irritating bile and pancreatic fluids to bypass the anastomosis line, thereby preventing esophageal regurgitation (Fig. 14-17). An alternate method of establishing continuity is a combination of a Roux-en-Y jejunojejunostomy and a jejunoesophagostomy (Fig. 14-18).

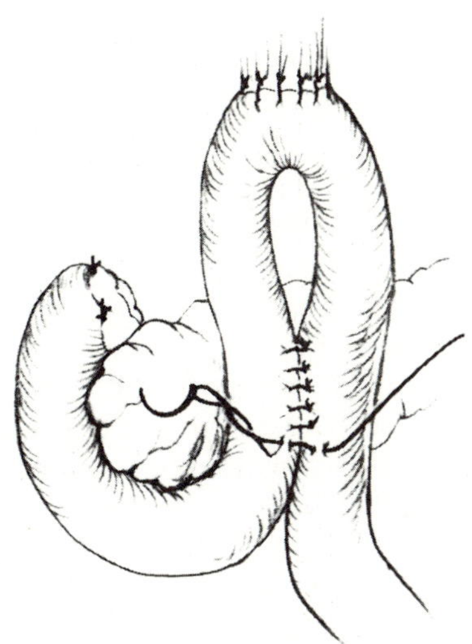

Fig. 14-17. Jejunojejunostomy performed to prevent regurgitation esophagitis. (From Wilder, J.R.: Atlas of general surgery, ed. 2, St. Louis, The C.V. Mosby Co.)

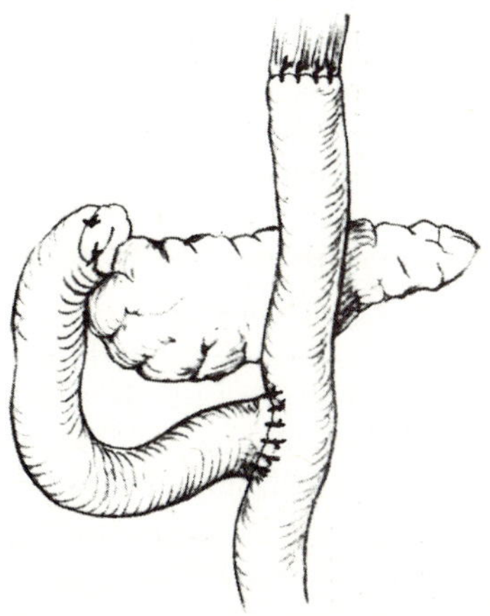

Fig. 14-18. Completed jejunoesophageal anastomosis with Roux-en-Y jejunojejunostomy. (From Wilder, J.R.: Atlas of general surgery, ed. 2, St. Louis, The C.V. Mosby Co.)

12. The abdominal wound is closed in layers. If retention sutures are used, they must be placed extraperitoneally due to the absence of omentum to protect the small bowel.

Gastric bypass

Definition. Creation of a small proximal gastric pouch by stapling, with bypass of the distal 90% of the stomach by a gastrojejunostomy. Alternative approaches are the Gomez fundoplasty, in which no anastomosis is performed, and gastric partitioning.

Considerations. Gastric bypass relies on the principle that early satiety in a morbidly obese person inhibits oral intake. Properly done, this operation creates a small stomach pouch with a controlled outlet obstruction through a small gastrojejunostomy. Given the usual morbidity and mortality that attend operations on obese patients, gastric bypass effectively produces weight loss comparable to that seen after jejunoileal bypass without producing the profound weakness and numerous metabolic complications seen after that operation. Although this procedure seems to be effective, long-term results are unavailable.

Setup and preparation of the patient. As described for gastrointestinal surgery with the addition of TA-90, TA-30, GIA, and LDS stapling instruments. The operation is greatly facilitated by the use of a Polytrac Gomez Abdominal Retractor.

Operative procedure

1. Through an upper abdominal vertical incision, the short gastric vessels are divided with the LDS stapler. A TA-90 stapler is passed from the greater curvature of the stomach through a small defect in the peritoneum to the right of the gastroesophageal junction, and the stapler is fired to create a gastric pouch measuring about 50 ml.

2. An antecolic gastrojejunostomy is performed distally on the greater curvature of the proximal gastric pouch with a GIA stapler to make the anastomosis. The resulting defect at the side of the anastomosis is closed with a TA-30 stapler, which is fired against a nasogastric tube passed through the anastomosis into the jejunum.

3. A Stamm gastrostomy (with a large Foley catheter) or a pyloroplasty is recommended by many to prevent excessive distention of the distal gastric pouch in the immediate postoperative period. In addition, some surgeons perform a jejunojejunostomy just distal to the gastrojejunostomy. Alternatively, some construct the gastrojejunostomy using a Roux-en-Y loop.

Vagotomy

Definitions

Truncal vagotomy. Identification of the two vagal trunks on the distal esophagus and resection of a segment of each, including any additional nerve fibers running separately from the trunks. It reduces the gastric acid secretion in patients with duodenal ulcers. When truncal vagotomy was initially performed alone, a high incidence of gastric stasis resulted from the loss of cholinergic innervation to the smooth muscle of the stomach; thus pyloroplasty or another gastric drainage procedure almost always accompanies truncal vagotomy. Truncal vagotomy deprives not only the stomach but also the liver, gallbladder, bile duct, pancreas, small intestine, and half of the large intestine of the parasympathetic nerve supply. Truncal vagotomy with antrectomy or drainage procedure is the most common operation for duodenal ulcers.

Selective vagotomy. Transection of each abdominal vagus at a point just beyond its bifurcation into the gastric and extragastric divisions. Thus, the hepatic branch of the anterior vagus and the celiac branch of the posterior vagus are preserved. It possesses theoretical advantages over truncal vagotomy because vagal innervation of the viscera other than the stomach is preserved. However, selective vagotomy also denervates the entire stomach, so the addition of a drainage procedure is still necessary. Selective vagotomy may cause less postvagotomy diarrhea than truncal vagotomy, but the incidence of dumping syndrome is probably the same or even higher. Both procedures are about equally effective in controlling duodenal ulcers.

Parietal cell vagotomy. Vagal denervation of just the parietal cell area of the stomach, a procedure only recently given widespread trial. The technique spares the main nerves of Latarjet but divides all vagal branches that terminate on the proximal two thirds of the stomach. The operation has also been called proximal gastric vagotomy or highly selective vagotomy. Since antral innervation is preserved, gastric emptying is unimpaired and a drainage procedure is unnecessary. Parietal cell vagotomy has not yet been sufficiently tested to ascertain its results. Preliminary reports suggest that recurrences are slightly more frequent than after the other procedures. The incidence of dumping and diarrhea following parietal cell vagotomy is much less frequent than after truncal or selective vagotomy.

Setup and preparation of the patient. Instrumentation is as follows: laparotomy short and long sets, basic thoracic set (if a thoracoabdominal incision is to be used), and an intestinal set, plus two blunt nerve hooks and two 10-inch vessel clip applicators with clips.

Operative procedure

1. A midline incision is made, and the esophagus is identified and retracted with Penrose drains.

2. The vagus nerves or their branches, depending on which type of vagotomy is being done, are identified, clamped, and resected with either a ligature or a hemostatic clip.

3. The wound is closed in layers.

Operation for Meckel's diverticulum

Definition. Removal of the diverticulum and establishment of bowel continuity.

Considerations. Meckel's diverticulum consists of an unobliterated congenital duct that is attached to the distal ileum (Fig. 14-19). The diverticulum may contain gastric mucosa, which may ulcerate, perforate, or bleed.

Setup and preparation of the patient. Laparotomy short and long sets and an intestinal set are required.

Operative procedure

1. The abdomen is opened, and the diverticulum is identified.

2. If it is long and narrow with a narrow base, the procedure is as for an appendectomy.

3. If the base is broad, the loop of bowel containing the diverticulum is isolated from the mesentery, and a limited small bowel resection is performed.

4. An anastomosis of the divided ends is completed with an inner continuous layer of chromic gut no. 3-0 and an interrupted outer layer of silk no. 4-0 sutures.

5. The wound is closed as in a laparotomy.

Appendectomy

Definition. Severance and removal of the appendix from its attachment to the cecum through a right lower quadrant muscle-splitting incision (McBurney) (Fig. 14-20).

Considerations. An appendectomy is performed to remove an acutely inflamed appendix, thereby controlling the spread of infection and reducing the danger of peritonitis. A normal appendix is sometimes removed when the abdomen is opened for another procedure.

Setup and preparation of the patient. Instrumentation is as for a laparotomy short set.

Operative procedure

1. A right lower quadrant muscle-splitting incision usually is made.

2. Muscles are retracted with Richardson or Parker retractors to expose the peritoneum.

3. The peritoneum is grasped with tissue forceps or Allis forceps, and a small incision is made with a scalpel and a no. 15 blade. A culture may be taken. The incision is completed with Metzenbaum scissors.

4. The mesoappendix is grasped near the tip with a Babcock forceps or a hemostat for gentle traction. The mesoappendix is dissected from the appendiceal wall by hemostats and ligated with silk no. 3-0. If a suture ligature is required, chromic suture no. 2-0 on a gastrointestinal needle is preferred.

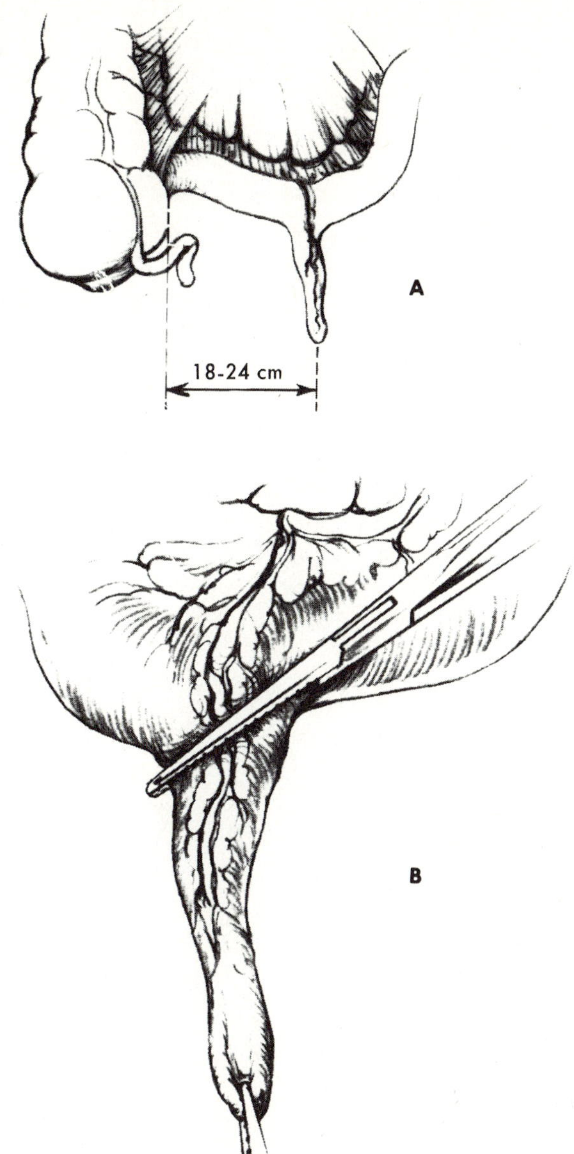

Fig. 14-19. A, Diagrammatic representation of usual location of Meckel's diverticulum. **B,** Ochsner clamp placed across base of diverticulum at its juncture with ileum. (From Wilder, J.R.: Atlas of general surgery, ed. 2, St. Louis, The C.V. Mosby Co.)

5A. The appendix is elevated as a purse-string suture of chromic no. 2-0 is placed in the cecal wall at its base.

a. The base of the appendix is crushed with a straight hemostat, a chromic no. 3-0 tie is placed over the crushed area, and a hemostat is placed above the ligature.
b. A basin for the specimen and discarded instruments is prepared.
c. Protective gauze sponges are placed over the cecum around the base of the appendix. The appendix is amputated between the clamp and chromic suture with a scalpel.
d. The appendiceal stump is inverted into the lumen of the cecum as the purse-string suture is tightened and tied by means of a fine straight hemostat and a small sponge on a holder. Soiled instruments are discarded in the basin.

5B. If the appendix has ruptured, the peritoneum is drained. A Penrose or suction drain may be inserted down to the appendix bed to allow continuous drainage. Deeper layers are closed leaving the subcutaneous tissue and skin open. The wound may then be packed open with wet fine-mesh gauze, and healing by secondary intent is permitted. This packing method may be used in any case in which bowel contamination or abscess formation is present. It allows clean healing and prevents pocketing of pus.

6. In cases in which there is no rupture, the abdomen is closed in the usual manner.

Resection of the small intestine

Definition. Excision of the diseased intestine through an abdominal incision that is made over the suspected site of the lesion (generally in the right lower quadrant) and completion of a suitable anastomosis.

Considerations. Resection of the small intestine is selected to remove certain tumors, a gangrenous portion of the intestine caused by strangulation from bands of adhesions, a herniation of the intestine, or a volvulus.

Setup and preparation of the patient. As described for gastrointestinal surgery.

Operative procedure

1. The abdominal wall is incised and retracted; the peritoneal cavity is explored and protected with moist packs.

2. The clamps are placed above and below the diseased segment of the bowel and mesentery. The involved area is removed with cautery or scalpel.

3. The continuity of the gastrointestinal tract is established by an end-to-end, an end-to-side, or a side-to-side anastomosis.

4. The wound is closed and dressed.

An alternative approach to a traditional suture anastomosis is the use of a mechanical stapling device (Fig. 14-21). The device allows the surgeon to perform an end-to-end, an end-to-side, or a side-to-side anastomosis. An enterotomy is made close to the anastomosis site. The stapler is inserted, and the distal bowel is secured between the anvil and the head of the stapler (Fig. 14-22). The anvil is then inserted into the proximal loop of bowel and secured to the center rod. The gap is closed, and the stapler fired. The stapler is extracted through the enterotomy. The integrity of the anastomosis is verified, and the enterotomy closed with sutures.

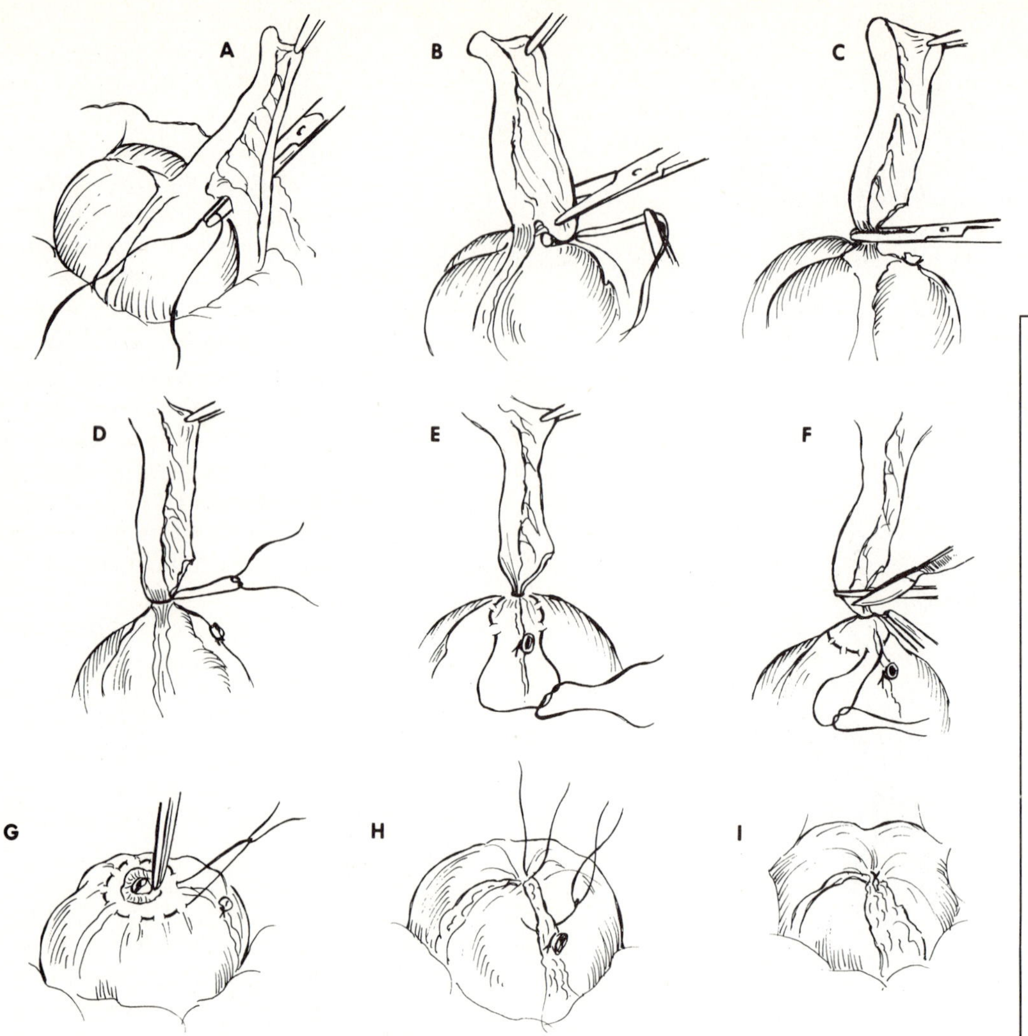

Fig. 14-20. For legend see opposite page.

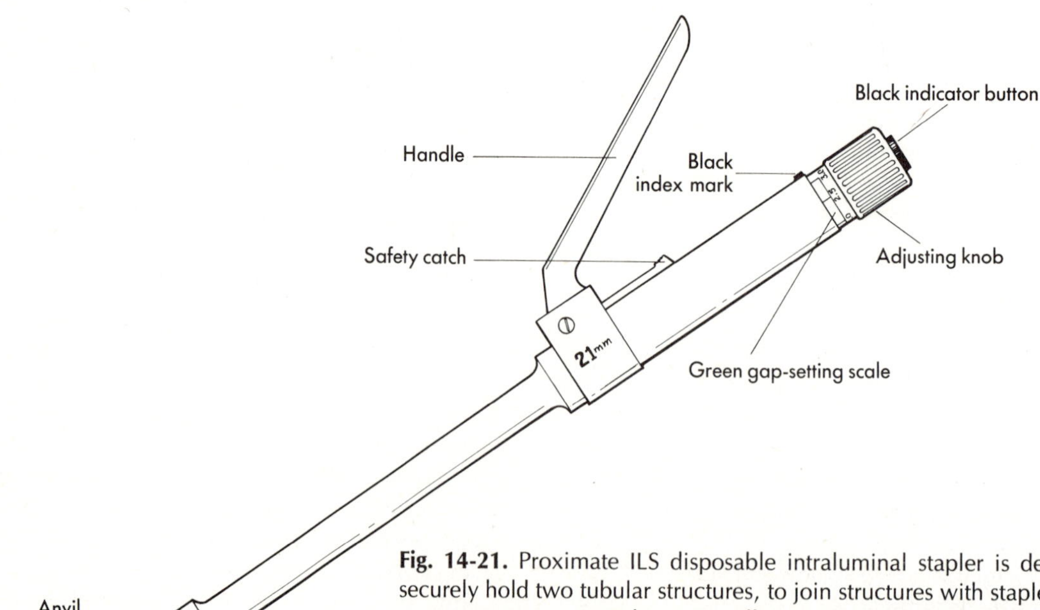

Fig. 14-21. Proximate ILS disposable intraluminal stapler is designed to securely hold two tubular structures, to join structures with staples applied at correct pressure, and to internally cut structures so that proper lumen is produced. Stapler may be introduced through enterotomy, gastrotomy, or colotomy site; through mouth into esophagus; or transanally. (Courtesy Ethicon, Inc., Somerville, N.J.)

Fig. 14-20. Appendectomy. **A,** Cecum is walled off, and ligature is passed through mesoappendix. **B,** Mesoappendix is ligated and cut. Multiple clamps may be used. **C,** Mesoappendix is separated, and clamp is placed at base of appendix. **D,** Crushing clamp is removed, and groove left in base is now ligated. **E,** Purse string suture at base. Appendix is ready for amputation. **F,** Clamp is placed distal to ligature. Appendix is amputated with knife. **G,** Appendiceal stump is inverted as purse-string suture is tied. **H,** Suture of ileocecal fat pad or mesentery protects stump. **I,** Operation is completed. Alternative method omits purse-string suture. (From Manual of operative procedures, Somerville, N.J., 1977, Ethicon, Inc.)

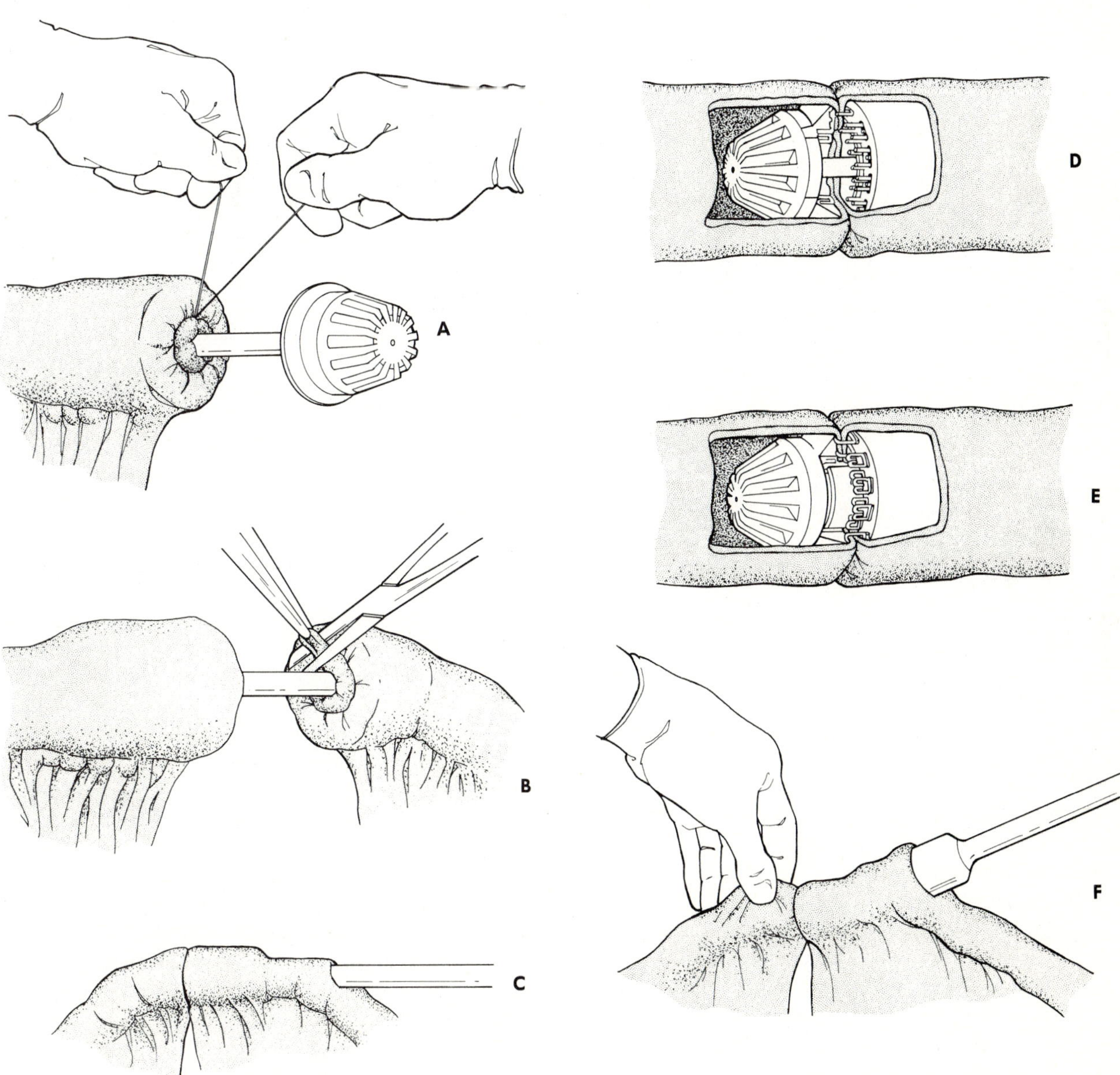

Fig. 14-22. Proximate ILS stapler. **A,** After purse-string suture is placed through distal portion of bowel, stapler is introduced through enterotomy. Distal bowel is secured between anvil and head of stapler. **B,** Anvil is then inserted into proximal loop of bowel and secured to center rod. **C,** Gap is closed, and stapler is fired. **D** and **E,** Staples are driven into tissue and formed against anvil, while knife blade advances to cut uniform stoma through tissue pulled around center rod. **F,** Stapler is extracted through enterotomy. *Continued.*

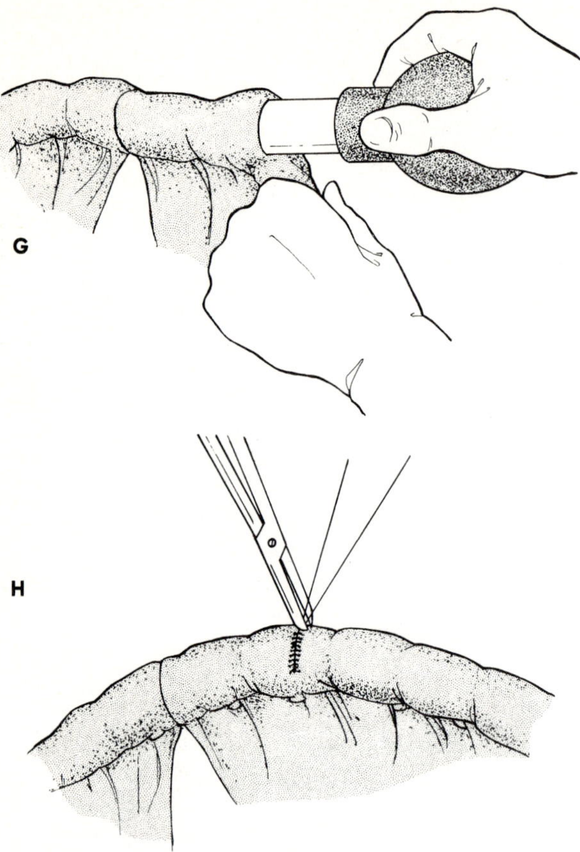

Fig. 14-22, cont'd. G, Integrity of anastomosis is verified. H, Enterotomy is closed with sutures. (Courtesy Ethicon, Inc., Somerville, N.J.)

Ileostomy

Definition. Formation of a temporary or permanent opening into the ileum.

Considerations. An ileostomy is generally done when an extensive lesion is present—to provide complete rest of the colon by means of diversion—or when all the large bowel is resected.

Setup and preparation of the patient. Laparotomy short and long sets and an intestinal set, plus a colostomy bag for the stoma, are required.

Operative procedure

1. Through a midline incision, the peritoneal cavity is explored and the pathological condition determined.

2. The ileum is mobilized with Metzenbaum scissors and hemostatic clamps; the mesentery is clamped, divided, and ligated with silk no. 3-0 sutures at the proposed site, usually about 15 cm from the ileocecal junction.

3. Two Payr intestinal clamps are placed on the bowel, and the ileum is divided with a scalpel between the two clamps.

4. The distal end of the ileum is closed with chromic no. 2-0 on a general closure needle.

5. The proximal end is brought out to the skin through an opening on the right side (held in place by clamps), making sure that the ileum is not overstretched or its blood supply compromised. The mesentery of the ileum is sutured to the parietal wall to eliminate a potential internal hernia. The abdomen is then closed.

6. The stoma is sutured to the skin after the ileum is everted to form a protective cover over the exposed ileal serosa.

7. A disposable colostomy bag is applied over the stoma to collect small bowel contents.

An alternative to a conventional ileostomy for selected patients is the Kock pouch, or continent ileostomy. The internal pouch is constructed of small intestine with an outlet to the skin. When functioning properly, no stool spontaneously exits from the stoma. A catheter is inserted into the stoma three or four times daily to evacuate the contents. This procedure obviates the need for an external appliance.

Colostomy

Definition. Mobilization of a loop of colon, through a right rectus incision to expose the transverse colon or through a left rectus incision to expose the descending sigmoid colon, and closure of the layers of the wound beneath or around it (Fig. 14-23).

Considerations. A colostomy is performed to treat an obstruction in the sigmoid colon resulting from a malignant lesion or an advanced inflammation or trauma that has caused a distention or obstruction of the proximal portion of the colon. A temporary colostomy is often done to decompress the bowel or to give the bowel a rest.

Setup and preparation of the patient. Laparotomy short and long sets and an intestinal set, plus stoma appliances as determined by the surgeon. These items may include a glass rod, rubber tubing, or loop ostomy bridge.

Operative procedure

First-stage loop colostomy

1. The abdomen is opened, and the wound edges are protected and retracted. The peritoneal cavity is opened and walled off with moist laparotomy packs, and appropriate retractors are inserted.

2. A small opening is made in the mesentery near the bowel with curved hemostats and Metzenbaum scissors. A piece of Penrose tubing is passed around the colon, and the two ends are held with a hemostat to maintain gentle traction.

3. The loop of colon is brought out through an incision made on the left side of the midline.

4. The abdomen is closed.

5. The Penrose tubing is removed after the glass rod is in place; a length of rubber tubing is then placed over the loop and securely attached to either end of the rod. A loop ostomy bridge may be used in place of the glass rod and rubber tubing.

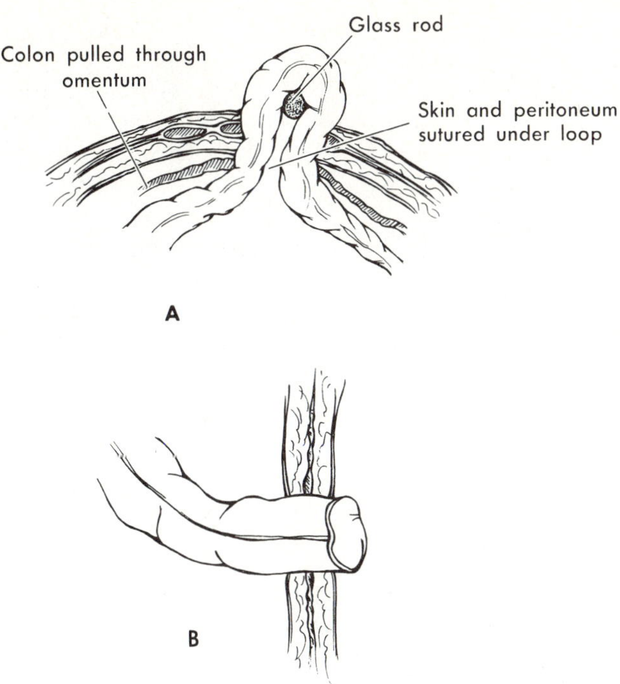

Fig. 14-23. A, Loop colostomy. **B,** Terminal colostomy.

6. The loop of intestine is dressed with petrolatum and 4 × 4–inch strips of gauze.

Second-stage loop colostomy. After 48 hours, the loop of colon is completely severed with a cautery. By this time, if there is no tension, healing has advanced sufficiently to make it safe to allow feces onto the wound. This procedure is very simple and painless and is usually performed in the patient's room or in a treatment room.

A transverse colostomy

1. A short incision, vertical or preferably transverse, is made to reach the transverse colon.
2. A loop of transverse colon, freed of omentum, is withdrawn. A glass rod or loop ostomy bridge passed through an avascular area of the mesocolon prevents the loop from returning to the peritoneal cavity. A mushroom catheter, which is held in place with a purse-string suture, brings about immediate decompression.
3. The bowel is opened 24 to 36 hours later.
4. The glass rod or bridge may be removed in about 10 days.

Closure of the colostomy

Definition. Reestablishment of internal intestinal continuity and repair of the abdominal wall (Fig. 14-24).

Considerations. When the loop has been completely divided, a closed or open anastomosis may be performed.

Setup and preparation of the patient. As described for colostomy operations.

Operative procedure

1. A circumferential incision is made around the colostomy to free the skin margin. Moist packs, a scalpel with a no. 20 blade, Metzenbaum scissors, and Crile hemostats are used as the layers of the abdominal wall are identified and dissected free.
2. An end-to-end anastomosis is completed in two layers, the inner with chromic gut no. 3-0 and the outer with silk no. 3-0 on an intestinal needle, using interrupted sutures.
3. The abdominal wound is closed in layers. A Penrose drain may be inserted, if indicated. A dressing is applied. The surgeon may elect to leave the subcutaneous tissue and skin open. The wound would be packed and permitted to heal by secondary intention.

Right hemicolectomy and ileocolostomy

Definition. Resection of the right half of the colon—including a portion of the transverse colon, the ascending colon, and the cecum—and a segment of the terminal ileum and mesentery through a right rectus abdominal incision. An anastomosis is done between the transverse colon and the ileum either end-to-end, side-to-side, or end-to-side (Fig. 14-25).

Considerations. A right hemicolectomy and ileocolostomy is performed to remove a malignant lesion of the right colon and, in some cases, to remove inflammatory lesions involving the ileum, cecum, or ascending colon.

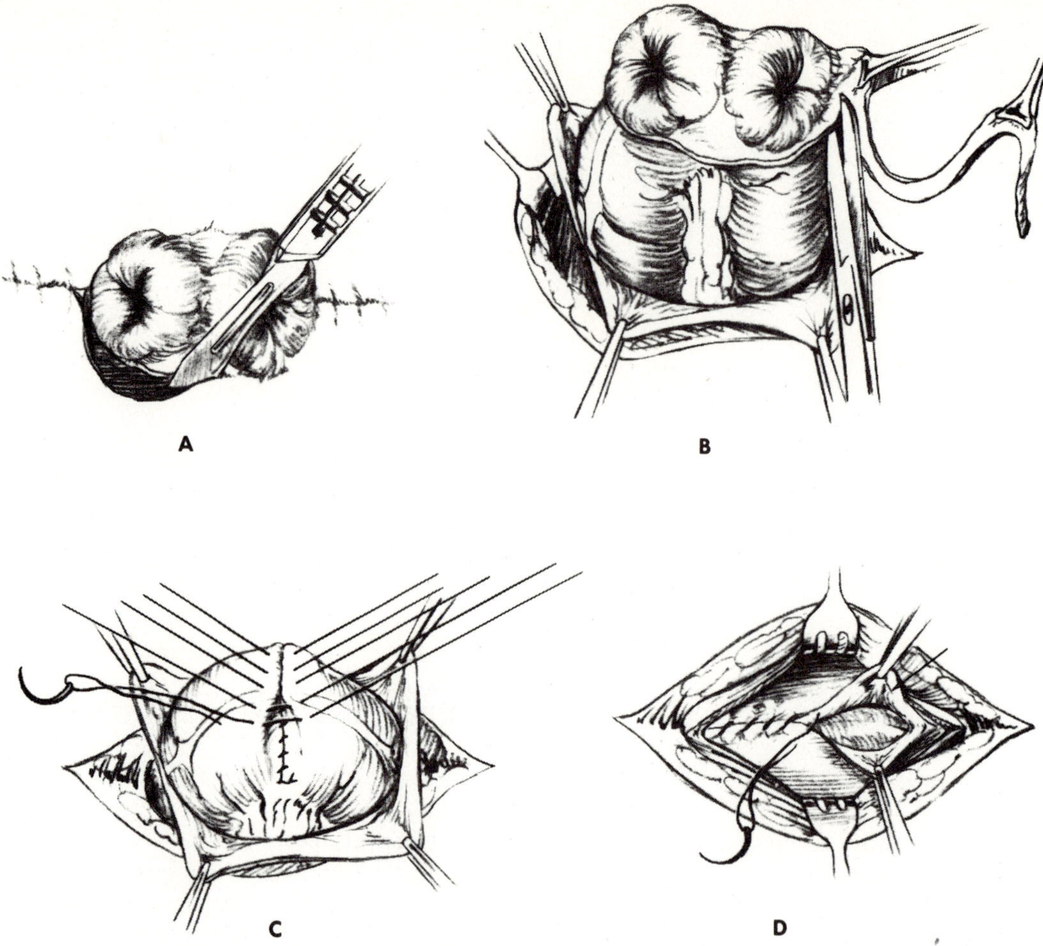

Fig. 14-24. Closure of colostomy. **A,** Skin incised close to colostomy bud. **B,** Scar tissue being excised. **C,** Bowel closed transversely with interrupted sutures of fine silk and replaced in abdomen. **D,** Wound closed completely with gut or wire sutures. (From Wilder, J.R.: Atlas of general surgery, ed. 2, St. Louis, The C.V. Mosby Co.)

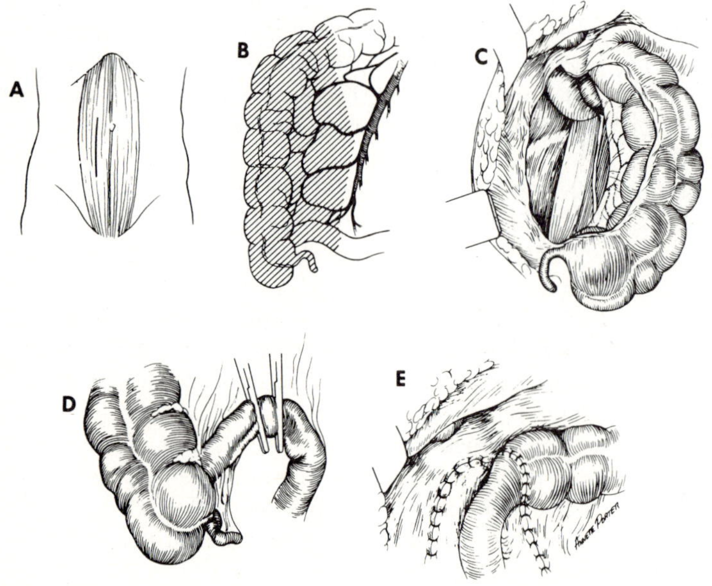

Fig. 14-25. Right hemicolectomy and ileocolostomy. **A,** Right paramedian incision. **B,** Specimen to be resected. **C,** Mobilization of right colon medially. **D,** Clamps on distal portion of ileum. **E,** End-to-end anastomosis of ileum and transverse colon. (Redrawn from Manual of operative procedures, Somerville, N.J., 1977, Ethicon, Inc.)

When a side-to-side anastomosis is carried out, the severed stumps of the ileum and the transverse colon are closed before the anastomosis is done. It is completed between the side portions of the ileum and the transverse colon. When an end-to-end anastomosis is performed, the layers of the severed stumps of the ileum and the transverse colon are sutured together.

Setup and preparation of the patient. Laparotomy short and long sets and an intestinal set are required.

Operative procedure

1. The abdomen is opened, and the peritoneal cavity is walled off, as described for laparotomy.

2. The mesentery of the transverse colon and the terminal ileum are incised at the points where the resection is to be done. Moist packs, Metzenbaum scissors, hemostats, and silk no. 3-0 ligatures are used.

3. The lateral peritoneal fold along the lateral side of the right colon is incised, and the right colon is mobilized medially. Metzenbaum scissors, hemostats, and sponges on holders are used. The ureter and duodenum are carefully identified.

4. The same procedure is done concerning the terminal ileum.

5. The mesenteric vessels are clamped and ligated with silk no. 2-0 ligatures.

6. The operative field is prepared for anastomosis. Resection clamps are placed on the transverse colon and ileum. Division is completed with a scalpel, and the specimen is removed.

7. An end-to-end anastomosis is completed between the severed ends of the terminal ileum and the transverse colon.

8. Contaminated instruments and supplies are discarded.

9. The mesentery and posterior peritoneum are closed with interrupted sutures of silk no. 3-0.

10. Retention sutures and a drain may be used. A dressing is applied.

Transverse colectomy

Definition. Excision of the transverse colon through an upper midline or transverse incision and reestablishment of continuity by an end-to-end anastomosis.

Considerations. A transverse colectomy is performed for malignant lesions of the transverse colon. A more radical procedure may be required when the lesion has perforated the greater curvature of the stomach. If the entire lesion is resectable, a partial gastrectomy may also have to be performed.

Setup and preparation of the patient. Laparotomy short and long sets and an intestinal set are required.

Operative procedure

1. The abdomen is opened, and the peritoneal cavity is explored to determine the extent of the pathological area.

2. Moist packs are used to wall off surrounding structures to expose the hepatic and splenic flexures.

3. The colon is mobilized by incising the lateral peritoneum on either side and transecting the transverse mesocolon. Hemostats, Metzenbaum scissors, and silk no. 3-0 ligatures are used.

4. The operative field is prepared for resection. Four Allen or Payr intestinal resection clamps are applied. Transection is completed with a scalpel, and end-to-end anastomosis is completed, as previously described.

5. Contaminated articles are discarded. Approximation of mesentery and lateral peritoneum is completed with silk no. 3-0 sutures.

6. The abdominal wound is closed. Retention sutures may be used. The wound is dressed.

Anterior resection of the sigmoid colon and rectosigmoidostomy

Definition. Removal of the lower sigmoid and rectosigmoid portions of the rectum, usually through a low left paramedian incision, and completion of an end-to-end anastomosis.

Considerations. This operation is selected to treat lesions in the lower portion of the sigmoid and rectum that permit excision with a wide margin of safety and still retain sufficient tissues with adequate blood supply for an accurate rectosigmoid end-to-end anastomosis.

Setup and preparation of the patient. Laparotomy short and long sets and an intestinal set are required.

Operative procedure

1. The abdomen is entered through a left paramedian incision. The peritoneal cavity is explored for metastasis and resectability of the lesion.

2. Before mobilizing the colon, the tumor-bearing segment is isolated by ligatures to the lymphovenous drainage (provided these structures are accessible).

3. A loop of sigmoid colon is elevated as the small intestines are walled off with moist packs; retractors are placed.

4. The peritoneum on the left side of the colon is incised with a long scalpel, scissors, hemostats, and sponge forceps. Traction sutures of silk no. 2-0 may be used as the peritoneum is reflected. Bleeding vessels are ligated with silk no. 2-0 or 3-0 ligatures.

5. The pelvic peritoneum is exposed and dissected free to form the left side of the reconstructed pelvic floor. Long dissecting instruments are used. Vessels are ligated with 24-inch silk ligatures. Extreme care must be exercised throughout to protect the ureters from injury.

6. The sigmoid colon is turned toward the left, and the same procedure as in step 4 is carried out on the right side of the pelvis. The two incisions are then curved and joined in front of the rectum.

7. The rectum is freed anteriorly and posteriorly from the adjacent structures.

8. The sigmoid colon is clamped with Payr or similar resection clamps after mobilization of the proximal portion. As the sigmoid colon is divided distal to the clamp, the severed rectal edges are grasped with Allis or Ochsner forceps, and the rectal opening is exposed. The diseased portion is removed, and the soiled instruments discarded.

9. Continuity is established by an end-to-end anastomosis of the proximal colon and the rectum.

10. The pelvic floor is reperitonealized, and drains may be placed.

11. The abdominal wound is closed in the routine manner, and a dressing is applied.

An alternative to traditional surgical anastomosis is the use of a stapling device. The device can be used intraabdominally through a colotomy approach or transanally (Fig. 14-26). Use of a stapling device may obviate the need for an abdominoperineal resection, since a very low anastomosis can be performed.

Abdominoperineal resection

Definition. Mobilization and division of the diseased segment of the lower bowel through a midline incision, extending from several centimeters above the umbilicus to the pubis. The proximal end of bowel is exteriorized through a separate stab wound as a colostomy. The distal

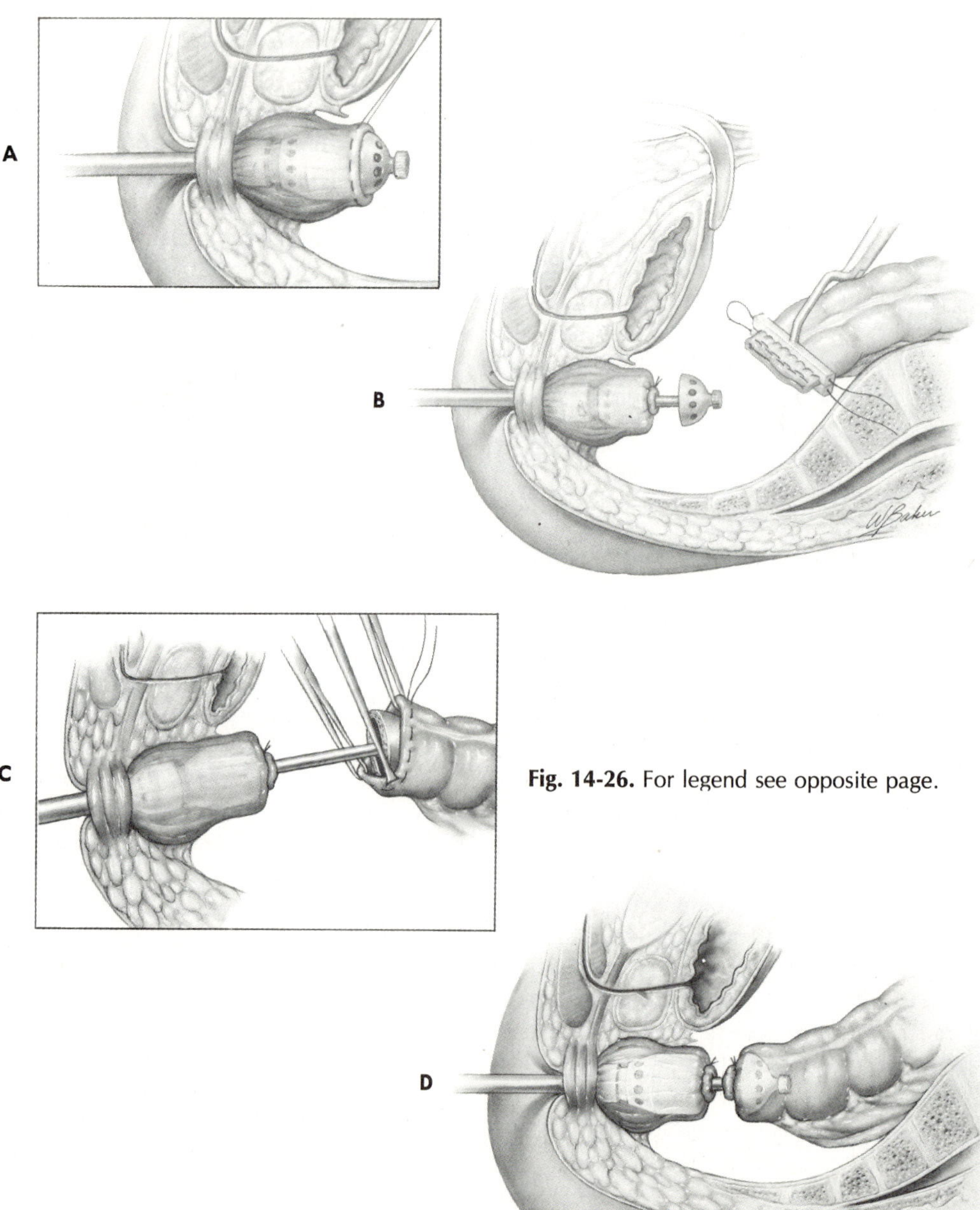

Fig. 14-26. For legend see opposite page.

end is pushed into the hollow of the sacrum and removed through the perineal route.

Considerations. An abdominoperineal resection is performed for malignant lesions and inflammatory diseases of the lower sigmoid colon, rectum, and anus. The choice of patient position depends on the surgeon. Some may prefer to start with the patient in the supine position and move the patient to the lithotomy position for the perineal portion of the operation. Others may originally place the patient in a modified lithotomy position; thus surgery may be performed simultaneously by two teams.

Setup and preparation of the patient. Laparotomy short and long sets, intestinal set, and a perineal set, plus a colostomy bag, are required. A Foley catheter is inserted after induction.

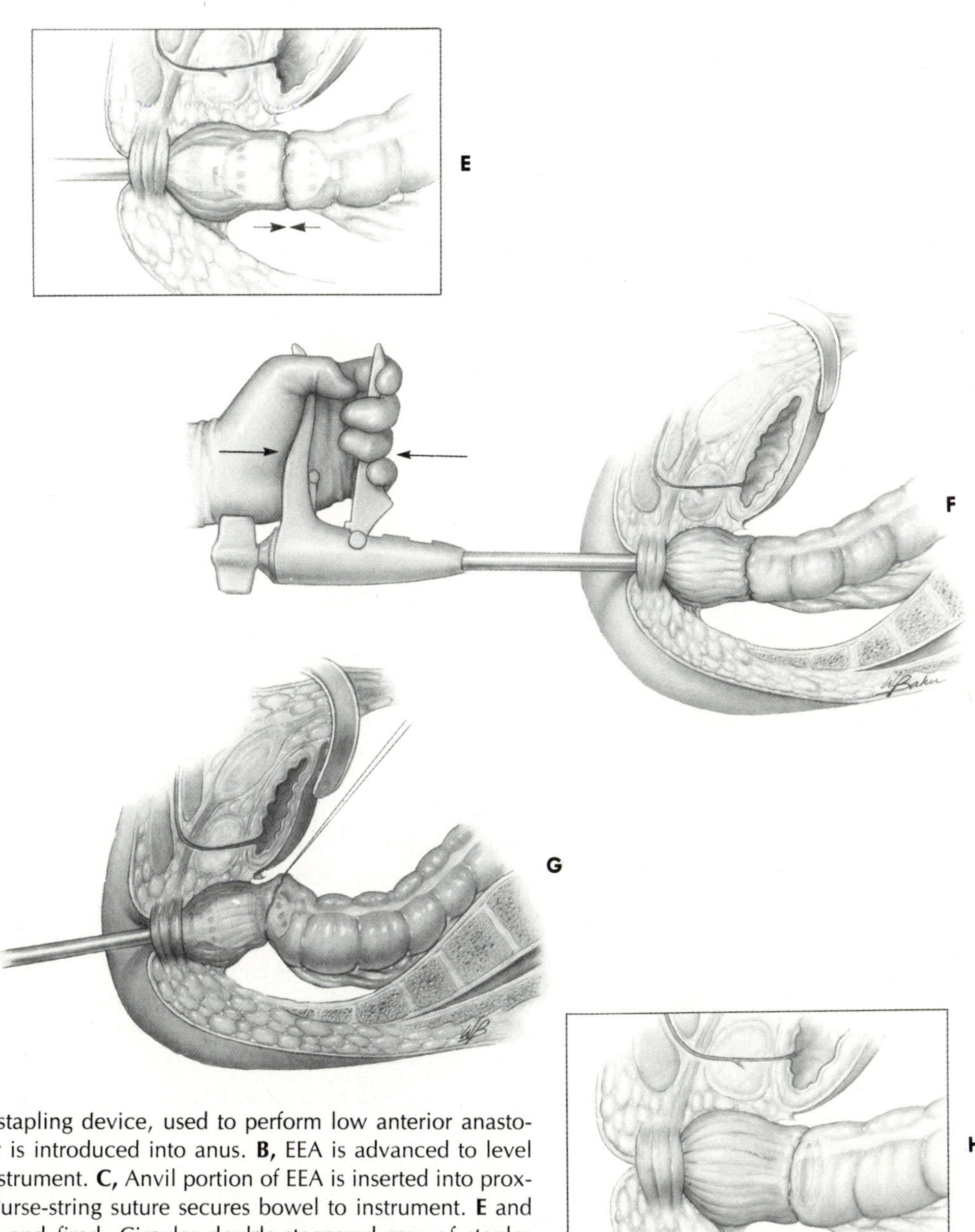

Fig. 14-26. EEA stapling device, used to perform low anterior anastomosis. **A,** Stapler is introduced into anus. **B,** EEA is advanced to level of purse-string instrument. **C,** Anvil portion of EEA is inserted into proximal colon. **D,** Purse-string suture secures bowel to instrument. **E** and **F,** EEA is closed and fired. Circular double-staggered row of staples joins bowel; simultaneously, circular blade in instrument cuts stoma. **G,** Instrument is gently removed. **H,** Resulting anastomosis is illustrated with bowel wall transparent to depict reconstruction. (Reprinted with the permission of U.S. Surgical Corporation © USSC 1974, 1975, 1980. All rights reserved.)

Operative procedure

1. A midline incision is made.

2. After thorough exploration of the abdominal cavity, the surgeon determines the extent and operability of the lesion.

3. If the resection is to be done, the surgeon retracts the sigmoid colon to the right side. The peritoneum on the left of the mesocolon is divided.

4. The incision into the peritoneum is made opposite the main branches of the inferior mesenteric vessels and is extended into the pelvis and around anterior to the rectum.

5. The pelvic peritoneum is mobilized by blunt dissection to form the left side of the new pelvic floor and to permit early visualization of the left ureter.

6. The peritoneum is incised on the right side until the incision connects with that made on the left. The right ureter is identified and protected.

7. The blood supply of the portion of intestine to be removed is isolated and ligated.

8. Care must be taken not to damage the left colic artery, since it will supply the blood to the colostomy.

9. The mesentery is tied to permit greater exposure in the operative field.

10. The surgeon frees the rectum, usually as low as the sacrococcygeal junction.

11. After the bowel is freed, the surgeon prepares the permanent colostomy.

12. The omentum is brought down into the pelvis, and the abdominal wound is closed. Many surgeons repair the pelvic peritoneum.

13. The patient is placed in the lithotomy position.

14. The surgical team changes gowns and gloves. New instrumentation is used for this portion of the procedure.

15. The perineal area is prepared, and the patient redraped.

16. To prevent contamination, the anus is often closed with a purse-string suture. An incision is made around the anus.

17. The anus is grasped with Allis forceps or Ochsner clamps and tipped upward to enable its attachment to the coccyx to be severed more readily.

18. The levator ani muscle is exposed, and while the finger of the surgeon is held beneath it, it is divided as far from the rectum as possible.

19. All bleeding points are clamped and tied.

20. The Foley catheter allows the surgeon to get as close to the bladder as possible without damaging it.

21. After the anococcygeal raphe is divided, the surgeon's hand is thrust up into the hollow sacrum to free the rectum by blunt dissection, grasp the upper end of the distal fragment, and bring the sigmoid colon into the wound.

22. Finally, the distal fragment with its tumor, the attached mesentery of the lower sigmoid colon, and all structures of the hollow of the sacrum are removed along with the rectum and anus.

23. When all bleeding is controlled, the incision is closed, usually around a drain.

Hemorrhoidectomy

Definition. Excision and ligation of dilated veins in the anal region to relieve discomfort and to control bleeding.

Considerations. Preoperative anal dilatation aids in exposing the vessels, as well as contributes to the patient's comfort in the immediate postoperative period. Many surgeons prefer to precede the operation with a sigmoidoscopy. Spinal or caudal anesthesia may be used.

Setup and preparation of the patient. A laparotomy short set, plus the following rectal instruments are required: two Hill retractors, one anoscope, one rectal speculum, one set of rectal dilators, Buie pile forceps, and a crypt hook.

Operative procedure

1. The patient is usually placed in the lithotomy or jackknife position.

2. The anal canal is dilated and inspected through an anoscope.

3. Four Allis forceps are applied several centimeters from the anal margin to expose the anus.

4. The base of the hemorrhoid and tissue are grasped with Allis forceps and held.

5. An intestinal suture of chromic gut no. 2-0 is placed and tied at the proximal end of the hemorrhoid, and a Buie pile forceps is applied across the base and above the proposed incision line. Excision is completed with a scalpel. Suturing is completed by loosely placed continuous stitches over the Buie forceps. The suture is tightened as the forceps is removed, and the suture ends are tied.

6. Traction may be maintained as hemostatic forceps are applied, and dissection is completed in segmental fashion. Suture ligatures of chromic gut no. 2-0 are used as each hemostat is removed.

7. Remaining hemorrhoids are excised in a similar manner.

8. Petrolatum gauze packing is placed in the anal canal. A dressing and a T binder are applied.

Excision of anal fissure

Definition. Dilatation and excision of the lesion.

Considerations. Anal fissures are benign lesions of the anal wall.

Setup and preparation of the patient. A laparotomy short set and rectal instruments, as listed previously, are required.

Operative procedure

1. The patient is placed in the lithotomy or jackknife position.

2. Dilatation of the anal sphincter is completed.

3. The fissure is excised, and bleeders are ligated or cauterized.

4. A drain or packing is inserted.

5. A dressing is applied.

Excision of pilonidal cyst and sinus

Definition. Excision of the cyst with sinus tracts from the intergluteal fold on the posterior surface of the lower sacrum.

Considerations. A pilonidal cyst and sinus, which may have a congenital origin, rarely becomes symptomatic until the individual reaches adulthood. Inflammatory reaction varies from the mild, irritating, draining sinus tract to an acute abscess with secondary recurrences. Treatment consists of drainage in the acute stage and total surgical excision during remission.

The excision of the cyst and sinus tracts must be complete to prevent recurrence. The defect resulting from recurrences may become too large for primary closure. In this case the wound is left open to heal by granulation.

Setup and preparation of the patient. A laparotomy short set and rectal instruments, as listed previously, are required.

Operative procedure

1. The patient is placed on the operating room table in a jackknife position.

2. The sinus tracts are identified with the probes.

3. An elliptical incision is made down to the fascia. A curette is used to remove gelatinous tissue. Excision of cyst and sinus tracts is completed.

4. Bleeding is controlled.

5A. If the wound is to be left open, it is then packed, and a pressure dressing is applied.

5B. If the wound is closed, 2-0 silk sutures are used for stay sutures on the deeper tissue, and fine silk is used on the skin.

SUGGESTED READINGS

Angelchik, J.P., and Cohen, R.: A new surgical procedure for the treatment of gastroesophageal reflux and hiatal hernia, Surg. Gynecol. Obstet. **148:**246, 1979.

Atkinson, L.J.: Trends in gastrointestinal surgery, Point of View **18**(3):4, 1981.

Atkinson, L.J., and Kohn, M.L.: Berry and Kohn's introduction to operating room technique, ed. 5, New York, 1978, McGraw-Hill Book Co.

Beyers, M., and Dudas, S.: The clinical practice of medical-surgical nursing, Boston, 1977, Little, Brown & Co.

Boehmer, V.W. and Turk, M.F.: Caring for the gastroplasty patient, AORN J. **34:**1036, 1981.

Bolinger, J., and others: Gastric bypass for morbid obesity, Nursing '81 **11:**54, 1981.

Bowden, T.A., Hooks, V.H., and Mansberger, A.R.: Intraoperative gastrointestinal endoscopy, Ann. Surg. **191:**680, 1980.

Brindley, G.V., and Hightower, N.C.: Surgical treatment of gastroesophageal reflux, Surg. Clin. North Am. **59:**841, 1979.

Brunner, L.S., and Suddart, D.S.: Textbook of medical-surgical nursing, ed. 4, Philadelphia, 1980, J.B. Lippincott Co..

Fazio, V.W.: Colorectal anastomosis using the EEA stapler, Curr. Surg. Tech. **3:**3, 1980.

Given, B.A., and Simmons, S.J.: Gastroenterology in clinical nursing, ed. 3, St. Louis, 1979, The C.V. Mosby Co.

Goligher, J.C.: Surgery of the anus, rectum and colon, ed. 4, London, 1980, Bailliére Tindall Publishers.

Gomez, C.A.: Gastroplasty in the surgical treatment of morbid obesity, Am. J. Clin. Nutr. **33:**406, 1980.

Griffen, W.O.: Gastric bypass for morbid obesity, Surg. Clin. North Am. **59:**1103, 1979.

Kaplan, J.: Pre- and postoperative care of the patient with cancer of the sigmoid colon, Point of View **18:**8, 1981.

Kelly, K.A.: Gastrointestinal and biliary conditions, Bull. Am. Coll. Surg. **66:**11, 1981.

MacArthur, R.I., and others: Revision of gastric bypass, Am. J. Surg. **140:**751, 1980.

MacClelland, D.C.: Kock pouch: a new type of ileostomy, AORN J. **32:**191, 1980.

Manteuffel, S.L., and McDonough, J.L.: Esophageal reconstruction with free jejunal grafts, AORN J. **30:**1059, 1979.

Mason, E.E., and others: Gastric bypass in morbid obesity, Am. J. Clin. Nutr. **33:**395, 1980.

Mittal, V.K., and Cortez, J.A.: New techniques of gastrointestinal anastomosis using the EEA stapler, Surgery **88:**715, 1980.

Nyhus, L.M., and Wastell, C.: Surgery of the stomach and duodenum, ed. 3, Boston, 1977, Little, Brown & Co.

Pace, W.G., and others: Gastric partitioning for morbid obesity, Ann. Surg. **190:**396, 1979.

Proximate ILS Disposable Stapler System: reference manual, Somerville, N.J., 1981, Ethicon, Inc.

Reiling, R.B.: Staplers in gastrointestinal surgery, Surg. Clin. North Am. **60:**381, 1980.

Sabiston, D.C., Jr., editor: Davis-Christopher textbook of surgery: the biological basis of modern surgical practice, ed. 11, Philadelphia, 1977, W.B. Saunders Co.

Schwartz, S.I., editor: Principles of surgery, ed. 3, New York, 1979, McGraw-Hill Book Co.

Shaw, L.M.: A teaching plan for Nissen fundoplication, AORN J. **34:**47, 1981.

Shaw, L.M.: Treating GI reflux with a prosthesis, AORN J. **35:**1303, 1982.

Simmons, S., and Given, B.: Nissen fundoplication for hiatal hernia repair, AORN J. **34:**35, 1981.

Stapling techniques in general surgery, ed. 2, Norwalk, Conn., 1980, United States Surgical Corp.

Stark, K.J.: Nursing care of the Kock pouch patient, AORN J. **32:**202, 1980.

Sweet, K.: Hiatal hernia: what to guard against most in postop patients, Nursing '77 **7**(8):36, 1977.

Wassner, J.D., Yohai, E., and Heimlich, H.J.: Complications associated with the use of gastrointestinal stapling devices, Surgery **82:**395, 1977.

Welch, C.E., and Malt, R.A.: Medical progress: abdominal surgery (pt. I), N. Engl. J. Med. **300:**648, 1979.

Welch, C.E., and Malt, R.A.: Medical progress: abdominal surgery (pt. II), N. Engl. J. Med. **300:**705, 1979.

Welch, C.E., and Malt, R.A.: Medical progress: abdominal surgery (pt. III), N. Engl. J. Med. **300:**765, 1979.

Wilpizeski, M.D.: Helping the osteomate return to normal life, Nursing '81 **11**(3):62, 1981.

Zollinger, R.M., and Zollinger, R.M., Jr.: Atlas of surgical operations, ed. 4, New York, 1975, Macmillan Publishing Co.

15 Genitourinary and transplant surgery

ANATOMY AND PHYSIOLOGY

The normal urinary tract comprises a pair of kidneys, which excrete urine and convey it to the bladder through the ureters, 25-cm–long muscular tubes. Urine is stored in the bladder, which serves as a reservoir until its full capacity is reached, and is eliminated from the body by way of the urethra (Fig. 15-1).

Kidneys. The kidneys are located in the retroperitoneal space along the lateral borders of the psoas muscle, one on each side of the vertebral column at the level of the twelfth thoracic to the third lumbar vertebrae. Usually, the right kidney is several centimeters lower than the left because the liver rests above and anterior to the right kidney (Fig. 15-1).

Each kidney is surrounded by a mass of fatty and loose areolar tissue known as *perirenal fat.* A capsule enclosing the renal space is known as fascia renalis or *Gerota's fascia.* These structures help keep the kidneys in their normal position. The anterior and posterior relationships of the kidneys are shown in Fig. 15-2.

On the medial side of each kidney is a concave area known as the *hilum* through which the renal artery and vein enter and leave. The *renal pelvis,* a funnel-shaped structure that lies posterior to the renal vascular pedicle, divides into several branches within the kidney called *calyces* (Fig. 15-3). When surgery is indicated in these structures, a posterior flank approach is preferred. In cases in which surgery for removal of a mass is anticipated, a transabdominal or thoracoabdominal incision is often chosen.

The kidneys are highly vascular organs that process approximately one fifth of the entire volume of blood at any one time. The blood supply of the kidney is conveyed through the renal artery, a large branch of the aorta (Fig. 15-4), and leaves the kidney through the renal vein. On entering the kidney, the renal artery divides into anterior and posterior sections that undergo further division into lobular arteries, which are smaller branches. Before several types of surgery, renal arteriography is performed to help identify the patient's particular vascular anatomy.

The renal lymphatic supply originates beneath the capsule of the kidney and empties into the lumbar lymph nodes at the junction of the renal vascular pedicle and aorta. The nerves of the autonomic (involuntary) nervous system come from the lumbar sympathetic trunk and from the vagus. Removal of the nerve pathways disrupts the ability to feel pain without impairing renal function. The artery and vein with their accompanying nerves and lymphatics are referred to as the pedicle of the kidney.

Ureters. Each ureter is a continuation of the renal pelvis. In the adult, the ureter extends from the renal pelvis to the base of the bladder and is approximately 25 to 30 cm long and 4 to 5 mm in diameter (Fig. 15-5). It is a fibromuscular cylindrical tube lined by transitional epithelium (urothelium). As urine accumulates in the renal pelvis, slight distension initiates a wave of muscular contraction. This peristaltic activity continues down the ureter, propelling urine into the bladder.

The ureter has three areas of narrowing in which calculi may become lodged and pose a potential problem with pain and obstruction: (1) the ureteropelvic junction, (2) the crossing of the ureter over the iliac vessels, and (3) the ureterovesical junction (Fig. 15-5). Urine may sometimes cause calculi to be washed down the ureter, producing severe ureteral colic. Of all renal calculi, 90% are spontaneously passed into the bladder. However, if they become lodged in the ureter, a ureterolithotomy may be indicated. In the female, during pelvic surgery, a ureteral catheter is often inserted because of the potential danger that the ureter might be inadvertently damaged or ligated.

Urinary bladder. The adult urinary bladder is a hollow muscular viscus that acts as a reservoir for urine until micturition occurs. It has an outer adventitial and inner urothelial layer. The floor of the bladder is composed of the trigone, which is triangular. The three corners of the trigone correspond to the orifices of the ureters and the bladder neck (opening of the urethra) (Fig. 15-6).

Physiologically, the bladder fills with urine, thereby expanding into the abdominal cavity. The extraperitoneal location is advantageous in that a suprapubic incision may be performed without violating the peritoneum and thus preventing potential intraperitoneal complications.

The main arterial supply of the bladder is derived from the branches of the internal iliac artery.

The bladder's size, position, and relation to the bowel, rectum, and reproductive organs vary according to the bladder's distension. In the female, the vagina lies dorsal to the base of the bladder and parallel to the urethra (Fig. 15-7). In the male, the prostate gland is interposed be-

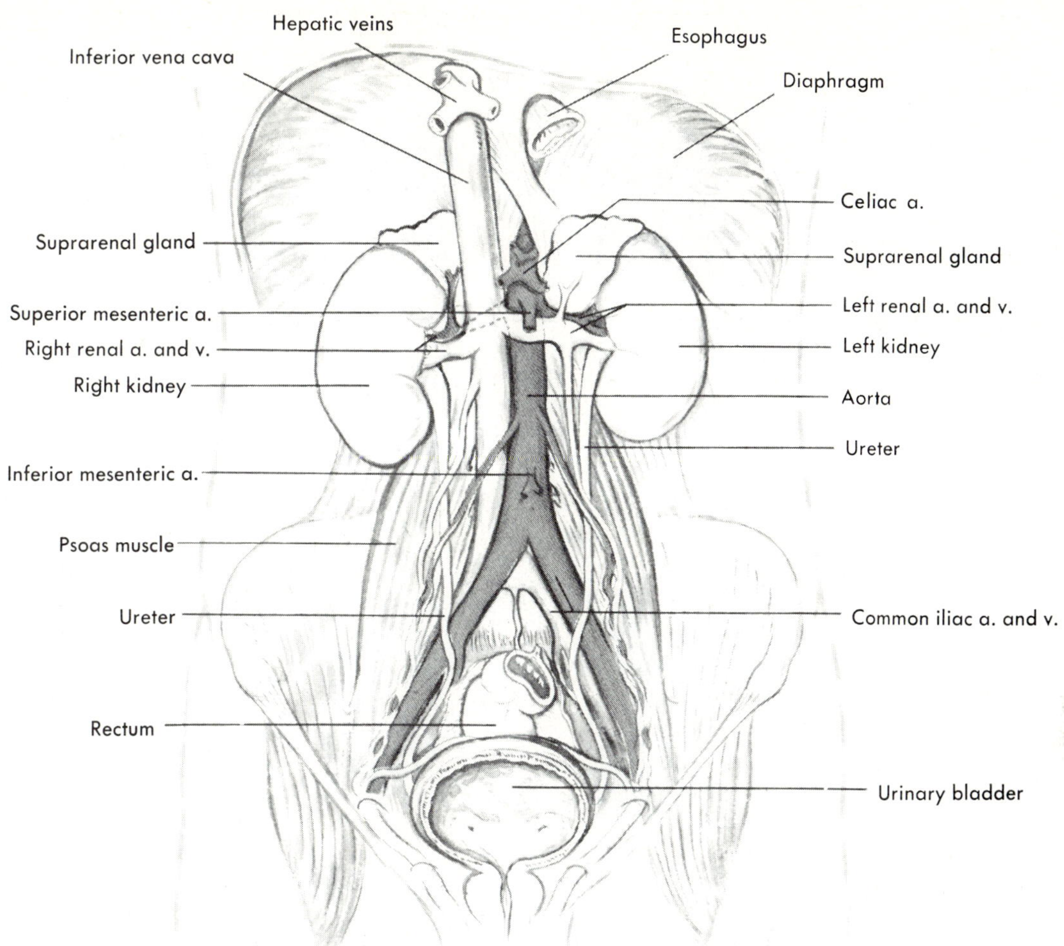

Fig. 15-1. Location of urinary system organs. (From Anthony, C.P., and Kolthoff, N.J.: Textbook of anatomy and physiology, ed. 9, St. Louis, 1975, The C.V. Mosby, Co.)

tween the bladder neck and the urethra (Fig. 15-8). These anatomical relationships are important during pelvic surgery.

The process of bladder evacuation appears to be initiated by nerve cells from the sacral divisions of the autonomic nervous system. These sacral reflex centers are controlled by higher voluntary centers in the brain. Stimulation of the sacral centers results in contraction of the bladder muscles and relaxation of the bladder outlet sphincters. Muscle tone maintains closure of the sphincters when the bladder is at rest, thus enabling continence.

Urethra. The *male urethra* normally 20 to 25 cm long, extends from the bladder neck to the tip of the penis and varies in diameter from 7 to 10 mm. It is subdivided into three portions: the prostatic, membranous, and penile urethra.

The prostatic urethra is approximately 2 to 4 cm long and is the widest portion of the urethra. On the floor of the prostatic urethra is the verumontanum, which contains the openings of the ejaculatory ducts.

The membranous urethra is the shortest portion, measuring approximately 2 cm long and extending from the external sphincter to the apex of the prostate (Fig. 15-9).

The penile or pendulous urethra lies within the corpus spongiosum. The urothelium of the urethra is continuous with that of the bladder.

The *female urethra* is a narrow membranous tube about 4 cm in length and 6 mm in diameter. The urethra lies behind and beneath the symphysis pubis. It passes through the internal and external sphincter and the urogenital diaphragm. Because of the shortness of the urethra, microorganisms find easy access to the bladder and subsequently cause infection.

Male reproductive organs. The male reproductive organs include several paired structures: the testes, epididymides, seminal ducts (vas deferens), seminal vesicles, ejaculatory ducts, and bulbourethral glands. Other organs of the reproductive tract are the penis, prostate gland, and urethra.

The *scrotum* is located behind the base of the penis

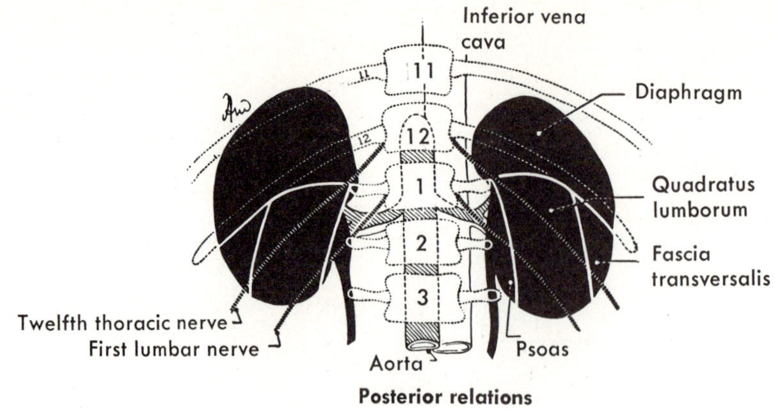

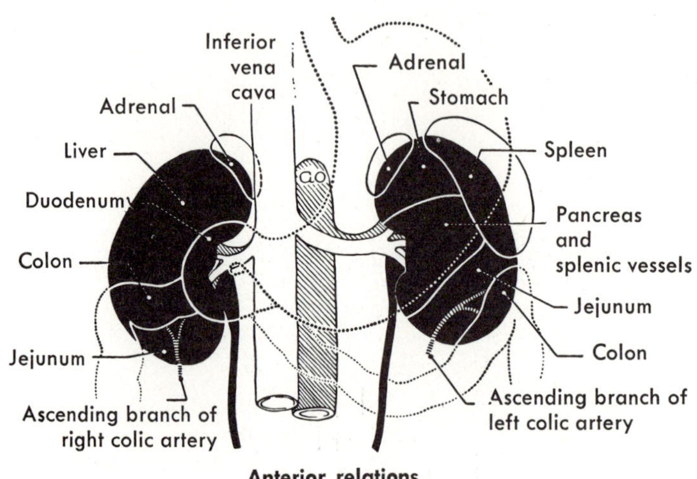

Fig. 15-2. Anterior and posterior relations of kidneys and ureters to organs in peritoneal cavity, to ureteral column posteriorly, and to main arteries and veins. (From Moseley, H.F., editor: Textbook of surgery, ed. 3, St. Louis, The C.V. Mosby Co.)

and in front of the anus. Each loose sac contains and supports the testis, the epididymis, and some of the spermatic cord. The two sides of the scrotum are separated from each other by a median raphe. Within the scrotum are two cavities or sacs that are lined with smooth and glistening tissue, the *tunica vaginalis*. Normally, a small amount of clear fluid is contained in the tunica vaginalis. The condition known as *hydrocele* denotes an abnormal accumulation of the fluid.

The *testes* manufacture the spermatozoa and also contain a specialized cell (Leydig) that produces the male hormone, testosterone. Each testis consists of many tubules in which the sperm are formed, surrounded by dense capsules of connective tissue. The tubules coalesce and continue into the adjacent epididymis, where the sperm mature and are stored.

The *epididymis* is a long convoluted duct located along the posterolateral surface of the testis. It is closely attached to the testicle by fibrous tissue and secretes seminal fluid, which gives the sperm a fluid medium in which to migrate. The *vas deferens* (ductus deferens, or seminal duct) is a distal continuation of the epididymis as it enters the prostate gland and conveys the sperm to the seminal vesicle.

The vas deferens lies within the *spermatic cord* in the inguinal region. The spermatic cord also contains veins, arteries, lymphatics, nerves, and surrounding connective tissue (cremaster muscle), which give support to the testes. The terminal portion of each vas deferens is called the *ejaculatory duct,* which passes between the lobes of the prostate gland and opens into the posterior urethra.

The accessory reproductive glands include the seminal vesicles, prostate gland, and bulbourethral gland. The seminal vesicles unite with the vas deferens on either side, are situated behind the bladder, and produce protein and fructose for the nutrition of the sperm cell. Sperm and prostatic fluid are discharged at the time of ejaculation.

The *prostate gland* is a fibromuscular organ located at the base of the bladder neck and the triangular ligament completely surrounding the urethra. The gland is about 4 cm at its base and about 2 cm in depth and weighs approximately 20 gm (Fig. 15-9).

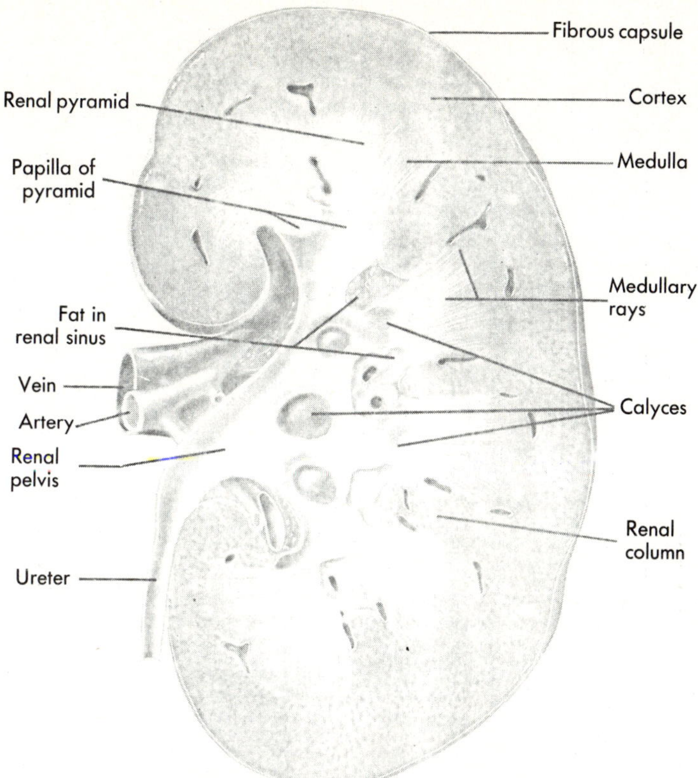

Fig. 15-3. Normal kidney. (Courtesy Burroughs Wellcome Co.)

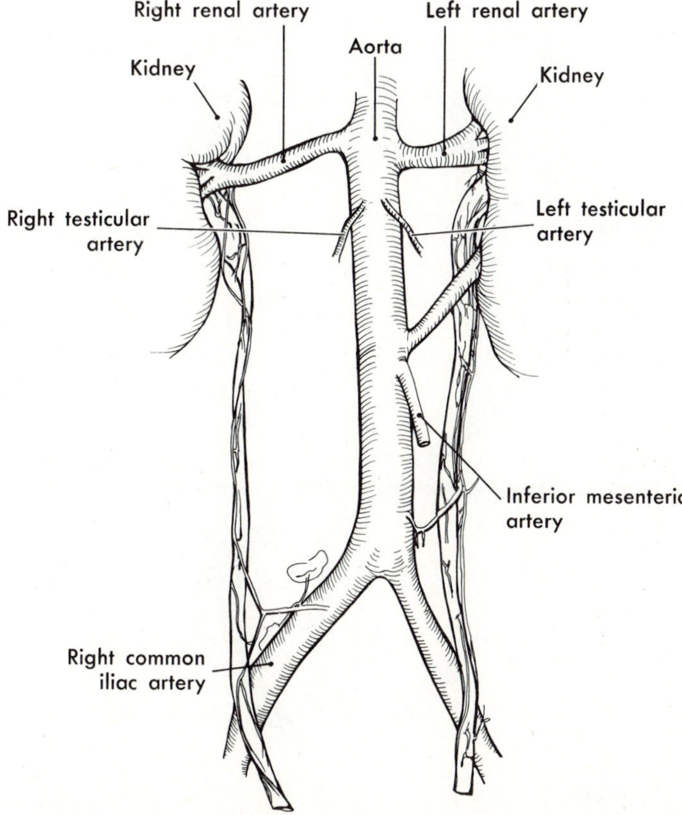

Fig. 15-4. Blood supply of kidneys. (Adapted by permission from J.C.B. Grant's Atlas of anatomy, 6th ed. Copyright © 1972, The Williams & Wilkins Co.)

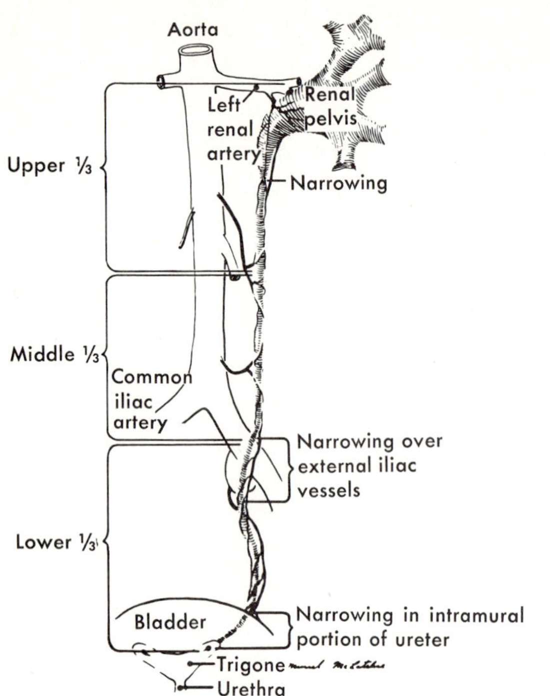

Fig. 15-5. Anatomy of ureter. (From Colby, F.H.: Essential urology, ed. 4, Baltimore, The Williams & Wilkins Co.)

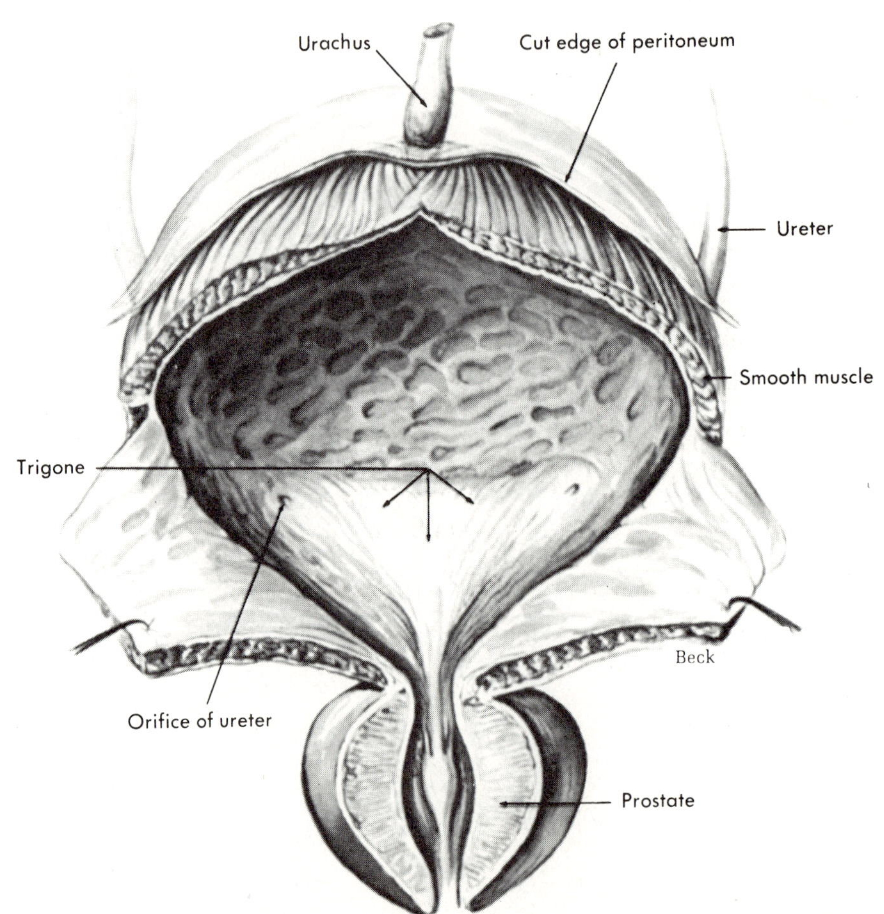

Fig. 15-6. Male urinary bladder cut to show interior. (From Anthony, C.P., and Kolthoff, N.J.: Anatomy and physiology, ed. 9, St. Louis, 1975, The C.V. Mosby Co.)

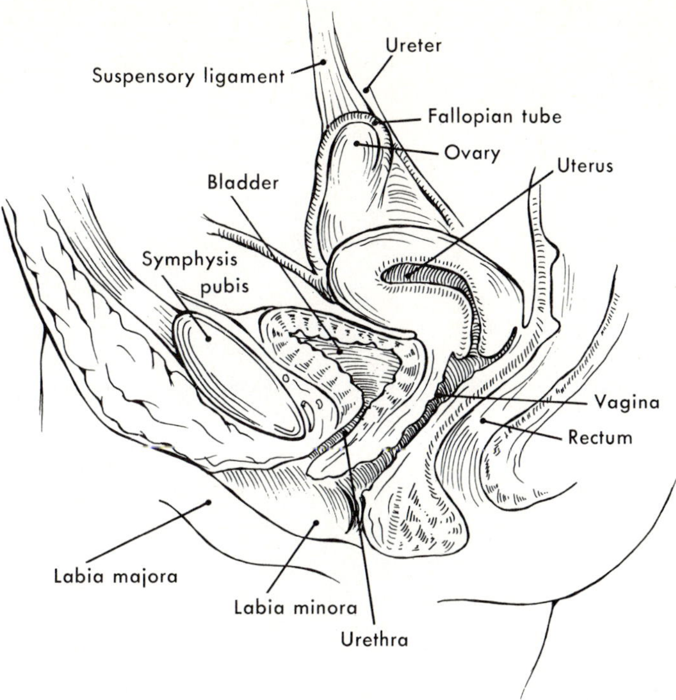

Fig. 15-7. Female genitourinary and reproductive anatomy. (Adapted from Keuhnelian, J., and Sanders, V.: Urologic nursing, New York, 1970, The Macmillan Co.)

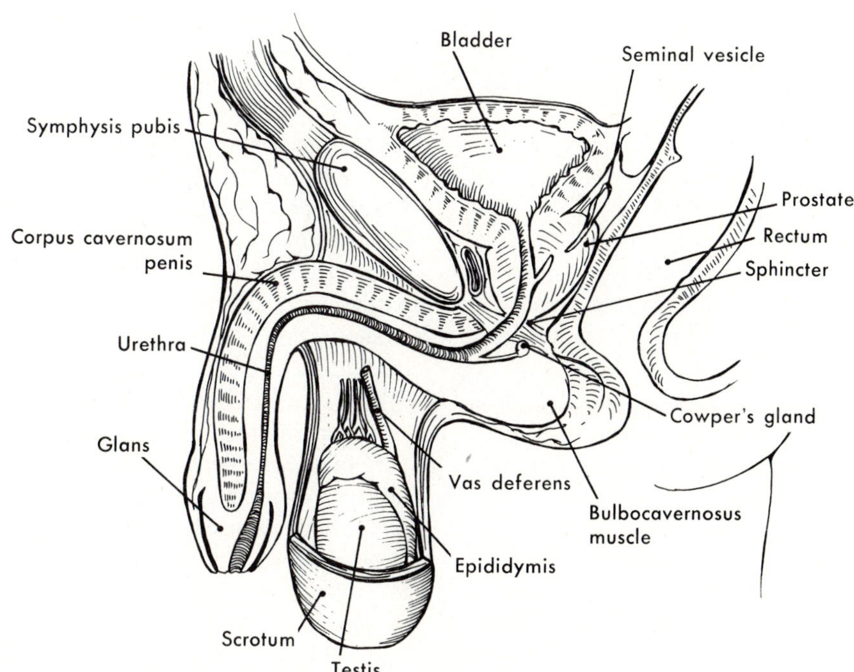

Fig. 15-8. Male genitourinary and reproductive anatomy. (Adapted from Keuhnelian, J., and Sanders, V.: Urologic nursing, New York, 1970, The Macmillan Co.)

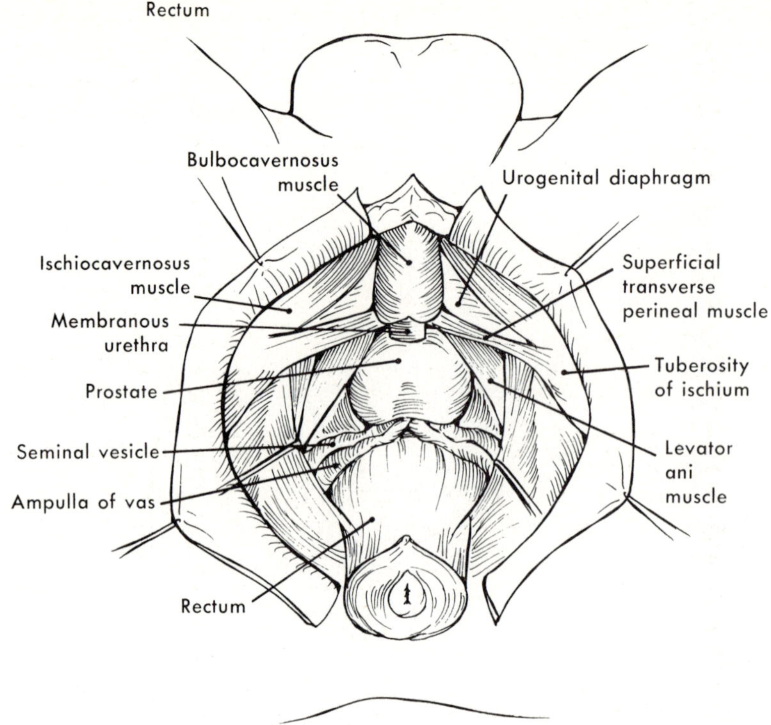

Fig. 15-9. Anatomy of male perineum and contiguous structures. (Adapted from Campbell, M.F., and Harrison, J.H., editors: Urology, vols. 1 to 3, ed. 3, Philadelphia, 1970, W.B. Saunders Co.)

The prostate consists essentially of six lobes: anterior, posterior, middle, subcervical, and right and left lateral. The posterior lobe is readily palpable during rectal examination and prone to cancerous degeneration.

Behind the prostatic capsule is a fibrous sheath known as the true prostatic capsule that separates the prostate gland and the seminal vesicles from the rectum. This fascia is of importance when perineal prostatectomy is contemplated.

The lobes of the gland secrete highly alkaline fluid that dilutes the testicular secretion as it is excreted by the ejaculatory ducts. These secretions are believed essential to the passage of spermatozoa and helpful in keeping them alive. The arterial supply to the prostate is derived from the pudendal, inferior vesical, and hemorrhoidal arteries.

Cowper's glands (bulbourethral glands) are located on either side of the membranous portion of the urethra. Each gland, by way of its duct, empties mucous secretions into the urethra.

The *penis* is suspended by the fascial attachments of the pubic arch and supported by the suspensory ligaments. The penis contains three distinct vascular sponge-like bodies: the two upper bodies are called the *right* and *left corpus cavernosum,* and the lower body, the *corpus spongiosum urethrae*. The tissue contains a network of vascular channels that fill with blood during erection. At the distal end of the penis, the skin is doubly folded to form the so-called prepuce, or foreskin, which serves as a covering for the glans penis (Fig. 15-8). The glans penis contains the urethral orifice.

Adrenal glands. The adrenal glands lie retroperitoneally beneath the diaphragm at the medial aspects of the superior pole of each kidney. On the right side, the gland is adjacent to the inferior vena cava; on the left side, the gland is posterior to the stomach and pancreas. Each adrenal gland has a medulla, which secretes adrenaline, and a cortex, which secretes steroids and other hormones. The glands are freely supplied with arterial branches from the phrenic and renal arteries and from the aorta. The venous drainage is accomplished on the right by the inferior vena cava and on the left by the left renal vein.

NURSING CONSIDERATIONS

Operating room nurses involved in genitourinary surgery must have comprehensive knowledge of the genitourinary system and special diagnostic studies and operative techniques used in this specialty. A thorough understanding of each proposed surgical procedure is essential to properly prepare the patient, room, equipment, and supplies.

Positioning. Thorough understanding of the urological operating room table and its functions is essential to provide optimum patient positioning required for each particular operative procedure. The position in which the patient is placed for surgery is determined by the particular operation to be performed. Urological operative procedures require the patient to be in the lateral, supine, or lithotomy position, which may be exaggerated to give optimum access to the organ involved. This is particularly true in radical surgery of the prostate and bladder. Considerable care must be taken to ensure that the patient position does not interfere with respiration or circulation. It is essential to avoid displacement of the joints and undue tension on neurovascular bundles or ligaments, particularly in the aged or debilitated patient.

A patient positioned laterally (flank position) for renal surgery has the spine extended for greater access to the retroperitoneal space. Padding and stabilized support with rubber-covered pillows, sandbags, and straps should be available for precise anatomical positioning and safety. If an electrosurgical unit is to be used, care must be taken to see that no part of the patient touches metal equipment other than the indifferent electrode (cautery pad) attached to the unit.

In some procedures involving stones of the kidneys or ureters, intraoperative x-ray examinations may be required. If x-ray films are to be taken, the patient must be on an operating table with a cassette holder. A cassette holder must be placed under the patient who is in the supine, prone, or lithotomy position before the procedure begins. If the patient is in the lateral position with the table flexed and kidney rest up, the cassette holder is placed under the patient at the time of x-ray exposure.

Aseptic techniques and safety measures. Aseptic techniques must be carefully maintained. Skin preparation and draping procedures (Chapter 5) vary depending on the surgery to be performed and individual hospital policy. Difficulty may be encountered in cleansing and preparing the perineal area. Gauze sponges on forceps are generally used to apply antimicrobial solution in perineal skin preparations.

Transurethral passage of instruments and catheters requires meticulous technique to prevent retrograde infections of the urinary system. The use of transurethral instruments is facilitated by darkening the room. Provision should be made for proper adjustments in lighting (Chapter 4).

Electrosurgical units and fiberoptic light sources are frequent adjuncts in urological surgery. The staff must be familiar with their use and with the precautions necessary to prevent fire or burns (Chapter 4).

Use of irrigating fluids. When the bladder is to be opened or manipulated, a continuous flow of sterile distilled irrigating fluid is administered to distend the bladder for effective visualization. Commercially prepared sterile irrigation solutions with appropriate closed administration sets are highly recommended. Such closed systems prevent the inherent risks of cross-contamination.

For simple observation cystoscopy, retrograde pyelography, and simple bladder tumor fulgurations, sterile distilled water may be used without complication. However, during transurethral resection of the prostate, venous sinuses may be opened, and varying amounts of irrigant are invariably absorbed into the bloodstream. Studies indicate that the use of distilled water for transurethral resection of the prostate may result in hemolysis of erythrocytes and possible renal failure. Other important complications include dilutional hyponatremia and cardiac decompensation.

Ideally, a clear, nonelectrolytic and isosmotic solution should be used. Recommended solutions include 5% mannitol, 1.8% urea, 4% glucose, and 1.5% glycine. Glycine, an aminoacetic solution, is the most widely used urological irrigating fluid. In a dilute solution (1.5%), glycine has several properties that make it particularly useful as an irrigating solution during transurethral prostatic surgery. At a concentration of 1.5%, which is slightly hypotonic, glycine does not induce hemolysis. Since the solution is also nonelectrolytic, it will not cause dispersion of high frequency with consequent loss of electrosurgical cutting capacity as occurs with normal saline.

Commercially prepared sterile irrigation solutions are available in collapsible plastic bags, as well as in rigid plastic containers. One advantage of the collapsible bag is that it is not dependent on air and may be hung in series, thus providing continuous irrigation without interruption (Fig. 15-10). Air bubbles, a problem that distorts visibility during the procedure, are also eliminated in this system.

Thorough knowledge of the potential hazards encountered intraoperatively during transurethral surgery is extremely important. Although complications are more prevalent in the postoperative stage, close observation during the intraoperative period may prove lifesaving. Symptoms such as sudden restlessness, apprehension, and irritability may suggest the transurethral resection syndrome, a shift of body fluids and electrolytes caused by a decrease of extracellular sodium. Serum electrolyte laboratory studies should be obtained without delay. Minimum amounts of fluids should be given. Irrigation fluid should be under as little pressure as possible, and the bladder emptied before it reaches full capacity to prevent intravesical pressure. Occasionally an operating room has the capacity to perform these crucial laboratory tests intraoperatively so that results are available for interpretation in a short time. If a low serum sodium value is reported, hypertonic sodium chloride is added to the intravenous line, or intravenous diuretics such as furosemide (Lasix) may be used. If the patient's reaction is severe, surgery may have to be terminated.

Endoscopic and ancillary equipment. Cystoscopic and ancillary equipment may vary from one institution to another. Therefore it is valuable to have a reference manual or Kardex system that illustrates and describes in detail the required instrumentation for each specific procedure.

The basic cystoscopy tray should include instruments and accessory items that are routinely used for all cystoscopy procedures. If ureteral catheterization is planned, catheterizing telescopes or an Albarrán bridge of the appropriate size, which can be packaged and gas sterilized separately, may easily be added to the basic cystoscopy setup. Trays for transurethral surgery and instruments for other special procedures may be wrapped and gas sterilized on a separate tray and available on request. This concept minimizes excessive handling of the delicate lensed instruments and ultimately reduces costly repairs.

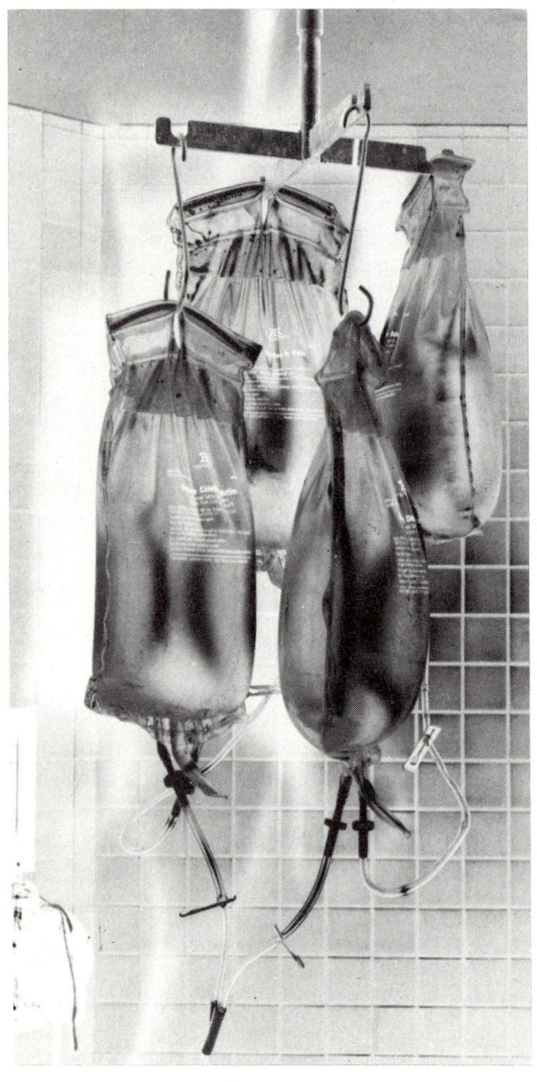

Fig. 15-10. Use of Y tube to convey irrigating solution without interruption. (Courtesy Travenol Laboratories, Deerfield, Ill.; from Morel, A., and Wise, G.J.: Urologic endoscopic procedures, ed. 2, St. Louis, 1979, The C.V. Mosby Co.)

In some instances during cystoscopic procedures, additional instrumentation is required. Instruments of various types and sizes, for example, a visual obturator, biopsy forceps, urethral sounds, Philips filiforms and followers, and Ellik evacuators may be packaged separately, sterilized, and available when needed.

Urethral and ureteral catheters. A variety of urethral and ureteral catheters are necessary in the management of urologic disease. Catheters are designed for specific procedures to meet the individualized needs of particular problems. Ureteral catheters are manufactured of polyvinyl or polyurethane material and are graduated so that the urologist may determine the exact distance the catheter has been inserted into the ureter. Ureteral catheters are available in both disposable and reusable forms. Many manufacturers provide the disposable catheters double-wrapped in a peel-open package to allow aseptic handling during ureteral insertion. Some indications for the use of ureteral catheters are to (1) perform retrograde pyelography, (2) identify the ureters during pelvic surgery, and (3) bypass partial or complete obstruction that may be present as a result of ureteral tumors, calculi, or strictures.

Frequently used ureteral catheters include the whistle tip, round, Braasch bulb, spiral, cone, and olive tip. The spiral Blasucci is useful when difficulty occurs in introducing a ureteral catheter past the ureterovesical junction. When a retrograde ureterogram is indicated, a Braasch bulb or cone-tip ureteral catheter may be helpful in effectively occluding the ureteral orifice to accurately accomplish the x-ray study (Fig. 15-11). When a ureteral catheter is left indwelling, a special adapter can be connected to the end of the ureteral catheter to facilitate connection to a closed urinary drainage system (Fig. 15-12).

Urethral catheters offer a multitude of functions, particularly in the operating room, for example, stents, drainage, and diagnostic studies. Urethral catheters are generally divided into two categories, plain and self-retaining, and range through different French sizes, most commonly 12 through 30. The Foley catheter is the most frequently used self-retaining catheter and is manufactured with a variety of balloon sizes, tip styles, lengths, and eye arrangements (Fig. 15-11, *C*).

After prostatic surgery, a three-way Foley catheter with a 30-cc balloon capacity may be left indwelling (Fig. 15-11, *D*). This type of catheter is preferred because it facilitates continuous bladder irrigation and aids in achieving hemostasis in the prostatic bed. At times the urologist may apply light traction on the Foley catheter, which causes pressure against the bladder neck and aids in hemostasis.

Diagnostic studies are also performed in the cystoscopy suite and require special catheters for specific studies. For example, the Davis female urethrographic catheter (Fig. 15-13, *A*) is used to diagnose lesions of the

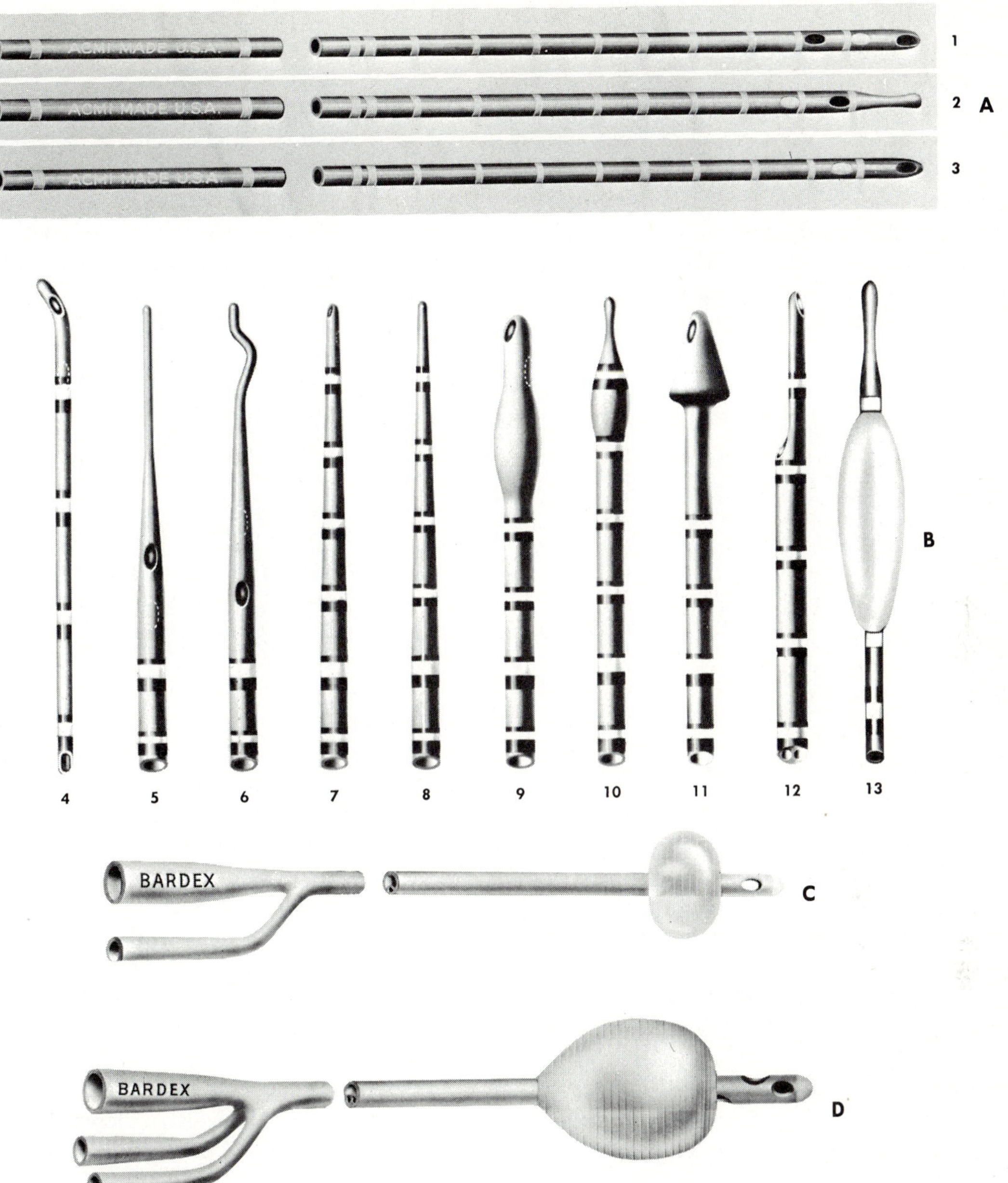

Fig. 15-11. A, X-ray graduated woven ureteral catheters are made of nylon or plastic material and have outer surfacing to provide flexibility, for easy entry without kinking. Eyes provide adequate high-flow rate. Catheter tips constructed for specific procedures as shown. *1,* Whistle tip; *2,* olive tip; *3,* round tip. **B,** X-ray graduated woven ureteral catheters and bougies. *4,* Wishard catheter, flat, coude tip; *5,* Blasucci catheter, flexible filiform tip; *6,* Blasucci catheter, flexible spiral filiform tip; *7,* Garceau catheter, tapered for dilatation, whistle tip; *8,* Garceau bougie, tapered for dilatation, conical tip; *9,* Braasch bulb catheter, whistle tip; *10,* Braasch bougie, bulb tip; *11,* Cone tip catheter (for ureteropyelography); *12,* Hyams double-lumen catheter; *13,* Dourmashkin dilator with inflation balloon, olive tip. **C,** Foley retention catheter. **D,** Bard three-way hemostatic catheter. (Courtesy American Cystoscope Makers, Inc., Stamford, Conn.)

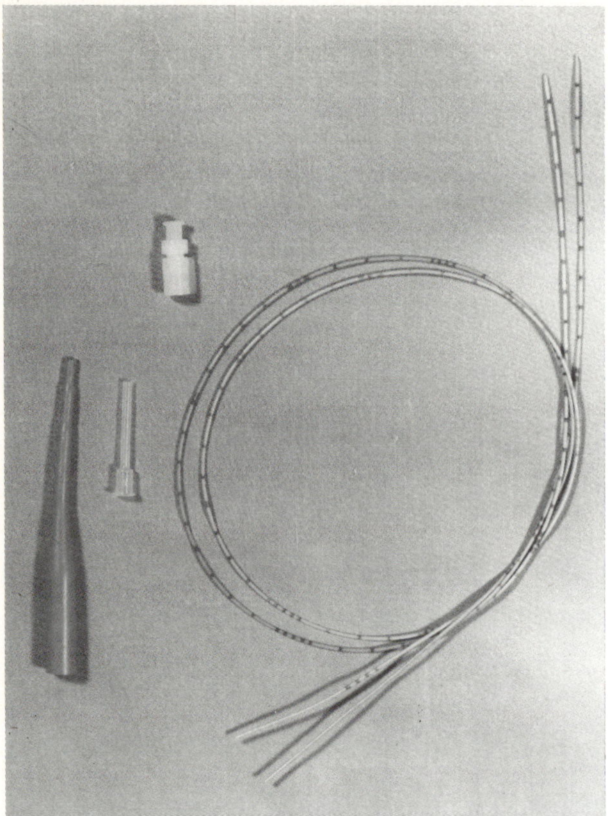

Fig. 15-12. Ureteral catheters and adaptors.

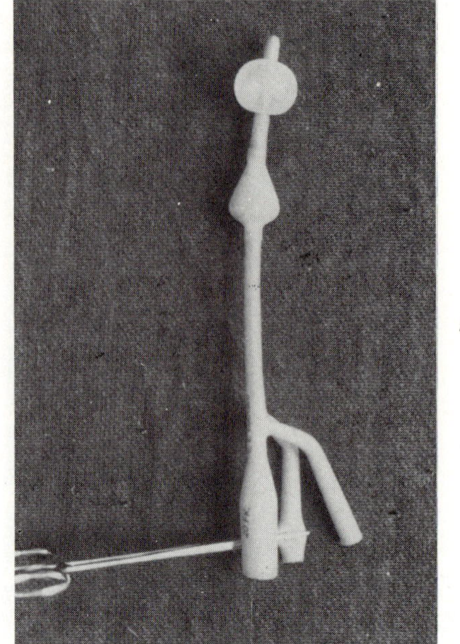

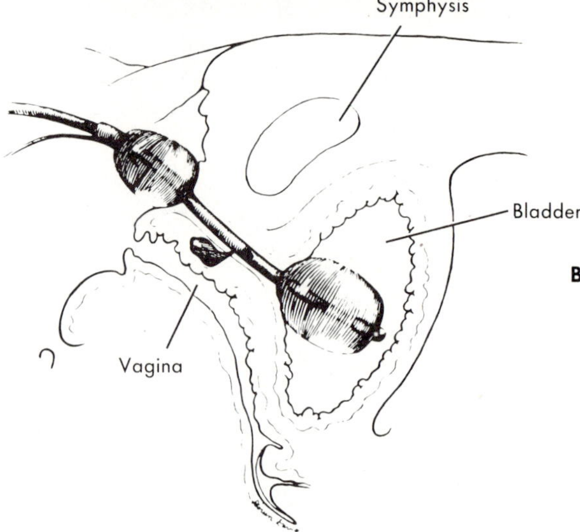

Fig. 15-13. A, Double-balloon Davis urethrographic catheter. **B,** Diagrammatic drawing of Davis urethrographic catheter in bladder.

female urethra, such as urethral strictures, diverticula, or fistulas. To accomplish female urethrography, the catheter is inserted through the urethra into the bladder; the two balloons on the catheter are inflated, effectively isolating the urethra; and contrast is injected to visualize the entire urethra (Fig. 15-13, *B*).

Another type of self-retaining catheter frequently used in the operating room is a Pezzer, also known as a "mushroom" catheter. It may be straight or angulated with a large single channel and preformed tip in the shape of a mushroom. The flexible mushroom tip helps keep the catheter in place. This catheter is primarily used to drain the bladder suprapubically, often for poor-risk patients who have uremia or possibly long-standing urinary retention. The catheter is inserted in the bladder through a midline or small transverse abdominal wall incision and secured to the abdomen with tape. The Malecot four-winged catheter is often used as a nephrostomy tube to provide temporary, and in some cases permanent, diversion of urine after kidney surgery and when renal tissue needs to be restored (Fig. 15-14). A Foley catheter of preferred size may also be used for this purpose. Nephrostomy tube replacement is accomplished by introducing the catheter into the surgical tract with a straight catheter guide and securing it in place by a nephrostomy retention disc, one size smaller than the nephrostomy tube being used. The flanges of the disc are then taped to the skin. The use of other variations of urethral catheters will be described later in the text.

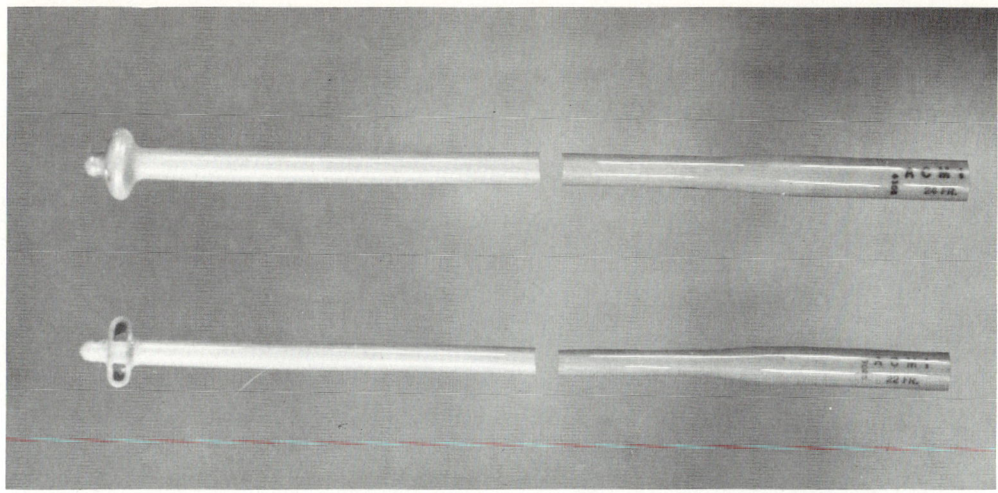

Fig. 15-14. Pezzer (mushroom) catheter and Malecot (bat-wing) four-winged catheter.

DIAGNOSTIC AND TRANSURETHRAL OPERATIONS

Cystoscopy

Definition. Endoscopic examination of the lower urinary tract, including visual inspection of the interior of the urethra, the bladder, and the ureteral orifices by means of the cystoscope, a versatile optical instrument with a variety of telescopic lenses. In the male patient, special attention is given to the examination of the verumontanum, the ejaculatory ducts, the bladder neck, and the median and lateral lobes of the prostate. In the female, the urethra, bladder neck, and bladder are thus examined.

Considerations. Cystoscopy is an important diagnostic tool that provides the urologist with valuable information concerning the patient's urological condition. Indications for cystoscopy include hematuria, urinary incontinence, urinary tract infection, tumors, fistulas, and vesical calculus disease.

Setup and preparation of the patient. Once in the cystoscopy suite, the patient should be greeted by name and identified by hospital number. The chart should be checked for operative consent and pertinent laboratory reports. Intravenous pyelograms and chest x-ray films should also be available for review.

It is customary to have each patient void before leaving the nursing unit or immediately before the procedure. This is of particular importance in ruling out residual urine in the bladder. The patient is then placed on the cystoscopy table. Correct positioning of the patient requires optimum relaxation of muscles of the legs and perineum. Proper positioning of the knee crutches on the cystoscopy table is a vital consideration for patient safety and comfort. When knee crutches are properly positioned, the curve of the yoke suspension should flow outward from the perineum, as do the patient's legs. This will relieve the pressure on the popliteal spaces. Padding the knee crutches is of further benefit. With the patient properly positioned, the table is tilted so that the patient's head is slightly higher than the buttocks. This will allow free drainage of the prep solution into the collecting pan. The pooling of prep solutions beneath the patient may cause skin reaction and at times severe irritation.

If the cystoscopic procedure requires the use of an electrosurgical unit, the lubricated cautery pad is placed on the patient in direct contact with the skin.

After proper positioning, the nurse or urologist dons gloves and prepares the entire pubic area, including the scrotum and perineum, with an antimicrobial solution. A sterile screen is placed over the drainage drawer on the cystoscopy table (Fig. 15-15). The patient is then draped according to hospital procedure. Adequate draping is important to ensure that aseptic technique is maintained during the urological procedure. If a general anesthetic is required, it is administered before prepping and draping. If a local anesthetic is preferred, it is instilled into the urethra of the male patient after prepping and draping but before instrumentation. In the female patient, a cotton applicator, dipped into the anesthetic solution, is placed in the urethral meatus. Lidocaine, 1% (Xylocaine) or 2% (Anestacon), is usually used.

The cystoscopy setup should include the following:

Prep set and solutions
Wappler cystourethroscope (Fig. 15-16)
2 Short bridges
1 Fiberoptic bundle
1 Lateral microlens telescope
1 Foroblique microlens telescope
1 Luer-Lok stopcock (for irrigation solution)
Lubricant, water-soluble
1 Calibrated container to measure residual urine
1 Test tube, screw-top, for urine specimens
Gauze sponges

Items in small emesis basin

1 Medicine glass for local anesthetic
Syringe, disposable 10 ml, to instill anesthetic
Penile clamp (to occlude urethra after local anesthetic is instilled)

Accessory items

Cystoscopy drape pack
Irrigation system
Gown and gloves

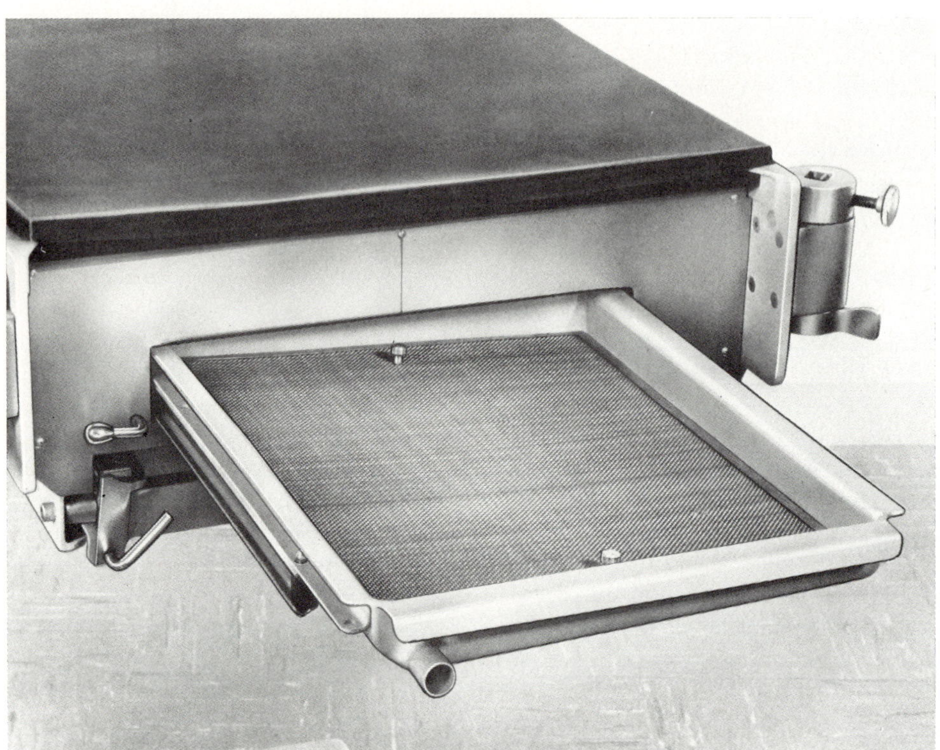

Fig. 15-15. Sterile screen placed over the drainage drawer on cystoscopy table.

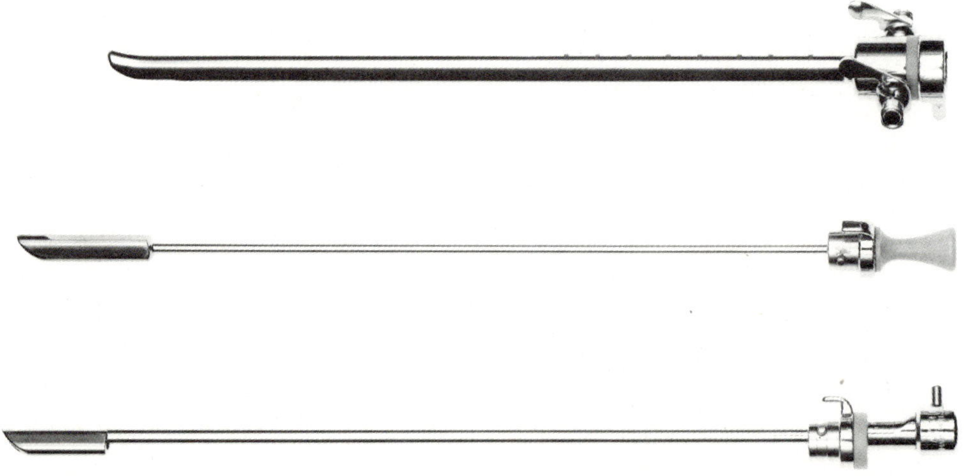

Fig. 15-16. Cystoscopy instrumentation. *Top to bottom,* Cystourethroscope, obturator, and visual obturator.

Several devices are available to support the urethroscope during the injection of radiopaque dye or while x-ray films are exposed. One such device is a "tite grip" towel holder, used by dentists, which can be easily adjusted to hold the instrument securely in place. The mechanism consists of a chrome chain with a clip on either end that is attached to the drape. The device can be packaged, sterilized, and reused.

Operative procedure

1. After the urologist has scrubbed, gowned, and gloved, the fiberoptic bundle is connected to the light source and tested for proper intensity. The irrigating system is set up, and, if required, the electrosurgical cord is connected to its power source.

2. The urethroscope is lubricated and introduced into the urethra, the obturator withdrawn, and residual urine obtained, provided the patient voided before the examination. The specimen may be saved for culture studies or cytological studies. The urethroscope is connected to the irrigating system, and the telescope inserted and locked in place. The urologist controls the flow and volume of fluid by adjusting the stopcock on the urethroscope. If difficulty is encountered during insertion, the visual obturator may be used to introduce the urethroscope under direct vision. This accessory is constructed to smooth the fenestral edges of the urethroscope and permits direct vision and irrigation during introduction.

3. Stone removal, bladder biopsy, or bladder fulguration may be performed by using special cystoscopic accessories such as the Hendrickson lithotrite, which is used to crush large bladder calculi (Fig. 15-17); Lowsley forceps; Wappler rigid cup forceps; and flexible foreign body forceps. Bladder fulguration (Fig. 15-18) requires the use of flexible stem electrodes available in various French sizes and tip configurations such as the ball, cone, dome, and bayonet tip (Fig. 15-19).

4. For retrograde ureteral catheterization and pyelography (Fig. 15-20), ureteral catheters are passed through the cystoscope sheath and directed by the Albarrán bridge deflector into the ureteral orifice and into the ureter. A radiopaque substance, such as 30% Renografin, is then injected, and an x-ray film exposed to outline the entire upper urinary collecting system.

Endoscope cleaning, maintenance, and sterilization. Sterilization, cleaning, and preventive maintenance of endoscopic equipment are important considerations in the care of fiberoptic lensed instruments. Ultimately, this process reduces costly repairs and ensures the availability of properly functioning instruments.

Protective padding should be placed on the countertop and on the bottom of the sink in the instrument decontamination area to prevent possible damage to lensed telescopes.

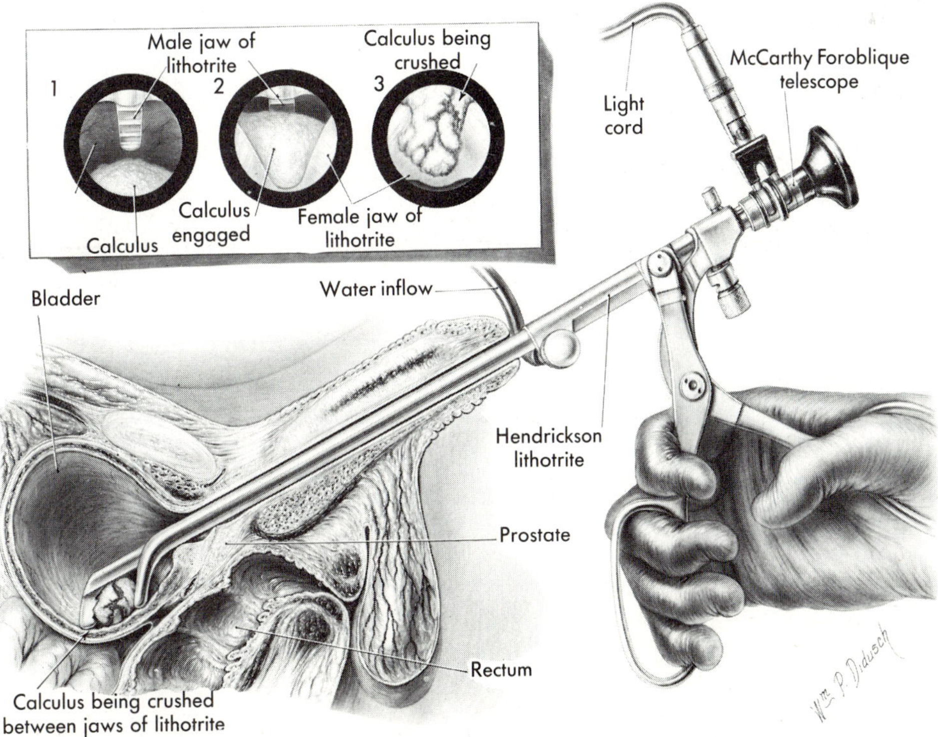

Fig. 15-17. Hendrickson lithotrite diagrammatic drawing. (Courtesy American Cystoscope Makers, Inc., Stamford, Conn.)

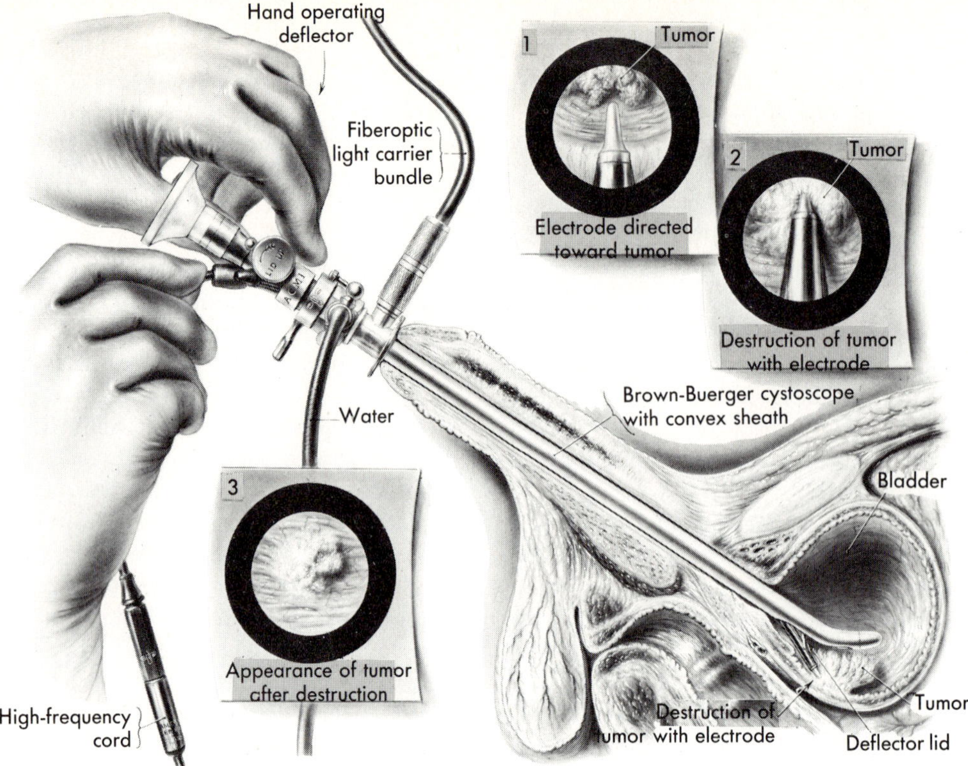

Fig. 15-18. Bladder fulguration diagrammatic drawing. (Courtesy American Cystoscope Makers, Inc., Stamford, Conn.)

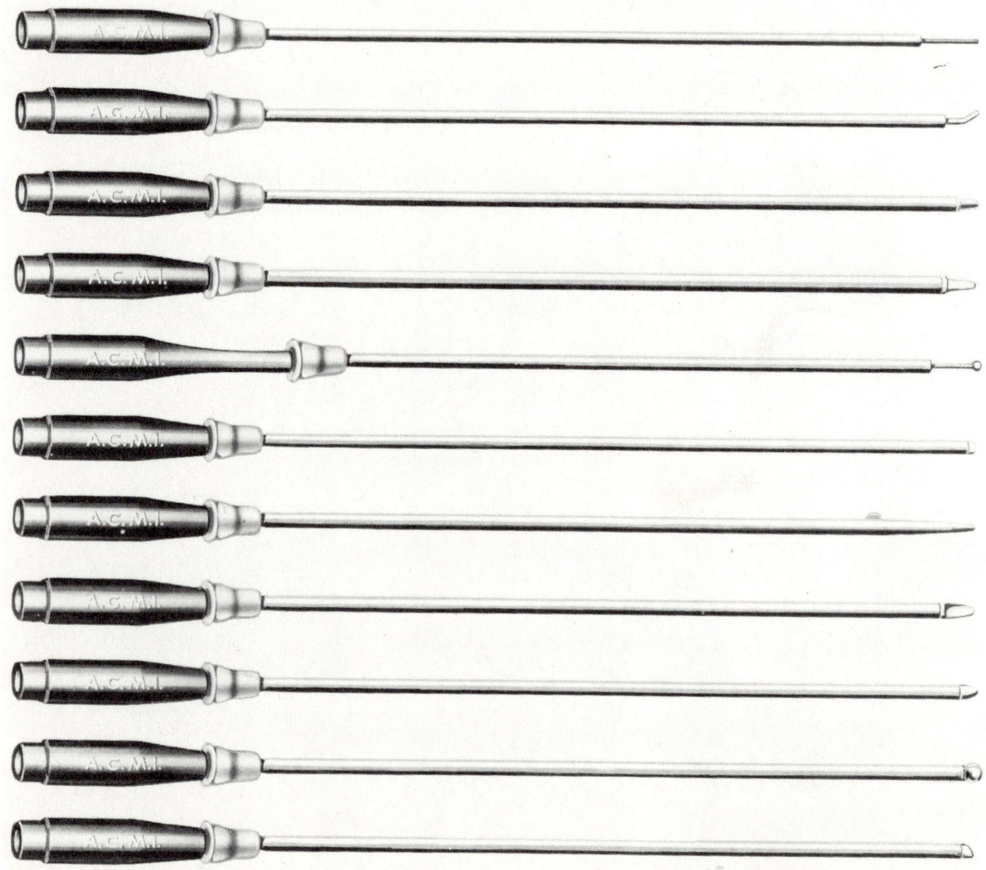

Fig. 15-19. Cystoscopic fulgurating electrodes with various types of tips. (Courtesy American Cystoscope Makers, Inc., Stamford, Conn.; from Morel, A., and Wise, G.J.: Urologic endoscopic procedures, ed. 2, St. Louis, 1979, The C.V. Mosby Co.)

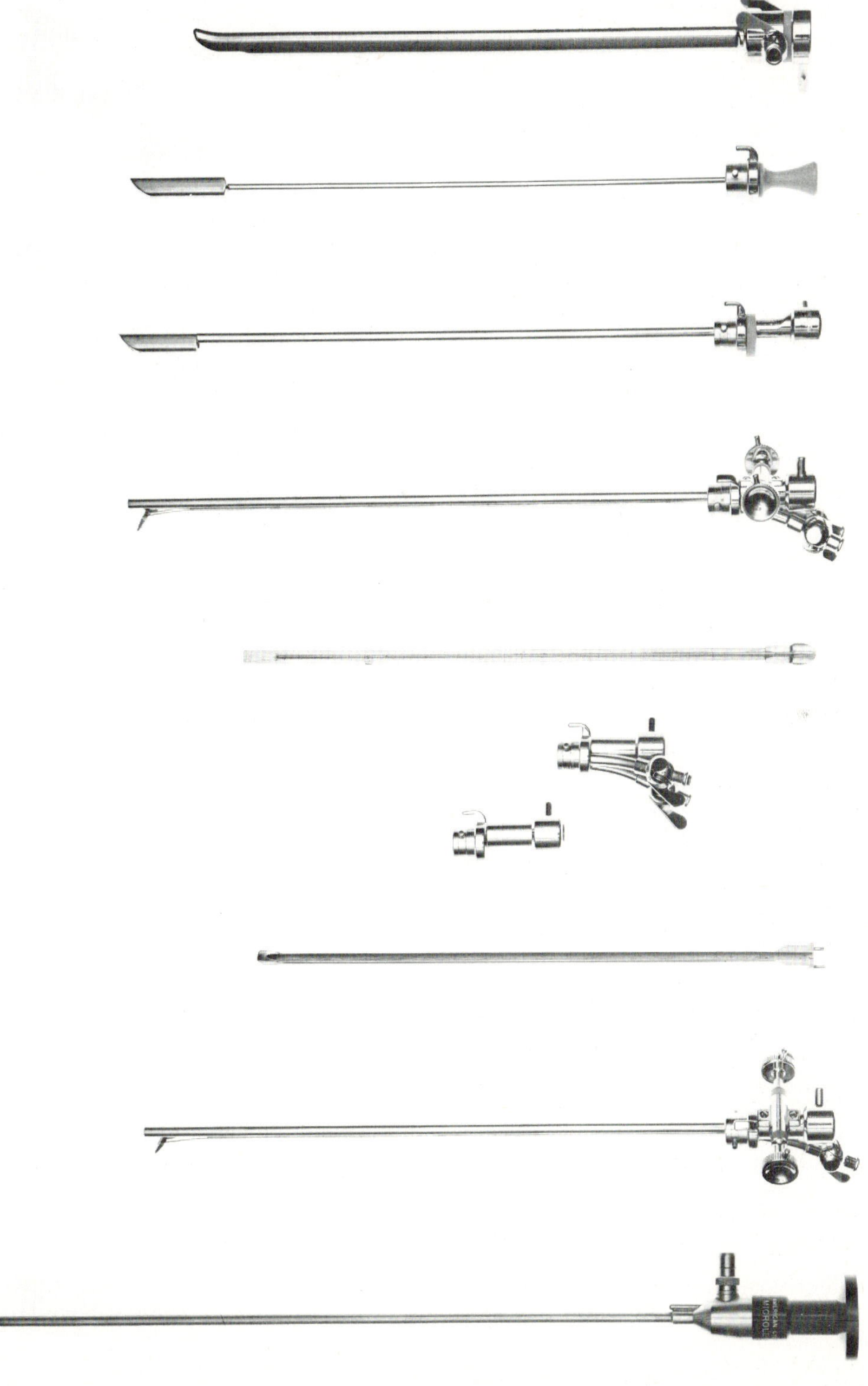

Fig. 15-20. Instruments for retrograde ureteral catheterization and pyelography. (Courtesy American Cystoscope Makers, Inc., Stamford, Conn.)

After each procedure, components of each cystoscopic set should be disassembled and soaked in a solution of warm water and germicidal detergent. All stopcocks and sheaths should be cleaned thoroughly with a soft brush to remove blood, dried lubricant jelly, or other debris. Instruments should then be rinsed in warm water, placed on protective padding, and allowed to dry. It is important that all moving parts be individually evaluated for mobility. A silicone instrument spray may be applied as required. The patency of all outlets must be maintained to ensure proper sterilization.

For gas sterilization, instruments should be assembled on a covered tray and protected with padding. Because the lens system is delicate and costly, a plastic covering available from the manufacturer may be used to protect the lens from breakage. Disinfection with glutaraldehyde solution is acceptable for urological endoscopic instruments. Fiberoptic light bundles *should not* be tangled, twisted, or sharply angulated.

Transurethral resection of the prostate gland

Definition. Removal of successive pieces of tissue from around the bladder neck by means of a resectoscope passed into the bladder through the urethra and resection of the lobes of the prostate gland itself, leaving the capsule intact. The resectoscope uses a stabilized cutting loop to resect tissue and coagulate blood vessels by means of electric current. The electric current that powers the electrode is supplied by a high-frequency electrosurgical unit. The current settings are as specified, and the urologist activates the cutting or coagulating current with a foot pedal as desired during the course of the procedure.

Considerations. Transurethral resection of the prostate is one of four acceptable surgical methods of treating obstructive enlargement of the prostate gland. Several factors influence the surgical approach: (1) size of the gland and location of the pathologic condition, (2) age and condition of the patient, and (3) presence of associated diseases.

Controversy continues in regard to the efficacy of prophylactic vasectomy to prevent the postoperative complication of epididymo-orchitis. If the procedure is to be considered, it should be performed immediately before instrumentation. It is important that the patient be well informed and have full understanding of the implications of the procedure. Operative consent is mandatory.

Setup and preparation of the patient. As described for cystoscopy with selection of necessary instruments. The four principal types of resectoscopes are (1) McCarthy, (2) Nesbit, (3) Iglesias, and (4) Baumrucker (Fig. 15-21). Adult resectoscopes range in size from 24 to 28 Fr and have the following components: (1) Foroblique microlens telescope, (2) operating element, (3) postresectoscope sheaths and obturators, and (4) cutting loops (Fig. 15-22). Supplementary instruments include a resectoscope adaptor and a lateral telescope.

A transurethral resection setup (Fig. 15-23) should include the following:

Resectoscope (multiple working elements)
Foroblique telescope
Stabilized cutting loops
Postresectoscope sheath with corresponding Timberlake obturator
Cystourethroscope
Fiberoptic bundle
Stopcock water adaptor
Active electrosurgical cord
Resectoscope adaptor
Short bridge

Accessory items (may be sterilized on tray or added)

Brush (to clean tissue from cutting loops)
Towel clamps
Plain forceps
Prep set and solutions
Toomey syringe
Syringe, 20 ml
Ellik evacuator
Van Buren sounds
Strainer
Lubricant, water-soluble
Foley catheter
Disposable urological drape with rectal sheath (Fig. 15-24)
Cystoscopic drape pack
Sterile gowns and gloves as required

Items ready in cystoscopy room

Sterile basin filled with glycine solution to be used with Ellik evacuator and Toomey syringe
Electrosurgical unit
Cautery pad

A continuous flow of isotonic and nonelectrolytic irrigating fluid is necessary to ensure transmission of electrical current and clear visualization throughout surgery. Irrigating solution such as 1.5% glycine, 3 to 6 liters, may be connected in tandem to provide a constant flow. At all times nursing personnel must be alert to replace the irrigation solution as required.

During transurethral prostatic surgery, return of irrigation fluid must be monitored, since bladder perforation may occur. The nurse should be cognizant of the early symptoms and measures employed to remedy this complication. The patient usually experiences significant respiratory changes and abdominal discomfort. Other important observations are rigidity and swelling of the lower abdomen coupled with changes in sensorium.

If bladder perforation with extravasation of irrigating fluid is evident, the surgical procedure is discontinued and a cystogram immediately obtained. The site of the perforation is radiographically determined, and surgical closure is accomplished through a cystotomy incision.

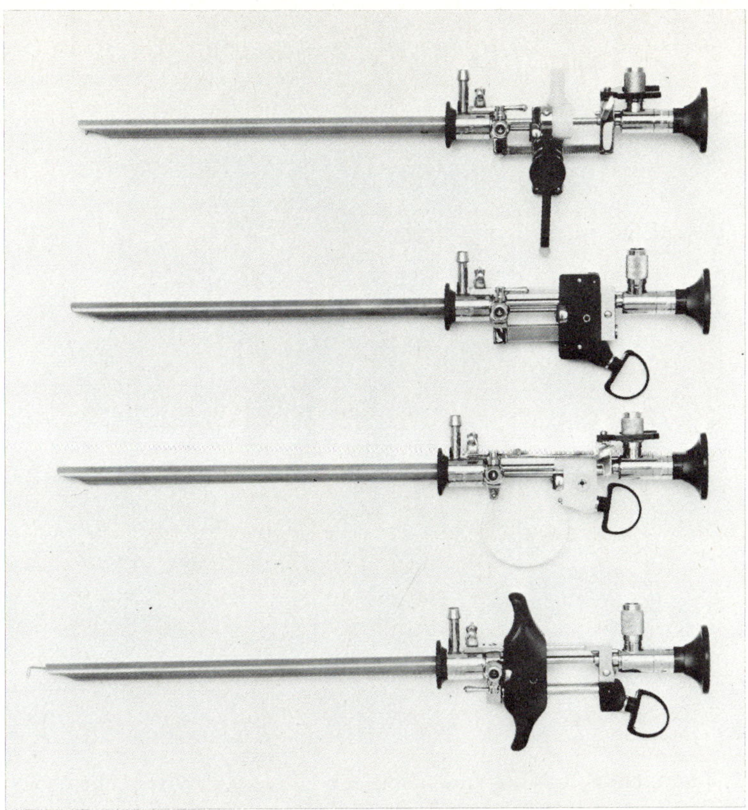

Fig. 15-21. Adult resectoscopes. *Top to bottom,* McCarthy, Nesbit, Iglesias, and Baumrucker.

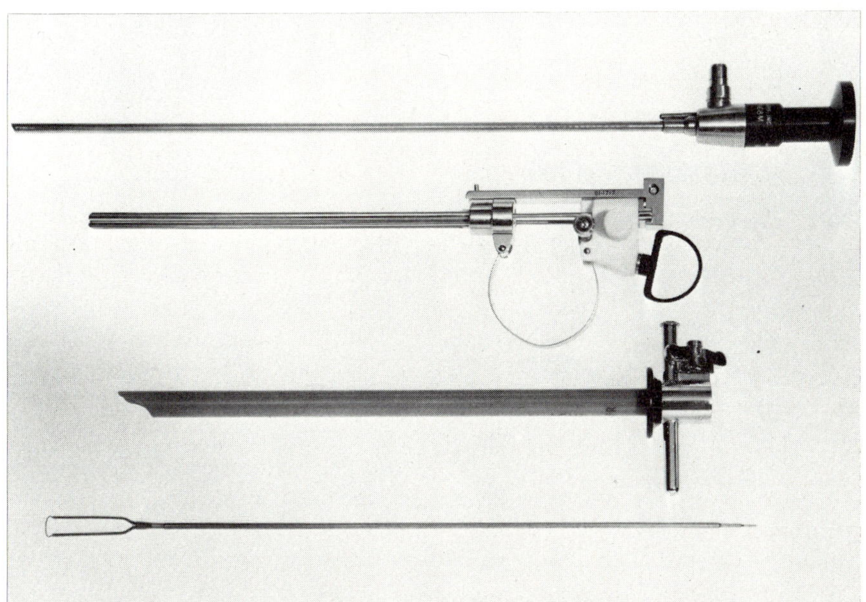

Fig. 15-22. Resectoscope components: Foroblique microlens, Iglesias operating element, postresectoscope sheath, and cutting loop. (Courtesy American Cystoscope Makers, Inc., Stamford, Conn.; from Morel, A., and Wise, G.J.: Urologic endoscopic procedures, ed. 2, St. Louis, 1979, The C.V. Mosby Co.)

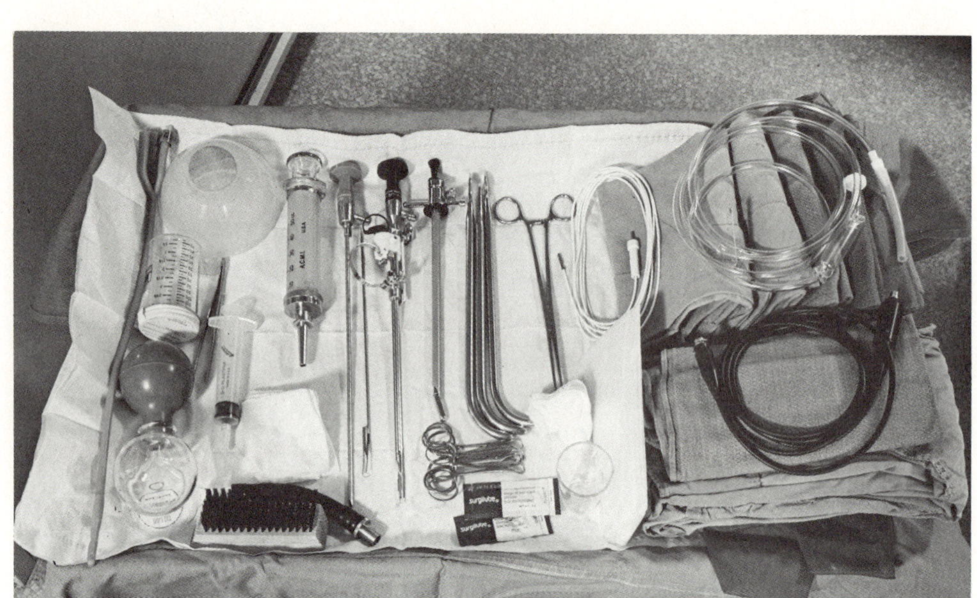

Fig. 15-23. Transurethral resection tray. (From Morel, A., and Wise, G.J.: Urologic endoscopic procedures, ed. 2, St. Louis, 1979, The C.V. Mosby Co.)

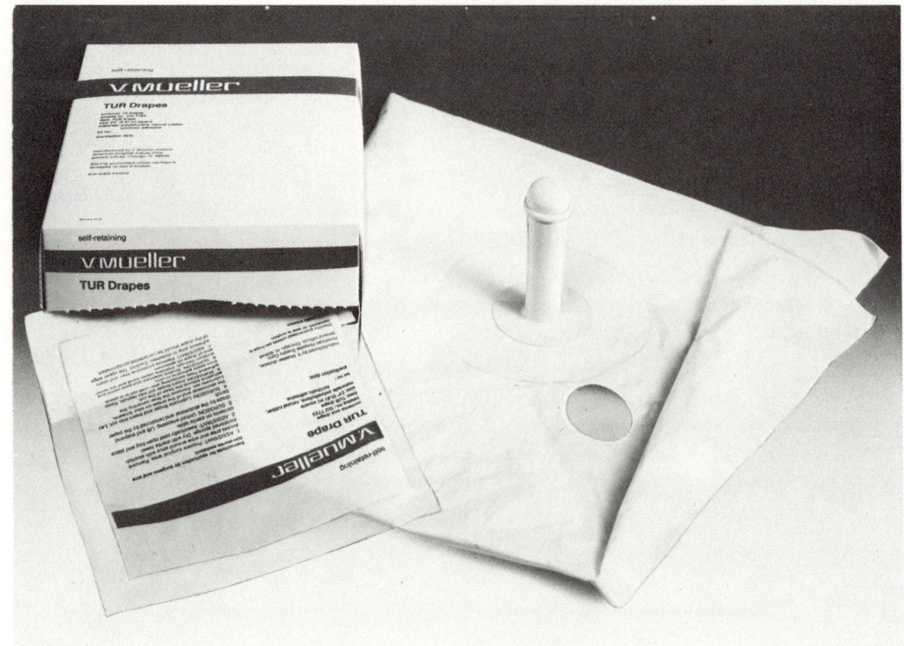

Fig. 15-24. Disposable urological drape with rectal sheath. (Courtesy American V. Mueller, Chicago, Ill.; from Morel, A., and Wise, G.J.: Urologic endoscopic procedures, ed. 2, St. Louis, 1979, The C.V. Mosby Co.)

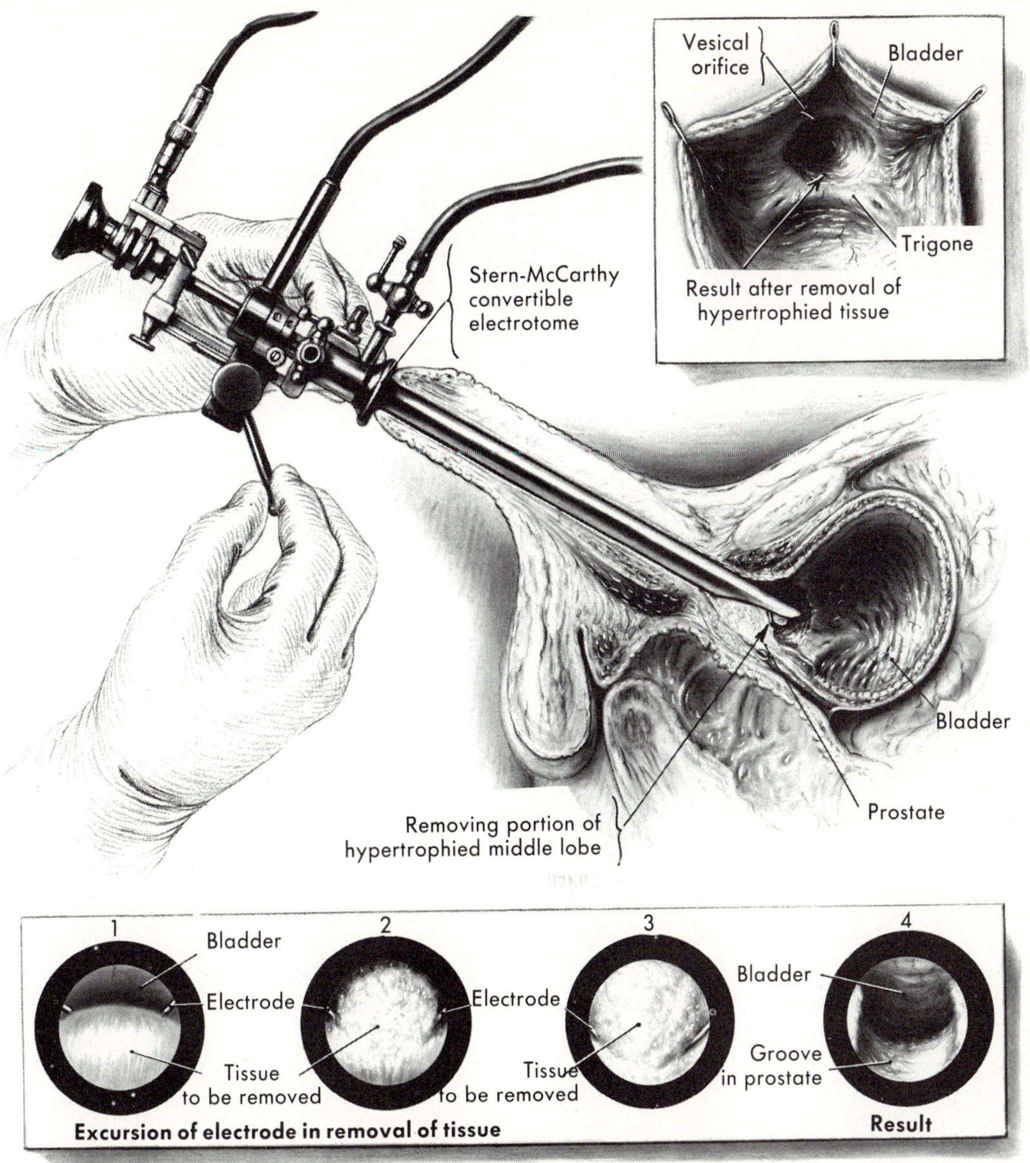

Fig. 15-25. Sectional view illustrating removal of portion of hypertrophied middle lobe of prostate gland with Stern-McCarthy resectoscope (TURP).

Operative procedure

1. The urologist checks the endoscopic instruments before performing the transurethral procedure. In transurethral prostatic surgery, the urethra is usually first dilated from 28 to 30 Fr with sounds.

2. Cystourethroscopy is performed to assess the degree of prostatic obstruction, as well as to inspect the bladder. Some urologists perform this diagnostic procedure several days before surgery, whereas others perform the examination in the operating room immediately before surgery.

3. A well-lubricated postresectoscope sheath with its fitted Timberlake obturator is passed into the urethra. The irrigation tubing, light cord, and electrosurgical cord are appropriately connected. The Timberlake obturator is removed, and the working element (resectoscope), assembled with the Foroblique telescope and cutting loop, is inserted through the sheath. Irrigation fluid is allowed to fill the bladder. Initial inspection of the prostatic urethra and bladder trigone is carried out. After determining the location of the ureteral orifice, the urologist initiates electrodissection, alternating cutting and coagulating currents as required (Fig. 15-25). At intervals, the bladder is drained, washing out prostatic tissue and small blood clots. At times it is necessary to employ the Ellik evacuator to more effectively remove resected prostatic tissue. To do this, the urologist must remove the working element of the resectoscope. The nozzle of the evacuator is fitted onto the resectoscope sheath, and by manual pulsatile pressure the bladder contents are removed. A basin of glycine solution with an Ellik evacuator and Toomey syringe should be readily available for manual irrigation.

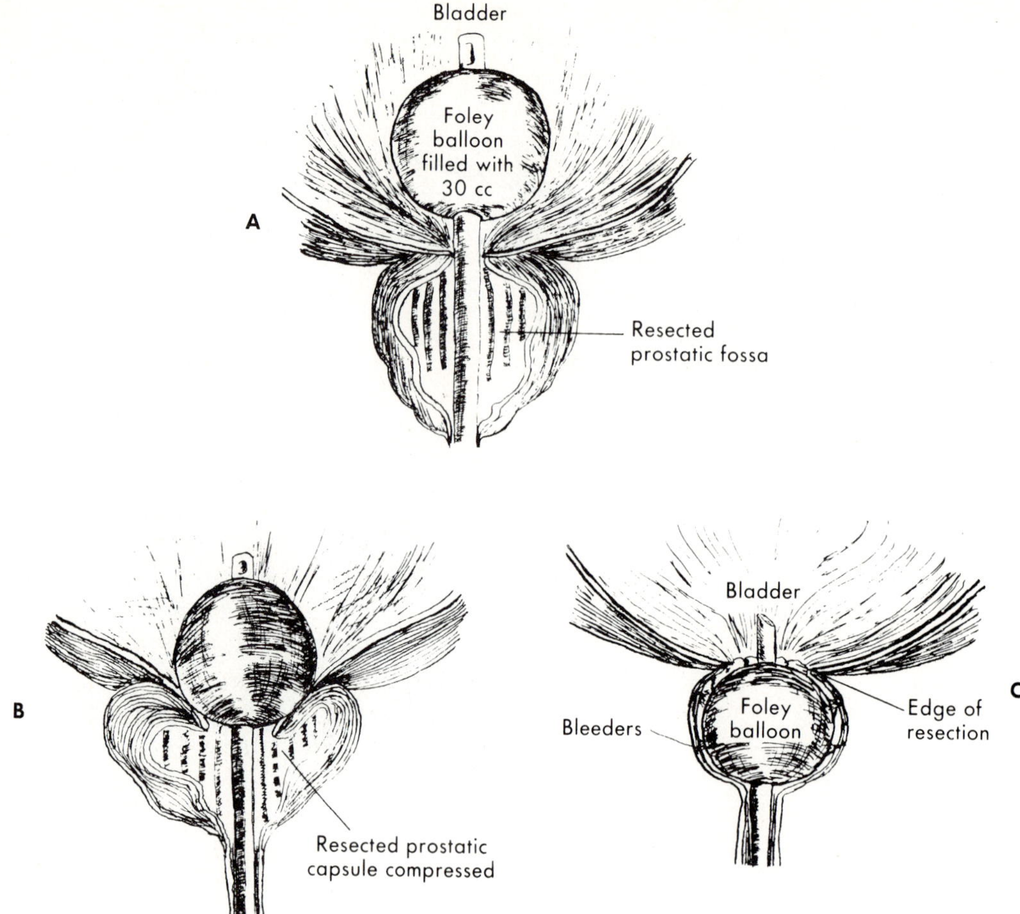

Fig. 15-26. A, Proper position for Foley catheter beyond prostatic capsule. **B,** Foley catheter balloon is inflated and pulled gently in traction at bladder neck. **C,** Foley balloon should not be inflated within prostatic fossa.

4. When the prostatic resection is completed, the prostatic fossa is inspected to ensure that all bleeding points have been coagulated. The resectoscope is then removed and a Foley catheter (22 or 24 Fr, two- or three-way, 30-cc balloon) is inserted into the bladder for urinary drainage. The balloon is inflated (Fig. 15-26, *A*) and pulled gently in traction against the bladder neck to help control venous bleeding (Fig. 15-26, *B*). It is important that the Foley balloon not be inflated within the prostatic fossa (Fig. 15-26, *C*), since this causes excessive bleeding from the resected prostatic capsule.

5. If desired, continuous irrigation with gravity drainage is initiated with normal saline as the bladder irrigant. Before the patient is transferred to the recovery room, the glycine irrigation must be discontinued and isotonic saline solution used in its place. A 2000-ml urinary drainage system is suggested to help minimize frequent emptying of the drainage bag.

OPERATIONS ON THE PENIS AND THE URETHRA

Hypospadias repair

Definition. Repair of a urethral meatus that is proximal to its normal glandular position at the tip of the penis.

Considerations. There are various degrees of hypospadias. The meatus may be on the ventral surface of the glans, on the corona, anywhere along the shaft, in the scrotum, or even in the perineum. The more proximal the opening, the greater the degree of chordee (ventral curvature of the penis). Chordee are fibrous bands that extend from the hypospadiac urethral meatus to the tip of the glans and represent the abnormally developed urethra and its investing layer of Buck's fascia, dartos, and skin.

Principles of hypospadias repair consist of release of chordee, thereby straightening the penis, and reconstruction of the urethra. Surgeons prefer to do a one-stage

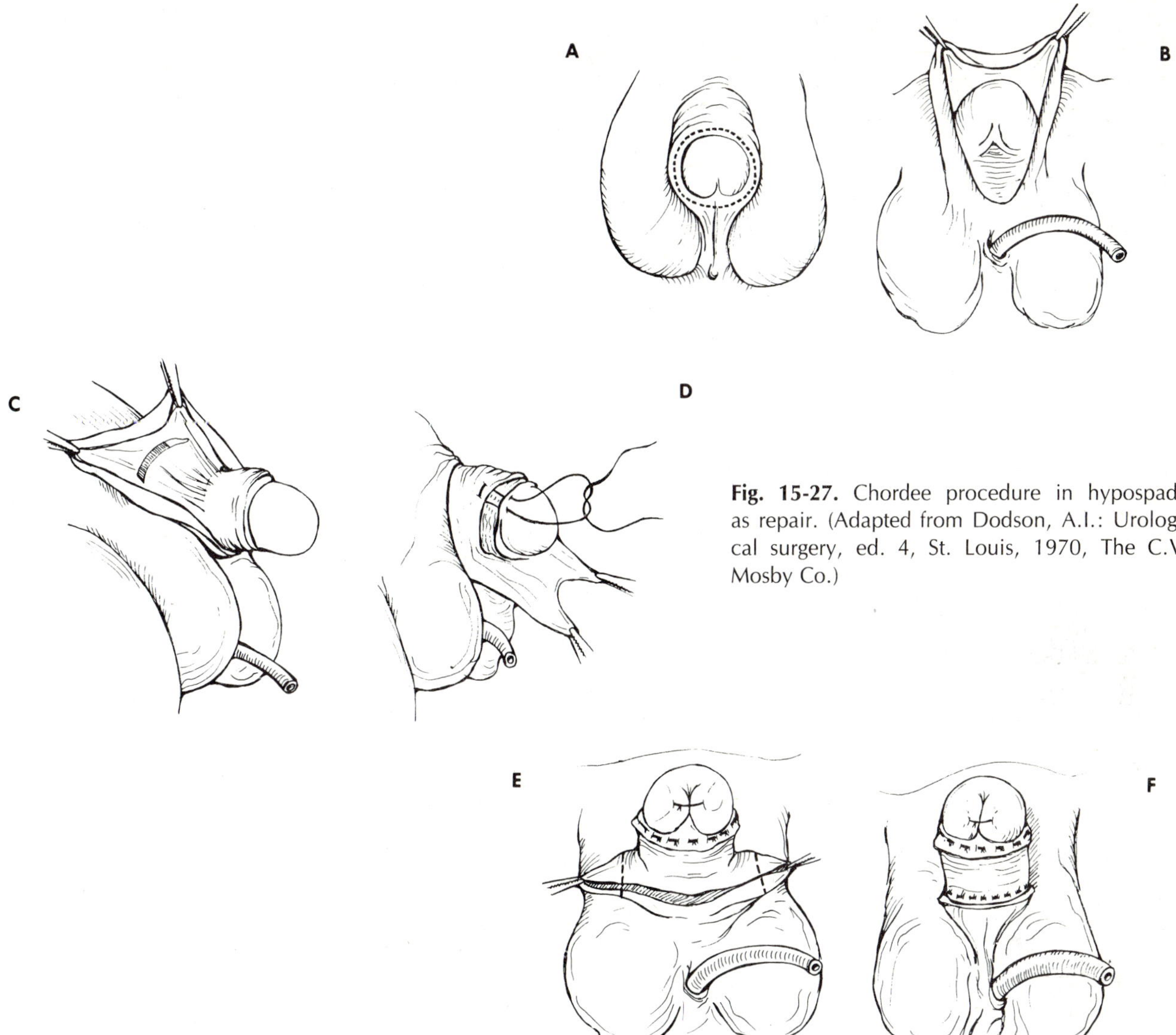

Fig. 15-27. Chordee procedure in hypospadias repair. (Adapted from Dodson, A.I.: Urological surgery, ed. 4, St. Louis, 1970, The C.V. Mosby Co.)

hypospadias repair in cases of distal penile hypospadias with minimal degrees of chordee. Recently, there has been a resurgence of interest in one-stage repairs.

One of the complications of hypospadias repair is urethral fistula formation, which can be repaired without much difficulty. Correction of strictures is more troublesome.

Setup and preparation of the patient. The patient is placed in the supine position with legs apart. The urine is diverted with a urethral catheter.

The instrument setup varies according to the surgeon's preference. However, a minor set with fine plastic instruments is generally required and sutures, polyethylene infant feeding tubes, silicone tubing or silicone Foley catheters, and drains may be desired. Owens gauze, Elastomull, Coban, and Elastoplast, as well as adhesive tape, are generally required for the dressing, which is an important part of the hypospadias repair.

Operative procedures

Chordee repair

1. An incision is made around the penis. The skin is stripped back from the phallus by subcutaneous dissection (Fig. 15-27, *A* and *B*).

2. Fibrous tissue on the ventral surface is removed, correcting the ventral curvature of the penis.

3. A buttonhole incision is made in the dorsal skin flap, and the glans penis is brought through the opening (Fig. 15-27, *C* and *D*).

4. The edges of the buttonhole incision are sutured to the skin adjacent to the corona. If skin is excessive at the extremities of the transverse suture, it may be trimmed (Fig. 15-27, *E*).

5. The skin flap distal to the buttonhole incision covers the denuded ventral surface of the penis and is sutured to the retracted skin margin (Fig. 15-27, *F*).

6. An indwelling catheter is placed, and the wound is dressed.

Urethral reconstruction

Many procedures are described for construction of a urethra. They may be divided into three general groups: (1) buried skin tube (Fig. 15-28), (2) buried skin flap (Fig. 15-29), and (3) free graft (Fig. 15-30). There are also many combinations of these procedures. In all the procedures some type of temporary urinary diversion, such as a perineal urethrostomy, is used.

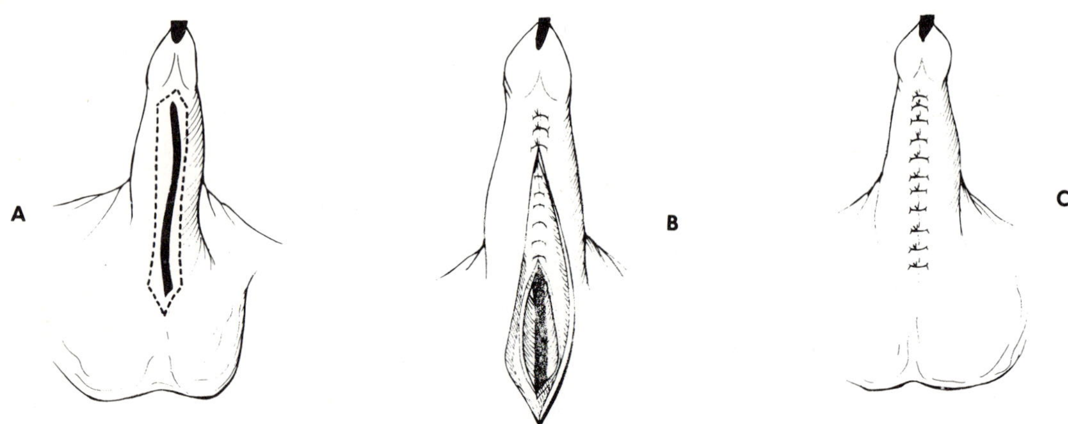

Fig. 15-28. Urethral reconstruction—buried skin tube. **A,** Parallel incisions, which meet as they encircle meatus proximally, made on ventral surface of shaft of penis. **B,** Medial edges of incision undermined so longitudinal skin flap can be sutured around catheter. **C,** Lateral edges undermined until sufficient relaxation and mobilization are obtained to suture them over catheter. (From Flocks, R.H., and Clup, D.A.: Surgical urology, 4th edition, Copyright © 1975 by Year Book Medical Publishers, Inc., Chicago. Used by permission.)

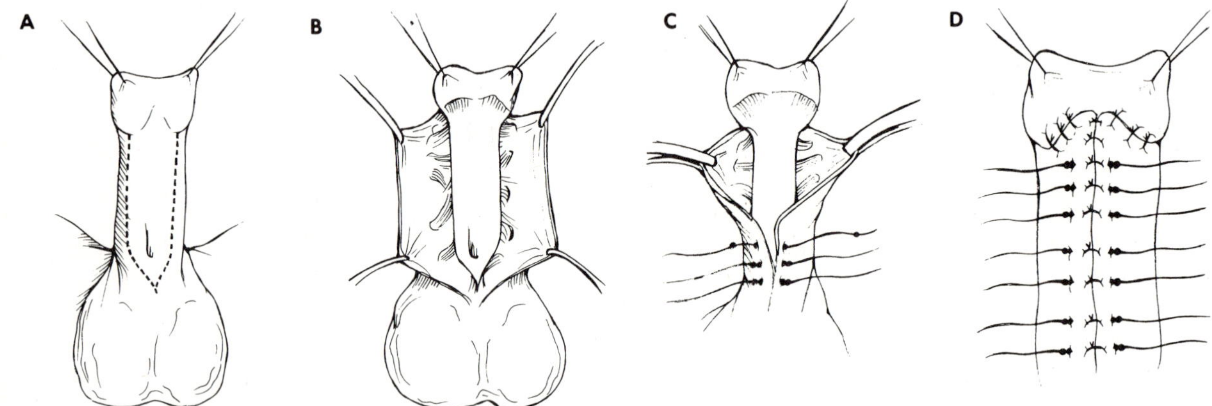

Fig. 15-29. Urethral reconstruction—buried skin flap. **A,** Incision made on ventral surface of penile shaft. **B,** Lateral edges of incision undermined. **C,** Lateral edges brought over rectangular flap of skin and sutured. No tube is formed. **D,** Sutures reinforced with wire tension sutures held in place with small lead shot. When healing, buried skin flap epithelializes in circular manner to form epithelial cyst that can be used as distal urethra. (From Flocks, R.H., and Clup, D.A.: Surgical urology, 4th edition. Copyright © 1975 by Year Book Medical Publishers, Inc. Chicago. Used by permission.)

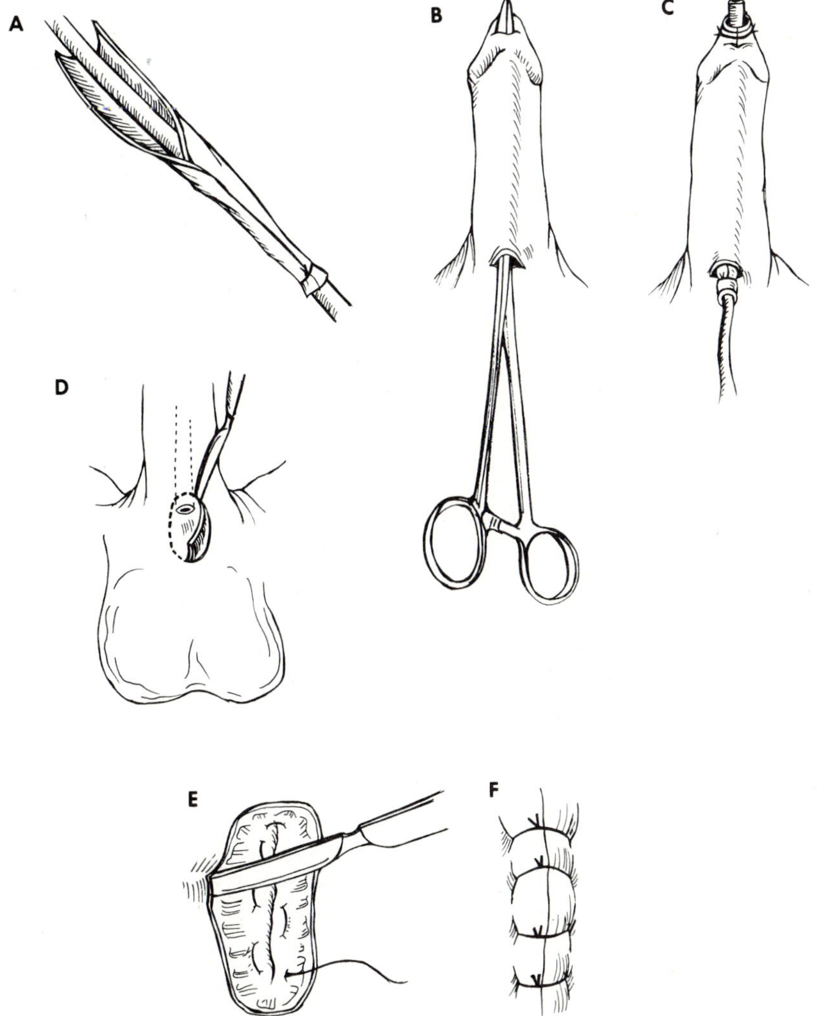

Fig. 15-30. Urethral reconstruction—free graft. **A,** Skin graft, which is taken from nonhair-bearing area such as inner aspect of upper arm, is wrapped around stiff catheter and anchored at each end. **B,** Bed for graft is prepared by making transverse incision in front of urethral meatus and bluntly dissecting to tip of glans penis. **C,** Catheter with graft pulled through channel with forceps. When graft is in place, both catheter and graft are anchored with sutures at both ends. **D,** Final closure of urethra is accomplished by incising skin around fistulous openings. **E,** Inner margins of incision are closed over catheter. **F,** Lateral margins of incision are undermined and closed in several layers. Catheter is then removed with diversion of urine flow through perineal urethrostomy or suprapubic cystostomy. (From Flocks, R.H., and Clup, D.A.: Surgical urology, 4th edition, Copyright © 1975 by Year Book Medical Publishers, Inc., Chicago. Used by permission.)

Epispadias repair

Definition. Correction of the absence of the dorsal wall of the urethra and the position of the corpora cavernosa, ventral to the urethra. The surgical procedures employed in the correction of epispadias depend on the extent of the deformity. In the mild incomplete defects, the repair is much the same as a simple hypospadias repair. The complete deformity is always associated with urinary incontinence because of little or no development of the bladder neck; thus the operation is much more involved.

Considerations. The least severe form of the exstrophy epispadias complex is balanitic epispadias, in which the urethra opens on the dorsum of the glans, or penile epispadias, in which the urethra opens on the shaft of the penis. The more severe variety, which occurs when the urethra opens on the proximal shaft or in the penopubic position, generally is associated with severe dorsal chordee and urinary incontinence.

Setup and preparation of the patient. As described for hypospadias repair.

Operative procedure

First-stage epispadias repair. A vertical incision is made distal to the epispadiac meatus and carried circumferentially to the dorsal coronal margin. The foreshortened dorsal urethral strip is lifted off the corpora cavernosa, and the ventral prepuce (foreskin) rotated dorsally to cover the dorsal skin defect created by penile straightening.

Second-stage epispadias repair

1. A vertical suprapubic incision is made, exposing the anterior bladder wall and widened vesical neck. A wedge section of the anterolateral prostatic urethra is removed on either side, so that when it is reconstructed a more normal caliber prostatic urethra is formed (Fig. 15-31, *A*).
2. The roof of the membranous urethra is removed (Fig. 15-31, *B*).
3. The prostatic urethra is closed, including muscle that is sutured together in the midline, with chromic catgut or Dexon sutures. The bladder is closed, leaving a suprapubic catheter indwelling. The abdomen is closed in layers (Fig. 15-31, *C*).
4. The anterior urethra is closed after outlining an appropriate sized octagonal strip or dorsal penile skin (Fig. 15-31, *D*).
5. The remainder of the repair, that is, the creation of the urethra, and its coverage with lateral penile skin is much like a second-stage hypospadias repair, except in reverse.

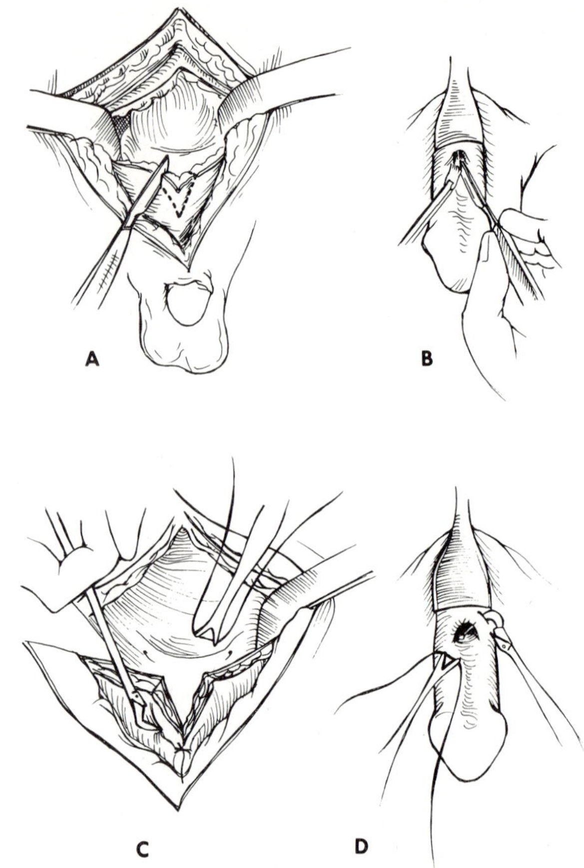

Fig. 15-31. Epispadias repair. (From Flocks, R.H., and Clup, D.A.: Surgical urology, 4th edition. Copyright © 1975 by Year Book Medical Publishers, Inc., Chicago. Used by permission.)

Bladder exstrophy repair

Definition. Repair of a more severe form of epispadias, in which the anterior bladder wall as well as the roof of the urethra is absent. Bladder exstrophy is always accompanied by wide separation of the recti muscles of the lower abdominal wall and by diastasis of the pubic bone with anterior displacement of the anus.

Considerations. Repair of bladder exstrophy requires an adequate sized bladder for ultimate continence to be achieved. This procedure is preferably performed in the neonatal period.

Setup and preparation of the patient. The infant is placed in a supine position, and the abdomen and thighs are prepared and draped. Instruments are as required for hypospadias repair.

Operative procedure

1. An incision is made around the exposed bladder medial to the paravesical neck mucosa. The incision is carried distally across the epispadiac urethra distal to the verumontanum. The paravesical mucosa is preserved for urethral lengthening. The bladder is then freed from the rectus fascia and the peritoneum. The dorsal chordee is released, and the mobilized paravesical mucosa apposed in the midline and sutured to the proximal urethra just distal to the verumontanum.

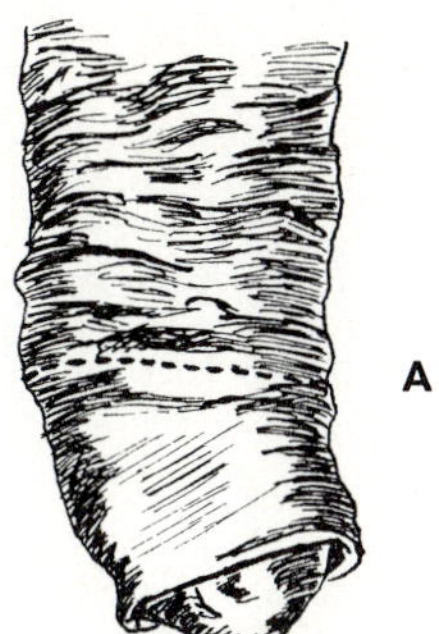

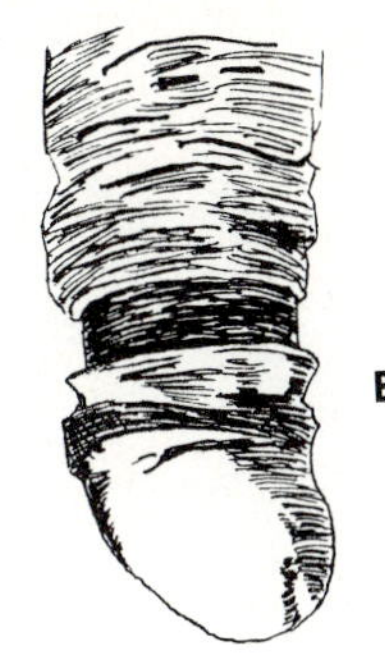

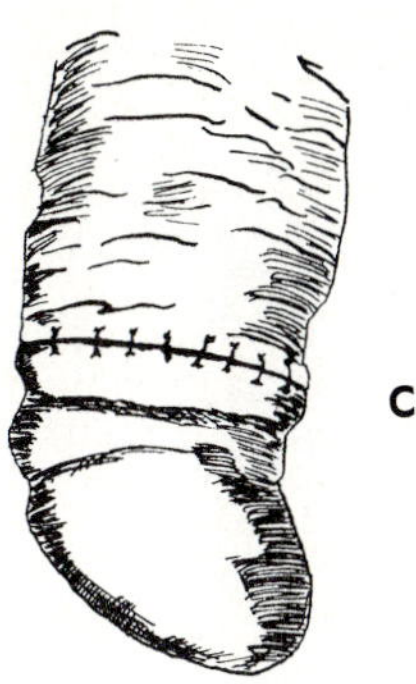

Fig. 15-32. Circumcision. **A,** Prepuce is incised toward coronal margin. **B,** Prepuce is completely separated from glans. **C,** Raw edges of skin incision are approximated to coronal cuff of mucosal prepuce.

2. The bladder wall is closed vertically in two layers with no. 3-0 chromic sutures, leaving a suprapubic tube for drainage.

3. The bladder neck is loosely reconstructed by approximating the interpubic ligament, which extends between the proximal end of the phallus and the pubic bone.

4. The symphysis pubis is approximated with a heavy no. 2 Prolene suture. During this step, the assistant rotates the iliac bones anteriorly.

Note: When closure of the bladder exstrophy is delayed beyond the neonatal period, bilateral iliac osteotomies are required to bring the symphysis pubis together in the midline. A vesical neck plasty is performed at a later date with bilateral ureteral reimplantation. The penis may be closed before, at the same time as, or some time after the vesical neck plasty.

Iliac osteotomy

Setup and preparation of the patient. The infant is placed in the prone position with a folded towel under the pelvis.

Operative procedure. A vertical incision is made 0.5 cm lateral to the sacroiliac joints. The iliac bone is exposed and osteotomy through both tables performed to bring the pubic bones together in the midline after reconstruction of the bladder.

Circumcision

Definition. Excision of the foreskin (prepuce) of the glans penis.

Considerations. Circumcision may be done prophylactically in infancy. The surgery may be performed for religious reasons, for example, as is required in the Jewish faith. Provision should be made in a hospital to observe the religious needs and preferences of Jewish parents.

Circumcision is also performed for the relief of phimosis, a condition in which the orifice of the prepuce is too small to permit easy retraction behind the glans. In addition, circumcision may be done to prevent recurrent paraphimosis, a condition in which the prepuce cannot be reduced easily from a retracted position. Circumcision is also indicated for recurrent balanitis.

Setup and preparation of the patient. Newborns are generally positioned on a specially constructed board that facilitates restraint by immobilizing the limbs and exposing the genitals. No anesthesia is used in this age group. Older children require anesthesia. Adults may be offered the option of local or general anesthesia.

For infants, the setup includes fine plastic instruments. A Gomco clamp of the appropriate size, a Plastibell, or the Hollister disposable circumcision device may be preferred. The Hollister device includes sutures that are sealed in a sterile packet ready for use. For older patients, a plastic instrument set is used. Petrolatum gauze for dressing should be available.

Operative procedure

1. If the prepuce is adherent, a probe or hemostat may be used to break up adhesions. The prepuce is clamped in the dorsal midline and incised toward the coronal margin (Fig. 15-32, *A*), leaving about 5 cm of coronal mucosa intact. A similar procedure is performed ventrally. The two incisions are then joined circumferentially. Alternately, a superficial, circumferential incision is made in the skin at the level of the coronal sulcus and the mucosa at the base of the glans with a scalpel. The redundant skin is undermined between the circumferential incisions and removed as a complete cuff (Fig. 15-32, *B*). Bleeding vessels are coagulated or clamped with mosquito hemostats and tied with fine catgut ligatures.

2. The raw edges of the skin incision are approximated to a coronal cuff of mucosal prepuce with no. 5-0 catgut sutures on atraumatic needles (Fig. 15-32, *C*). The wound is usually dressed with petrolatum gauze.

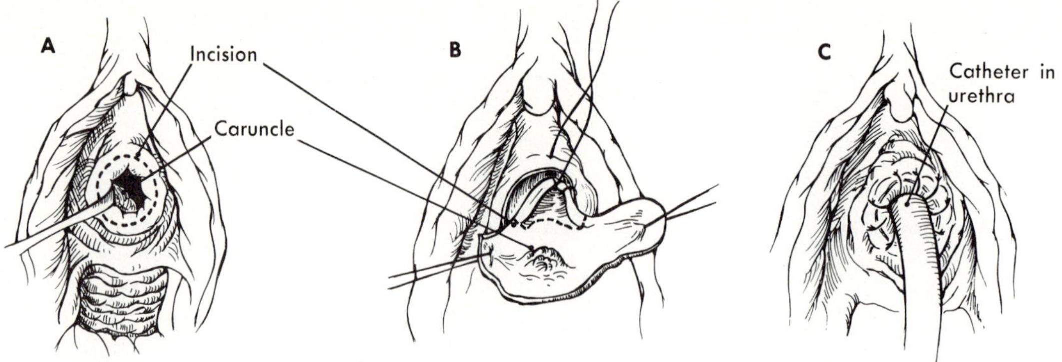

Fig. 15-33. Excision of sessile growth. **A,** Incision around urethral meatus and caruncle. **B,** Urethra freed from caruncle, meatus dissected back to healthy tissue, and caruncle excised. **C,** Reanastomosis of mucocutaneous junction, and catheter inserted. (From Flocks, R.H., and Clup, D.A.: Surgical urology, 4th edition. Copyright © 1975 by Year Book Medical Publishers, Inc., Chicago. Used by permission.)

Excision of urethral caruncle

Definition. Removal of papillary or sessile tumors of the urethra.

Considerations. A urethral caruncle is a benign lesion or inflammatory prolapse of the external urinary meatus in the female.

Setup and preparation of the patient. The patient is placed in the lithotomy position. A minor or plastic set, an electrosurgical unit, and a local anesthetic are used. A urethral catheter of an appropriate size may be required if the distal urethral prolapse is severe.

Operative procedure. With a small Metzenbaum scissors, the growth is exposed and excised within a wedge of ventral urethral tissue. Figure-of-eight no. 4-0 chromic sutures at the edge of the incision are usually sufficient to achieve good hemostasis (Fig. 15-33).

Urethral meatotomy

Definition. Incisional enlargement of the external urethral meatus.

Considerations. Relief of stenosis or stricture at the external meatus that may be congenital or acquired.

Setup and preparation of the patient. The male patient is placed in the supine position. Skin preparation and draping is as described for urethral catheterization. For the female patient, the lithotomy position is used. Local anesthesia is generally employed. A plastic instrument set is needed. A petrolatum gauze dressing is usually applied.

Operative procedure. A straight hemostat is placed on the ventral surface of the meatus. An incision is made along the frenum to enlarge the opening and overcome the stricture. Bleeding vessels are clamped and ligated with fine plain surgical gut sutures. The mucosal layer is sutured to the skin with fine plain gut sutures. A dressing of petrolatum gauze may be applied.

Urethral dilatation and internal urethrotomy

Definition. Gradual dilatation and lysis of a urethral stricture to provide relief of distal lower urinary tract obstruction.

Considerations. Urethral strictures or narrowing of the urethra may be caused by a congenital malformation that is usually found at the external urinary meatus. Infection or trauma may also contribute to stricture of the membranous and pendulous urethra. One method of treating urethral stricture disease is by periodic dilatation with Philips filiforms and followers or Van Buren sounds.

Setup and preparation of the patient. The male patient may be placed in a supine position for routine urethral dilatation but in lithotomy position for other procedures. Skin preparation and draping is as required for male catheterization. A local anesthetic such as lidocaine (Xylocaine gel or Anestacon) should be used. For the female, the patient is placed in the lithotomy position. A cotton-tipped applicator dipped in the local anesthetic is placed in the urethral opening. Female urethral dilatation is performed with short straight metal dilators or with hollow McCarthy dilators, through which a catheterized urine specimen can also be obtained.

The setup includes the following:

Urethrotomes (Fig. 15-34)
Direct viewing telescope and bridge for ureteral catheters
Resectoscope working element, sheath, obturator, and cold knives
Urethral dilators

Accessory items

Philips filiforms and followers
Van Buren sounds
Irrigation system
Prep set and solutions
Silicone Foley catheter
Syringe, 20 ml
Lubricant, water-soluble
Fiberoptic light cord
Luer-Lok water adaptor
Cystoscopy drape pack
Sterile gown and gloves
Cystoscopy setup, if required

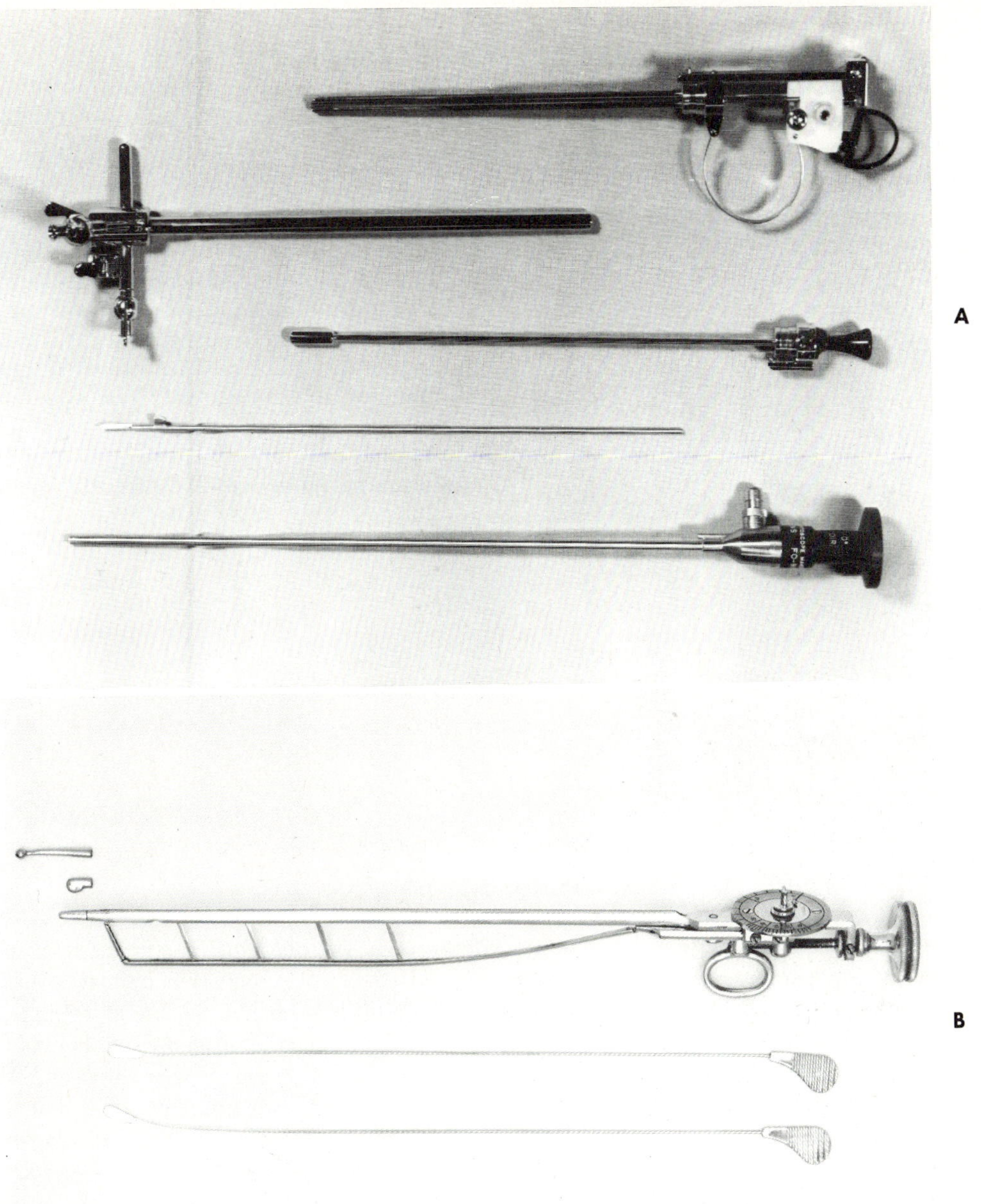

Fig. 15-34. A, ACMI internal urethrotome. **B,** Otis urethrotome.

Operative procedures

Gradual dilatation. In the male patient, the urethra is lubricated and anesthetized with a viscous anesthetic that is injected into the urethra with a 10-ml plastic syringe. A penile clamp occludes the penile urethra at the coronal sulcus and keeps the anesthetic within the urethra. Philips filiforms of various tips and sizes are first introduced in an attempt to pass an instrument beyond the urethral stricture. Followers of gradual increased size will be attached to the filiforms and passed through the strictured area of the urethra, stretching the scarred area (Fig. 15-35). Slow dilatation is also achieved with a small catheter or filiform left in the urethra. This will lead to softening of the stricture over the course of several days. Before use and/or sterilization, the filiforms and followers should be carefully inspected for damaged or weak points, particularly around the screw thread end. Van Buren sounds may also be used for urethral dilatation.

Internal urethrotomy. Under direct vision, the assembled visualizing urethrotome is inserted into the urethra. When necessary, a filiform or ureteral catheter is fed into the catheterizing channel to help identify the patent portion of the urethra. The urethrotome is advanced to the desired position, and the blade is used to incise the urethral scar. The normal urethra must be increased 1 cm proximally and distally beyond the stricture to achieve good results. A silicone Foley catheter is usually left in place for 3 to 5 days after surgery.

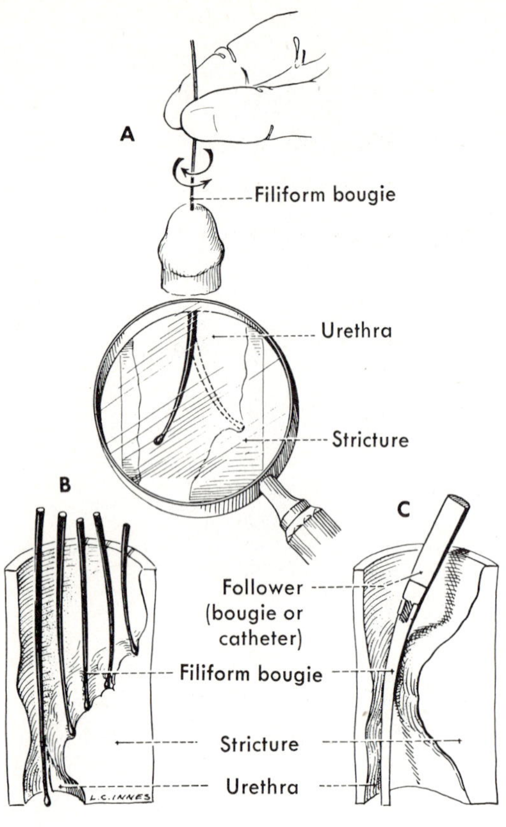

Fig. 15-35. Method of using coude-tipped bougie for passing stricture. **A,** Bougie withdrawn 1 to 2 cm each time obstruction is met; bougie is rotated and then is passed inward again. **B,** Method of using multiple bougies to pass through urethral stricture. Pocket is filled with bougie tips; this displaces one to opening through stricture. **C,** Philips filiform and follower. Follower is screwed onto end of filiform. Filiform passed through stricture guides follower through. (From Barnes, R.W., and Hadley, H.L.: Urological practice, St. Louis, The C.V. Mosby Co.)

Urethroplasty

Definition. Reconstructive surgery of the urethra.

Considerations. Strictures, or narrowing of the urethral lumen, are congenital, inflammatory, or traumatic in origin. Various surgical techniques are described in the surgical treatment of stricture disease.

Setup and preparation of the patient. The patient is placed in the exaggerated lithotomy position. Routine draping procedures are employed with precautions for protecting the anus (that is, use of impervious plastic adherent drape). The instrument setup includes a minor instrument set with fine plastic instruments for dissection and plastic repair. Strictures may be deeply located, requiring special instruments such as Turner-Warwick needles and retractors (Fig. 15-36). A Dennis-Brown ring is also helpful (Fig. 15-37). Fiberoptic lighting is desirable, and an electrosurgical unit may be required.

Operative procedure

First-stage Johanson urethroplasty

1. An inverted U incision is made in the perineum from the inner borders of the ischial tuberosities up to and including the base of the scrotum. A Van Buren sound is passed into the urethra up to the stricture. The bulbocavernosus muscle is dissected and retracted laterally.

2. An incision is made in the urethra over the strictured area and is extended at least 1 cm beyond the diseased area into the urethra in each direction (Fig. 15-38, *A*).

3. The abnormal scar tissue is excised or simply incised, since scrotal skin ultimately increases the lumen (Fig. 15-38, *B*). A no. 28 sound is passed through the proximal and the distal urethral lumina to rule out further stricture. The remaining urethral mucosa is sutured with fine chromic catgut to the scrotal skin (Fig. 15-38, *C*). A cystotomy tube to divert the urinary stream may be left indwelling and removed in 5 to 7 days.

Approximately 3 months after the first stage, if there is adequate voiding and healing of the operative site, a second-stage procedure is undertaken.

Second stage Johanson urethroplasty

1. A Robinson catheter is temporarily inserted into the bladder through the proximal urethral stoma. The skin is incised along prolongitudinal lines, and flaps of skin are developed to construct a new urethra.

2. The flaps are brought together in the midline and closed with a continuous or interrupted fine catgut suture to a predetermined caliber.

3. Layers of subcutaneous tissue are dissected free, then sutured over the newly constructed urethra with interrupted plain catgut sutures.

4. A bulky pressure dressing is applied. Suprapubic cystotomy drainage is an option, but a urethral catheter usually suffices.

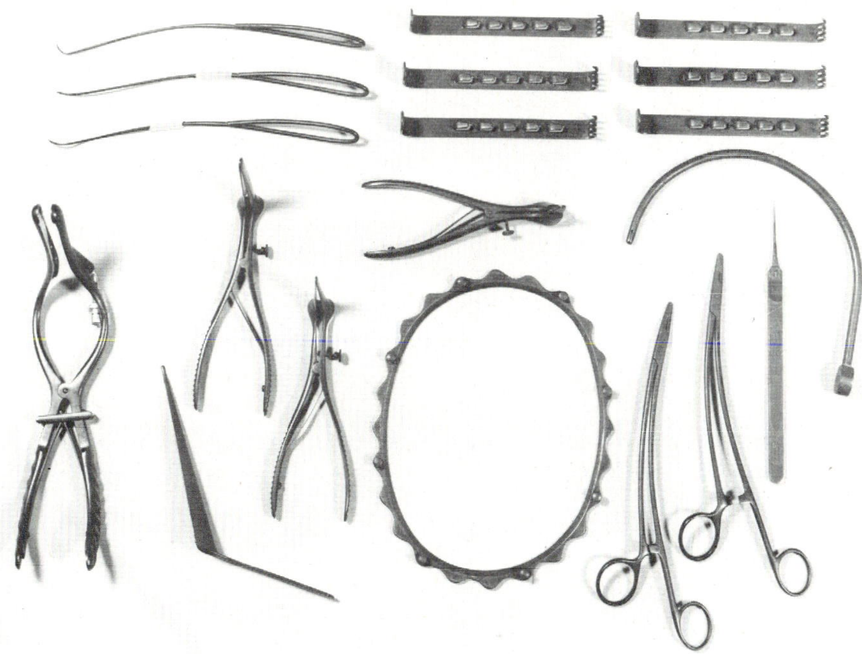

Fig. 15-36. Turner-Warwick urethroplasty instruments.

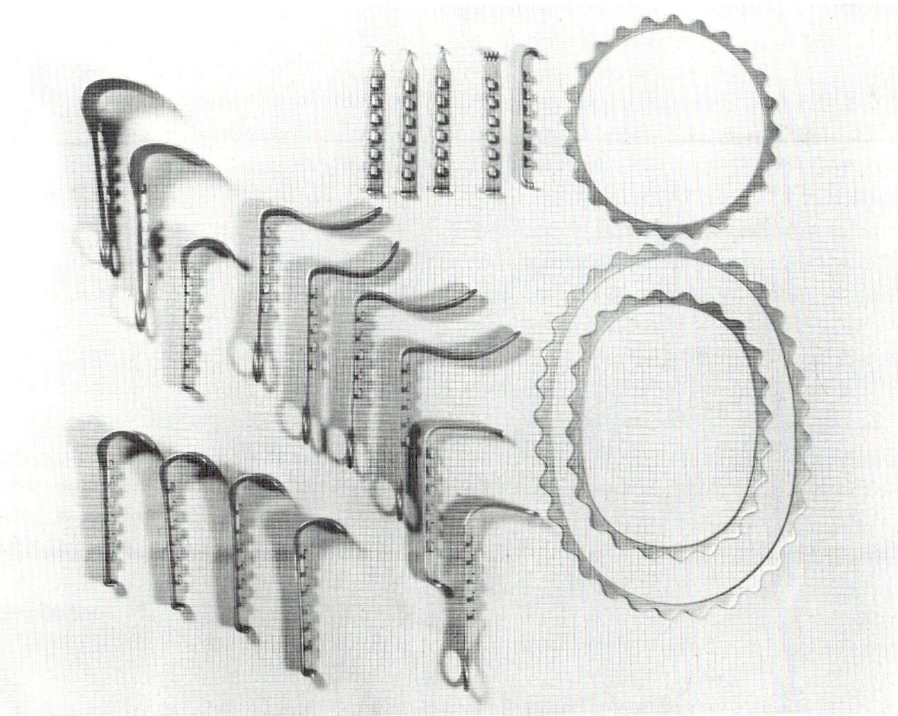

Fig. 15-37. Dennis-Brown self-retaining ring retractor.

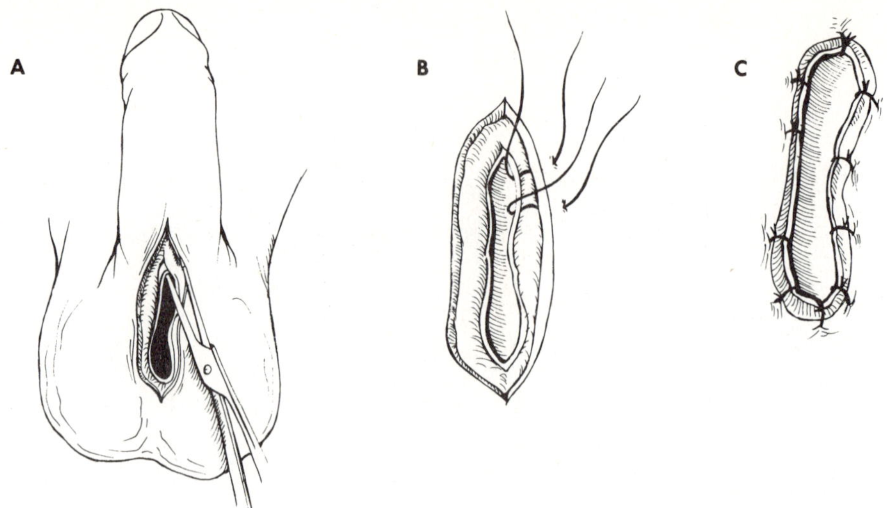

Fig. 15-38. Urethroplasty. (From Flocks, R.H., and Clup, D.A.: Surgical urology, 4th edition. Copyright © 1975 by Year Book Medical Publishers, Inc., Chicago. Used by permission.)

Penile implant

Definition. Insertion of a penile prosthesis for treatment of organic sexual impotence.

Considerations. The insertion of a prosthesis is considered in relieving sexual impotence caused by (1) diabetes mellitus, (2) priapism, (3) Peyronie's disease, (4) penile trauma, (5) pelvic surgery, (6) neurological disease (in selected cases), and (7) idiopathic impotence (in carefully screened cases). The penile implant serves as a stent to enable vaginal penetration for sexual intercourse.

Setup and preparation of the patient. Regional or general anesthesia is required. The supine or lithotomy position may be employed. Skin preparation and draping is carried out according to hospital policy. A no. 14 or 16 Foley catheter may be inserted to identify the urethra intraoperatively. Electrosurgery may be required.

The instrument setup includes a minor set with fine instruments, plus the following:

Hegar dilators
Penile prosthesis of urologist's choice (Fig. 15-39)
Calipers
Blunt nerve hooks
Dennis-Brown retractor

A disastrous complication is infection of the prosthesis, so careful draping is essential. The anus should be isolated in the perineal approach. The use of an antibiotic irrigant and systemic antibiotics may be required.

Operative procedure

1. A hemicircular incision is made on the dorsal surface of the penis (Fig. 15-40, *A*).
2. The tunica albuginea is incised over the corpus in a longitudinal manner (Fig. 15-40, *B*), and the corpus is dilated distally and proximally (Fig. 15-40, *C* and *D*) with Hegar dilators. Care must be taken not to perforate the urethra.
3. The prosthesis is inserted in the corpus (Fig. 15-40, *E* and *F*). Proper placement is evident immediately by change in the configuration of the penis with no buckling of the glans (Fig. 15-40, *G*). The tunica albuginea is then closed with a no. 2-0 Dexon continuous suture; no. 3-0 chromic interrupted sutures are used for skin closure.
4. Petrolatum gauze or 2-inch Kling tube gauze may be used for the dressing.
5. A Foley catheter is inserted, and the amount and color of urine are noted.

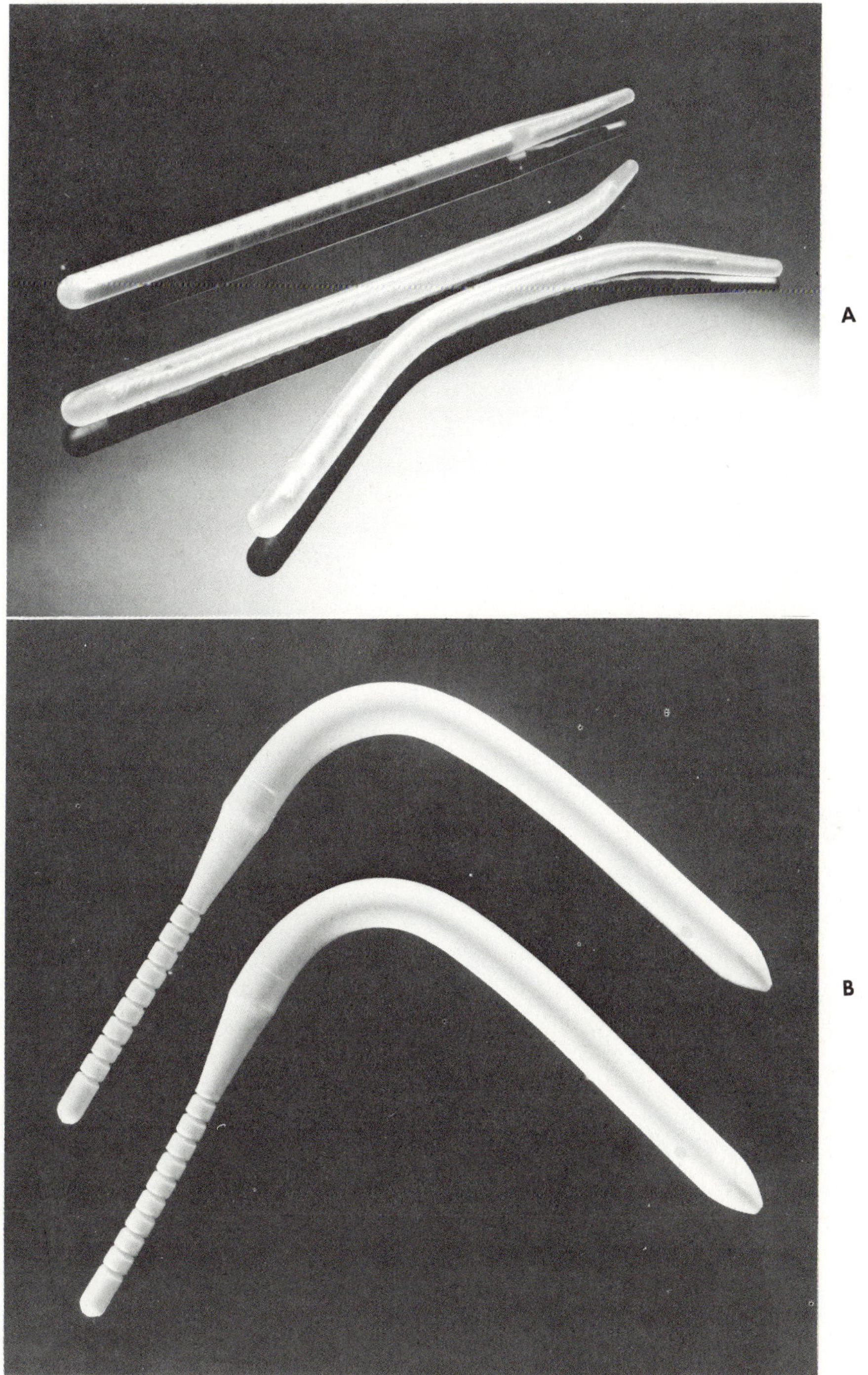

Fig. 15-39. Penile prostheses. **A,** Jonas silicone silver penile prosthesis. **B,** Flexirod penile prosthesis.

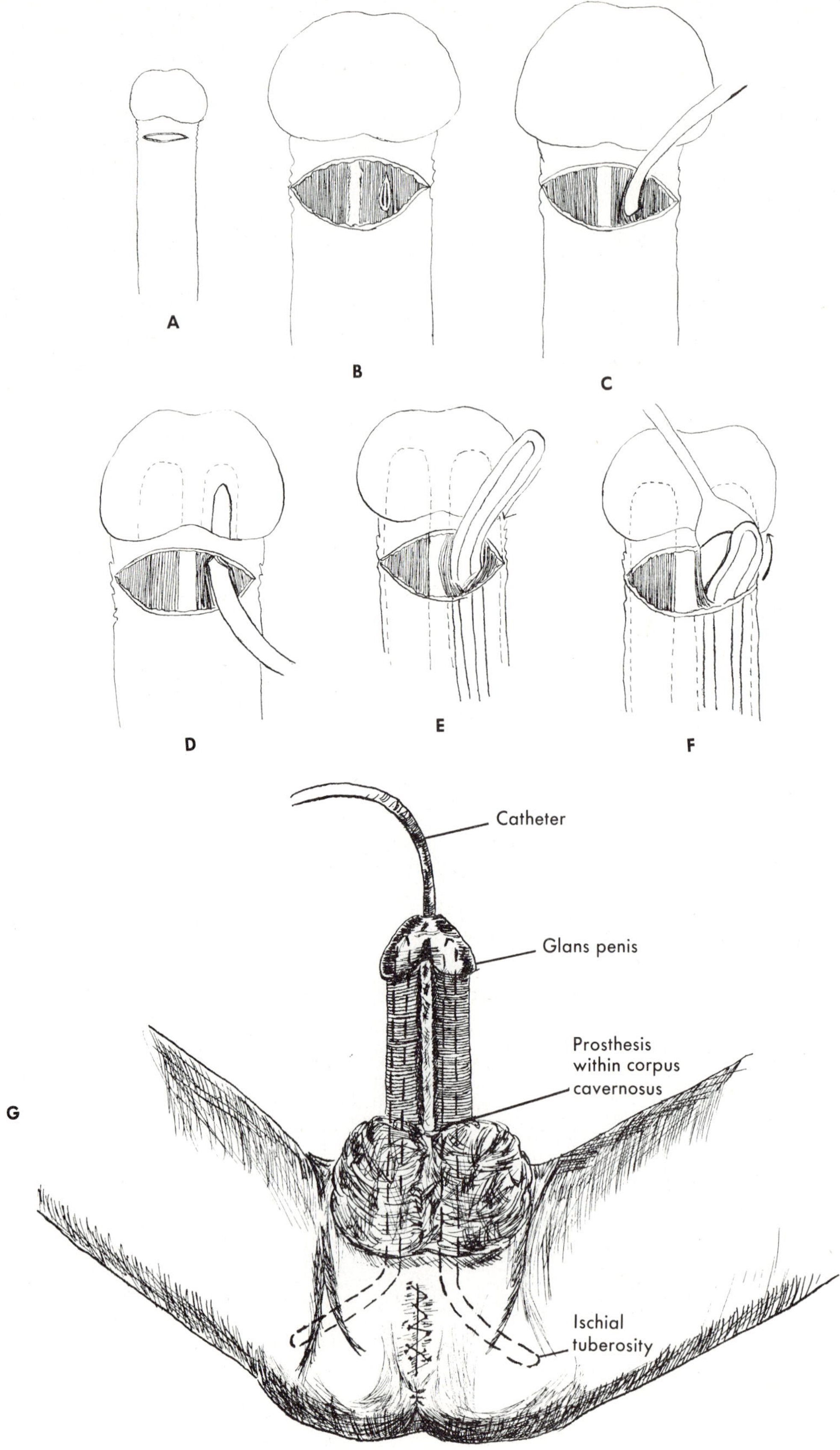

Fig. 15-40. Penile implant. **A,** Hemicircular incision of dorsal surface of penis. **B,** Opening of tunica albuginea. **C,** Dilatation of corpus down to crura. **D,** Dilatation down glans. **E,** Prosthesis being inserted. **F,** Distal prosthesis tip inserted with eyelid retractor to lift corpus. **G,** Penile prostheses in place.

OPERATIONS ON THE SCROTUM

Hydrocelectomy

Definition. Excision of the tunica vaginalis of the testis to remove an enlarged, fluid-filled sac.

Considerations. A hydrocele is an abnormal accumulation of fluid within the scrotum. The fluid is contained within the tunica vaginalis. Excessive secretion or accumulation of hydrocele fluid may be the result of infection or trauma.

Setup and preparation of the patient. The patient is placed in the supine position (Chapter 6). Preparation and draping of the patient include routine cleansing of the external genitals and draping of the patient with a fenestrated sheet. A minor instrument set is required, including a small Penrose drain, 30-ml syringe, 20-gauge 2-inch aspirating needle, and suspensory dressing.

Operative procedure

1. An anterolateral incision is made in the skin of the scrotum over the hydrocele mass by a scalpel with a no. 20 blade. Bleeding is controlled with Crile hemostats, and vessels are ligated with no. 3-0 plain gut ligatures (Fig. 15-41, *A*).

2. Small retractors may be placed, after which the fascial layers are incised to expose the tunica vaginalis (Fig. 15-41, *B*). With fine scissors, forceps, and blunt dissection, the hydrocele is dissected free and delivered (Fig. 15-41, *C*). The sac is opened, and fluid contents aspirated.

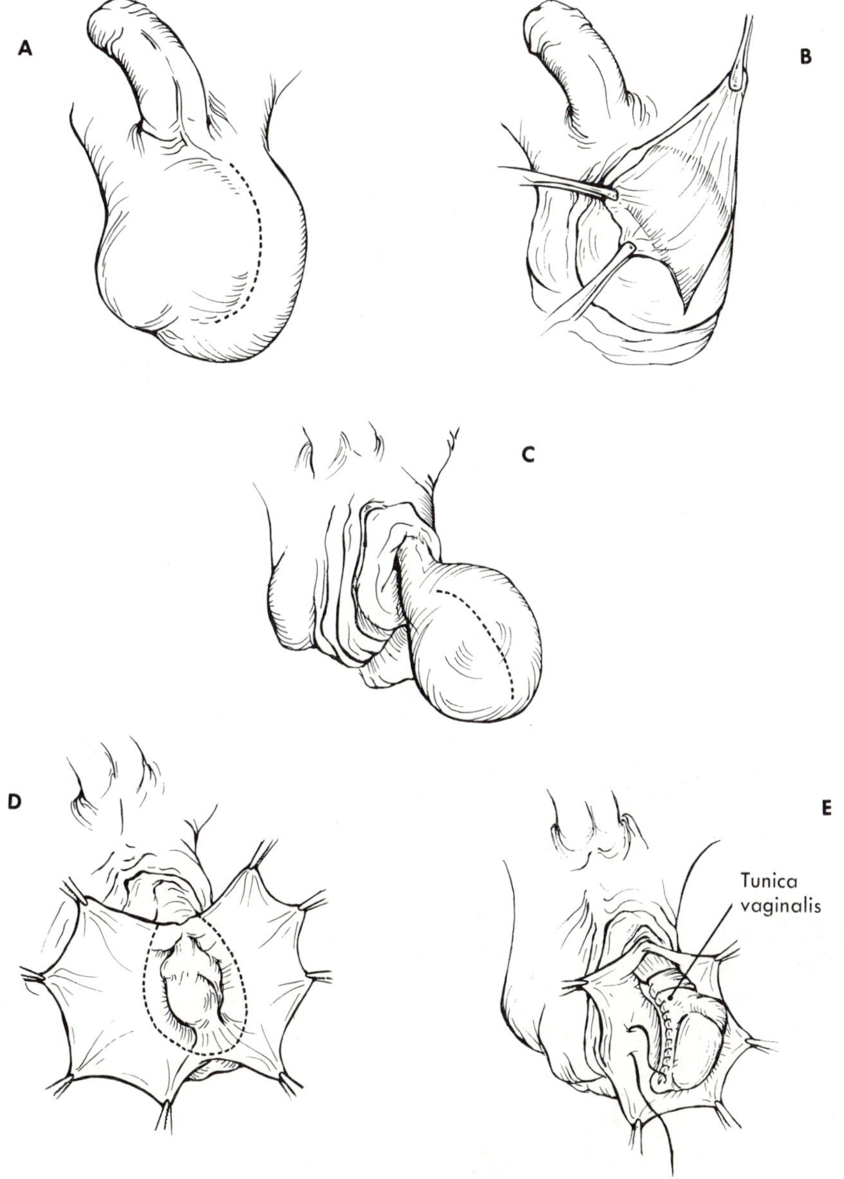

Fig. 15-41. Hydrocelectomy. (From Dodson, A.I.: Urological surgery, ed. 4, St. Louis, 1970, The C.V. Mosby Co.)

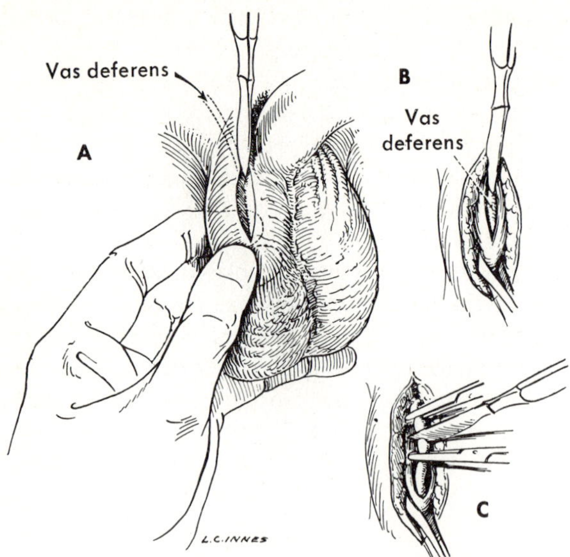

Fig. 15-42. Vasectomy (vas ligation). **A,** Vas grasped between surgeon's thumb in front and first and second fingers behind. Incision 2 cm long made over vas. **B,** Vas grasped with Allis clamp, and incision deepened into it. **C,** Vas clamped with two hemostats and incised between them. (From Barnes, R.W., and Hadley, H.L.: Urological practice, St. Louis, The C.V. Mosby Co.)

3. The sac is inverted so that it surrounds the testis, epididymis, and distal cord. Excess tunica vaginalis is excised, and the edges of the remaining tunica sutured with a continuous no. 4-0 chromic suture. The testicle is "bottled" by the inverted tunica vaginalis, and the testis may then be returned to the sac (Fig. 15-41, *D* and *E*).

4. A Penrose drain is placed within the scrotum and brought out through a stab wound in the most dependent portion of the scrotum. The scrotal incision is closed in layers with no. 3-0 chromic sutures. The skin is closed with interrupted no. 4-0 chromic sutures. A fluff compression dressing contained in a scrotal support aids in reducing postoperative scrotal edema.

Vasectomy

Definition. Excision of a section of the vas deferens.

Considerations. Vas ligation, or vasectomy, involves interruption of the vas deferens (Fig. 15-42). The operation is performed electively as a permanent method of sterilization and also before prostatectomy to prevent possible postoperative bacterial epididymitis. Because of the serious implications of permanent sterilization, particular attention must be paid to acquiring informed consent.

Setup and preparation of the patient. The patient usually lies in the supine position, although the operation may be performed in the lithotomy position before transurethral prostatectomy. The procedure may be accomplished under local or general anesthesia. A minor instrument set, collodion dressing, and scrotal suspensory are needed.

Operative procedure

1. The vas is located by digital palpation of the upper part of the scrotum. A small incision is made in the skin over the vas (Fig. 15-42, *A*).

2. An Allis clamp is inserted into the scrotal incision to grasp the vas and deliver it to the surface of the wound (Fig. 15-42, *B*). The vas is denuded of surrounding tissues, and straight clamps are placed on either side of the Allis forceps to crush the vas.

3. The vas is cut between the clamps (Fig. 15-42, *C*), and a section is removed. The cut ends are ligated with no. 0 chromic ties. The cut ends of the vas may also be fulgurated by electrocautery, and the severed ends of the vas are allowed to return to the scrotum.

4. The skin incision is closed with no. 4-0 chromic interrupted sutures. The patient is instructed to wear a scrotal support of the appropriate size for approximately 3 to 4 days.

Epididymectomy

Definition. Excision of the epididymis from the testis.

Considerations. Epididymectomy is rarely performed today but may be indicated to treat degenerative cystic disease or fungating tuberculous infection of the epididymis.

Setup and preparation of the patient. The patient is placed in the supine position with the legs slightly abducted. A general anesthetic is required. Setup is as described for hydrocelectomy, plus an electrosurgical unit, if desired.

Operative procedure

1. An anterolateral incision is made over the testis in the scrotum to expose the tunica vaginalis.

2. The tunica is incised to expose the testis and overlying epididymis.

3. An incision is made between the upper pole of the epididymis, which is then sharply dissected from the testis. A portion of the vas deferens may also be excised.

4. Bleeding is controlled by electrocautery and chromic ties. The skin wound is closed with no. 4-0 chromic sutures. A small Penrose drain may be left intrascrotally for 24 to 48 hours.

Spermatocelectomy

Definition. Removal of a spermatocele.

Considerations. A spermatocele, a lobulated intrascrotal cystic mass attached to the upper pole of the epididymis, is usually caused by an obstruction of the tubular system that conveys the sperm. An epididymovasostomy (side-to-side anastomosis between the vas deferens and the epididymis) may be attempted after excision of the mass to maintain continuity of the ductal system. Usually, this type of procedure requires the operative microscope for an accurate anastomosis.

Setup and preparation of the patient. As described for hydrocelectomy, plus the following:

1 Syringe, 10 ml
1 Needle, blunt, no. 20
Methylene blue solution
Hydrogen peroxide
Polyethylene tubing, 20 Fr or other size as desired
Silk sutures or fine wire
Chromic sutures, no. 4-0 or 5-0, on fine plastic curved needles
Lead shot
Isotonic saline solution
Microscope and slides, if desired

Operative procedure

1. The mass is approached through a scrotal incision as described for hydrocelectomy (Fig. 15-41).

2. The structures of the testis and spermatic cord are identified (Fig. 15-8), and the cystic structure is dissected free. Bleeding is controlled with electrocautery.

3. The wound is closed and dressed as described for hydrocelectomy.

Varicocelectomy

Definition. High ligation of the gonadal veins of the testes.

Considerations. Varicocelectomy is done to reduce congestion of the venous plexus around the testes and to improve spermatogenesis. When surgery for this condition was first devised 70 years ago, the veins of the pampiniform plexus were ligated and divided individually.

This condition occurs more frequently on the left side, since the gonadal vein of the left testis unites retroperitoneally with the renal vein at a 90-degree angle and is consequently under greater back pressure. As a result of this unusual back pressure, the pampiniform plexus of the spermatic cord becomes tortuous and engorged, resembling what is frequently referred to as a "bag of worms."

Setup and preparation of the patient. As described for hydrocelectomy.

Operative procedure

1. The incision may be made low in the inguinal canal or in the upper portion of the scrotum. The structures of the spermatic cord are identified, and the vessels dissected free from the vas deferens (Fig. 15-43, *A*).

2. The abnormal vessels in the inguinal canal are clamped and ligated (Fig. 15-43, *B*). The redundant portions are excised. To support the testicle, the remaining structures are sutured either to the external oblique fascia above the external inguinal ring or to the internal oblique muscle near the inguinal ring, depending on the approach used (Fig. 15-43, *C*).

3. A Penrose drain may be placed. The incision is closed in layers.

Orchiectomy

Definition. Removal of the testis or testes.

Considerations. Removal of both testes is castration and renders the patient sterile and deficient of the hormone *testosterone,* which is responsible for development of secondary sexual characteristics and potency. Because of legal implications, this operation, like vasectomy, requires particular attention in acquiring informed consent for surgery. Bilateral orchiectomy is usually performed to control symptomatic metastatic carcinoma of the prostate gland. A unilateral orchiectomy may be indicated because of testicular cancer, trauma, or infection. In many situations, a prosthesis may be implanted for cosmetic or psychological reasons. Prostheses are usually made of silicone rubber gel to approximate normal testicular consistency.

Setup and preparation of the patient. The patient is placed in the supine position and draped according to hospital procedure. A minor instrument setup is required, plus a testicular prosthesis, if specified.

Operative procedure

1A. For benign conditions, the incision is made over the anterolateral surface of the midportion of the scrotum. The skin incision is carried through the subcutaneous and fascial layers through the tunica vaginalis, exposing the testicle. Retractors are placed, and bleeding vessels are clamped and tied. The spermatic cord is divided into two or three vascular bundles. Each vascular bundle is double-clamped, cut, and ligated—first with no. 0 chromic suture ligature and then with a proximal free no. 0 chromic tie. The vas is separately ligated with a no. 0 chromic tie. The testis is removed.

1B. For malignant conditions, the incision is begun just above the internal ring, extending downward and inward over the inguinal canal to the external inguinal ring.

The inguinal canal is exposed, and the spermatic cord is dissected free, cross-clamped, and divided into vascular bundles at the internal ring. Gentle forward traction is applied to the cord, which is dissected from its bed. The testis is everted into the wound from the scrotum and excised.

2. Bleeding is controlled with electrocautery. A small Penrose drain may be placed in the empty hemiscrotum, if desired. The external oblique fascia is reapproximated with no. 2-0 chromic interrupted sutures. Subcutaneous tissue, including Scarpa's fascia, is closed with no. 4-0 chromic catgut sutures. The skin is reapproximated with stainless steel surgical staples.

Radical lymphadenectomy

Definition. Bilateral resection of retroperitoneal lymph nodes. Dissection usually includes lymph nodes, channels, and fat around both renal pedicles, the vena cava, and the aorta, including the bifurcation of the aorta.

Considerations. Lymph node dissection is performed for treatment of nonseminomatous testicular tumors. The procedure is performed after radical inguinal orchiectomy.

Setup and preparation of the patient. The patient is placed in the supine position. If the dissection is unilateral, the patient is supine with the operative side tilted upward. Routine skin preparation from nipples to midthigh and draping procedures are carried out. Long fine dissection instruments along with basic laparotomy instruments are required.

Operative procedure

1. A midline abdominal incision is made from the xiphoid process to the symphysis pubis. The abdominal contents are explored to determine the degree of gross nodal involvement. The colon is either packed within the abdominal cavity or mobilized and kept moist outside the abdomen.

2. The posterior peritoneum is opened between the aorta and the vena cava.

3. By blunt and sharp dissection, the lymphatic structures and fat are removed en bloc from around both renal pedicles, the vena cava, and the aorta from above the renal hilum to beyond the bifurcation of the iliac vessels on the side of the original testicular neoplasm.

4. The spermatic vessels of the affected side are re-

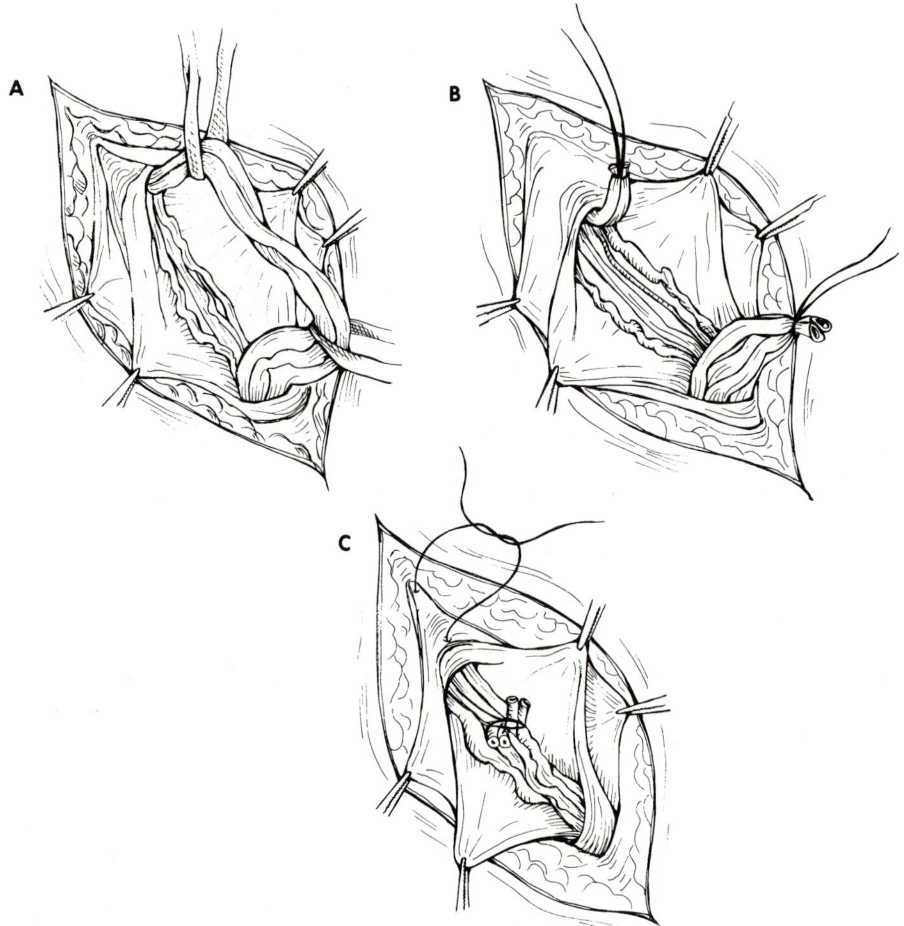

Fig. 15-43. Varicocelectomy. (Adapted from Dodson, A.I.: Urological surgery, ed. 4, St. Louis, 1970, The C.V. Mosby Co.)

moved down to and including the stump of the previous orchiectomy.

5. The inferior mesenteric artery may be sacrificed if technically necessary, but the superior mesenteric artery is not disturbed. The ureter on the affected side is skeletonized to remove any perilymphatic tissue.

6. If reperitonealization is desired, the posterior peritoneum is closed with a no. 2-0 chromic continuous suture. The viscera are returned to the abdominal cavity, and the wound is closed with a one-layer no. 0 Prolene interrupted suture, usually without placement of a drain.

Orchiopexy

Definition. Surgical placement and fixation of the testicle in a normal anatomical position in the scrotal sac.

Considerations. If the testis fails to descend into the scrotum during gestation, it is considered undescended. A truly undescended testis becomes arrested somewhere along its normal path of descent. If it is palpable in a position other than its normal path of descent, its position is considered to be ectopic.

A retractile testis is one in which the testis has fully descended into the scrotum but that retracts out of the scrotum as a result of contraction of the cremaster muscle. Gentle manipulation allows replacement of the testis in the most dependent portion of the scrotum. Retractile testes require no surgical or hormonal treatment.

All testes that are undescended after 1 year, including those which are unresponsive to hormone injections, require surgical placement in the scrotum for optimum maturation.

Setup and preparation of the patient. As described for hydrocelectomy. General anesthesia is required. Preparation and draping include the lower abdomen, genitals, and thighs. Since this operation is usually performed on children, a setup containing small, delicate instruments and sutures is required.

Operative procedure

1. An inguinal incision is generally employed for exploration of undescended testes (Fig. 15-44, *A*). Most undescended testes are located in the superficial inguinal pouch or inguinal canal.

2. The external oblique aponeurosis is opened through the external inguinal ring, exposing the inguinal canal; the gubernacular attachments of the undescended testis are freed (Fig. 15-44, *B*).

3. All adhesions and the associated inguinal hernial sac are freed to lengthen the cord. The hernia sac is transected, twisted, and ligated with sutures (Fig. 15-44, *C*).

4. A scrotal pocket is created (Fig. 15-44, *D*), and the testis is anchored in the scrotum in a normal anatomical position (Fig. 15-44, *E*).

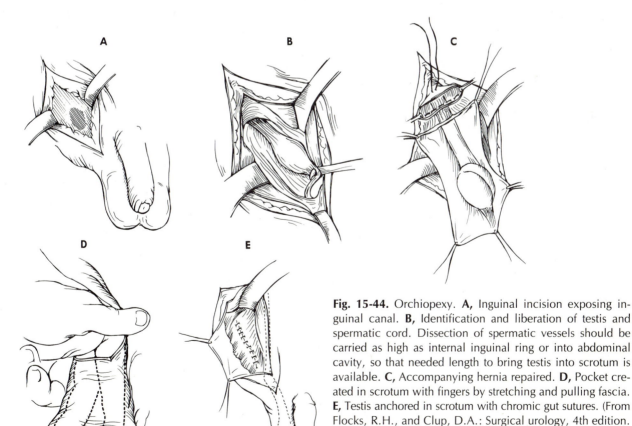

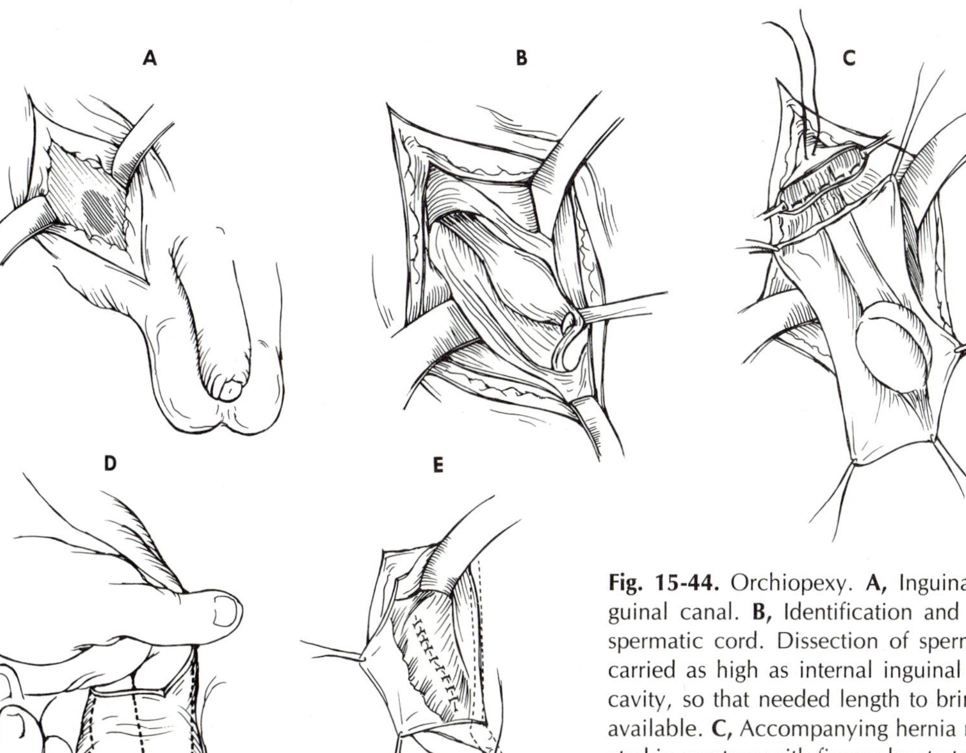

Fig. 15-44. Orchiopexy. **A,** Inguinal incision exposing inguinal canal. **B,** Identification and liberation of testis and spermatic cord. Dissection of spermatic vessels should be carried as high as internal inguinal ring or into abdominal cavity, so that needed length to bring testis into scrotum is available. **C,** Accompanying hernia repaired. **D,** Pocket created in scrotum with fingers by stretching and pulling fascia. **E,** Testis anchored in scrotum with chromic gut sutures. (From Flocks, R.H., and Clup, D.A.: Surgical urology, 4th edition. Copyright © 1975 by Year Book Medical Publishers, Inc., Chicago. Used by permission.)

Orchiopexy may be accomplished by several surgical methods. The dependent portion of the undescended testis may be sutured to the base of the scrotum with absorbable or nonabsorbable sutures brought out through the scrotal wall and tied over a peanut dissector or pledget. The most popular method used is anchoring the testis into a dissected subdartos pouch. In this procedure a small midtransverse scrotal incision is made, and space between the skin and the dartos muscle dissected. The testis is then brought through a small hole in the dartos into the subdartos pouch and anchored in position by the traction suture. The overlying skin of the subdartos pouch is closed with fine catgut. The inguinal incision is repaired in layers with no. 3-0 chromic sutures. The skin is closed with a subcuticular suture; collodion and Steri-strips are used for dressing.

OPEN OPERATIONS ON THE PROSTATE GLAND

Considerations. Glandular hyperplasia of the prostatic urethra usually manifests itself after the age of 55. Prostatic enlargement may occur in one or more lobes of the prostate but most frequently occurs in the lateral or median lobes. Progressive growth of the hyperplastic gland compresses the remaining normal prostatic tissue, forming what is called a "surgical capsule." Slowly, the growth of adenomatous tissue encroaches on the prostatic urethral lumen, causing obstruction to urinary outflow.

Prostatic enlargement may be benign or malignant. In benign prostatic hypertrophy, only the periurethral adenomatous portion of the gland is removed (Fig. 15-8). Operable prostatic malignancy requires radical prostatectomy, which includes removal of the entire prostate gland along with the seminal vesicles. Before prostatic surgery, it is necessary to obtain a determination of the prostatic serum acid phosphatase level. If the prostatic fraction of this test is elevated, the patient probably has metastatic carcinoma of the prostate. In such instances, a bone scan and skeletal survey will be necessary for confirmation. If these tests are negative, however, the possibility of hemolytic anemia, Gaucher's disease, or Paget's disease of the bone must be considered. If these tests are positive, a transrectal needle biopsy or Franzen transrectal aspiration biopsy may be performed to confirm the diagnosis.

Three open approaches are possible in removing the benign hyperplastic obstructive prostate gland: the retropubic prostatectomy, the suprapubic prostatectomy, and the perineal prostatectomy. An endoscopic (closed) approach, the transurethral prostatectomy, may be employed. If the prostate gland is cancerous, a radical retropubic or radical perineal prostatectomy is performed.

Several factors must be taken into account to determine the best route for removal of the prostatic obstruction: (1) the age and medical condition of the patient, (2) the size of the gland and location of the pathological condition, and (3) the presence of associated medical disease.

Retropubic prostatectomy

Definition. Enucleation of hypertrophic prostatic tissue through an incision in the anterior prostatic capsule by an extravesical approach.

Considerations. The retropubic approach is the most frequently used technique for open prostatectomy. It offers ideal exposure to the prostate bed and vesical neck; hence an opportunity for excellent hemostasis is afforded, and, consequently, intraoperative and postoperative bleeding is minimized.

Setup and preparation of the patient. The patient is placed in a supine and slight Trendelenburg position with a bolster under the pelvis and the legs slightly abducted. Routine skin preparation is carried out. Electrosurgery is usually employed.

The draping procedure conforms to individual operating room policy. Following is a suggested method for draping:

1. The first towel with a cuff is placed under the scrotum.
2. The next three towels are placed around the lower abdominal incision site, followed by a sterile plastic sheet, which is placed from the scrotum to the bottom of the table.
3. A bottom sheet, laparotomy sheet, and arm drape follow.
4. A fifth towel, folded in half, is placed over the penis and scrotum below the retropubic incision site and secured with two towel clamps.

The instrument setup includes a basic laparotomy set and bladder and prostatic instruments (Figs. 15-45 and 15-46). The following supplies should be readily available:

Jackson-Pratt or 1-inch Penrose drains
Surgilube, sterile
Syringe, 30 ml
Urinary drainage set
Robinson coude catheter, no. 18 Fr
Foley catheter, no. 22 or 24, 30-cc balloon
Pezzer or Malecot catheter

Operative procedure

1. Through a Pfannenstiel incision, the anterior rectus sheath is incised along with portions of the internal and external oblique muscles. The rectus abdominis muscles are retracted laterally to expose the space of Retzius.
2. The anterior portion of the prostatic capsule is incised transversely (Fig. 15-47, *A*), and the prostatic adenoma may be dissected or finger enucleated from the "surgical capsule" (Fig. 15-47, *B*).
3. Care is taken to place hemostatic chromic sutures at the 5 and 7 o'clock positions, encompassing the vesical neck and prostatic capsule in order to ligate the primary blood supply to the prostate (Fig. 15-47, *C*). Other bleeding points within the capsule may be suture ligated with no. 2-0 chromic sutures.

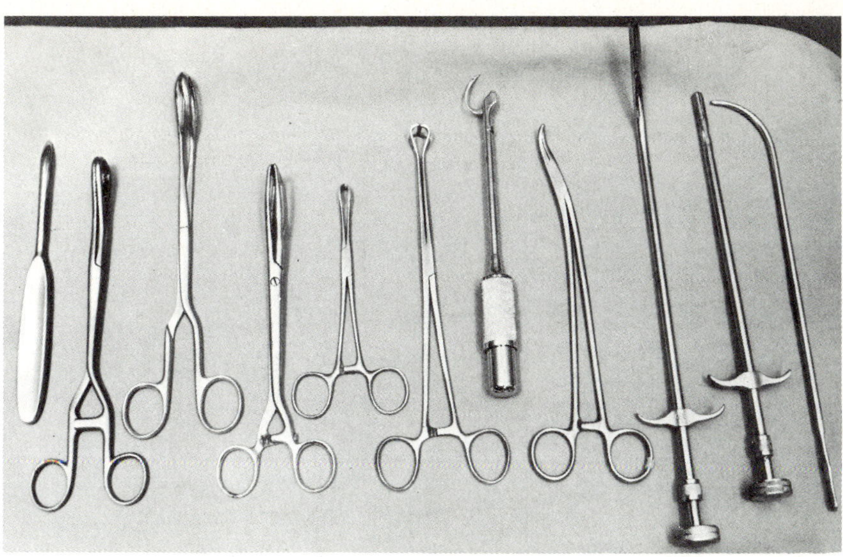

Fig. 15-45. Prostatic instruments. *Left to right,* Prostatic enucleator, prostatic lobe forceps, Leahy clamp, long Babcock forceps, boomerang, Heaney needle holder, Lowsley prostatic tractors, urethral sound.

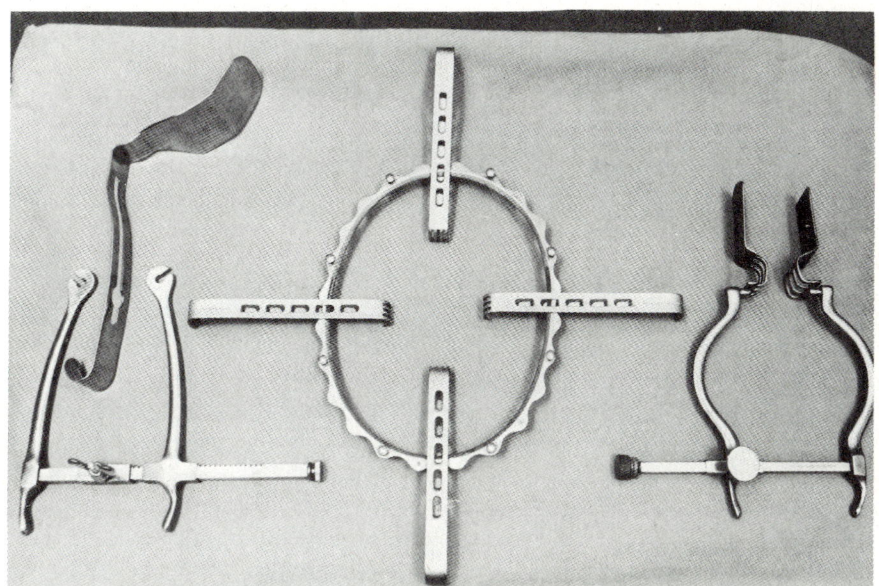

Fig. 15-46. Retractors for prostatectomy. *Left to right,* Millin retropubic bladder retractor, Dennis-Brown ring retractor (perineal), Mason-Judd bladder retractor (suprapubic).

4. A Foley catheter is inserted in the urethra and through the bladder neck and inflated within the bladder. Frequently, a three-way catheter is used to afford continuous bladder irrigation.

5. The prostatic capsule incision is closed with either a continuous or an interrupted no. 0 chromic suture (Fig. 15-47, *D*). A Penrose drain is placed in the space of Retzius and brought out through the fascia and skin through a separate stab incision. The abdominal incision is then closed in layers, and the wound is dressed.

6. If continuous bladder irrigation is to be used, normal saline solution irrigation is initiated through a 4000-ml closed irrigation system.

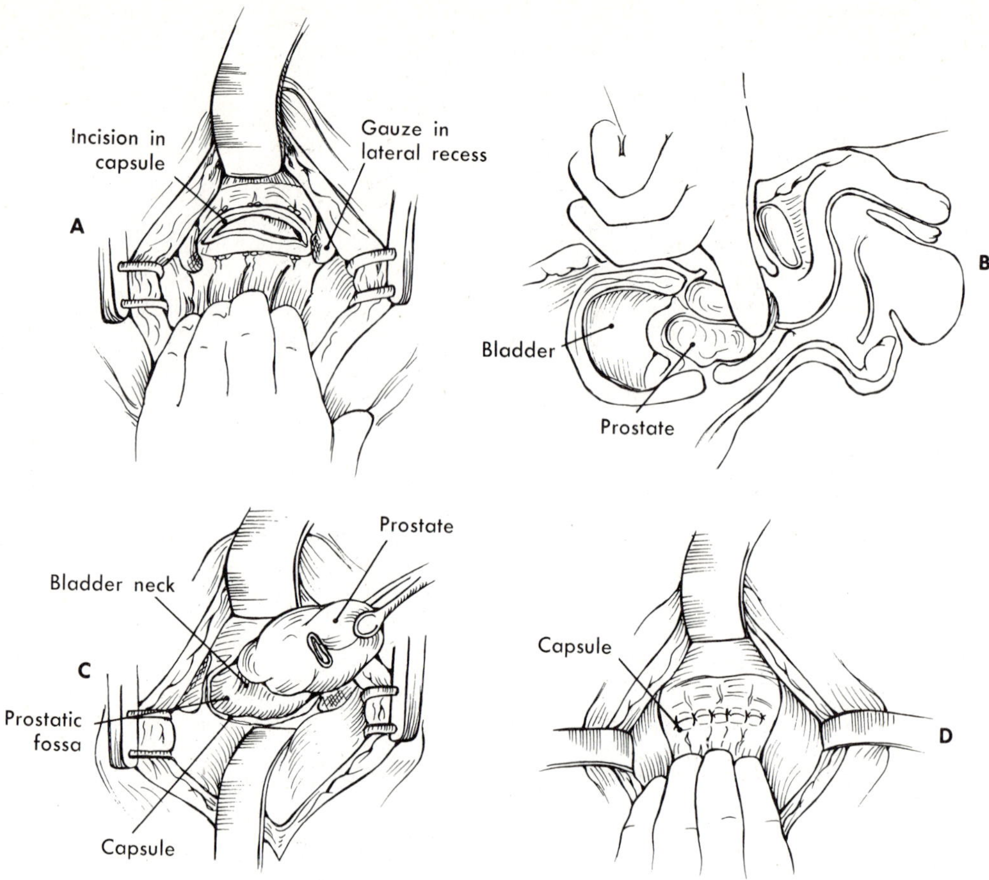

Fig. 15-47. Retropubic prostatectomy. (Adapted from Dodson, A.I.: Urological surgery, ed. 4, St. Louis, 1970, The C.V. Mosby Co.)

Suprapubic prostatectomy

Definition. Removal, by a suprapubic approach, of benign periurethral glandular tissue obstructing the outlet of the urinary tract.

Considerations. One of the advantages of the suprapubic approach is that it allows access to surgical correction of any existing bladder condition such as vesical calculi or vesical diverticula.

Control of bleeding is a major consideration in any prostatectomy and is one disadvantage of the suprapubic approach. Since the prostate is located beneath the symphysis pubis, ligation of bleeding capsular vessels is exceedingly difficult. However, control of hemmorrhage and replacement of blood loss coupled with skilled nursing care and early mobilization of the patient has greatly minimized complications.

Setup and preparation of the patient. Spinal, epidural, or general anesthesia are equally acceptable. The patient is placed in a slight Trendelenburg position with a bolster under the buttocks and the legs abducted. Skin preparation, draping, and instrumentation are as described for retropubic prostatectomy. Bilateral vasectomy is frequently considered to reduce the incidence of postoperative epididymo-orchitis.

Operative procedure

1. Bilateral vasectomy may be performed to decrease the postoperative incidence of epididymitis and orchitis. A meatotomy may also be required if the penile meatus is too small to accommodate a Foley catheter.
2. A Robinson catheter is inserted through the urethra into the bladder, and the bladder inflated with a preferred irrigating fluid. This maneuver facilitates identification of the bladder.
3. A transverse lower abdominal incision is made through the skin and the two layers of superficial fascia. The external and internal oblique muscles are cut along the lines of the original incision. Bleeding vessels are clamped, cauterized, or tied with fine plain catgut ties on a roll.
4. The rectus muscles are separated in the midline and retracted laterally.
5. The bladder is opened at the dome with a scalpel. Liquid contents are aspirated, and the bladder incision enlarged. The bladder is visually and manually explored for calculi, a tumor, or diverticuli.

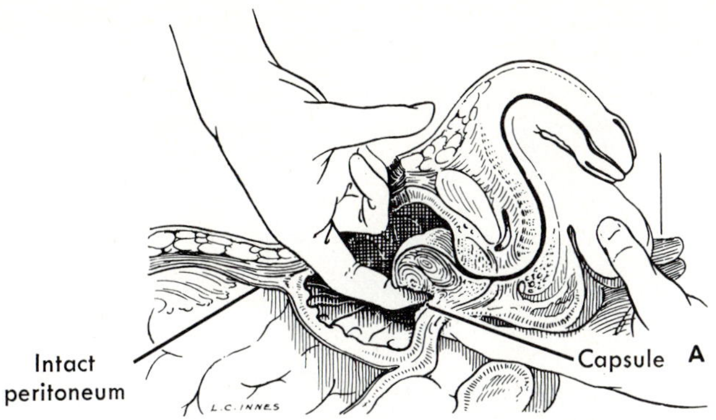

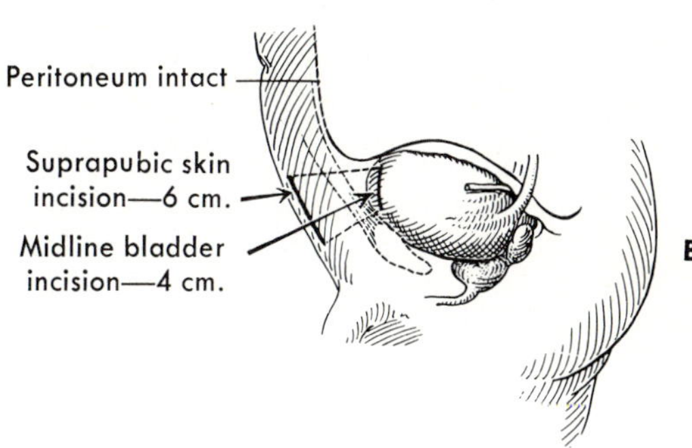

Fig. 15-48. A, Enucleation of prostate by suprapubic approach. **B,** Anatomical delineation. (From Barnes, R.W., and Hadley, H.L.: Urological practice, St. Louis, The C.V. Mosby Co.)

6. The tip of the index finger of the operating hand is inserted through the vesical neck into the prostatic urethra, and the adenomatous tissue is enucleated. If difficulty is experienced with the enucleation, a finger may be placed in the rectum to elevate the prostate gland (Fig. 15-48). This is accomplished with the use of a sterile rectal sheath.

7. After enucleation is completed, attention is directed to maintaining good hemostasis. This is achieved by suture ligation of the vesical neck at the 5 and 7 o'clock positions. Other significant bleeding points may also be ligated.

8. A suprapubic catheter of the urologist's choice is placed into the bladder lumen through a small stab incision. A no. 22 or 24 Fr three-way Foley catheter with a 30-cc balloon is inserted into the urethra, and the balloon inflated to a size that will prevent the catheter from falling or being pulled into the prostatic fossa (Fig. 15-49). The cystostomy incision is then closed with interrupted no. 0 chromic sutures. A 1-inch Penrose drain is left along the cystotomy incision, brought out through a separate stab wound, and secured to the skin with a silk suture. The muscles, fascia, and subcutaneous tissues are closed in layers, and a dressing is applied.

9. Normal saline irrigation solution is connected to the Foley catheter to provide through and through irrigation to the bladder to reduce clot formation and maintain catheter patency. Continuous irrigation may be initiated during closure.

Perineal prostatectomy

Definition. Removal of a prostatic adenoma through a perineal approach. Radical perineal excision for prostatic carcinoma may also be performed by the perineal approach and involves removal of the entire gland, its capsule, and seminal vesicles.

Considerations. A perineal approach to the prostate gland is most suitable when open prostatic biopsy is desired and, after receiving pathological confirmation, radical excision is to follow. Other advantages include preservation of the bladder neck, improved urethrovesical anastomosis, and easier control of bleeding. Following are several surgical disadvantages:

1. Inability to perform biopsy of the iliac and obturator nodes for extension of disease
2. Incidence of urinary incontinence compatible with other radical prostatic procedures
3. Loss of sexual potency
4. Urethrorectal fistulas

Setup and preparation of the patient. The patient is placed in an exaggerated lithotomy position with a bolster beneath the sacrum, placing the perineum as parallel to the operating table as possible. Stirrups should be well padded to protect the popliteal fossa. Routine skin preparation is carried out. Special draping is as follows:

1. A towel folded in half is placed over the pubic area.

2. Two leggings, with points down, are placed over the legs.

3. One towel folded in half (lengthwise) is placed below the anus.

4. A large sheet open fully with a large cuff is placed across from one stirrup to the other and secured by towel clamps.

5. A laparatomy sheet follows, with the short end to the floor.

6. A large sheet is placed over each leg.

7. One towel is folded in half and then in thirds and attached to a drape made to hold cautery and suction.

The instrument setup is as described for suprapubic prostatectomy, omitting abdominal self-retaining retractors and adding the following:

Curved and straight Lowsley tractors (Fig. 15-50)
Roux retractors
Jackson retractors, short and long blades
Doyen vaginal retractors
Perineal prostatic retractors (Fig. 15-51)
Sauerbrach retractors, narrow and wide

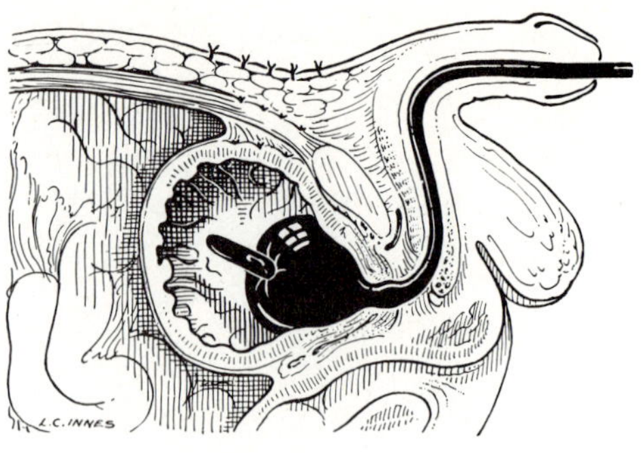

Fig. 15-49. Hemostatic bag (Foley), which can be deflated and removed through urethra. It is used after most prostatectomies by any approach. (From Barnes, R.W., and Hadley, H.L.: Urological practice, St. Louis, The C.V. Mosby Co.)

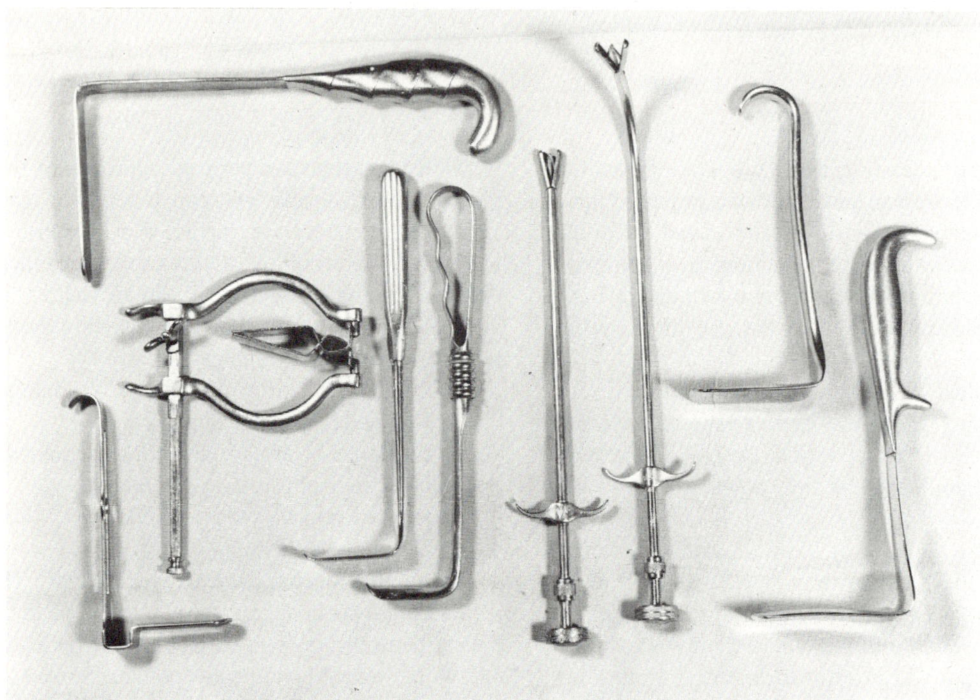

Fig. 15-50. Perineal and suprapubic prostatectomy instruments.

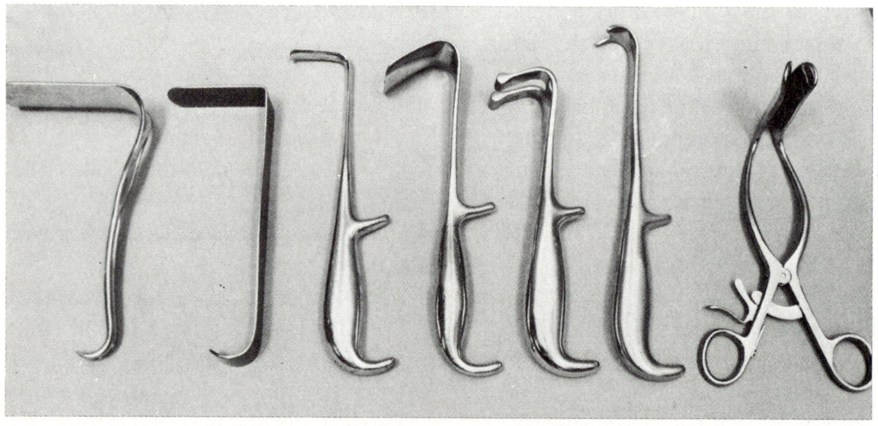

Fig. 15-51. Perineal prostatectomy retractors. *Left to right,* Three prostatic lateral retractors, prostatic anterior retractor, two prostatic bifurcated retractors, self-retaining retractor.

Operative procedure

1. A curved Lowsley tractor (Fig. 15-45) is placed through the urethra into the bladder and held back by the second assistant, causing the prostate to be pushed down toward the perineum.

2. An inverted U-shaped incision is made from one ischial tuberosity to another, curving just anterior to the anus (Fig. 15-52, *A*).

3. The posterior drapes are clipped to the posterior lip of the incision, draping the anus out of the sterile field.

4. Subcutaneous bleeders are clamped with straight mosquitoes and cauterized or tied with no. 3-0 plain catgut.

5. The central tendon is isolated, clamped, and cut, and the levator ani muscle exposed and retracted superiorly (Fig. 15-52, *B*). The prostate gland is then exposed.

6. The prostate may be biopsied for pathological confirmation. If the results are negative, the prostatic adenoma is removed. If the frozen section reveals malignancy, the urologist may choose to do a radical prostatectomy at this time.

7. If simple enucleation is to be performed, the curved Lowsley tractor is removed from the urethra, and the straight Lowsley inserted into the incision (Fig. 15-52, *C* and *D*).

8. Two empty sponge sticks are used to grasp the prostatic lobes. The straight Lowsley tractor is removed, and the adenoma is manually enucleated from the "surgical capsule" (Fig. 15-52, *E*).

9. A no. 22 Foley catheter with a 30-cc balloon is inserted through the urethra into the bladder (Fig. 15-52, *F*).

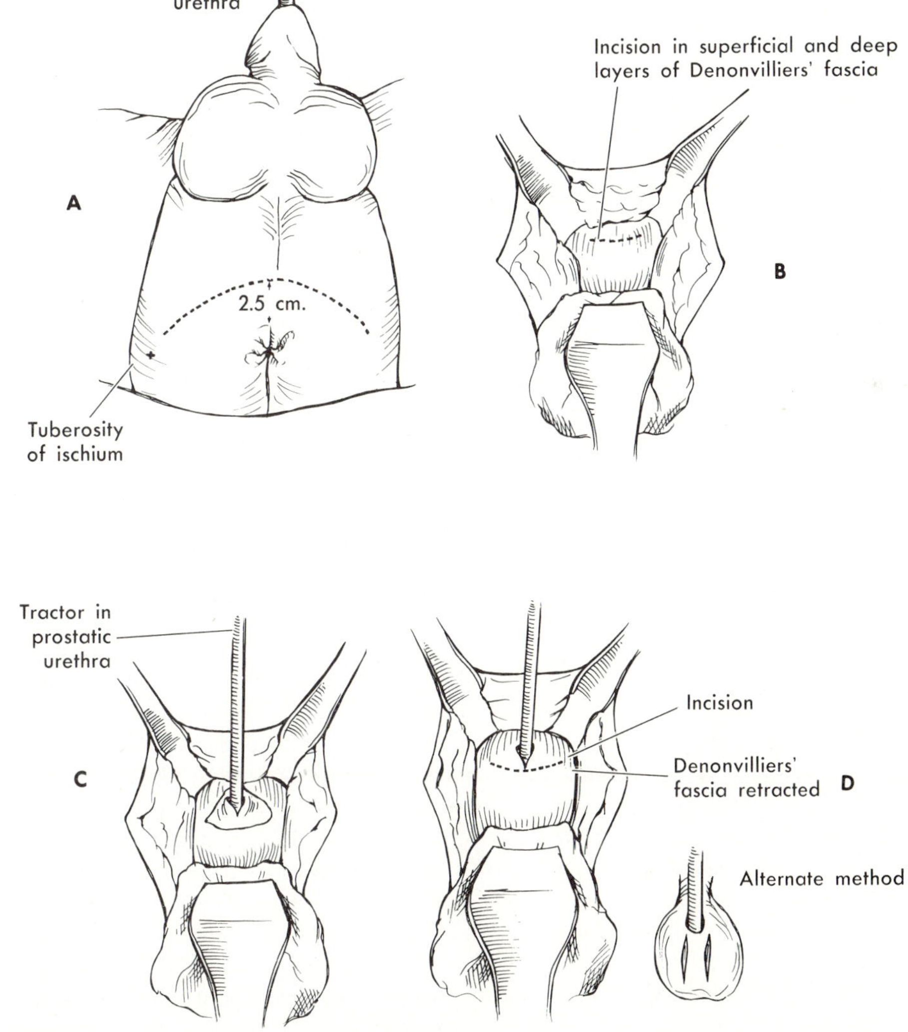

Fig. 15-52. Perineal prostatectomy. **A,** Proposed incisional site. **B,** Rectourethral muscle has been incised and pushed downward from central tendon, and levator ani muscles on each side have been divided; incision in superficial and deep layers of Denonvilliers' fascia is shown. **C,** Urethrotomy in prostatic urethra. **D,** Incision in prostatic capsule. *Continued.*

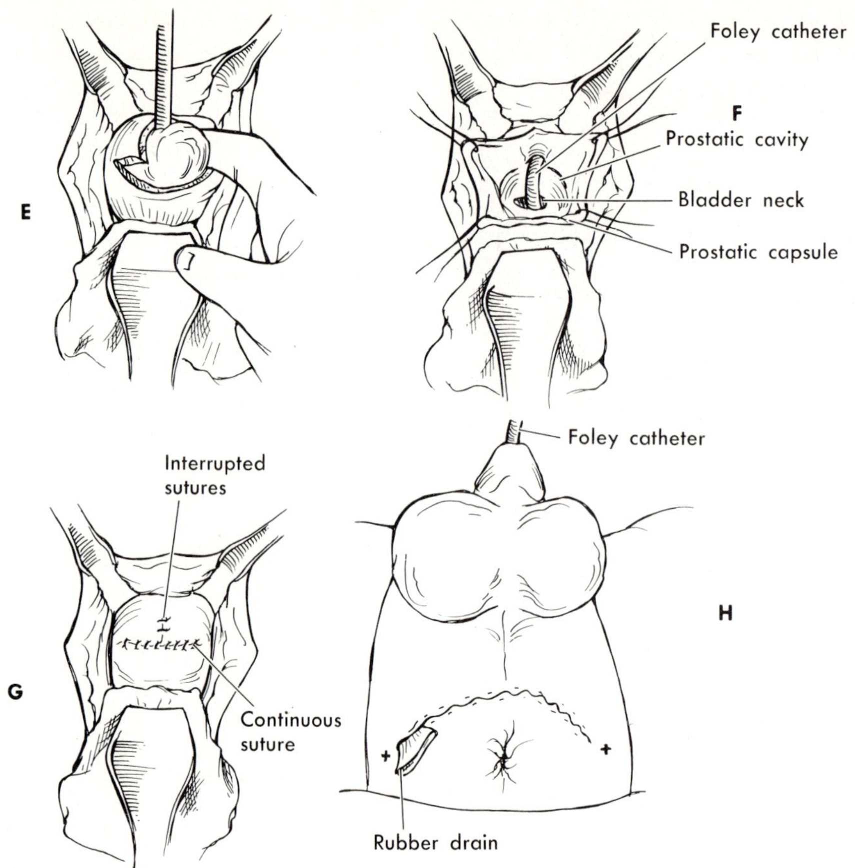

Fig. 15-52, cont'd. E, Enucleating entire prostate with aid of finger. **F,** Catheter in urethra and bladder; exposure of prostatic bed. **G,** Closure of inverted-T incisions. **H,** Closure of perineal wounds. (Adapted from Dodson, A.I.: Urological surgery, ed. 4, St. Louis, 1970, The C.V. Mosby Co.)

10. The capsulotomy incision is repaired with a continuous suture of no. 0 chromic catgut (Fig. 15-52, *G*). A Penrose drain is left in place at the level of the capsulotomy incision.

11. The subcutaneous tissue is reapproximated with no. 3-0 chromic catgut. The skin incision is reapproximated with no. 2-0 silk mattress sutures (Fig. 15-52, *H*).

12. The wound is dressed with Telfa, 4 × 8–inch gauze pads, and tape.

13. A vasectomy may be performed.

OPERATIONS ON THE BLADDER

Considerations. Operations on the urinary bladder may be performed by an open abdominal incision or through the transurethral route. Special transurethral instruments such as the lithotrite may be used to manually crush vesical calculi. An electrohydraulic cystolithotriptor may be also used to fragment the stone within the bladder by using shock waves initiated by electric current (Fig. 15-53). Stones may also be removed from the bladder through a suprapubic incision (cystolithotomy). Bladder tumors, diverticula, congenital defects, or trauma may necessitate an open abdominal approach. A thorough diagnostic workup and endoscopic examination will help determine the appropriate surgical approach to be employed. Radical procedures, such as total cystectomy, are performed for the treatment of invasive carcinoma of the bladder and require permanent urinary diversion.

Setup and preparation of the patient. For most open bladder surgery the patient is placed in the supine position with a bolster under the pelvis. The Trendelenberg position may be desired, since it tilts the head down, allowing the viscera to fall cephalad. This affords excellent exposure of the pelvic organs, including the bladder. The patient is draped as described for routine suprapubic prostatectomy, using a disposable waterproof drape that is placed immediately below the bladder incision. A catheter of choice may be inserted into the urethra and the bladder distended with sterile saline at the start of surgery for easy identification. Electrosurgery may be desired. The instrument setup for open bladder operations requires a basic laparotomy set, plus the following (Fig. 15-46):

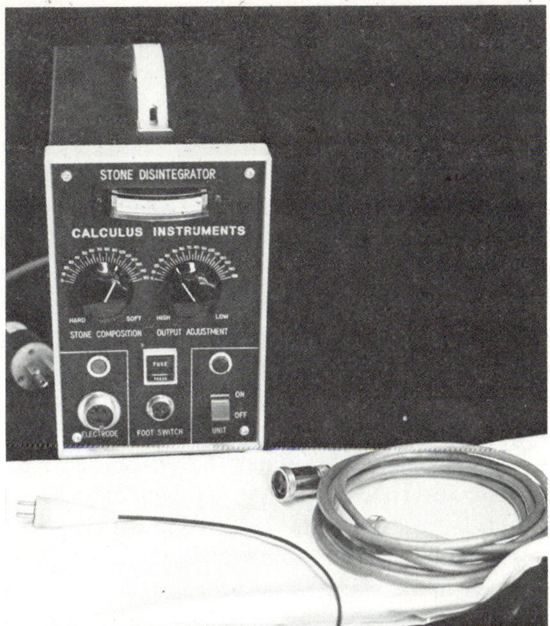

Fig. 15-53. Stone disintegrator. (Courtesy Calculus Instruments; from Morel, A., and Wise, G.J.: Urologic endoscopic procedures, ed. 2, St. Louis, 1979, The C.V. Mosby Co.)

2 Mason-Judd bladder retractors
9 Van Buren urethral sounds, sizes 14 to 30 Fr
3 Thyroid traction forceps, long
3 Thyroid traction forceps, short
2 Prostatic enucleators
2 Retropubic needle holders or other long needle holders as desired
1 Trocar (optional)
Closed wound suction or Penrose drains
Assorted Foley, Pezzar, and Malecot catheters in available sizes
Vessel loops
Catheter stylet
Electrosurgical unit

Suprapubic cystotomy and cystostomy

Definition. Opening into the urinary bladder made through a low abdominal incision for exploration and/or insertion of a drainage tube.

Operative procedure

1. A vertical or Pfannenstiel incision (transverse) is used (Fig. 15-54, *A*). The surgical approach is as described for retropubic prostatectomy.

2. The bladder is distended with saline solution, instilled with an Asepto syringe through a Robinson catheter. The dome of the bladder is then dissected free with Metzenbaum scissors. The wall of the bladder is grasped on either side of the midline with Allis clamps. Two traction sutures may be placed through the bladder wall and held with straight hemostats (Fig. 15-54, *B*). The bladder is then incised with a scalpel in a downward direction. Bleeding vessels in the bladder wall are clamped and ligated. The bladder contents are aspirated with a Poole suction.

3. The bladder opening may be extended if the bladder is to be explored for diverticula or calculi. A large-sized Malecot or Pezzar catheter is introduced into the bladder.

4. The incision is closed snugly about the catheter with chromic sutures to render the closure watertight about the cystostomy tube (Fig. 15-54, *C*). The abdominal muscle, fascia, and subcutaneous tissue are closed with chromic or Dexon, and the skin with staples or nonabsorbable material. The cystostomy tube is further secured to the skin with a heavy black silk suture to prevent it from being inadvertently dislodged from the bladder. A drain such as the Jackson-Pratt may be left in the prevesical space.

5. The wound is dressed, and the cystostomy tube connected to a straight urinary drainage system.

Trocar cystostomy

Definition. Opening of the bladder, drainage by puncture with needles or trocar, and insertion of a catheter.

Setup and preparation of the patient. A minor set of instruments, which includes the following:

Cutting instruments

1 Knife handle no. 4 with blade no. 20
2 Knife handles no. 3 with blades nos. 11 and 15
2 Mayo scissors, straight and curved, 6¼ inches
1 Metzenbaum scissors, curved, 7½ inches

Holding instruments

4 Towel clamps, 5¼ inches
4 Towel clamps, 3 inches
2 Babcock forceps, 6 inches
2 Tissue forceps with teeth, 5½ inches
2 Tissue forceps without teeth, 5½ inches
2 Adson forceps with teeth
2 Adson forceps without teeth

Clamping instruments

16 Mosquito hemostats, straight and curved, 5½ inches
8 Crile hemostats, straight and curved, 6½ inches
4 Allis forceps, 6½ inches
4 Ochsner forceps, 6½ inches

Exposing instruments

2 Cushing vein retractors
2 Green fenestrated retractors, blunt
4 Richardson retractors, 2 pair small and medium
2 Army-Navy retractors

Suturing items

2 Crile needle holders
Sutures and needles, as needed

Accessory items

1 Silver probe
1 Grooved director
1 Anthony suction tube and tubing
1 Trocar
Catheters, as required

A local anesthesia setup may be used.

Operative procedure. The skin at the site of the puncture is nicked with the scalpel, and the trocar is inserted into the bladder. The trocar obturator is withdrawn, and a catheter is passed into the bladder over a catheter guide. The cannula is withdrawn, and the catheter is sutured to the wound edges. The wound is dressed.

Suprapubic cystolithotomy

Definition. Removal of calculi from the bladder through a suprapubic incision.

Considerations. Obstruction, such as prostatic enlargement, or foreign bodies are common causes of bladder calculi and may be corrected at the time of surgery.

Setup and preparation of the patient. The instrument setup for open bladder operations is used, plus the following:

2 Millin T-shaped stone forceps
2 Millin capsule forceps
1 Lewkowitz lithotomy forceps

Repair of vesical fistulas

Definition. Repair of fistula occurring between the bladder and the intestines or vagina.

Considerations

1. Vesicointestinal fistula may be caused by ulcerative colitis, diverticulitis, or neoplasms of the colon or rectum. A colostomy proximal to the fistula may be performed to protect the repaired segment of bowel. The communicating area of bladder and bowel is totally resected. Generally, an end-to-end bowel resection is performed after excision of the involved intestinal segment. The bladder is then repaired in three layers.
2. Vesicovaginal fistula may be a complication of radiotherapy for cervical cancer or endoscopic procedures involving surgery of the trigone or vesical neck. Such fistulas are also caused by obstetrical injuries and hysterectomies. If the fistula is at the dome of the bladder, the approach will be extraperitoneal. A suprapubic tube is usually left in the bladder in these cases. If the fistula is in the trigone of the bladder, a vaginal approach may be employed.

Setup and preparation of the patient. As described for open bladder operations. An intestinal resection setup (Chapter 14) is also necessary for vesicointestinal fistulas. For vesicovaginal fistulas, vaginal preparation and a colporrhaphy set (Chapter 16) with colostomy or ileostomy instruments are used.

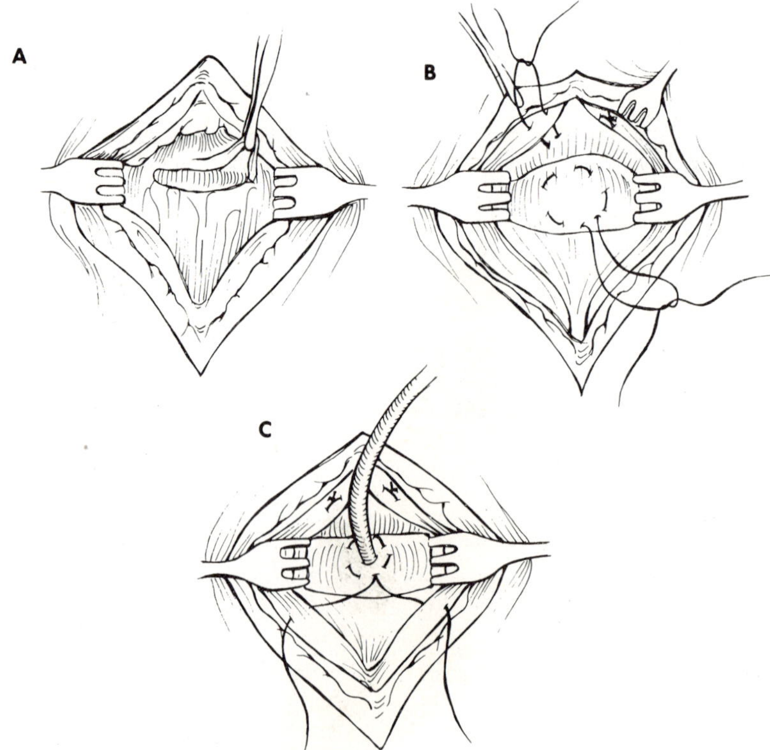

Fig. 15-54. Suprapubic cystostomy. **A,** Incision. **B,** Purse-string suture in preparation of stab wound in bladder. **C,** Catheter in bladder. (Adapted from Dodson, A.I.: Urological surgery, ed. 4, St. Louis, 1970, The C.V. Mosby Co.)

Cystectomy

Definition. Total excision of the urinary bladder and adjacent structures.

Considerations. Cystectomy is a surgical consideration when a vesical malignancy has not invaded the muscular wall of the entire bladder or when frequent recurrences of widespread papillary tumors do not respond to endoscopic or chemotherapeutic management. The patient should be medically able to withstand surgery with the expectation of reasonable longevity. Total cystectomy necessitates permanent urinary diversion into an ileal or colonic conduit. Conservative measures such as radiotherapy or chemotherapy may be used when the neoplasm is far advanced.

In the male patient, the prostate gland, seminal vesicles, and distal ureters are removed with the bladder and its peritoneal surface. In the female, the bladder, urethra, distal ureters, uterus, cervix, and proximal third of the vagina are removed.

Setup and preparation of the patient. The patient is placed in the supine position. Instruments are as described for major abdominal procedures. For the male, if the prostate and seminal vesicles are to be removed, prostatectomy instruments should be added. For the female, major vaginal plastic instruments should be added.

Operative procedure

1. A midline incision from the epigastrium to the symphysis pubis, curving to the left of the umbilicus, is generally preferred.
2. The incision is deepened, the rectus muscles retracted laterally, and the peritoneum opened. At this point, long instruments will be necessary.
3. In the male, the bladder dome is lifted at its peritoneal surface. Dissection proceeds laterally on either side with ligation of the major vesical arteries. The bladder is then retracted to expose the prostate and seminal vesicles, which are dissected free in continuity with the bladder. The vas deferens is divided, and the urethra cut at the level of the pelvic diaphragm.
4. The surgical specimen consisting of the bladder, distal ureters, seminal vesicles, and distal vas is removed en bloc. The urethra is ligated with absorbable suture.
5. Lap pads are placed in the denuded pelvis, and pressure applied to reduce lost blood from oozing.
6. Urinary diversion by isolated ileal or colonic conduit may be performed. Direct anastomosis of the ureters to the colon may be performed by ureterosigmoidostomy.
7. The surgical approach for total cystectomy in the female patient is as described for the male patient, but the urethra is removed in continuity with the bladder and internal reproductive organs.

Radical cystectomy and lymphadenectomy

Definition. Total excision of the urinary bladder and contiguous organs as well as pelvic lymph nodes (iliac and obturator).

Considerations. Radical cystectomy and lymphadenectomy is indicated when larger tumors penetrate the full thickness of the bladder wall and invade perivesical fat. Urinary diversion is also performed in this slightly more extensive surgery.

Setup and preparation of the patient. As described previously in this chapter.

Bladder neck operation (Y-V–plasty)

Definition. Open plastic revision of a strictured bladder neck.

Consideration. Y-V–plasty is performed to overcome contracture of the bladder neck caused by primary or secondary stricture.

Setup and preparation of the patient. The patient is placed in a modified Trendelenburg position. Epidural, spinal, or general anesthesia may be used. Instrumentation is as described for open bladder operations.

Operative procedure

1. The bladder is approached through a transverse Pfannenstiel incision in the same manner as in retropubic prostatectomy. A self-retaining retractor is employed to achieve exposure.
2. Traction sutures of fine silk on small, fine, cutting-edge needles (cleft palate type) are placed at the base and on either side of the urethra to start the pattern for the plastic dissection.
3. With the aid of the traction sutures and an Allis forceps, the anterior bladder wall, bladder neck, and urethra are visualized. A Y incision is made in the anterior bladder wall with its distal end extending through the vesical neck and prostate at the 12 o'clock position (Fig. 15-55, *A*). Bleeding vessels in the wall of the bladder and bladder neck are ligated. The broad-based V flap is developed, and the length of the Y arm is determined by how far the stricture extends beyond the vesical neck.
4. The apex of the V is mobilized so that it fits into the leg of the Y incision (Fig. 15-55, *B*). In this manner, the vesical outlet is greatly increased in diameter. A catheter is placed in the urethra as a guide. A suture is taken through the apex of the V and into the prostatic urethra to the base of the Y and tied. The closure of the plastic repair is completed with mattress sutures on atraumatic needles (Fig. 15-55, *C*).
5. A cystostomy tube is placed in the bladder, and the bladder and abdominal wall are closed in the usual manner for cystostomy.

Vesicourethral suspension (Marshall-Marchetti operation)

Definition. Elevation of the pubococcygeal muscle surrounding the urethra and bladder neck for the correction of stress incontinence caused by an abnormal urethrovesical angle.

Setup and preparation of the patient. The patient

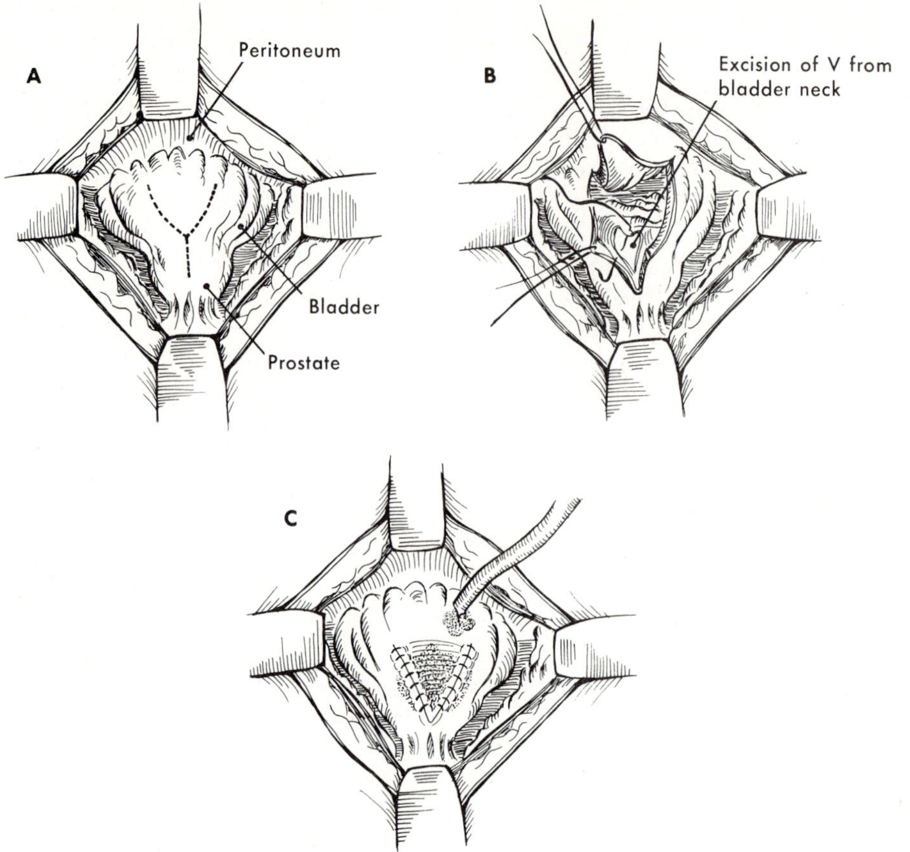

Fig. 15-55. Bladder neck operation. **A,** Y incision. **B,** Conversion of Y incision to V closure. **C,** V closure. (From Flocks, R.H. and Clup, D.A.: Surgical urology, 4th edition. Copyright © 1975 by Year Book Medical Publishers, Inc., Chicago. Used by permission.)

is usually placed in a supine and moderate Trendelenburg position. Legs are placed in frog-leg position with supports under each knee to allow for intraoperative vaginal manipulation. Abdominal and vaginal preparation is required. A Foley catheter is inserted into the urethra at the beginning of surgery.

The basic laparotomy set is used, and the following instruments are added:

1 Mason-Judd bladder retractor
2 Extra-long needle holders, retropubic needle holders, or Heaney needle holders
Chromic sutures, no. 0 or 1, swaged to ⅝-circle needles

Operative procedure

1. A Foley catheter is inserted in the bladder through the urethra. A suprapubic transverse incision is made to expose the prevesical space of Retzius. The Millin retractor is positioned with small moist lap pads in place.

2. The bladder and urethra are freed from the posterior surface of the rectus muscle and symphysis pubis by gentle blunt manipulation.

3. The second assistant places two fingers into the vagina and lifts the urethra upward against the symphysis pubis so that the periurethral musculofascial structures are more easily repaired by the surgeon.

4. A heavy nonabsorbable atraumatic suture on a Heaney needle holder is placed through the supporting fascia of the vaginal wall on each side of the urethra. The suture is then passed through the symphysis pubis, providing support to the urethra and bladder neck.

5. Generally, a row of three such sutures is placed on each side of the urethra, the most proximal being located just at the vesical neck.

6. The area is drained with a Penrose or Jackson-Pratt drain, and the wound is closed in layers and dressed.

7. The vagina may be packed with 2-inch packing. This packing should be removed in 24 to 36 hours. The Foley catheter is connected to a closed urinary drainage system.

Stress incontinence in males may also be treated surgically with perineal prostheses, for example, the Kaufman prosthesis.

OPERATIONS ON THE KIDNEY AND THE URETER

General considerations. Stones, infections, and tumors are the most common causes of urinary tract obstruction necessitating surgery to prevent renal obstruction and subsequent failure. Obstruction may also result from congenital malformations or previous operations on the urinary tract (Fig. 15-56).

Although the causes of many kidney stones are obscure, certain conditions such as obstruction, stasis, or imbalance of metabolism predispose their formation. Stones may form from various elements: calcium oxalate, calcium phosphate, magnesium ammonium phosphate, uric acid, calcium carbonate, or cystine. All stones removed during surgery are usually subjected to chemical analysis. Stones obtained as surgical specimens should be submitted in a dry jar. Fixative agents such as formalin invalidate the results of the analysis.

Stones in the renal pelvis may fall into the ureteropelvic junction and obstruct the flow of urine. However, calculi less than 1 cm in diameter may pass down the ureter and lodge at a more distal location, such as where the ureter crosses the iliac vessels or at the ureterovesical junction. A stone may remain in a renal calyx and continue to enlarge, eventually filling the entire renal collecting system (staghorn stone).

Hydroureteronephrosis, infection, and destruction of renal parenchyma frequently result from unrelieved obstruction.

Hypothermia is useful in renal stone surgery as a means of prolonging the safe period of renal ischemia during extensive parenchymal manipulation. This method is also employed for surgery in the renal artery. Several methods enable renal cooling: (1) ice slush or cold saline solution, (2) surface cooling coils, (3) perfusion of cold solutions through the renal artery, or (4) a variation of these basic techniques, for example, perfusion of the renal pelvis with saline that has been cooled by a coil immersed in ice slush.

Saline slush for renal surgery may be prepared in several ways:

1. Sterile Mason jars are filled with sterile normal saline solution and double-wrapped in a sterile plastic bag. Each bag should be individually wrapped and secured with a twist tie. The Mason jars are placed for 2 to 3 hours in a bucket of ice to which 2 pints of isopropyl alcohol and two boxes of salt are added and mixed. When the saline is ready for use, the circulating nurse will remove the Mason jar from the ice, open the first plastic bag by sterile technique, and hand it to the scrub nurse. The scrub nurse shakes the contents of the Mason jar to cause crystallization of the saline. The slush is removed from the Mason jar with a sterile spoon. (For an alternate method, refer to the *Journal of Urology* **122:**287, 1979.)

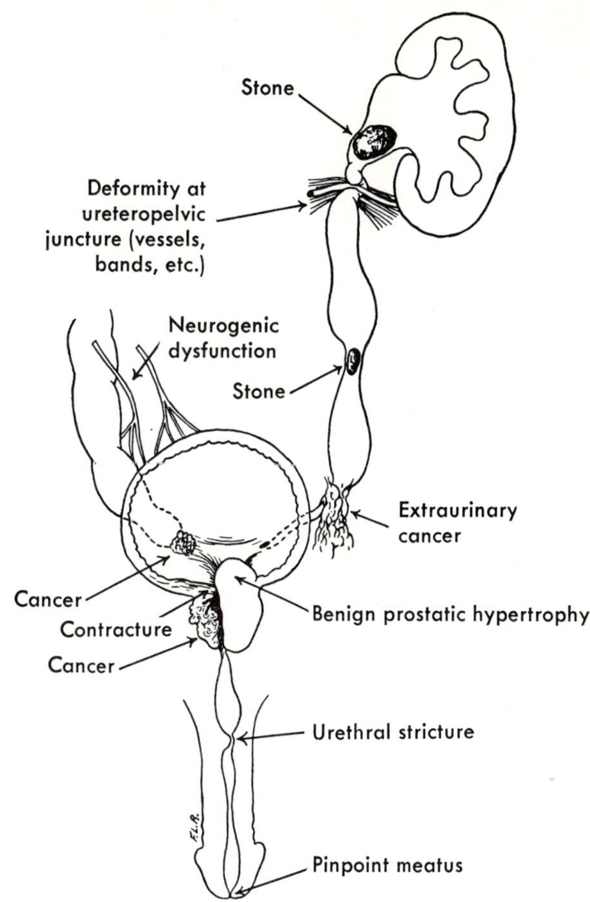

Fig. 15-56. Some common causes of obstruction vary in location and nature, but all can destroy renal function, usually in presence of infection. (From Marshall, V.F.: Textbook of urology, ed. 2, New York, Harper & Row, Publishers.)

2. A rigid plastic container of 1000 ml of normal saline irrigation solution may be placed on its side in the freezer several hours before surgery. To prevent the solution from solidifying, the container should be rotated one half turn every 20 to 30 minutes. Sterile "slush" may then be poured directly into a sterile basin as required.

Surgical approaches to the kidney. Surgical approach in renal surgery is predicated on (1) the patient's somatotype, (2) the need for exposure to a part or all of the kidney, and (3) the surgical procedure to be performed. In the case of renal masses, attention is directed toward control of the vascular pedicle. For this reason, patient position and surgical exposure are of prime consideration. There are three principal surgical approaches to the kidney:

1. The lumbar or simple flank incision is most frequently used and may include removal of the eleventh or twelfth rib. The incision begins at the posterior axillary line and parallels the course of the twelfth rib. It extends

forward and slightly downward between the iliac crest and the thorax (Fig. 15-57).

2. The transthoracic, transdiaphragmatic exposure is employed primarily for large upper pole renal neoplasms. The tenth and eleventh ribs are usually removed, and the chest cavity opened, collapsing the lung. The leaves of the diaphragm are separated to expose the kidney. A large retractor, such as a Finochietto, and chest drains are required.

3. For the transabdominal transperitoneal incision, the patient is placed in a supine position with bolsters under the flank and lower thorax. This effectively places the flank in an oblique position, causing the abdominal viscera to fall away from the operative incision. This approach is used for renal neoplasms and affords an excellent approach to the renal pedicle.

Nephrectomy

Definition. Surgical removal of a kidney.

Considerations. Nephrectomy is performed as a means of definitive therapy for a number of renal problems, such as congenital ureteropelvic junction obstruction with severe hydronephrosis, renal tumors, renal trauma, calculous disease with infection, cortical abscess, pyelonephrosis, and renovascular hypertension.

Setup and preparation of the patient. In routine renal surgery, the patient is placed in the lateral position with the loin directly over the kidney rest. The operative flank is uppermost with the patient's back brought to the edge of the operating table. The upper arm is supported on a rest, and the lower arm flexed at the elbow so that the hand rests on or under the head pillow. The patient's legs are positioned by placing a pillow between them and flexing the lower leg at the knee. The upper leg remains extended. The kidney rest is then raised; when the desired position is achieved, 3-inch adhesive tape is used to stabilize the patient throughout surgery. Routine skin preparation and draping procedures are carried out.

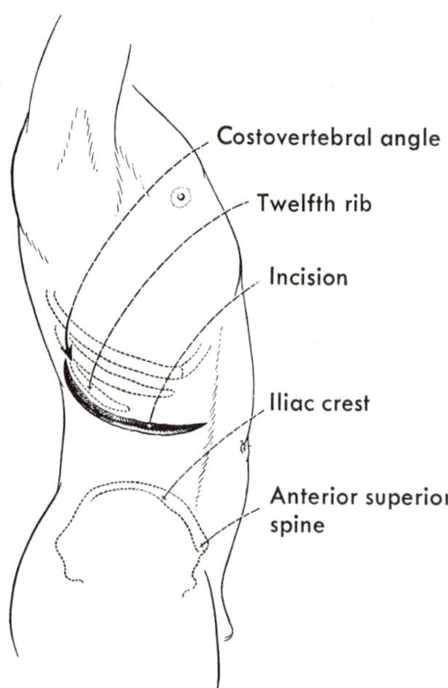

Fig. 15-57. Incision for lumbar approach to kidney. It is made parallel to twelfth rib and 1 cm below it, extends from costovertebral angle to point 3 cm above anterosuperior iliac spine. (From Barnes, R.W., and Hadley, H.L.: Urological practice, St. Louis, The C.V. Mosby Co.)

The instrument setup includes the routine laparotomy setup, plus kidney instruments (Fig. 15-58). The nephrectomy setup includes the following:

2 Satinsky, Herrick, or Mayo pedicle clamps
1 Lewkowitz lithotomy forceps
5 Randall stone forceps, varied sizes
1 Silver probe (Bakes dilators may be used)
Rubber catheter, size 8 or 10 Fr
Asepto syringe
Penrose drains
Pezzar or Malecot catheter
Closed wound drainage system
Vessel loops

In certain operations, the chest or the gastrointestinal tract is opened. If the chest is opened, appropriate instruments, drainage, and suction are needed. When the gastrointestinal tract is opened, precautions must be taken in the anastomosis and closure techniques. For rib resection, the following is added to the basic setup:

1 Finochietto rib retractor, large
1 Matson costal periosteotome
1 Alexander costal periosteotome
2 Doyen rib raspatories, right and left
1 Bethune rib cutter
1 Double-action duckbill rongeur
1 Bailey rib approximator
1 Langenbeck periosteal elevator

Operative procedure (lumbar approach)

1. The incision is carried through the skin, fat, and fascia (Fig. 15-59, *A*). Bleeding vessels are clamped with hemostats and ligated.

2. The external oblique, internal oblique, and transversalis muscles are sequentially exposed and incised in the direction of the initial skin incision.

3. If necessary, a rib or ribs (eleventh or twelfth) may be resected to provide better access to the kidney. The periosteum is stripped with an Alexander costal periosteotome and Doyen rib raspatory.

4. A scalpel and heavy scissors may be used to cut through the lumbocostal ligaments. The rib is grasped with an Ochsner clamp and cut with rib shears, removing the portion necessary to expose the kidney.

5. Gerota's fascia is identified and incised with Metz-

enbaum scissors (Fig. 15-59, *B*). The incision is extended, and the kidney and perirenal fat are exposed by blunt and sharp dissection. *Note:* All perirenal fat that is removed during surgery may be saved in a small basin of normal saline. Perirenal fat may later be used as a bolster to stop bleeding.

6. The ureter is identified, separated from its adjacent structures, doubly clamped, divided, and ligated with absorbable no. 0 chromic catgut (Fig. 15-59, *C*).

7. The kidney pedicle containing the major blood vessels is isolated and doubly clamped; each vessel is triply ligated with heavy chromic or silk ties (Fig. 15-59, *D*). Each vessel is then severed, leaving two ligatures remaining on the pedicle, and the kidney is removed (Fig. 15-59, *E*).

8. The renal fossa is explored for bleeding, and necessary hemostasis achieved. The fossa is then irrigated with normal saline, and the irrigant removed by suction. A Penrose drain, which may be provided with a gauze wick, or a wound suction drain such as a Jackson-Pratt is placed in the empty fossa and brought out through a separate stab incision in the skin.

9. The fascia and muscles are closed in layers with interrupted, chromic sutures. If necessary, retention sutures may be used in obese or chronically ill individuals in whom wound healing may be a problem. The skin edges are approximated with interrupted sutures of silk or with skin staples.

10. The drain is secured, and the wound dressed with gauze sponges, abdominal pads, and adhesive strips.

Radical nephrectomy

Definition. Excision of kidney, perirenal fat, adrenal gland, Gerota's capsule (fascia), and contiguous periaortic lymph nodes.

Considerations. Radical nephrectomy is performed for parenchymal renal neoplasms. A lumbar, transthoracic, or transabdominal approach to the kidney is performed, depending on the size and location of the lesion. The transthoracic or transabdominal approach is preferred because the blood vessels of the kidney can be more easily reached and ligated before the tumor is mobilized, thus decreasing the possibility of tumor embolization into the bloodstream.

Setup and preparation of the patient. As described for nephrectomy.

Operative procedure

1. In general, the procedure is as described for nephrectomy with two exceptions:
   a. The renal pedicle is ligated before the kidney is mobilized.
   b. Gerota's capsule is not incised but is removed en bloc with the kidney.
2. Involved lymph nodes surrounding the renal pedicle are excised.
3. A chest tube is inserted if the transthoracic approach is used.

Heminephrectomy

Definition. Removal of a portion of the kidney.

Considerations. Heminephrectomy is usually indi-

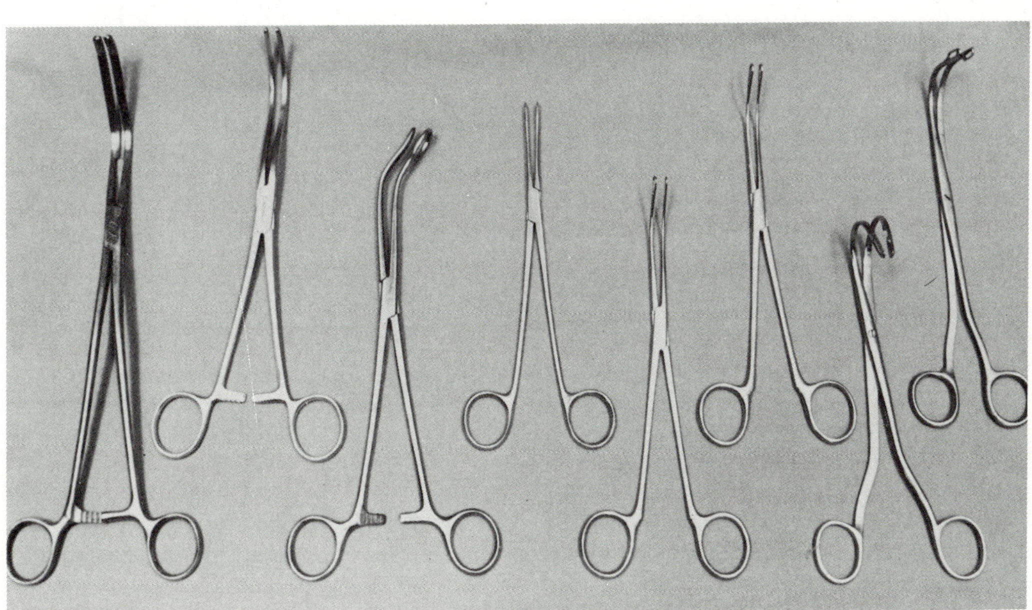

Fig. 15-58. Kidney instruments. *Left to right,* Satinsky pedicle clamp, Mayo pedicle clamp, Lewkowitz lithotomy forceps, set of five Randall stone forceps.

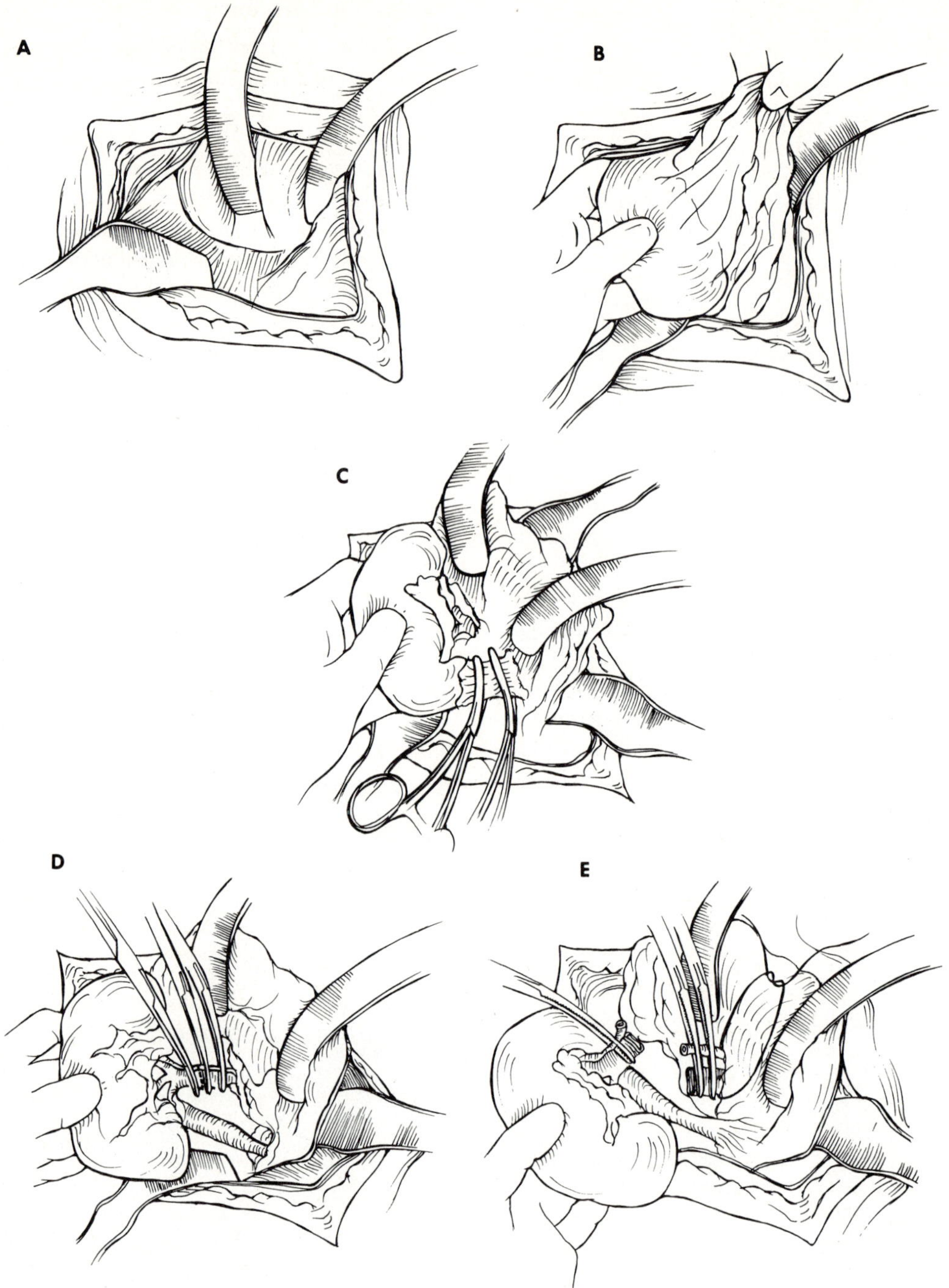

Fig. 15-59. Nephrectomy. **A,** Incision. **B,** Gerota's fascia. **C,** Clamping of ureter. **D,** Clamping of renal vein and artery. **E,** Excision of kidney. (From Dodson, A.I.: Urological surgery, ed. 4, St. Louis, 1970, The C.V. Mosby Co.)

cated for conditions involving the lower or upper pole of the kidney, such as calculous disease, or trauma limited to one pole of a kidney. In rare instances in which a patient has only one kidney, such surgery may be used for renal neoplasms to prevent the need for dialysis and subsequent renal transplantation.

Setup and preparation of the patient. As described for nephrectomy.

Operative procedure

1. The kidney and its pedicle should be completely mobilized as described for nephrectomy.

2. The main vessels may be temporarily occluded for only 20 to 30 minutes, after which progressive renal damage may occur. Local hypothermia may be indicated to prolong ischemic operating time.

3. The renal capsule is incised and stripped back. A

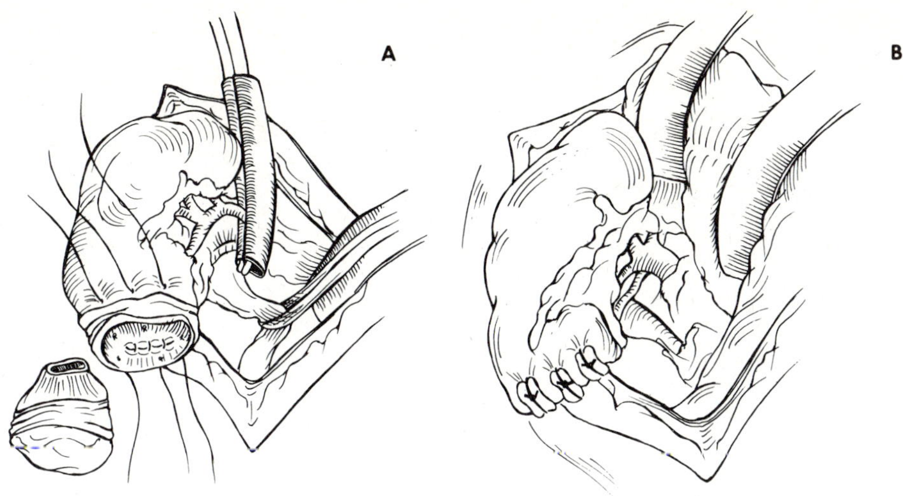

Fig. 15-60. Heminephrectomy. **A,** Resection of diseased kidney tissue. **B,** Suture line. (From Dodson, A.I.: Urological surgery, ed. 4, St. Louis, 1970, The C.V. Mosby Co.)

wedge of kidney tissue containing the diseased or damaged cortex is excised (Fig. 15-60, *A*). Interlobar fat or arcuate and interlobular arteries are clamped with Hopkin's clamps and suture ligated with no. 4-0 chromic or Dexon on urological needles.

4. The open collecting system is reapproximated with a continuous no. 4-0 chromic suture.

5. Perirenal fat is placed in the area in which tissue was excised, and the renal parenchyma is reapproximated with horizontal mattress sutures (Fig. 15-60, *B*). If possible, the renal capsule is reapproximated with a continuous no. 2-0 chromic suture.

Procedures for opening the kidney

Definitions

nephrotomy Incision into the kidney, usually over a collecting system containing a calculus.

pyelotomy Incision into the renal pelvis used as an access to stones in the renal pelvis or collecting system.

pyelostomy Opening made in the renal pelvis for temporarily or permanently diverting the flow of urine (Fig. 15-61).

pyelolithotomy Removal of a calculus through an opening in the renal pelvis.

nephrostomy Opening into the kidney to maintain temporary or permanent urinary drainage. A nephrostomy is used to correct an obstruction of the urinary tract and to conserve and permit physiological functioning of renal tissue. It is also used to provide permanent urinary drainage when a ureter is obstructed or temporary urinary drainage immediately following a plastic repair on the kidney or renal pelvis (Fig. 15-61).

Operative procedures

Pyelotomy or pyelostomy. The pelvis of the kidney is incised with a small scalpel blade. Traction sutures of no. 4-0 chromic catgut swaged on needles may be placed at the edges of the incision for gentle retraction while the pelvis and calyces are explored. In pyelostomy a small Malecot catheter is placed through the incision into the renal pelvis (Fig. 15-62). Pyelotomy should be used only for very short periods of renal drainage, since tubes tend to easily dislodge from the renal pelvis.

Nephrostomy. A curved clamp or stone forceps is passed through a pyelotomy incision into the renal pelvis and then out through the substance of the renal parenchyma via a lower pole minor calyx. The tip of a Malecot or Pezzar catheter is drawn into the renal pelvis, and the pyelotomy incision is sutured closed. The distal end of the nephrostomy tube is brought out through a separate stab incision in the flank. A two-way Foley catheter is frequently used for this purpose. A Penrose drain is placed at the level of the pyelotomy incision, and all layers closed in the regular manner.

Pyelolithotomy and nephrolithotomy. The renal pelvis is opened, and the pelvic calculus gently removed (Fig. 15-62). The pelvis and collecting systems are thoroughly irrigated with saline using an Asepto syringe to dislodge the small remaining calculi and remove them from the kidney. Nephrolithotomy is employed when calculi are locked in the calyceal system and cannot be removed through a pyelotomy incision. In such cases, the renal parenchyma above the calculus is incised and the calculus removed. In many instances such a situation is associated with a calyceal diverticulum. After removal of the calculus, the collecting system is closed and the renal cortex reapproximated with deep hemostatic no. 2-0 chromic sutures.

A nephroscope is sometimes used to localize and remove calyceal calculi (Fig. 15-63). It is also useful in staghorn calculi nephroscopy to completely remove residual fragments in the pelvic portion of the calculus.

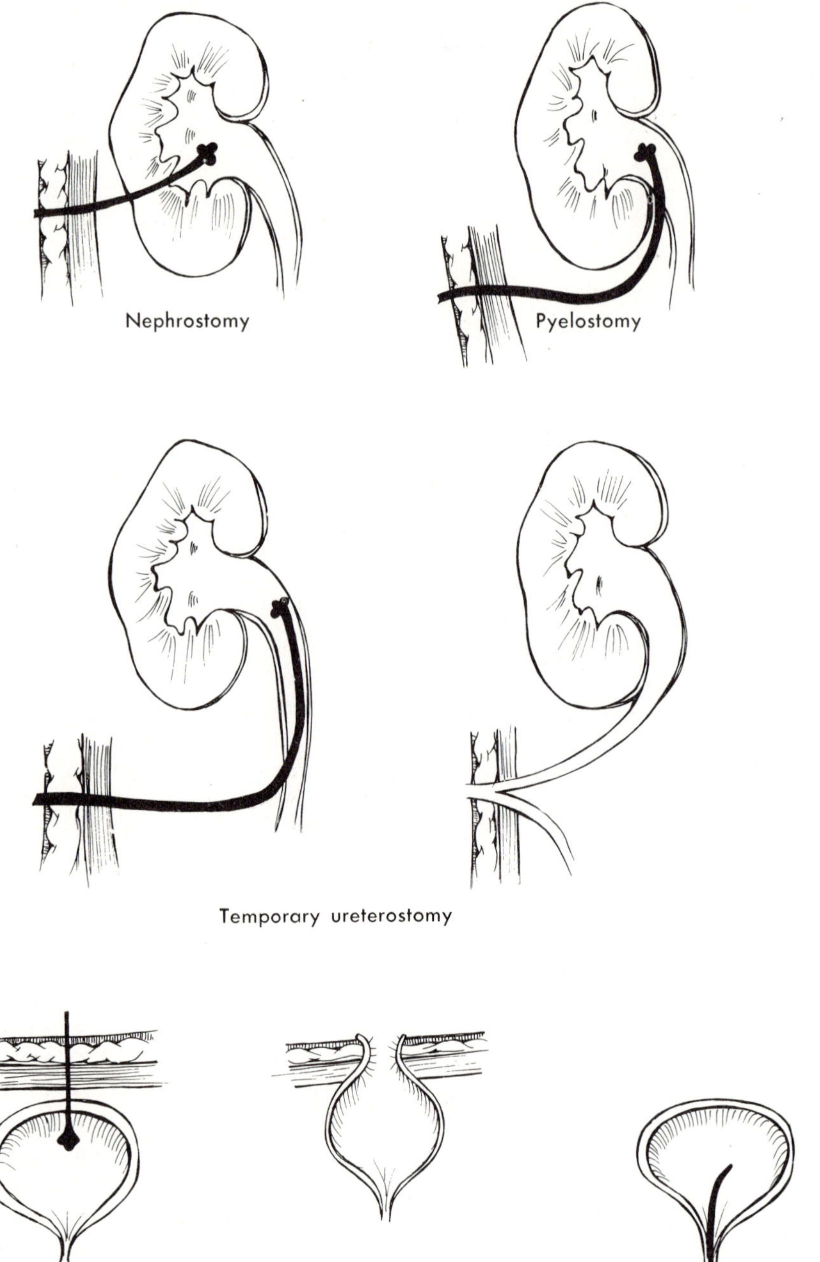

Fig. 15-61. Types of urinary diversions. (From Sabiston, D.C., Jr., editor: Davis-Christopher textbook of surgery: the biological basis of modern surgical practice, ed. 12, Philadelphia, 1981, W.B. Saunders Co.)

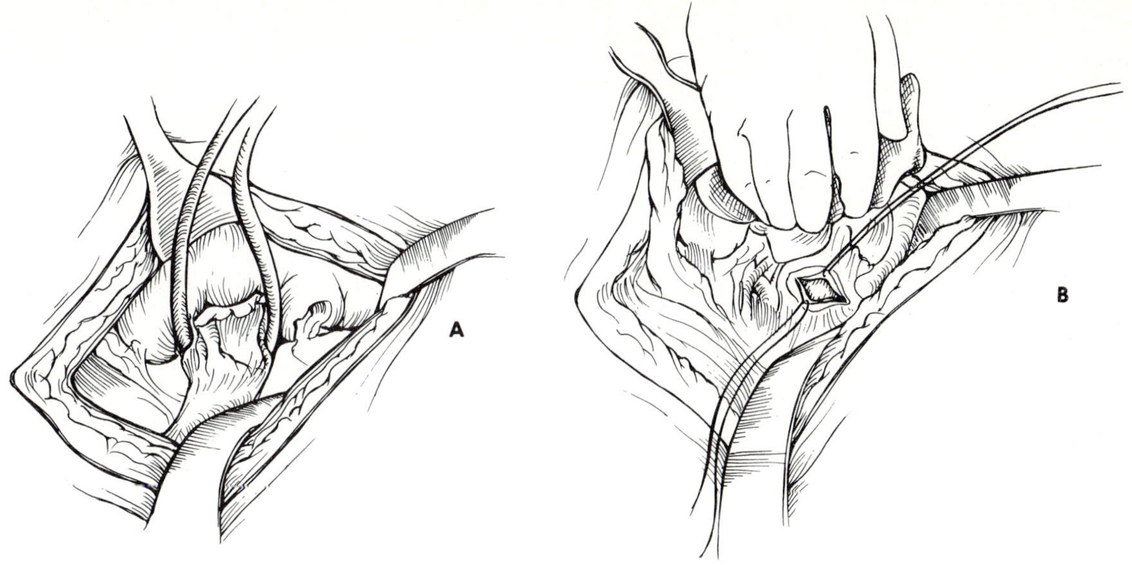

Fig. 15-62. Pyelolithotomy. **A,** Exposing renal pelvis. **B,** Incision into renal pelvis. (Adapted from Dodson, A.I.: Urological surgery, ed. 4, St. Louis, 1970, The C.V. Mosby Co.)

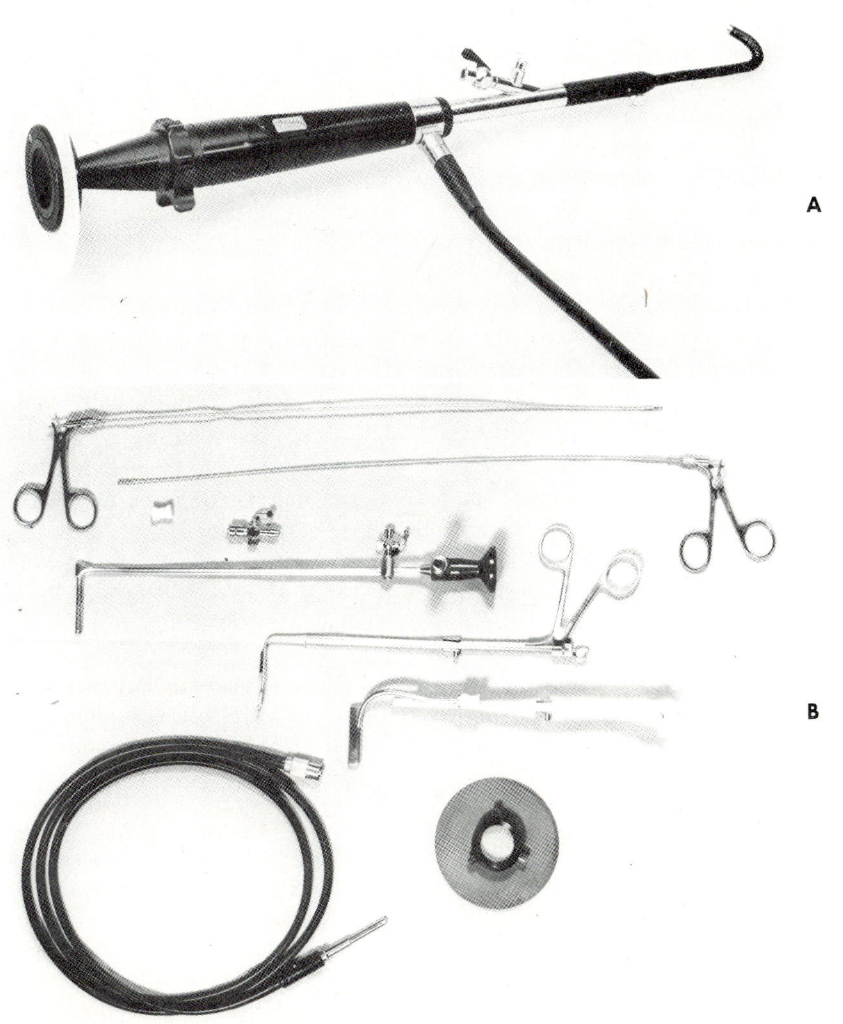

Fig. 15-63. A, Flexible nephroscope. **B,** Nephroscope set. (**A** courtesy American Cystoscope Makers, Inc., Stamford, Conn.)

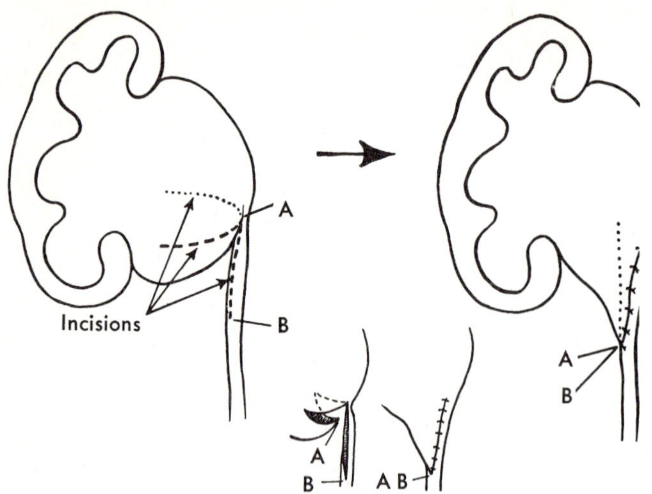

Fig. 15-64. Plastic Y-V repair (Foley type) for ureteropelvic obstruction at outlet of renal pelvis. This is actually conversion of Y incision in three dimensions into two-dimensional V incision. Nephrostomy and splinting catheter through anastomosis are usually employed. (From Marshall, V.F.: Textbook of urology, ed. 2, New York, Harper & Row, Publishers.)

Closure. An incision in the renal pelvis may be closed with no. 4-0 chromic catgut swaged on needles. The renal fossa is drained and closed, as for nephrectomy. Reinforced absorbent dressings are useful since there is generally some urinary leakage for 3 to 4 days after surgery.

Nephroureterectomy

Definition. Removal of a kidney and its entire ureter.

Considerations. Nephroureterectomy is indicated for hydroureteronephrosis of such a degree that reconstructive repair is impossible. It is also employed for collecting system tumors of the kidney and ureter.

Setup and preparation of the patient. This procedure usually requires two separate incisions: exposure and delivery of the kidney, which requires a flank incision, and a lower hemisuprapubic incision to free the lower portion of the ureter from the bladder. Only one instrument set is required, but a second skin preparation setup and set of sterile drapes are necessary.

Operative procedure

1. The patient is placed in a lateral position. The kidney and upper ureter are exposed, as described for nephrectomy. Simple nephrectomy is performed as previously described. The kidney is placed in a plastic bag to prevent possible spillage of tumor cells. The ureter is not cut at this time but is mobilized as far distally as possible.

2. The operating table is adjusted so that surgery on the lower ureter may proceed. The abdomen is prepared, sterile drapes are applied, and an abdominal incision is made to expose the lower ureter and bladder on the operative side. These structures are identified and mobilized. The ureter and a small cuff of the bladder are removed in continuity, and the bladder repaired with a single layer of no. 2-0 chromic catgut interrupted sutures.

3. The ureter and cuff of bladder may be pulled superiorly into the flank incision, where the intact kidney and ureter may be removed from the surgical field.

4. A no. 18 or 20 Fr Foley catheter is left in the bladder, and a Penrose placed behind the bladder. Both incisions are closed in sequence in the usual manner.

Reconstructive operations on the kidney

Definitions

pyeloplasty Revision or plastic reconstruction of the renal pelvis.

ureteroplasty Reconstruction of the ureter distal to the ureteropelvic junction.

Foley-Y-V pyeloureteroplasty Combined correction of a redundant renal pelvis and resection of a stenotic portion of the ureteropelvic junction (Fig. 15-64).

Considerations. Pyeloplasty is done to create a better anatomical relationship between the renal pelvis and the proximal ureter and to allow proper urinary drainage from the kidney to the bladder. A temporary nephrostomy is usually included in such surgery to protect the plastic reconstruction of the ureteropelvic junction. Usually, tissue healing has occurred in 10 to 12 days, and the nephrostomy is removed once ureteral patency is demonstrated.

Setup and preparation of the patient. The instrument setup is as described for nephrectomy, plus the following:

1 Schnidt gall duct forceps, small
1 Metzenbaum dissecting scissors, small, straight, and fine
1 Metzenbaum dissecting scissors, small, curved, and fine
1 Iris scissors, curved
2 Vascular tissue forceps, plain, 7 inches
2 Vascular tissue forceps with teeth, 7 inches
2 Vascular needle holders, 7 inches
12 Mosquito hemostats, straight and curved, 5 inches
Ureteral catheter for splinting
Red rubber catheters, 8 and 10 Fr
5 Randall stone forceps
Chromic sutures, fine, on atraumatic needles

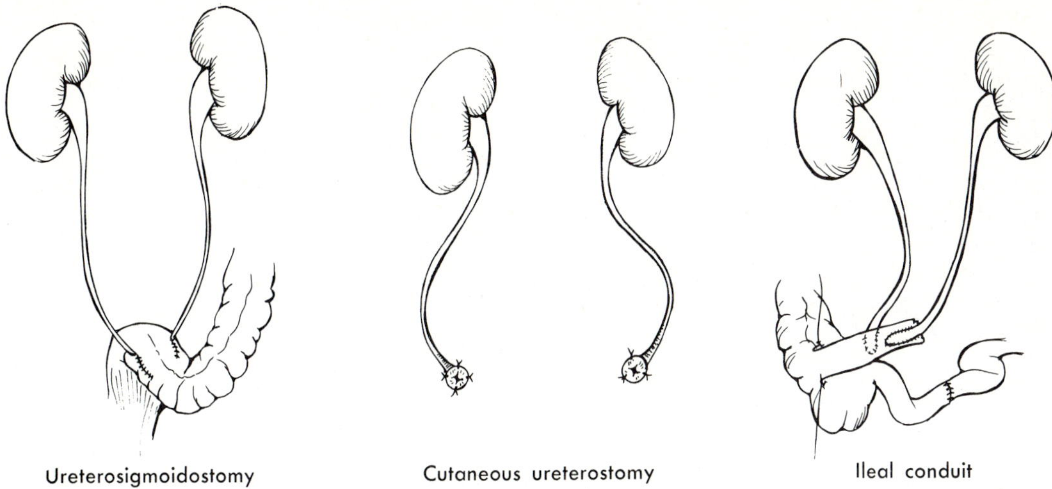

Fig. 15-65. Methods of permanent urinary diversion. (From Keuhnelian, J.G., and Sanders, V.E.: Urologic nursing, New York, 1970, The Macmillan Co.)

Operative procedure

1. The kidney and upper ureter are exposed, as described for single nephrectomy, by the desired surgical approach.

2. The renal pelvis and ureter are incised, trimmed, and shaped to the desired contour with fine forceps and scissors. A caliper and a ruler may be used for establishing more precise relationships when plastic repair is undertaken. Anchoring sutures or soft rubber drains may be used for traction during reconstruction of the renal pelvis. All suture material used in such repairs is absorbable.

The Foley Y-V–plasty technique may be followed as shown in Fig. 15-65. It converts a Y-shaped surgical incision of the renal pelvis into a V as described in the illustrations. This provides a larger funnel-shaped ureteropelvic junction. Interrupted no. 4-0 or 5-0 are used in the repair.

3. A Silastic tubing may be used to stent the repaired pelvis until adequate healing has occurred. A nephrostomy tube is also placed within the pelvis to divert urine safely while the edema in the area of the plastic repair resolves.

4. A Penrose drain is placed where the pelvis was reconstructed, and the surgical incision is closed in layers.

Diversionary surgery on the ureter

Definitions

ureterostomy (ureterotomy) Opening the ureter for continued drainage from it into another part.

cutaneous ureterostomy Diversion of the flow of urine from the kidney, through the ureter, away from the bladder, and onto the skin of the lower abdomen (Fig. 15-65). A suitable urinary collecting device is placed over the ureteral stoma to keep the patient dry.

ureterectomy Complete removal of the ureter. This procedure is generally employed in collecting system tumors and includes nephrectomy and the excision of a cuff of bladder.

ureterolithotomy Incision into the ureter and removal of an obstructing calculus.

ureteroureterostomy Segmental resection of a diseased portion of the ureter and reconstruction in continuity of the two normal segments.

ureteroenterostomy Diversion of the ureter into a segment of the ileum (ureteroileostomy) or into the sigmoid colon (ureterosigmoidostomy). The common terms used in describing these procedures are *ileal urinary conduit* and *ureterosigmoidostomy* (Figs. 15-65 and 15-66).

ureteroneocystostomy (ureterovesical anastomosis) Division of the distal ureter from the bladder and reimplantation of the ureter into the bladder with a submucosal tunnel.

Considerations. Reconstructive operations may be indicated because of a pathological condition of the bladder or lower ureter that interferes with normal drainage. Conditions requiring urinary diversion or reconstruction of the urinary tract include malignancy, cystitis, stricture, trauma, and congenital ureterovesical reflux. Invasive vesical malignancy requiring surgical removal of the bladder necessitates urinary diversion.

Setup and preparation of the patient. The site of the incision and position of the patient depend on the nature of the proposed surgery. The patient may be placed in the supine position for abdominal surgery, in modified Trendelenburg's position for low abdominal or pelvic surgery, or in the lateral position for high or midureteral obstructing calculi.

Instruments include the nephrectomy set, plus plastic instrumentation for pyeloplasty. Additional instruments may be required, depending on the type of operation and the surgical approach used.

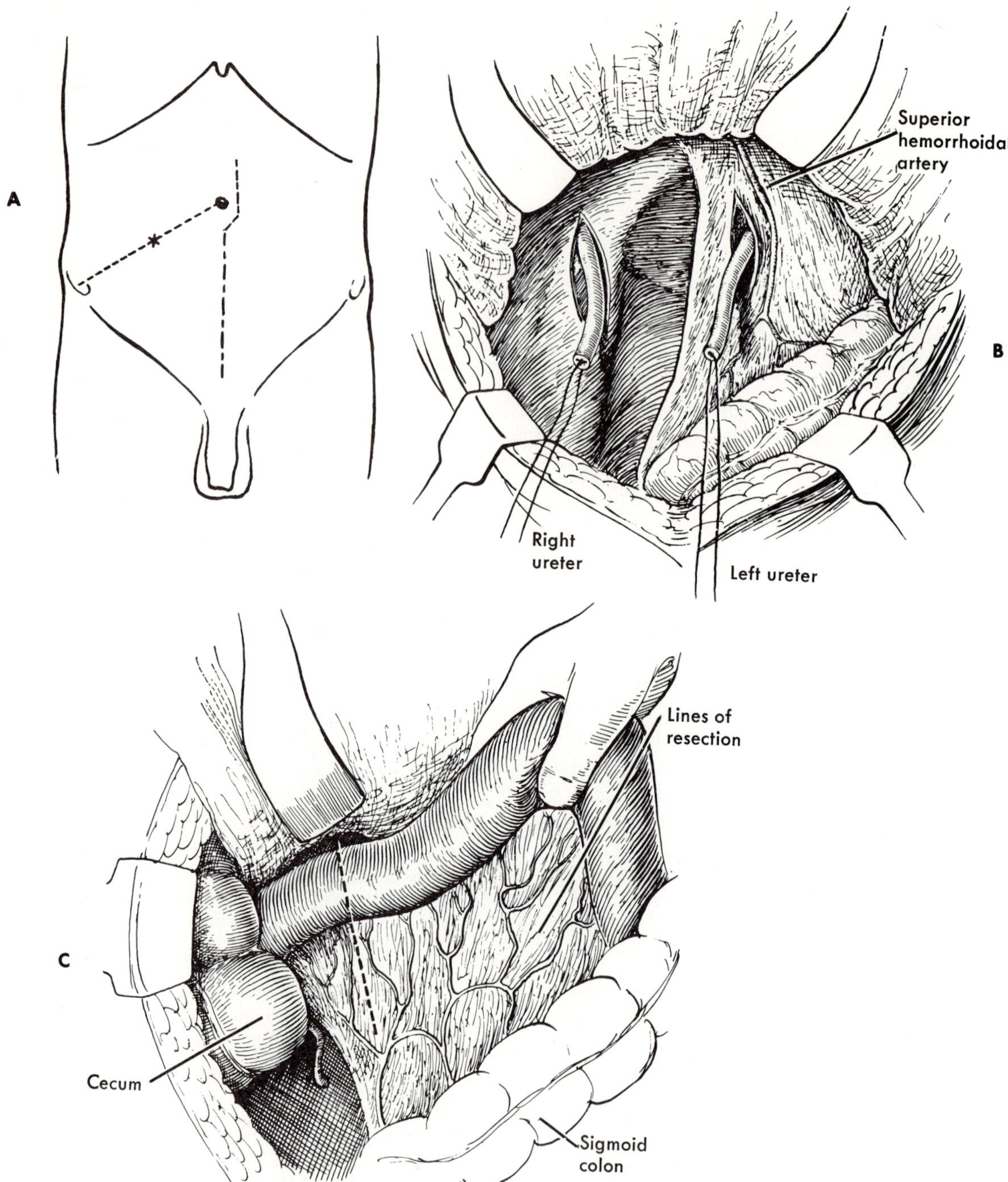

Fig. 15-66. Major steps of operation for ileal conduit, urinary diversion. **A,** Location of ileal stoma. **B,** Ureters freed. Left ureter brought under base of mesosigmoid colon. **C,** Location of ileal segment.

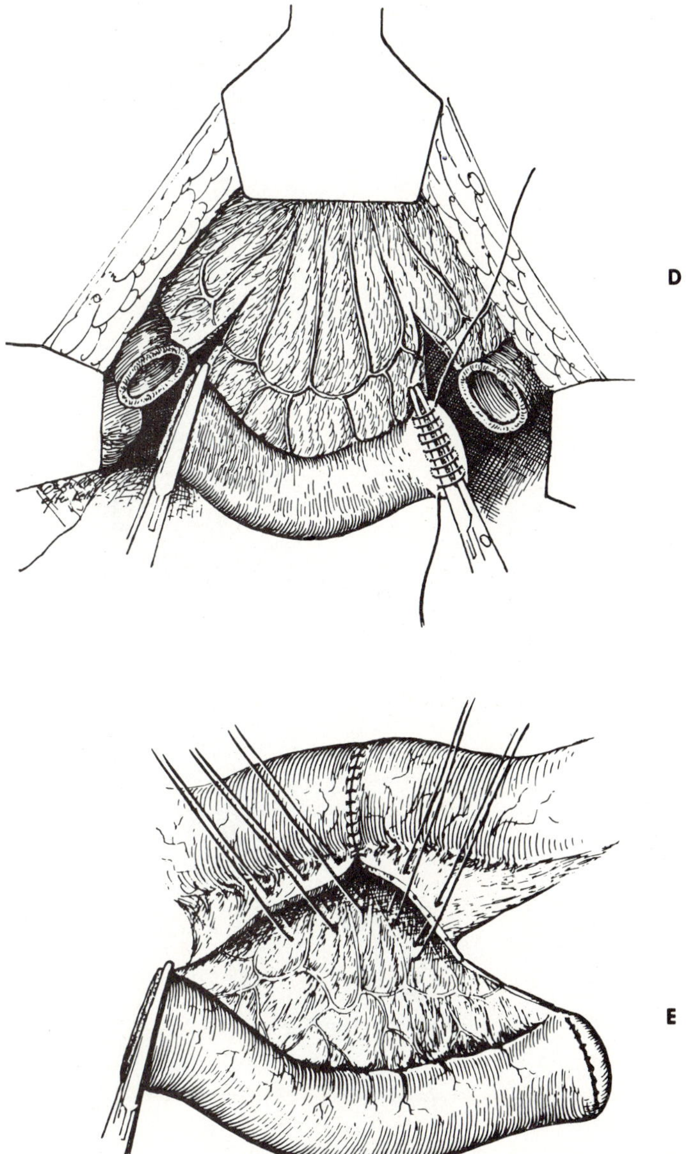

Fig. 15-66, cont'd. D, Closure of proximal end of segment. **E,** Closure of opening at base of mesentery of segment showing transverse approximation. *Continued.*

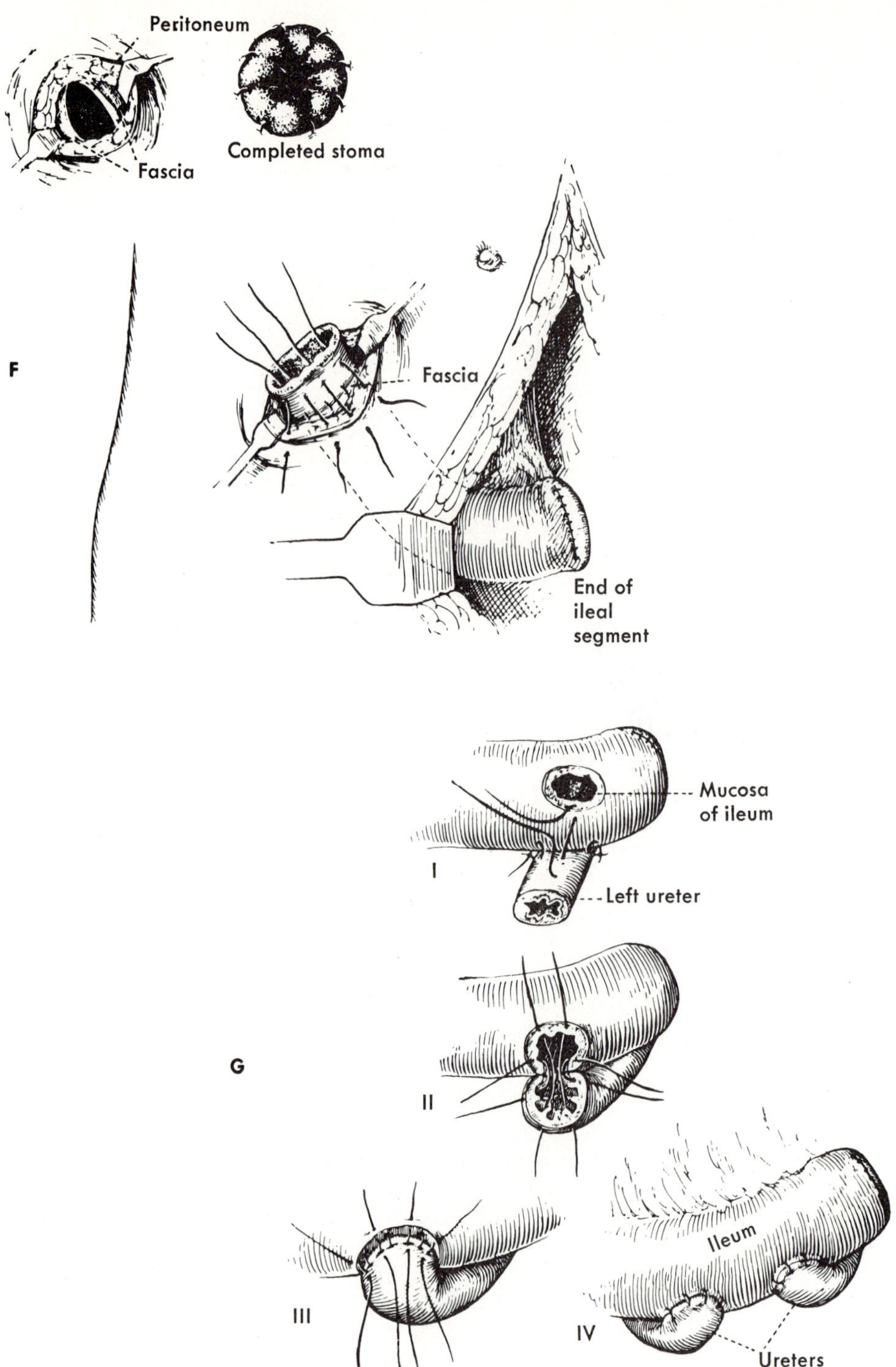

Fig. 15-66, cont'd. F, Preparation of stoma. **G,** Ureteroileal anastomosis.

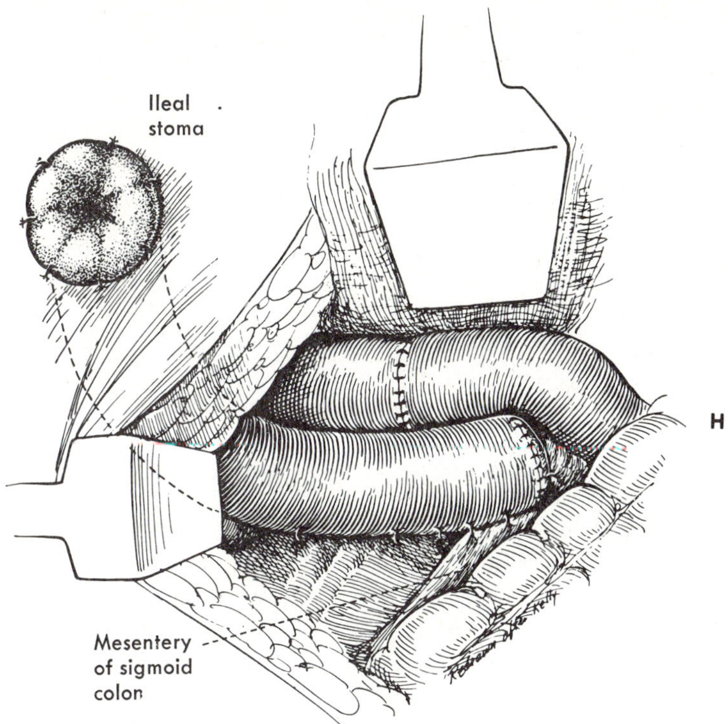

Fig. 15-66, cont'd. H, Completed segment. (From Cordonnier, J.J.: Surgery of the ureter and urinary conduits. In Campbell, F.M., and Harrison, J.H., editors: Urology, ed. 3, Philadelphia, 1970, W.B. Saunders Co.)

Operative procedures

Ureteral anastomosis

1. The ureter is exposed through the desired incision, which is determined by the location of the ureteral reimplantation. A ureteral catheter, passed retrogradely, may be used to facilitate identification and isolation of the ureter. The ureter is identified and dissected free with long forceps and scissors.
2. The ureter is picked up with fine traction sutures, freed from the surrounding tissues, and severed at the desired level.
3. The distal end of the ureter is ligated, and the proximal stoma is transferred to the site of anastomosis. The anastomosis is accomplished with fine dissection instruments and fine swaged-on sutures.
4. A soft splinting catheter is usually left in place until healing has taken place and free drainage is ensured.
5. The wound is closed in layers and dressed in the routine manner.

Ureterolithotomy. A kidney, ureter, and bladder x-ray film should be taken immediately before surgery to determine the exact location of the stone. The surgeon may also schedule a cystoscopic examination preoperatively and may attempt to remove the calculus endoscopically if the stone is in the most distal portion of the ureter.

The location of the calculus determines the surgical approach. A calculus high in the ureter will require a flank incision with possible removal of the twelfth rib; a more distal ureteral calculus requires a lower abdominal incision. Both of these have been described previously in some detail. After exposure of the ureter, the calculus may be kept stationary with Babcock clamps or vessel loops applied above and below the calculus. With a no. 15 blade, the incision in the ureter is made directly over the calculus. The calculus may then be easily removed with a Randall stone forceps. A no. 10 Fr Robinson catheter is passed proximally up and distally down the ureter while irrigating with saline to check for ureteral patency and to dislodge any remaining fragments of calculus. The ureter is closed with fine chromic sutures no. 4-0 or 5-0. All urological stones should be placed in dry receptacles and sent to the chemistry laboratory for analysis. Either of the approaches described requires routine layer surgical closure.

Ureterocutaneous transplant, ureterosigmoid anastomosis, and ileal conduit are urinary diversionary procedures performed when the bladder is no longer functional as a proper urine reservoir. Following are etiologic factors in causing irreparable vesical dysfunction: chronic inflammation (tuberculosis or interstitial cystitis), neurogenic bladder, exstrophy, trauma, tumor, or infiltrative disease (amyloidosis).

Ureterocutaneous transplant (anastomosis). The surgical approach is the same as for a low ureterolithotomy, and the ureter is divided as far distally as possible. The severed ureter is passed retroperitoneally through the lower abdominal wall and is sutured to the skin with an everting suture of no. 4-0 chromic gut on an atraumatic needle to form a stoma. The ureter is handled gently with plastic instruments, fixation forceps, and iris scissors. A small Silastic stenting catheter is passed up into the ureter and is left in situ for 48 to 72 hours, during which time ureteral edema subsides. The patient will require a urine-collecting device after surgery.

Ureterosigmoid anastomosis

1. The abdomen and peritoneal cavity are entered in the routine manner through a lower left paramedian incision. The major portion of the large bowel is protected with packs. Deep retractors are placed in position, and with long forceps and scissors the posterior peritoneum is incised.

2. The ureters are identified and divided close to the bladder. The ureters are mobilized and brought through the posterior peritoneal incision to lie near the sigmoid. Traction sutures and smooth tissue forceps are used to handle the ureters.

3. The sigmoid colon is mobilized to prevent tension on the ureteroenteric anastomosis. The sigmoid colon is sutured with no. 3-0 silk to the pelvic peritoneum at a point where the ureter falls easily on the bowel. Using a scalpel with a no. 15 blade, an incision is made into the tenia of the sigmoid down to the mucosal layer. The edges of the tenia are undermined to create two parallel flaps.

4. The ureter is laid on the bowel mucosa, and a small slit is made through the mucosa into the lumen of the colon.

5. With fixation forceps and iris scissors, the ureter is beveled to lie flat in the tunical incision. The distal ureter is anchored to the bowel mucosa with no. 4-0 chromic, ureteral sutures on atraumatic needles. The other ureter is anastomosed in the same manner in a position slightly above the first.

6. The tunicae are then loosely reapproximated over the ureter with no. 4-0 Dexon, creating an antireflux anastomosis.

7. The posterior peritoneum is closed with fine silk sutures. Drainage is achieved with Penrose or Jackson-Pratt drains brought out retroperitoneally.

Ileal conduit

Definition. The ileal conduit is one method by which the urine flow is diverted to an isolated loop of bowel. One end of the isolated loop is brought out through the skin so that the urine can be collected in a pouch, which is intermittently emptied.

Considerations. The stoma site should be carefully selected preoperatively by the surgeon and/or enterostomal therapist. The selected site, usually in the right lower quadrant of the abdomen (Fig. 15-66, *A*), is marked with a fine needle dipped in methylene blue to prevent erasure during skin preparation. The surgeon's goal is to create a round protruding stoma without wrinkles in the skin to prevent urine leakage under the collecting device. Puckering around the stoma is minimized by using a subcuticular technique when suturing the stoma in place.

Setup and preparation of the patient. The patient is placed in the supine position. A prostatectomy or hysterectomy may also be done at the time of surgery.

Operative procedure

1. The bladder is decompressed with a Robinson catheter. Through a midline abdominal incision, the abdomen is entered. A self-retaining abdominal retractor is placed so that the viscera are excluded from the region of dissection.

2. The ureters are identified and mobilized by severing them 1 to 1½ inches from the bladder (Fig. 15-66, *B*). A retroperitoneal tunnel is made so that the left ureter lies close to the right ureter.

3. The distal ileum and mesentery are inspected to identify the bowel's blood supply. A Penrose drain is passed through the mesentery, midway between the two main arterial arcades adjacent to the ileum at the proximal and distal ends of the selected segment. This segment usually comprises 15 to 20 cm of the terminal ileum, a few centimeters from the ileocecal valve (Fig. 15-66, *C*).

4. Care is exercised to preserve the ileocecal artery and adequate circulation to the isolated ileal segment. The peritoneum is incised over the proposed line of division of the mesentery. Dennis or Gavin Miller intestinal clamps are placed across the ileum, and the bowel is divided flush with the clamps (Fig. 15-66, *D*). By gastrointestinal technique (Chapter 14), the proximal end of the isolated ileal segment is closed first with a layer of chromic sutures and then with a second layer of interrupted no. 2-0 silk sutures. The proximal and distal segments of ileum are reanastomosed end to end in two layers.

5. The mesenteric incision is closed with interrupted silk sutures (Fig. 15-66, *E*).

6. The closed proximal end of the conduit segment is fixed to the posterior peritoneum. The ureters are implanted in the ileal segment by fine instruments and ureteral sutures of chromic no. 4-0 on atraumatic needles (Fig. 15-66, *F* and *G*). The peritoneum and muscle of the abdominal wall lateral to the original incision is separated by blunt dissection. The abdominal opening for the stoma is made. The distal opening of the ileal conduit is then drawn through a fenestration in the muscle, fascia, and skin. The ileum is fixed to the fascia with quadrant sutures of no. 2-0 chromic catgut. A rosebud stoma is constructed at the same time the ileum is sutured to the skin with fine no. 3-0 subcuticular chromic catgut (Fig.

15-66, *H*). A ureteral stent is usually left in the stoma, and a urinary collecting pouch is placed over the rosebud stoma to collect urine. The wound is drained with two Jackson-Pratt drains. The abdominal incision is closed with no. 0 Prolene. The skin is reapproximated with skin staples.

Cystectomy may be performed before or after this procedure, depending on the patient's condition and diagnosis. In some cases the surgeon may choose not to remove the bladder rather than to subject a debilitated patient to further surgery. In cases of bladder carcinoma, the surgeon may elect to treat the patient with radiation in an attempt to decrease the size of the tumor and "sterilize" the regional lymph nodes before performing a cystectomy.

OPERATIONS ON THE ADRENAL GLANDS

Adrenalectomy

Definition. Partial or total excision of one or both adrenal glands.

Considerations. Adrenalectomy may be performed for several reasons: hypersecretion of adrenal hormones, neoplasms of the adrenal gland, or secondary treatment of neoplasms elsewhere in the body that are dependent on adrenal hormonal secretions, such as carcinoma of the prostate and breast.

Setup and preparation of the patient. For unilateral adrenalectomy, the patient may be placed in the lateral kidney or supine position (Chapter 6). More often, however, both glands are explored, and the supine or prone position is selected.

Lateral approach. As described for nephrectomy, including rib resection instruments, vascular instruments, and vessel clips and applicators.

Abdominal approach. As described for laparotomy, including vascular instruments, extra-long scissors, tissue forceps, Rochester-Pean forceps, Mixter forceps, and needle holders. Penrose tubing is needed for retraction. Vessel clips and applicators may also be needed, as well as various sizes of silk sutures.

Operative procedures

Lateral approach

1. A flank incision is performed as described for nephrectomy. The twelfth and sometimes the eleventh ribs are resected for optimum exposure of the upper pole of the kidney.
2. An opening is made through the transverse fascia with scissors. The pleura and diaphragm are protected with wet packs, and Gerota's capsule is incised to expose the kidney and adrenal gland.
3. The gland is identified and dissected free from the upper pole of the kidney by scissors and Babcock forceps. The blood supply of the gland is identified, clamped or clipped, and divided. Bleeding vessels are ligated. To release the glands, the left adrenal vein, a branch of the left renal vein, is separated by clamping and cutting. The right adrenal vein, a tributary of the vena cava, is also divided. Fine vascular sutures may be required to repair inadvertent injury to the vena cava.
4. When hemostasis has been ensured, the wound is closed sequentially in layers: muscle, fascia, subcutaneous tissue, and skin.

Abdominal approach

1. The abdominal wall is incised with an upper abdominal incision, and the peritoneal cavity is opened and explored. Bleeding vessels are clamped and ligated.
2. The abdominal wound is retracted, and the surrounding organs protected with laparotomy packs, using instruments and sutures as described for routine laparotomy.
3. The retroperitoneal area near the diaphragm is opened on the left side, exposing the renal fascia.
4. The renal fascia is opened to reveal the left kidney and adrenal gland.
5. The adrenal gland is freed from the kidney by sharp and blunt dissection, clamping and ligating all bleeding vessels with no. 3-0 silk suture.
6. After all bleeding is controlled, the kidney is gently replaced in the renal fascia, which is closed with interrupted no. 0 chromic sutures.
7. The peritoneum is closed over the left kidney and renal fascia.
8. The abdominal retractors are rearranged to give access to the peritoneum over the right kidney and adrenal gland. Care must be taken to prevent trauma to the liver.
9. The same procedure is repeated on the right side taking care to carefully clamp and ligate the short adrenal vein.
10. The abdomen is inspected for bleeding vessels, which are ligated.
11. The wound is closed as in routine laparotomy.

Prone position. The prone position is especially useful for debilitated patients with an advanced neoplasm because the position is relatively atraumatic; since the abdominal cavity is not entered, ileus does not usually occur. Thus patients may resume eating and ambulating the next day.

KIDNEY TRANSPLANT

Definition. Transplantation of a living related or cadaveric donor kidney into the recipient's iliac fossa (Fig. 15-67).

General considerations. A kidney transplant is performed in an effort to restore renal function and thus maintain life in a patient who has end-stage renal disease.

Transplant from a living donor

Considerations. It is essential that the kidney donor be in perfect health. A complete workup verifies the presence of two normal kidneys. Blood type, tissue type, and lymphocyte cross matching determine donor-recipient

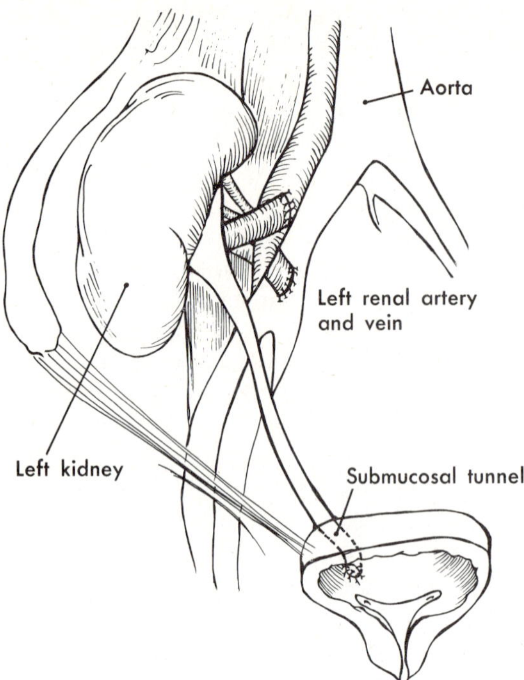

Fig. 15-67. Transplanted kidney in recipient's iliac fossa. (From Flocks, R.H., and Clup, D.A.: Surgical urology, 4th edition. Copyright © 1975 by Year Book Medical Publishers, Inc., Chicago. Used by permission.)

compatability. An arteriogram visualizes the renal arterial status and rules out the presence of renal lesions. A kidney with a single renal artery is preferred, but kidneys with double and triple arteries may be used if necessary.

The ideal living donor is an identical twin, although any immediate family member (usually a sibling or parent) may be a donor if the person is medically acceptable.

Setup and preparation of the patient. Two adjacent operating rooms are prepared for the procedures; surgery on the donor and recipient proceeds simultaneously.

A Foley catheter is inserted and left in the donor's bladder to accurately measure urinary output and prevent bladder distension from the increased urine production induced by diuretics. The donor is placed in the lateral position, prepared from midchest to midthigh, and draped in the usual manner, exposing the flank area.

Required instruments and equipment are identical to the nephrectomy setup, plus the following for the sterile perfusion table (Fig. 15-68):

1 IV pole
1 Bottle electrolyte solution (Collins or Sachs) (in iced bucket until needed)
2 Intravenous extension tubes, sterile
1 Kidney basin with cold (4° C) intravenous saline solution
1 Stopcock, three-way
1 Needle catheter (Medicut), 18-gauge
6 Mosquito clamps
2 Vascular forceps, fine, 3 inches
1 Metzenbaum scissors, fine
1 Suture scissors, fine
1 Kelly clamp

Operative procedure

1. The donor nephrectomy procedure is as described in for nephrectomy; however, the renal vein and artery require meticulous dissection. Particular care must be taken to remove the maximum length of renal vein and artery. To obtain the maximum length of a right renal vein sometimes requires partial occlusion of the inferior vena cava with a Satinsky clamp and dissection of a portion of the inferior vena cava. Repair of the inferior vena cava is made with a no. 4-0 or 5-0 continuous vascular suture. To reduce warm ischemia time, the surgeon may double-clamp the vein and the artery, enabling the kidney to be removed quickly and immediately perfused with Collins or Sachs solution while another surgeon ligates the renal vessels. Warm ischemia time (from the clamping of renal vessels to a point at which the kidney is perfused with cold electrolyte solution) should be kept to a minimum to prevent acute tubular necrosis and to obtain maximum renal function after transplantation.

2. Five minutes before the surgeon clamps the renal vessels, 5000 units of heparin sodium is systemically administered to the patient to prevent intravascular clotting. Immediately after the kidney is removed from the donor, 50 mg of protamine sulfate is given intravenously to reverse the heparinization. Furosemide, mannitol, and intravenous fluids are administered to the donor to maintain adequate urinary output from the donor's remaining kidney.

3. Particular care must also be given to the ureter. Maximum length is achieved by dividing at or below the pelvic brim if possible. To preserve adequate ureteral vascularization, the surgeon is cautious not to skeletonize the ureter.

4. Gentle handling of the kidney is essential. Team members must prevent undue traction on the vascular pedicle, since this may induce vasospasm and reduce perfusion of the kidney.

5. After being excised, the kidney is placed in cold saline solution on a sterile back table, where it is flushed with cold Sachs or Collins solution. Equipment and solutions must be immediately available to avoid unnecessary warm ischemia time (Fig. 15-68).

6. Mosquito clamps and fine vascular forceps are used to expose the renal artery to permit insertion of a needle catheter, for example, a Medicut. The cold electrolyte solution passes through the intravenous tubing and the needle catheter, flushing any remaining donor's blood from the kidney. This also decreases the kidney's metabolic rate by lowering its temperature. Flushing time is usually 2 to 5 minutes. It may be necessary after flushing to trim

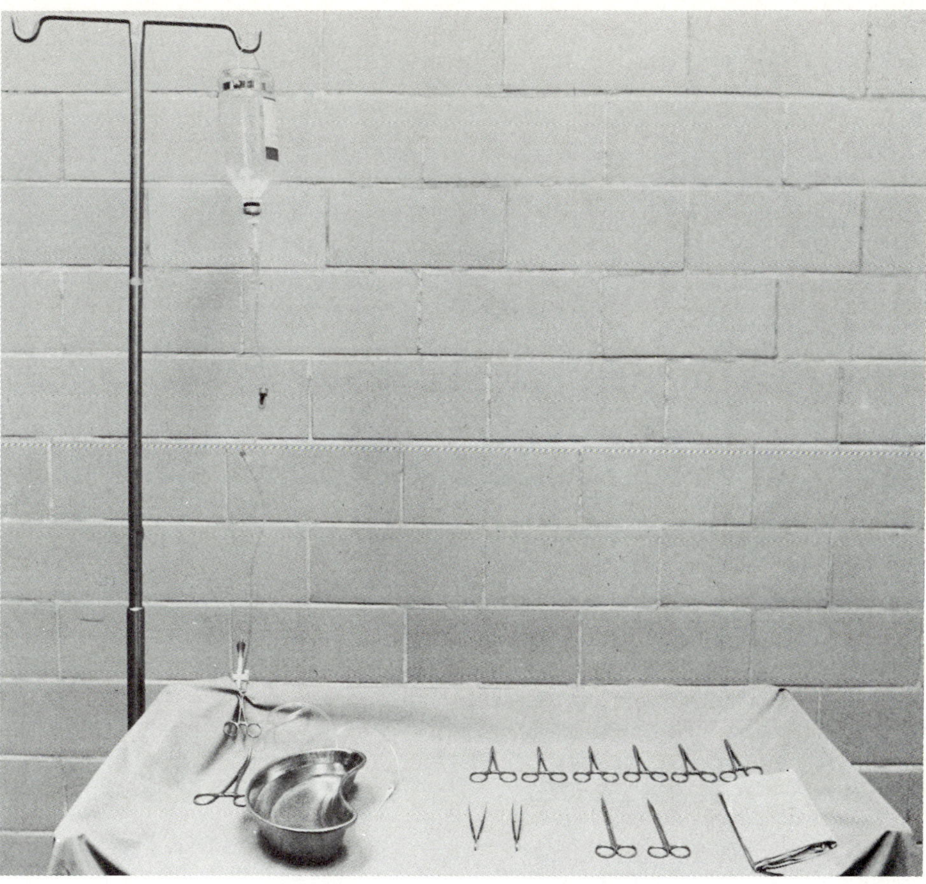

Fig. 15-68. Kidney perfusion table setup.

the vessels of adventitia to facilitate the vascular anastomosis to the recipient's iliac vessels.

7. The kidney, in cold saline solution, is covered with sterile drapes and taken by the surgeon to the room in which the recipient's iliac vessels have been exposed.

8. Wound closure for the donor is as described for nephrectomy.

Transplant from a cadaveric donor

Considerations. The ideal cadaveric donor is young, free of infection and cancer, normotensive until a short time before death, and under hospital observation several hours before death. Permission to harvest the donor kidney must be obtained from the family and/or medical examiner, after brain death has been unequivocally established. It is advisable to be aware of existing state legislation in this complex area.

Setup and preparation of the patient. After death has been established, the body is taken to the operating suite with respiratory and cardiac function being maintained mechanically. The patient is placed in the supine position and is prepared for a laparotomy. Anticoagulant and alpha adrenergic blocking agents are administered systemically during the procedure. Adequate renal perfusion and function is maintained with intravenous fluids and diuretics.

Instruments and equipment are the same as for the nephrectomy setup, excluding the rib instruments and adding the following:

Cutting instruments

1 Metzenbaum scissors, 9¼ inches
1 Suture scissors, 9¼ inches
1 Metzenbaum scissors, fine
1 Suture scissors

Holding instruments

2 Vascular forceps, fine
2 DeBakey forceps, 4, 7, and 10 inches

Clamping instruments

12 Dean hemostatic forceps
12 Mosquito hemostats
6 DeBakey clamps, angled
2 Metal clip applicators with medium and large clips
6 Bulldog clamps
4 Vascular clamps, angled, large

Exposing instruments

2 Deaver retractors, extra wide
2 Harrington splanchnic retractors, small and large

Suturing instruments

4 Vascular needle holders, 2 short and 2 long

Accessory items

1 Bottle electrolyte solution (Sachs or Collins), cold (in iced bucket until needed)
1 IV pole
2 Intravenous extension tubes, sterile
1 Kidney basin with cold (4° C) intravenous saline solution
1 Stopcock, three-way
1 Needle catheter (Medicut), 18-gauge
1 Centimeter ruler
1 Electrosurgical unit
Perfusion machine or kidney transplant equipment and ice

Operative procedure

1. A midline incision is made from the xiphoid process to the symphysis pubis with bilateral supraumbilical transverse extensions through the skin, subcutaneous layer, fascia, and muscle.

2. Hemostasis is obtained with clamps, ties, suture ligatures, and electrocautery.

3. The kidney, renal vessels, and ureter are carefully dissected with Metzenbaum scissors, DeBakey forceps, and Dean hemostatic forceps.

4. Heparin sodium, 15,000 units, is given intravenously 5 to 10 minutes before clamping the renal vessels.

5. One method of resection is en bloc resection (harvesting of donor kidneys) (Fig. 15-69), which involves the removal of sections of the inferior vena cava and aorta with both kidneys in continuity. An incision is made along the route of the small bowel mesentery up to the esophageal hiatus. The entire gastrointestinal tract, spleen, and inferior portion of the pancreas are mobilized by dividing the celiac axis and the superior mesenteric artery, exposing the entire retroperitoneal region. The inferior vena cava and aorta are clamped below the renal vessels with vascular clamps, and the vessels are divided. Lumbar tributaries are secured with metal clips and are divided. The kidneys and ureters are freed from their surrounding soft tissues. The ureters are divided distally at the pelvic brim. The suprarenal aorta and inferior vena cava are clamped and divided at the level of the diaphragm. The vessels and kidneys are severed from the surgical field, and the aorta and vena cava are ligated.

6. After removal of the kidneys, immediate perfusion with cold (4° C) electrolyte solution is carried out as in steps 5 and 6 for a donor kidney.

7. The kidneys are placed in a container of cold saline solution and surrounded by saline slush in an insulated carrier or placed on a hypothermic pulsatile perfusion machine for transport (Fig. 15-70).

8. While kidney perfusion is begun, the abdominal lymph nodes and spleen are removed for use in tissue typing.

9. The incision is closed with interrupted sutures.

10. Artificial life support systems are terminated.

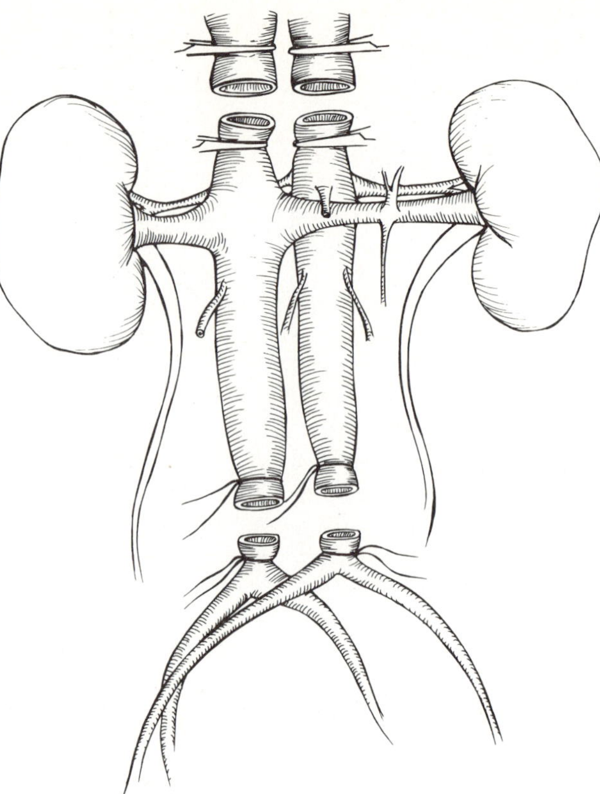

Fig. 15-69. En bloc resection.

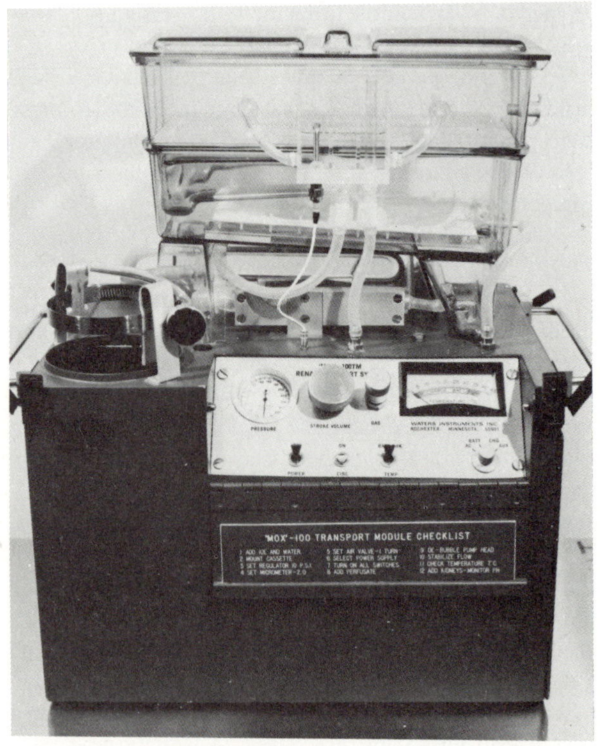

Fig. 15-70. Waters perfusion machine.

Transplant recipient

Considerations. Each potential recipient is judged individually in regard to kidney transplantation. Most persons below the age of 55 years are acceptable; however, older patients are less tolerant of postoperative complications. Transplantation in infants is still experimental. Contraindications for renal transplantation include (1) systemic disease that precludes major surgery, (2) oxalosis, (3) active cancer, and (4) Fabry's disease. If required, a patient may need to undergo bilateral nephrectomy before renal transplantation for the following reasons: (1) to control hypertension; (2) to remove infected, bleeding, or polycystic kidneys; and (3) to remove the ureters if vesicoureteral reflux exists. A splenectomy may also be performed at this time to decrease the leukopenic and thrombocytopenic effects of immunosuppressive drugs.

Setup and preparation of the patient. The patient is placed in the supine position. A Foley catheter with an attached Silastic stenting catheter is inserted in the bladder by sterile technique. From 50 to 75 ml of 1% neomycin sulfate is instilled in the bladder through a sterile catheter tip syringe, allowed to remain for 20 minutes, and drained. The patient is prepared from nipples to knees and is draped in the routine manner.

Instruments and equipment to assemble are the routine laparotomy setup, plus the following:

Cutting instruments

1 Metzenbaum scissors, 9¼ inches
1 Suture scissors, 9¼ inches
1 Metzenbaum scissors, fine
1 Suture scissors, fine
1 Potts scissors, angled

Holding instruments

2 DeBakey forceps, 4, 7, and 10 inches
2 Vascular forceps, fine, 3 inches

Clamping instruments

12 Dean hemostatic forceps
12 Mosquito hemostats, straight
6 Mosquito hemostats, curved
6 DeBakey clamps, angled
2 Metal clip applicators with medium and large clips
3 Bulldog clamps, curved
3 Bulldog clamps, straight

Exposing instruments

2 Harrington splanchnic retractors, small and large

Suturing instruments

4 Vascular needle holders, 2 long and 2 short

Accessory items

2 Asepto syringes
1 Centimeter ruler
1 Needle catheter (Medicut), 18 gauge on 10-ml syringe
1 Closed wound suction
Electrosurgical unit
1 Pediatric feeding tube, 5 Fr
1 Stockinette, 3 × 10 inches
Heparin sodium solution (1:1000)
Intravenous saline solution, cold (4° C)

Operative procedure

1. A curved, lower quadrant incision is made through the skin, subcutaneous layer, fascia, and muscle. Bleeding is controlled with clamps, ties, and electrocautery.

2. The inferior epigastric vessels are divided between suture ligatures of no. 2-0 silk. A retroperitoneal dissection is performed by mobilizing the peritoneum superiorly and medially. A Balfour self-retaining retractor is placed in the wound for exposure, and a wide Deaver retractor is inserted to reflect the peritoneum superiorly and medially.

3. With the use of the 9½-inch Metzenbaum scissors and the DeBakey forceps, dissection is made along the entire length of the external and common iliac arteries to the bifurcation of the aorta and continuing down the internal iliac artery. The internal iliac artery is ligated distally and divided, with proximal control maintained by a vascular clamp. The iliac vein is dissected free by ligating and dividing the internal iliac venous branches with no. 3-0 silk sutures or metal clips.

4. The donor kidney is brought into the operative field and placed in cold (4° C) intravenous saline solution.

5. Mosquito hemostats, 4-inch DeBakey forceps, and curved and straight fine scissors are used to make the necessary alterations on the donor kidney vessels to facilitate the anastomoses.

6. The donor kidney is returned to the cold intravenous saline solution until the time of the anastomosis.

7. Two angled DeBakey vascular clamps are placed on the internal iliac vein. A no. 11 blade is used to make a 1-cm incision in the iliac vein between the clamps. The vessel is rinsed with heparin sodium solution (10 units/mm) in the Asepto syringe. An angled Potts scissors is used to extend the incision to accommodate the donor renal vein.

8. The donor kidney is placed in the 3 × 10–inch, cold saline-soaked stockinette, with the renal vessels exiting from a hole in the side. Use of the stockinette prevents direct contact with the kidney and therefore trauma. The renal vein is anastomosed to the side of the recipient's iliac vein with no. 5-0, double-armed, Prolene sutures. In like manner the renal artery is anastomosed end to end with the proximal portion of the internal iliac artery using no. 5-0 Prolene sutures. The vessels are irrigated proximally and distally with heparin sodium solution by using the 10-ml syringe attached to the Medicut catheter before placing the final sutures.

9. The stockinette is removed for adequate visualization of the entire kidney.

10. The angled DeBakey clamps are removed from the venous vessels, and the anastomosis is checked for leakage. Immediately afterward, the clamps on the internal iliac artery are released, and the anastomosis is checked. Meticulous inspection is made of the hilum and surface of the kidney for bleeding and infarction. Diuretics are given intravenously as needed.

11. Attention is now directed to the ureter and bladder. Two long Allis clamps are used to grasp the anterior bladder wall. With a no. 20 knife blade, a 4-cm incision is made anteriorly. Two narrow Harrington retractors and one narrow Deaver retractor are inserted in the bladder for exposure. The ureter is passed through the bladder wall and tunneled suburothelially for 2 to 2.5 cm. The spatulated end of the ureter is then sutured into the bladder urothelium with four to six no. 4-0 absorbable sutures on a small atraumatic needle, creating a ureteroneocystostomy.

12. A no. 5 Fr pediatric infant feeding tube is passed through the ureteroneocystostomy, up to the renal pelvis, and out through the urethra with the Foley catheter. This stenting catheter will remain in place for 36 to 48 hours to ensure ureteral patency during a period in which ureteral edema may occur.

13. Retractors are removed, and the bladder is closed in three layers:
   a. Continuous no. 4-0 chromic urothelial closure
   b. Interrupted no. 2-0 chromic closure of bladder muscles
   c. An imbricating layer of no. 2-0 Tevdek to bury the suture line

14. The bladder is irrigated with normal saline to check for leaks.

15. The renal anastomoses are again checked for bleeding.

16. Three metal clips are placed on the superior, inferior, and lateral aspects of the kidney to radiographically measure renal size and determine postoperative swelling.

17. Retractors are removed from the incision.

18. Closed wound suction drains are inserted into the wound, brought through the skin laterally, and secured with no. 2-0 silk on a cutting needle.

19. Muscle and fascial layers are closed with a single layer of no. 0 nonabsorbable sutures on a large atraumatic needle. The subcutaneous layer is closed with no. 3-0 absorbable sutures on an atraumatic needle. Skin closure is accomplished with skin staples.

20. Dressings are applied.

21. The bladder is irrigated with 50 to 75 ml of 1% neomycin sulfate to prevent infection and to free any blood clots.

SUGGESTED READINGS

Anthony, C.P., and Thibodeau, G.A.: Textbook of anatomy and physiology, ed. 10, St. Louis, 1979, The C.V. Mosby Co.

Badenoch, A.W.: Manual of urology, ed. 2, Chicago, 1974, Year Book Medical Publishers, Inc.

Berci, G., editor: Endoscopy, New York, 1976, Appleton-Century-Crofts.

Blandy, J.: Operative urology, Philadelphia, 1978, J.B. Lippincott Co.

Brunner, L.S., and others: The Lippincott manual of nursing practice, Philadelphia, 1974, J.B. Lippincott Co.

Dodson, A.I., Jr.: Urological surgery, ed. 4, St. Louis, 1970, The C.V. Mosby, Co.

Ehrlich, R.: Modern techniques in surgery, Mt. Kisco, N.Y., 1980, Futura Publishing Co., Inc.

Flocks, R.H.: Radical retropubic prostatectomy in prostatic carcinoma: a photographic seminar presented by Warner-Chilcott Laboratories, Urol. Proc. **1**(2), 1972.

Glenn, J.F., editor: Urologic surgery, ed. 2, New York, 1975, Harper & Row, Publishers.

Hudson, P.B., and Stout, A.P.: An atlas of prostatic surgery, Philadelphia, 1962, W.B. Saunders Co.

Jameson, R.M., and others: Management of the urological patient, New York, 1976, Churchill Livingstone.

Jonas, U., and Jacobi, G.H.: Silicone-silver penile prosthesis: description, operative approach and results, J. Urol., **123:**865, 1980.

Karafin, L., and Kendall, A.R.: Urology, vol. 1, New York, 1973, Harper & Row, Publishers.

Karafin, L., and Kendall, A.R.: Urology, vol. 2, New York, 1972, Harper & Row, Publishers.

Keuhnelian, J.G., and Sanders, V.E.: Urologic nursing, New York, 1970, Macmillan Publishing Co.

Marshall, V.F.: Textbook of urology, ed. 2, New York, 1964, Harper & Row, Publishers.

Marshall, V.F.: The Marshall-Marchetti-Krantz procedure for the correction of stress incontinence, Urol. Proc. **1**(1), 1972.

Morel, A., and Wise, G.J.: Urologic endoscopic procedures, ed. 2, St. Louis, 1979, The C.V. Mosby Co.

Netter, F.H.: Kidneys, ureters and urinary bladder, vol. 6, Summit, N.J., 1975, Ciba Pharmaceutical Co.

Phipps, W.J., Long, B.C., and Woods, N.F.: Shafer's medical-surgical nursing, ed. 7, St. Louis, 1980, The C.V. Mosby Co.

Rob, C., and Smith, R.: Operative surgery, Philadelphia, 1970, J.B. Lippincott Co.

Small, M.: Small-Carrion urethroplasty for the management of bulbous and membranous urethral strictures, Urol. Proc. **3**(2), 1974.

Smith, D.R.: General urology, ed. 8, 1972.

Turnbull, R.B., and Weakley, F.L.: Atlas of intestinal stomas, St. Louis, 1967, The C.V. Mosby Co.

Whitehead, E.D.: Current operative urology, New York, 1975, Harper & Row, Publishers.

Whitehead, S.L.: Nursing care of the adult urology patient, New York, 1970, Appleton-Century-Crofts.

Winter, C.C., and Morel, A.: Nursing care of patients with urologic diseases, ed. 4, St. Louis, 1977, The C.V. Mosby Co.

16 Gynecological surgery and cesarean section

A general understanding of the anatomy and physiology of the female pelvis, reproductive organs, and associated structures is necessary for the operating room nursing staff. Knowledge of anatomy is extremely important in positioning the patient for surgery, in selecting the proper instruments for a specific type of operation, and in understanding the plan of surgery.

ANATOMY AND PHYSIOLOGY

The female reproductive organs and their relationships are shown in Fig. 16-1. The adult female structures, as associated with the process of reproduction, are the bony pelvis, the associated ligaments and muscles, the soft tissues and contents of the pelvic cavity, the external organs (vulva) (Figs. 16-2 and 16-3), and the breasts (mammary glands).

Bony pelvis. The Latin word *pelvis* means basin. The pelvis is the part of the trunk below and behind the abdomen. The bony pelvis is made up of the ilium, symphysis pubis, ischium, sacrum, and coccyx (Fig. 16-2). The so-called pelvic brim divides the abdominal false portion from the true portion of the pelvis. The abdominal false pelvis is the part above the arcuate line (Fig. 16-2). The true pelvis is the part below this line. It forms the passageway through which the infant passes during parturition.

The true pelvis may be considered as having three parts: the inlet, cavity, and outlet. The muscles lining the pelvis facilitate movement of the thighs, give form to the pelvic cavity, and provide firm elastic lining to the bony pelvic framework. All organs located in the pelvis are covered by pelvic fascia (Fig. 16-4). The fascia covering some muscles is dense and firm, whereas that covering other organs is thin and elastic. The nerves, blood vessels, and ureters coursing through the anatomical structures are closely associated with muscular and fascial structures.

The *pelvic fascia* may be divided into three general groups: parietal, diaphragmatic, and visceral. The parietal pelvic fascia covers the muscles of the true pelvic wall and the perineum. The diaphragmatic fascia covers both sides of the pelvic diaphragm, which is made up of the levator ani and coccygeal muscles (Fig. 16-5). The visceral fascia is thin, flexible fascia, which covers the pelvic organs. The *floor of the pelvis,* known as the *pelvic diaphragm,* gives support to the abdominal pelvic viscera in this region. The pelvic diaphragm, consisting of the levator ani and coccygeal muscles with their respective fascial coverings, separates the pelvic cavity from the perineum (Fig. 16-5).

The *levator ani muscles,* varying in thickness and strength, may be divided into three parts: the iliococcygeal, the pubococcygeal, and the puborectal muscles (Fig. 16-5). The fibers of the levator ani muscles blend with the muscle fibers of the rectum and vagina. The fibers (pubovaginal) of the pubococcygeal part of the levator ani muscles, lying directly below the urinary bladder, are involved in the control of micturition. The pubococcygeal fibers of the levator ani muscles control and pull the coccyx forward and assist in the closure of the pelvic outlet. The fibers pull the rectum, vagina, and bladder neck upward toward the symphysis pubis in an effort to close the pelvic outlet and are responsible for the flexure at the anorectal junction. Relaxation of the fibers during defecation permits a straightening at this junction. During parturition, the action of the levator ani muscles directs the fetal head into the lower part of the passageway.

The uterus gains much of its support by its direct attachment to the vagina and by indirect attachments to nearby structures such as the rectum and pelvic diaphragm (Fig. 16-6). On each side of the uterus are the broad, round, cardinal (transverse cervical), and uterosacral ligaments and levator ani muscles.

Female pelvis

The *uterus,* which occupies a central place in the pelvis, is a pear-shaped organ situated between the bladder and the rectum. Its upper lateral points, the uterine cornua, receive the uterine tubes (Fig. 16-1). The fundus of the uterus is the upper rounded portion situated above the level of the tubal openings and just below the pelvic brim. Below, the body of the uterus joins the cervix, from which it is separated by a slight constriction canal, called the *isthmus*. The cervix lies at the level of the ischial spines. The body of the uterus communicates with the cervical canal at the internal orifice, called the *internal os* (Fig. 16-1). The constriction (canal) ends at the vaginal portion of the cervix at the external orifice, called the *external os*. This is a small oval aperture situated between two lips.

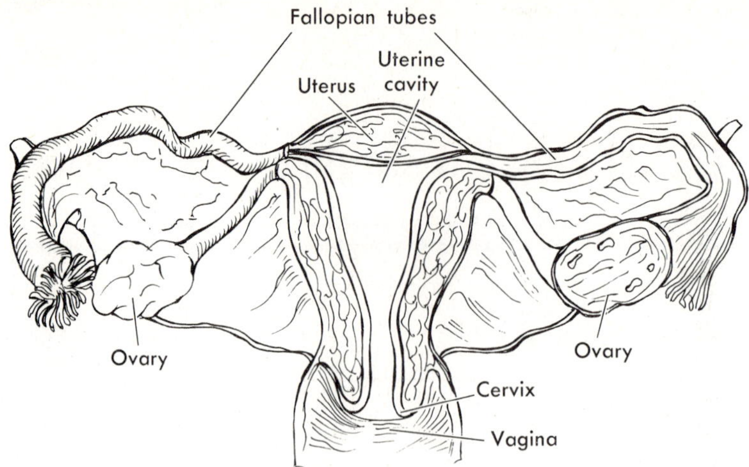

Fig. 16-1. Female reproductive organs.

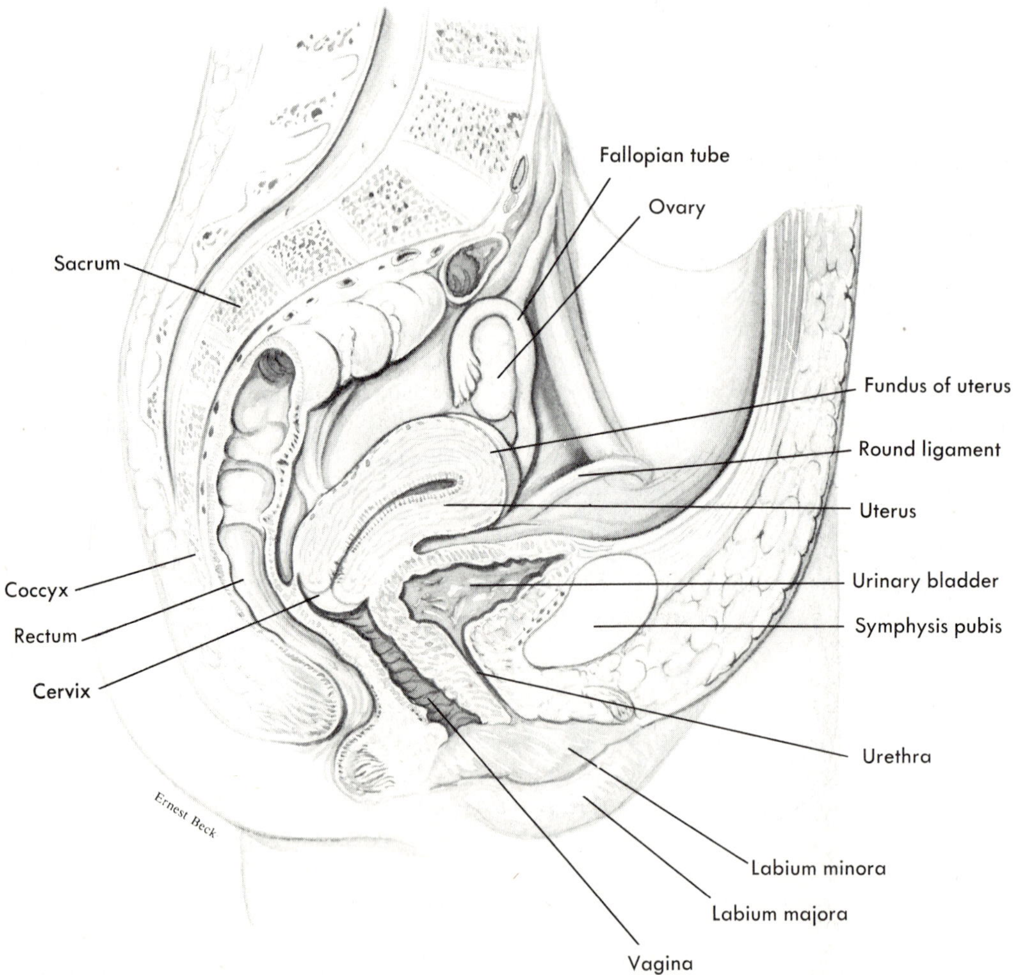

Fig. 16-2. Female pelvic organs as reviewed in median sagittal section. (From Anthony, C.P., and Kolthoff, N.J.: Textbook of anatomy and physiology, ed. 9, St. Louis, 1975, The C.V. Mosby Co.)

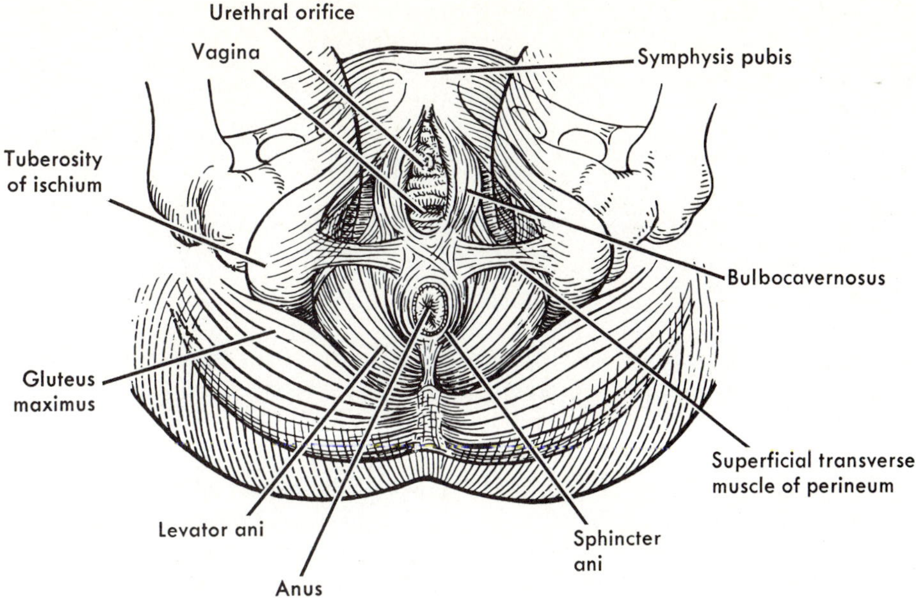

Fig. 16-3. Topographical anatomy of important perineal structures. (From Greenhill, J.P.: Surgical gynecology, Chicago, Year Book Medical Publishers, Inc.)

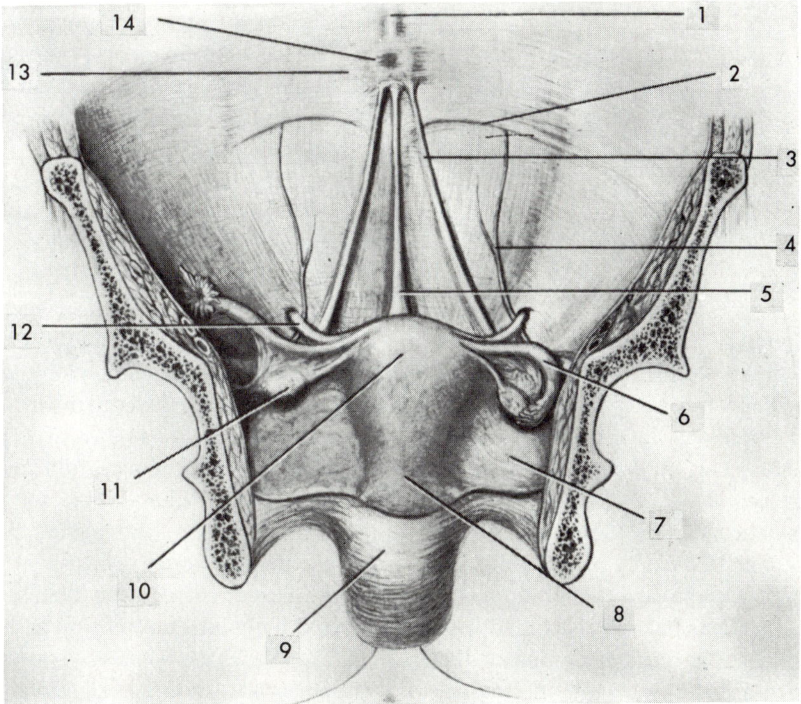

Fig. 16-4. Relationship of female sexual organs to anterior abdominal wall. *1,* Round ligament and liver; *2,* semicircular line of Douglas; *3,* lateral umbilical ligament; *4,* inferior epigastric artery; *5,* medial umbilical ligament; *6,* fallopian tube; *7,* broad ligament; *8,* cervix; *9,* vagina; *10,* uterine corpus; *11,* ovary; *12,* round ligament; *13,* umbilical fascia; *14,* umbilicus. (From Rubin, I.C., and Novak, J.: Integrated gynecology, New York, McGraw-Hill Book Co.)

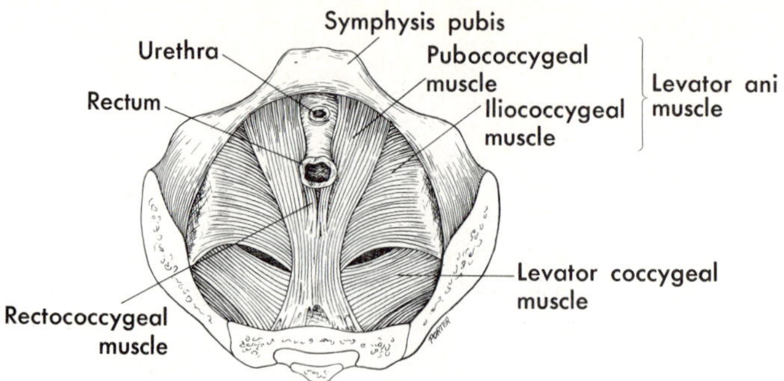

Fig. 16-5. Perineal musculature. (Redrawn from Anthony, C.P., and Kolthoff, N.J.: Textbook of anatomy and physiology, ed. 9, St. Louis, 1975, The C.V. Mosby Co.)

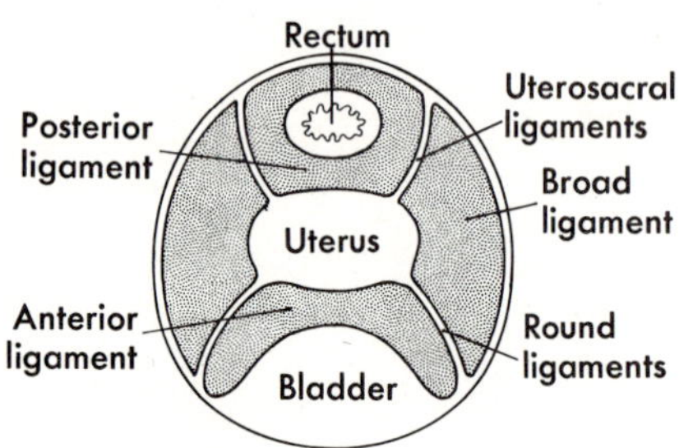

Fig. 16-6. Scheme to show relative positions of eight uterine ligaments formed by folds of peritoneum: two broad ligaments, double folds extending from uterus to side walls of pelvic cavity; two uterosacral ligaments, fold-like extensions of peritoneum from uterus to sacrum; posterior ligament, fold between uterus and rectum; and two round ligaments, folds from uterus to deep inguinal ring. (Redrawn from Anthony, C.P., and Kolthoff, N.J.: Textbook of anatomy and physiology, ed. 9, 1975, St. Louis, The C.V. Mosby Co.)

Structure of the uterus. The Greek word for uterus is *hystera*. The uterus lies posterior to the bladder and anterior to the rectum. The uterine body has three layers: (1) the outer peritoneal, or serous, layer, which is a reflection of the pelvic peritoneum; (2) the myometrium, or muscular layer, which houses involuntary muscles, nerves, blood vessels, and lymphatics; and (3) the endometrium, or mucosal layer, which lines the cavity of the uterus.

The *cervix* consists of a supravaginal and a vaginal portion. The supravaginal portion is closely associated with the bladder and the ureters. The vaginal portion of the cervix projects downward and backward into the vaginal vault.

Uterine (fallopian) tubes. The Greek word *salpinx*, meaning trumpet or tube, is used in referring to the uterine tube (Fig. 16-1). Bilateral tubes, each consisting of a musculomembranous channel about 4 to 5 inches long, form the canals through which the ova from either ovary are conveyed to the uterus. Each uterine tube leaves the upper portion of the uterus, passes outward toward the sides of the pelvis, and ends in fringe-like projections, called *fimbriae*. These fimbriae, or projections, are situated just below the ovaries. How the ova are transported from the ruptured follicles into the uterus is unknown. One theory is that transfer is accomplished through vascular changes, which together with contraction of the smooth muscle fibers of the tube and the peristaltic movements of the tube push the ova toward the uterus. The outer surfaces of the tubes are covered by peritoneum. Each tube receives its blood supply from the branches of the uterine and ovarian arteries.

The right tube and ovary are in close relationship to the cecum and appendix, and the left tube and ovary to the sigmoid flexure. Their close proximity to the ureters should be noted.

Ovaries. The ovaries are situated at the sides of the uterus. Each ovary lies within a depression (ovarian fossa) on the lateral wall of the pelvic cavity and above the broad ligament (Fig. 16-1). The ovary is attached to the posterior surface of the broad ligament by the mesovarium and is suspended by the ovarian ligament.

The ovary, a small, almond-shaped organ, is composed of an outer layer, known as the *cortex*, and an inner vascular layer, known as the *medulla*. The cortex contains ovarian (graafian) follicles in different stages of maturity. After ovulation, the corpus luteum arises from the graafian follicle that expelled the ovum. The medulla, lying within the cortex, consists of connective tissue containing nerves, blood, and lymph vessels. The ovary is covered by epithelium, not by peritoneum.

The ovaries are homologous with the testes of the male. They produce ova after puberty and also function as endocrine glands, producing hormones. The hormone estrogen is secreted by the ovarian follicles. It controls the development of the secondary sexual characteristics and initiates growth of the lining of the uterus during the menstrual cycle. The hormone progesterone, which is secreted by the corpus luteum, is essential for the implantation of the fertilized ovum and for the development of the embryo.

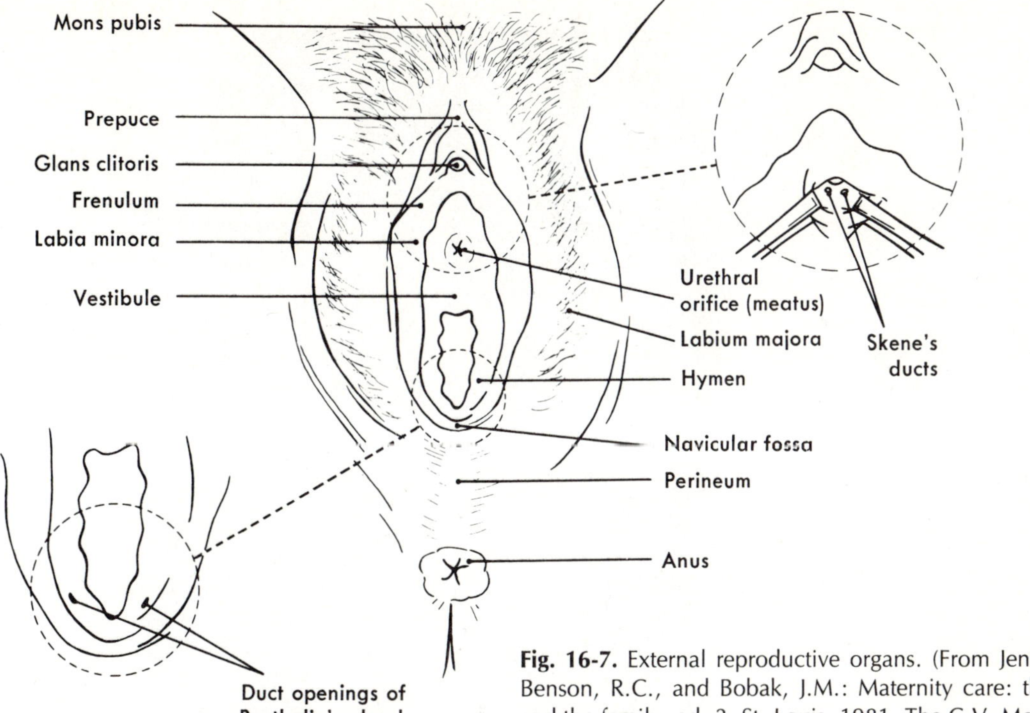

Fig. 16-7. External reproductive organs. (From Jensen, M., Benson, R.C., and Bobak, J.M.: Maternity care: the nurse and the family, ed. 2, St. Louis, 1981, The C.V. Mosby Co.)

Ligaments of the uterus. The uterine ligaments are the broad, round, transverse cervical (cardinal), and uterosacral (Figs. 16-4 and 16-6).

Broad ligaments. From each side of the uterus, the pelvic peritoneum extends laterally, downward, and posteriorly. A double fold of pelvic peritoneum forms the layers of the broad ligament, enclosing the uterus (Fig. 16-4). These layers separate to cover the floor and sides of the pelvis. The uterine tube is situated within the free border of broad ligament. The part of the broad ligament lying immediately below the uterine tube is termed the *mesosalpinx* (Fig. 16-1). The ovary lies behind the broad ligament.

Round ligaments. Round ligaments are fibromuscular bands that are attached to the uterus (Figs. 16-2 and 16-4). Each round ligament passes forward and laterally between the layers of the broad ligament to enter the deep inguinal ring.

Transverse cervical ligaments. Transverse cervical ligaments are cardinal ligaments composed of connective tissue masses with smooth muscle fibers that are strong support for the uterus.

Uterosacral ligaments. Uterosacral ligaments are a posterior continuation of the peritoneal tissue, which forms the cardinal ligaments. The ligaments pass posteriorly to the sacrum on either side of the rectum (Fig. 16-6).

Vagina. The vagina is a collapsed tube-like structure. It functions as the organ for copulation, the excretory duct for products of menstruation, and the birth canal. The anterior wall measures 6 to 8 cm in length, and the posterior wall 7 to 10 cm in length (Figs. 16-1 and 16-2). The anterior wall of the vagina is in close contact with the bladder and urethra. The lower posterior wall is anteriorly adjacent to the rectum. The upper portion of the vagina lies above the pelvic floor and is surrounded by visceral pelvic fascia. The lower half is surrounded by the levator ani muscles. The walls of the vagina are lined with mucous membrane.

Fornices. The projection of the cervix into the vaginal vault divides the vault into four regions, called *fornices:* anterior and posterior and right and left lateral.

The posterior fornix is in close contact with the peritoneum of the pouch of Douglas or cul-de-sac. The rectovaginal septum lies between the vagina and rectum. The dense connective tissue separating the anterior wall of the vagina from the distal urethra is termed the *urethrovaginal septum.*

Female external genital organs (vulva)

The external organs are referred to collectively as the *vulva* and occupy the central portion of the perineal region. The mons veneris, urethra, and Skene glands are in proximity to the vulva (Fig. 16-7).

The *mons veneris* of the vulva is a rounded elevation of tissue covered by skin and, after puberty, by hair. It is situated in front of the symphysis pubis, beneath which are located the labia majora.

The *labia majora* are two folds of skin that extend

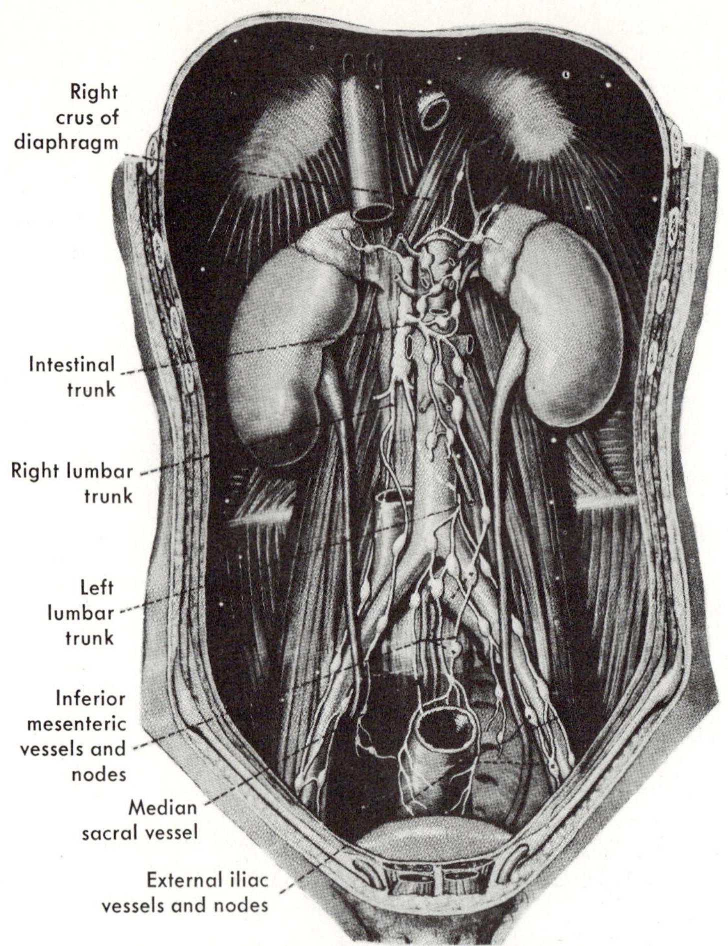

Fig. 16-8. Lymphatic system of abdomen and pelvis. (Adapted from Hamilton, W.J., editor: Textbook of human anatomy, ed. 2, St. Louis, 1976, The C.V. Mosby Co.)

downward and backward. They unite below and behind to form the posterior commissure and in front to form the anterior commissure. Bartholin's glands are situated on each side of the vaginal orifice.

The *labia minora* comprise the two delicate folds of skin that lie within the labia majora (Fig. 16-7). Each labium minus splits into lateral and medial parts. The lateral part forms the *prepuce of clitoris,* and the medial part forms the *frenulum.* The posterior folds of the labia are united by a delicate fold extending between them. This forms the fossa navicularis.

The *clitoris* is the homologue of the penis in the male. It hangs free and terminates in a rounded glans (small sensitive vascular body). Unlike the penis, the clitoris does not contain the urethra.

The *vestibule* is a smooth area surrounded by the labia minora, with the clitoris at its apex and the fossa navicularis at its base. It contains openings for the urethra and the vagina.

The *urethra,* which is about 4 cm long, is in close relationship with the anterior vaginal wall and connects the bladder with the urinary meatus. At each side of the urinary meatus lie two small ducts, termed the *paraurethral ducts,* which drain small *urethral (Skene's) glands* (Fig. 16-7).

The *vaginal orifice* lies below the urethral meatus. This opening extends through the hymen, which was originally a septum. The configuration and size of the opening varies and cannot be used as a determinate of a virginal state.

Bartholin's glands and ducts lie one at each side of the lower end of the vagina. They are homologues of the bulbourethral glands in the male. These narrow gland ducts open into the vaginal orifice on the inner aspects of the labia minora.

Vascular, nerve, and lymphatic supplies of the reproductive system

The *blood supply* of the female pelvis is derived from the internal iliac branches of the common iliac artery and is supplemented by the ovarian, superior rectal, and median sacral arteries—branches of the aorta.

The *nerve supply* of the female pelvis comes from the autonomic nerves, which enter the pelvis in the superior hypogastric plexus (presacral nerve).

The *lymphatics* of the female pelvis either follow the course of the vessels to the iliac and preaortic nodes or empty into the inguinal glands (Fig. 16-8).

NURSING CONSIDERATIONS

Operations on the structures of the reproductive system in the female are performed for diagnostic or therapeutic purposes, for conditions such as abnormal bleeding from any of the female reproductive organs, for suspected malignant or benign neoplasms, or for infertility. Procedures are also done to remove or repair weakened anatomical structures.

Because of the potential for altered body image and threatened sexuality in gynecological surgical patients, it is important to emphasize nursing considerations. The gynecological patient needs reassurance and emotional support for effective management of anxiety levels.

Principles and methods for positioning patients for different types of operations are described in Chapter 6. The patient is placed in the lithotomy position for most vaginal and perineal surgery. For abdominal surgery, the supine with the Trendelenburg position may be used. Care should be taken to protect the patient from nerve injury and provide for adequate circulatory, renal, and respiratory functions.

Skin preparation and routine draping procedures are described in Chapter 5. A basic vaginal instrument setup is needed for vaginal surgery. A laparotomy setup is needed for an abdominal operation. Instrument preferences by surgeons may vary, and the following setups are not meant to be all inclusive.

Because pelvic and vaginal procedures involve manipulation of the ureters, bladder, and urethra, indwelling urinary drainage systems are frequently established before or during operations. Either the urethral Foley catheter or the suprapubic cystostomy (Silastic) cannula directly into the bladder may be used, depending on the surgeon's preference and the type of procedure. The size of sutures, needles, and drains also varies depending on surgeon's preference.

BASIC VAGINAL INSTRUMENT SETUP

The sterile setup for the vaginal approach includes the following:

1 Graves vaginal speculum
1 Urethral catheter, 16 or 18 Fr
1 Boseman dressing forceps
3 Sponge-holding forceps
Gauze sponges
2 Towels
Antimicrobial solutions, as desired

Accessory unsterile items

Prep table
Kick buckets
Stools

The vaginal instrument setup includes the following:

Cutting instruments

3 Bard-Parker knife handles nos. 4 and 3, with blades nos. 20 and 10
2 Mayo uterine scissors, 1 curved and 1 straight, 6¾ inches (Fig. 16-9)
1 Metzenbaum scissors, curved or flat, 7 inches
1 Suture scissors, straight
1 Kelly scissors, curved on flat, 6¾ inches
1 Mayo scissors

Holding instruments

4 Foerster sponge-holding forceps, 9½ inches
6 Backhaus towel clamps, 5¼ inches
2 Tissue forceps with 2 and 3 teeth, 5½ inches
1 Tissue forceps with 2 and 3 teeth, 10 inches
2 Tissue forceps without teeth, 5½ inches
8 Allis-Adair tissue forceps, 6 inches
4 Allis forceps, 6 inches
2 Kocher forceps, 5½ inches
1 Bozeman dressing forceps (Fig. 16-10)
1 Jacobs vulsellum forceps (Fig. 16-10)
4 Babcock forceps (2 long)
1 Uterine tenaculum (Fig. 16-10)
1 Staude uterine tenaculum (Fig. 16-10)

Clamping instruments

12 Crile hemostats, straight, 6¼ inches
12 Kelly hemostats, curved, 5 inches (optional)
2 Mayo-Pean hemostats, curved, 6¼ inches
4 Kocher hemostats, straight, 8 inches (optional)
4 Heaney hysterectomy forceps, 8 inches
8 Rochester-Oschner hysterectomy forceps, 8 inches
4 Rogers vascular hysterectomy forceps

Exposing instruments (Fig. 16-11)

1 Self-retaining vaginal speculum
1 Jackson vaginal retractor
2 Heaney retractors
2 Deaver retractors
1 Uterine sound, graduated
1 Auvard speculum, weighted
1 Doyen vaginal retractor

Suturing instruments

1 Mayo-Hegar needle holder, 7 inches
2 Heaney needle holders (Fig. 16-9)
3 Crile-Wood needle holders, 6¼ inches

Accessory items (Figs. 16-12 and 16-13)

Indwelling urinary drainage items: Foley catheter or suprapubic cystostomy (Silastic) tube
Asepto syringe, 2 oz (optional)

Metal tray for surgeon's lap (optional)
Specimen containers
Lubricant, water-soluble
Electrocautery unit, if desired
Suction tip and tubing
1 Lithotomy drape pack
1 Sheet, small
1 Vaginal supply pack
1 Penrose drain (optional)
1 Goodell dilator
6 Hank uterine dilators
1 Uterine sound
2 Deschamp ligature carriers
Hegar dilators
1 Gaylor biopsy forceps
6 Blunt uterine curettes
6 Sharp uterine curettes
1 Endometrial biopsy suction curette

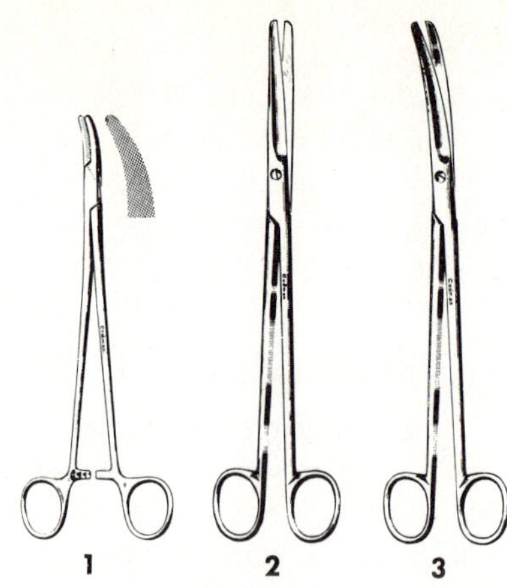

Fig. 16-9. Abdominal gynecological instruments: cutting and suturing. *1,* Heaney needle holder; *2,* Mayo uterine scissors (straight, 7¼ inches); *3,* Mayo uterine scissors (curved, 7¼ inches). (Courtesy Codman & Shurtleff, Inc., Randolph, Mass.)

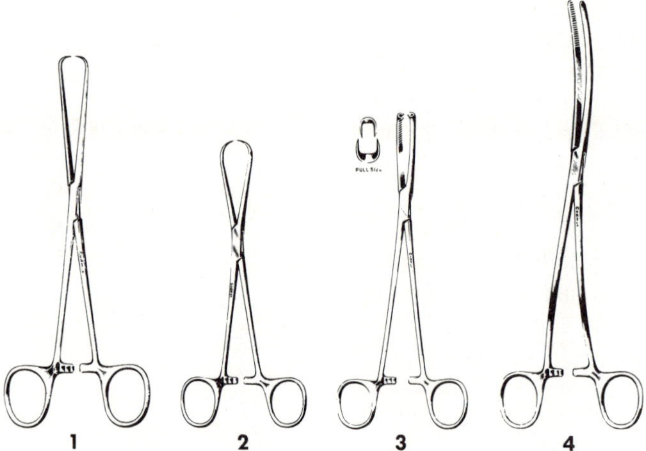

Fig. 16-10. Vaginal instruments: holding. *1,* Uterine tenaculum; *2,* Staude uterine tenaculum; *3,* Jacobs vulsellum forceps; *4,* Bozeman dressing forceps. (Courtesy Codman & Shurtleff, Inc., Randolph, Mass.)

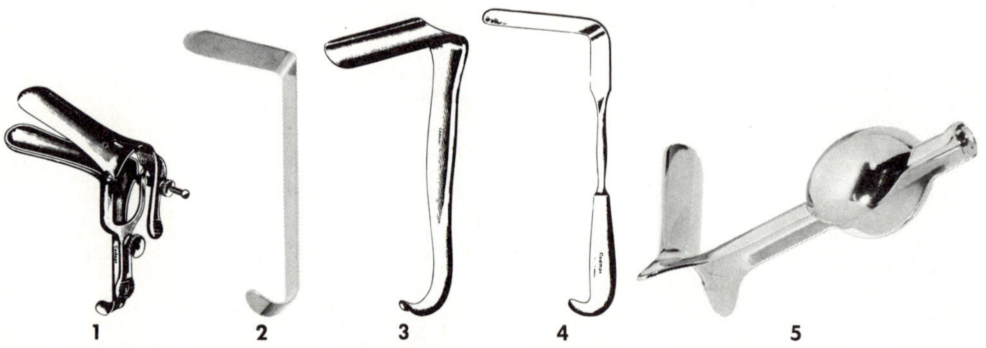

Fig. 16-11. Vaginal instruments: exposing. *1,* Graves vaginal speculum; *2,* Heaney hysterectomy retractor; *3,* Doyen vaginal retractor; *4,* Glenner vaginal retractor; *5,* Auvard vaginal speculum (weighted). (Courtesy Codman & Shurtleff, Inc., Randolph, Mass.)

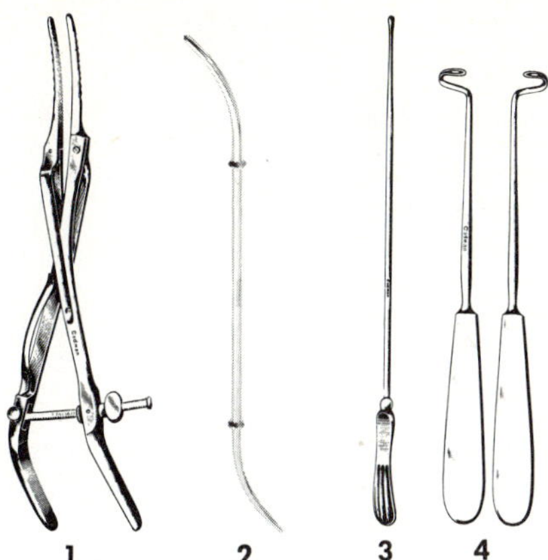

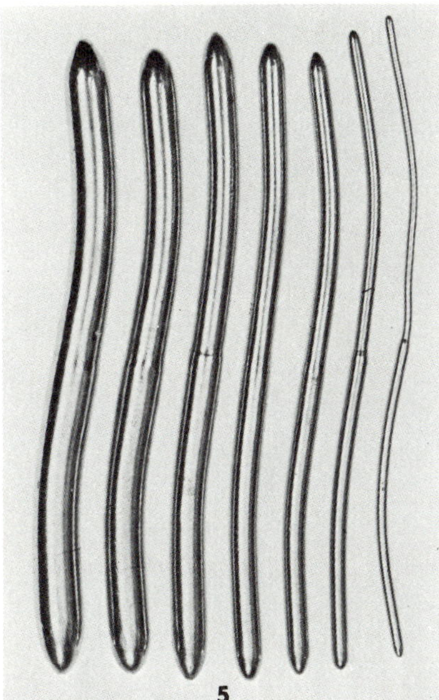

Fig. 16-12. Vaginal instruments: accessories. *1,* Goodell uterine dilator; *2,* Hank uterine dilator; *3,* uterine sound (graduated); *4,* Deschamp ligature carriers (right and left); *5,* Hegar dilators. (Courtesy Codman & Shurtleff, Inc., Randolph, Mass.)

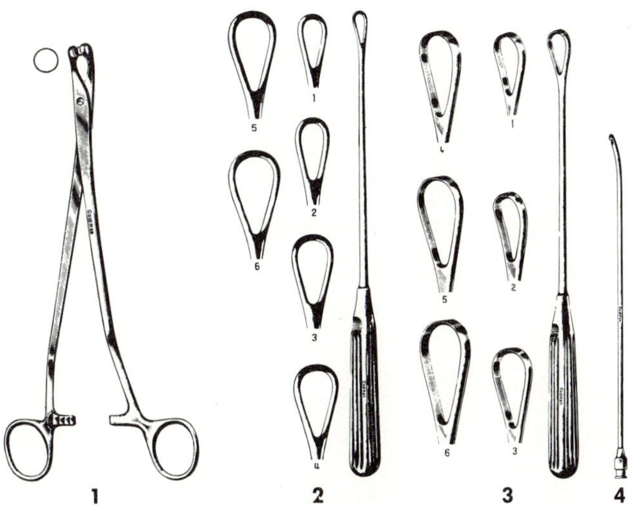

Fig. 16-13. Uterine instruments: cutting. *1,* Gaylor biopsy forceps; *2,* uterine curettes (blunt); *3,* uterine curettes (sharp); *4,* endometrial biopsy suction curette. (Courtesy Codman & Shurtleff, Inc., Randolph, Mass.)

BASIC ABDOMINAL INSTRUMENT SETUP

The standard instrument setup for the abdominal approach (oophorectomy, salpingectomy, hysterectomy, excision of ovarian cyst, and cesarean section) includes the basic laparotomy setup (Chapter 10) and the major vaginal repair set, plus the following:

Cutting instrument

1 Jorgenson scissors

Holding instruments

1 Somer uterine elevating forceps (Fig. 16-14)
2 Tenacula, single tooth
1 Tenaculum, two teeth

Exposing instruments (Fig. 16-15)

1 Martin or O'Sullivan-O'Connor universal retractor with lateral and center blades
1 Balfour retractor
1 Balfour extender

Suturing items

2 Mayo-Hegar needle holders, long

For most abdominal gynecological procedures, a dilatation and curettage setup should be available (Figs. 16-12 and 16-13).

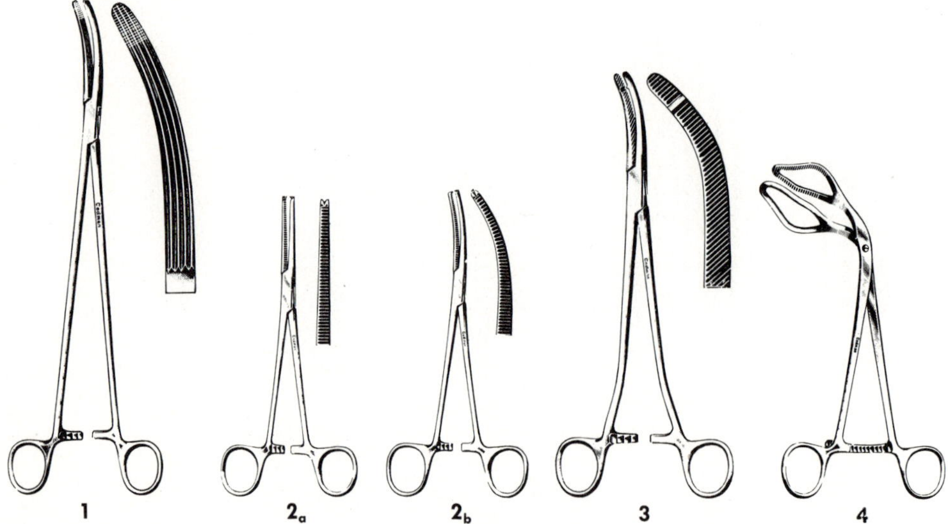

Fig. 16-14. Abdominal gynecological instruments: clamping. *1,* Rochester-Pean forceps; *2_a,* Rochester-Ochsner (straight); *2_b,* Rochester-Ochsner (curved); *3,* Heaney hysterectomy forceps; *4,* Somer uterine elevating forceps. (Courtesy Codman & Shurtleff, Inc., Randolph, Mass.)

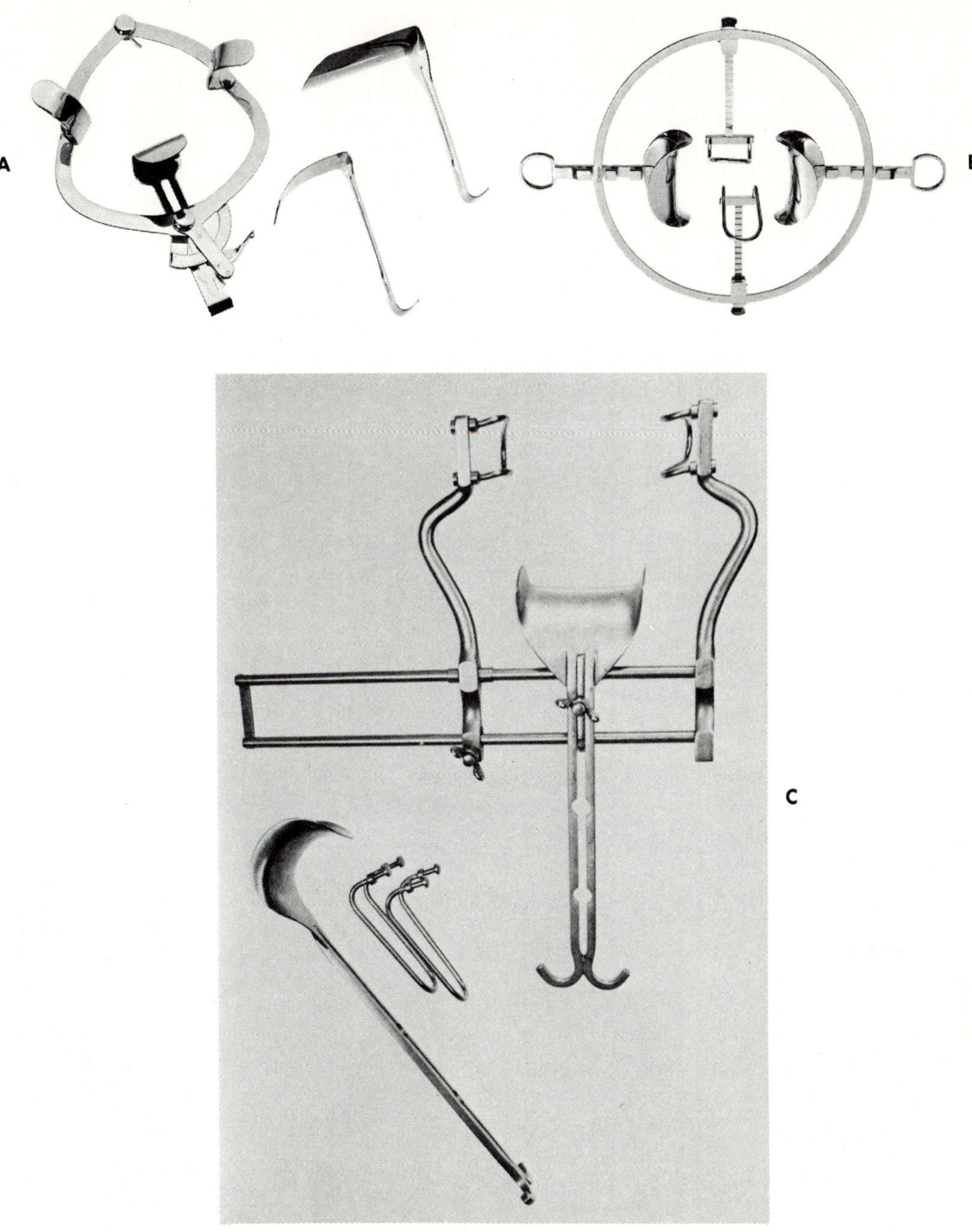

Fig. 16-15. Abdominal gynecological instruments: exposing. **A,** O'Sullivan-O'Connor self-retaining abdominal retractor. **B,** Martin self-retaining abdominal ring retractor. **C,** Balfour retractor. (Courtesy Codman & Shurtleff, Inc., Randolph, Mass.)

VULVAR SURGERY

The treatment of early malignant disease of the vulva is accomplished by a skinning technique, local wide excision, or, in more multicentric or extensive lesions, simple vulvectomy. These procedures may also be accomplished by use of a laser.

Simple vulvectomy

Definition. Removal of the labia majora and labia minora, possibly but not preferably the glans clitoris, and occasionally the perianal area, with a plastic closure.

Considerations. A simple vulvectomy is usually done for the treatment of carcinoma in situ of the vulva when it is multicentric or for treatment of Bowen's or Paget's disease. Occasionally it is necessary for the treatment of either leukoplakia or intractable pruritus, especially when a skinning procedure is impractical or has failed.

Setup and preparation of the patient. The patient is anesthetized and placed in the lithotomy position, as described in Chapter 6. The operative site is cleansed, and the patient is draped as described previously. The basic vaginal set is used, plus an electrosurgical unit, if desired.

Operative procedure

1. The affected skin is incised, usually starting anteriorly above the clitoris. The incision is continued laterally to the labia majora, to the midline of the perineum, and around the anus, if it is involved (Fig. 16-16, *A*). A knife, forceps, gauze sponges on holders, tissue forceps, and Allis forceps are needed. Bleeding vessels are clamped. Bleeding is also controlled by use of the electrosurgical unit or sutures.

2. Periurethral and perivaginal incisions are made. Bleeding of this vascular area can be controlled by means of Kelly or Crile hemostats and the electrosurgical unit. Ligation of blood vessels should be minimal. Allis-

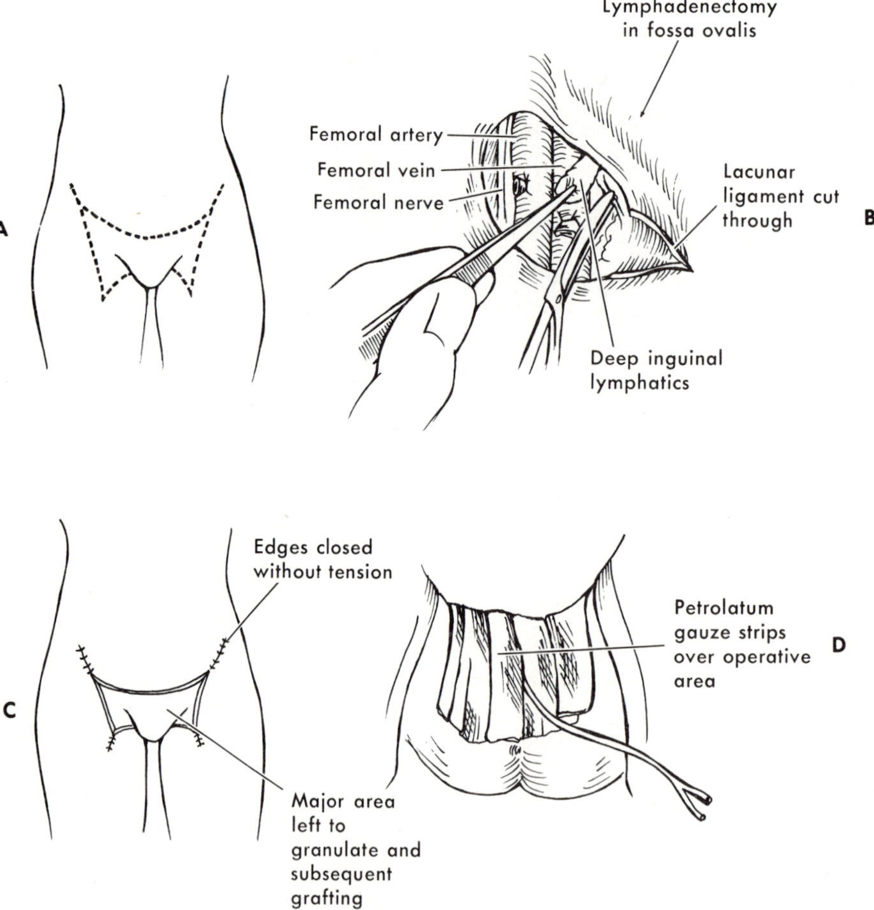

Fig. 16-16. A, Outline of incisional lines for simple or radical operations for vulval cover. **B,** Dissection is completed, involving nerves, saphenous veins, and muscles, when dissection of distal half of femoral canal has been completed. **C,** Upper edges of abdominal incisions may be partially closed. **D,** With indwelling catheter in bladder, wound is dressed with layers of gauze and held in place with light pressure dressing. (From Ball, T.L.: Gynecologic surgery and urology, ed. 2, St. Louis, The C.V. Mosby Co.)

Adair forceps are used for holding diseased tissues.

3. All skin and subcutaneous tissues are undermined and mobilized with curved dissecting tissue forceps, scissors, Allis forceps, and sponges on holders.

4. The wound is closed, usually by simple bilateral Z-plasty or other plastic closure. In some cases, an excision of the skin is made around the anus to accomplish a sliding skin flap.

5. Drains or continuous suction sometimes is placed in the dependent areas, an indwelling system of urinary drainage is established, and gauze packing may be placed in the vagina. Gauze dressings are applied and held in place with plastic tape and a binder.

Skinning vulvectomy

Definition. For superficial malignant lesions or multicentric benign lesions, the simple removal of the external skin from the affected area, which has been previously identified with a stain such as toluidine blue.

Considerations. The main purpose of this procedure is to preserve the underlying structures of the external genitals. A skinning procedure may be done to treat leukoplakia, intractable pruritus, or other types of skin lesions, such as kraurosis, vitiligo, and chronic venereal granulomas.

Setup and preparation of the patient. As described for simple vulvectomy.

Operative procedure. Simple excision of the external skin from the affected area.

Radical vulvectomy and groin lymphadenectomy

Definition. En bloc dissection comprising the following structures: a large segment of skin from the abdomen and groin, the labia majora, labia minora, clitoris, mons veneris, and terminal portions of the urethra, vagina, and other vulval organs, as well as the superficial and/or deep inguinal nodes, portions of the round ligaments, portions of the saphenous veins, and the lesion itself. It also involves reconstruction of the vaginal walls and pelvic floor and closure of the abdominal wounds (Fig. 16-16). Later, placement of full-thickness pinch or split-thickness grafts may be done if the denuded area of the vulva appears too large for normal granulation (Chapter 21).

Considerations. A radical vulvectomy and groin lymphadenectomy involve abdominoperineal dissection and groin dissection, which may be performed as a one- or two-stage operation. When performed as a one-stage operation, it is optimally conducted by a four-person team.

Setup and preparation of the patient. The patient lies supine and may be placed in Trendelenburg's and low lithotomy positions, as required for the various stages. The skin preparation includes both the abdomen and vulva, and the skin of the thighs is usually prepared down to the knees. As in other radical surgery, the nursing team should be prepared to measure blood loss and anticipate procedures to combat shock.

The setups include a basic gynecological abdominal setup, plus additional incisional instruments. A minor vaginal setup is also required.

Groin lymphadenectomy (dissection). The basic laparotomy setup, plus the following:

Clamping instruments

8 Schnidt gall duct forceps, full-curved, right-angled (Chapter 7)
1 Set silver clips and holders

Accessory items (optional)

Drains:
2 Latex rubber catheters, 14 Fr
4 Pieces Penrose tubing, 12 × ⅝ inch
Gauze packing
2 Closed wound drainage systems

Vulvectomy. The basic vaginal instrument setup, plus the following:

Exposing instruments

2 Richardson retractors, small
2 Richardson retractors, narrow, long blades
2 Volkmann rake retractors, three-pronged, dull

Accessory items (optional)

Drains:
4 Pieces Penrose tubing, 12 × ⅝ inch
2 Closed wound drainage systems

Operative procedures

Groin lymphadenectomy

1. The first skin incision is made on the side opposite the primary lesion. The end of the incised skin is grasped with Allis forceps. The incision is carried down to the aponeuroses of the external oblique muscle.

2. The fascia over the inguinal ligament and the fascia lata of the upper thigh are exposed, separated, and freed with retractors, knife, scissors, hemostats, and sponges.

3. Bleeding vessels are clamped and ligated, including the superficial iliac artery and vein, the epigastric artery and vein, and the superficial external pudendal artery and vein. The smaller bleeding vessels are controlled by electrocautery.

4. The fibers of the inguinal, hypogastric, and femoral nerves are resected by Metzenbaum or Harrington scissors, tissue forceps without teeth, and long-bladed retractors.

5. The lymphatic node beds may be identified with silk or metal clips. Fine, long, sharp dissection scissors are needed.

6. The large tissue surfaces are exposed for complete dissection by means of retractors and are protected by

warm, wet laparotomy packs. High saphenous vein ligation is performed with scissors, forceps, and hemostats and should be doubly tied with nonreactive suture.

7. The femoral canal is cleaned of its lymphatics; the round ligament is clamped, cut, and ligated.

8. The peritoneum is freed from the muscles; the fascia is dissected free; deep lymphatic nodes and areolar tissue are removed; and vessels and their attachments are clamped, cut, and ligated, using long curved scissors, long tissue forceps, hemostats, and ligatures (Fig. 16-16, *B*).

9. The lesion is removed. In deep pelvic lymphadenectomy, the ureter may be exposed and the area drained.

10. The inguinal canal is reconstructed, and the wound is partially closed with a nonabsorbable suture (Fig. 16-16, *C*). An indwelling system of urinary drainage is established, and the wound is dressed (Fig. 16-16, *D*).

Radical vulvectomy

1. The skin incisions of the abdomen and thigh join with those for vulvectomy. The incisions in the vulva encircle the urethra.

2. In the vulval dissection, terminal portions of the urethra and vagina, the mons veneris, the clitoris, the frenulum, the prepuce of the clitoris, Bartholin's and Skene's glands, and fascial coverings of the vulva are removed with the specimen.

3. Reconstruction of the vaginal walls and the pelvic floor is completed. An indwelling system of urinary drainage is established, suction drains are placed in the denuded area, and the wound is dressed with a gauze pressure dressing (Fig. 16-16).

VAGINAL SURGERY

Vaginal plastic operation (anterior and posterior repair)

Definition. Reconstruction of the vaginal walls, the pelvic floor, and the muscles and fascia of the rectum, urethra, bladder, and perineum.

Considerations. A vaginal repair is done to correct a cystocele or a rectocele and to reestablish the support of the anterior vaginal wall, which will restore the bladder to its normal position.

A *cystocele* is a herniation of the bladder causing the anterior vaginal wall to bulge downward. A defect in the anterior vaginal wall is usually caused by obstetrical or surgical trauma, age, and/or an inherent weakness. A large protrusion may cause a sensation of pressure in the vagina or present a mass at, or through, the introitus; it may also cause voiding difficulties (Fig. 16-17).

A *rectocele* is formed by a protrusion of the anterior rectal wall (posterior vaginal wall) into the vagina. In general, the anterior rectal wall forms a bulging mass beneath the posterior vaginal mucosa (Fig. 16-17). As the mass pushes downward into the lower vaginal canal, the rectum may be torn from the fascial and muscular attachments of the urogenital diaphragm and the pelvic wall.

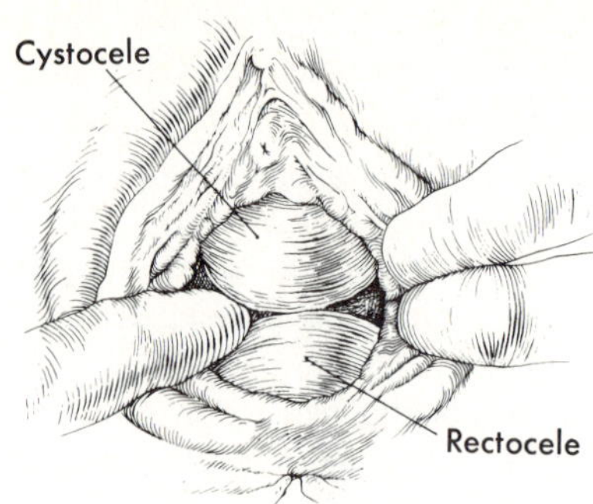

Fig. 16-17. Cystocele and rectocele resulting from unrepaired tears of muscles of pelvic floor and those under bladder, usually resulting from childbirth, surgical trauma, age, and/or inherent weakness. (From Crossen, R.J.: Diseases of women, ed. 10, St. Louis, The C.V. Mosby Co.)

The levator ani muscles become stretched or torn (Fig. 16-5). The symptomatic signs are a mass protruding from the vagina, difficulty in evacuating the lower bowel, hemorrhoids, and a feeling of pressure.

An *enterocele* is a herniation of Douglas' cul-de-sac and almost always contains loops of the small intestine. An enterocele herniates into a weakened area between the anterior and posterior vaginal walls.

Setup and preparation of the patient. The patient is anesthetized and placed in the lithotomy position. Vaginal preparation, including cleansing of the vaginal vault and vulva and draping, is completed. The bladder is usually drained after vaginal preparation, depending on the surgeon's preference. Instruments are as described for major vaginal repair, plus the setup described for uterine dilatation and curettage (Figs. 16-12 and 16-13).

Operative procedures

1. Dilatation and curettage may be done.

2. Vaginal retractors are used for exposure. The labia may be sewn back if the exposure is inadequate.

Anterior wall repair

1. The bladder may be drained, or an indwelling urinary or suprapubic cystostomy catheter may be established, according to the surgeon's preference. Areolar tissue between the bladder and vagina at the bladder reflection is exposed. The full thickness of the vaginal wall is separated up to the bladder neck by a knife, curved scissors, tissue forceps, Adair or Allis forceps (Fig. 16-18, *A*), and gauze sponges. Bleeding vessels are clamped and tied with ligatures or cauterized.

2. The urethra and bladder neck are freely mobilized with a knife, gauze sponges, and curved scissors (Fig. 16-18, *B*).

3. Sutures are placed adjacent to the urethra and bladder neck in such a manner that, after they have been tied, a narrowing of the bladder neck and a delineating of the posterior urethrovesical angle occurs (Fig. 16-18, *C*).

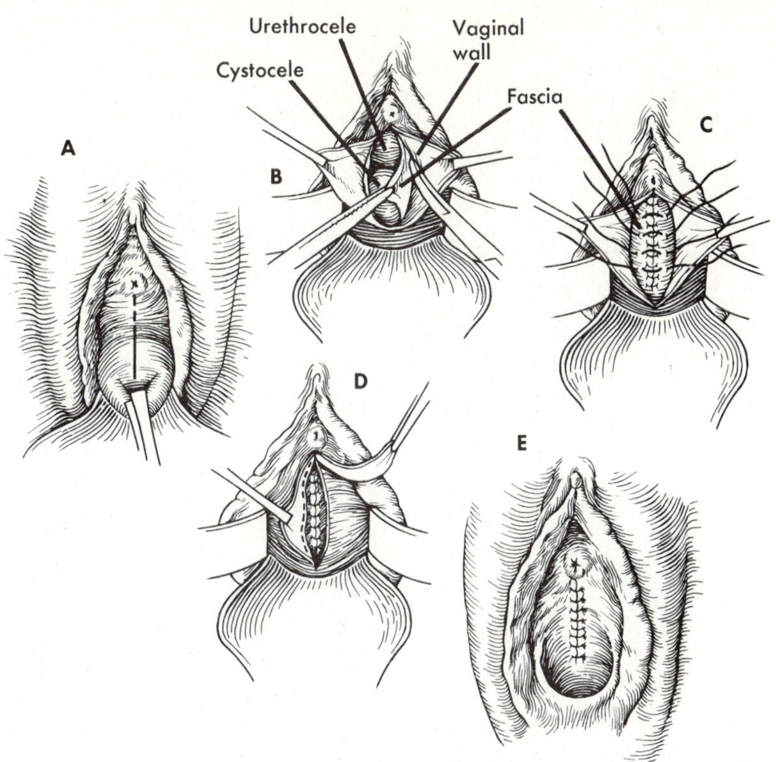

Fig. 16-18. Correction of cystourethrocele. **A,** Cervix pulled down as far as possible with tenaculum. Vertical incision made entirely through to vaginal wall. **B,** Vaginal flaps further dissected upward. Urethral meatus and pubocervical fascia separated from vaginal wall with Mayo scissors. **C,** Fascia brought together with continuous suture, beginning at lowest point and ending near external urethral meatus. A few interrupted sutures placed secondarily. **D,** Excess portion of vaginal wall carefully removed, leaving sufficient amount to be closed with tension. **E,** Completed operation, maintaining bladder and urethra in normal position. (From Counseller, V.S.: In Lowrie, R.J., editor: Gynecology: surgical techniques, Springfield, Ill., Charles C Thomas, Publisher.)

4. The connective tissue on the lateral aspects of the cervix is sutured into the cervix to shorten the cardinal ligaments.

5. Allis-Adair tissue forceps are applied to the edges of the incision, and the left flap of the vaginal wall is drawn across the midline. Edges are trimmed according to the size of the cystocele (Fig. 16-18, *D*). This process is repeated on the right flap of the vaginal incision.

6. The anterior vaginal wall is closed in a manner resulting in reconstruction of an anterior vaginal fornix (Fig. 16-18, *E*).

Posterior wall repair

1. Allis forceps are placed posteriorly at the mucocutaneous junction on each side, at the hymenal ring, and just above the anus (Fig. 16-19, *A*).

2. Skin and mucosa are incised and dissected from the muscles beneath with a knife, tissue forceps, curved scissors, and gauze sponges.

3. Allis-Adair forceps are placed on the posterior vaginal wall, scar tissue (from obstetrical trauma) is removed, and dissection is continued to the posterior vaginal fornix and laterally, depending on the size of the rectocele (Fig. 16-19, *A* and *B*).

4. The perineum is denuded by sharp dissection, and the trimming of the posterior vaginal wall is carried out with Allis forceps, curved scissors, and gauze sponges.

5. The rectal wall proximal to the puborectal muscle is strengthened by placement of sutures (Fig. 16-19, *C*).

6. Bleeding is controlled, and the vaginal wall is closed from above, downward to the anterior edge of the puborectal muscle. The rectocele is repaired from the posterior fornix to the perineal body (Fig. 16-19, *D* and *E*). Remains of the transverse perineal and bulbocavernous muscles are used to build up the perineum. The anterior edge of the levator ani muscle may be approximated.

7. The mucosa and skin are trimmed, and the remaining closure is effected by interrupted sutures.

8. The vagina may be packed with 2-inch vaginal packing. An indwelling urinary or suprapubic cystostomy catheter is established, according to the surgeon's preference.

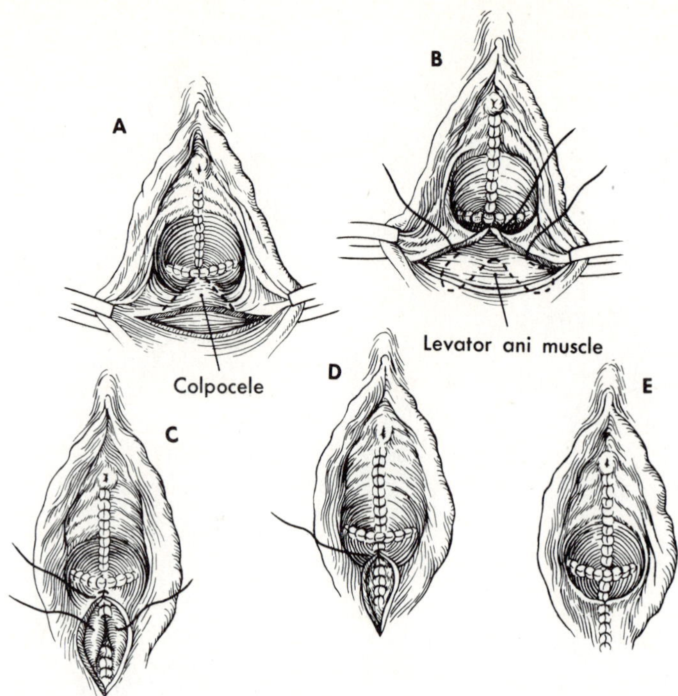

Fig. 16-19. Repair of rectocele. **A,** Exposure of perineum and portion of posterior vaginal wall excised. **B,** Excess skin and excess portion of posterior vaginal wall excised up to vaginal vault. First suture placed in vaginal vault. **C,** Levator ani muscles brought together with interrupted stitches; Colles' fascia brought together over perineum. **D,** Perineum restored and Colles' fascia repaired with interrupted sutures. **E,** Skin of perineum closed. (From Counseller, V.S.: In Lowrie, R.J., editor: Gynecology: surgical techniques, Springfield, Ill., Charles C Thomas, Publisher.)

Enterocele repair. Setup is as described for anterior and posterior repair; the procedure is illustrated in Fig. 16-20. The peritoneal sac must be carefully dissected from the underlying rectum or the overlying bladder, or both, so that the prolonged peritoneal tissues are completely freed from the surrounding structures. The sac is opened to establish true identification and is then closed as high as possible by permanent purse-string sutures. The portion of peritoneal tissue distal to the purse-string ties is then excised, and the area is reinforced locally by transverse suture closures of whatever supportive tissues may be available. This technique is done to prevent recurrence.

Perineal repair. Basic vaginal setup and procedure as illustrated in Fig. 16-21.

Vesicovaginal fistula repair

Definition. Through the vaginal outlet, free dissection of the mucosal tissue of the anterior vaginal wall, closing of the vagina, repair of the fascial attachments between the bladder and vagina, and establishment of urinary drainage (Fig. 16-22).

Considerations. Fistulas vary in size from a small opening that permits only slight leakage of urine into the vagina to a large opening that permits all urine to pass into the vagina (Fig. 16-22).

Fistulas may result from radical surgery in the management of pelvic cancer, from radium therapy without surgery, from chronic ulceration of the vaginal structures, from penetrating wounds, or from obstetrical trauma.

A *urethrovaginal fistula* usually causes constant incontinence or difficulty in retaining urine. This condition occurs after damage to the anterior wall and bladder or following radiation surgery or parturition. A *ureterovaginal fistula* develops as a result of injury to the ureter. In some cases, reimplantation of the ureter in the bladder or ureterostomy may be done.

Vaginal approach

Setup and preparation of the patient. As described for vaginal plastic repair, plus the following:

1 Kelly fistula scissors
1 Adson dressing forceps, 7⅛ inches
2 Probes, pliable
1 Frazier suction set
2 Hooks, fine and blunt
2 Ureteral catheters
1 Foley indwelling or suprapubic cystostomy catheter

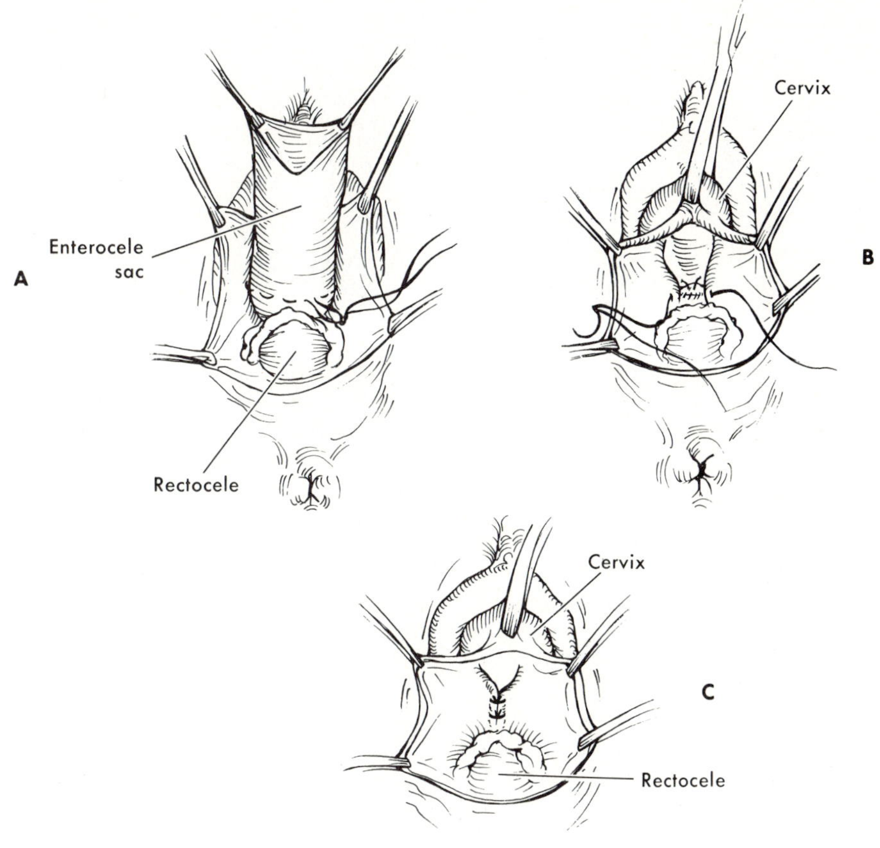

Fig. 16-20. Repair of enterocele. **A,** Transverse incision has been made at mucocutaneous border, as in operation for rectocele. Then posterior vaginal wall mucosa is divided in midline up to cervix. Sac of peritoneum has been excised completely, then opened, and contents pushed into peritoneal cavity. Purse-string suture of no. 1 chromic has been placed about neck of sac. **B,** Uterosacral ligaments that have been exposed are approximated with no. 1 chromic sutures. First suture bites into posterior surface of cervix and also retracted remainder of neck of sac. **C,** Two sutures that bite into posterior surface of cervix have been tied. (Adapted from TeLinde, R.W., and Mattingly, R.F.: Operative gynecology, ed. 4, Philadelphia, 1970, J.B. Lippincott Co.)

1 Asepto syringe, 2 oz
Gauze dressings, if desired
Distilled, sterile water, if desired
1 Penrose drain (optional)
Electrocautery unit

Operative procedure

1. Traction sutures are placed about the fistulous tract; tissues are grasped with Adair forceps and plain tissue forceps.

2. The scar tissue around the fistula is excised, cleavage between bladder and vagina is located, and clean flaps are mobilized with scissors, forceps, and gauze sponges.

3. The bladder mucosa is inverted toward the interior of the bladder with interrupted sutures. The sutures are passed through the muscularis of the bladder down to the mucosa.

4. A second layer of inverting sutures is placed in the bladder and tied, thereby completely inverting the bladder mucosa toward the interior.

5. The vaginal wall is closed with interrupted sutures in the direction opposite to the closure of the bladder wall.

6. The bladder is distended with distilled, sterile water to determine any leaks. A urinary catheter is left in place; dressings are applied and held in place with plastic tape and a binder.

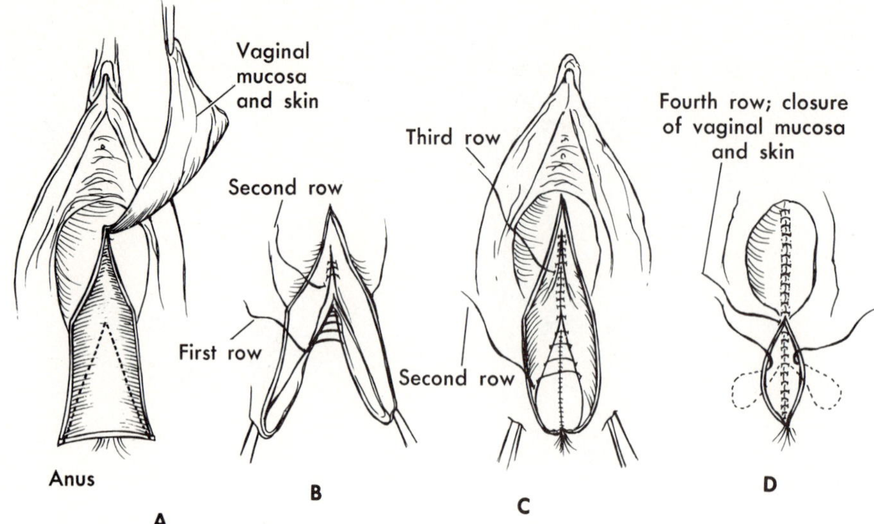

Fig. 16-21. Repair of complete lacerations of the perineum. **A,** Lower margins of incision. **B,** Placement of first and second rows of sutures. **C,** Second and third rows of sutures. **D,** Fourth row of sutures. (Adapted from Counseller, V.S.: In Lowrie, R.J., editor: Gynecology: surgical techniques, Springfield, Ill., Charles C Thomas, Publisher.)

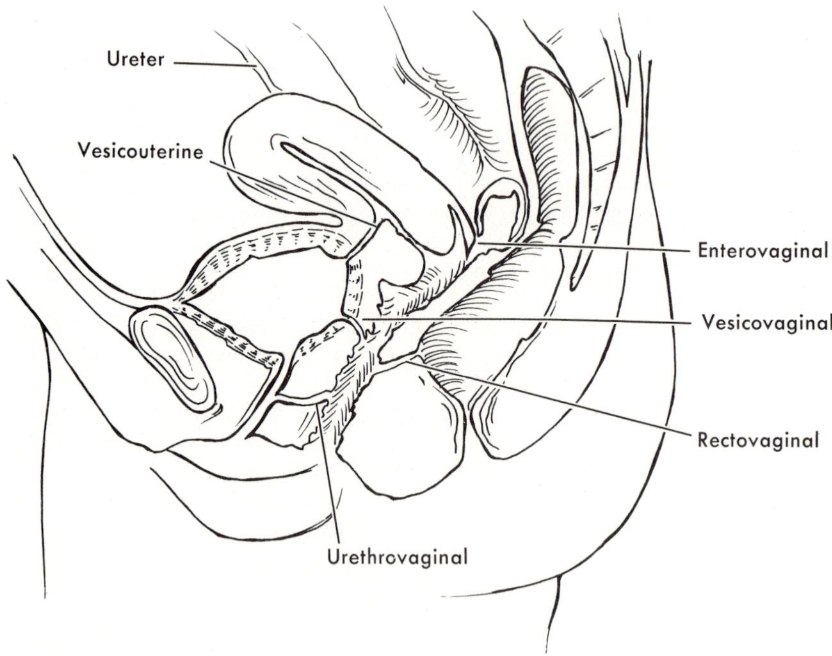

Fig. 16-22. Types of genital fistulas. Urogenital fistula is communication between urethra, bladder, or one of ureters and some part of genital tract. Urethrovaginal, vesicovaginal, or ureterovaginal fistulas, most common types, empty into vaginal canal. (Adapted from Huffman, J.W.: Gynecology and obstetrics, Philadelphia, W.B. Saunders Co.)

Transperitoneal approach

Considerations. In the presence of a high vesicovaginal fistula, a suprapubic incision is used. The opening from the bladder into the vagina is closed, and the fascial attachments are repaired.

Setup and preparation of the patient. The patient is placed in slight Trendelenburg's position. Ureteral catheters may be introduced just before surgery (Chapter 15). The vagina is cleansed and packed with moist gauze saturated with an antibiotic or antimicrobial solution. The abdominal operative site is cleansed, and the patient is draped.

The instrument setup required is as described for laparotomy (Chapter 10).

Operative procedure

1. A midline abdominal incision is usually made, as described for laparotomy.
2. The fistulous tract is identified; the vaginal vault and the adjacent adherent bladder are separated with scissors, forceps, and sponges.
3. The vesicovaginal septum is dissected down to the healthy tissue beyond the site of the fistula.
4. The fistulous tract is mobilized. The bladder site of the fistula is inverted into the interior of the bladder with two rows of inverting sutures. The muscularis and mucosa layers of the vagina are inverted into the vaginal vault by means of two rows of sutures.
5. The flaps of peritoneum are mobilized, both from the bladder and from the adjacent vaginal vault, and are closed to form a new vesicovaginal reflection of peritoneum below the site of the old fistulous tract.
6. The wound is closed in layers, as for laparotomy. Abdominal dressings are applied and held in place with adhesive or plastic tape, and an indwelling catheter is left in the bladder.

Rectovaginal fistula repair

Vaginal approach

Definition. Vaginal repair of the perineum, fascia, and muscle-supporting structures between the rectum and vagina, thereby closing the fistula formed between the rectum and the vagina (Fig. 16-23).

In the presence of a large rectovaginal fistula, as in patients who suffer from incurable cancer, a colostomy may be done (Chapter 14).

Setup and preparation of the patient. The patient is placed in the lithotomy position and prepared as described for vaginal repair. The instruments and other items needed are as described for vaginal plastic repair.

Operative procedure

1. The scar tissue and tract between the rectum and vagina are excised; edges of fresh tissue are approximated with absorbable sutures (Fig. 16-24).
2. The rectum and vaginal walls are mobilized; the rectum is closed with inversion of the mucosa into the rectal canal.

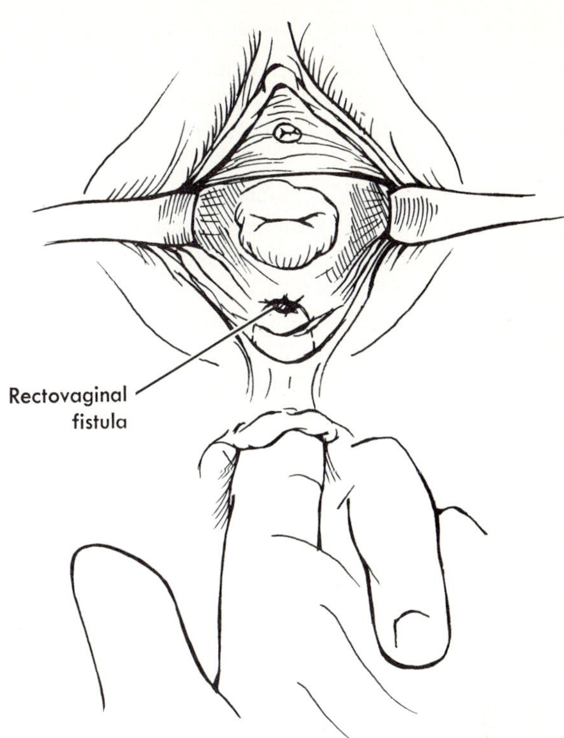

Fig. 16-23. Rectovaginal fistula. Examiner's finger puts tension on rectovaginal septum. (Adapted from Huffman, J.W.: Gynecology and obstetrics, Philadelphia, W.B. Saunders Co.)

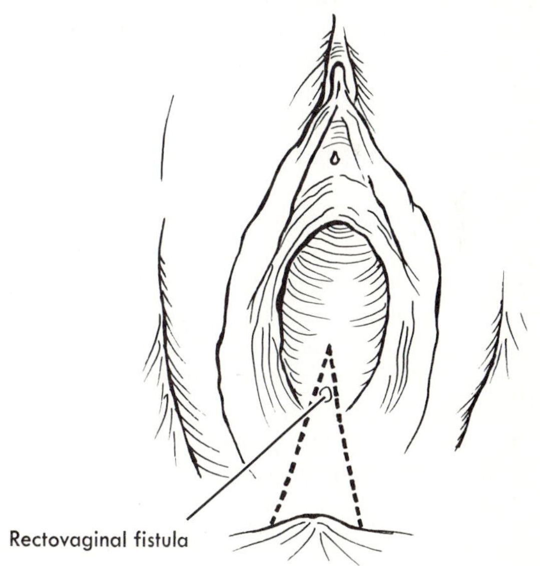

Fig. 16-24. Repair of rectovaginal fistulas of all types essentially same as shown here. Portion of scar tissue to be excised is included in dotted line; repair is as described for complete lacerations of perineum (Fig. 16-21). (Adapted from Counseller, V.S.: In Lowrie, R.J., editor: Gynecology: surgical techniques, Springfield, Ill., Charles C Thomas, Publisher.)

3. The vagina is closed transversely or in a sagittal plane different from that of the rectal canal. The vaginal mucosal layer is inverted into the vaginal wall; an indwelling urinary drainage system is established.

Operations for urinary stress incontinence

Definition. Through a vaginal or abdominal approach, repair of the fascial supports and the pubococcygeal muscle surrounding the urethra and the bladder neck (Fig. 16-5).

Considerations. The proper operative approach for the treatment of stress incontinence must be selected specifically for each patient. Normal micturition depends on a finely coordinated group of voluntary and involuntary movements. As a result of volitional impulses, voiding may be inhibited or stopped by the intrinsic muscles of the bladder neck and proximal urethra and the puborectalis division of the levator ani muscle (Chapter 15).

The type of operation selected depends on the severity of stress incontinence, the extent of the lesion causing it, the patient's ability to use the anatomical mechanism for voluntary inhibition of urination, and the operations that have previously been performed. Stages of stress incontinence are classified in relation to frequency and degree of incontinence, the presence of other diseases, and the function of pubococcygeus muscle (levator ani) (Figs. 16-3 and 16-5).

Previous pelvic operations may have resulted in scarring and distortion, with displacement of the bladder neck to an unfavorable position for proper functioning. Conditions such as uterine prolapse, cystocele, urethrocele, cystourethrocele, or urogenital fistulas following radiation therapy may be associated with stress incontinence.

The aim of any operation for urinary stress incontinence is to improve the performance of a dislodged or dysfunctional vesical neck, to restore normal urethral length, and to tighten and restore the anterior urethral vesical angle.

Setup and preparation of the patient. *For vaginal approach,* as described for vaginal plastic repair. However, vaginal plastic surgery requires careful preoperative planning and patient education. *For partial vaginal vesicourethrolysis and plication,* as described for anterior and posterior vaginal repair. *For combined vaginal and abdominal approach,* as described for anterior vaginal plastic repair and suprapubic cystectomy (Chapter 15).

Operative procedures

Vaginal approach

1. An indwelling urinary or suprapubic cystostomy catheter is established, according to the surgeon's preference. The posterior vaginal wall is retracted, and an incision is made through the anterior vaginal wall down to the urethra and bladder.

2. The vaginal wall is dissected from the bladder and urethra; the neck of the bladder is sutured together. The wound is closed, as described for vaginal repair.

Vesicourethral suspension. See the Marshall-Marchetti procedure (Chapter 15).

1. Through a suprapubic abdominal incision, the space of Retzius is entered, and the bladder and urethra are freed from the underlying structures.

2. Mattress sutures are inserted through the perivaginal fascia on either side of the vesicourethral angle area and preferably at right angles to the long axis of the urethra and the bladder. These are then passed through the central portion of the undersurface of the symphysis pubis under direct vision. The application of the sutures to the perivaginal connective tissue is done with the operator's hand in the vagina to ensure that the permanent suture material is not passed through the vaginal mucosa (Figs. 16-2 and 16-3).

3. The wound is closed and may be drained if the vascularity of the area warrants. An abdominal dressing is applied.

Excision of fibroma of the vagina

Definition. Removal of a lesion through a transverse or longitudinal incision of the wall of the vagina.

Considerations. Small cysts or small benign tumors that distort the vagina or those which are ulcerated and infected are treated surgically.

Setup and preparation of the patient. As described for simple vaginal surgery, plus six Halsted hemostats.

Operative procedure

1. The vaginal vault is retracted with lateral retractors. Sutures may be placed on each side of the tumor. The posterior lip of the cervix is grasped with a tenaculum and is drawn anteriorly to expose the operative site.

2. The vaginal wall is incised, and the edges are grasped with traction sutures on curved, taper-point needles or with Allis forceps.

3. The base and its capsule are excised by a knife and curved scissors; bleeding vessels are clamped and ligated with Halsted forceps and fine sutures.

4. The vaginal incision is closed with interrupted sutures.

Construction of a vagina

Definition. Two basic technical approaches for repairing or overcoming a congenital or surgical defect of the vagina: the taking of a skin graft, which is applied to a mold and placed in the area of vaginal reconstruction, and a simple opening of the area of vaginal reconstruction and the placing of a mold to permit the spontaneous epithelialization of the area.

Setup and preparation of the patient. The patient is placed in the lithotomy position. The instrument setups include the following:

Skin grafting (Chapter 21)

Cutting instruments

1 Mayo scissors, straight, 6¼ inches
1 Skin-grafting set
2 Iris scissors, 1 straight and 1 curved

Holding instruments

2 Fixation forceps

Clamping instruments

12 Halsted mosquito hemostats, 6 curved and 6 straight, 5 inches

Accessory items

Metal or plastic slab for spreading and handling skin
Xeroform gauze dressing
1 Fenestrated sheet
1 Vaginal supply pack

Vaginal construction. The vaginal plastic repair setup and dilatation and curettage setup, plus the following:

Cutting instruments

2 Iris scissors, 1 straight and 1 curved

Holding instruments

2 Fixation forceps
2 Skin hooks

Clamping instruments

12 Halsted mosquito hemostats, 6 straight and 6 curved, 5 inches

Exposing instruments

2 Kocher appendectomy retractors, right-angled, 2-inch blade
2 Pryor-Pean retractors, right-angled, 4-inch blade

Suturing instruments

2 Crile-Wood needle holders

Accessory items

Metal ruler
Mold compound, plastic, or other substance as requested

Operative procedure

1. Skin is taken from the abdomen or anterior thighs. The donor sites are dressed in the routine manner with pressure dressings over nonadherent gauze.

2. A vaginal orifice is created by sharp dissection. Great care must be taken to prevent damage to the rectum or bladder. A mold is then adapted from the plastic material that is available. This mold is used to apply the donor skin or simply to hold the dissected area open to permit spontaneous epithelialization.

Trachelorrhaphy

Definition. Removal of torn surfaces of the anterior and posterior cervical lips and reconstruction of the cervical canal.

Considerations. Trachelorrhaphy is done to treat deep lacerations of a cervix that is relatively free of infection.

Setup and preparation of the patient. As described for vaginal plastic repair, plus an electrocautery unit with a cone type of electrode, if desired. A retention catheter may be introduced into the bladder, depending on the surgeon's preference.

Operative procedure

1. The labia are retracted with Allis-Adair tissue forceps or sutures. The cervix is grasped with a tenaculum.

2. The infected tissue of the exocervix is denuded with a knife. The flaps are undermined by means of a knife and curved scissors. Bleeding vessels are clamped and ligated. The musosa is dissected from the cervix.

3. A small distal portion of the cervical canal is coned to remove infected tissue by means of a knife. Bleeding vessels are clamped and ligated.

4. The denuded and coned areas are covered by suturing the mucosal flaps of the exocervix transversely, using interrupted sutures. Tissue forceps, hemostats, and gauze sponges are needed. The sutures are placed in such a manner that the fibromuscular tissue of the cervix is included, thereby eliminating dead space where a hematoma may form and providing a complete reconstructed cervical canal.

5. The wound is cleansed, and a vaginal pack may be used.

Removal of pedunculated cervical myoma

Definition. Removal of the tumor by the snare method or by dissection from the cervical canal with a knife or with cold-knife conization.

Considerations. Cervical polyps (small pedunculated lesions) stem from the endocervical canal and consist almost entirely of columnar epithelium with or without squamous metaplasia. They may vary in size and are soft, red, and friable. Bleeding may result from the slightest trauma. Usually, the surgeon performs an endometrial and endocervical curettage, and a cytological smear is taken.

Setup and preparation of the patient. As described for dilatation and curettage, adding a tonsil snare and medium snare wire, smear slides, and an electrocautery unit, including a pencil knife.

Operative procedure

1. The anterior lip of the cervix is grasped with a Jacobs vulsellum forceps or a tenaculum. The canal is sounded and dilated to either visualize or palpate the base of the pedicle.

2. If the pedicle of the tumor is thin, a tonsil snare may be placed over the body of the tumor, permitting the snare to crush the base of the tumor and to control bleeding. If the tumor is large, its base is dissected out with a knife. Bleeding may be controlled by the use of warm, moist gauze sponges.

3. Uterine packing may be introduced into the cervical os. Then the tenaculum is removed from the cervix, and the retractors are withdrawn. A vaginal pack may be also used for hemostasis.

Dilatation of the cervix and curettage

Definition. Introduction of instruments through the vagina into the cervical canal and then into the uterus and, in some cases, removal of substances and blood. Dilatation of the cervix can also take place by inserting a laminaria tent into the cervical os 24 hours before surgery.

Considerations. Dilatation and curettage is done either for diagnostic purposes or as a form of therapy for a variety of pelvic conditions such as incomplete abortion, therapeutic abortion, abnormal uterine bleeding, or primary dysmenorrhea. Dilatation and currettage may also be performed when carcinoma of the endometrium is suspected, in the study of infertility, or before amputation of the cervix or an operation for prolapse of the uterus.

Setup and preparation of the patient. The patient is placed in the lithotomy position, and the vagina and cervix are cleansed. Draping of the patient is as described for vaginal plastic repair. A urinary catheter may be used. The instrument setup includes the following items:

Exposing instruments (Figs. 16-11 and 16-12)

1 Auvard weighted vaginal speculum, if desired
2 Jackson retractors
2 Eastman retractors
1 Uterine sound
1 Set Hegar or Hank dilators
1 Goodell uterine dilator

Holding instruments (Fig. 16-9)

2 Barrett tenaculi
1 Jacobs vulsellum forceps
2 Foerster sponge-holding forceps
2 Backhaus towel clamps
1 Boseman uterine forceps
2 Allis forceps
1 Tissue forceps, plain, 7¼ inches
2 Fletcher-Van Doren polyp forceps
1 Tissue forceps, one and two teeth, 5½ inches
1 Tenaculum, single tooth

Cutting instruments (Fig. 16-10)

1 Knife handle no. 3 with blade no. 10
2 Scissors, 1 curved and 1 straight
1 Set Sims uterine curettes, sharp
1 Set Thomas uterine curettes, blunt
1 Gaylor biopsy forceps

Clamping instruments

2 Crile hemostats
2 Mayo-Pean hemostats

Suturing items

1 Needle holder
1 Suture of surgeon's preference

Accessory items

1 Specimen container
Uterine and vaginal packing, as desired
1 Ampule muscular action drug, if desired
1 Urethral catheter, if desired

Operative procedure

1. A Kelly or Auvard retractor is placed posteriorly in the vagina. A Sims or Kelly retractor is placed anteriorly to expose the cervix. The anterior lip of the cervix is grasped with a tenaculum (Fig. 16-25).
2. The direction of the cervical canal and the depth of the uterine cavity are determined by means of a blunt probe or graduated pliable uterine sound.
3. The cervix is gradually dilated by means of graduated Hegar or Hank dilators and possibly a Goodell uterine dilator.
4. Exploration for pedunculated polyps or myomas may be done with a polyp forceps.
5. The interior of the cervical canal and the cavity of the uterus are curetted to obtain either a fractional or a routine specimen. For specific identification of the site of specimens, the endocervix is scraped with the curette first, and the specimen is separated from the curettings of the uterine endometrium. In a routine curettage, all curettings are sent together for identification of tissue cells.
6. Fragments of endometrium or other dislodged tissues may be removed with warm, wet gauze sponges on holders or collected on Telfa.
7. Multiple punch biopsies of the cervical circumference (at the 12, 3, 6, and 9 o'clock positions) may be taken with the Gaylor biopsy forceps to supplement the diagnostic workup.
8. Retractors are withdrawn; iodoform or plain gauze packing may be inserted into the uterus, using dressing forceps. The tenaculum is removed from the cervix. A vaginal pack may be used.

Suction curettage

Definition. Vacuum aspiration of the contents of the uterus.

Considerations. Aspiration has proved to be a safe and effective method for early termination of pregnancy and for use in missed and incomplete spontaneous abortions. Advantages are smaller dilatation of the cervix, less damage to the uterus, less blood loss, less chance of uterine perforation, and reduced danger of infection. A laminaria tent may be used for approximately 4 to 24 hours before removal of the uterine contents.

Setup and preparation of the patient. The patient is placed in the lithotomy position, and a local or general anesthetic is used. An external and internal vaginal prep is done, and the patient is draped. The setup includes the following:

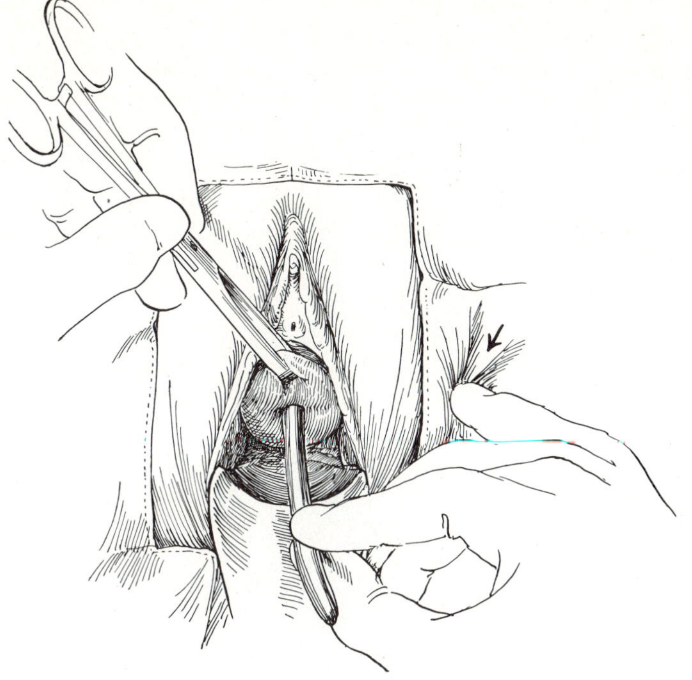

Fig. 16-25. Dilatation of cervix and curettage. Vaginal wall retracted; cervix held by tenaculum; cervix dilated with dilator. Uterine cavity curetted with sharp curettes. (From Ball, T.L.: Gynecologic surgery and urology, ed. 2, St. Louis, The C.V. Mosby Co.)

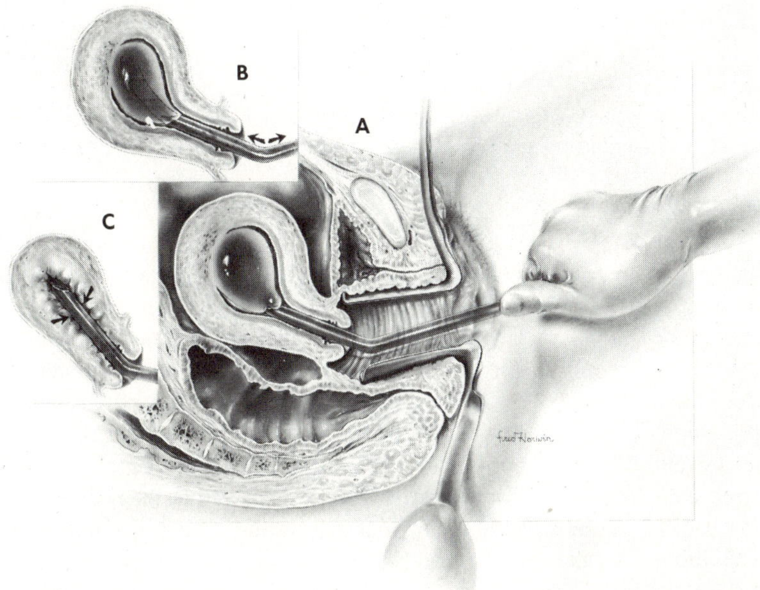

Fig. 16-26. Suction curettage. **A,** Insertion of cannula. **B,** Gentle suction motion to aspirate contents. **C,** Uterine contents evacuated. (From Eaton, C.J.: Technic of uterine aspiration, Berkeley, Calif., Bio-Engineering, Inc.)

Dilatation and curettage set
Controlled suction apparatus
Vacuum aspirator
Sterile cannulas and aspirating tubing
Surgical gel, sterile
Oxytocic drugs

Operative procedure

1. The cervix is exposed with an Auvard weighted speculum and an anterior retractor; then the cervix is grasped with a sharp tenaculum and is drawn toward the introitus (Fig. 16-26).

2. The laminaria tent is removed, and the cervix can be further dilated in the routine manner, allowing 1 mm of cannula diameter for each week of pregnancy.

3. The appropriate sized cannula is inserted into the uterus until the sac is encountered. The vacuum is turned on with immediate disruption and aspiration of the contents. Continued gentle motion of the cannula will remove the entire uterine contents (Fig. 16-26).

4. Retractors and tenaculum are withdrawn.

5. The specimen is contained in the vacuum bottle, from which it is removed for laboratory examination.

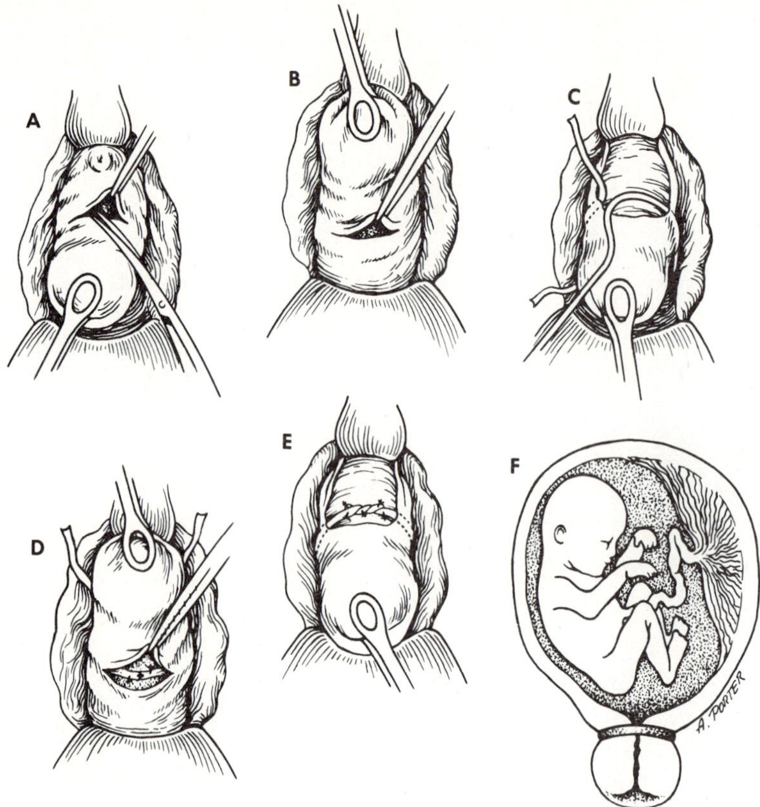

Fig. 16-27. Principles of Shirodkar operation for treatment of incompetent internal cervical os during pregnancy. (From Taylor, E.S.: Essentials of gynecology, ed. 2, Philadelphia, Lea & Febiger.)

Shirodkar operation (postconceptional)

Definition. Placement of a collar-type ligature of Mersilene, Dacron tape, heavy nylon suture, or plastic-covered braided steel suture at the level of the internal os to close it (Fig. 16-27).

Considerations. Incompetence of the cervix is a condition characterized by habitual midtrimester spontaneous abortions. The operation is designed to prevent cervical dilatation that results in release of uterine contents.

Setup and preparation of the patient. The lithotomy position is used, and gentle vaginal preparation is carried out. The instrument setup includes the basic vaginal setup, plus a few hemostats and the following:

1 Needle holder, short, fine
2 Ligature carriers
1 Basic needle set
2 Trocar needles
Sutures as noted plus the surgeon's preference for closure of mucosa

Operative procedure

1. Anterior and posterior vaginal retractors are placed, and the cervix is pulled down with smooth ovum or sponge forceps. With smooth tissue forceps and dissecting scissors, the mucosa over the anterior cervix is opened to permit the bladder to be pushed back (Fig. 16-27).

2. The cervix is lifted, and the posterior vaginal mucosa is similarly incised at the level of the peritoneal reflection. The corners of the anterior and posterior incisions are bilaterally approximated in the area of the lateral mucosa with curved tonsil or Allis forceps.

3. The prepared ligature is placed at the desired level by passage of the material through the approximated tissue and is drawn tight posteriorly to close the cervix. The suture material for the ligature is then tied. It is not necessary to suture the ligature to the underlying tissues. The suture material used for this ligation is 0.5-cm prepared Dacron or Mersilene tape. The anterior and posterior mucosal incisions are usually closed with Dexon or Vicryl no. 2-0 suture to complete the procedure.

Conization and biopsy of the cervix

Definition. Removal of diseased cervical tissue to treat strictures of the cervix, chronic cervicitis, epithelial dysplasia, and carcinoma in situ (Fig. 16-28). The conization may be performed by scalpel resection and suturing, by the application of cutting electrocautery current with an active electrode inserted into the cervical canal, or by use of the laser.

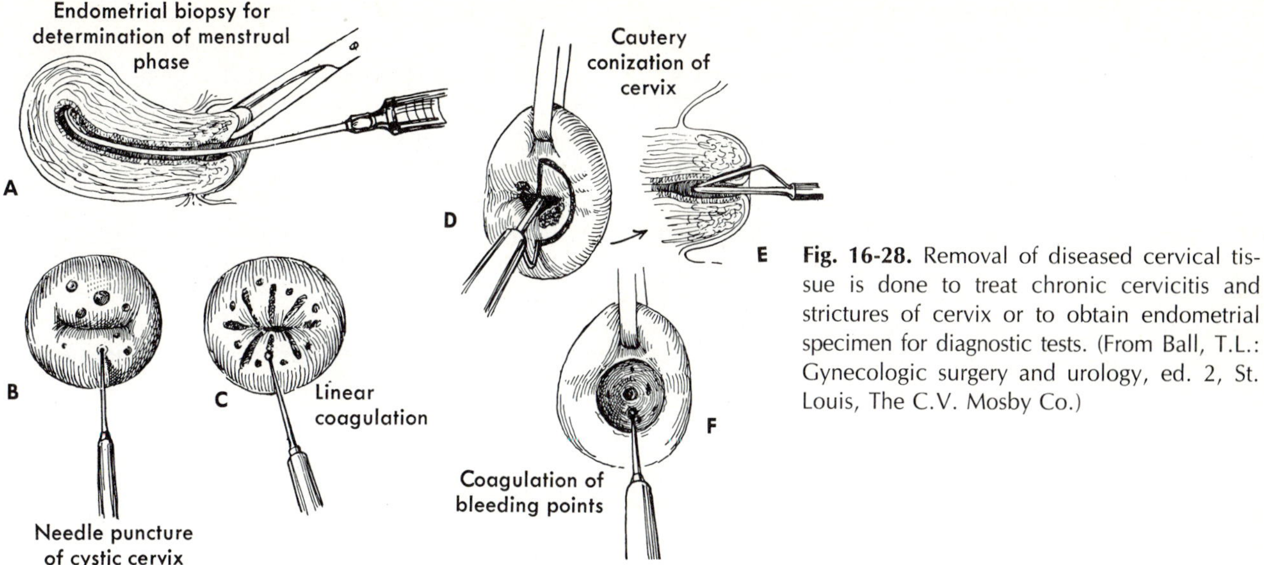

Fig. 16-28. Removal of diseased cervical tissue is done to treat chronic cervicitis and strictures of cervix or to obtain endometrial specimen for diagnostic tests. (From Ball, T.L.: Gynecologic surgery and urology, ed. 2, St. Louis, The C.V. Mosby Co.)

Considerations. Endometrial biopsy is done to determine the menstrual phase and carry out histological study of the endometrium. Scalpel conizations are done for diagnostic purposes, such as when a patient has a positive Papanicolaou (Pap) smear. Conization of the cervix, instead of hysterectomy, may be done in some cases to preserve reproductive function. It may also be done for benign or malignant diseases of the cervix and in cases in which total hysterectomy is not feasible.

Setup and preparation of the patient. As described for vaginal surgery. The instruments include a dilatation and curettage set, minor vaginal set, 1-ml syringe, curved metal cannula, and the appropriate scalpel or an electrocautery unit with conization and ball-tip electrodes.

Operative procedure (Fig. 16-28)

1. The posterior vaginal wall is retracted by a speculum, and the anterior vaginal wall by lateral retractors. The outer portions of the cervix are grasped with a tenaculum, and the cervix is drawn toward the introitus; then the anterior speculum is removed. Cystic cervix may be treated with a needle electrode. Endometrial biopsy may be done (Fig. 16-28, *A*). Bleeding points may be coagulated.

2. For cauterization the electrode is passed into the cervical canal, and the diseased membrane is removed.

3. The cervical canal is cleansed with an antiseptic solution. If a wide conization is performed, the cervix may be sutured and vaginal packing may be used. An indwelling urinary catheter may be inserted.

Cesium insertion for cervical and endometrial malignancy

Definition. Insertion of cesium into the cervix or endometrium for treatment of malignancy.

Considerations. Cesium has generally replaced radium insertions for malignancy of the cervix and endometrium.* The patient is brought to surgery for insertion of the applicators; the cesium is inserted later in the radiation department, or in the patient's room under controlled conditions in which the nursing personnel are monitored by use of the dosimeter.

Setup and preparation of the patient. As described for vaginal surgery. Aseptic technique must be maintained. The bladder is drained with a retention catheter. The retention bag is inflated with a radiopaque medium for radiographic visualization after insertion of the cesium. Various cesium applicators may be used according to the surgeon's preference and the area of malignancy.

Interstitial therapy. Cesium needles are available in various lengths with small diameters for insertion into the tissue surrounding the cervix. They are inserted vaginally with a needle applicator and are used as a supplement to intravaginal or intrauterine sources. To facilitate removal, the needles have wires or threads attached to their distal ends.

Culdoscopy

Definition. Visualization of pelvic structures through a tubular instrument similar to a cystoscope, which is introduced through a small incision in the posterior vaginal cul-de-sac.

Considerations. Culdoscopy is a diagnostic procedure most frequently used to investigate infertility. Direct observation of the passage of dye from the uterus through the fimbriated ends of the tube is possible with the cul-

*If radium is to be used, we recommend that the reader review Chapter 15 of Rhodes, M.J., Gruendemann B.J., and Ballinger, W.F.: Alexander's care of the patient in surgery, ed. 6, St. Louis, 1978, The C.V. Mosby Co.

doscope to help determine tubal patency. Culdoscopy may also be employed to determine the presence of an ectopic pregnancy, unexplained abdominal or pelvic pain, and the nature of pelvic masses and to evaluate normal functioning of the genital tract. This examination may enable the surgeon to avoid unnecessary pelvic surgery for the patient.

Setup and preparation of the patient. The patient is prepared as for vaginal operation. A local or regional anesthetic may be employed. When a general anesthetic is administered, the patient is intubated. The patient is usually placed in a knee-chest position, kneeling on the footboard with a kneestrap around the thighs, the chest supported on pillows, and the arms comfortably flexed above the head (Chapter 6). Instruments may be placed on a small accessory table; the surgeon may require no assistance. The instrument setup includes the following:

- 1 Culdoscopy set
- 2 Syringes, 5 ml and methylene blue (optional)
- 1 Piece plastic tubing
- 2 Barrett tenaculum forceps
- 1 Jacobs vulsellum forceps
- 2 Sponge-holding forceps
- 2 Retractors, 1 anterior and 1 posterior
- 2 Deaver or Doyen retractors, narrow blade
- 1 Vaginal dressing forceps

The lens of the scope, if introduced when cold, may become foggy because of body heat. Thus the tip of the scope should be dipped in warm water and wiped dry before it is handed to the surgeon.

Operative procedure

1. The trocar of the culdoscope is inserted into the posterior fornix; the trocar is then introduced into the pelvis between the two uterosacral ligaments (Fig. 16-29).

2. The trocar is withdrawn from the sheath; the sterile culdoscope is inserted through the sheath. The culdoscope does not touch the vaginal mucous membrane, thus reducing to a minimum the possibility of infection.

3. The uterus, tubes, ovaries, broad ligaments, uterosacral ligaments, rectal wall, sigmoid, and small intestine may be visualized through manipulation of the scope (Fig. 16-30).

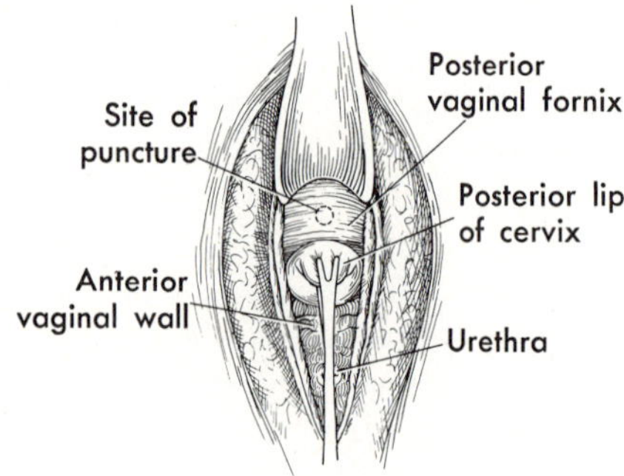

Fig. 16-29. Culdoscopy. View of vagina, with patient in knee-chest position showing site of puncture. (From TeLinde, R.W., and Mattingly, R.F.: Operative gynecology, ed. 4, Philadelphia, 1970, J.B. Lippincott Co.)

4. In a study of infertility, a self-retaining screw-lipped cervical cannula is introduced into the cervical canal and connected by a plastic tube to a syringe containing a dye. If the tube is patent, the dye solution is seen dripping from the fimbriated end.

5. The culdoscope and sheath are withdrawn. The vaginal wound is not sutured. The patient is returned to bed.

Culdocentesis and posterior colpotomy (culdotomy)

Definitions

needle culdocentesis Insertion of an aspirating needle through the posterior fornix of the vagina.

posterior colpotomy (culdotomy) Incision through the vagina and peritoneum and the removal of pus and blood.

Considerations. Diagnostic needle culdocentesis is done to diagnose ectopic pregnancy and to detect intraperitoneal bleeding or cul-de-sac hematoma. Posterior colpotomy is done to carry out definitive operative procedures: various kinds of tubal ligations, aspiration or the removal of ovarian cysts, the occasional management of an ectopic pregnancy, and exploratory diagnostic operative procedures.

Setup and preparation of the patient. As described for simple vaginal repair, plus the following:

- 2 Aspirating needles, 15 gauge, 3½ inches
- 1 Rochester-Pean hemostat, 10 inches
- 2 Culture tubes
- 2 Scissors, angulated blades, right and left
- 2 Drains

An abdominal setup should also be available.

Operative procedure

1A. *For needle culdocentesis,* a 15-gauge needle attached to a syringe is inserted through the posterior fornix of the vagina. Suspected intraperitoneal bleeding is confirmed if dark or red blood flows freely into the syringe. Failure to obtain blood does not rule out the possibility of intraperitoneal bleeding.

1B. *For posterior colpotomy,* a transverse incision is made through the posterior vaginal wall with the curved scissors. This incision is carried into the peritoneum, behind the cervix at the superior point of the posterior fornix. Allis clamps are used to facilitate exposure, and hemostasis is obtained by placing a number of sutures in the corners or angles of the wound. The posterior vaginal wall is held open with a heavy, weighted retractor that can have a long blade added. In case of infection in the cul-de-sac, the opening is enlarged enough to permit drainage from the cul-de-sac. The cavity is explored; drains may be inserted.

2. In either procedure, bleeding of the vaginal wall is controlled by sutures, and in the case of posterior colpot-

omy the peritoneum and the vaginal mucosa are closed with a running lock suture. Vaginal packing or an indwelling urinary catheter may also be used in culdocentesis or posterior colpotomy.

Marsupialization of Bartholin's duct cyst or abscess

Definition. Through the vaginal outlet, removal or incision of the cyst and drainage of the area.

Considerations. A cyst in Bartholin's gland usually follows acute infection and is treated by marsupialization when it is quiescent. Such cysts are non-neoplastic and result from retention of glandular secretions caused by blockage somewhere in the duct system.

Setup and preparation of the patient. As described for minor vaginal surgery, including dilatation and curettage setup, plus the following:

1 Syringe, 10 ml
1 Needle, 15 gauge, long
2 Culture tubes
2 Smear slides
1 Iodoform gauze packing

Operative procedure

1. The labia minora may be sutured to the perineal skin on each side to expose the vaginal introitus.

2. An elliptical incision is always made in the mucosa, which is distended over the cyst.

3. The cyst wall is dissected, and removal of the gland is completed with blunt-pointed scissors. A drain may be inserted, and a dressing is applied.

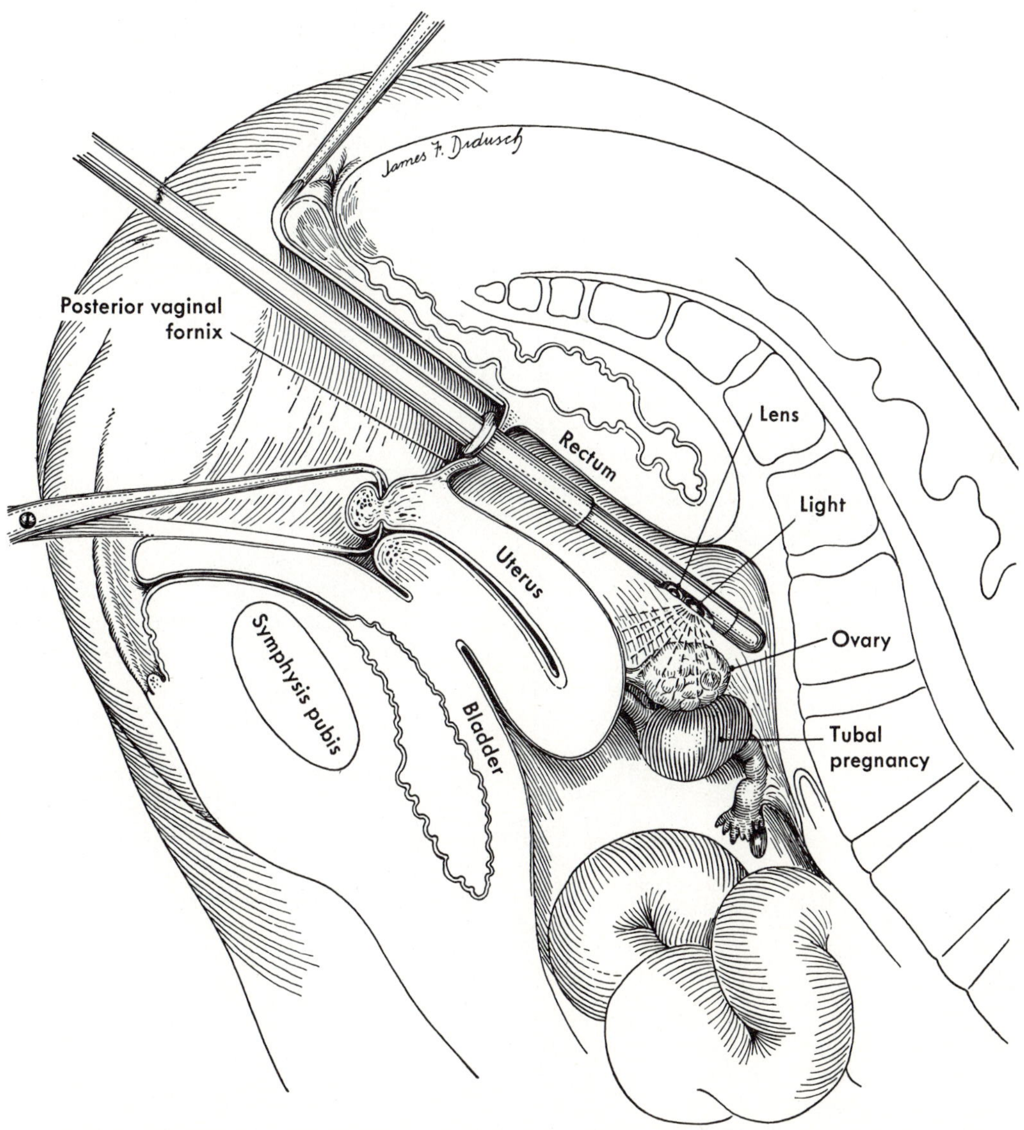

Fig. 16-30. Culdoscopy. Sagittal section showing culdoscope viewing pelvic viscera. (From TeLinde, R.W., and Mattingly, R.F.: Operative gynecology, ed. 4, Philadelphia, 1970, J.B. Lippincott Co.)

Vaginal hysterectomy

Definition. Removal of the uterus through an incision made in the vaginal wall and the pelvic cavity.

Considerations. The uterus may be removed through the vaginal outlet, except in the case of pelvic malignancy or when a large uterine tumor is present. The vaginal approach is contraindicated in pelvic malignancy because of an associated inflammatory process involving the uterine tubes and ovaries. Vaginal plastic surgery can be undertaken at this time.

Setup and preparation of the patient. Instruments include the major vaginal repair setup and the dilatation and curettage setup, plus two needles, 22 gauge × 3 inches, and two syringes, 10 ml.

To facilitate dissection and to decrease bleeding, the vaginal walls may be infiltrated with normal saline solution or local anesthetic (vasoconstrictors are optional). A laparotomy setup should also be available but not opened.

Operative procedure

1. The labia may be retracted with sutures. A vaginal retractor is inserted to retract the vaginal wall.
2. Dilatation and curettage may be performed, as previously described (Fig. 16-25).
3. A Jacobs vulsellum forceps, tenaculum, or suture ligature is placed through the cervical lips to permit traction on the cervix (Fig. 16-31, *A*).
4. The vaginal wall is incised with a knife. The incision is made anteriorly through the full thickness of the wall. The bladder is freed from the anterior surface of the cervix by sharp blunt dissection. The bladder is then elevated to expose the peritoneum of the anterior cul-de-sac, which is entered by sharp incision (Fig. 16-31, *B*).
5. The peritoneum of the posterior cul-de-sac is identified and entered by sharp incision.
6. The uterosacral ligaments containing blood vessels are clamped, cut, and ligated. The ends of the ligatures are left long and are tagged with a clamp (Fig. 16-31, *C*).
7. The uterus is drawn downward and the bladder held aside with retractors and moist, small laparotomy packs (Fig. 16-31, *D*).
8. The cardinal ligament on each side is clamped, cut, and ligated. The uterine arteries are doubly clamped, cut, and ligated.
9. The fundus is delivered through the anterior or posterior route; occasionally the aid of a uterine tenaculum is necessary.
10. When the ovaries are to be left, the round liga-

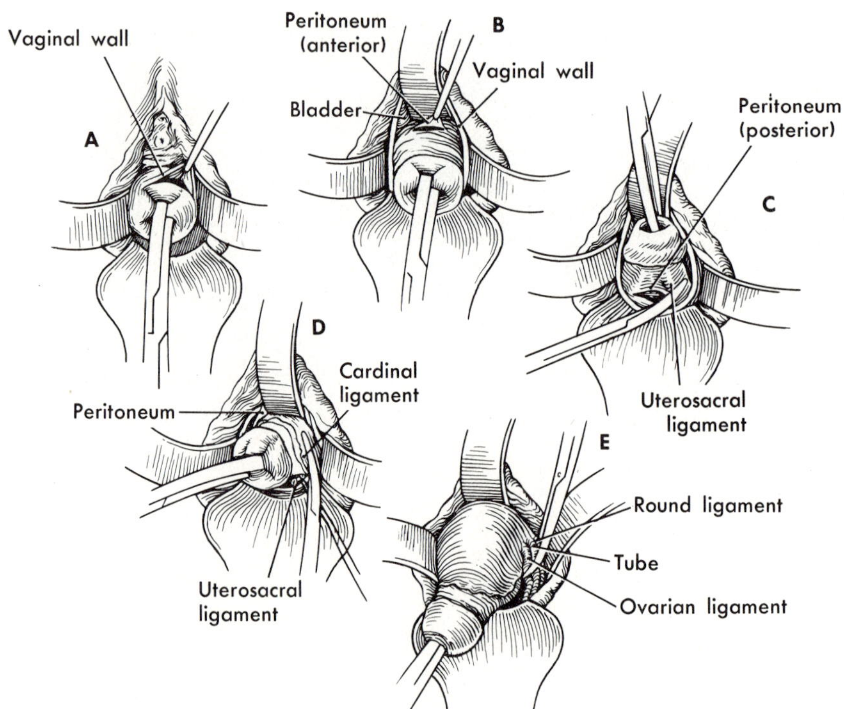

Fig. 16-31. Vaginal hysterectomy. **A,** Incision of vaginal wall around cervix. Anterior vaginal wall slightly elevated. **B,** Deaver retractor on each side; one Deaver retractor under bladder. Peritoneum opened. **C,** Posterior cul-de-sac opened. Heaney clamp applied to left uterosacral ligament. **D,** Left uterosacral ligament cut and tied. Clamp applied to left cardinal ligament. **E,** Clamps applied to ovarian ligament, round ligament, and fallopian tube. Reconstruction of vaginal vault.

ment, the uterovarian ligament, and the fallopian tube are clamped together and cut, and the uterus is removed. These pedicles are then ligated (Fig. 16-31, *E*).

11. The peritoneum between the rectum and vagina is approximated with a continuous suture. The retroperitoneal obliteration of the cul-de-sac is done by sutures that pass from the vaginal wall through the infundibulopelvic ligament and round ligament, through the cardinal ligament, and out the vaginal wall. The suture is tied on the vaginal aspect of the new vault (Fig. 16-31, *F* and *G*). The round, cardinal, and ureterosacral ligaments may be individually approximated for additional support.

12. Any existing rectocele and the perineum are repaired, as described for vaginal plastic repair (Figs. 16-19 and 16-21). In the presence of prolapse, reconstruction of the pelvic floor may be required.

13. An indwelling system of urinary drainage is established. The vagina may be packed, and a Penrose drain may be used.

ABDOMINAL GYNECOLOGICAL SURGERY

Laparoscopy (peritoneoscopy, celioscopy)

Definition. Endoscopic visualization of the peritoneal cavity through the anterior abdominal wall after the establishment of a pneumoperitoneum.

Considerations. Laparoscopy provides the gynecologist the same anatomical view of the pelvic organs as is seen at the diagnostic laparotomy. Pathological conditions can be seen, and ancillary procedures such as aspiration of cysts, adhesolysis, tissue biopsies, and sterilization can be performed. Hemostasis can be obtained readily by using the active electrode probe. This procedure may enable the surgeon to avoid unnecessary pelvic surgery for the patient.

Setup and preparation of the patient. The patient is placed in the lithotomy position, a local or general anesthetic is administered, the skin is prepared as for a laparotomy, and the bladder is drained. A Hulka forceps or cervical suction cannula may be introduced into the cervix after vaginal preparation. This is used to manipulate the pelvic organs to afford the surgeon better visibility. The patient is placed in extreme Trendelenburg's position. Instruments may be placed on a small table. The setup includes the following:

1 Dilatation and curettage set
1 Hulka forceps
1 Cervical suction cannula
1 Suction tubing
1 Laparoscope set (scope, fiberoptic cord, manipulative probe, biopsy forceps, cautery probe, cautery hook, suction tip) (Fig. 16-32)
1 Syringe, 5 ml
1 Knife handle no. 3 and blade no. 15 or 11
6 Towel clamps
2 Allis forceps, 6 inches
2 Kelly clamps, 5¼ inches
1 Metzenbaum scissors, 5½ inches
1 Needle holder, 6 inches
2 Adson forceps with teeth
2 Skin hooks, single
1 Suture for skin closure
1 Piece rubber tubing, 3 ft
Electrosurgical unit
Fiberoptic power source
Gas source for pneumoperitoneum

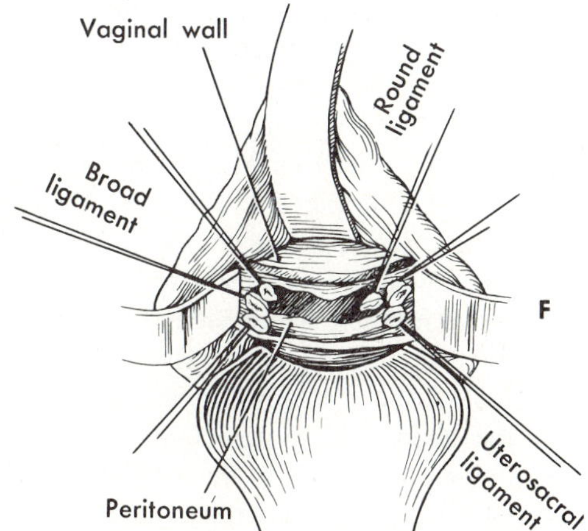

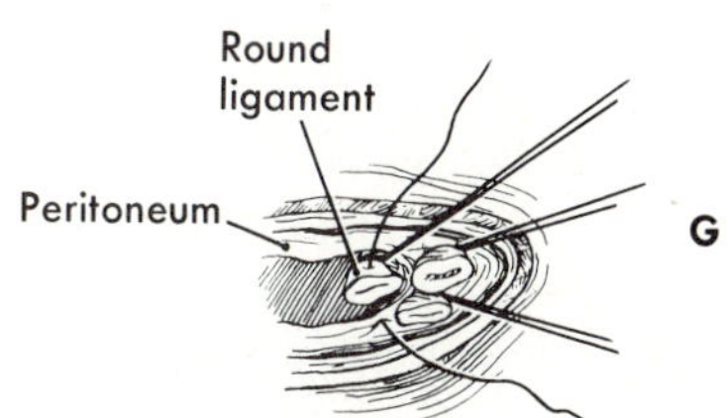

Fig. 16-31, cont'd. F, Uterosacral ligament, broad ligament, and round ligament shown in their respective normal positions. **G,** Peritoneum closed and cardinal broad ligament and uterosacral ligaments reattached to angle of vagina. Left uterosacral and broad ligaments anchored. (From Counseller, V.S.: In Lowrie, R.J., editor: Gynecology: surgical techniques, Springfield, Ill., Charles C Thomas, Publisher.)

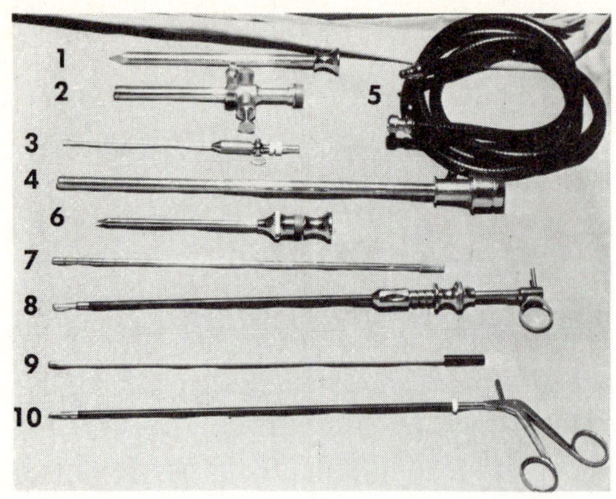

Fig. 16-32. Laparoscope. *1,* Trocar; *2,* valved cannula; *3,* pneumoperitoneal needle; *4,* Foroblique vision laparoscope, 180 degrees; *5,* fiberoptic cord; *6,* secondary trocar and cannula; *7,* graduated probe; *8,* Palmer forceps within sheath; *9,* cautery probe; *10,* biopsy forceps. Not shown are fiberoptic power source, cautery cord, and cautery unit.

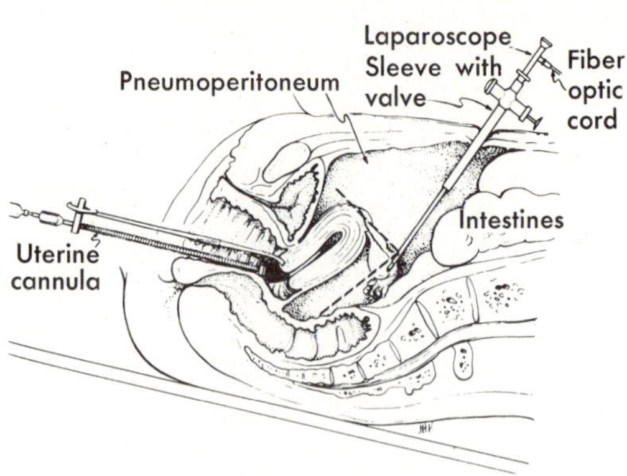

Fig. 16-33. Technique of laparoscopy. (From Cohen, M.R.: J. Obstet. Gynecol. **31:**310.)

The lens of the laparoscope may be wiped with sterile pHisoHex and soaked in warm water 37.2° C (99° F) to prevent fogging in the warmth of the peritoneal cavity. If fogging occurs after the lens is introduced into the peritoneal cavity, touching the lens to the peritoneum may clear it.

Operative procedure

1. A 1-cm incision is placed below or to the left of the umbilicus.

2. Elevating the skin with towel clamps and suturing or grasping below the umbilicus with a 4 × 4 gauze sponge for traction, the surgeon inserts a Verres (pneumoperitoneal) needle through the layers of the abdominal wall into the peritoneal cavity. Approximately 3 liters of carbon dioxide gas is then passed into the peritoneal cavity. Care must be taken to prevent overdistension of the abdomen. The trocar and valve sleeve are inserted boldly through the remaining layers of the abdominal wall into the peritoneal cavity. The angle taken by the trocar is approximately 45 degrees toward the concavity of the pelvis.

3. The patient is then placed in Trendelenburg's position, the laparoscope is introduced, and inspection is begun (Fig. 16-33). Should the biopsy or cautery forceps be needed, it is introduced by trocar through a separate small incision on the lower abdomen.

4. Gas is allowed to escape from the sleeve, then the scope is withdrawn. Subcuticular closure of the skin is followed by the application of a Band-Aid dressing.

Total abdominal hysterectomy

Definition. Through an abdominal incision, opening of the peritoneal cavity and removal of the entire uterus, including the corpus and the cervix. Removal of both adnexae at the same time is a *bilateral salpingo-oophorectomy,* termed by common usage as panhysterectomy or complete hysterectomy.

Considerations. Total hysterectomy may be performed for symptomatic pelvis relaxation or prolapse, pain associated with pelvic congestion, pelvic inflammatory disease, endometriosis, recurrent ovarian cysts, fibroids (myomas), bleeding with no apparent cause in postmenopausal women, adenomyosis, or dysfunctional bleeding. Total hysterectomy, usually with bilateral salpingo-oophorectomy, is also indicated in anatomical disease, malignancy, premalignant states, and high-risk conditions of malignancy potential or recurrency rate. Total hysterectomy can also be used to accomplish sterilization.

Setup and preparation of the patient. The patient is prepared as described for vaginal and abdominal surgery. Diagnostic dilatation and curettage usually have already been performed. However, a setup should be readily available. Before the abdominal skin preparation, an internal and external vaginal preparation is done. A retention catheter is inserted to provide constant bladder drainage during the operation. Supine and Trendelenburg's positions are used. Instrumentation includes the abdominal gynecological set. Provisions are made to remove from the abdomen and field those instruments used in separating the cervix from the vagina, thereby avoiding vaginal contamination of the pelvis. In performing the abdominal hysterectomy, instrument tables are arranged in relation to the side of the operating table from which the surgeon works.

Operative procedure

1. In case of an obese patient or for exploration of the upper abdominal cavity, a left rectus or midline incision may be made. For simple hysterectomy, a Pfannenstiel incision may be used. The abdominal layers and the peritoneum are opened as described for laparotomy.

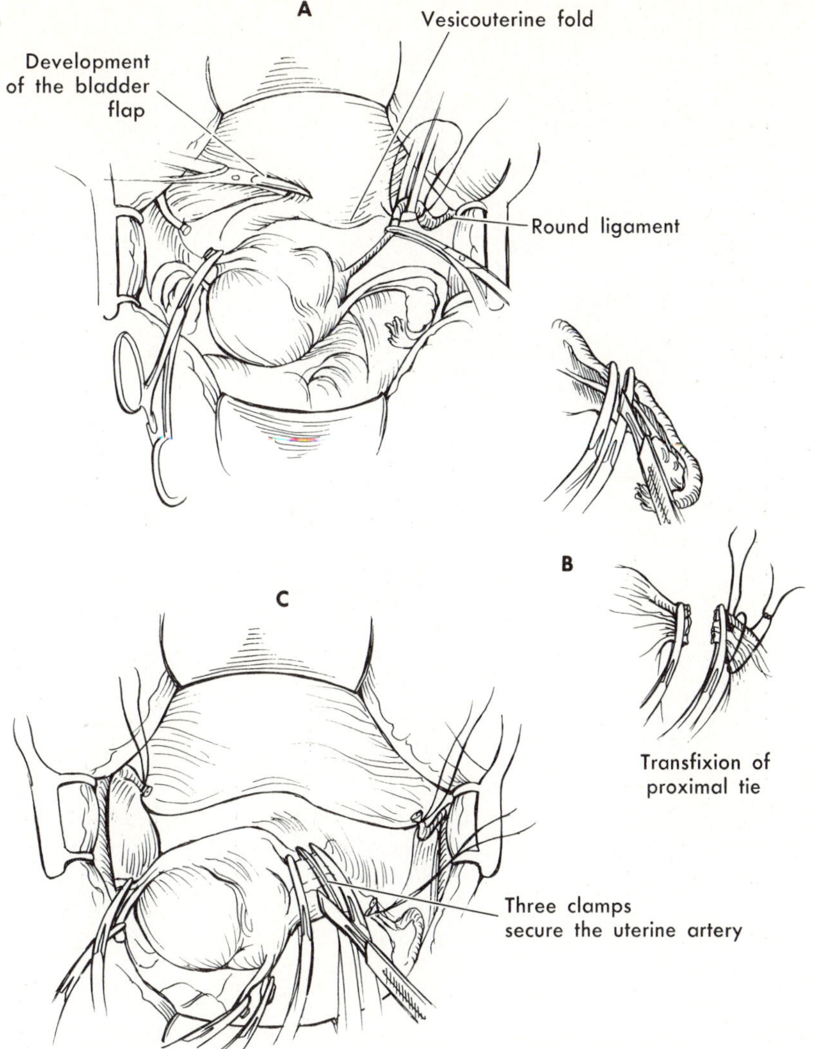

Fig. 16-34. Abdominal hysterectomy for simple fibroid uterus. **A,** Peritoneal cavity retracted with self-retaining retractors, and organs protected with laparotomy packs saturated in warm normal saline solution. Transverse incision made through uterine peritoneum and carried to each side of uterine attachments of round ligaments. Bleeding vessels clamped and ligated. Round ligament grasped, ligated, and cut. **B,** Tube and ovarian ligaments clamped, cut, and sutured. **C,** Uterus pulled forward, posterior sheath of broad ligaments divided, and uterine artery and veins secured by three heavy curved clamps. Pedicle divided, leaving two hemostats in proximal pedicle. *Continued.*

2. As the peritoneal cavity is opened, the patient is placed in the desired position for pelvic surgery (usually Trendelenburg's).

3. The round ligament is grasped with forceps, clamped, and ligated with sutures on long needle holders. Pedicles are cut with Metzenbaum scissors; sutures are tagged with a hemostat to be used as traction later. This procedure is done on both sides (Fig. 16-34, *A*).

4. By use of the surgeon's fingers, the layer of the broad ligament close to the uterus is separated on each side, bleeding vessels are clamped and ligated, and a moistened laparotomy pack is inserted behind the flap. The fallopian tube and the utero-ovarian ligaments are double-clamped together, incised, and double-tied with suture ligatures (Fig. 16-34, *B*).

5. The uterus is pulled forward to expose the posterior sheath of the broad ligament, which is incised with a knife or Metzenbaum scissors. Ureters are identified. The uterine vessels and uterosacral ligaments are double-clamped, divided by sharp dissection at the level of the internal os, and ligated with suture ligatures (Fig. 16-34, *C*).

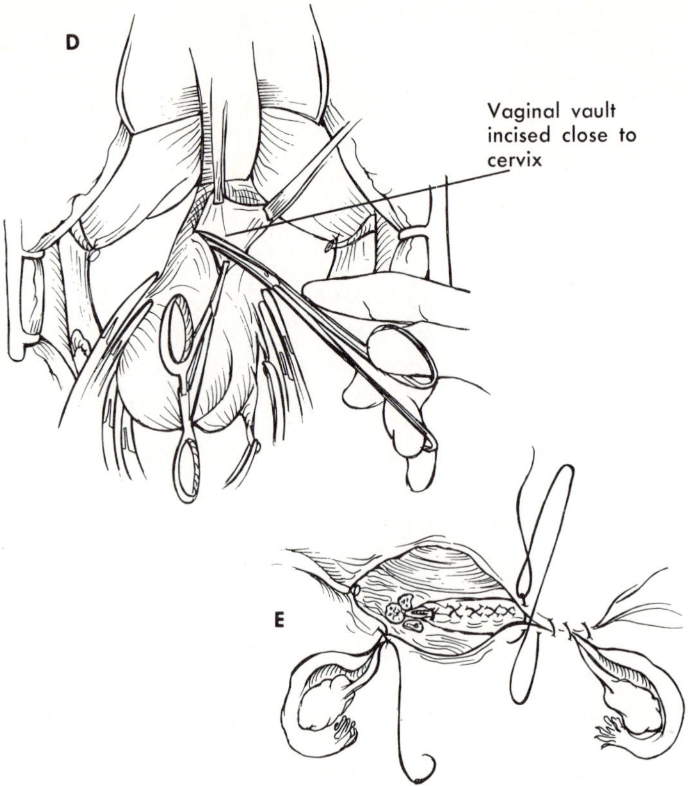

Fig. 16-34, cont'd. D, Bladder separated from cervix and upper vagina. Vaginal vault opened and grasped with Allis forceps. Allis forceps placed on anterior lip of cervix, and dissection of cervix is carried out, to complete its amputation from vagina. **E,** Three connective tissue thickenings anchored to vaginal vault, vaginal mucosa approximated, and vault closed. As shown, peritoneum closed with continuous suture. (From Ball, T.L.: Operative gynecology and urology, ed. 2, St. Louis, The C.V. Mosby Co.)

6. The severed uterine vessels are bluntly dissected away from the cervix on each side with the aid of sponges on holders, scissors, and tissue forceps.

7. The bladder is separated from the cervix and upper vagina with sharp and blunt dissection assisted by sponges on holders.

8. The bladder may be retracted with a moist laparotomy pack and a retractor with an angular blade. The vaginal vault is incised close to the cervix with a knife or scissors (Fig. 16-34, *D*).

9. The anterior lip of the cervix is grasped with an Allis, Kocher, or tenaculum forceps. With scissors, the cervix is dissected and amputated from the vagina. The uterus is removed. Potentially contaminated instruments used on the cervix and vagina are placed in a discard basin and removed from the field (including sponge forceps and suction). Bleeding is controlled with hemostats and sutures.

10. The vaginal vault is reconstructed with interrupted sutures. Angle sutures anchor all three connective tissue ligaments to the vaginal vault. The pedicles, tube, and ovarian ligament are left free of the vault.

11. Vaginal mucosa is approximated with a continuous suture on a long needle holder. The muscular coat of the vagina may be closed with figure-of-eight sutures to make the vault of the vagina firm and provide resistance against prolapse. A Penrose drain may be placed in the vagina.

12. The peritoneum is closed over the bladder, vaginal vault, and rectum (Fig. 16-34, *E*). The laparotomy packs are removed, and the omentum is drawn over the bowel.

13. The abdominal wound is closed, as described for abdominal closure (Chapter 10).

Abdominal myomectomy

Definition. Removal of fibromyomas from the uterine wall through an abdominal incision and opening of the peritoneal cavity.

Considerations. Myomectomy is usually done in young women who have symptoms that indicate the presence of tumors and who wish to preserve their potential fertility. Also, tumors may be removed because of infertility or habitual abortion or because of distortion of the bladder and other organs. Myomectomy may be performed as a prophylactic measure in conjunction with other abdominopelvic surgery.

Setup and preparation of the patient. As described for vaginal preparation and possible dilatation and curettage. The patient is placed in Trendelenburg's position. A basic abdominal gynecological setup is used, plus Bonney's myomectomy clamp.

Operative procedure

1. The patient is prepared as described for abdominal hysterectomy. A midline or Pfannenstiel incision is used, and the uterus is exposed.
2. To contract the musculature of the uterine wall, a suitable drug may be injected into the fundus.
3. The fibroid tumor is grasped with a tenaculum. The broad ligament may be opened with curved hemostats and Metzenbaum scissors to determine the course of the ureter or to free the bladder.
4. Each tumor is shelled out of its bed, using blunt and sharp instruments. Bleeding vessels are clamped and ligated or cauterized.
5. The uterus is reconstructed with interrupted or continuous sutures.
6. The perimetrium is closed over the operative site. The abdominal wound is closed, as described for laparotomy closure.

Radical hysterectomy (Wertheim)

Definition. Through an abdominal incision, opening of the peritoneum and en bloc dissection with careful removal of all recognizable lymph nodes in the pelvis, together with wide removal of the uterus, tubes, ovaries, supporting ligaments, and upper vagina. Extensive dissection of the ureters and of the bladder is also involved. Therefore ureteral catheters may be inserted before the procedure.

Considerations. Radical abdominal hysterectomy is performed in the presence of cervical carcinoma, with or without attendant radiation therapy. Abdominal exploration determines lymph node involvement. If there is no lymph node involvement, a wide-cuff hysterectomy is performed. The uterus, tubes, and ovaries, together with most of the parametrial tissues and the upper portion of the vagina, are dissected en bloc. Dissection of the ureters from the paracervical structures takes place so that the ligaments supporting the uterus and vagina can be removed. Radical abdominal hysterectomy can also be used in certain cases of endometrial carcinoma. Careful estimating of blood loss and calculation of urinary output is needed throughout the operative procedure.

Setup and preparation of the patient. As described for total hysterectomy. The following are added to the abdominal instrument set:

8 Schnidt tonsil hemostats
6 Lahey gall duct forceps, 9 inches
2 Cushing vein retractors
2 Vascular, fine-tissue forceps, plain, 12 inches
Hemostatic clips and applicator (optional)
Kitner sponges
2 Closed wound drainage systems

Operative procedure

1. The skin is incised, and the abdominal layers are opened, as described for laparotomy.
2. The peritoneum is cut at its reflection on the anterior surface of the uterus between the round ligaments (Fig. 16-35, *A*). By blunt dissection, the bladder surface is freed from the cervix and vagina.
3. The right round and infundibulopelvic ligaments are clamped, cut with Metzenbaum scissors, and ligated with sutures to expose the external iliac artery. The ureter is identified and retracted with a vein retractor (Fig. 16-35, *B*).
4. The lymph and areolar tissues are dissected from the iliac artery, obturator fossa, and ureter with Lahey forceps, Kitner sponges, and Metzenbaum scissors. A complete lymph gland dissection removes the tissue from Cloquet's node to the bifurcation of the iliac arteries bilaterally. The uterine artery and vein are clamped, cut, and doubly ligated.
5. The uterus is elevated, the cul-de-sac is opened (Fig. 16-35, *C*), and the uterosacral and cardinal ligaments are clamped, cut with scissors, and doubly ligated with suture ligatures. The pararectal and paravesical areolar tissues are dissected free to skeletonize the upper vagina, and the paraurethral tissues are removed as near to the pelvic walls as possible.
6. The upper third of the vagina is cross-clamped with Heaney forceps (Fig. 16-35, *D*) and divided with a long no. 4 knife handle and no. 20 blade. The uterus and surrounding tissues are removed. Electrocoagulation is useful in minimizing venous oozing from small venules and capillaries. Lowering the head of the operating table 15 degrees has also been helpful in further reducing the oozing of blood and serum. Careful apposition of the skin edges with interrupted, mattress, on-end sutures must take place to prevent overlapping of the skin edges and a resulting delay in healing.
7. The vagina is sutured open with a running locked stitch, and closed wound drainage is provided from above (Fig. 16-35, *E*). The pelvis is peritonealized with a continuous suture.
8. The abdominal wound is closed (retention sutures may be used) and dressed in the usual manner. Vaginal packing and drains may be used. All packs, sponges, and towels must be accounted for at the end of the procedure.

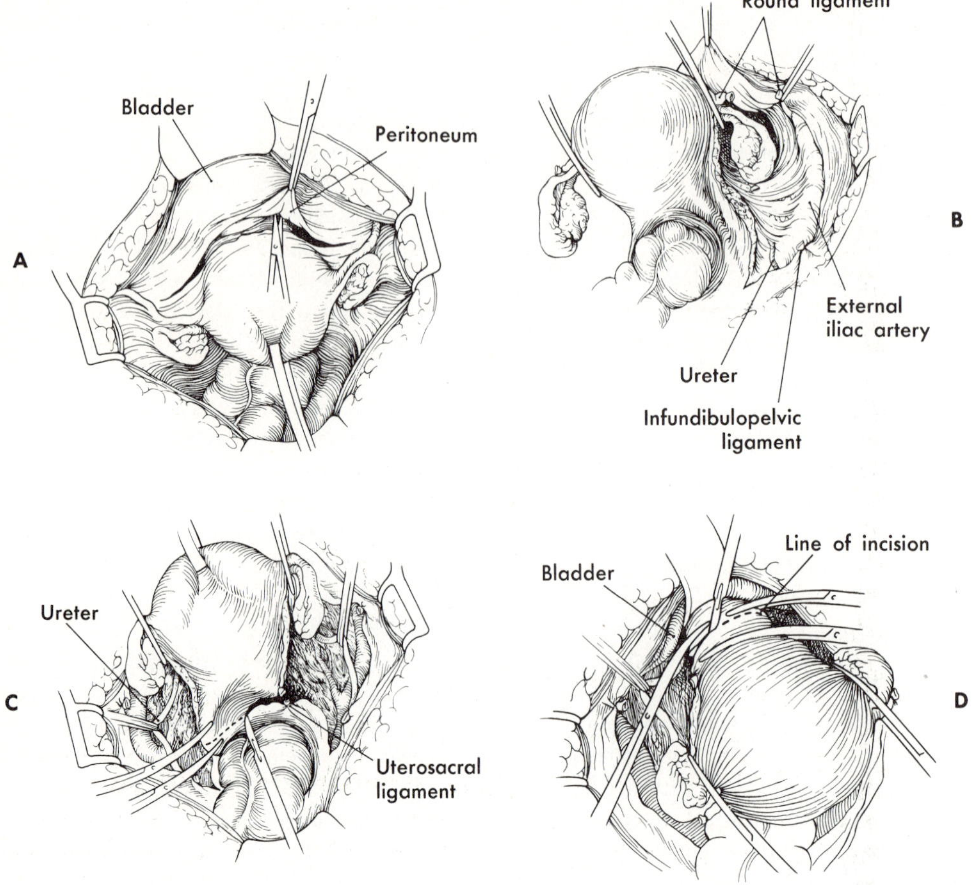

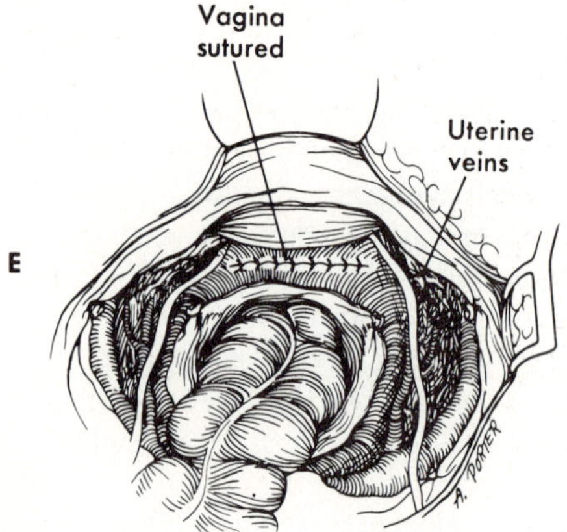

Fig. 16-35. Wertheim type of radical hysterectomy. **A,** Applying upward traction on uterus, peritoneum is incised from round ligament to round ligament. **B,** Right round ligament and right infundibulopelvic ligaments ligated and cut, thus exposing right external iliac artery. **C,** Uterus is held upward and forward, exposing cul-de-sac, which is incised as shown by dotted line. **D,** After dissection is completed, vagina is doubly clamped preparatory to transection, after which entire specimen will be lifted out en masse. **E,** Vagina is closed. Peritoneum remains to be reperitonealized. (Redrawn from TeLinde, R.W. and Mattingly, R.F.: Operative gynecology, ed. 4, Philadelphia, 1970, J.B. Lippincott Co.)

DEEP PELVIC SURGERY

The success of modern deep pelvic surgery for malignant abdominoperineal lesions is attributable to increased knowledge regarding aseptic and surgical techniques, anesthesia, transfusions, intravenous antibiotic therapy, and the pathophysiology of involved organs. Current therapeutic techniques evolved after determination of the modes of metastasis, resective possibilities, and means of reestablishing modified physiological function.

PELVIC EXENTERATION

Definition. En bloc "removal of the rectum, distal sigmoid colon, the urinary bladder and the distal ureters, the internal iliac vessels and their lateral branches, all pelvic reproductive organs and lymph nodes, and the entire pelvic floor with the accompanying pelvic peritoneum, levator muscles, and perineum."* Bricker's technique is described here. A partial exenteration, either anterior or posterior, may be performed, depending on the origin of the carcinoma and the extent of local tissue invasion.

Considerations. Pelvic exenteration is the preferred treatment for recurrent or persistent carcinoma of the cervix after radiation therapy; it is also applicable to carcinomas of the endometrium or rectum. Exenteration is considered only after a thorough investigation of the patient and disease status to determine if there is a reasonable chance of cure and of return to a productive lifestyle. Determination of the chance of resectability with cure can be made with finality at the time of abdominal exploration by the surgeon.

The need for creation of urinary and bowel diversion must also be considered, together with the patient's ability to cope with these diversions postoperatively. Total pelvic exenteration has been advocated as being the definitive procedure of choice in a critical clinical situation.

Setup and preparation of the patient. Psychological preparation of the patient and family by the physician is a prime requisite. Nursing care should be directed toward supporting the patient during the course of therapy and helping the patient maintain personal dignity.

Preoperative cleansing of the bowel with antibiotics and enemas is done. A nasogastric tube, urinary catheter, and rectal tube are inserted before or during surgery. Antiembolic stockings are placed on both legs. Constant cardiac and central venous pressure monitoring are carried out.

A general endotracheal anesthetic with muscle relaxants is usually administered. The patient is placed in the supine position with legs elevated in a modified lithotomy position to allow access to the perineum without disruptive position changes.

*From Bricker, E.M.: Pelvic exenteration. In Welch, C.E., editor: Advances in surgery, Chicago, 1970, Year Book Medical Publishers, Inc., p. 14.

The circulating and scrub nurses must be alert to fluid and blood loss, irrigation solutions must be accurately measured, laparotomy packs must be weighed to assess blood volume loss, and the anesthetist and surgical team must be apprised of the measurement.

Two separate instrument setups are required for the abdominal and perineal approaches. Extra drapes, gowns, and gloves should be available.

Abdominal approach. As described previously for abdominoperineal resection (Chapter 14), plus the following:

1 Metzenbaum scissors, 12 inches
8 Schnidt tonsil hemostats
6 Lahey gall duct forceps, 9 inches
6 Allis forceps, 9¼ inches
8 Pean hysterectomy forceps, 9½ inches
4 Right-angled clamps, large, 12 inches
2 Stille kidney clamps, 9 inches
2 Cushing vein retractors
2 Vascular, fine-tissue forceps, plain, 12 inches
2 Needle holders, 12 inches
Instruments for removal of reproductive organs of the male or female
Electrosurgical unit (optional)
Red rubber catheters, assorted French sizes
Ileostomy bag
Colostomy bag
Hemoclips (optional)
Sutures: various sizes of silk (long and short), steel wire, 28-gauge, and other sutures of surgeon's preference
1 Central venous pressure line

When the colon is transected or ureteral drainage is diverted into an ileosegment, the gastrointestinal technique as described in Chapter 14 should be followed.

Perineal approach. As described for abdominoperineal resection (Chapter 14). Antiseptic skin preparation includes the abdomen, thighs, and perineum, including the internal vaginal vault. At this time, the bladder is drained, and the catheter removed; the anus is tightly closed with a running silk suture on a cutting needle.

Operative procedure

1. A long midline incision from the symphysis pubis to the umbilicus is made, and the abdomen is opened in the usual manner. A second incision within the perineum encircling the vestibule and anus is also made.

2. The peritoneal cavity is explored for metastasis to the liver, the nodes of the celiac axis, the superior mesenteric artery, and the paraaortic tissues.

3. The pelvis is explored, and the peritoneum along the brim of the pelvis examined for lymph node involvement. Frozen sections may be indicated. The obturator fossa and the region of the uterosacral ligaments are explored. On negative findings at exploration, retractors are placed, and the small bowel is packed off with moist laparotomy packs (Fig. 16-36).

4. The sigmoid mesocolon is freed and sectioned by means of Payr clamps and a scalpel. The proximal end is exteriorized through an opening in the left side of the abdomen; an intestinal clamp is left across the lumen until later, when the permanent colostomy will be secured to the skin.

5. The remaining sigmoid mesentery is clamped with Rochester-Pean forceps, cut, and ligated down to and including the superior hemorrhoidal vessels. Long instruments and sutures are used to facilitate reaching the deep pelvic structures.

6. The distal sigmoid colon is closed with an inverting suture. The sigmoid colon and rectum are freed from the sacrococcygeal area by blunt and sharp dissection.

7. The lateral pelvic peritoneum is cut along the iliac vessels; the ovarian vessels and round ligaments on each side are clamped with Rochester-Pean forceps, cut, and doubly ligated.

8. The peritoneum is incised over the dome of the bladder with a long knife and Metzenbaum scissors, and the bladder is separated from the symphysis pubis down to the urethra.

9. The ureters are identified and divided 2 to 3 cm below the brim of the pelvis. The proximal end is left open to allow urinary drainage while the distal end is ligated.

10. The hypogastric artery, the internal iliac vein, and the superior and inferior gluteal vessels are exposed, clamped with hemostats, doubly ligated, and cut. The external iliac vein is retracted to allow evacuation of the contents of the obturator fossa, leaving the obturator nerve intact. Care must be taken in dissection not to damage the sacral plexus and sciatic nerve.

11. The internal pudendal vessels are isolated, ligated with transfixion sutures, and cut. The remaining soft tissue attachments of the pelvis are clamped and cut. Steps 10 and 11 are then performed on the opposite side.

12. The perineum is incised by an elliptical incision that includes the clitoris and anus. The ischiorectal fat is incised up to the area of the levator muscle.

13. The coccygeal attachment of the rectum is severed. The levator muscles are severed at their lateral attachments by means of a long no. 4 knife handle with no. 20 blade; hemostasis is maintained by pressure and traction.

14. The paravesical and paravaginal tissues are resected from the periosteum of the symphysis pubis and superior pubic rami by means of a knife. The specimen is completely freed and removed from the pelvis (Fig. 16-37).

15. After residual bleeding vessels are identified and controlled by transfixing ligatures, the subcutaneous tissue is closed by interrupted sutures. A drain is placed in the wound, and the skin is closed.

16. In the abdomen, further residual bleeding vessels are controlled. Gauze pads may be left in the pelvis to be removed through the perineum after 48 hours.

17. The ileosegment is then fashioned and the ureters anastomosed to it in the manner described in Chapter 15. The external stoma of the ileosegment is placed on the right side of the abdomen.

18. A red rubber, multieyed tube, size 16 Fr, is inserted into the proximal jejunum for the length of the jejunum and the ileum to aid in postoperative bowel decompression. It is sutured to the bowel with a purse-string suture and brought out to the skin, where it is sutured in place.

19. A gastrostomy tube is placed in the stomach in the same manner.

20. Hemostasis is checked. The small intestines are carefully placed into the pelvis. Packs and retractors are removed (Fig. 16-38).

21. The peritoneum, rectus muscles, and fascial sheaths are closed with interrupted figure-of-eight sutures of 28-gauge wire. The skin is closed with interrupted sutures.

22. The colostomy stoma is prepared by removing the intestinal clamp from the sigmoid colon, opening the colon, and suturing the stoma to the skin edges (Fig. 16-39).

23. The abdominal wound and tube sites are dressed in the usual manner. Drainage bags are applied to the colostomy and ileostomy stomas. A perineal dressing is secured by means of a T binder.

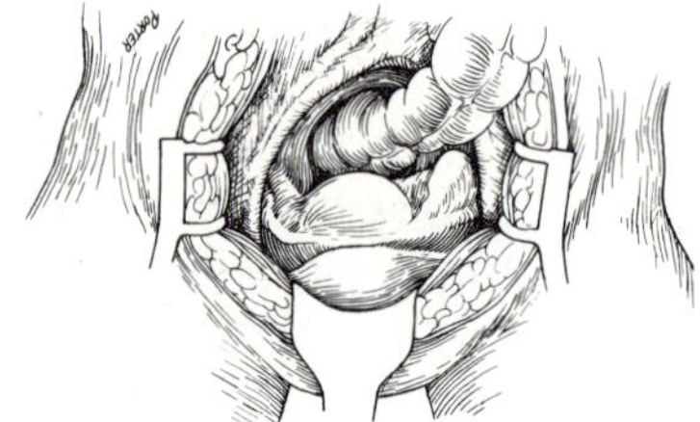

Fig. 16-36. Pelvic exenteration. Pelvic viscera in situ as viewed from operating surgeon's vantage point after retractors are placed and small bowel is packed off. (Redrawn from Lindenauer, S.M., and others: Arch. Surg. **96**:493.)

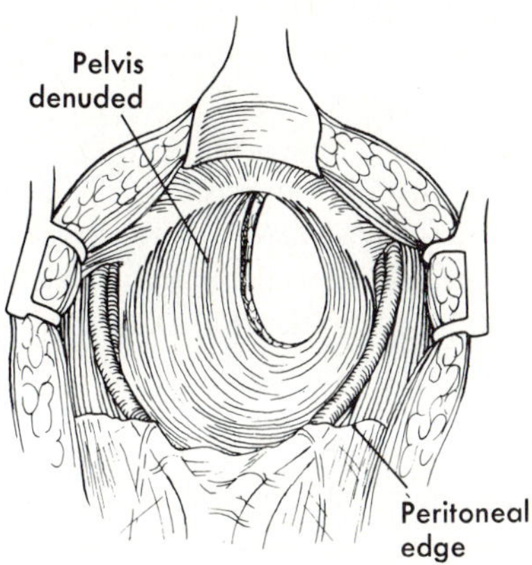

Fig. 16-37. Pelvic exenteration, continued. Empty pelvis after dissection of paravesical and paravaginal tissues and removal of specimen en bloc. (Redrawn from Lindenauer, S.M., and others: Arch. Surg. **96**:493.)

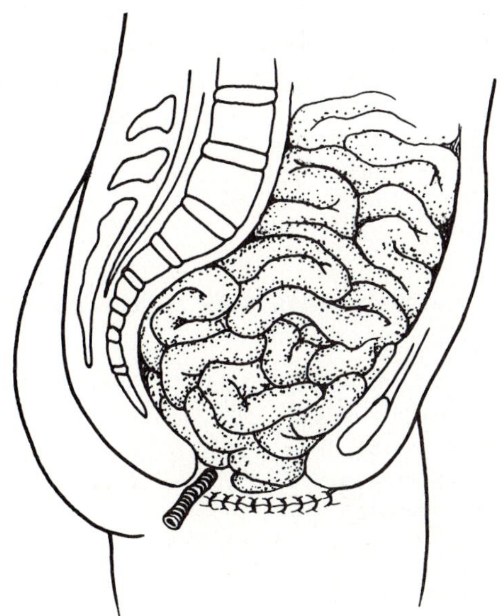

Fig. 16-38. Pelvic exenteration, continued. Sagittal view of small bowel above pelvic defect. Perineal packing and/or drain may be used. (Redrawn from Lindenauer, S.M., and others.: Arch. Surg. **96**:493.)

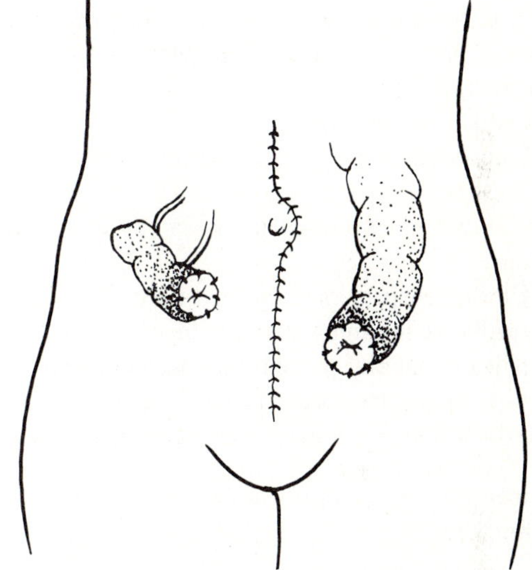

Fig. 16-39. Pelvic exenteration, continued. After closure of abdominal wall, colostomy and ileostomy stomas are sutured to skin edges. (Redrawn from Lindenauer, S.M., and others.: Arch. Surg. **96**:493.)

SURGERY FOR CONDITIONS THAT AFFECT FERTILITY

Uterine suspension

Definition. Through an abdominal incision and opening of the peritoneum, shortening the ligaments of the uterus and positioning them retroperitoneally by traction. The ligaments are then sutured to the undersurface of the abdominal fascia in the corners of the transverse incision bilaterally.

Considerations. Uterine suspension is done today as part of a conservative surgical treatment of pelvic inflammatory disease or endometriosis and in any other situation in which the uterus is bound down in the cul-de-sac. It is also used in most cases of tuboplasty and for the correction of the symptoms of uterine retroversion. Frequently, presacral neurectomy is performed at the same time.

Setup and preparation of the patient. The vaginal preparation is done as described for vaginal surgery. The laparotomy preparation and a laparotomy setup, as described for myomectomy, are used.

Operative procedure

1. The abdomen is opened, as described for myomectomy.

2. The wound is closed in layers, as described for laparotomy.

3. Uterine suspension may also be used in cases of uterine prolapse in young women, in which case a strip of Mersilene material is retroperitoneally placed in a manner to elevate the uterus at the level of the internal os posteriorly and to correct the prolapse into the vagina.

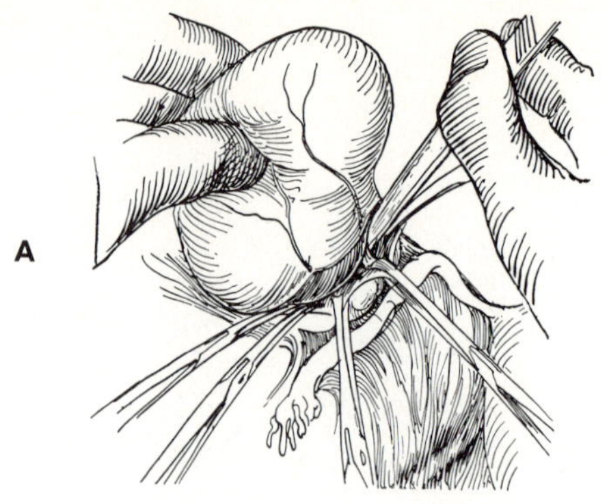

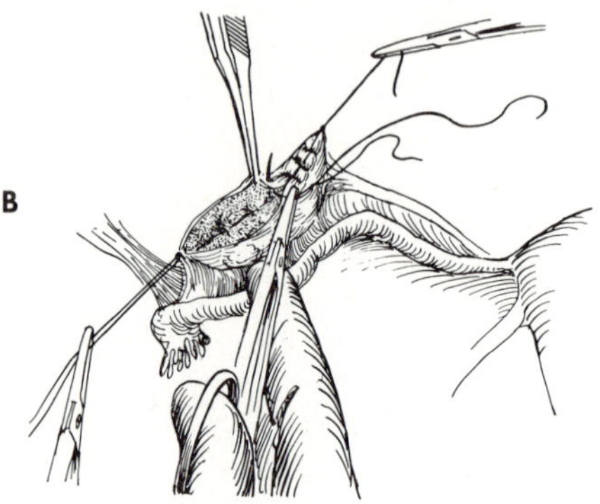

Fig. 16-40. Resection of small cyst from ovary. **A,** Incision made around ovary near junction of cyst wall and normal ovarian tissue. Knife handle is convenient instrument for shelling out cyst. **B,** Wound in ovary closed. (From Ball, T.L.: Operative gynecology and urology, ed. 2, St. Louis, The C.V. Mosby Co.)

Oophorectomy and oophorocystectomy

Definitions

oophorectomy Removal of an ovary.
oophorocystectomy Removal of an ovarian cyst (Fig. 16-40).

Considerations. Functional cysts comprise the majority of the ovarian enlargements. Follicle cysts are the most common. Functional cysts develop in the corpus luteum. Corpus luteum cysts are usually larger than other functional cysts. The true ovarian epithelial tumors, serous cystadenomas and pseudomucinous cystadenomas, are prone to malignant change.

The choice of operation depends on the patient's age and symptoms, findings during physical examination, and direct examination of the adnexa during exploration. If the ovarian tumor is recognized as benign, only the visibly diseased portions of the adnexa are removed. In the presence of dermoid, follicle, and corpus luteum cysts, the cyst is usually enucleated, and most of the ovarian parenchyma is preserved. In tubal pregnancy, the pregnant tube is usually removed and, in some cases, the ovary also.

Setup and preparation of the patient. As described for laparotomy, plus the following:

1 Trocar and cannula with tubing
1 Abdominal suction set
4 Babcock forceps
1 Metzenbaum scissors, 7¼ inches
6 Mayo hemostats, curved
1 Syringe, 10 ml, with 21-gauge needle

Operative procedure

1. The abdominoperitoneal cavity is opened, as described for laparotomy.

2A. *For removal of a large ovarian cyst,* a purse-string suture may be placed in the cyst wall, and a trocar is introduced in its center; the suture is placed around the trocar as the fluid is aspirated. The trocar is removed, and the purse-string suture is tied. All normal ovarian tissue is preserved.

2B. *For removal of a dermoid cyst,* the field is protected with laparotomy packs, since the contents of such cysts produce irritation if they are spilled into the peritoneal cavity. An incision is made along the base of the cyst between the wall and normal ovarian tissue. The cystic wall is dissected away. The ovary is closed with interrupted or continuous sutures.

2C. *For decortication of the enlarged ovary and wedge resection,* a large segment of the ovarian cortex opposite the hilum is removed. The cysts are punctured with a needle point and collapsed. A wedge of ovarian stroma, extending deep in the hilum, is resected with a small knife; the cortex of the ovary is closed with interrupted or continuous sutures.

3. To prevent prolapse of the tube into the cul-de-sac, it may be sutured to the posterior sheath of the broad ligament.

4. The abdominal wound is closed, as described for laparotomy.

Salpingo-oophorectomy

Definition. Removal of a fallopian tube and all or part of the associated ovary.

Considerations. Unilateral salpingo-oophorectomy may be done in some young women who are anxious to have children after all other methods of treatment have failed to cure chronic salpingo-oophoritis, in patients with ectopic tubal gestation, or in those with tuberculosis of the adnexa or large adnexal cysts. If both tubes and ovaries are diseased, they are removed with total hysterectomy.

Setup and preparation of the patient. As described for myomectomy; in some cases, as described for total hysterectomy.

Operative procedure

1. The abdominal wall and peritoneal cavity are opened, as described for laparotomy.

2. The affected tube is grasped with Allis or Babcock forceps. The infundibulopelvic ligament is clamped with Mayo hemostats, cut, and ligated.

3. The mesosalpinx is grasped with Kelly hemostats and divided with the suspensory ligament of the ovary.

4. The cornual attachment of the tube is excised with a knife or curved scissors. Bleeding vessels are clamped and ligated.

5. The edges of the broad ligament are peritonealized from the uterine horn to the infundibulopelvic ligament, as described for total hysterectomy.

6. The wound is closed, as described for laparotomy; dressings are applied and held in place with adhesive or plastic tape.

Tuboplasty

Definition. Removal of the obstructed portion of the uterine (fallopian) tube and opening of the remaining portion of the tube for the possibility of fertilization. This can be accomplished by anastamosis or reconstruction of the tube or by tubal implantation, in which the muscularis of the fallopian tube is brought into position with the muscularis of the uterine cornu. Microsurgical correction of tubal failure is becoming the most successful way to perform tuboplasties and may be employed in all abovementioned methods.

Considerations. These procedures are done to restore fertility in two basic categories of patients: the woman who has a fixed uterus and palpable disease of the reproductive tract and the woman who has no palpable evidence of disease but who has cornual occlusion.

Setup and preparation of the patient. *For vaginal insertion of cannula,* a Kahn, Calvin, Rubin set, Hui, or Humi; one Schroeder single-pronged tenaculum; one sponge forceps; one Auvard vaginal weighted speculum; two Sims vaginal retractors; and assorted cannulas (as preferred by the surgeon) are needed.

For abdominal procedure, a complete microsurgical unit, including a needle tip for hemostasis using electrocautery, and a basic abdominal gynecological setup, are required, plus the following:

2 Iris scissors, 1 curved and 1 straight
2 Razor blades
2 Adson forceps
12 Halsted mosquito hemostats, 6 straight and 6 curved
1 Crile hemostat, rubber-shod, curved
1 Probe
2 Crile-Wood needle holders, light with fine tips
Microsurgery instruments

Accessory items

Microscope or operative loupes
Suction tube and tubing
Eyedropper with small rubber bulb
Polyethylene tubing
Plastic tubing and connectors
Pieces of Dacron cloth material
Complete suction setup with syringes for constant bathing of tissues with saline solution

Operative procedure. Operative procedures for correction of postsurgical tubal occlusion are usually done under the operating microscope. Other reconstructive procedures vary according to the nature of the tubal pathological condition and may be done by use of the operative loupes.

In microsurgery, the surgeon must make sure that virtually no instruments are used in contact with the fallopian tube except those necessary to carry out the surgical technique.

Tubal ligation

Definition. Interruption of uterine (fallopian) tube continuity, resulting in sterilization of the patient.

Considerations. In general, the indication for sterilization depends entirely on the desire of the patient. Certain medical indications and concern for the psychosocial needs of the patient are factors, and occasionally an obstetrical indication exists, such as inherited fetal deformity. However, at least in the United States, sterilization is entirely a voluntary procedure. In many of the states, a sterilization permit does not have to be signed by the husband. Good presurgical counseling is needed for the patient and her husband, since this procedure is not predictably reversible.

The optimum time for sterilization is approximately 24 hours after vaginal delivery. This method does not delay the normal discharge time. An objection to this is that the danger of hemorrhage still exists soon after delivery. With a normal delivery, tubal ligation is done on the first to third postpartum day. If a cesarean section is done, the tubes may be ligated at that time.

Setup and preparation of the patient. The patient is placed in a supine position. A catheter is inserted in the bladder. The abdomen is prepared and draped as described for laparotomy. Instrumentation includes the basic laparotomy setup.

Operative procedures. There are many new surgical methods and techniques. The objective of each method is to achieve complete closure of the fallopian tube so that conception is prevented. When a segment of each fallopian tube is excised, it is preserved for pathological examination. General surgical considerations are directed to excising a section of each fallopian tube, ligating the severed ends, achieving hemostasis and incorporating the proximal stump within layers of the mesosalpinx.

Laparoscopic tubal occlusion

1. A 1-cm intraumbilical or periumbilical incision is made.

2. An accessory suprapubic incision may be made for the occluding instrument.

3. Sterilization can take place by the use of electrocoagulation or thermal coagulation or by the placement of a tubal clip or plastic ring, once the tube has been identified and isolated in the grasping forceps.

Vaginal approach (posterior colpotomy)

1. Operative procedure is the same as for posterior colpotomy.

2. Sterilization can take place by the placement of a tubal clip, by fimbriectomy, or by ligation of the proximal portion of the fallopian tubes with a permanent suture.

Minilaparotomy approach. A small 2-cm transverse incision is made above the pubic hairline, and a large bivalved speculum is placed through it and into the peritoneal cavity. The large Graves bivalve speculum serves as a small abdominal retractor and permits easy access to the tubes, at which time either tubal clips can be applied or a Pomeroy method of ligation can be carried out.

CESAREAN SECTION

Definition. Delivery of the fetus or fetuses through an abdominal incision.

Considerations. In general, cesarean section is employed whenever it is believed that further delay in delivery would seriously compromise the fetus, the mother, or both, yet vaginal delivery cannot be safely accomplished. Once delivery has been effected by cesarean section, delivery in subsequent pregnancies is usually performed the same way. In recent years, the use of cesarean section has increased, as a result of fetal monitoring, fetal scalp blood sampling for pH determination, and the widespread emphasis on recognition of actual or suspected impairment of fetal well-being if delivery were delayed or vaginal delivery attempted. Reasons for cesarean section include malposition-malpresentation, cephalopelvic disproportion, abruptio placentae, toxemia, fetal distress, uterine dysfunction, placenta previa, prolapsed cord, previous pelvic surgery, cervical dystosia, active herpes progenitalis, diabetes, and previous cesarean section.

Considerations. Patients about to undergo cesarean sections need careful assessment and emotional support. Because cesarean sections frequently involve emergency situations, the patient may express grave concern for the infant's well-being. If the patient has participated in childbirth classes, she may feel she has failed in some way. When the mother chooses regional anesthesia, the father may be permitted to enter the operating room and witness the birth. This should only occur if the father has had adequate preparation during the pregnancy and if hospital policy permits. The father helps provide emotional support and can be included in the bonding that takes place at birth. The mother, if awake, will be shown and allowed to touch the infant. The nurse will be caring for two patients: the mother and the infant.

The patient should be in a supine position with an elevation of the right side to ensure adequate venous return during preparation and surgery. If a general anesthetic is to be employed, *all* preparations, including skin preparation, bladder drainage, draping, suction connection, counts, and gowning and gloving of personnel involved in the operative procedure, must be done before induction. Personnel from the nursery must be notified when the cesarean section is scheduled so that they are in attendance for the delivery. The nursery personnel generally provide a bassinet with a warmer (Fig. 16-41) and usually do the immediate postdelivery care of the infant in the operating room.

Setup and preparation of the patient. Hair is shaved from the abdominal wall from above the umbilicus to below the level of the mons pubis and laterally to about the level of the iliac crests. The skin is prepared for abdominal surgery. The vagina is not prepared. The bladder is emptied through an indwelling catheter with continuous drainage during and after the procedure. Instrumentation includes the basic abdominal gynecological set, plus the following (Fig. 16-42):

Cutting instrument

1 Lister bandage scissors

Holding instruments

4 Ring forceps, 8 inches
6 Pennington forceps

Clamping instruments

2 Cord clamps

Exposing instruments

1 DeLee retractor
1 Jackson right-angled retractor

Obstetrical instruments

1 Pair delivery forceps

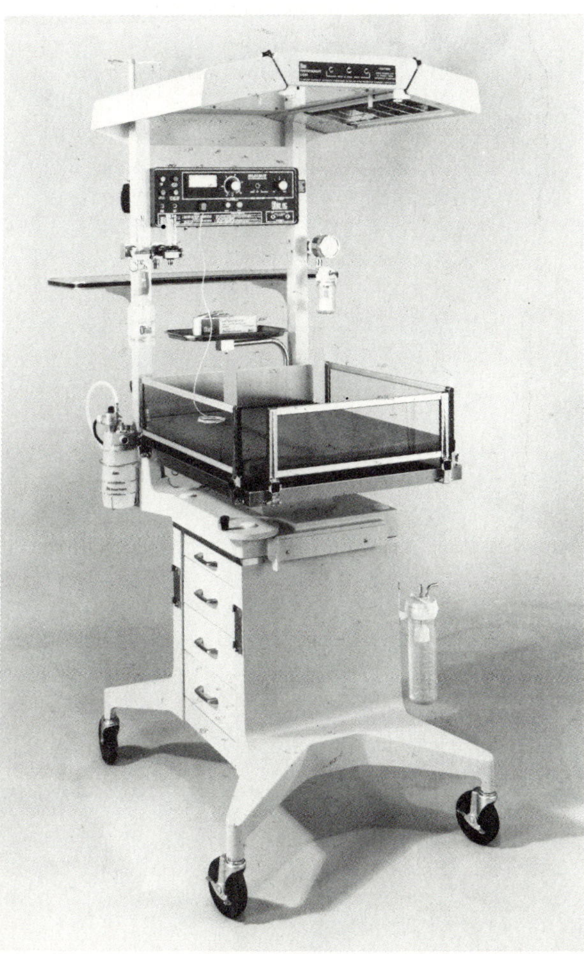

Fig. 16-41. Neonatal intensive care unit. (Courtesy Ohio Medical Products, Madison, Wis.)

Accessory items

2 Laboratory tubes for cord blood
1 Penrose drain (optional)
1 Bulb syringe
4 Sponge-holding forceps, 10 inches

Operative procedure

1. An infraumbilical vertical incision or lower transverse Pfannenstiel incision is made. The incision should be long enough to allow the infant to be delivered without difficulty, but no longer. Therefore the length of the incision will vary with the estimated size of the fetus.
2. The abdominal wall is opened in layers. The rectus and pyramidalis muscles are separated in the midline by sharp and blunt dissection to expose the underlying transversalis fascia and peritoneum.
3. The peritoneum is elevated with two Crile hemostats about 2 cm apart. The peritoneum between the two clamps is palpated to rule out the inclusion of bowel, omentum, or bladder. The peritoneum is opened, and the abdominal cavity entered.
4. Bleeding sites anywhere in the abdominal incision may be clamped but not ligated until later unless the clamps obstruct exposure.
5. The uterus is quickly but carefully palpated to determine the size and presenting part of the fetus as well as the direction and degree of rotation of the uterus.
6. The reflection of peritoneum (serosa) above the upper margin of the bladder and overlying the anterior lower uterine segment is gently separated by sharp and blunt dissection.
7. The developed bladder flap is held downward beneath the symphysis with a bladder retractor such as the DeLee.
8. The uterus is opened with a knife through the lower uterine segment about 2 cm above the detached bladder. Once the uterus is opened, the incision can be extended by cutting laterally with large bandage scissors or by simply spreading the incision by means of lateral pressure applied with each index finger when the lower uterine segment is thin.
9. The presenting membranes are incised. Suction is imperative here, and many surgeons prefer no suction tip (only the large open end of the suction tubing) during the expulsion and suctioning of fluid.
10. All retractors are removed. The fetal head is gently elevated, either manually or by use of obstetrical forceps, through the incision, aided by transabdominal fundal pressure. The pressure helps expel the fetus.
11. As soon as the head is delivered, a bulb syringe is used to aspirate the exposed nares and mouth to minimize aspiration of amniotic fluid and its contents (Fig. 16-43).
12. As soon as the shoulders are delivered, about 20

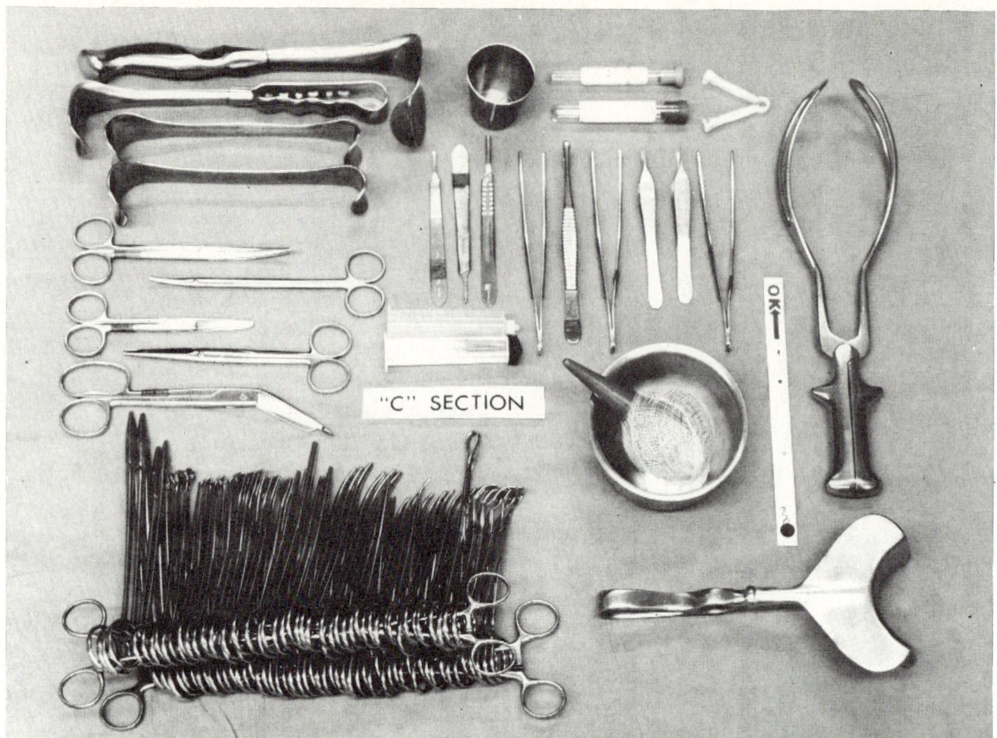

Fig. 16-42. Instrument setup for cesarean section. (Courtesy Edward Weck & Co., Research Triangle Park, N.C.)

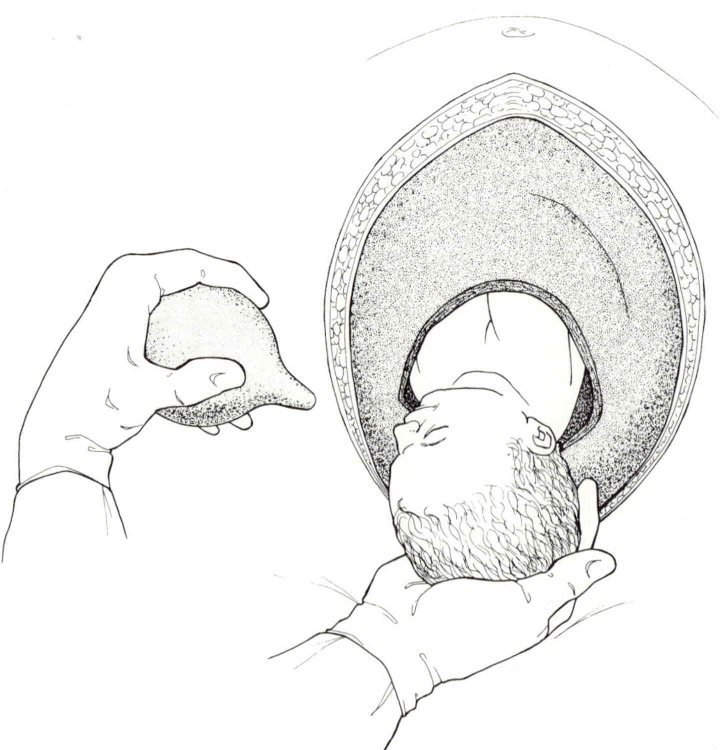

Fig. 16-43. Cesarean section. Delivery of head; suction bulb used to clear nares and mouth of amniotic fluid.

units of oxytocin per liter of fluid are administered intravenously so that the uterus contracts; this minimizes blood loss and aids expulsion of the placenta and membranes.

13. On delivery of the entire infant, the cord is clamped and cut and the infant given to the member of the team who is responsible for resuscitation efforts as needed. A sterile receptacle (gown or sheet) should be provided for this individual so that there is no break in aseptic technique during transferral of the infant.

14. The edges of the uterine incision are promptly clamped with Pean forceps, ring forceps, or Pennington clamps.

15. The placenta is delivered and placed in a large receptacle provided from the back table. Fundal massage or manual removal may be employed to hasten delivery of the placenta and reduce bleeding.

16. One or two separate layers of suture may be used to close the uterine incision.

17. Following determination of no further bleeding after closure of the uterine incision, the cut edges of the serosa overlying the uterus and bladder are approximated with a continuous suture.

18. The gutters on each side of the uterus are checked and clots of blood removed. The fallopian tubes and ovaries are also inspected. Tubal ligation may be carried out at this point. Moist laparotomy pads saturated with warm normal saline solution are generally used extensively during the procedure from the time the peritoneum has been opened until it is closed.

19. The peritoneum and each abdominal layer are closed, with suture preference determined by the surgeon.

SUGGESTED READINGS

Baggist, M.S.: High-power-density carbon dioxide laser therapy for early cervical neoplasia, Am. J. Obstet. Gynecol. **136:**1, Jan. 1980.

Benedet, J.L., and others: Squamous carcinoma of the vulva: results of treatment, 1938 to 1976, Am. J. Obstet. Gynecol. **134:**2, May 1979.

Benedet, J.L., and others: Radical hysterectomy in the treatment of cervical cancer, Am. J. Obstet. Gynecol. **137:**2, May 1980.

Buchsbaum, H.J., and Sciarra, J.J.: Gynecology and obstetrics, vol. 4, Gynecologic oncology, New York, 1980, Harper & Row, Publishers.

Butts, P.: Meeting the special needs of your hysterectomy patient, Nursing '79 **9:**40, Nov. 1979.

Chatman, D.L.: Laparoscopic Falope Ring sterilization, Am. J. Obstet. Gynecol. **131:**3, June 1978.

Depp, R., Eschenbach, D.A., and Sciarra, J.J.: Gynecology and obstetrics, vol. 3, Maternal and fetal medicine, New York, 1980, Harper & Row, Publishers.

DiSaia, P.J., and others: An alternate approach to early cancer of the vulva, Am. J. Obstet. Gynecol. **133:**7, April 1979.

Douglas R.G., and Stromme, W.B.: Operative obstetrics ed. 3, New York, 1976, Appleton-Century-Crofts.

Gerbic, A.B., and Sciarra, J.J.: Sciarra gynecology and obstetrics, vol. 2, Obstetrics, New York, 1980, Harper & Row, Publishers.

Gray, H.: Anatomy of the human body, ed. 29, Philadelphia, 1973, Lea & Febiger. (Edited by C.M. Goss.)

Gunning, J.E., and others: Laparoscopic tubal sterilization using thermal coagulation, Obstet. Gynecol. **54:**4, Oct. 1979.

Hartgill, J.: Wertheim's hysterectomy, Nurs. Times **74:**2061, 1978.

Kibrick, S.: Herpes simplex infection at term, J.A.M.A. **243:**2, 1980.

Kistner, R.W.: Gynecology principles and practice, ed. 3, Chicago, 1979, Year Book Medical Publishers, Inc.

McElin, T.W., and Sciarra, J.J.: Sciarra gynecology and obstetrics, vol. 1, Gynecology, New York, 1980, Harper & Row, Publishers.

Neutra, R.R., and others: Effects of fetal monitoring on cesarean section rates, Obstet. Gynecol. **55:**2, Feb. 1980.

Pelosi, M.A., and others: The "intra-abdominal version technique" for delivery of transverse lie by low segment cesarean section, Am. J. Obstet. Gynecol. **135:**8, Dec. 1979.

Phillips, J.M.: Microsurgery in gynecology, St. Louis, 1977, Christian Board of Publications.

Pitkin, R.M., and Scott, J.R.: The year book of obstetrics and gynecology, Chicago, 1977, Year Book Medical Publishers, Inc.

Pritchard, J.A., and MacDonald P.C.: Williams obstetrics, ed. 16, New York, 1980, Appleton-Century-Crofts.

Webb, M.J., and Symmonds, R.E.: Radical hysterectomy: influence of recent conization on morbidity and complications, Obstet. Gynecol. **53:**3, March 1979.

Woods, N.F.: Human sexuality in health and illness, ed. 2, St. Louis, 1979, The C.V. Mosby Co.

17 Thoracic surgery

ANATOMY

The skeletal framework of the thorax is formed anteriorly by the sternum and costal cartilages, laterally by the twelve pairs of ribs, and posteriorly by the twelve thoracic vertebrae (Figs. 17-1 and 17-2). This airtight compartment is enclosed in the root of the neck by Sibson's fascia and is separated from the abdomen by the diaphragm.

The sternum, or breast bone, forms the anterior thoracic wall in the midline. It consists of three parts: (1) the upper part, or manubrium; (2) the body, or gladiolus; and (3) the lower cartilage, or xiphoid process. The manubrium articulates with the clavicles and the first two ribs on each side; the gladiolus articulates with the remaining true ribs by separate costal cartilages; and the xiphoid fuses with the gladiolus in early development and is attached to the diaphragm by the substernal ligament (Figs. 17-1 and 17-3).

Normally, the lateral walls of the thorax are formed by the twelve pairs of ribs. Posteriorly, each pair of ribs articulates with its corresponding thoracic vertebrae (Fig. 17-2). Anteriorly, the first seven ribs articulate with the sternum. The eighth, ninth, and tenth ribs articulate with the costal cartilages of the rib above; however, the eleventh and twelfth are not fixed to the costal arch.

The muscles of each hemithorax (Figs. 17-3 and 17-4) include the eleven external and eleven internal intercostal muscles, which fill the spaces between the ribs.

An intercostal artery, vein, and nerve accompany each intercostal muscle. The arteries communicate with the internal thoracic artery anteriorly and with the aortic branches posteriorly. The intercostal veins follow the course of the arteries and communicate with the mammary veins anteriorly and with the axygos and hemiazygos veins posteriorly.

During surgery, great care is taken to prevent injury to the intercostal nerve, which passes forward and alongside the posterior intercostal artery and which shares with the superior branch of the artery the intercostal groove on the inferior edge of the corresponding rib. When the nerve must be disturbed, an anesthetic agent may be injected to prevent postoperative pain.

The chest cavity is subdivided into the right and left pleural cavities, which contain the lungs and are separated by the mediastinum, which lies medially between the two pleural membranes (Fig. 17-5). The *parietal pleura,* the membrane that lines the inner surface of the thorax, is adjacent to the inner surfaces of the ribs posteriorly and with the mediastinum medially and covers the surface of the diaphragm, except at the central portion. Part of the parietal membrane is reflected back at the root of each lung to form a sac around it. This reflection is called the *visceral pleura.* A serous secretion existing between these two membranes acts as a lubricant to minimize friction.

The lungs are the essential organs of respiration.The base of each lung rests on the diaphragm, whereas its apex (upper end) projects into the base of the neck at a level above the first rib. The bronchus, the nerves, the lymphatics, and the pulmonary and bronchial vessels enter and leave the lung on the mediastinal surface in a structure known as the hilum, or root, of the lung. Deep fissures divide the spongy, porous lung into lobes. The primary bronchi divide, then subdivide in each lobe and eventually become bronchioles. The right lung has an upper, middle, and lower lobe, and the left lung has only an upper and lower lobe. However, the lungs are similar in that each is composed of ten major segments. Each segment extends to the pleural surface, expanding in volume from its center to its peripheral edges. Each segment also has its own bronchus and branches of the pulmonary artery and vein.

The bronchial arteries, arising from the aorta, supply nourishment to the lungs. They vary in their number and course. The arrangement may include two branches to the left lung and one branch to the right lung, which later branches into two, or there may be one branch for each lung or two branches for each lung. The pulmonary arteries carry the blood to the pulmonary parenchyma, and the pulmonary veins transport the oxygenated blood to the left atrium.

The nerves of the lungs are a part of the autonomic nervous system (Chapter 24). They regulate constriction and relaxation of the bronchi and of the blood vessels within the lungs.

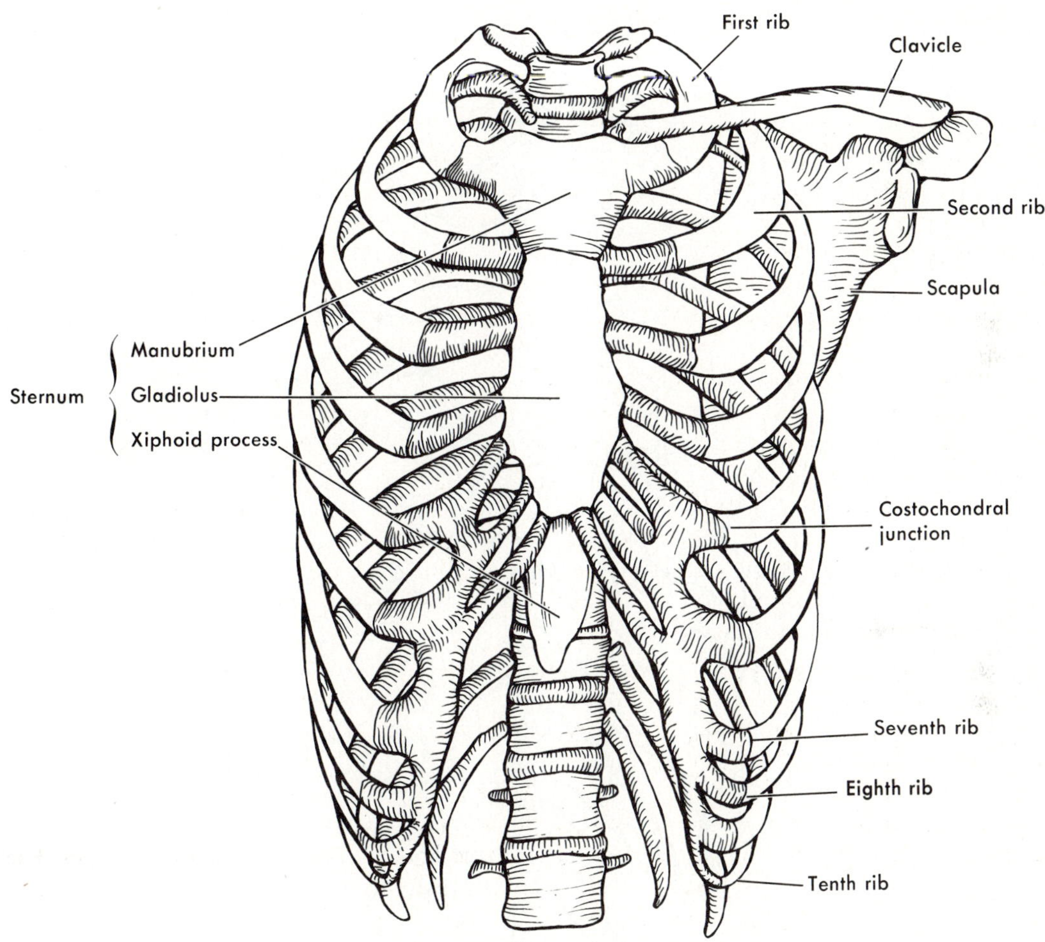

Fig. 17-1. Bony thorax.

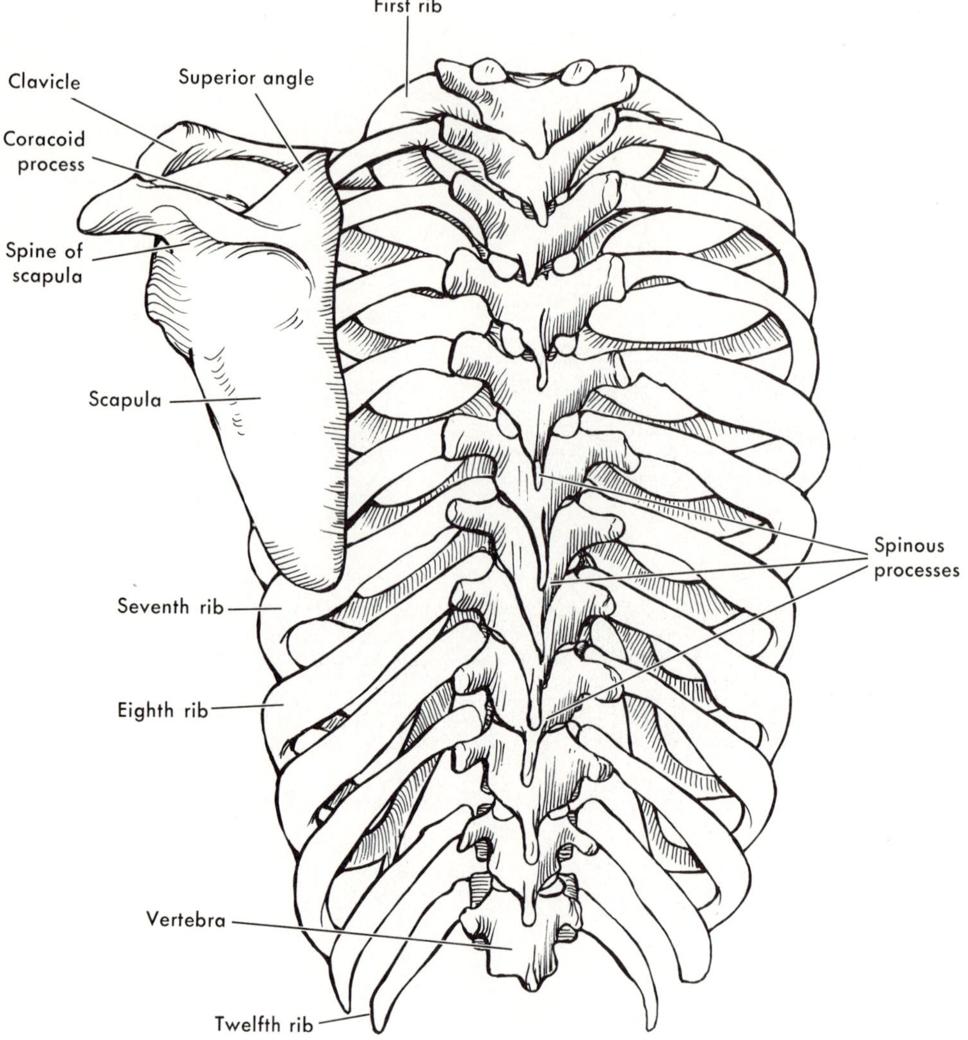

Fig. 17-2. Posterior view of bony thorax.

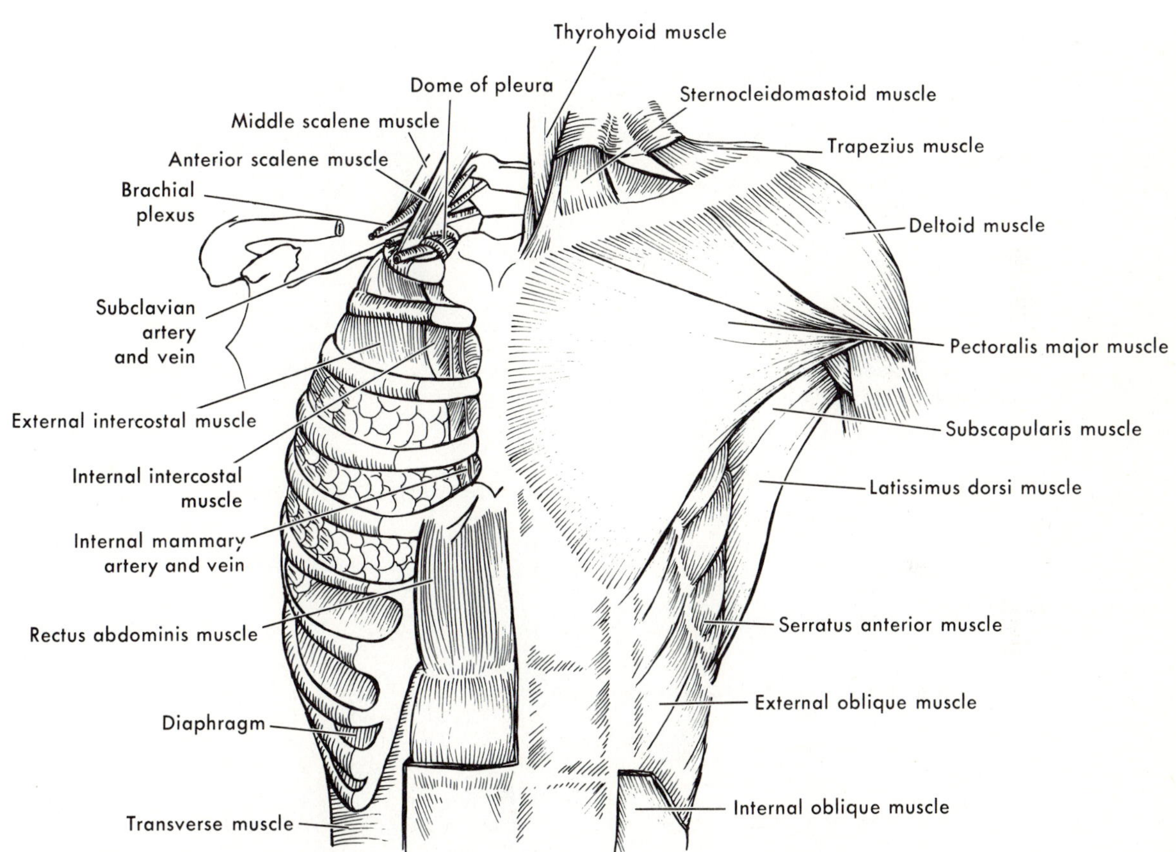

Fig. 17-3. Anterior view of thorax and contiguous portions of base of neck and anterior abdominal wall. *Right half,* Superficial layer of muscles and fascia; *left half,* relations of deep muscles of neck and abdomen to rib cage, intercostal muscles, diaphragm, and internal mammary vessels; relations of muscles, nerves, and vessels with first rib; and anterior relations of lung.

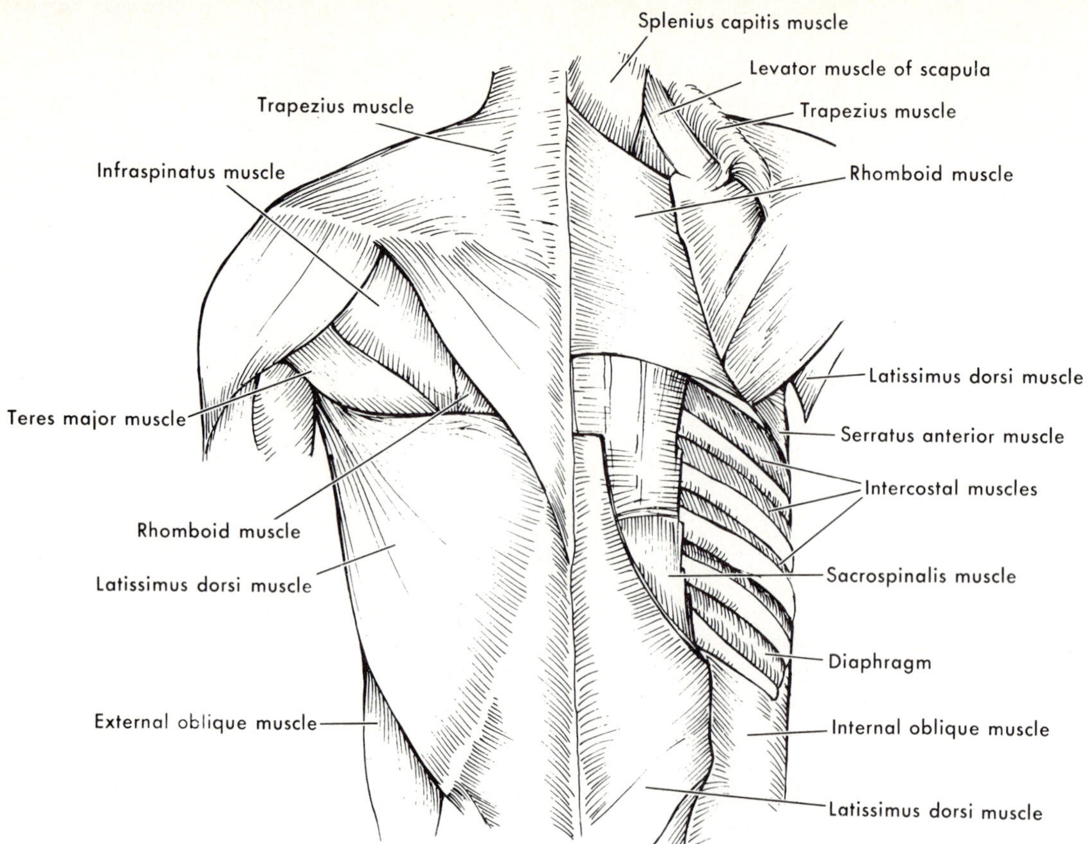

Fig. 17-4. Posterior view of thorax and contiguous portions of neck and abdominal wall. *Left half,* Superficial muscles; *right half,* deeper muscles.

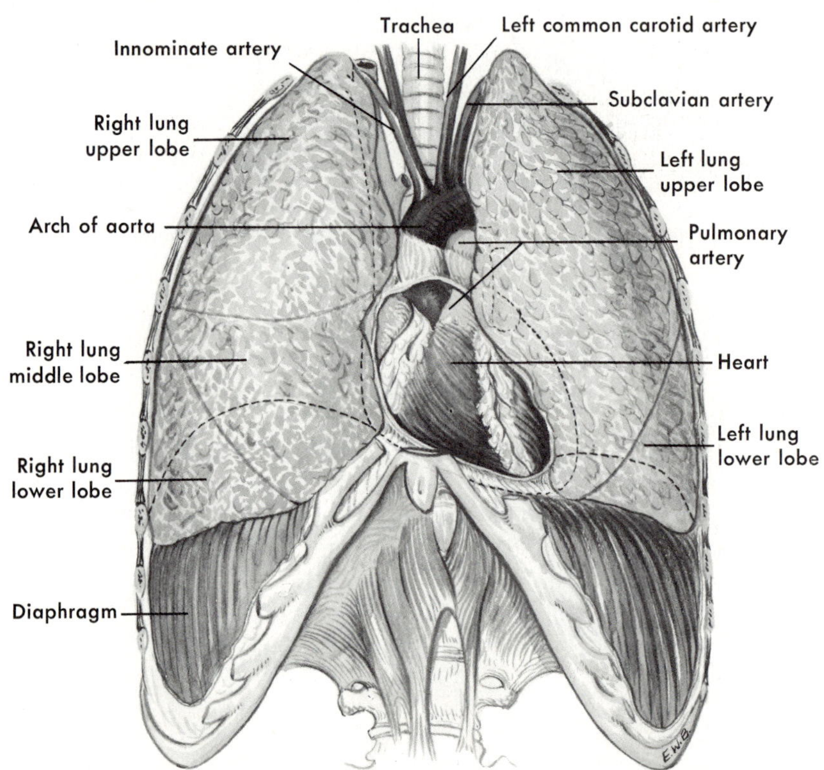

Fig. 17-5. Organs of thoracic cavity. Part of pericardium has been removed to expose heart. (From Schottelius, B.A., and Schottelius, D.D.: Textbook of physiology, ed. 18, St. Louis, 1978, The C.V. Mosby Co.)

PHYSIOLOGY

Although the thoracic cavity is an airtight space, the lungs inspire outside air through the nasal passages, trachea, and bronchi. The main function of the lungs is to provide a means for the exchange of carbon dioxide for oxygen. Normally, as the thorax expands, the lungs also expand and draw air in; as the thorax relaxes and compresses the lungs, air is forced out. Inspiration normally takes place when the intrathoracic pressure is slightly below atmospheric pressure (76 cm Hg or 760 mm Hg) and when a partial vacuum exists between the parietal and visceral pleural (intrathoracic) surfaces. As the muscles of inspiration contract to enlarge the chest cage, the lungs passively follow the diaphragm and chest wall because of decreased intrathoracic pressure. The acts of inspiration and expiration are the result of air moving in and out so that the pressure equalizes that of the atmosphere at the end of expiration (Fig. 17-6).

The normal intrapleural pressure varies from −9 to −12 cm H_2O during inspiration, and from about −3 to −6 cm H_2O during expiration. The greatest amount of air that can be expired after a maximum inspiration is termed the *vital capacity*. Size, age, and sex of the patient and presence of pulmonary disease in the patient influence vital capacity. Any condition that interferes with the normally negative intrapleural pressure generally has a serious effect on respiratory function.

Respiratory complications. In the presence of restrictive and obstructive pulmonary disease, the lung may not fully expand or contract, causing a reduction in alveolar ventilation with resultant hypoxia. Other conditions that interfere with respiratory function are mucus or a foreign body in a bronchus, pleural effusion, pulmonary edema, pneumonia, closed pneumothorax (simple and tension types), open pneumothorax, hemothorax, and multiple rib injuries that produce paradoxical motion of the thoracic cage (Fig. 17-7).

As previously mentioned, the normal function of the "pulmonary bellows" is caused by the elasticity of the lungs and by the negative intrapleural pressure. If the lung is not adherent to the chest wall, collapse of the normal lung will follow any condition that reduces or eliminates the negative intrapleural pressure. When the pleural space is filled with air, reducing the negative pressure, the lung collapses. This action may cause a complete collapse if the pressure within the intrathoracic (pleural) space becomes positive.

Also, a diminished negative pressure or the occurrence of actual positive pressure in one pleural space may cause a shift of the mediastinum toward the opposite side. When this happens, not only does the affected lung collapse because of a positive pressure in the pleural space, but the function of the lung on the opposite side may also be impaired as a result of compression by the shifted me-

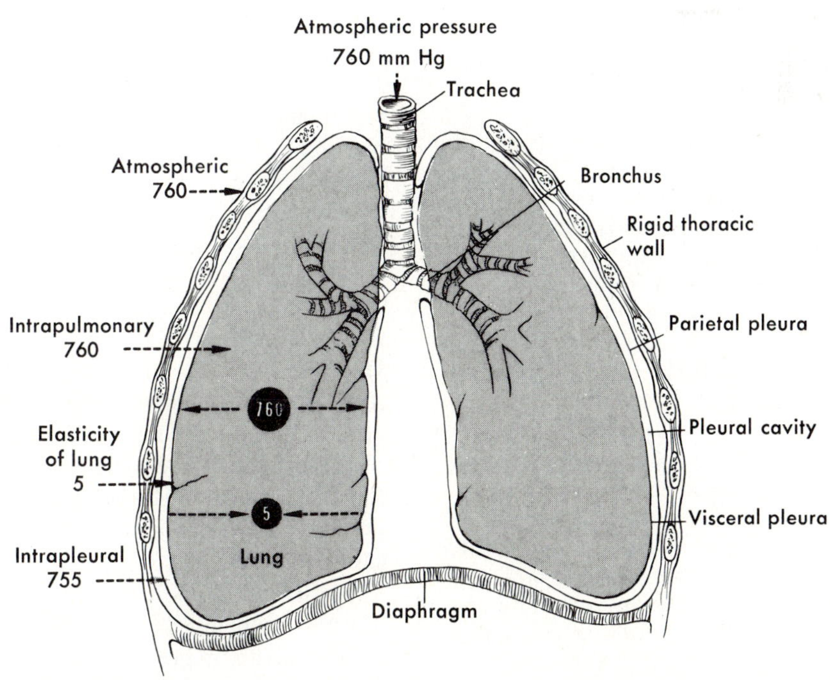

Fig. 17-6. Illustration of thoracic cavity structures showing intrapulmonary and intrapleural pressures with chest wall in resting position. (From Schottelius, B.A., and Schottelius, D.D.: Textbook of physiology, ed. 18, St. Louis, 1978, The C.V. Mosby Co.)

diastinum. Tension pneumothorax can produce serious effects as air continues to escape from the lung into the intrapleural space. The air is unable to return to the bronchi to be exhaled, thereby increasing the intrapleural pressure. When a large opening in the chest wall allows direct communication of the pleural space with atmospheric pressure, it may cause death if the mediastinum becomes mobile. The exposure of the pleural space to atmospheric pressure collapses the affected lung. Also, the positive pressure is transmitted to the mediastinum, which, in turn, shifts toward the opposite side and may cause the opposite lung to collapse.

Paradoxical motion of the chest results from severe instability of the chest wall because of multiple and often bilateral rib fractures; with inspiration partial collapse of the thoracic space occurs. This may result in severe, life-threatening hypoxia. Treatment is described later.

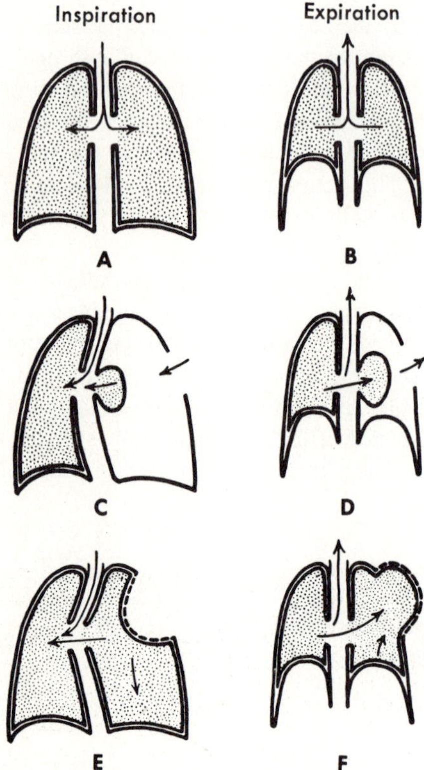

Fig. 17-7. Pathophysiology of severe chest injuries. **A** and **B,** Normal physiology of inspiration and expiration. **C** and **D,** Open (sucking) wound of thorax. On inspiration, air at atmospheric pressure rushed in through defect, **C,** collapsing lung. Next, positive pressure causes mediastinum to shift, compressing opposite lung. On expiration, **D,** air from lung on uninjured side reenters collapsed lung and is rebreathed in next inspiration. Impaired cardiopulmonary function in presence of sucking wound of chest is caused by (1) collapse of lung on injured side; (2) partial collapse of opposite lung; (3) increased functional dead space, caused by rebreathing of unoxygenated air from collapsed lung; and (4) diminished venous return to right side of heart. **E** and **F,** Primary effect of paradoxical motion resulting from flail or stove-in chest is diminution of pulmonary ventilation and extensive rebreathing from one lung to the other. Venous return to right side of heart is impaired. Appropriate treatment requires intubation of trachea and use of volume-limited ventilator. (From Johnson, J., and Kirby, C.K.: Surgery of the chest, ed. 4, Chicago, Year Book Medical Publishers, Inc.)

NURSING CONSIDERATIONS

In addition to the routine nursing measures that apply to all surgical patients, some considerations pertain to those involved in caring for the patient who is undergoing thoracic surgery. Preoperative assessment and teaching is important in planning the intraoperative care of the thoracic surgical patient and in contributing to a successful patient outcome. In addition to the usual preoperative instructions, the thoracic patient and family should be instructed on the presence and purpose of the chest tube or tubes and water-seal bottles.

Preoperative chest x-ray films should be obtained and available in the operating room during surgery.

The electrocardiogram is monitored during thoracic procedures. Nurses should be familiar with the correct method of placing the electrodes for the specific electrocardiography monitor being used. Arterial pressure, central venous pressure, and occasionally pulmonary artery pressure are also monitored with increased frequency.

Most thoracic surgery patients receive a general anesthetic administered by way of an endotracheal tube with an inflated cuff to ensure an airtight system. Since the pleura is opened in the majority of procedures and a pneumothorax results when the negative intrapleural pressure is lost, the closed endotracheal system ensures adequate ventilation. Suction equipment must be available for the aspiration of mucus, blood, or other fluids and secretions.

A defibrillator with internal and external paddles should be readily available. It is essential that nurses fully understand the purpose and use of the equipment. A supply of various medications that might be necessary in an emergency situation, such as hypovolemic shock or cardiac arrest, should also be available. This might include such drugs as sodium bicarbonate, epinephrine, digitalis, calcium chloride, calcium gluconate, potassium chloride, isoproterenol, furosemide, dopamine, and nitroprusside.

Positioning. The principles of good positioning are followed, as outlined in Chapter 6.

The patient is placed on the operating table in a position that provides adequate exposure of the operative site, efficient ventilatory and circulatory functions, and good body alignment. Pulmonary mechanics and return of blood to the right side of the heart are influenced by the position of the patient. Proper support and elimination of undue pressure areas are important. Abrupt changes of position should be avoided to prevent hypotension.

The lateral position permits a full posterolateral thoracotomy incision (Fig. 17-8), which gives the surgeon access to both the anterior and posterior surfaces of the lung and blood vessels.

The supine position is used for median sternotomy (Fig. 17-9) and bilateral anterior transpleural incisions. The sternum may be split vertically or transected horizontally. The arms may be extended and supported on arm-

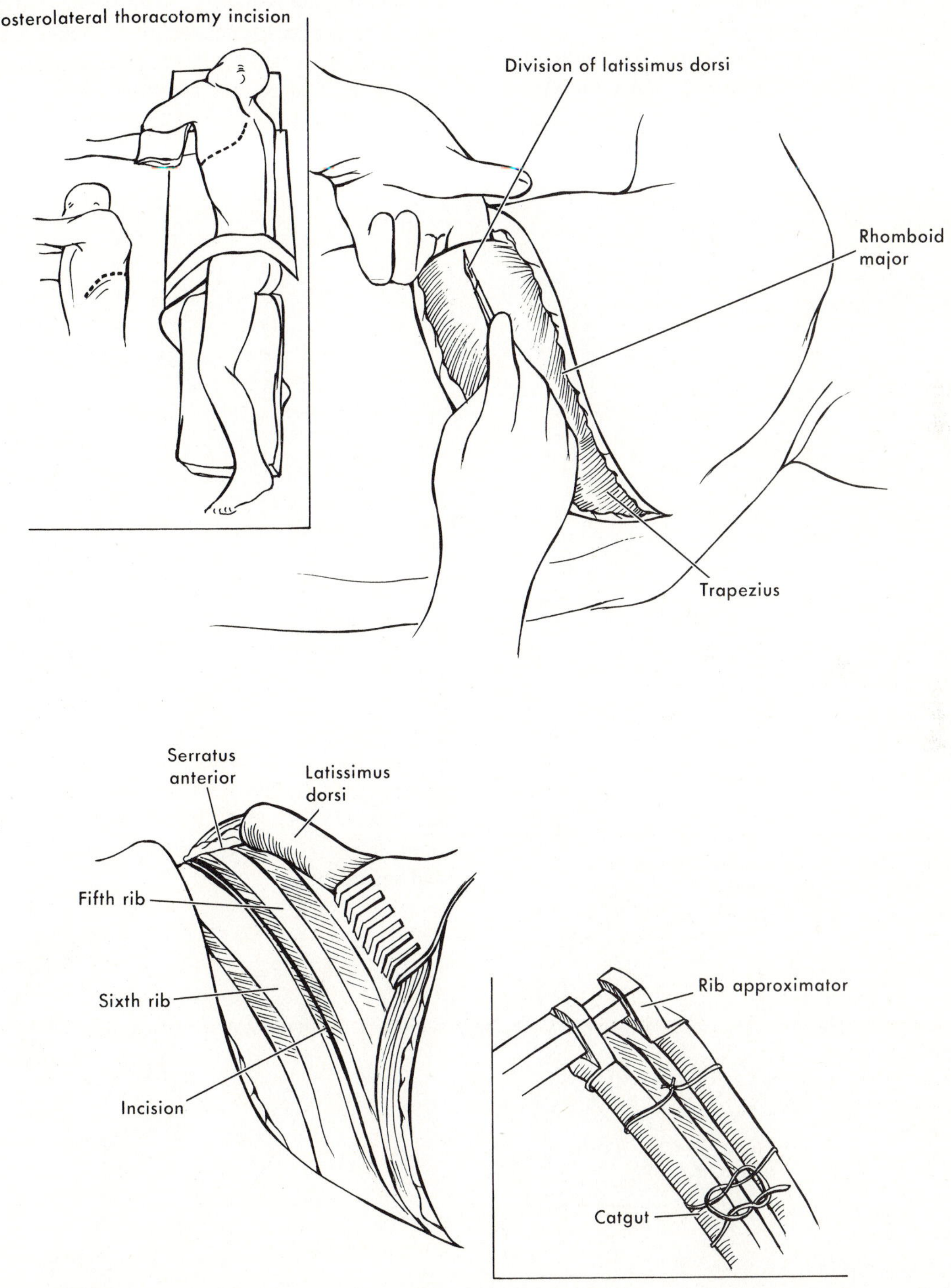

Fig. 17-8. Posterolateral thoracotomy. Wide exposure is dependent on adequate division of trapezius.

boards, or they may be positioned at the patient's side. In either case, the principles of physiological and safe positioning are employed to protect the patient from injury.

For an anterolateral thoracotomy, the operative side may be slightly elevated with a sandbag or towels placed under the scapula. The arm on the operative side is padded and usually extended on an overhead armboard.

Skin preparation and draping. Procedures are followed as described in Chapter 5.

Provisions for blood replacement. Before the operation begins, blood should be made available for replacement.

Chest drainage. One or more chest tubes may be used for postoperative closed chest drainage. The chest tubes provide a conduit for drainage of blood and other fluid from the intrapleural or mediastinal space and/or reestablishment of a negative pressure in the intrapleural space. The chest tubes are clamped until connected to a sterile, water-seal drainage system. When a persistent air leak cannot be controlled by drainage alone, water-seal suction may be necessary. Traditionally, a two- or three-bottle system has been used to accomplish this. Several compact, disposable units are available. These units are preferable because they are easier and safer to use. The

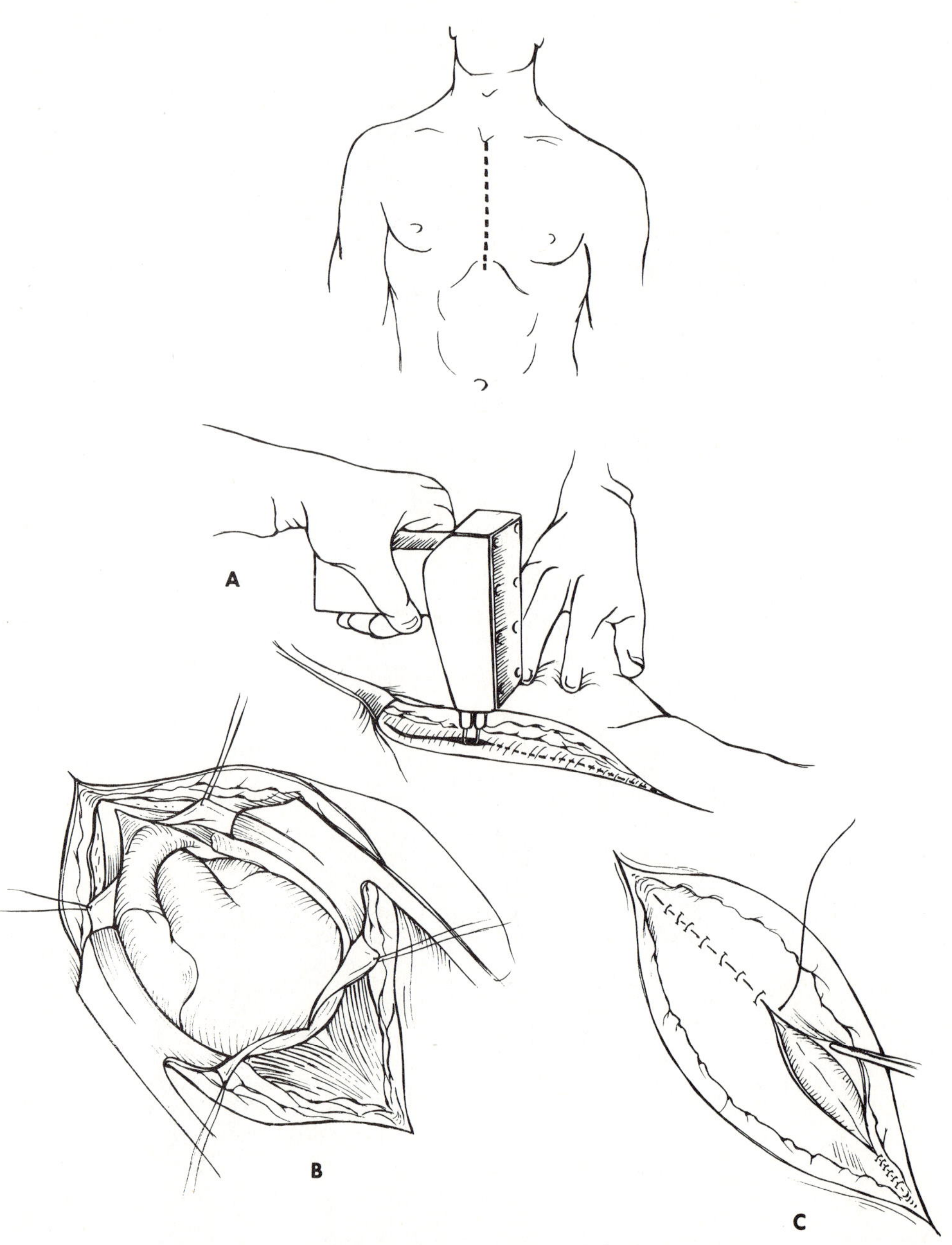

Fig. 17-9. Median sternotomy. Sternum divided with power-driven saw.

principles of operation, however, remain the same and can be described more easily by using the bottle system as a model (Fig. 17-10). The first bottle collects the drainage from the intrapleural space, the second bottle provides the water seal, and the third provides the suction control.

If two chest tubes are inserted, they may be connected by a Y connector to a single drainage unit, or they may be attached, individually, to two separate units. All connections should be banded or otherwise secured to ensure an intact system. Regardless of the type of closed drainage system selected, it is imperative that it be sterile and that it always be maintained at a position lower than the patient's body to prevent reentrance of air and fluid into the chest cavity. Clamps for the tubing should always be available as a precautionary measure against accidental interruption of the closed system.

Instrumentation. The thoracic setup includes the basic laparotomy instrument setup (Chapter 7) and surgical pack with an appropriate fenestrated drape or individual medium sheets to surround the incision. The thoracic setup also might include the following specialty instruments (Figs. 17-11 to 17-13):

Cutting instruments

2 Nelson scissors, curved, 10 inches (Fig. 17-11)
1 Potts tenotomy scissors, 7½ inches
1 Potts dissecting scissors, angulated 60-degree, 7½ inches
1 Wire cutter

Holding instruments

14 Backhaus towel clamps, 5 inches
2 Potts-Smith vascular forceps, smooth, 7 inches
2 Potts-Smith vascular forceps, fine-toothed, 7 inches
6 Rumel thoracic clamps, 9 inches (Fig. 17-11)
4 Duval lung-grasping forceps (Fig. 17-11)
1 Semb forceps, 9¼ inches

Clamping instruments

6 Right-angled clamps, assorted lengths and angulations
4 Sarot or Lees bronchus clamps, right and left for resection (Fig. 17-11)

Vascular instruments

2 Crafoord coarctation clamps
4 Patent ductus clamps, 2 angulated and 2 straight
2 Satinsky clamps
2 Cooley clamps

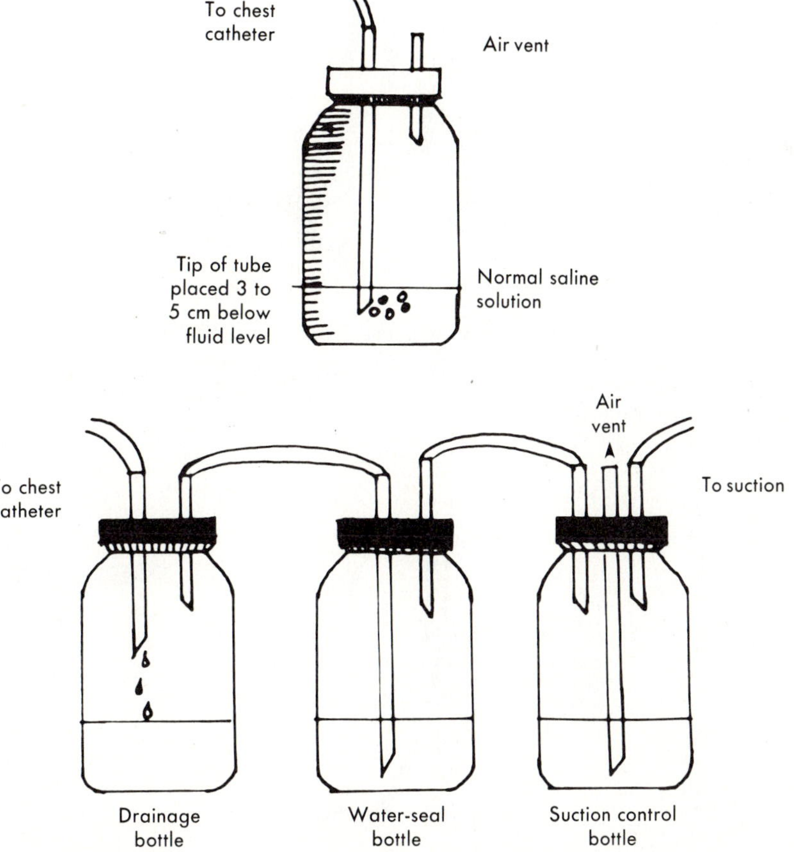

Fig. 17-10. Methods of draining pleural space, using bottle system as model. Disposable units, using same principles, are also available.

Bone instruments (Figs. 17-12 and 17-13)

1 Alexander periosteotome
1 Overholt elevator
2 Doyen rib raspatories and elevators, 1 right and 1 left
1 Liston-Stille bone-cutting forceps
1 Bethune rib shears
1 Sauerbruch rib rongeur, double-action, square jaw
1 Stille-Luer bone rongeur, multiple action

Median sternotomy instruments

1 Sternal saw (Sarns electric) (Fig. 17-12)
1 Lebsche sternal knife (Fig. 17-12)
1 Mallet
1 Sternum spreader
1 Sternum approximator
2 Bone tenacula, single-hook
1 Bone punch or awl with fenestrated tip

Retractors

2 Volkmann rake retractors, dull, six- or eight-pronged
2 Kelly retractors, large
1 Burford-Finochietto rib retractor with 2 sets blades (Fig. 17-13)
3 Finochietto retractors, assorted sizes (Fig. 17-13)
2 Bailey rib contractors (Fig. 17-13)
1 Davidson scapula retractor (Fig. 17-13)

Suturing instruments

6 Sarot needle holders, 10 inches and 12 inches

Accessory items

Electrocautery unit
2 Plastic chest catheters, selected sizes (with appropriate connectors)
1 Bone wax
2 Asepto syringes
1 Closed drainage set (Fig. 17-10)
2 Suction tubings, 6-ft lengths
6 Pieces umbilical tape, 18 inches

Thoracic surgery arrangement of items on the instrument table and Mayo stand should be determined by the nursing staff, depending on an effective standard method that applies principles of work simplification and thorough knowledge of procedure.

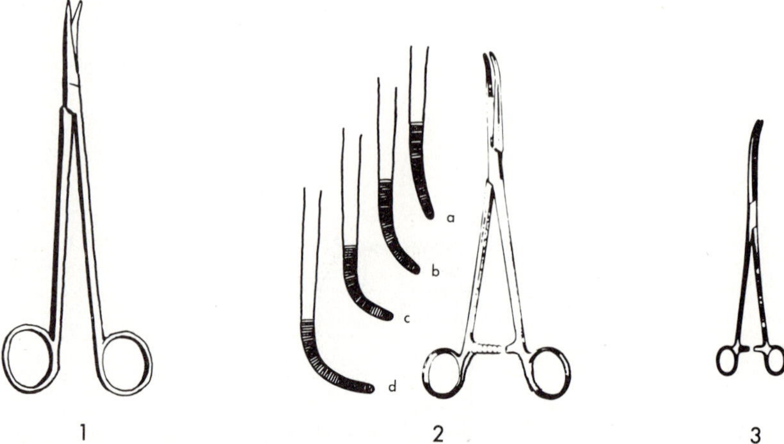

Fig. 17-11. Instruments for lobectomy and pneumonectomy. *1,* Nelson scissors; *2,* Rumel thoracic forceps, *a* to *d*; *3,* Harrington forceps; *4,* Willauer-Allis thoracic tissue forceps; *5,* Duval lung-grasping forceps; *6,* Sarot bronchus clamps, right and left. (Courtesy Codman & Shurtleff, Inc., Randolph, Mass.)

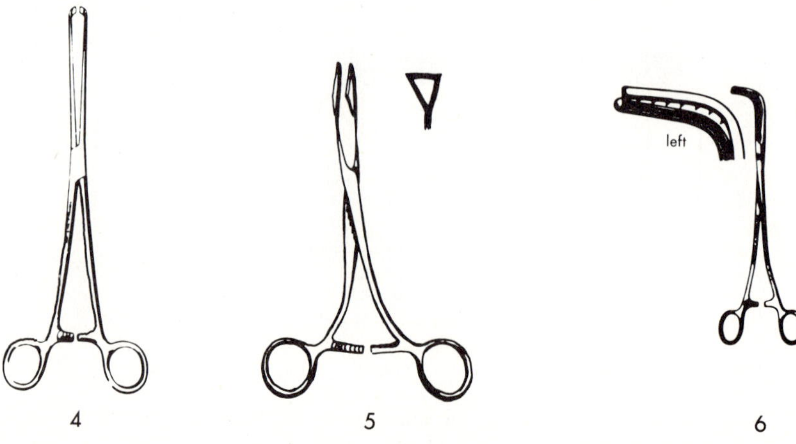

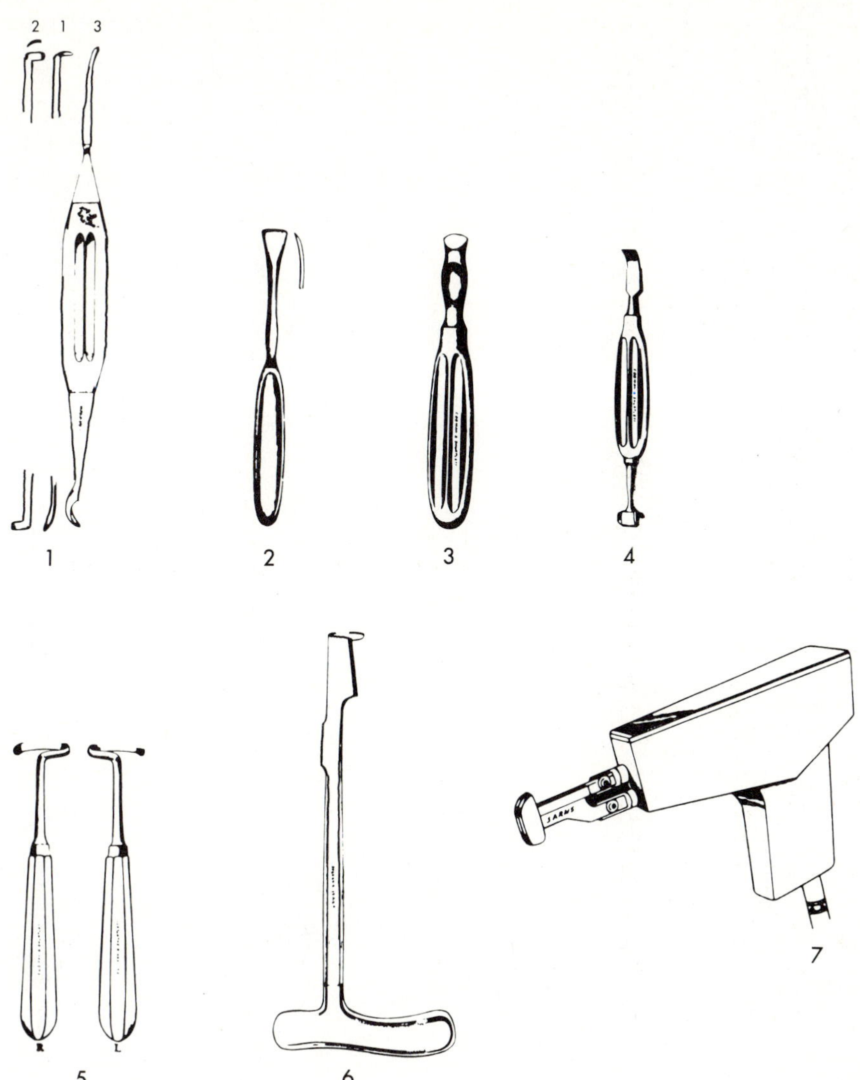

Fig. 17-12. Instruments for thoracotomy. *1,* Overholt elevators, nos. 1, 2, and 3; *2,* Langenbeck periosteal elevator; *3,* Kermission periosteal raspatory; *4,* Alexander costal periosteotome; *5,* Doyen rib raspatories, right and left; *6,* Lebsche sternum knife; *7,* Sarns sternal electric saw. (*1* courtesy American V. Mueller, Chicago, Ill.; *2* to *6* courtesy Codman & Shurtleff, Inc., Randolph, Mass.; *7* courtesy Sarns, Inc., Ann Arbor, Mich.)

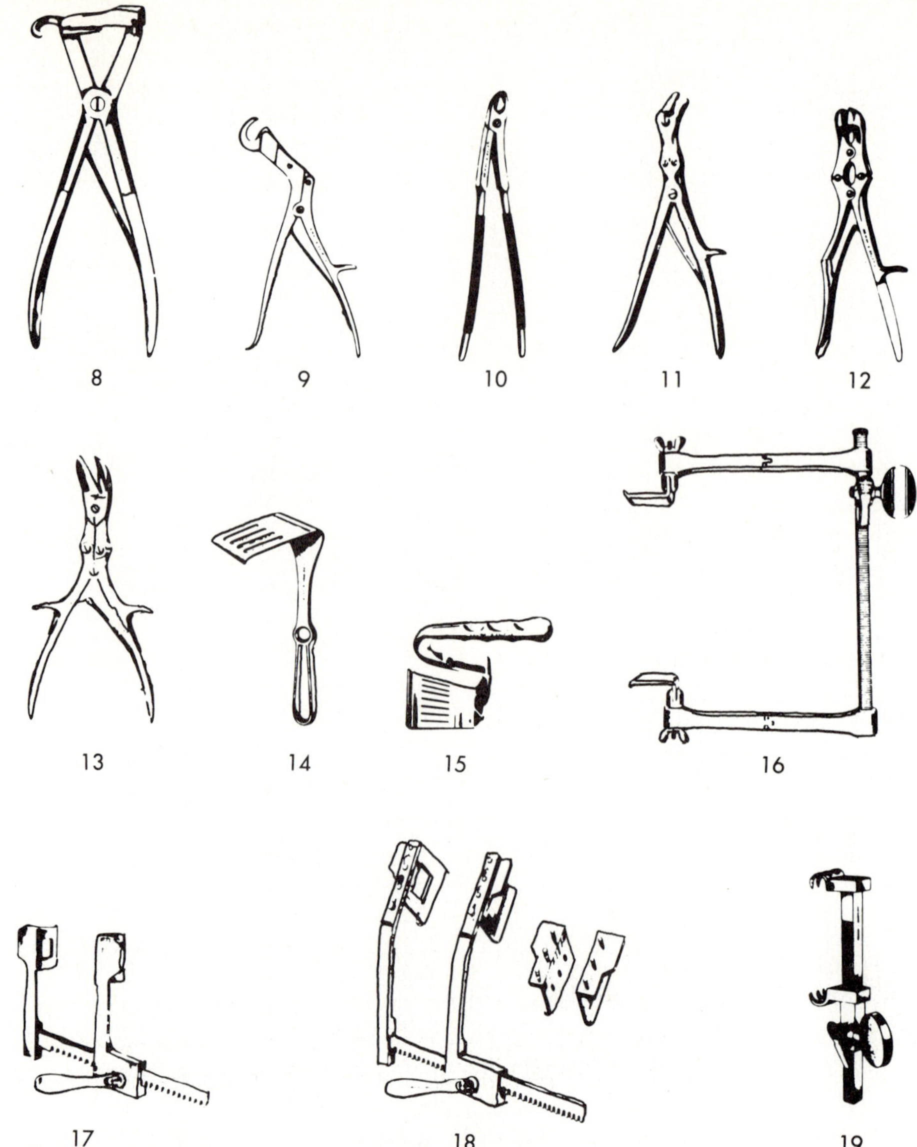

Fig. 17-13. Instruments for thoracotomy, continued. *8,* Shoemaker rib shears; *9,* Stille-Giertz rib shears; *10,* Bethune rib shears; *11,* Stille-Luer bone rongeur; *12,* Sauerbruch rib rongeur; *13,* Liston-Stille bone-cutting forceps, straight; *14,* Coryllos retractor, large size; *15,* Davidson scapula retractor; *16,* Himmelstein sternal retractor with hinged arms; *17,* Finochietto rib retractor; *18,* Burford-Finochietto rib retractor with two sets detachable blades; *19,* Bailey rib contractor. (*8* to *11* and *15* to *19* courtesy Codman & Shurtleff, Inc., Randolph, Mass.; *12* to *14* courtesy American V. Mueller, Chicago, Ill.)

OPERATIONS

Types of incisions

The type of incision is determined by the operative procedure planned. In thoracic surgery there are three basic approaches, which have been mentioned previously: (1) median sternotomy, (2) anterolateral thoracotomy, and (3) posterolateral thoracotomy. Transsternal bilateral thoracotomy is a fourth type of incision, but it is rarely used.

The most frequently used incision is the posterolateral thoracotomy (Fig. 17-8), which provides the surgeon with good visualization and relatively easy access to the lung and hilum. Procedures that are usually performed through a posterolateral thoracotomy include lobectomy, pneumonectomy, decortication, talc poudrage, and drainage of empyema.

The incision is made over the selected rib or interspace and is carried through the subcutaneous tissue and muscle. Bleeding vessels are controlled with hemostats, nonabsorbable or chromic ligatures, and electrocautery.

The periosteum is incised, and the intercostal muscles are freed from the rib with a periosteal elevator, Doyen raspatory, and/or scissors. A segment of rib is then removed with the bone shear. The bone edges are trimmed with a rongeur, and bone wax may be applied for hemostasis. In some procedures, a rib may not be removed.

In an anterolateral thoracotomy, an inframammary incision is made from the anterior midline or the sternal border to the midaxillary line. Muscles are divided as described above. The internal mammary vessels may be ligated. A rib may be resected. This incision is usually used for less complex thoracic procedures, such as a lung biopsy.

A median sternotomy is usually performed when surgery involving the mediastinum is planned, such as resection of mediastinal tumors or lymph nodes or thymectomy (Fig. 17-9). The skin incision is carried from the manubrium to the xiphoid process. Hemostasis is achieved with hemostats and ligatures or electrocautery.

The sternum is usually transected with an electric or air-driven saw. A Lebsche sternal knife and a mallet may be used if a saw is not available. Hemostasis of the sternal edges is obtained with electrocautery and bone wax.

In transsternal bilateral thoracotomy, the incision for anterolateral thoracotomy is made bilaterally. In addition, the sternum is transected horizontally with an electric or air-driven saw or a Gigli saw. The internal mammary vessels are ligated.

ENDOSCOPIC PROCEDURES

The term *endoscopy* refers to the examination of body cavities by means of instruments that permit visual inspection of the contents and the walls of the cavities.

Endoscopic procedures pertinent to thoracic surgery are (1) bronchoscopy, (2) esophagoscopy, and (3) mediastinoscopy. These can be used as diagnostic and therapeutic procedures.

Each endoscopist has preferences regarding the type of endoscope, the positioning of the patient, and the type of anesthetic to be administered.

Preparation of the patient. The patient is not permitted food or fluids for at least 8 hours before examination.

The teeth are brushed just before sedation. The patient's dentures must be removed, and, before examination, any loose teeth may be removed. Psychological preparation of the patient by the physician and assistants is as important as the drug preparation, since examinations may be performed under topical anesthesia.

Drug preparation makes the examination easier for the patient. Endoscopy is not done unless the patient is sufficiently relaxed. For routine procedures, the patient is usually given a sedative orally at bedtime. An hour before examination, the patient is given a sedative. A tranquilizer, such as diazepam (Valium), is often used to provide sedation and patient cooperation when the endoscopy is performed under local anesthesia.

Administration of anesthetic agents. Topical or general anesthetics may be used. The topical (local) anesthetic setup should include the following:

- 1 Head light
- 2 Laryngeal mirrors, various sizes
- 1 Lingual spatula
- 2 Sprays with straight and curved cannulas and anesthetic drugs, as ordered
- 1 Laryngeal syringe with straight and curved cannulas
- 1 Jackson cross-action forceps
- 1 Schindler pharyngeal anesthetizer, if desired
- 2 Medication cups
- 1 Emesis basin
- 1 Basin, small, with very warm water
- 1 Luer-Lok syringe, 10 ml, and needles, 20 and 22 gauge, for transtracheal injection
- 6 Gauze sponges, 4 × 4 inches
- 1 Box paper tissues
- 1 Adjustable stretcher
- 1 Footstool

The anesthetic drugs frequently used are lidocaine (Xylocaine), procaine (Novocain), and tetracaine (Pontocaine) with epinephrine. Epinephrine reduces the rapidity of systemic absorption of the local anesthetic. The traditional drug has been cocaine in a 0.5% or 0.25% solution; however, because of its relatively high reaction risk, it has been replaced by less toxic agents. Cetacaine may be also used.

Pauses of 3 to 4 minutes are taken between applications of the agent to the tongue, palate, and pharynx, and then to the larynx and to the trachea. The anesthetic agent is applied by means of a spray or laryngeal syringe with a straight or curved cannula.

Some physicians prefer to have the patient sit upright and gargle with the topical anesthetic mixture, rinse it around in the mouth, and then expectorate it, thereby producing a partial anesthesia of the buccal mucosa and pharynx.

For direct bronchoscopy, a long metal cannula attached to a syringe is generally used to apply the anesthetic agent to the surface of the vocal cords; then the agent is injected through the anesthetized glottis into the trachea. This act causes the patient to produce a sharp, sudden cough.

For intrabronchial anesthesia, a portion of the anesthetic agent is introduced through the bronchoscope.

Positioning. The principles of providing comfort, safety, proper ventilation, and adequate exposure are discussed in Chapter 6.

For bronchoscopy. The patient is placed in a dorsal recumbent position with shoulders flat on the table at a precise point to permit proper overhanging of the head and neck during the examination. The proper position of the patient is shown in Fig. 17-23.

For esophagoscopy. One of several positions may be selected. For direct esophagoscopy, the supine or the lateral position may be used. When the lateral position is used, the person who will hold the patient's head may sit on a high stool behind the patient's head.

Draping. The patient's eyes are draped with a towel, and long hair is enclosed in a disposable cap. Aseptic techniques are used during endoscopy.

Instruments

Instruments are designed for direct inspection and observation of the larynx, trachea, bronchi, esophagus, or mediastinum and to facilitate the removal of secretions, washings, and tissue for bacteriological and cytological studies. They are also designed to remove foreign bodies (Fig. 17-14).

Bronchoscope. The standard bronchoscope is a rigid speculum for observation of the tracheobronchial tree. A fiberoptic light carrier is inserted into the bronchoscope to provide illumination at the distal opening. A side channel has been incorporated into the bronchoscope to permit aeration of the other lung with oxygen or anesthetic gases (Fig. 17-15). An additional device, the Sanders Venturi System, is available to the anesthesiologist. This system provides adequate patient observation and ventilation during bronchoscopies or laryngoscopies. Fiberoptic telescopes provide visualization of the upper, middle, and lower lobe bronchi (Fig. 17-15).

Esophagoscope. One of several models of esophagoscopes—the Schindler, Holinger, Jesberg (Fig. 17-16), and Jackson—is used to examine the oropharynx and hypopharynx, esophagus, and proximal portion of the fundus of the stomach.

The Jesberg oval esophagoscope is a rigid tube with the light carrier channel built into the wall of the instrument (Fig. 17-16).

The fiberoptic esophagoscope permits visual observation and simultaneous photography of the selected parts of the esophagus, stomach, and duodenum with minimal patient discomfort (Fig. 17-17).

Mediastinoscope. The mediastinoscope is used to view lymph nodes or tumors in the superior mediastinum. The instrument is a hollow tube with a fiberoptic light carrier (Fig. 17-18).

A fiberoptic illuminator with a rheostat switch provides power and control of the illumination (Fig. 17-19).

Light carriers, cord, and illuminator. Each standard scope requires a fiberoptic light carrier, cord, and illuminator. Duplicates of each along with the appropriate light bulbs for the illuminator should be available for immediate use.

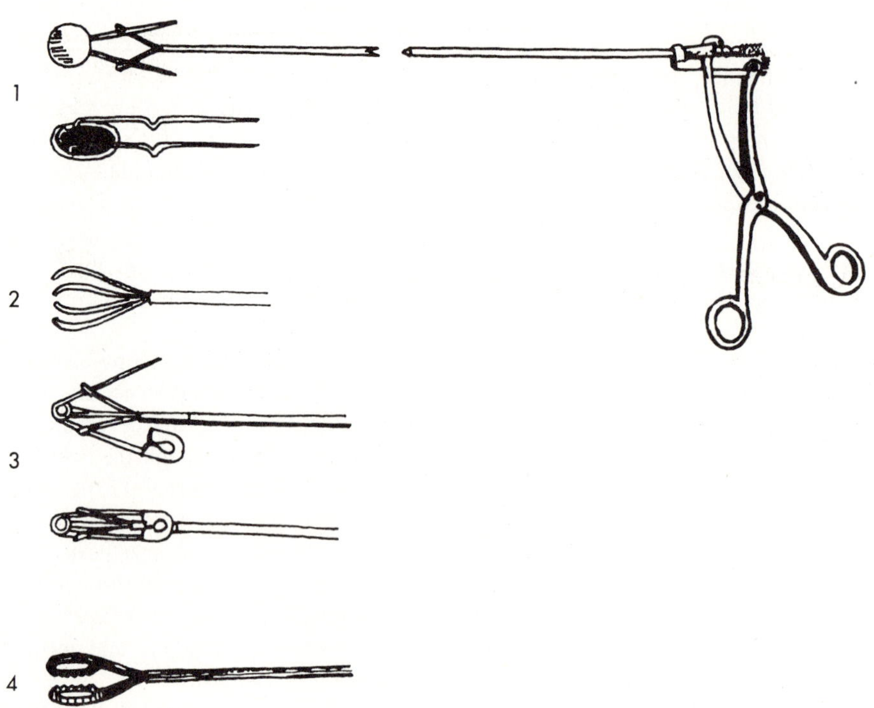

Fig. 17-14. Instruments used in foreign body removal. *1,* Jackson approximation forceps; *2,* Gordon bead forceps; *3,* Clerf-Arrowsmith safety pin closer; *4,* Jackson fenestrated meat-grasping forceps. (Courtesy Pilling Co., Fort Washington, Pa.)

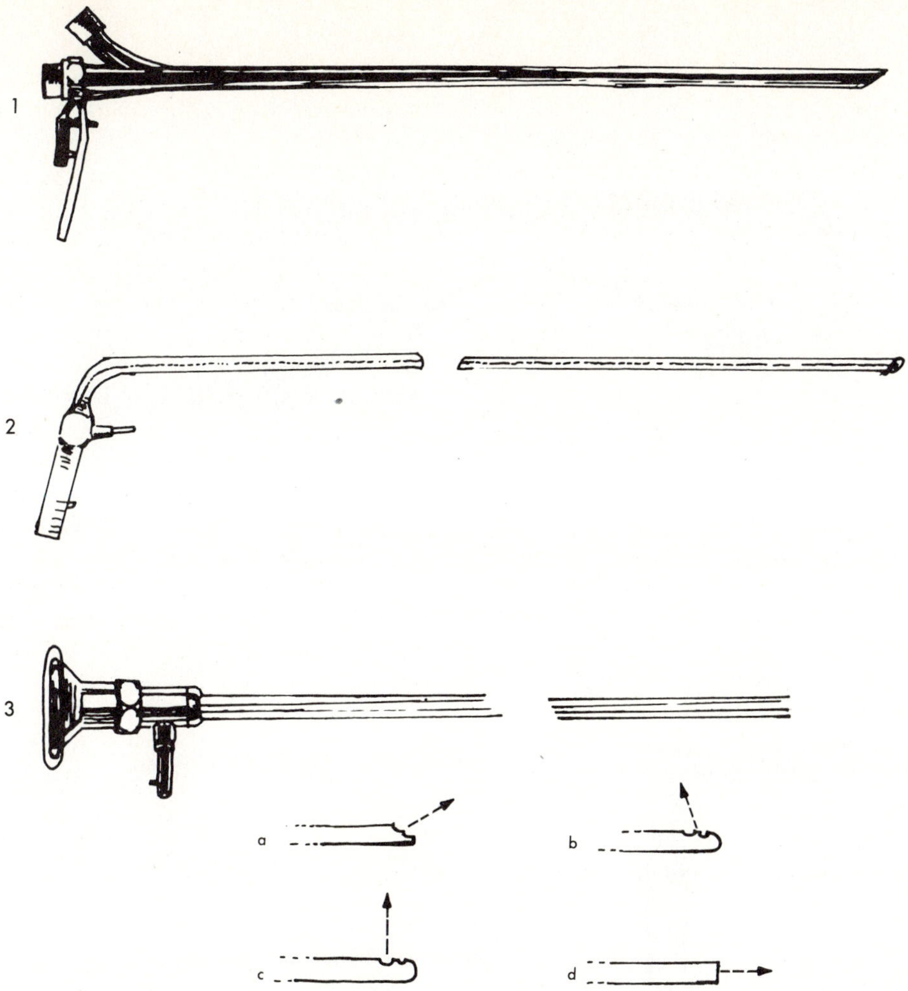

Fig. 17-15. Instruments for bronchoscopy. *1,* Holinger ventilating fiberoptic bronchoscope; *2,* fiberoptic light carrier; *3,* fiberoptic bronchoscopic telescopes: *a,* Foroblique; *b,* retrospective; *c,* right angle; *d,* forward. (Courtesy Pilling Co., Fort Washington, Pa.)

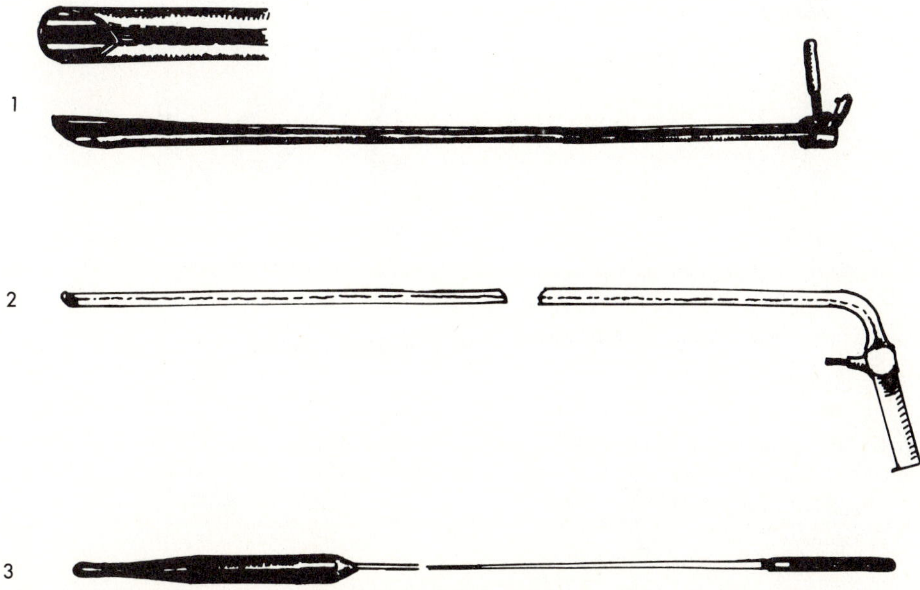

Fig. 17-16. Instruments for esophagoscopy. *1,* Jesberg oval esophagoscope; *2,* fiberoptic light carrier; *3,* Jackson esophageal bougie. (Courtesy Pilling Co., Fort Washington, Pa.)

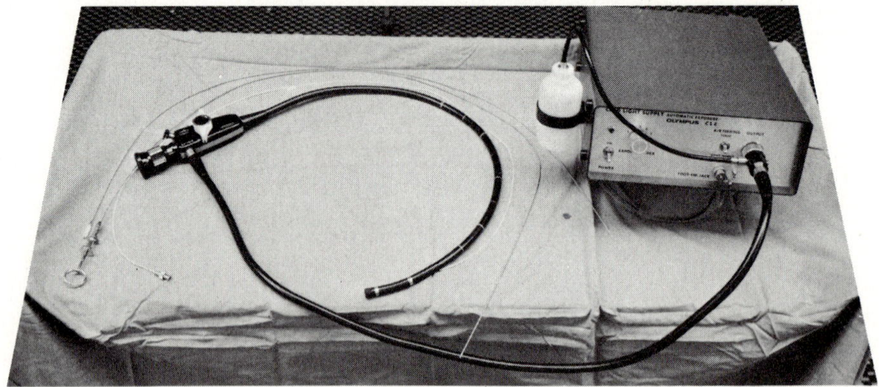

Fig. 17-17. Cold light source; fiberoptic esophagoscope. (Courtesy Olympus, New Hyde Park, N.Y.)

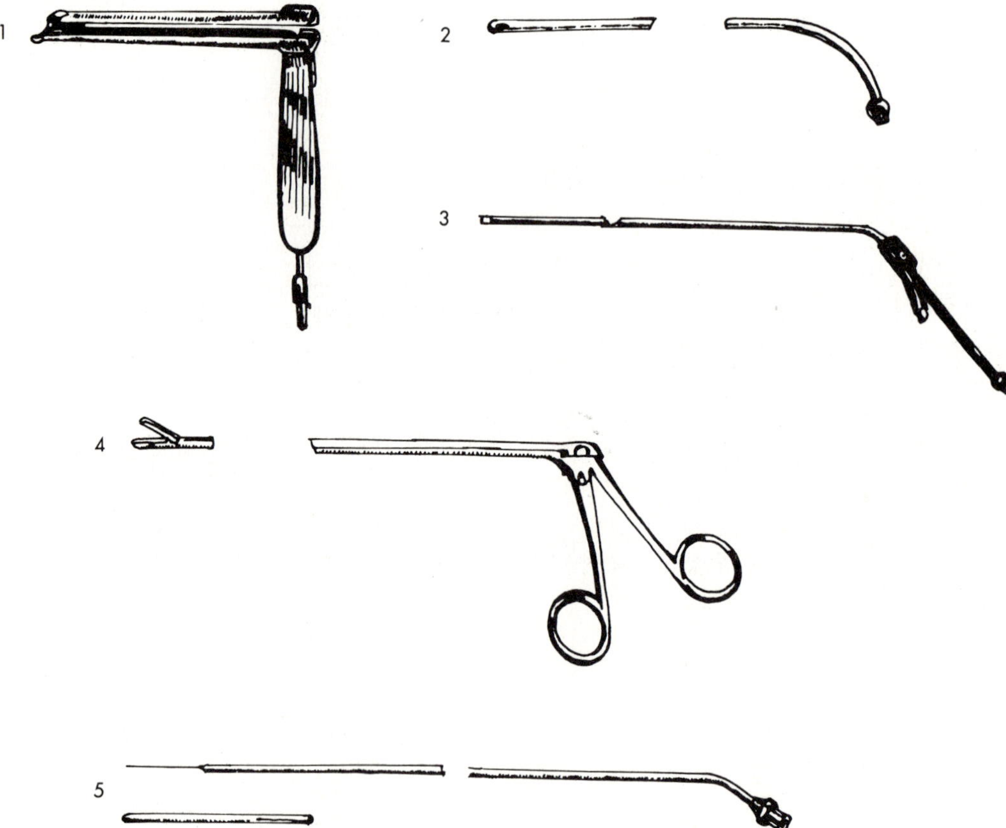

Fig. 17-18. Instruments for mediastinoscopy. *1,* Carlens mediastinoscope; *2,* Holinger aspirating tube; *3,* insulated suction tip; *4,* Jackson laryngeal forceps; *5,* aspirating needle. (Courtesy Pilling Co., Fort Washington, Pa.)

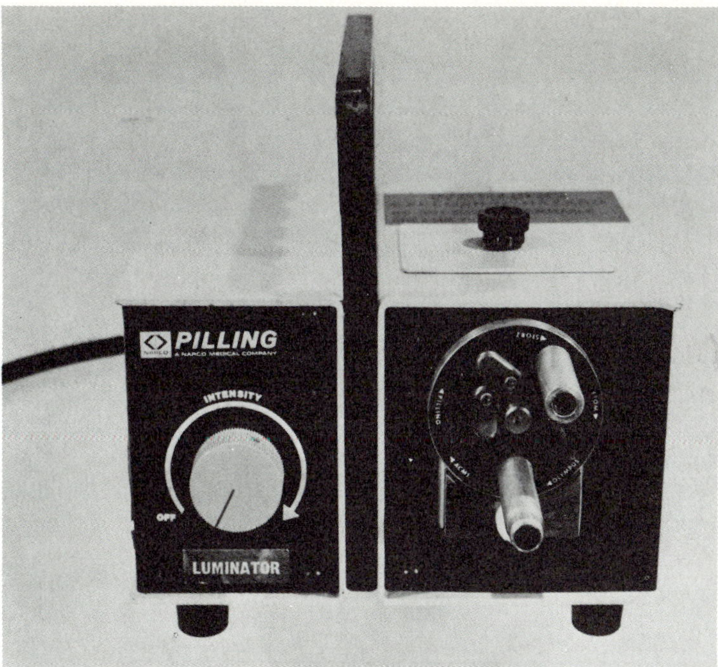

Fig. 17-19. Fiberoptic illuminator with multipurpose adaptor. (Courtesy Pilling Co., Fort Washington, Pa.)

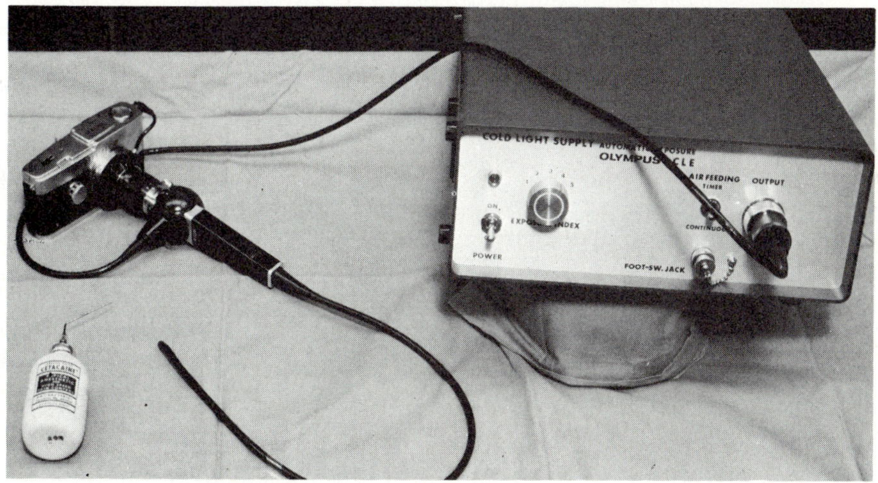

Fig. 17-20. Cold light source. (Courtesy Olympus, New Hyde Park, N.Y.)

The power supply unit (Figs. 17-19 and 17-20) should be tested periodically and also immediately before use.

Sponge carriers and sponges. The metal sponge carrier (Fig. 17-21) consists of two parts: an inner rod, which has two jaws protruding from its distal end, and an outer band, which is screwed down on the inner rod so that the sponge is held securely within the jaws. The small gauze sponges are used to keep the field dry, remove secretions, or apply a topical anesthetic agent.

Specimen collectors. Cytological specimen collectors, such as the Clerf (Fig. 17-21) or Lukens, are used to hold the secretions as they are obtained.

Aspirators. Aspirating tubes of different lengths and designs (Fig. 17-21) are used to remove secretions and collect material for microscopic examinations. The straight aspirating tube with one or two openings at the distal end is used to remove material from the pharynx, larynx, and esophagus. The curved aspirating tube with a flexible tip is used to remove secretions from the upper and dorsal orifices of the bronchi.

Forceps. Various types of forceps are designed to remove foreign bodies or tissues for histological study. In bronchoscopy, a biting tip forceps may be used to secure tissue for study. A forceps with jaws that veer laterally at about a 45-degree angle from the instrument's axis provides visualization during the biopsy maneuver. A bronchoesophageal forceps (Fig. 17-22) consists of a stylet, a cannula with a handle, a screw, a lock nut, and a set screw. Noncannulated forceps for laryngeal and bronchial regions are designed to remove tissue specimens.

Bougies. Flexible bougies of various sizes are used either as lumen finders or to dilate an esophageal stricture (Fig. 17-16). The bougie is passed through the esophagoscope.

Handling, terminal disinfection, and care

Handling of instruments. To ensure long life of the optical system of endoscopes, each instrument should be kept straight at all times when not in use. Flexible endoscopes should never be severely bent, except during introduction into or passage within the patient.

Only the instrument manufacturer should replace a part of the scope. When a telescopic scope is sent for repair, it must be properly packed in a padded instrument case and placed within a padded carton to ensure protection of the lens system during transportation. A direct blow can break the objective window or lenses of modern telescopic endoscopes. The junction of the flexible and rigid portions of the scope is the most vulnerable point.

During use, the patient might bite down while the flexible portion of the scope is being passed. The sheath covering the flexible part may become perforated after contact. When a new covering is needed, the instrument should be sent to the manufacturer.

Cleaning endoscopes. Rigid endoscopes can be cleaned in the ultrasonic cleaner or with soap and water. Terminal disinfection should be accomplished with activated glutaraldehyde or by steam sterilization. The man-

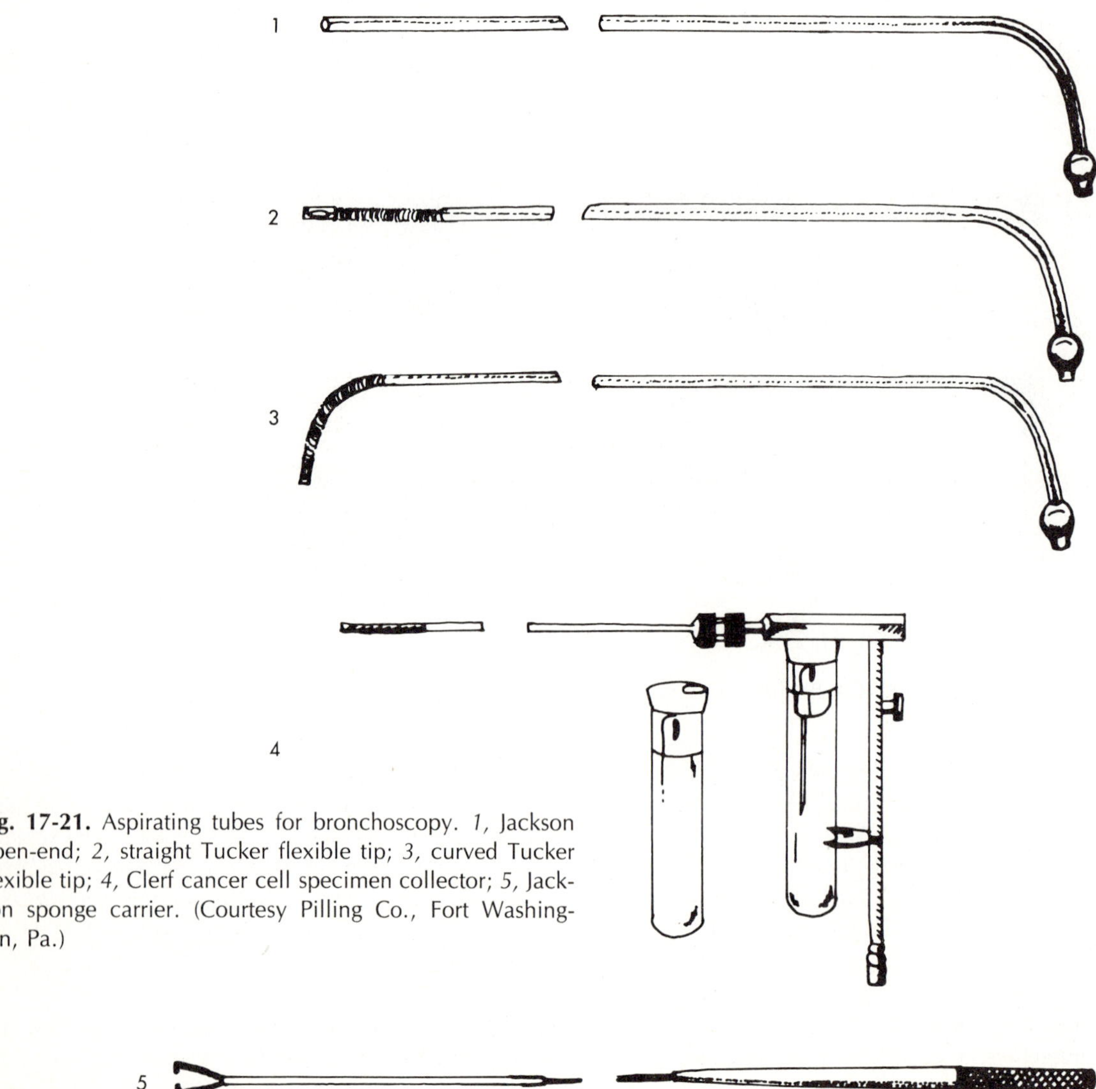

Fig. 17-21. Aspirating tubes for bronchoscopy. *1,* Jackson open-end; *2,* straight Tucker flexible tip; *3,* curved Tucker flexible tip; *4,* Clerf cancer cell specimen collector; *5,* Jackson sponge carrier. (Courtesy Pilling Co., Fort Washington, Pa.)

ufacturer's procedures for cleaning, terminally disinfecting, or terminally sterilizing flexible endoscopes should be followed. Usually, the fiberoptic scopes can be washed with soap and water, then soaked in activated glutaraldehyde or an iodophor concentrate germicide. If feasible, they should be gas sterilized.

Cleaning a telescopic endoscope. The scope is held vertically by its ocular end and is wiped repeatedly with downward strokes using gauze sponges or a soft brush saturated with surgical soap and water. Special attention is given to surface joints and crevices that may retain mucus. The scope is then dried thoroughly with clean gauze sponges.

Optical telescopes should never undergo boiling or steam sterilization. Sterilization could be accomplished in a noncorrosive bactericidal solution or with ethylene oxide.

Cleaning aspirating tubes and sponge carriers. These instruments are cleaned in an ultrasonic cleaner or with soap and water and are flushed and sterilized by means of saturated steam or gas. Special care must be given to spiral-tipped aspirators. All bent or broken-tipped aspirators should be sent to the manufacturer for repair.

The collar of sponge carriers must be unscrewed before it is cleansed. After sterilization, the threads of the carrier are oiled. The carrier is reassembled and stored lying straight on the shelf.

Cleaning forceps. The forceps may be placed in an ultrasonic cleaner. After cleaning, each forceps is taken apart, one at a time, by unscrewing the nut and removing the stylet. All parts are examined carefully, and noncorrosive solvent oil is applied to the crotch of the forceps. Each forceps is reassembled and its action tested; then it is stored in a cabinet with jaws open. In perfect forceps (1) the jaws are close together in parallel position; (2) the handles just touch when the jaws are closed; (3) the jaws go into the cannula when the forceps is closed and protrude widely without expanding the spring when it is open; (4) the end nut, located in the stylet, is in place; (5) the side screw is tight; and (6) the distal end and jaws' edges are smooth on finger examination.

Setting and testing the illumination. To test the fiberoptic light carrier and telescope, the instrument should be held vertically by its ocular end. The endoscope should always be tested immediately before its passage into the patient. The rheostat should be set at the proper voltage, as specified by the manufacturer. The light source should be switched on and off to test its function.

Standard (rigid) bronchoscopy

Definition. Direct visualization of the mucosa of the trachea, the main bronchi and their openings, and most of the segmental bronchi and removal of material for microscopic study if necessary.

Considerations. Bronchoscopy is an integral part of the examination of patients with pulmonary symptoms such as persistent cough or wheezing, hemoptysis, obstruction, or abnormal roentgenographic changes. Common causes of bleeding (hemoptysis) are bronchiectasis, carcinoma, and tuberculosis. Congenital anomalies and suspected presence of a foreign body, especially in infants and children, are responsible for emergency examinations of the respiratory tract.

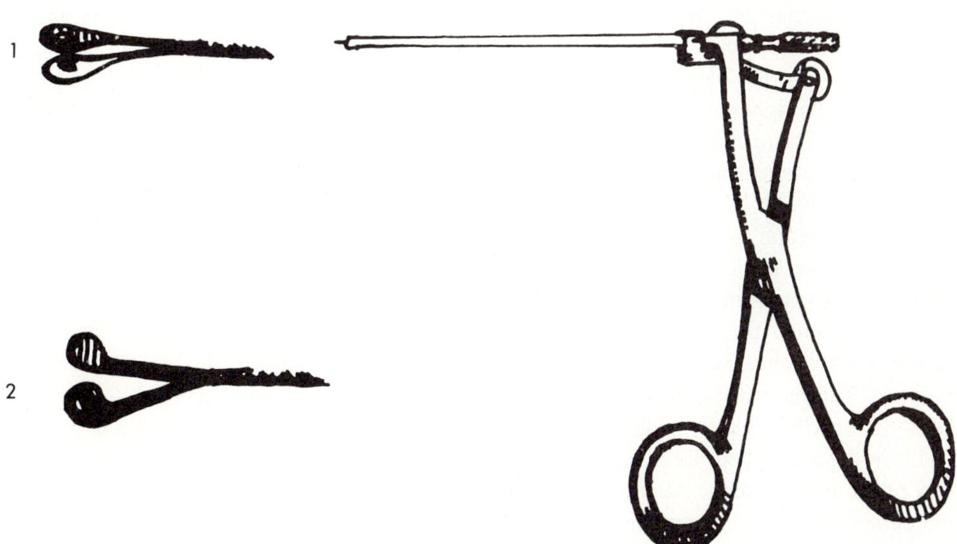

Fig. 17-22. Forceps for bronchoscopy. *1,* Jackson forward grasping forceps with serrated, cupped jaws; *2,* Jackson side-curved grasping forceps. (Courtesy Pilling Co., Fort Washington, Pa.)

Bronchoscopy is done to determine whether a lesion is present in the tracheobronchial passages, to identify and localize that lesion accurately, and to observe periodically the effects of therapy. In suspected carcinoma, the aspirated secretions obtained by bronchoscopy may contain malignant cells that were not observed microscopically in expectorated sputum.

Setup and preparation of the patient. As described previously, including the following:

1 Bronchoscope and telescopes, desired type, with power supply and cords (Fig. 17-15)
1 Suction tubing
2 Aspirating tubes (Fig. 17-21)
2 Specimen collectors (Fig. 17-21)
Sponge carriers (Fig. 17-21)
2 Forceps, desired types (Figs. 17-14 and 17-22)
1 Bronchial spray and cannula
1 Lubricating jelly tube
1 Topical anesthesia set, if desired
1 Emesis basin
6 Gauze sponges
1 Round basin with sterile saline solution

The bronchoscopist is exposed to a definite risk of contamination in the presence of communicable diseases. For this reason, the endoscopist and assistants should wear face masks. The endoscopist should also wear eyeglasses or an opaque disc, which is attached to a headband. Strict aseptic technique is used to prevent any possibility of cross-contamination from one patient to another.

Procedure

1. The patient is placed (Fig. 17-23) with the head positioned to the left by the head holder when the right bronchi are inspected and to the right when the left bronchi are inspected. The head may be lowered when the right middle lobe orifices are inspected.

2. The bronchoscope is inserted over the surface of the tongue, usually through the right corner of the mouth. The patient's lip is retracted from the upper teeth with the finger of the endoscopist's left hand. The epiglottis is identified and elevated with the tip of the bronchoscope.

3. The distal end of the scope is passed through the true vocal cords of the larynx; the upper tracheal rings are viewed. At this time, a small amount of anesthetic solution may be sprayed through the tube on the carina of the trachea and into the bronchus by means of a bronchial atomizer or spray. The patient's head is moved to the left to obtain a view of the right bronchi. A right-angle telescope, with its light adjusted previously, is inserted into the head of the bronchoscope. A few seconds are allowed for the optical system to become free of precipitated moisture.

4. The segmental bronchial orifices of the upper right lobe bronchi are viewed. The telescope is removed. Suction and aspirating tubes are used to provide a clear dry field of vision (Fig. 17-24).

5. The scope is advanced to inspect the middle lobe branches by means of insertion of an oblique 30-degree–angle telescope or right-angle telescope. The patient's head may be lowered so that the right middle lobe orifices can be viewed or the head turned to the right so that the left main bronchus can be viewed.

6. Aspiration of secretions for study is done, if necessary. Using suitable forceps, the surgeon may obtain a biopsy for histological diagnosis of a thoracic disorder. Foreign bodies are removed by means of forceps.

7. The bronchoscope is removed. The patient's face is cleansed. The patient is permitted to sit up on the table for a few minutes before being transported to the stretcher. An emesis basin and sponges must be available.

Flexible bronchoscopy

Flexible bronchoscopy may be performed in addition to a standard rigid bronchoscopy or as an independent procedure. If performed separately, the patient may remain on the transporting stretcher.

Setup and preparation of the patient. The setup for flexible bronchoscopy includes the following:

Fiberoptic light source
Fiberoptic bronchoscope
Flexible biopsy forceps
Flexible brush (optional); if used, slides and alcohol are necessary to collect specimen
Saline solution
Culture jar for biopsy specimen
Syringe for wash
Suction tubing with Luki tube attached to collect wash specimen
Lubricant for fiberoptic bronchoscope
Gauze sponges

Procedure. If the procedure is performed under a general anesthetic, a swivel adaptor is given to the anesthetist to connect to the endotracheal tube. After the patient is asleep and intubated, the anesthetist indicates that the procedure may begin.

1. The light source is turned on, and the lubricated fiberoptic bronchoscope is passed to the surgeon. The surgeon passes the bronchoscope through the adaptor into the endotracheal tube, which is held secure by the anesthetist.

2. If bronchial washings are desired as the bronchoscope is being passed, the assistant should be in position with a suction tip that has a Luki tube attached. When the surgeon indicates, the assistant should attach suction to the bronchoscope, being sure the tube is held securely between the little and index fingers. The tube should always be in an upright position; otherwise the specimen will be lost through the suction tubing.

3. A syringe with 50 ml of saline solution should be ready. The suction tube is disconnected, and about 5 ml of saline solution is injected into the channel. Suction is quickly reapplied. This may be done several times.

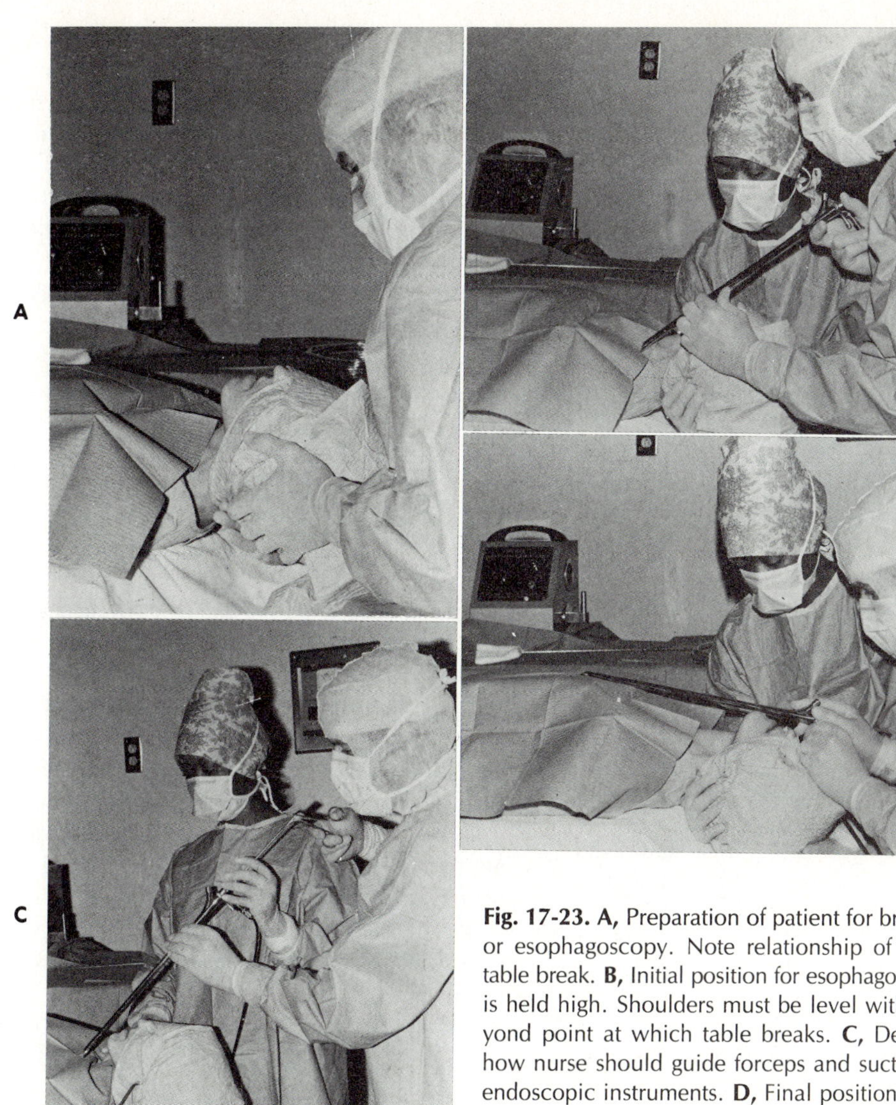

Fig. 17-23. A, Preparation of patient for bronchoscopy or esophagoscopy. Note relationship of shoulder to table break. **B,** Initial position for esophagoscopy. Head is held high. Shoulders must be level with or just beyond point at which table breaks. **C,** Demonstrating how nurse should guide forceps and suction tips into endoscopic instruments. **D,** Final position that will be assumed in esophagoscopy. Head holder raises or lowers head slowly on direction of endoscopist.

4. If a biopsy is taken, a flexible forceps is passed through the same channel. The assistant should be sure the forceps is closed at the tip before passing. To close, the finger is pulled; to open, the fingers are pushed forward.

After the procedure is finished, all washings, cultures, and specimens are put in proper containers and labeled.

Esophagoscopy

Definition. Direct visualization of the esophagus and the cardia of the stomach and removal of tissue or secretions for study.

Considerations. Esophagoscopy is done to aid in the diagnosis of esophageal cancer, diverticula, hiatus hernia, stricture, benign stenosis, or varices; to obtain additional information by means of a tissue biopsy; or to clarify the roentgenographic findings. Patients with suspected obstruction, symptoms of bleeding, or regurgitation may require endoscopy. To perform direct therapeutic manipulations, such as removal of a foreign body or insertion of an esophageal bougie, esophagoscopy is done.

Setup and preparation of the patient. As described previously (Fig. 17-23). The setup includes the following:

Esophagoscopes, desired type, size, and length (Figs. 17-16 and 17-17)
Suction tubing
Fiberoptic light source and cords
Bougies, if desired
Forceps, desired types and lengths
Aspirating tubes
Specimen containers
Lubricating jelly
Topical anesthesia set
6 Gauze sponges
1 Round basin with sterile saline solution

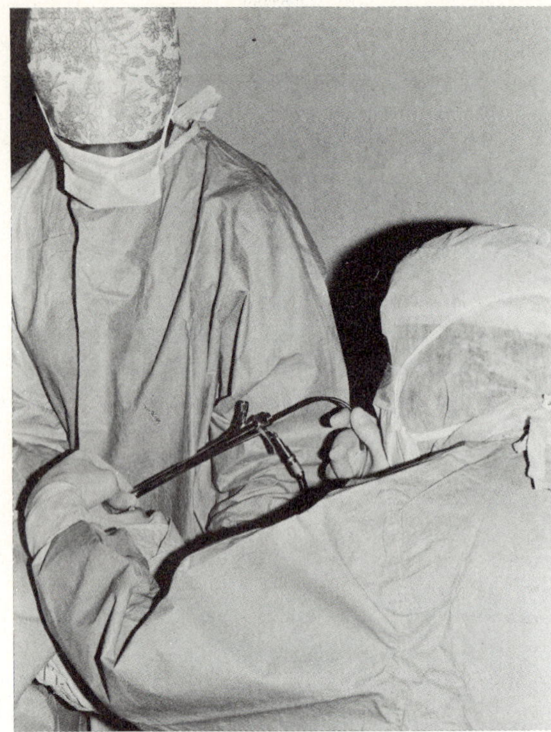

Fig. 17-24. Introduction of bronchoscope without laryngoscope. Fingers and thumb of endoscopist's left hand fix bronchoscope lightly against upper teeth, while right hand introduces metallic aspirating tube. Sometimes aspirating bronchoscope with integral aspirating canal is used.

Procedure

1. The indirect or direct technique may be followed. When the indirect method is used, the obturator within the scope is passed through the cricopharyngeal lumen and then removed. When the direct technique is used, the esophagoscope with the light carrier is thinly lubricated. With the patient in correct position, the suction is turned on. The scope is passed into the mouth. The tongue, epiglottis and laryngeal aditus, and cricopharyngeal lumen are identified. The head holder may tip the patient's head backward while extending the neck anteriorly. If the endoscope is passed to the side of the tongue, the patient's head is turned slightly to the opposite side.

2. When the scope has passed the inferior constrictors, the patient's head is moved so that all areas of the esophageal wall can be examined.

3. Specimens of secretions from the esophageal lumen may be obtained by aspirating tube and suctioning apparatus. In some cases, saline solution may be injected through the endoscope's aspirating channel, and the fluid withdrawn immediately for histological study. A biopsy of tissue may be taken using forceps with jaws at a 45-degree angle.

4. The esophagoscope is removed.

Mediastinoscopy

Definition. Direct visualization of lymph nodes or tumors at the tracheobronchial junction, under the carina of the trachea, or on the upper lobe bronchi and biopsy.

Considerations. Mediastinoscopy may precede an exploratory thoracotomy in known cases of lung carcinoma. Patients with positive findings may be treated with radiation or chemotherapy, as indicated.

Setup and preparation of the patient. As described previously, including the following:

Minor set of instruments
2 Mediastinoscopes, desired type with power supply and cords
1 Suction tubing
2 Aspirating tubes
1 Biopsy forceps
Electrocautery unit
Endocardiac needle, 20 gauge, 8 inches

The patient is placed under endotracheal anesthesia and positioned as for a tracheostomy.

Operative procedure

1. A short transverse incision is made above the suprasternal notch, and the pretracheal fascia is exposed.

2. By blunt dissection the plane beneath the pretracheal fascia is developed into the mediastinum.

3. The mediastinoscope is passed under direct vision into this fascial plane and is advanced along the anterior tracheal surface toward the mediastinum.

4. The surgeon manipulates the scope to visualize the tracheal bifurcation, bronchi, aortic arch, and associated lymph nodes.

5. Lymph nodal tissue to be biopsied is located, and a needle aspiration done to positively identify a nonvascular structure.

6. A biopsy forceps is inserted through the scope, and a tissue specimen excised. A bronchus sponge on a holder may be used to apply pressure to the excisional site. The mediastinum is again inspected.

7. The mediastinoscope is withdrawn.

8. The subcutaneous tissue is closed with chromic sutures on a taper needle; the skin is closed with silk sutures on a cutting needle. A small dressing is aplied.

PROCEDURES INVOLVING THE LUNG

Open lung biopsy

Definition. Resection of a small portion of the lung for diagnosis.

Considerations. Lung biopsy is usually performed through a small anterolateral thoracotomy incision without rib resection, unless it is performed secondarily in the course of a lobectomy or pneumonectomy.

Setup and preparation of the patient. The patient is placed in the supine position, with the anterior thorax slightly elevated as described. The complete thoracic setup is not required; usually only the following instruments are used:

1 Basic laparotomy setup
1 Nelson scissors (Fig. 17-11)
4 Duval lung-grasping forceps (Fig. 17-11)
1 Finochietto retractor, small (Fig. 17-13)

Operative procedure

1. A small, anterolateral thoracotomy is performed on the affected side.

2. A portion of the lung is secured with a lung clamp, and the biopsy is obtained.

3. A stapling device may be used to insert one or more rows of stainless steel staples proximal to the biopsy site, or the lung tissue is reapproximated with a continuous chromic suture.

4. A chest tube is placed in the pleural space during closure of the chest. It is usually connected to suction.

5. If the chest tube is left in place after the procedure, a closed drainage system is used. The tube is secured to the skin with sutures, and all connections of the drainage system are taped or otherwise secured.

6. Dressings are applied.

Segmental resection

Definition. Removal of individual bronchovascular segments of the pulmonary lobe, ligation of segmental branches of the pulmonary vein and artery, and division of the segmental bronchus.

Considerations. Segmental resection of the lung is performed to remove a chronic, localized, pyogenic lung abscess; to excise congenital cysts or blebs; to remove a benign tumor; or to save the undiseased portion of the lobe in pulmonary tuberculosis or bronchiectasis.

Setup and preparation of the patient. The basic thoracic setup is required.

The patient is placed on the operating table in a position that would facilitate the removal of the affected segment. A right or left lateral position, with the affected side uppermost, is the usual position.

Operative procedure

1. A posterolateral incision is made.

2. The parietal pleura is incised with a scalpel and long curved scissors, and adhesions are divided.

3. The bronchus of the diseased segment is identified, using Rumel or fine right-angled cystic duct forceps. The segmental pulmonary vein and segmental branches of the pulmonary artery are ligated.

4A. The bronchus is clamped with a Sarot bronchus clamp (Fig. 17-25), and the lung is inflated. The line of demarcation quickly confirms the proper placement of the clamp; the bronchus is divided with a scalpel or angled scissors.

4B. Alternatively, a thoracic stapling instrument may be used, as described in the lobectomy operative procedure, step 4B (Fig. 17-26).

5. The visceral pleura is completely incised around the diseased segment, beginning at the hilum and progressing toward the periphery. Narrow malleable retractors facilitate exposure. The intersegmental vessels are clamped with thoracic hemostats and are ligated.

6A. The segmental bronchus is transected with a knife or scissors, and the bronchus is closed with interrupted mattress sutures on swaged-on needles.

6B. The surgeon may follow step 4B of the lobectomy procedure. Contaminated items are discarded.

7. The parietal pleural flap may be placed over the bronchial stump.

8. The lung is reinflated; bleeding vessels are controlled. The operative field is prepared for closure, and the thoracic wall is examined for ragged bone edges.

9. For closed drainage, catheters are inserted in the pleural space through a stab wound and are secured to the skin with sutures.

10. The thoracotomy incision is closed, as described for lobectomy. Dressings are applied, and closed drainage is established.

Wedge resection

Definition. Excision of a small, wedge-shaped section from the peripheral portion of a lobe.

Considerations. A wedge resection is preferred in certain cases of peripherally located, benign primary tumors of the lung. No effort is made to isolate and ligate separately the pulmonary vessels or to secure the bronchi individually.

Setup and preparation of the patient. As described for segmental resection.

Operative procedure

1. A posterolateral or anterolateral thoracotomy is performed.

2. The ribs are protected by moist sponges, and a Finochietto rib retractor is placed.

3A. Hemostatic clamps are applied, and the lung is resected in a wedge fashion. The lung edges, held within the clamps, may be sutured continuously and checked for air leaks.

3B. If the thoracic stapling instrument is used, the lobe containing the lesion is grasped with a lung clamp, and the instrument is applied to the parenchymal portion of the lung, along the limits of the wedge that is being excised. The staples are released, and a scalpel is used to cut between the staples and the thoracic stapling instrument. The instrument is removed and reloaded. It is then reapplied to the other side of the lesion adjoining the already applied staples, and another line of staples is applied (Fig. 17-26).

4. The specimen is removed.

5. Hemostasis is maintained by ligatures and electrocautery.

6. The chest tube is inserted and connected to closed drainage.

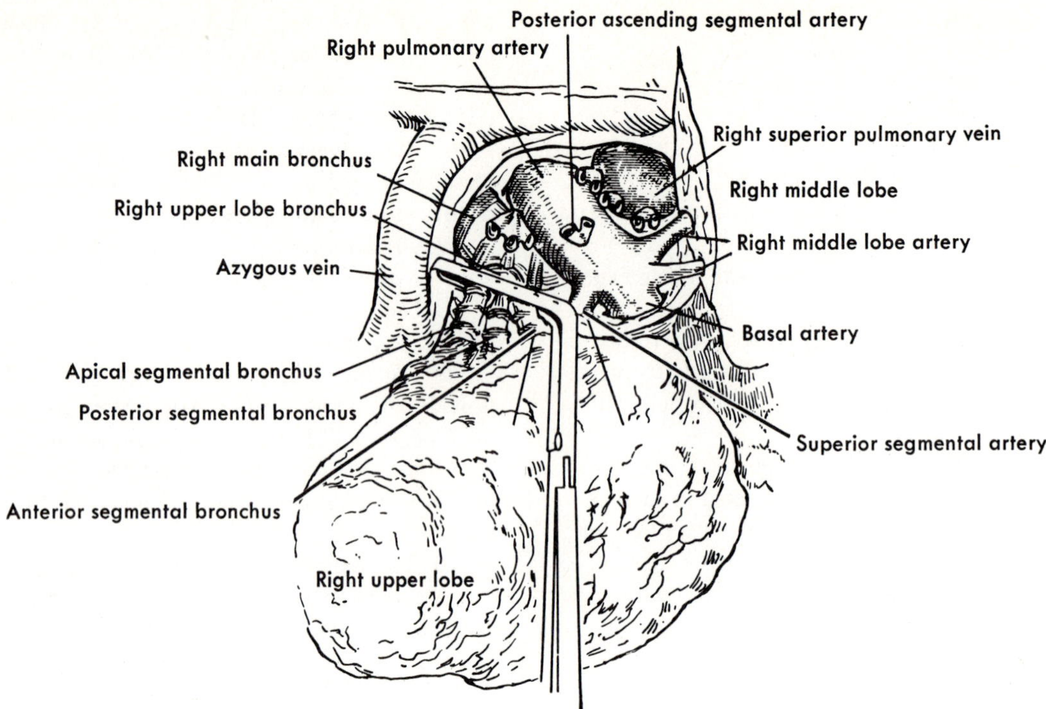

Fig. 17-25. Bronchus clamp applied to bronchus of right upper lobe. (From Reed, W.A., and Allbritten, F.F., Jr.: In Gibbon, J.H., Jr., editor: Surgery of the chest, Philadelphia, W.B. Saunders Co.)

7. The thoracotomy is closed, as described for lobectomy.

8. Dressings are applied. The chest tube is anchored to the chest wall with sutures, and the connections are secured.

Lobectomy

Definition. Excision of one or more lobes of lung.

Considerations. This operation is performed through a right or left posterolateral thoracotomy to treat a wide variety of pulmonary diseases.

Setup and preparation of the patient. Setup and preparation are as previously described for basic thoracic surgery. The lateral position is usually used for this procedure.

Operative procedure

1. A posterolateral thoracotomy is performed.

2. The pleura is entered, and adhesions are freed. Suction is used as exploration is carried out, and location of the pathological area is determined.

3. The visceral pleura is incised and dissected free from the hilum of the involved lobe. The branches of the pulmonary artery and vein of the involved lobe are isolated, clamped, ligated, and divided. Fine right-angled and vascular clamps are used.

4A. The bronchus is doubly clamped with selected bronchus clamps (Fig. 17-25), and the lung is inflated to identify the line of demarcation. Division of the bronchus is completed with a scalpel or heavy angled scissors. Bronchial secretions are aspirated. Closure of the bronchus is completed with mattress sutures of nonabsorbable material on swaged-on needles. Contaminated items are discarded.

4B. Alternatively, the thoracic stapler loaded with bronchus staples may be applied to the bronchus. The staple is released, and a scalpel is used to complete the division of the bronchus. The jaws of the stapling device are loosened after transection (Fig. 17-26).

5. Incomplete fissures are divided between hemostats with fine Metzenbaum scissors. Raw edges are closed with a continuous, intestinal type of suture of fine chromic gut.

6. The specimen is removed, and the bronchus suture line is covered with a pleural flap (Fig. 17-26).

7. The pleural cavity is irrigated thoroughly with normal saline, and the adequacy of hemostasis is checked. The remaining lobes are inflated to check for the presence of air leaks and to assess the degree of expansion of the remaining lobes.

8. A large pleural drainage catheter (28 to 30 Fr) is brought out through the eighth or ninth interspace, near the anterior axillary line. If indicated, an upper tube is also inserted to evacuate leaking air. Tubes are connected to a closed drainage system (Fig. 17-10).

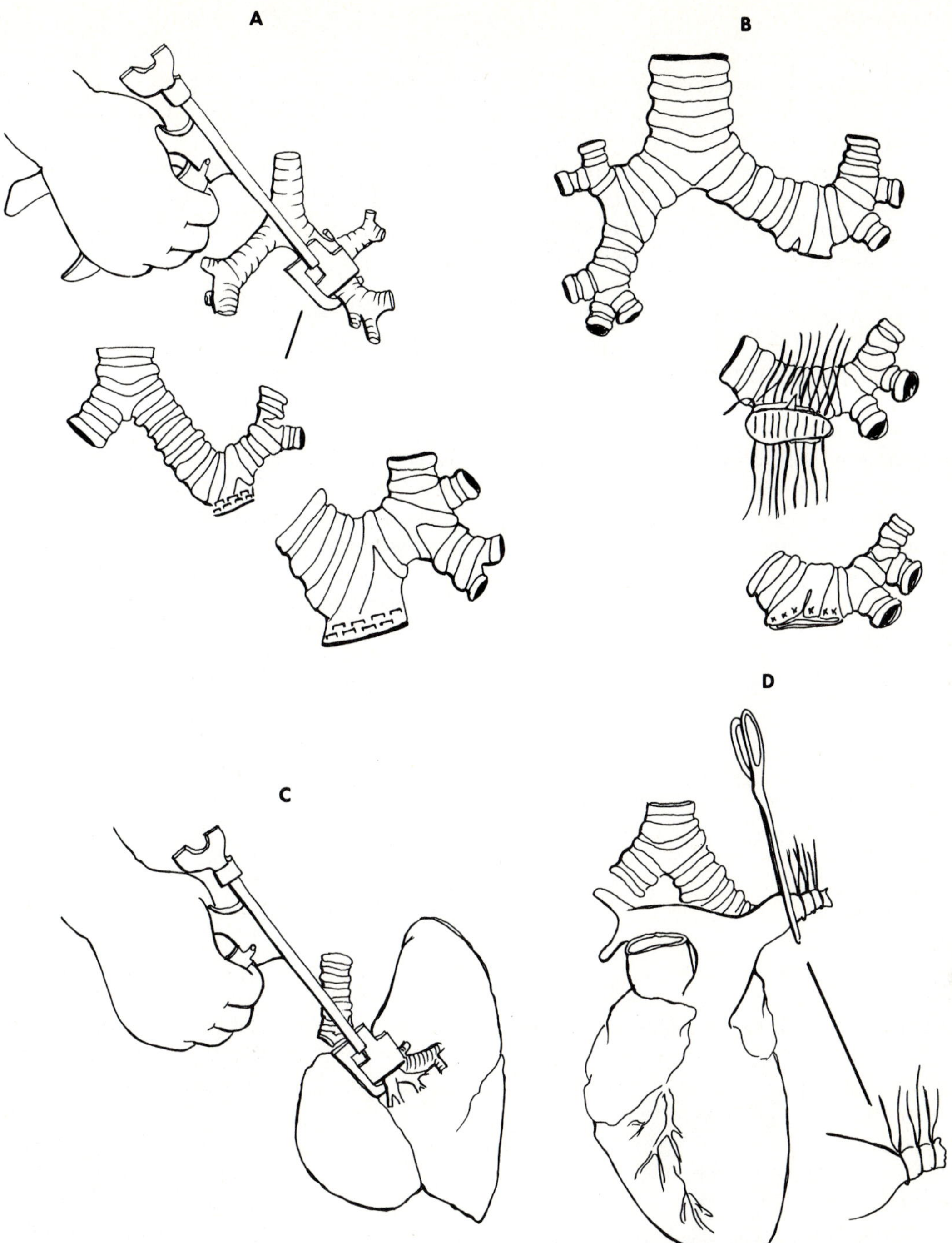

Fig. 17-26. A, Staple suturing of bronchus. **B,** Conventional suturing of bronchus. **C,** Staple suturing of pulmonary vessels. **D,** Conventional suturing of pulmonary vessels. (Redrawn from Dehnel, W.: Staple suturing vs. conventional suturing, AORN J. **18:**296, 1973.)

9. Interrupted, chromic gut sutures are used to reapproximate the ribs. A Bailey rib contractor (Fig. 17-13) is inserted, and sutures are tied in place. The periosteum may be closed with a continuous chromic gut suture.

10. The muscles, superficial fascia, and subcutaneous tissue are closed in layers with chromic gut sutures. Nonabsorbable, interrupted or continuous skin sutures or surgical staples may be used.

11. Dressings are applied. Drains are anchored to the chest wall with sutures, and connections are secured.

Pneumonectomy

Definition. Removal of the entire lung.

Considerations. Pneumonectomy is done to treat malignant neoplasms of the lung or an extensive unilateral bronchiectasis involving the greater part of one lung; to drain an extensive, chronic pulmonary abscess involving portions of one or more lobes; to remove selected benign tumors; or to treat extensive tuberculosis, main stem endobronchial tuberculosis, or any extensive unilateral lesion (Fig. 17-27).

Setup and preparation of the patient. The basic thoracic setup is used.

A posterolateral approach is used, and the patient is placed on the operating table in a lateral position.

Operative procedure

Opening of the chest cavity. The chest wall is opened, the pleura incised, and the hilum exposed, as described for lobectomy. The mediastinal pleura is opened.

Resection of the right lung

1. All lymph nodes and fat are dissected from the trachea, esophagus, and superior vena cava. The vagus nerve is divided.

2. The right main pulmonary artery and superior pulmonary vein are identified, doubly clamped, ligated, and divided (Fig. 17-27).

3. The inferior pulmonary ligament is identified and divided at its insertion in the diaphragm.

4. The right main bronchus is clamped and divided near the tracheal bifurcation; then the bronchial stump is sutured or stapled.

5. After bronchial closure, the lung is removed from the chest. The pleural space is flooded with normal saline to check for air leaks during positive pressure inspiration.

6. A pleural flap is created and sutured over the bronchial stump.

7. Hemostasis is secured in the pleural space.

8. The pleural space is closed, without drainage, according to the surgeon's preference. Dressings are applied.

Decortication of the lung

Definition. Removal of the fibrinous deposit or restrictive membrane on the visceral and parietal pleurae that interferes with pulmonary ventilatory function.

Considerations. Since one of the major objectives is to return the chest wall to as near normal function as possible, an intercostal incision is preferred; however, rib resection may be necessary to permit adequate exposure.

Setup and preparation of the patient. As described for lobectomy.

Operative procedure

1. The incision is carried through skin, superficial fascia, deep fascia, and muscles; wound edges are protected, as described for lobectomy.

2. One rib—usually the fifth or sixth—is resected, if necessary.

3. Ribs are protected by moist gauze, and a Finochietto rib retractor is placed. The rib retractor is opened slowly to achieve exposure.

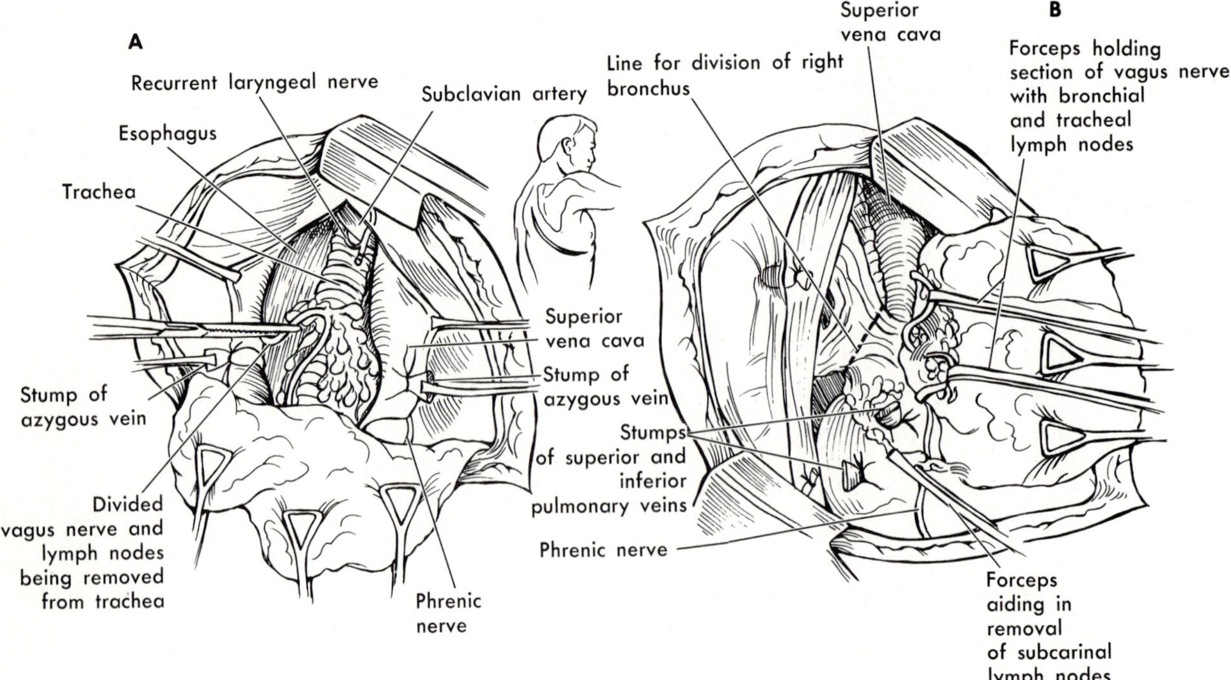

Fig. 17-27. Right radical pneumonectomy. **A,** Early-stage dissection. **B,** Late-stage dissection. (Adapted from Gibbon, J.H., Jr., Stokes, T.L., and McKeown, J.J., Jr.: The surgical treatment of carcinoma of the lungs, Am. J. Surg. **89:**484.)

4. The parietal adhesions to margins of the lung, mediastinal surface, and pericardium are divided, if necessary. Long curved thoracic scissors, forceps, hemostats, moist sponges on holders, and long ligatures are needed.

5. The fibrous membrane of the chest wall is incised and peeled away from visceral pleura, using blunt and sharp dissection. Gentle handling is imperative to prevent damage to the lung as thickened outside layers are removed.

6. During its liberation, the lung is expanded by positive pressure through the closed anesthesia system. The lung assumes its normal relation to the chest, and the negative pressure in the pleural cavity is stabilized by an airtight wound closure.

7. Bronchiolar openings are repaired, as necessary with sutures on taper point needles.

8. The drainage of serous material in the pleural space and the removal of air are accomplished by insertion of two chest catheters.

9. The wound is closed in layers as described for lobectomy. Drainage apparatus is connected, and dressings are applied.

Talc poudrage

Definition. Liberal application of sterile talcum powder to the visceral and parietal pleural surfaces to stimulate the growth of adhesions between the pleurae.

Considerations. The creation of pleural adhesions is indicated in the presence of recurrent idiopathic spontaneous pneumothorax or as a palliative measure in the presence of excessive pleural effusions related to inoperable malignancies.

Setup and preparation of the patient. The basic thoracic setup and talcum powder are required. The patient is usually placed in the lateral position, with the affected side uppermost.

Operative procedure. As described for open thoracotomy. Talc is sprinkled on the lung or spread on a wet sponge and then wiped on the lung surface.

Drainage of empyema

Before the existence of chemotherapeutic agents and antibiotics, acute empyema usually developed as a complication of lobar pneumonia, streptococcal infections, or tuberculosis. Anaerobic infections are presently found to be associated with the greatest mortality and morbidity of empyema. Infection is usually associated with a lung abscess and pneumonia.

In *chronic empyema,* the pleural membranes become thick and rigid as a result of a prolonged intrapleural infection. The chest wall becomes rigid and smaller, thus distorting the lungs. The fibrous pleural pocket may extend over a part of all of the lung and chest wall. Chronic empyema creates additional complications such as mediastinal shift, difficulties in swallowing, deformity of the chest, and respiratory limitations.

Closed thoracostomy (intercostal drainage)

Definition. Insertion of a catheter through an intercostal space and establishment of closed drainage.

Considerations. Closed thoracostomy is done to provide continuous aspiration of an infectious fluid from the pleural cavity and to prevent an ingress of air at a time when the lung may collapse. This procedure is used when an open thoracostomy might result in the collapse of a lung.

Setup and preparation of the patient. Instrumentation includes the basic general surgery instruments, plus the following:

- 1 Local anesthesia set, including syringes, needles, and anesthetic
- 2 Patterson or Davidson trocars and cannulas to fit catheters or disposable catheters with trocars
- 1 Luer-Lok syringe, 30 ml
- 2 Aspirating needles, 16 gauge, 3½ inches
- 2 Culture tubes
- 1 Water-seal drainage set (Fig. 17-10)

The patient is placed in a lateral or sitting position (Chapter 6).

During the operation, air is prevented from entering the cavity by having the catheter fit snugly, by clamping the catheter as it is inserted into the cavity, and then by attaching the catheter to the drainage set.

Operative procedure

1. The prepared operative site is anesthetized. An aspirating needle, attached to a syringe, is introduced into the chest cavity to verify the presence of pus.

2. The trocar and cannula are introduced through the puncture wound, into the intercostal space, and then into the pleural cavity.

3. A catheter of the desired size, which has been marked for its correct length, is introduced into the cavity immediately after withdrawal of the trocar obturator. The free end of the catheter is clamped to prevent the ingress of air.

4. When the cannula is withdrawn and a second clamp is placed between the end of the cannula and the patient, the terminal clamp is removed, so that the cannula can be slipped off the distal end of the catheter.

5. The skin edges are sutured, and the free ends of the suture are tied around the catheter to prevent its accidental withdrawal.

6. A dressing is then applied to the wound.

7. For continuous drainage without the entrance of air into the pleural cavity, the free end of the catheter is attached to a water-seal system, with or without suction (Fig. 17-10).

Open thoracostomy (partial rib resection)

Definition. Partial resection of a selected rib or ribs to treat empyemic lesions by the establishment of continuous drainage, with eventual healing and reexpansion of the lung.

Setup and preparation of the patient. The basic thoracic setup is required.

The patient is usually placed in the lateral position, with the affected side uppermost, although the sitting position may be used. Local anesthesia may be used.

Operative procedure

1. A posterolateral thoracotomy incision is made.
2. The pleura is incised. Suction is available. Cultures are obtained, and the cavity is evacuated.
3. A large drainage tube is inserted through the pleural opening, and the margins of the wound are fitted snugly to prevent leakage at this point.
4. A suture of heavy material on a cutting needle is passed through both sides of the incision and tied around the tube.
5. Tubes are clamped until connected with drainage bottles, and connections are secured.
6. The intercostal muscles, fascia, and skin are approximated in layers, using chromic gut interrupted sutures for muscle and fascia and nonabsorbable sutures or staples for skin closure.
7. Dressings are applied over the wound.

Posterolateral thoracoplasty

Definition. Resection of several ribs.

Considerations. Thoracoplasty is done to induce a permanent collapse of the underlying lung. This operation is selected for patients with a productive, unilateral fibrocavernous type of pulmonary tuberculosis, when therapeutic pneumothorax, phrenic nerve paralysis, and drug therapy have failed to control the disease.

An extrapleural thoracoplasty is performed in one or two stages. The initial stage includes the complete resection of the first through the fifth ribs; the second stage may include the resection of portions of the next four to five ribs.

Setup and preparation of the patient. Instrumentation includes the basic thoracic setup, minus drainage tubes and lung-resection instruments. The lateral position is used for a posterolateral approach.

Anterior thoracoplasty

Definition. Excision of the ribs and their costal cartilages, which prevents collapse of the remaining residual cavities following extensive posterolateral thoracoplasty.

Setup and preparation of the patient. As described for thoracoplasty. The patient is placed on the operating table in a supine position, with the affected side slightly elevated. The arm is positioned to permit access to the lateral edge of the incision. Skin preparation and draping are completed.

Repair of penetrating thoracic wounds with hemothorax

Definition. Control of hemorrhage and establishment of drainage of pleural cavity.

Considerations. Hemothorax may be produced by an injury to the intercostal vessels, the vessels within the lung, or the major vessels in the mediastinum. When blood accumulates in the thoracic cavity, the increased pressure displaces the lung and the mediastinum and may cause circulatory and respiratory problems.

Setup and preparation of the patient. For hemorrhage of major vessels of the lung, a thoracotomy setup is required.

Operative procedure

1. Aspiration (thoracocentesis), which is the procedure of choice, is performed.
2. Progressive hemorrhage is stopped (thoracotomy).
3. A compressed and constricted lung is expanded (decortication).

With fracture of numerous ribs, injury to the chest wall may be so severe that the integrity of the chest wall is destroyed. Segments may reveal paradoxical respiration and require stabilization.

Operative fixation of multiple fractures is neither feasible nor necessary. Tracheostomy is beneficial because it removes tracheal secretions and provides a mode of positive pressure ventilation. It is the single best mode of effective therapy for a flail chest.

OPERATIONS ON THE MEDIASTINUM

Excision of tumors in the upper anterior mediastinum

Definition. Excision of the cysts most frequently found in the mediastinum: the "clear water," the dermoid, and the bronchogenic cysts. The solid tumors of the mediastinum may be benign or malignant.

Setup and preparation of the patient. The basic thoracic setup, the sternal cutting instruments, and the thyroid instruments are used.

The patient is prepared on the operating table, as described for thyroidectomy (Chapter 12) or for median sternotomy (Fig. 17-9).

Operative procedure

1. Median sternotomy is carried out, as previously described.
2. The tumor is dissected free.
3. Bleeding is controlled with ligatures and electrocautery.
4. Chest catheter may or may not be inserted, depending on the entry into the pleural space and the surgeon's preference.
5. The sternum is reapproximated and closed with heavy wire.
6. The subcutaneous tissue is closed with chromic gut suture, and the skin with interrupted, nonabsorbable sutures or surgical staples.
7. If a chest catheter is used, it is anchored to the chest wall with sutures, and connections are secured.
8. Dressings are applied.

Thymectomy

Definition. Removal of the thymus gland.

Considerations. An attempt to alleviate the severity of symptoms in a patient with myasthenia gravis is a frequent indication for the removal of the thymus gland.

Setup and preparation of the patient. Basic thoracic setup and sternum-cutting instruments are used.

Operative procedure. Median sternotomy gives the best exposure for excision of the thymus gland. Dissection of the gland is carried out, and blood vessels are clamped and ligated. If either pleural space has been inadvertently opened during dissection, the anesthetist maintains full expansion of the lung during the closure of the incision with chromic gut to prevent any subsequent respiratory embarrassment. Closure is effected as in the procedure for excision of anterior mediastinal tumors.

Operations on the posterior mediastinum

Definition. Removal of segments of rib or ribs, removal of a tumor, drainage of an abscess, or exposure of the esophagus through an incision made in the mediastinum.

Setup and preparation of the patient. The major thoracic setup is required.

A posterolateral incision with the patient in a lateral position is used.

Operative procedure

1. The thoracic wall is opened as for posterolateral thoracoplasty. The pleura is freed from the posterior mediastinum, and retractors are placed.

2. The great blood vessels and intercostal arteries are identified and isolated. Bleeding vessels are ligated.

3. If the pleura is opened inadvertently, it is closed before the abscess is drained. The abscess, if present, is aspirated and drained. If a tumor is present, it is resected, and bleeding is controlled.

4. The intercostal muscles, rib periosteum, overlying muscles, fascia, and skin are closed in layers, as for thoracoplasty.

5. Dressings are applied.

Funnel chest operation (correction of pectus excavatum)

Definition. Correction of a structural deformity of the anterior thoracic wall: depression of the sternum and costal cartilages.

Considerations. Many theories have been proposed regarding the cause of funnel chest—fetal position in utero, upper respiratory tract obstruction, inherited tendency, or obstruction in breathing that necessitates an increased amount of pull by the diaphragm, thereby increasing the negative pressure. The deformity is characterized by a posterior depression of the sternum, which has its deepest depression at the junction of the xiphoid process with the gladiolus. The sternal ends become elongated and depressed in a posterior direction, forming a narrow inverted cone- or funnel-shaped configuration. This causes a mild compression of the thoracic viscera. The lower end of the sternum may push the mediastinum back against the anterior surface of the vertebral bodies, thus occasionally causing cardiac symptoms.

The funnel chest operation is performed for cosmesis and to establish normal circulatory function with exercise, by eliminating the abnormal inward inclination of the sternum and by straightening the attachments of the cartilages to the sides of the sternum. An anterior midline incision may be made through the level of the second rib to a point halfway between the xiphoid process and umbilicus (Fig. 17-9), or a bilateral inframammary incision may be preferred.

Setup and preparation of the patient. The patient is placed on the operating table in a supine position, the upper half of the chest slightly elevated with a rolled sheet (Chapter 6). Instrumentation is as described for the basic thoracic setup and median sternotomy, omitting lung resection instruments and long hemostatic clamps and adding the following:

Periosteal elevator
Gigli saw set (optional)
Circular blade for Stryker saw
Osteotomes
Bone hooks
Bone-holding forceps
Stainless steel wire sutures or heavy suture material

Since the procedure is frequently performed on children, smaller instruments may be required.

Operative procedure

1. The selected incision is carried through the skin to the fascia. Bleeding points are controlled with electrocautery and silk ligatures. The wound edges are protected with towels; moist packs and retractors are placed.

2. The fascial insertions of the greater pectoral muscles into the sternum are cut and retracted. Dissecting scissors, Pean hemostats, and suture ligatures are used. Rib cartilages are freed from the sternum with an elevator and knife.

3. A transverse incision is made, separating the xiphoid process from the sternum and dividing the substernal ligament and extension of abdominal muscles. A knife, periosteal elevator, sternal knife (Gigli saw or chisel may be preferred), and heavy scissors are used.

4. The xiphoid process is grasped with bone forceps as the anterior mediastinum is entered. With sharp and blunt dissection, the pericardium is freed from the sternum.

5. The posterior cartilages are cut with heavy scissors to free the depressed bone. (This allows the pleura and pericardium to drop back posteriorly and the heart to shift to a normal position.)

6. A wedge-shaped, transverse osteotomy is made with

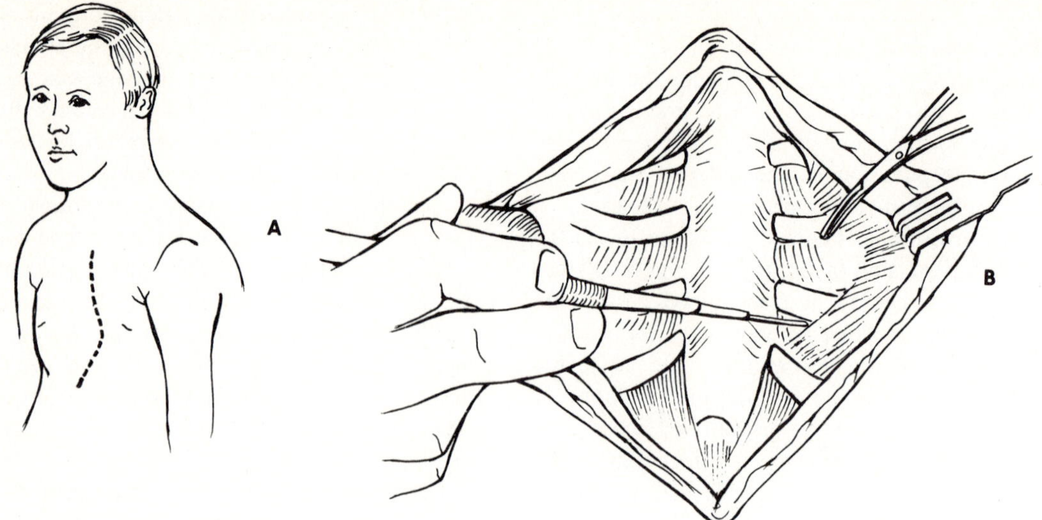

Fig. 17-28. Operation for correction of funnel chest (pectus excavatum). **A,** Deformity and line of incision. **B,** Sternum has been divided.

a knife in the outer table of the sternum at a point where the deformity begins (Fig. 17-28).

7. The sternum is trimmed by rongeur and shears; cartilages are shortened or resected so that the new surfaces fit flat against each other. The depressed sternum is bent forward, so that it may assume a normal position.

8. The sternum is maintained in the corrected position by mattress sutures that are placed across the osteotomy. (The special sternal osteotomy sutures with swaged-on needles are well suited for this purpose.) The pectoral muscles are sutured back to the sternum, the intercostal muscles are sutured to the undersurface of the sternum, and the xiphoid process is left free.

9. The wound is closed with interrupted silk or synthetic sutures after pleural drainage has been established.

10. Dressings are applied.

SUGGESTED READINGS

Anthony, C.P., and Thibodeau, G.A.: Textbook of anatomy and physiology, ed. 10, St. Louis, 1979, The C.V. Mosby Co.

Birch, A.A., and Tolmie, J.D.: Anesthesia for the uninterested, Baltimore, 1976, University Park Press.

Bricker, P.L.: Chest tubes: the crucial points you mustn't forget, RN **43:**21, Nov. 1980.

Cameron, M.: What patients need most before and after thoracotomy, Nursing '78 **8**(5):28, 1978.

DeWeese, D.D., and Saunders, W.H.: Textbook of otolaryngology, ed. 6, St. Louis, 1982, The C.V. Mosby Co.

Edwards, E.A., Malone, P.D., and Collins, J.J.: Operative anatomy of the thorax, Philadelphia, 1972, Lea & Febiger.

Effler, D.B., editor: Blade's surgical diseases of the chest, St. Louis, 1978, The C.V. Mosby Co.

Erickson, R.: Chest tubes: they're really not that complicated, Nursing '81 **11**(5):34, 1981.

Glenn, W.W.L., Liebow, A.A., and Lindskog, G.E.: Thoracic and cardiovascular surgery with related pathology, New York, 1976, Appleton-Century-Crofts.

Hinshaw, H.C., and Murray, J.F.: Diseases of the chest, Philadelphia, 1980, W.B. Saunders Co.

Mattox, K.L.: Management of penetrating chest trauma, Hosp. Med. **13:**8, June 1977.

Palmer, E.D., and Boyce, H.W.: Techniques of clinical gastroenterology, Springfield, 1975, Charles C Thomas, Publisher.

Pinet, F., and others: Selective bronchography and bronchial brushing, New York, 1979, Springer-Verlag New York, Inc.

Ravitch, M.: Congenital deformities of the chest wall and their operative correction, Philadelphia, 1977, W.B. Saunders Co.

Saum, M.: Taking the mystery out of chest tubes, AORN J. **32:**86, 1980.

Schottelius, B.A., and Schottelius, D.D.: Textbook of physiology, ed. 18, St. Louis, 1978, The C.V. Mosby Co.

Schwartz, S., editor: Principles of surgery, New York, 1979, McGraw-Hill Book Co.

Zollinger, R.M., and Zollinger, R.M., Jr.: Atlas of surgical operations, New York, 1975, Macmillan Publishing Co.

18 Cardiac surgery

Continued refinements in diagnostic techniques, advances in anesthesia and monitoring methods, and improved cardiopulmonary bypass techniques give surgeons increasing opportunities to perform a greater variety of cardiac procedures. For example, in pediatric cardiac surgery, many defects now can be corrected at the first operation rather than treated in a palliative manner.

Many factors are involved in the selection of the procedure, including the experience and skill of the surgical team, patterns of nursing care, and availability of ancillary facilities and equipment. The decision as to the need for surgery and the type of procedure to be performed is primarily made by correlating the patient's history, cardiac catheterization, and other diagnostic data.

ANATOMY AND PHYSIOLOGY

The standard textbooks of anatomy and physiology should be consulted for detailed description and function of the circulatory structures. Certain facts are presented here as they relate to surgical procedures and operating room nursing.

The heart, a hollow muscular organ that acts as a power pump for the circulatory system, is enclosed in the pericardial sac forming the middle subdivision of the lower part of the mediastinum (Fig. 18-1). The heart lies in the region between the lungs, anterior to the esophagus and the descending portion of the aorta. The large blood vessels enter and leave the heart at its base. Two thirds of the heart lies to the left of the midline, and the remaining third to the right. The right chambers of the heart are in an anterior position.

The heart wall is composed of three layers: the *epicardium,* the outer lining; the *myocardium,* or muscular layer, which is the important functional layer; and the *endocardium,* the inner lining.

The heart is divided into right and left halves. Each half contains an upper and a lower communicating chamber. The upper chambers are called the *atria,* and the lower chambers the *ventricles.* The atria receive blood from the systemic and pulmonary veins. The right atrium has three orifices through which blood enters from the superior and inferior venae cavae and from the coronary sinus. The left atrium has four orifices through which the blood enters from the four pulmonary veins, two from each lung. The ventricles discharge the blood into the arteries. The left ventricle sends the blood through the aorta and its numerous branches to the head, upper extremities, abdominal organs, and lower extremities. This system is termed the *systemic* or greater circulatory system. The right ventricle discharges the venous blood into the lungs by means of the main pulmonary artery, which divides into right and left pulmonary arteries. These subdivide into arterioles and eventually form the capillaries in the lungs. This system is called the lesser or *pulmonary* circulatory system (Fig. 18-2). In both the systemic and pulmonary systems, metabolic exchange occurs only in *capillary beds.* Oxygen is given off into the tissues, and carbon dioxide is taken in by the red blood cells. The capillaries empty into the veins, which bring the blood back to the right atrium.

The membranous valves of the heart open and close with the cyclic fluctuations in the blood pressure that occur during systole and diastole. The valves allow blood to flow in one direction only. The heart chambers have four valves: two atrioventricular valves and two semilunar valves. The two atrioventricular valves are located between the atrium and ventricle of each side of the heart. The right atrioventricular valve, commonly called the *tricuspid valve,* is composed of three leaflets of endocardium, while the left atrioventricular valve, known as the *mitral valve,* has only two leaflets. Fine chordae tendinae (Fig. 18-2) prevent the valves from being turned back into the atria during ventricular contraction. The semilunar valves are located at the outlets of the left and right ventricles. These valves are known as the *aortic* and *pulmonic* valves, respectively.

The pumping cycle of the heart has two phases, *systole* and *diastole.* During systole the ventricles contract; the atrioventricular valves close, preventing reflux of blood into the atria; and the semilunar valves are forced open, allowing the blood to flow into the aorta and the pulmonary artery.

During diastole, the ventricles relax and the atria contract, pumping blood through the atrioventricular valves into the ventricles.

When disease deforms the valves, the leaflets become fibrous and stiff, and their margins uneven and adherent to one another. Such abnormalities impair their mechanical functions and compound the work load of the heart. When a valve loses its ability to close tightly, that is,

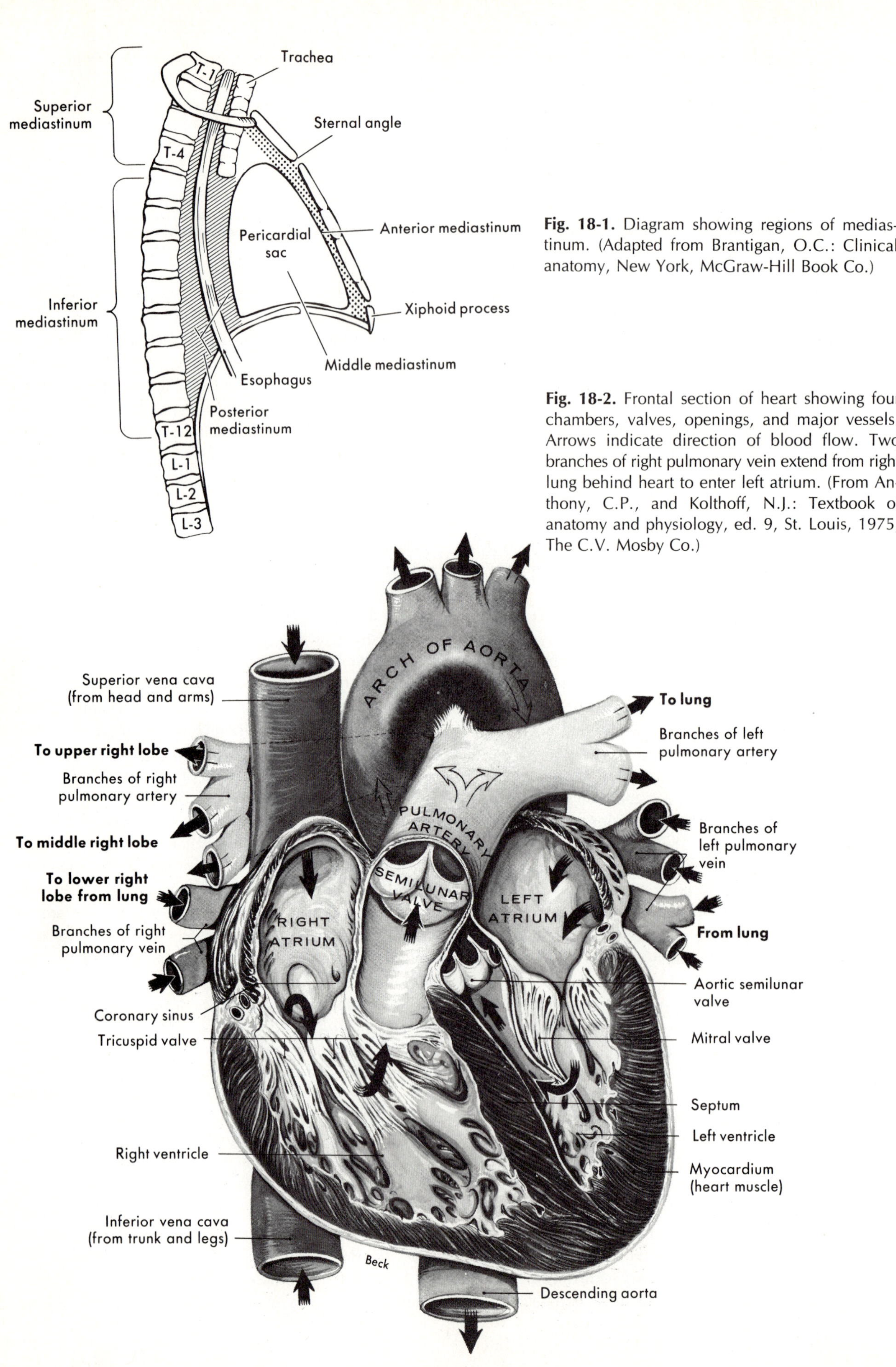

Fig. 18-1. Diagram showing regions of mediastinum. (Adapted from Brantigan, O.C.: Clinical anatomy, New York, McGraw-Hill Book Co.)

Fig. 18-2. Frontal section of heart showing four chambers, valves, openings, and major vessels. Arrows indicate direction of blood flow. Two branches of right pulmonary vein extend from right lung behind heart to enter left atrium. (From Anthony, C.P., and Kolthoff, N.J.: Textbook of anatomy and physiology, ed. 9, St. Louis, 1975, The C.V. Mosby Co.)

when there is a valvular insufficiency, the blood flows back through the diseased valve into its originating chamber. This condition is known as *regurgitation*. In rheumatic heart disease, the mitral valve frequently becomes narrowed, obstructing the passage of blood from the atrium to the left ventricle and causing enlargement of the left atrium. This condition is called *mitral stenosis*. The aortic valve can also be affected. The pulmonic valve is more often affected by *congenital stenosis*.

The myocardium of the heart receives its blood supply from two branches arising from the aorta, the left and right coronary arteries (Fig. 18-3). Their function is to carry blood to the cardiac muscle cells. Acute obstruction of the blood supply results in myocardial ischemia and may cause a loss of myocardial contractility.

The middle cervical nerve, composed of sympathetic fibers, and the vagus nerve, composed of parasympathetic fibers, carry nerve impulses to the heart from the medulla oblongata (Chapter 24). The sympathetic nerves promote an increase in the force and rate of the heartbeat, and the parasympathetic fibers cause a decrease in the rate.

Certain areas of the heart muscle tissue are modified to form a conducting system. This system comprises the *sinoatrial (SA) node,* which is located at the junction of the superior vena cava and the right atrium, and the *atrioventricular (AV) node* with extending fibers (bundle of His), which are located medial to the entrance of the coronary sinus into the right atrium (Fig. 18-4). The extending fibers (Purkinje fibers) proceed down the posterior and inferior portion of the membranous interventricular septum to form right and left branches. The strands of these branches end in the papillary muscles and muscle wall. The excitation wave passes from the SA node to the AV node throughout the conducting system, which stimulates the ventricles to contract (Fig. 18-4).

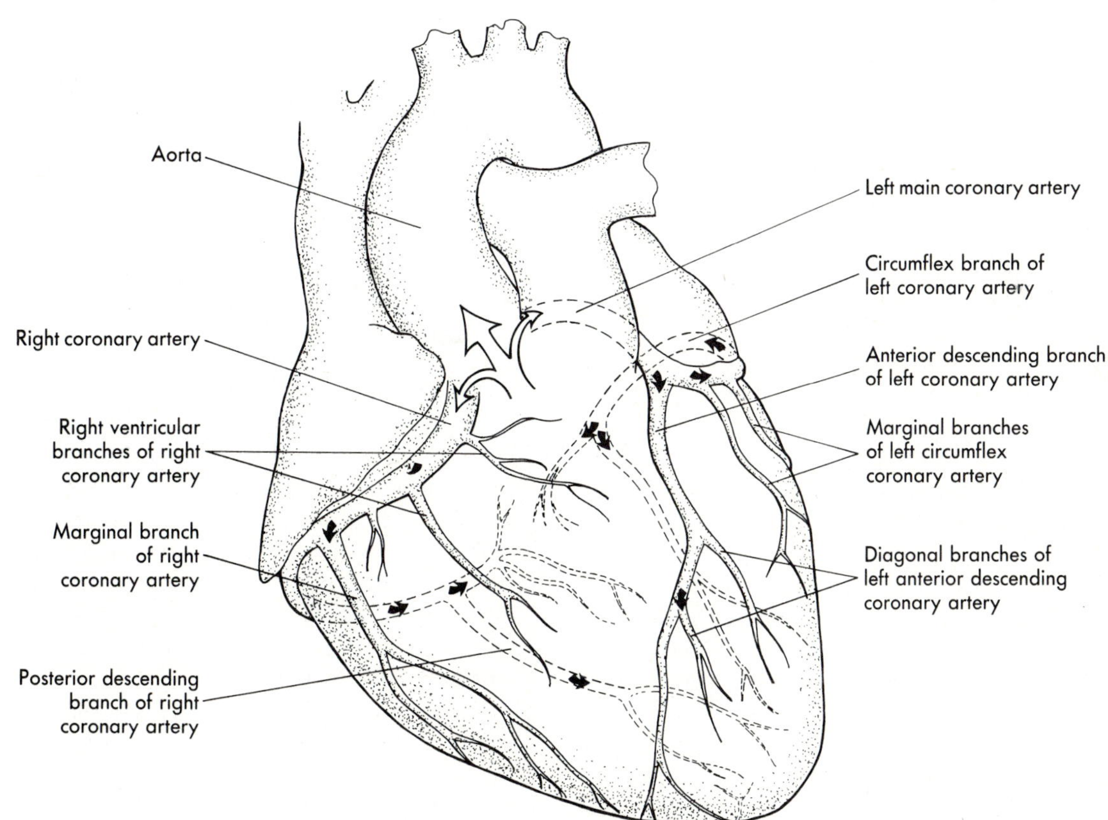

Fig. 18-3. Diagram of coronary artery system.

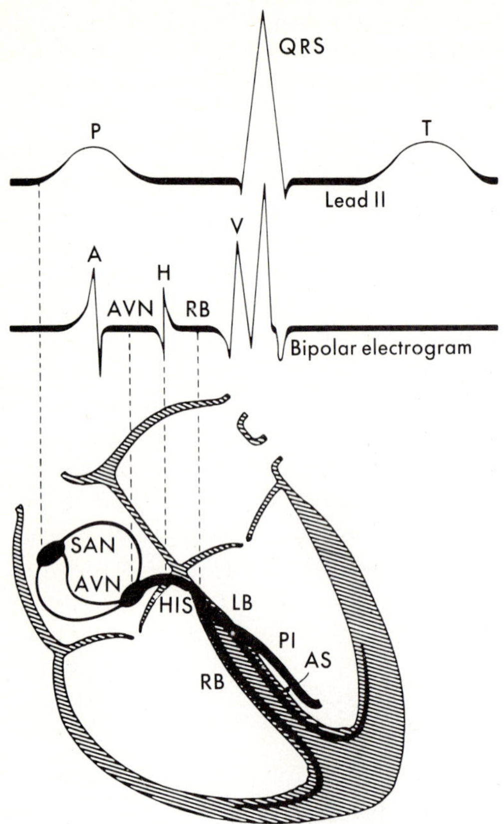

Fig. 18-4. Conducting system of heart muscle tissue. *Top,* limb lead; *middle,* His bundle electrogram; *bottom,* sites of origin of various complexes. *SAN,* Sinoatrial node; *AVN,* atrioventricular node; *H,* His deflection; *V* ventricular deflections; *RB,* right bundle; *LB,* left bundle; *PI,* posteroinferior ramus of *LB; AS,* anterosuperior ramus of *LB.* (From Effler, D.B.: Blades' surgical diseases of the chest, ed. 4, St. Louis, 1978, The C.V. Mosby Co.).

NURSING CONSIDERATIONS

All specialized nursing considerations that are indicated for thoracic operations (Chapter 17) also apply to cardiac surgery.

Preoperative assessment of patients can be particularly useful because of the complex symptoms that frequently result from the acute and chronic hemodynamic changes that are present. The treatment for many patients can be equally complex and multifaceted.

Some considerations, other than those previously mentioned, that can be useful in implementing the nursing care plan for patients undergoing cardiac surgery are discussed in this chapter.

Special facilities

The operating room must be of sufficient size that bulky, highly specialized equipment can be accommodated without interference in maintenance of aseptic technique. For open heart surgery, the facilities must include multiple isolated electrical outlets, auxiliary lighting, a water supply for the heat exchanger in the pump-oxygenator, and multiple suction outlets.

Cardiac catheterization

Angiocardiography provides significant information in regard to the anatomical structure and functional capability of the heart. This information serves as a definitive guide in determining the need for surgery and in selecting the operation of choice.

Definition. Insertion of a radiopaque plastic catheter into the right or left side of the heart via a percutaneous puncture or a cutdown to the brachial or femoral vessels. Pressure determinations in the chambers and large vessels, determination of oxygen saturation and cardiac output, and injection of contrast media to demonstrate certain anatomical structural defects can be accomplished with this technique.

Considerations. Cardiac catheterization is usually performed in a separate department and may or may not directly involve the operating room nursing staff.

Nursing responsibilities however, include supervision of the preparation of instruments, solutions, and supplies for the sterile procedure and the maintenance of standby emergency equipment, that is, the pacemaker, defibrillator, emergency drugs, and resuscitation apparatus. The nurse might also assist the physicians during the procedure, monitoring the patient's vital signs and providing physical and emotional support, as required.

Local anesthesia is used at the site of the puncture wound or cutdown. Electrocardiographic monitoring is continued throughout the procedure.

Operative procedure. The physiological reference point is determined for pressure readings (Fig. 18-5), the skin is prepared, and sterile drapes are applied. Local infiltration is completed, and the catheter is introduced into the brachial or femoral artery and vein through puncture wounds or a cutdown. As the catheter is advanced, perfusion with saline solution to which heparin has been added prevents blood from clotting in the lumen. Fluoroscopy is used to follow the progress of the catheter. The course of the catheter across or through a normal or abnormal pathway, such as an atrial septal defect or stenosis of a valve, is noted.

Injection of dye, generally on the right side of the heart, is used to plot an indicator dye-dilution curve. The concentration of dye in the systemic vessels with respect to time is used to determine the cardiac output. This can be used to determine the amount of blood shunted across abnormal openings in the ventricular or atrial systems.

Intracardiac pressure measurements are made, from which a diagnosis of valvular stenosis or incompetence may be determined (Fig. 18-6). Oxygen analysis aids in determining the presence of shunts. Selective angiocar-

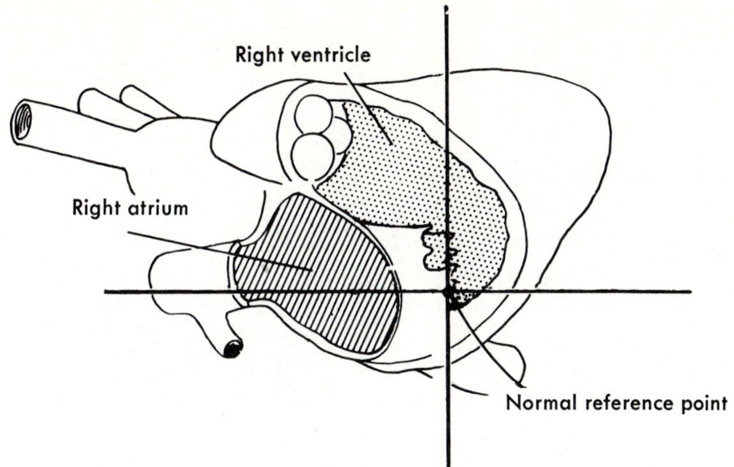

Fig. 18-5. Location at tricuspid valve of physiological reference point for venous pressure measurements. (From Guyton, A.C.: Circulatory physiology: cardiac output and its regulation, Philadelphia, 1971, W.B. Saunders Co.)

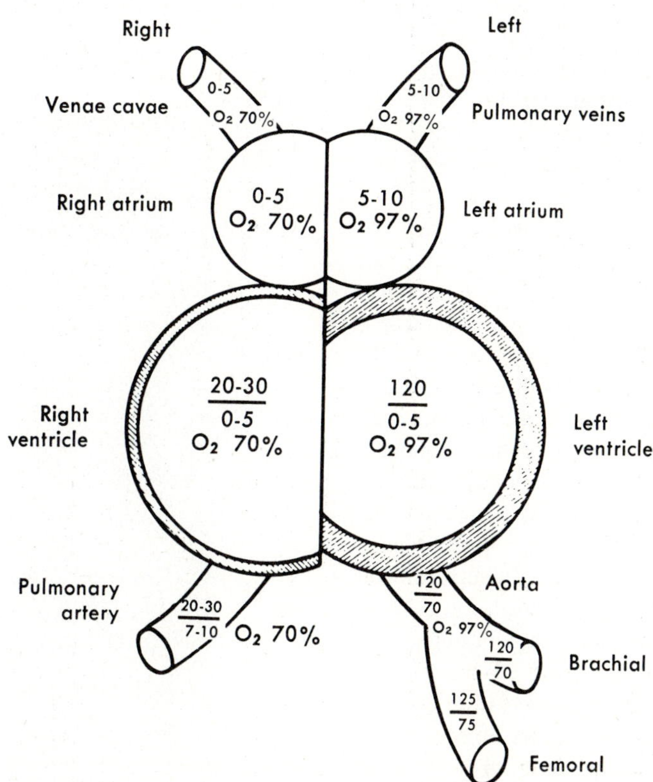

Fig. 18-6. Cardiac catheterization data. Schematic representation of pressure and oxygen saturation in great vessels and cardiac chambers. (From Effler, D.B.: Blades' surgical diseases of the chest, ed. 4, St. Louis, 1978, The C.V. Mosby Co.)

diography, rapid serial x-ray films, or cine movies of a specific area with radiopaque material are useful in isolating structural and functional defects.

The left side of the heart may be approached retrogradely through the aortic valve by a peripheral artery or transeptally from the right atrium.

Preoperative assessment

Because the severity of the pathological changes varies among patients, it is especially important that an understanding of each patient's hemodynamic and general physiological status be obtained by reviewing the chart, communicating with the surgeon, and inverviewing the patient and family.

Patients awaiting cardiac surgery are likely to exhibit more anxiety and stress than many other types of patients, and nurses should anticipate and prepare for this.

Intraoperative care

The patient is positioned on an operating room bed with a thermia blanket.

Anesthesia induction can be one of the most critical times during the intraoperative period. This is especially true for patients with ventricular ischemia from either acquired or congenital disease.

Pressure monitoring catheters are usually inserted after the patient has been anesthetized and intubated. Arterial, venous, or left atrial pressures are usually monitored directly by means of a transducer and oscilloscope. The nurse may be required to assist with the preparation and placement of these lines.

For a direct arterial pressure reading, a catheter is usually inserted into the radial artery. Occasionally, the dorsalis pedis or femoral artery is used. This catheter is connected by an extension tubing to a transducer (Fig. 18-7). The transducer senses fluid pressure changes and converts these to an electrical signal, which is displayed on the oscilloscope. A regulated, pressurized flush system of heparinized intravenous solution is used with this pressure line to keep it patent.

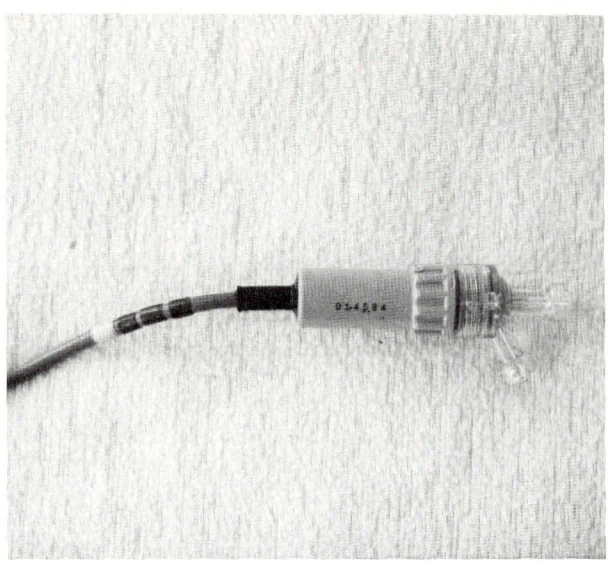

Fig. 18-7. Pressure tranducer.

The central venous pressure (CVP) line is usually inserted into a jugular or subclavian vein. This catheter may be connected to either a transducer, in the same manner as the arterial line, or to a water manometer. This line is also connected to some type of flush system.

Left atrial pressure is monitored with increasing frequency during cardiac surgery. This is accomplished directly, or indirectly by measurement of the pulmonary wedge pressure. If the direct method is used, a catheter is inserted after the chest is open, usually before the cessation of a cardiopulmonary bypass. For indirect measurements, a balloon-flotation pulmonary artery catheter (Fig. 18-8) is used. This is inserted through a jugular or subclavian vein and is advanced through the right side of the heart into a distal pulmonary artery. When it is in position and the balloon is inflated, the pressure distal to the balloon is measured. The pulmonary artery wedge pressure is a good index of the left atrial pressure (Fig. 18-9).

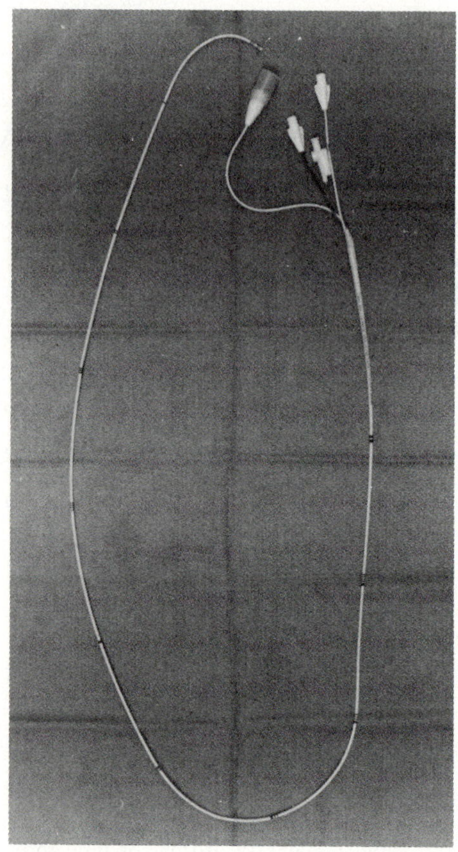

Fig. 18-8. Swan-Ganz balloon-flotation pulmonary artery catheter.

Since these pressure lines are usually left in place for a number of days, strict aseptic technique is required for their placement, including the recommended methods for the care of indwelling intravascular catheters.

A urinary catheter is inserted for monitoring renal function, especially during and after cardiopulmonary bypass.

Several thermistor temperature probes may also be placed, usually in the esophagus, nasopharynx, or rectum.

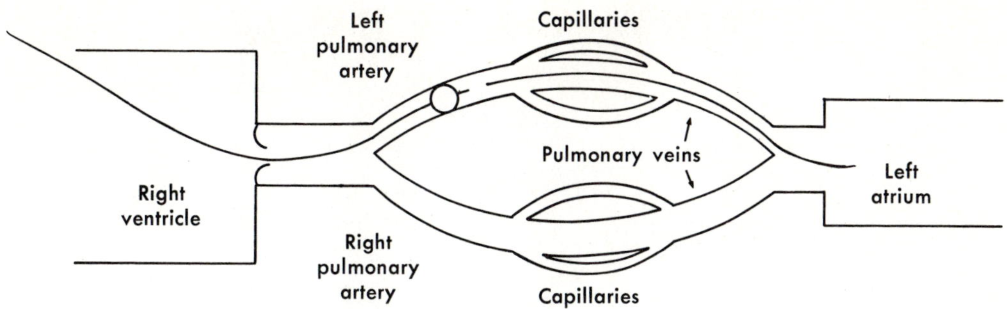

Fig. 18-9. Transmission of atrial pressure. Left atrial pressure is transmitted retrograde to tip of catheter because no valves are interposed.

It is the circulating nurse's responsibility to ensure that blood is available before the procedure begins.

Positioning is as described in Chapter 6.

Commonly used drugs

Heparin sodium is used as an anticoagulant. Dosage is calculated according to the weight of the patient. The patient is heparinized before extracorporeal perfusion. The fluid used to prime the pump-oxygenator also may contain heparin, and it may be added to an intravenous saline solution for irrigation of the lumen of blood vessels during anastomosis.

Protamine sulfate is used to neutralize the action of heparin, and its dosage is calculated according to the amount of heparin previously given.

Lidocaine (Xylocaine), 1%, is used to treat ventricular arrhythmias. It controls premature ventricular contractions and ventricular tachycardia and can prevent the development of ventricular fibrillation.

Epinephrine (Adrenalin) is used as a short-acting cardiac stimulant. A dilute solution of epinephrine 1:10,000 (1 to 2 ml) may be given.

Calcium chloride is used to increase the force of contractions in the weakly beating heart. It increases the tone of the myocardium and opposes the effect of potassium.

Sodium bicarbonate is a buffer that is used to prevent or correct metabolic acidosis.

Dopamine is an inotropic agent that increases cardiac output but produces little peripheral vasoconstriction and therefore preserves renal blood flow.

Isoproterenol (Isuprel) is an adrenergic drug that accelerates the heart rate and lowers pulmonary vascular resistance.

Nitroprusside (Nipride) is a hypotensive agent that acts by relaxing the smooth muscle of the vascular wall.

Extracorporeal circulation

Reliable equipment and established methods now exist that make the temporary substitution of a pump-oxygenator for the heart and lungs a safe clinical procedure. When this equipment is used in combination with varying degrees of hypothermia, the surgeon has sufficient time to complete more complicated and lengthy procedures under direct vision in a relatively dry, motionless field.

Equipment. Many types of pump-oxygenators are available. Generally, one of the following two methods of gas exchange (that is, removal of carbon dioxide and subsequent oxygenation) is used:

1. *Bubble method,* in which oxygen is bubbled through a column of venous blood
2. *Membrane method,* in which the oxygen is diffused through a gas-permeable membrane that separates the oxygenating gas and the venous blood

The bubble oxygenators are the most commonly used type. Many different models are available, and the primary appeal is simplicity of design, low priming volume, and disposability (Fig. 18-10).

Some disposable membrane oxygenators are available for clinical use. The trend may be toward this method of oxygenation, since it is the only method that does not employ a direct blood-gas interface, which is inherently destructive to the formed elements of the blood.

The roller pump has important basic features and is commonly used. It propels the blood through flexible plastic tubing and, with careful calibration and judicious use, can provide relatively atraumatic blood flow. Arterial blood flow with any roller pump, however, is "nonpulsatile" and will be manifested by a "mean" arterial wave form on the oscilloscope during total cardiopulmonary bypass.

Methodology. To place a patient on total heart-lung bypass, the venous blood is drained, by gravity, to the oxygenator through cannulas placed in the inferior and superior venae cavae. The catheters are inserted through small incisions in the right atrium. For some procedures, a single catheter in the right atrium may be sufficient. The oxygenated blood is returned from the pump to the systemic arterial circulation through the arterial cannula. The ascending aorta is usually selected, although the

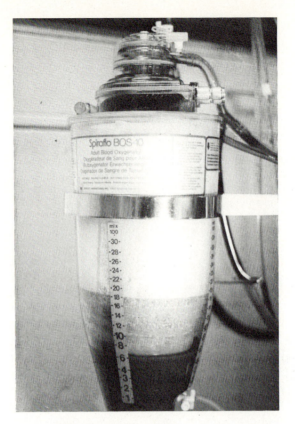

Fig. 18-10. Disposable oxygenator.

common femoral artery may also be used.

Gas exchange and some filtration take place in the oxygenator. The blood usually then passes through a heat exchanger for temperature control, although most bubbler oxygenators have the heat exchanger as an integral part of the unit. The blood also may be pumped through a filter before it is returned to the patient. This is to remove any gaseous or particulate microemboli that may be present in the blood (Fig. 18-11).

Two or more suction lines are ordinarily used during cardiopulmonary bypass to return lost blood directly to the oxygenator (Fig. 18-11). These lines are usually a combination of conventional hand-held suction tips (Fig. 18-12, *1*) and ventricular decompression lines or sumps.

Occasionally, separate perfusion to the coronary arteries may be required, as in an aortic valve replacement. If blood perfusion is to be used, this is accomplished by means of a line coming from the main arterial line of the extracorporeal circuit. Many surgeons prefer to use an infusion of cold potassium cardioplegic solution into the aortic root or directly into the coronary arteries. This produces profound local hypothermia of the myocardium as well as a quiet, flaccid heart. Infusion into the coronary arteries is usually accomplished through a standard intravenous set under pressure, with special tips for the coronary ostia (Fig. 18-12, *2*).

The entire extracorporeal circuit, as well as the tubing and cannulas, must be "primed," or rendered free of air, before the initiation of cardiopulmonary bypass to prevent air emboli. The priming solution is usually a combination of colloid and crystalloid fluids. The colloid component may be blood, albumin, or plasma fraction, and the crystalloid component is usually lactated Ringer's solution or 5% dextrose and water. Most, if not all, institutions today employ the technique of hemodilution, meaning that crystalloid solutions are predominately used to prime the pump in an attempt to reduce the amount of bank blood being used. This has the advantage of reducing cost, the number of homologous serum reactions, and the incidence of hepatitis, as well as providing better perfusion of the capillary beds because of reduced blood viscosity.

The amount and kind of drugs used in the priming solution vary among institutions, but heparin and calcium are used almost routinely, according to the amount of whole blood, if any, that has been added to the priming solution.

Arterial blood flow rates are calculated according to the patient's body surface area and are adjusted during bypass, depending on the arterial and venous pressure values as well as the results of blood gas determinations.

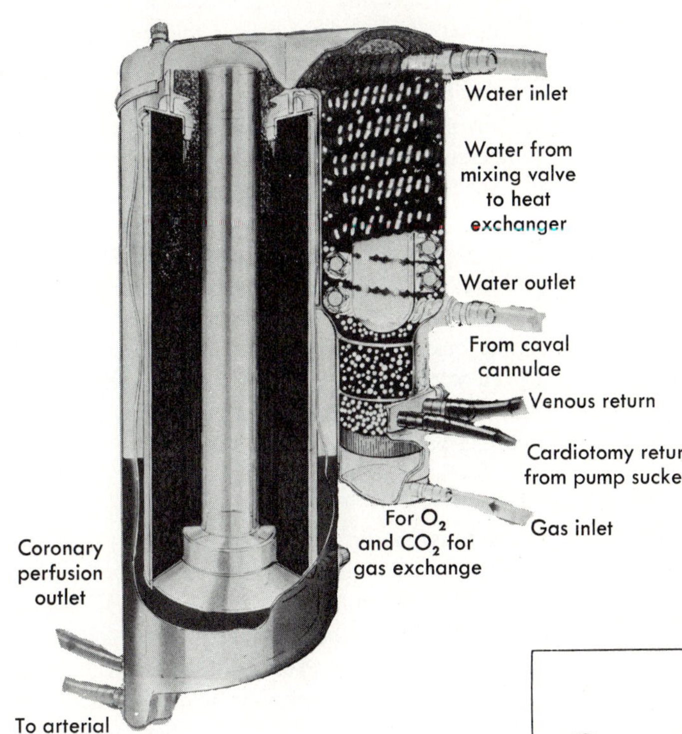

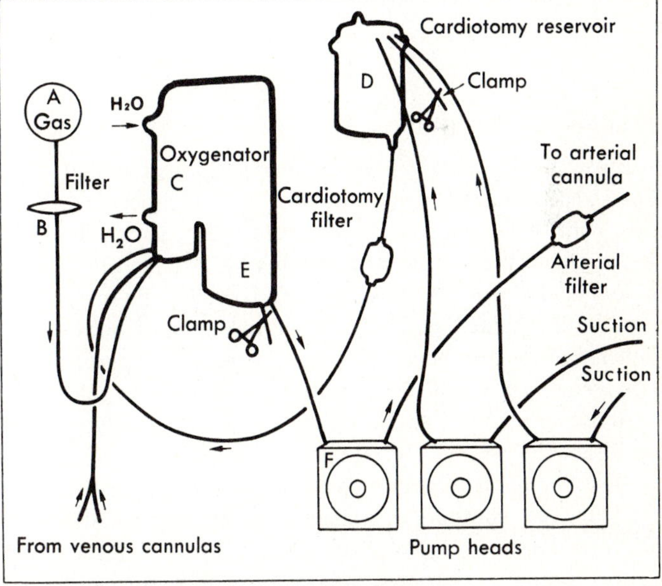

Above diagram is for orientation of equipment set-up only.

•The use of blood filtration during cardiopulmonary bypass has been implicated in the reduction of the risk of tissue and organ dysfunction related to particulate matter and gas emboli present in the extracorporeal circuit.

Fig. 18-11. Representative pump circuit with Shiley oxygenator. *A,* Pressurized gas source with flowmeters for oxygen and carbon dioxide; *B,* bacterial and particulate matter filter, screen size 0.2 μm; *C,* bubble column (blood and gas) with integral heat exchanger; *D,* cardiotomy reservoir with filter to remove particulate matter; *E,* arterial reservoir from which oxygenated blood is pumped to patient; *F,* roller pump head, which drives oxygenated blood to patient. (Courtesy Shiley Sales Corp., Irving, Calif.)

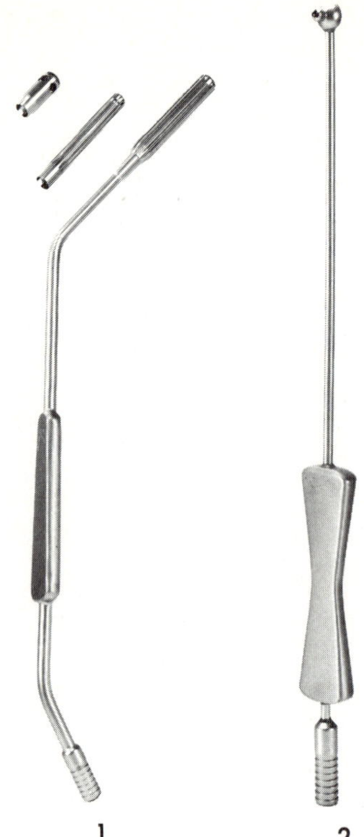

Fig. 18-12. *1,* Intracardiac suction with interchangeable tips; *2,* coronary perfusion cannula with malleable shaft, size 4-, 5-, or 6-mm diameter for ¼-inch tubing. (Courtesy Sarns, Inc., Ann Arbor, Mich.)

Hypothermia

Most cardiac surgical procedures performed today employ some degree of hypothermia. This is especially true in the field of pediatric cardiac surgery, in which total circulatory arrest in conjunction with profound hypothermia (14° to 18° C) may be used. Hypothermia may be generally defined as the deliberate reduction of body temperature for therapeutic purposes. A moderate degree of hypothermia, to 28° C, permits reduction of oxygen consumption by 50%. At 20° C, there is a further reduction of about 25%.

Hypothermia is used in surgery to lengthen the period of circulatory interruption, ischemia, or hypoperfusion, with little danger of neurological or other organ damage, thus permitting the surgeon sufficient time to repair cardiac lesions under direct vision. Total body hypothermia can be achieved by surface cooling, application of a cooling blanket, or the heat exchanger of the heart-lung machine. Except for small infants, in whom surface cooling may be accomplished before the surgical procedure, the cooling and rewarming processes are accomplished during cardiopulmonary bypass.

There are two principal dangers inherent in the use of hypothermia. First, frostbite can occur with surface cooling during which an infant is covered with plastic bags of ice. Usually, wrapping the extremities is effective in preventing frostbite. Second, ventricular fibrillation can occur during the cooling process. This is usually not a problem, since the patient is ordinarily on total cardiopulmonary bypass. It can be a real concern with infants who are undergoing surface cooling before surgery. Ventricular fibrillation is unusual at temperatures above 32° C, but in children with cyanosis it can occur at higher temperatures.

Specific nursing measures are aimed at prevention of frostbite, as previously mentioned, maintenance of the correct temperature when the cooling blanket is being used, and prevention of pressure areas from the blanket itself.

Another method of accomplishing local hypothermia of the heart is to use saline slush. With this technique, frozen sterile saline is crushed and mixed with liquid saline to form a slushy mixture. This is poured directly over the pericardial sac.

Intraaortic balloon pump

The intraaortic balloon pump (IABP) is a device that is used as an adjunct in the treatment of patients with acute left ventricular failure. Basically, it consists of an inflatable balloon that is placed in the descending aorta via a femoral artery. This balloon is attached by a connecting line, to the pumping module, which uses either helium or carbon dioxide as the inflating gas.

Balloon inflation occurs during ventricular diastole, thus augmenting coronary blood flow, and deflation occurs during systole, which reduces the work load of the left ventricle. The principle on which the IABP operates is termed "counterpulsation," since it pumps during diastole.

To insert the balloon, instruments are needed for a femoral cutdown, as well as peripheral vascular clamps and a short (10 mm) vascular graft.

Suture materials

A variety of nonabsorbable cardiovascular sutures with swaged-on needles are available from most suture manufacturers. Synthetic sutures of Teflon, Dacron, polyester, or polypropylene are usually selected for insertion of prostheses and for vascular anastomoses. Most sutures will be double-armed with a needle on each end.

Basic instrument setup

The basic setup described for thoracic procedures (Chapter 17) is used, along with some specialized cardiovascular instruments and equipment (Figs. 18-13 and 18-14). Additional items may also be required:

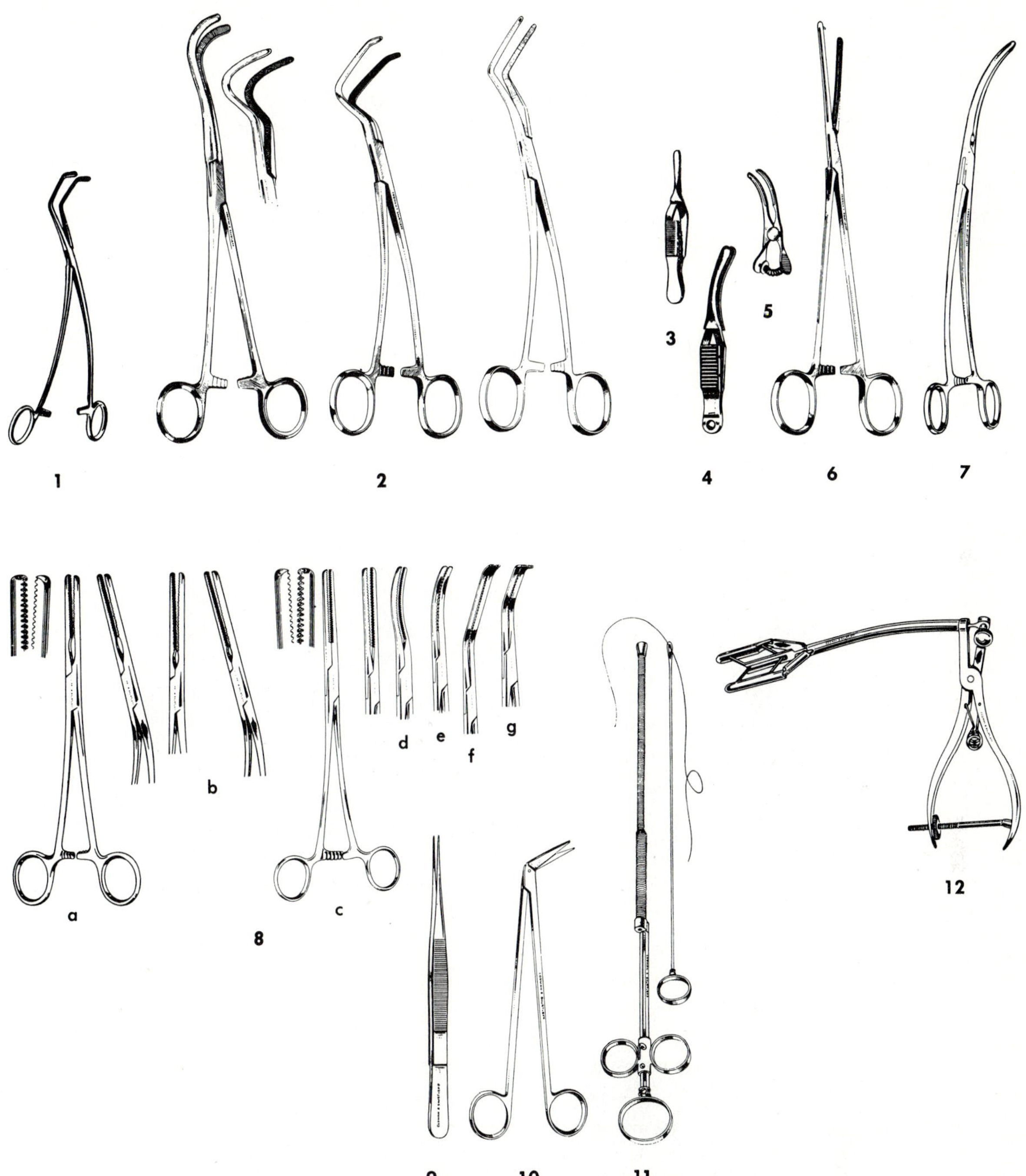

Fig. 18-13. Cardiothoracic instruments. *1,* Satinsky vena cava clamp; *2,* Harken auricle clamps, various sizes; *3* to *5,* bulldog clamps, straight, curved, and adjustable spring type; *6,* Gross coarctation occlusion clamp; *7,* Crafoord coarctation clamp; *8,* vascular clamps: *a,* patent ductus, straight and curved; *b,* coarctation, straight and curved; *c,* anastomosis, straight; *d,* spoon; *e,* curved; *f,* aortic; *g,* appendage; *9,* Potts thumb forceps, fine; *10,* Potts 60-degree angled scissors; *11,* Rumel tourniquet; *12,* Gerbode mitral valvulotome for retrograde insertion. (Courtesy Codman & Shurtleff, Inc., Randolph, Mass.)

Electric fibrillator
DC defibrillator
External pulse generator (pacemaker) available
Fiberoptic head light
Thermia unit

For bypass cannulations, the following are also required:

Intracardiac suctions and vents (Fig. 18-12)
Obturators for inserting cannulas (optional)
Perfusion cannulas or catheters (Fig. 18-15)
Perfusion tubing, lengths and sizes determined by particular institution and type of extracorporeal apparatus
Adapters and connectors for securing cannulas to perfusion tubing
Plastic ties and tie gun (optional)
Saline irrigating solution containing heparin

Vascular clamps, which are designed to partially or completely occlude blood flow, must be maintained in good condition if they are to prevent fracture of the delicate intima of the blood vessels and still retain their specific holding qualities. There are many variations in construction of vascular instruments. The jaws may consist of single or double rows of fine, sharp, or blunt teeth or special cross-hatching or longitudinal serrations. The working angles of the clamps also vary. All clamps are designed to hold the vessels securely but without trauma (Fig. 18-13).

Prosthetic materials

Intracardiac patches, heart valves, and synthetic grafts should be handled with care to prevent damage or the introduction of foreign materials.

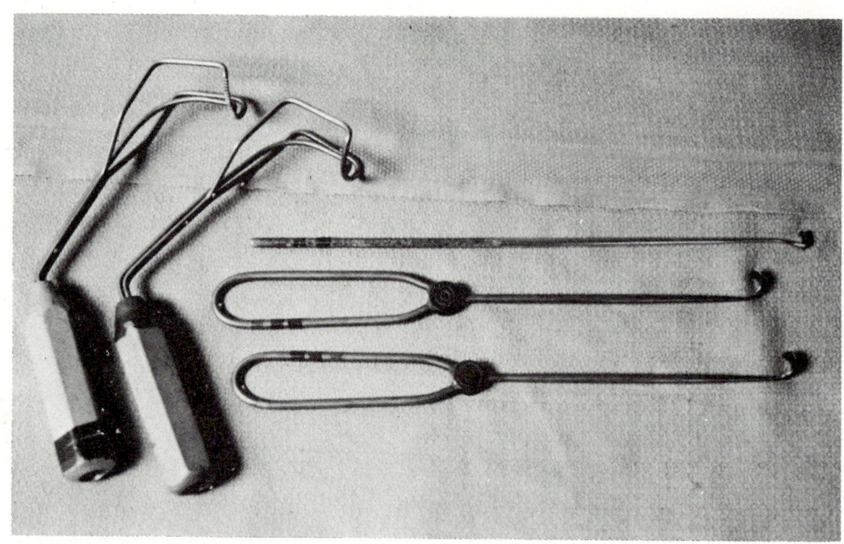

Fig. 18-14. Atrial and leaflet retractors.

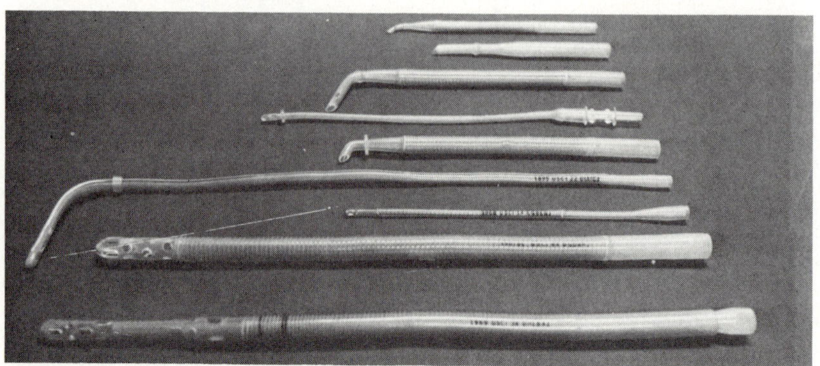

Fig. 18-15. Polyvinyl perfusion catheters. (Courtesy Harvey Cardiopulmonary Division, C.R. Bard, Inc., Santa Ana, Calif.)

Teflon, a fluorocarbon fiber, and Dacron, a polyester fiber, are available in a variety of meshes, fabrics, felts, tapes, and sutures and are also combined with other materials in prosthetic heart valves.

Teflon patches (Fig. 18-16) are made in a variety of forms for intracardiac and outflow tract use. Varying degrees of firmness, thickness, and porosity are available for specific uses. Low reactivity, retention of strength, and tissue acceptance are important properties to be considered in the selection of such patches.

Dacron arterial grafts are usually used in cardiac surgery, although a new material, reinforced expanded polytetrafluorethylene (PTFE) is being used with increasing frequency. There are two types of Dacron grafts: knitted and woven. Woven prosthetic grafts are usually used when the patient has been given heparin, since the interstices are tighter and bleeding is usually reduced. Knitted grafts do not fray as readily as woven grafts when cut. The grafts are available in sizes suitable for straight arterial grafts, as well as for aortic bifurcated grafts (Fig. 18-17).

Valve prostheses are selected according to their hemodynamics, thromboresistance, and ease of insertion. Most mechanical prostheses employ a cage-and-disc or a tilting disc design. These valves allow complete closure with slight regurgitation to prevent stasis of blood (Fig. 18-18).

In addition, porcine heterograft prostheses (Fig. 18-19) are in use. The valve consists of an aortic valve from the pig, which is sutured to a Dacron-covered stent. The advantage of using this valve is that long-term anticoagulants are not necessary in most patients.

Another type of biologic valve uses pericardium and offers the advantage of improved flow characteristics (Fig. 18-20).

Valve sizers and holder for insertion of valve prostheses are shown in Fig. 18-21.

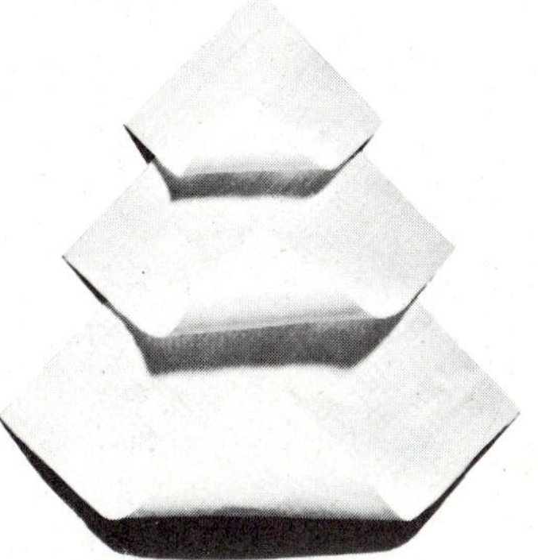

Fig. 18-16. Teflon intracardiac patches, for closure of intracardiac septal defects. (Courtesy C.R. Bard, Inc., Murray Hill, N.J.)

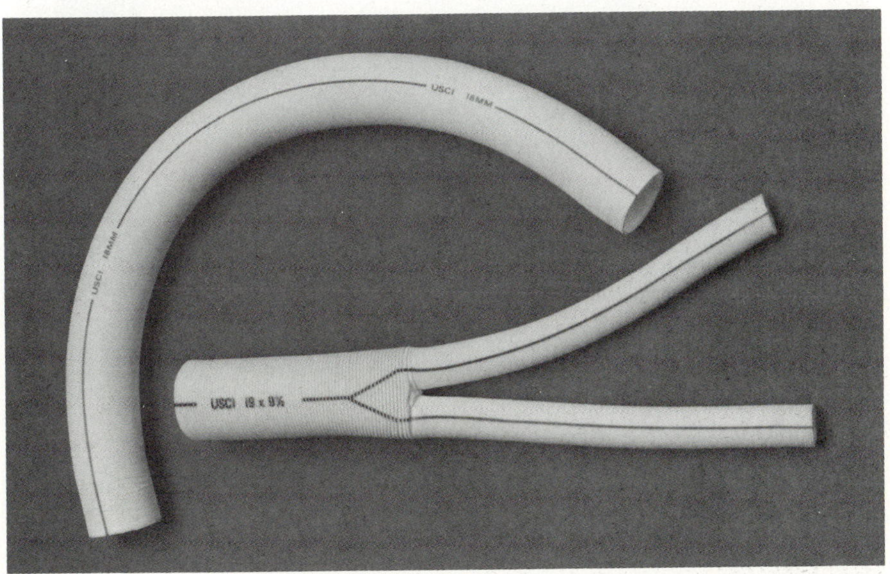

Fig. 18-17. Low-porosity woven Dacron arterial grafts. (Courtesy Bard Implants Division, C.R. Bard, Inc., Billerica, Mass.)

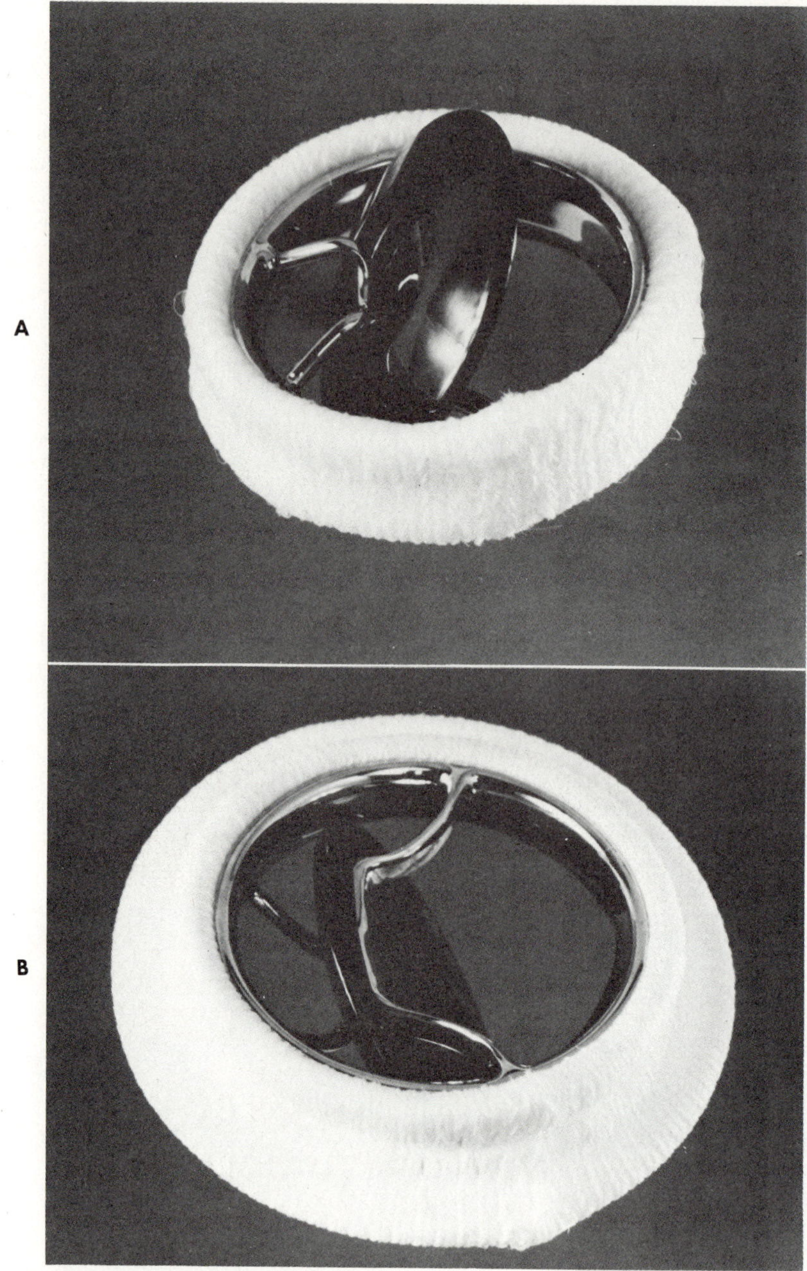

Fig 18-18. A, Bjork-Shiley mitral valve prosthesis. **B,** Bjork-Shiley aortic valve prothesis. (Courtesy Shiley Laboratories, Irvine, Calif.).

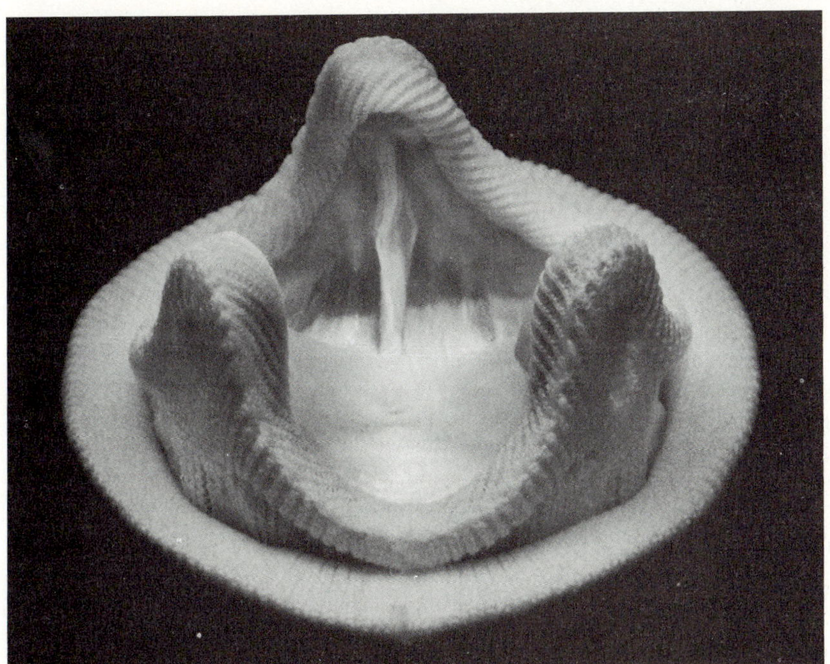

Fig. 18-19. Hancock aortic bioprosthesis aortic-outflow aspect. (Courtesy Hancock Laboratories, Inc., Anaheim, Calif.)

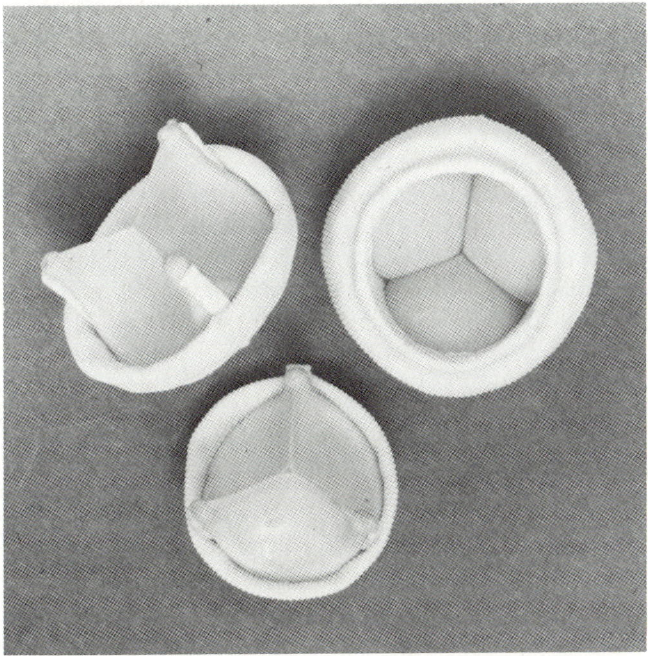

Fig. 18-20. Ionescu-Shiley pericardial xenograft. *Clockwise from 11 o'clock position:* Profile, inflow, and outflow views. (Courtesy Shiley Laboratories, Irvine, Calif.).

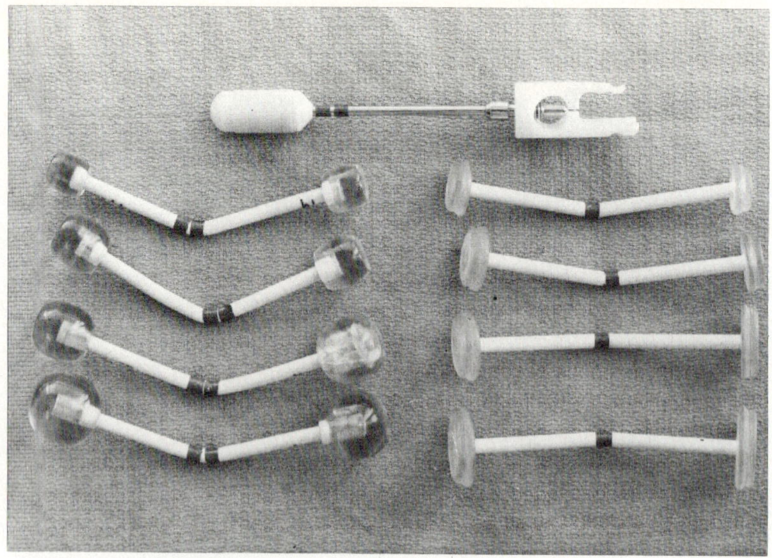

Fig. 18-21. Assorted valve sizers and holder.

EXTRACORPOREAL CIRCULATION PROCEDURES (Fig. 18-22)

Types of incisions. The heart is usually approached through a median sternotomy or a posterolateral thoracotomy. Occasionally, an anterolateral thoracotomy may be used. All of these approaches are described in detail in Chapter 17.

Procedure for cannulation

1. A longitudinal pericardial incision is made, and the pericardial edges are sutured to the chest wall.

2. The aorta, if it is to be cannulated for arterial blood return to the patient, is dissected free, as are the venae cavae.

3. Each vena cava is encircled with an umbilical tape, the loose ends of which are threaded with a stylet through a ¼ × 2–inch red rubber or plastic tubing tourniquet and held taut by a hemostat. Compression on the vena cava may be accomplished by tightening the tourniquet and repositioning the hemostat.

4. Purse-string sutures are placed in the aorta and venae cavae for the eventual placement of the perfusion cannulas.

5. The ascending aorta is cannulated for the arterial blood return. A partial occlusion clamp is used to isolate a segment of the aortic wall. The wall is incised, the cannula is inserted, and the purse-string suture is secured with a tourniquet. It is important to have the distal end of the cannula clamped before it is inserted into the aorta. The arterial cannulation is always performed before the caval cannulations so that direct access for blood replacement is available if needed.

6. For the venous return to the pump-oxygenator, the inferior and superior venae cavae are cannulated. An incision is usually made in the atrial appendage for the inferior caval cannula, and a transverse incision through the atrial wall is made for the superior caval cannula. Each incision is made over a curved partial occlusion vascular clamp and the cannula is inserted. The purse-string suture is secured with a tourniquet, and the catheter is permitted to partially fill with blood before the occluding clamp is applied.

7. Occasionally, only the right atrium is cannulated for the venous return to the pump. This is most commonly done in procedures in which the heart need not be completely empty of blood, such as an aortic valve replacement or coronary artery bypass procedures.

Procedure for femoral cutdown for arterial cannulations. To save time, a second team may simultaneously be preparing the arterial return site if the femoral artery is selected for cannulation.

A vertical or oblique incision is made in the femoral triangle, and the femoral artery is exposed. Umbilical compression tapes are passed around the vessel above and below the proposed arteriotomy. (Two vascular clamps may also be applied to the vessel.) An incision is made into the vessel, and the perfusion catheter is inserted retrogradely into the artery as the proximal clamp or tourniquet is released. After the cannula is in place, the proximal tourniqet is tightened to prevent bleeding from the arteriotomy. Here again, it is important to have a clamp on the distal end of the perfusion cannula before it is inserted into the artery.

Procedure for pump-oxygenator preparation. While the surgical team prepares the cannulations for connection to the pump-oxygenator, the perfusionist tests and completes assemblage of the equipment.

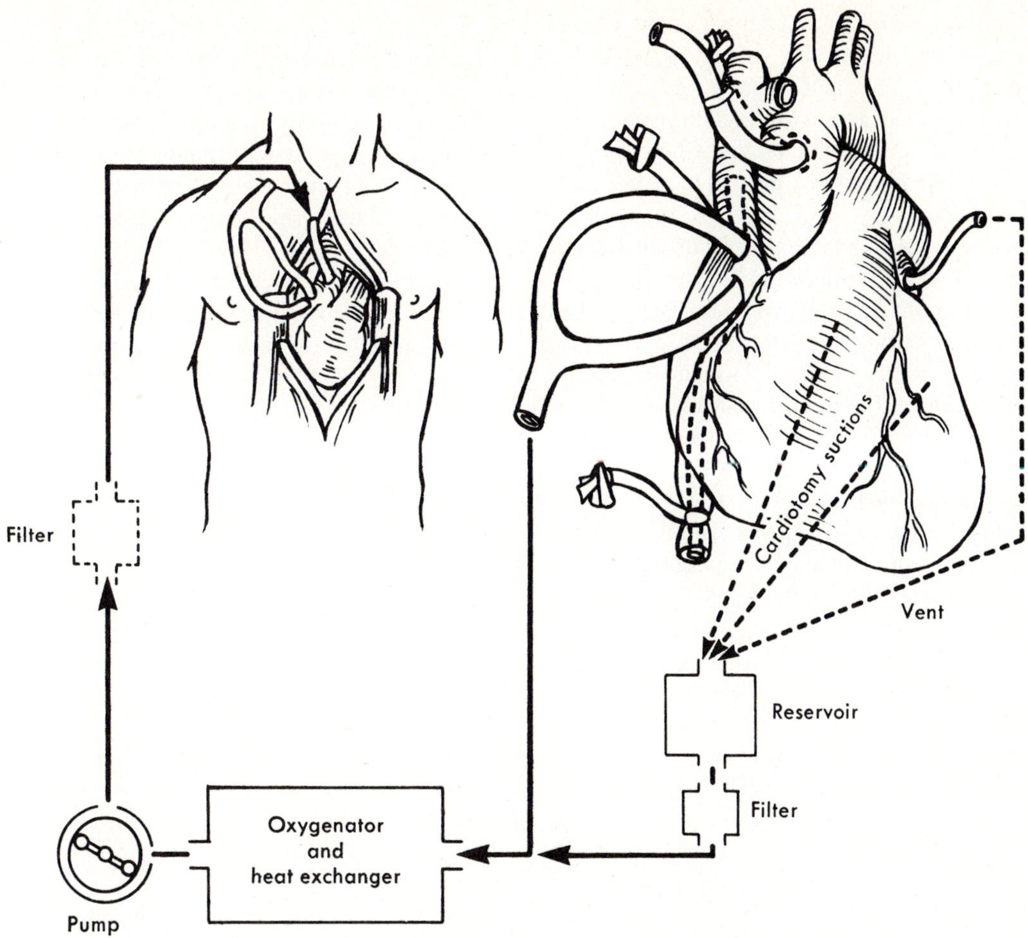

Fig. 18-22. Diagram of extracorporeal circulation.

1. Before the incision is made, the tubing is passed to the perfusionist after the proximal ends have been secured to the drapes.

2. After the venous and arterial lines are connected to the pump-oxygenator, blood is pumped through the lines to displace air in the tubing. To prevent air emboli, caution is exercised particularly as the arterial connection is completed. This connection is usually made under a saline drip.

3. When all connections are properly secured and the pump-oxygenator is ready, partial bypass is begun. After the flow is in balance, the tapes around the venae cavae are tightened, and total cardiopulmonary bypass is achieved. The perfusion rate is adjusted as the operation proceeds.

Procedure for termination of bypass

1. After the intracardiac procedure has been completed, the heart is closed with continuous, synthetic cardiovascular sutures. All air is evacuated from the left ventricle.

2. Defibrillation may be spontaneous with removal of an aortic cross clamp, if used, or rewarming, if hypothermia was induced. If not, electrical defibrillation will be necessary.

3. Compression tapes around the venae cavae are released, and venous flow to the pump is reduced. Arterial flow is also reduced to equal the venous return. When heart action is sufficient and systemic arterial blood pressure is stabilized, venous return is further reduced, and the patient is taken off bypass by clamping all lines and stopping the pump.

4. As the cannulation catheters are removed, the pursestring sutures are tightened and tied. Additional sutures may be required for tight closure.

5. Protamine sulfate, a heparin antagonist, is administered.

6. The pericardium is usually left open for drainage.

Drainage. Catheters may be inserted into the pericardium, the anterior mediastinum, or either or both pleurae. They are connected by straight or Y connectors to a water-seal collection system (Chapter 17).

Closure of chest

1. *For posterolateral and anterolateral thoracotomy.* Ribs are approximated by the application of rib approxi-

mators and the insertion of interrupted pericostal sutures of chromic gut or other absorbable suture materials. Sutures are tied in place, and approximators are removed. Continuous or interrupted sutures are used throughout for muscle and subcutaneous tissue closures. Continuous or interrupted nonabsorbable sutures may be used for skin closure.

2. *For median sternotomy*. Corresponding holes are punched or drilled on each side of the sternum to facilitate placement of wire sutures. The wire sutures are twisted, cut, and buried into the sternum. A layer of interrupted, synthetic sutures is placed to approximate the muscle over the sternum. The subcutaneous tissue is closed with absorbable suture. Continuous or interrupted synthetic sutures may be used for skin closure.

Closure of femoral incision

1. The femoral catheter is removed, and the arteriotomy is closed with nonabsorbable cardiovascular suture. Compression tapes and bulldog clamps, if used, are removed.

2. The wound is closed with absorbable sutures, and the skin is closed with interrupted or continuous nonabsorbable suture.

3. Dressings are applied to all wounds.

Postoperatively, the patient is usually transferred directly to the surgical intensive care unit, although the recovery room is occasionally used. The nurse in the postoperative unit should be notified with a report on the patient's condition and an estimated time of arrival.

SURGERY FOR ACQUIRED LESIONS

Pericardiectomy

Definition. Partial excision of the adhered, thickened fibrotic pericardium to relieve constriction of compressed heart and large blood vessels.

Considerations. Myocardial contractility is restricted by the adhered portions of the scarred, thickened pericardium. As the pericardial space is obliterated and calcification of the pericardium occurs, the heart is further compressed. Ascites, elevated venous pressure, decreased arterial pressure, edema, and hepatic enlargement result. This condition is usually caused by chronic pericarditis, which may be of tubercular, rheumatic, viral, or neoplastic origin.

Setup and preparation of the patient. The patient is placed in a supine position. The setup is as described previously. Occasionally, cardiopulmonary bypass may be requested on a standby basis, but usually the supplies and instruments for bypass are not needed.

Operative procedure

1. A median sternotomy is performed to expose the pericardium (Chapter 17).

2. The lungs are displaced laterally, and the phrenic nerves are identified and carefully protected. The pericardium is incised.

3. The atria and the ventricles are freed. The outer thickened pericardium is removed, as indicated. The cartilage scissors may be used. The fibrous adherent portions are carefully dissected with dry dissectors and Metzenbaum scissors. Caution is exercised to prevent perforation of the atria and right ventricle. Rather than cause perforation, small areas of adherent pericardium may be retained.

4. Dissection is continued, and the large blood vessels are exposed and freed as indicated.

5. Adequate drainage of the pericardial wound is facilitated by catheters placed near the heart or through the pleural spaces. Connections to closed drainage sets are established as described in Chapter 17.

6. Hemostasis is carefully controlled.

7. The chest wound is closed as described for median sternotomy. A dressing is applied.

Operations on the mitral valve

General considerations. Mitral stenosis, the most common acquired valvular lesion, is usually caused by rheumatic fever. The normal opening in the cone-like valve is about 5 cm^2. As the disease progresses, the mitral valve becomes a narrow slit in a fibrotic plaque, severely limiting blood flow into the left ventricle (Fig. 18-23). Mitral stenosis causes a rise in pressure and dilatation of the left atrium. This pressure is transmitted throughout the pulmonary vascular bed, with subsequent right ventricular hypertrophy and pulmonary hypertension.

The major symptoms are dyspnea, fatigue, and orthopnea. A characteristic diastolic murmur is heard, and atrial fibrillation is not unusual. An embolism may result from clots in the atrial appendage. Later findings are severe pulmonary congestion and right ventricular failure.

The surgeon's selection of the procedure (open or closed commissurotomy or valve replacement) is determined by the stage of disease, presence or absence of calcification, history of thromboembolism and heart rhythm, and any associated pathological defects. Usually the open approach, using cardiopulmonary bypass, is preferred.

Closed commissurotomy for mitral stenosis

Definition. Separation of the adherent leaflets of the mitral valve.

Setup and preparation of the patient. Instrumentation is as described, without items for cardiopulmonary bypass, plus a Gerbode or Tubbs dilator and tourniquets.

A supine position with the left thorax slightly elevated is used for the left anterior thoracotomy approach, or a lateral position is used for a left posterolateral thoracotomy approach. Preparation and draping are as described for thoracic surgery.

Operative procedure. The major steps and items used for a left lateral approach are as described in Chapter 17.

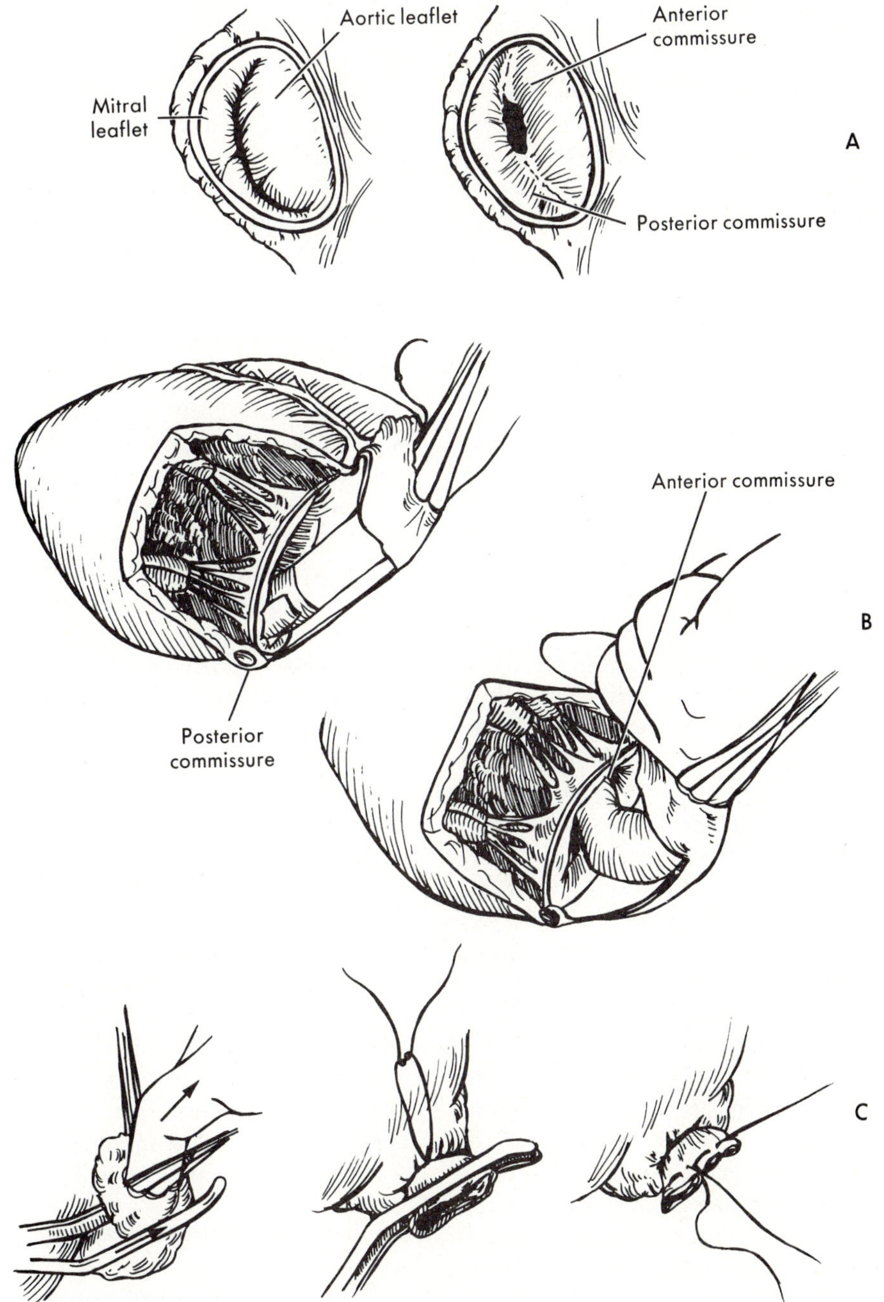

Fig. 18-23. A, *Left,* Normal mitral valve; *right,* fusion and thickening of valve leaflets in center and surrounding area. **B,** Finger fracture of valve. **C,** Closure of atrial appendage. (From Johnson, J., and Kirby, C.K.: Surgery of the chest, ed. 4, Chicago, 1970, Year Book Medical Publishers, Inc.)

1. The pleura is opened with a knife and dissecting scissors. A small Finochietto retractor is placed, with blades over moist sponges to protect the wound edges, and opened for desired exposure.

2. As the pericardium is incised, using scissors and fine forceps, the phrenic nerve is protected. The pericardial stay sutures are placed.

3. A purse-string suture is placed about the base of the atrial appendage. The swaged-on needles are cut off, and the suture ends threaded through a Rumel tourniquet.

4. An angled vascular clamp is applied to the base of the appendage, and the tip of the appendage is partially amputated with scissors and long forceps.

5. Trabeculae within the atrial appendage are divided with a fine forceps and scissors.

6. Superficial thrombi, if present, are removed by momentary release of the clamp. Clamps are applied to the cut edges of the appendage.

7. The appendage traction clamps are elevated, the purse-string suture is held taut, the surgeon introduces a finger into the atrium, and the curved vascular clamp is slowly released. The clamp is kept on the field for reapplication if necessary.

8. The pathological condition is noted as the valve is explored. The adherent leaflets are separated by finger pressure, first laterally, and then medially (Fig. 18-23).

9. Another method of separating the leaflets is a *retrograde procedure*. A purse-string or mattress suture with felt pledget is placed in the left ventricle, and a ventriculotomy is made with a scalpel, using a no. 11 blade. A Gerbode or Tubbs valve dilator is introduced, the tips of which are guided into the left atrium by the right index finger. The blades are adjusted to the desired opening, and dilatation with separation of the adherent leaflets of the valve is completed. The instrument is removed, and the purse-string suture is secured. Additional fine sutures with felt pledgets are used to complete hemostasis.

10. The finger is removed, and the atrial purse-string suture is tied (Fig. 18-23). The appendage is closed with cardiovascular suture.

11. A pleural cavity drainage catheter is inserted through a stab wound in the lateral interspace and anchored to the skin with silk sutures.

12. The chest catheter is connected to a closed water-seal drainage system.

13. Closure of the chest is accomplished. Dressings are applied.

Open commissurotomy for mitral stenosis

Setup and preparation of the patient. The patient is placed in a supine position for a median sternotomy. The setup is as described for open heart procedures, with mitral valve instruments (Fig. 18-13).

Operative procedure

1. A median sternotomy is performed, and cardiopulmonary bypass begun as described.

2. The left atrium is incised, and the valve is inspected.

3. Fused leaflets are separated with vascular forceps and scissors.

4. The valve is again inspected for any resultant insufficiency and, if necessary, annular plication may be performed.

5. The left atrium is closed with a continuous cardiovascular suture.

6. Cardiopulmonary bypass is discontinued, and the sternum closed as described.

Mitral valve replacement

Definition. Excision of the mitral valve leaflets, chordae tendinae, and papillary muscles and replacement with a mechanical prosthesis or heterograft.

Setup and preparation of the patient. The patient is usually placed in the supine position. The setup is as described for open heart procedures, plus the following: atrial and leaflet retractors and valve scissors (Fig. 18-13), valve prostheses, holders, and sizers (Figs. 18-18 to 18-21).

Operative procedure

1. A median sternotomy is performed, and cardiopulmonary bypass begun as described.

2. The aorta is cross-clamped with a curved vascular clamp such as a Crafoord or DeBakey. Fibrillation may then occur spontaneously, as a result of coronary ischemia, or may be electrically induced.

3. The left atrium is incised, blood is suctioned away, and the incision is enlarged to expose the mitral valve for subsequent replacement (Fig. 18-24).

4. The pathological condition is determined, and the valve leaflets are excised with the papillary muscles and chordae tendinae (Fig. 18-24). Selection of the cutting instrument depends on the degree of calcification present and the method of excision. A small margin of the valve annulus is retained for insertion of fixation sutures to the valve. The ventricle is inspected, and all loose debris is removed.

5. The valve sizer is used to determine the correct size of the prosthesis.

6. Nonabsorbable cardiovascular sutures (about twenty) are first placed in the retained margin of the valve with the ends tagged with mosquito clamps and are then placed into the sewing ring of the prosthesis.

7. The sutures are held taut as the prosthesis is guided into position and secured, and the sutures are tied and cut.

8. Continuous sutures are used to close the atriotomy. The patient is placed in reverse Trendelenburg's position.

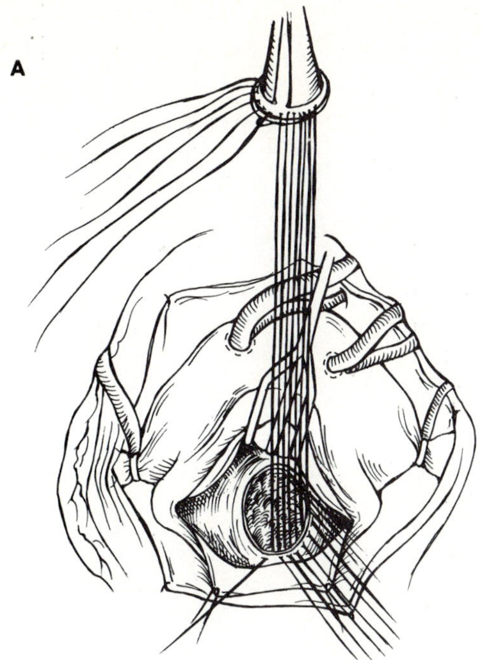

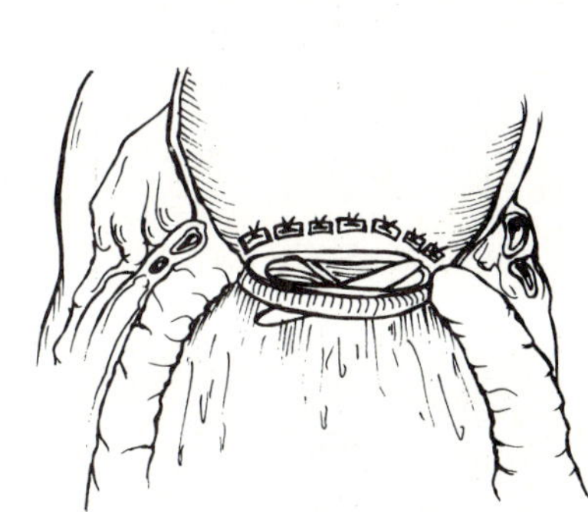

Fig. 18-24. Mitral valve replacement.

Air is aspirated from the left ventricle through a hypodermic or vent needle, and the atrial closure is completed. It is important that evacuation of air be completed before the heart resumes beating and the cross clamp is removed.

9. Cardiopulmonary bypass is discontinued, and the sternum closed as described.

Operation on the aortic valve

General considerations. Obstruction to left ventricular outflow is usually caused by valvular stenosis, a condition in which the valve leaflets are fused. This causes a smaller opening than normal during ejection and results in a reduction of flow, a large pressure difference across the stenotic valve, or both. Obstruction caused by subvalvular and supravalvular stenosis is rare.

Aortic valvular stenosis may be of congenital origin, but it is more frequently an acquired lesion resulting from complications of rheumatic fever. Extensive fibrosis and heavily calcified deposits make it difficult to release the fused leaflets and restore normal function (Fig. 18-25.)

In most patients, symptoms are not evident in early life. Fatigue and dyspnea during exertion are prominent symptoms that may not appear until the late teens. Late findings of angina pectoris, syncope, and congestive failure attributable to aortic stenosis present a grave prognosis. Sudden death is not uncommon.

A systolic aortic murmur is present, and electrocardiograms and catheterization studies reveal left ventricular hypertrophy and pressure gradients across the aortic valve. Surgical procedures are designed to improve valvular function, which may be accomplished by meticulous separation of the commissures or repair of individual leaflets; but, most often, total excision of the valve and replacement with a prosthesis is necessary (Figs. 18-26 and 18-27).

Aortic valvulotomy and aortic valve replacement

Definition. Separation of the fused leaflets or excision of the valve and replacement with a mechanical prosthesis or heterograft.

Setup and preparation of the patient. The patient is placed in the supine position. The instrument setup is as described for open heart surgery, plus the following:

Valve scissors
Aortic valves, sizers, and holders (Figs. 18-19 and 18-21)
Complete set coronary artery perfusion cannulas (surgeon's preference)

Operative procedure

1. A median sternotomy is performed, and cardiopulmonary bypass is begun as described.

2. Venting of the left ventricle is begun while the patient's temperature is being lowered.

3. The aorta is cross-clamped, a transverse aortotomy is completed, and coronary ostia are identified. These may be cannulated for perfusion, or cardioplegia may be induced with cold potassium solution.

4A. The valve is inspected, and the extent of the pathological defect confirmed. Separation of the commis-

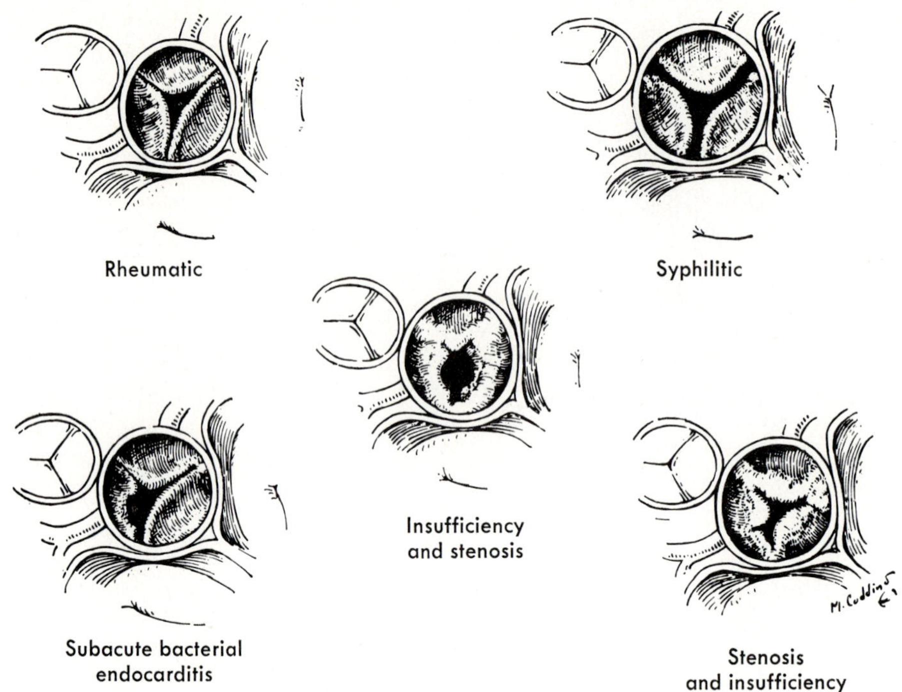

Fig. 18-25. Diagram showing pathological patterns of aortic insufficiency. (From Blades, B., editor: surgical diseases of the chest, ed. 3, St. Louis, 1974, The C.V. Mosby Co.)

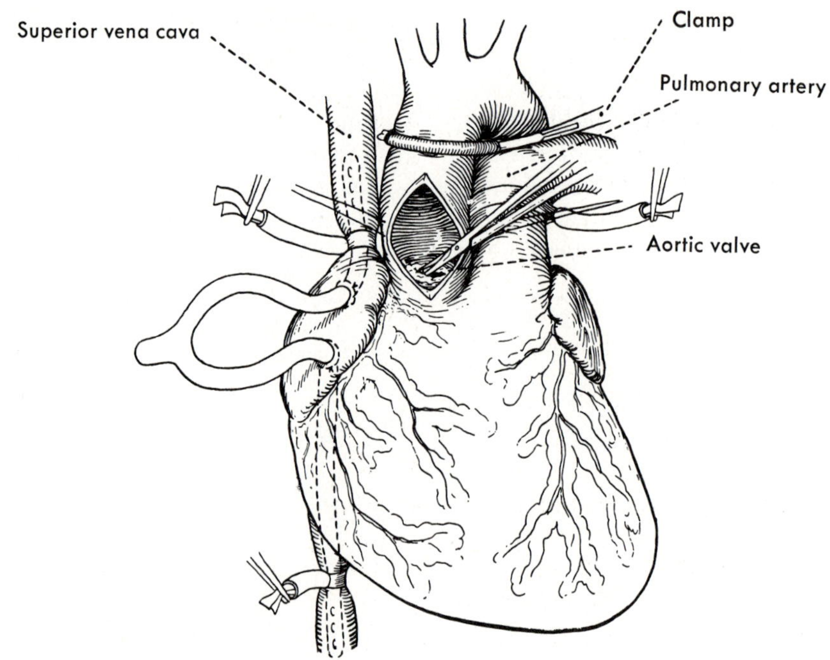

Fig. 18-26. Technique of open aortic valvulotomy. Scissors are used to open fused commissures. Compression tapes are shown around both venae cavae and pulmonary artery. Aorta is cross-clamped. (From Holswade, G.R., and Arditi, L.I.: The diagnosis and surgical correction of aortic stenosis, Surg. Clin. North Am. **41**:463, 1961.)

sures is completed by sharp dissection, if indicated (Fig. 18-26). Calcium deposits are removed as carefully as possible to prevent damage to underlying structures and permit mobilization of the leaflets. Narrow packing may be used in the left ventricle to confine small, loose, calcified fragments that could subsequently embolize.

4B. The valve is inspected; the pathological condition is confirmed. Total excision of the valve is completed. The proper size of prosthesis is selected. Insertion is completed by a technique similar to that previously described for mitral valve replacement (Fig. 18-27).

5. The left side of the heart is flushed to remove air, and the aortotomy is closed with nonabsorbable suture. The aortic clamp is removed, and rewarming of the heart is begun.

6. The venting catheter is removed from the left atrium or ventricle.

7. Cardiopulmonary bypass is discontinued, and the sternum closed as described.

Thoracic aortic aneurysmectomy

Definition. Excision of an aneurysmic portion of the thoracic aorta and replacement with a prosthetic graft.

Considerations. Obliterative arterial disease is the most common cause of death in the United States. Two important acquired pathological conditions may be found, together or separately. The term *atherosclerosis* refers to a lesion of large and medium sized arteries, with deposits in the intima of yellowish plaques containing cholesterol, lipoid material, and lipophages. *Arteriosclerosis* is defined as a condition marked by loss of elasticity, thickening, and hardening of the arteries. Further degeneration and destruction may lead to aneurysm formation. Any artery may become involved. Surgical intervention becomes necessary when the presenting symptoms indicate a compromise in circulation or danger of rupture of an aneurysm; however, medical management with hypotensive agents is the preferred initial treatment.

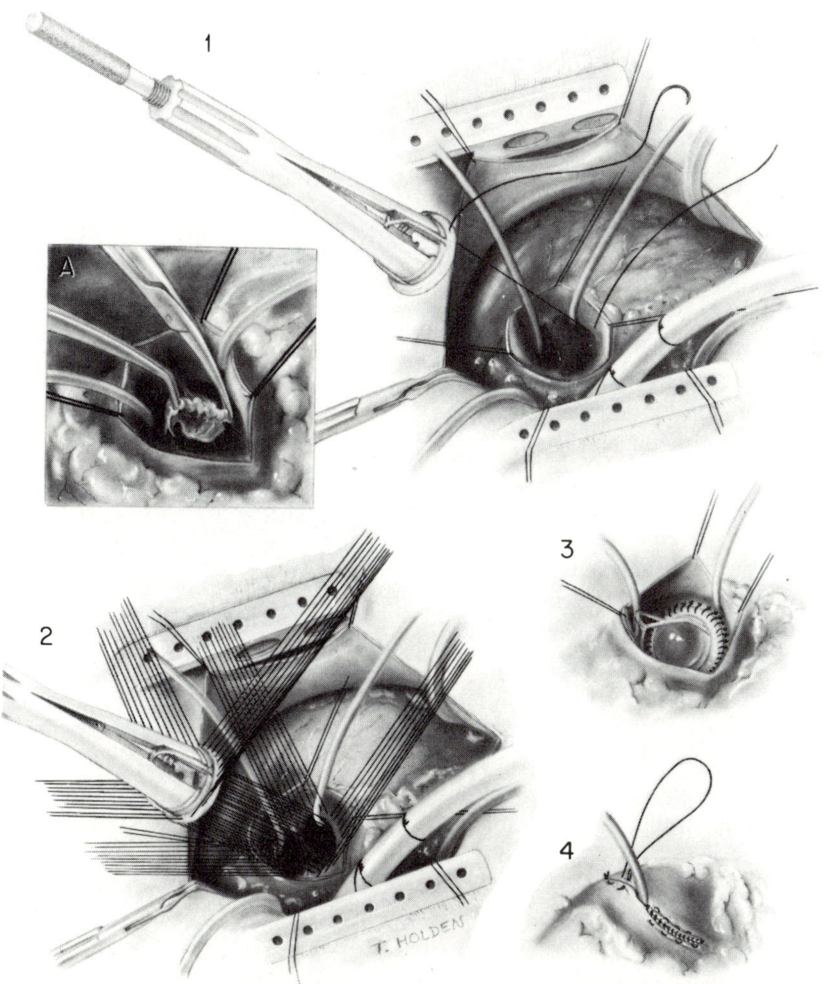

Fig. 18-27. Diseased aortic valve is completely excised, and overlapping fixation sutures are placed before valve is lowered into place. Hollow titanium ball is not replaced until valve chassis is firmly seated. (From Harken, D.E.: Mitral and aortic valve surgery. In Cooper, P., editor: Craft of surgery, ed. 2, Boston, 1971, Little, Brown & Co.)

Aneurysms may be caused by atherosclerosis, arteriosclerosis, trauma, or infection. The congenital type is very uncommon and usually associated with other anomalies. Pathologically, aneurysms can be classified as true or false. The true type usually results from a weakness in the arterial wall, and the sac includes one or all the layers of the artery. The false type usually results from trauma, with development of a hematoma, which increases in size and eventually becomes a well-organized, pulsating blood clot.

Aneurysms are also categorized morphologically as follows: (a) saccular—a sac type of formation with a narrowed neck projecting from the side of the artery, (2) fusiform—a spindle-shaped formation with complete circumferential involvement of the artery, and (3) dissecting—a splitting of the intima of the aorta, permitting blood to pass between the layers of the wall to form a false channel; as the channel extends and enlarges, the blood flow is obstructed.

Setup and preparation of the patient. The patient is positioned for either a median sternotomy or a left posterolateral thoracotomy. The setup is as described for open heart surgery, plus available assorted sizes of grafts and shunt devices.

The shunt is used to divert the flow of arterial blood around the aneurysm. It is inserted in the aorta, proximal and distal to the aneurysm.

Operative procedure. Several methods of surgical treatment are available, including replacement of the root and ascending aorta and aortic valve or reinforcement of the aneurysm by wrapping it.

A recently developed device is being used in a limited number of procedures. It consists of a woven Dacron intraluminal prosthesis with rigid rings at either end. The prosthesis is placed in the true aortic lumen, and the aortic wall is ligated at each end around the rings.

Circumferential suturing of the proximal area of dissection is performed.

Aortic valve replacement in conjunction with resection of the aneurysmal portion of the aortic root may occasionally be performed. This necessitates reimplantation of the coronary arteries into the prosthetic graft.

Various types of cardiopulmonary bypasses can be performed for these operative procedures, if a shunt cannot be used. These include total bypass, femoral artery partial bypass, and left heart bypass. The last two allow the heart to maintain perfusion to the systemic arteries proximal to the aneurysm.

Operations for coronary artery disease

Definition. Bypass of obstructed portions of coronary arteries, using autologous saphenous veins or an internal mammary artery.

Considerations. Coronary artery disease continues to affect a large segment of the population. Risk factors such as heredity, hypertension, high cholesterol levels, smoking, excessive drinking, and lack of regular aerobic exercise have all been implicated in the formation of atheromatous plaques in the coronary arteries. Coronary bypass surgery can revascularize ischemic areas of the ventricular myocardium and improve function, as well as relieve angina pectoris, but the underlying causes of the disease must still be addressed.

Setup and preparation of the patient. The patient is placed in a supine position. The instrument setup is as described for open heart surgery, plus coronary artery instruments (Fig. 18-28).

Operative procedures

Aortocoronary saphenous vein bypass (Fig. 18-29)

1. A median sternotomy is performed as described and the necessary length of saphenous vein is harvested from one or both legs.
2. The distal end of the vein is identified to place the vein in a reversed position so that the semilunar valves will not interfere with the flow of blood. The vein is kept in heparinized blood.
3. The aortic anastomosis of the vein can be performed before or after the coronary anastomosis and can be done with or without the aid of cardiopulmonary bypass.
4. Cardiopulmonary bypass is instituted, as previously described. Usually, mild to moderate hypothermia is employed.

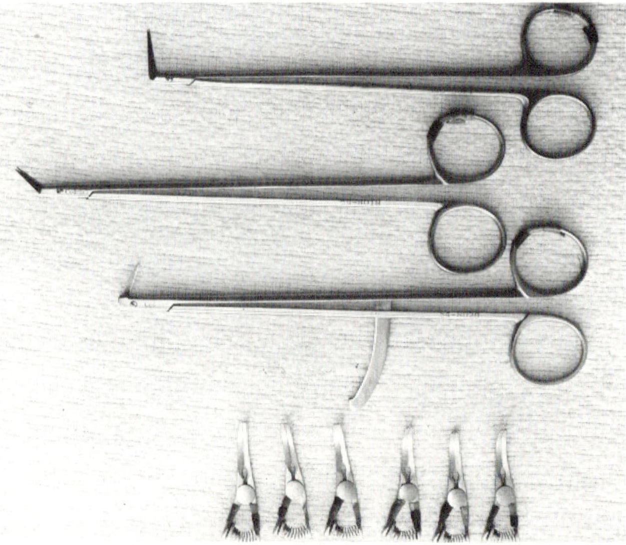

Fig. 18-28. Diethrich coronary artery instruments.

5. Aortic anastomosis

a. The aorta is partially occluded with an angled vascular clamp, such as a Beck, Reynolds, or Cooley clamp, and a small segment is resected, approximately the diameter of the vein graft.

b. The vein is anastomosed, end to side, to the aorta with fine vascular sutures (Fig. 18-30). If this anastomosis is performed before the coronary anastomosis, the distal end of the vein is clamped with a small bulldog clamp. Then the partial occlusion clamp is removed, allowing the proximal portion of the vein to fill with blood.

6. Coronary anastomosis

a. The aorta is usually cross-clamped. Alternatively, suture tourniquets may be placed proximal and distal to the site of anastomosis to prevent bleeding during suturing, or the aorta may be cross-clamped to accomplish the same purpose.

b. A small incision is made into the coronary artery, and the vein is beveled to approximate the incision.

c. The anastomosis is made with fine cardiovascular suture. Before the anastomosis is completed, the distal coronary artery may be probed to ensure patency.

d. If the coronary anastomosis is performed before the aortic anastomosis, a small bulldog clamp is placed on the proximal portion of the vein prior to reestablishing blood flow through the coronary artery.

7. The aortic anastomoses of the vein grafts are usually marked with clips or rings for future identification.

8. Cardiopulmonary bypass is discontinued, and the sternum is closed as described.

Internal mammary artery bypass (Fig. 18-31)

1. A median sternotomy is performed.

2. A special retractor, such as the Favallaro retractor, can be used to expose the internal mammary artery. It is dissected, subcostally, until the necessary length is obtained. Clips are used for hemostasis.

3. The anastomosis of the internal mammary artery to the coronary artery is done on cardiopulmonary bypass and in the same manner as described for the anastomosis of the saphenous vein graft to the coronary artery. No aortic anastomosis is required, since the internal mammary artery remains intact at its takeoff from the subclavian artery.

4. The remainder of the procedure is as described for a saphenous vein graft.

Pulmonary embolectomy

Definition. Opening of the pulmonary artery and removal of the emboli. This procedure is being performed with less frequency, since the preferred method of treatment at this time is with intravenous heparin. Enzyme thrombolyzing agents may also be used.

Setup and preparation of the patient. The patient is placed in the supine position. The preferred method of pulmonary embolectomy requires the use of cardiopulmonary bypass. Setup is as described for open heart procedures, plus Fogarty embolectomy catheters.

Operative procedure. The patient may be placed on cardiopulmonary bypass as an emergency procedure. This may be done by way of a femoral vein–femoral artery partial bypass before performing the median sternotomy, if the patient is in circulatory collapse.

A median sternotomy is performed, and the partial bypass is converted to total bypass. The aorta is cross-clamped, the pulmonary artery is opened, and the emboli are removed. Fogarty catheters may be used. The artery is then closed, and the aortic clamp is removed. Cardiopulmonary bypass is terminated, and the sternum is closed as described previously.

Ventricular aneurysmectomy

Definition. Excision of an aneurysmic portion of the left ventricle and reinforcement with synthetic patch material.

Considerations. An aneurysm of the left ventricle occasionally develops after a severe myocardial infarction in which part of the myocardium is replaced by thin scar tissue. The scar may stretch as a result of the left ventricular pressure, thus forming an aneurysm. The aneurysm is usually adherent to the pericardium, and it may not be possible to dissect it free until cardiopulmonary bypass has been established.

Setup and preparation of the patient. The patient is placed in the supine position. The setup is as described for open heart surgery, plus Teflon felt pledgets and no. 0 cardiovascular sutures on a large needle.

Operative procedure

1. A median sternotomy is performed, and cardiopulmonary bypass is begun as described.

2. The scar tissue of the ventricle is excised and any clot removed carefully.

3. A cuff of scar tissue is left, through which heavy cardiovascular sutures reinforced with Teflon felt pledgets are passed.

4. Cardiopulmonary bypass is discontinued, and the sternum closed as described.

Heart transplantation (Fig. 18-32)

Considerations. Cardiac transplantation is now a clinical reality; its therapeutic value will be tested by the passage of time. Transplantation of the heart has been surgically feasible since 1960, when the surgical method was developed. Important considerations are "recipient" selection and the immune response.

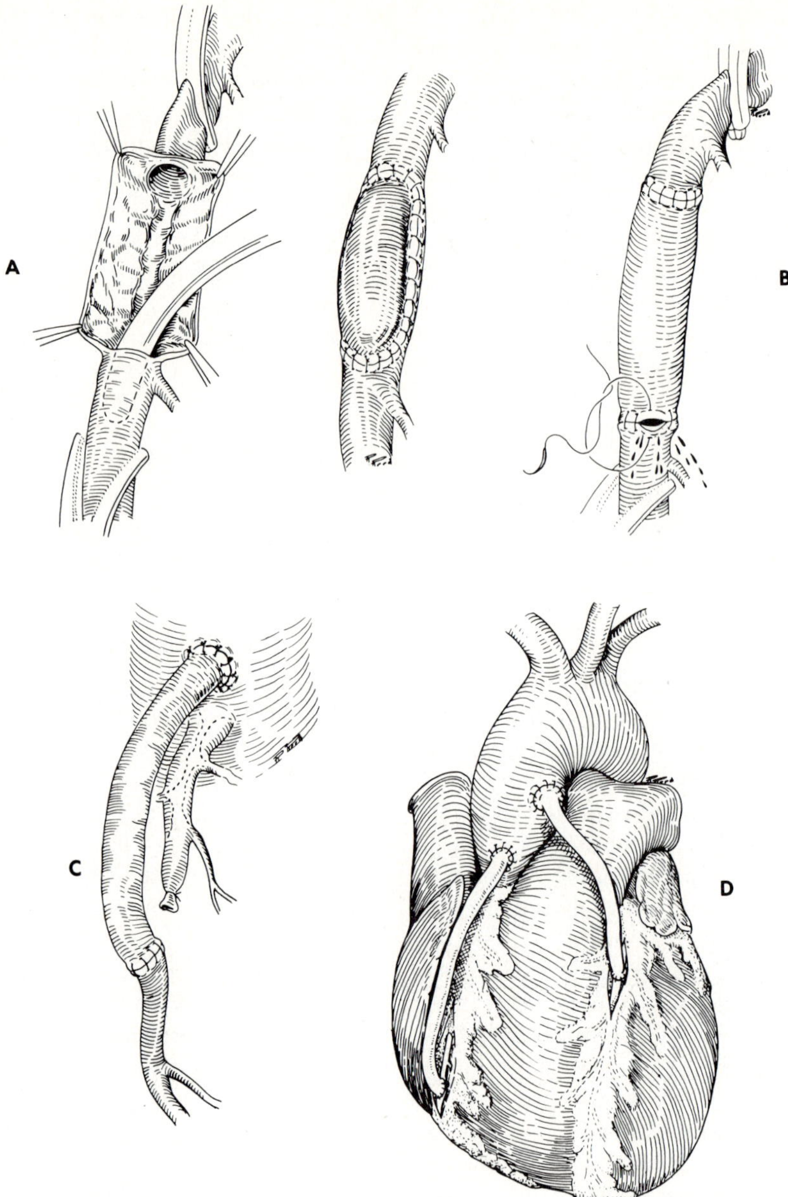

Fig. 18-29. Current form of venous autograft. Aortocoronary bypass graft can reach any of the three major coronary vessels. (From Blades, B., editor: Surgical diseases of the chest, ed. 3, St. Louis, 1974, The C.V. Mosby Co.)

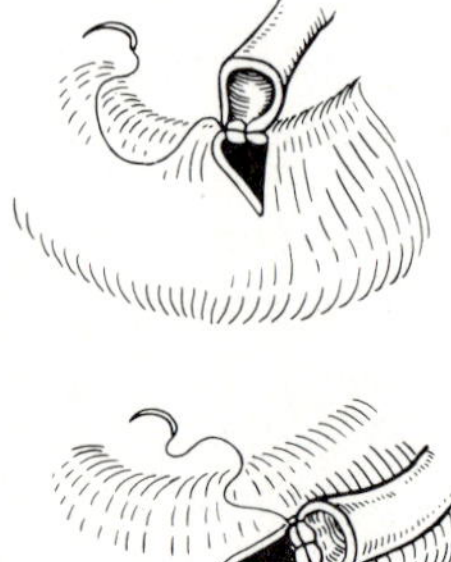

Fig. 18-30. Proximal or aortic anastomosis. Triangular wedge of aortic wall has been excised. Graft is sutured into aorta by interrupted or continuous suturing technique. Strictures at aortic ostium are virtually eliminated when segment of wall is removed. (From Blades, B., editor: Surgical diseases of the chest, ed. 3, St. Louis, 1974, The C.V. Mosby Co.)

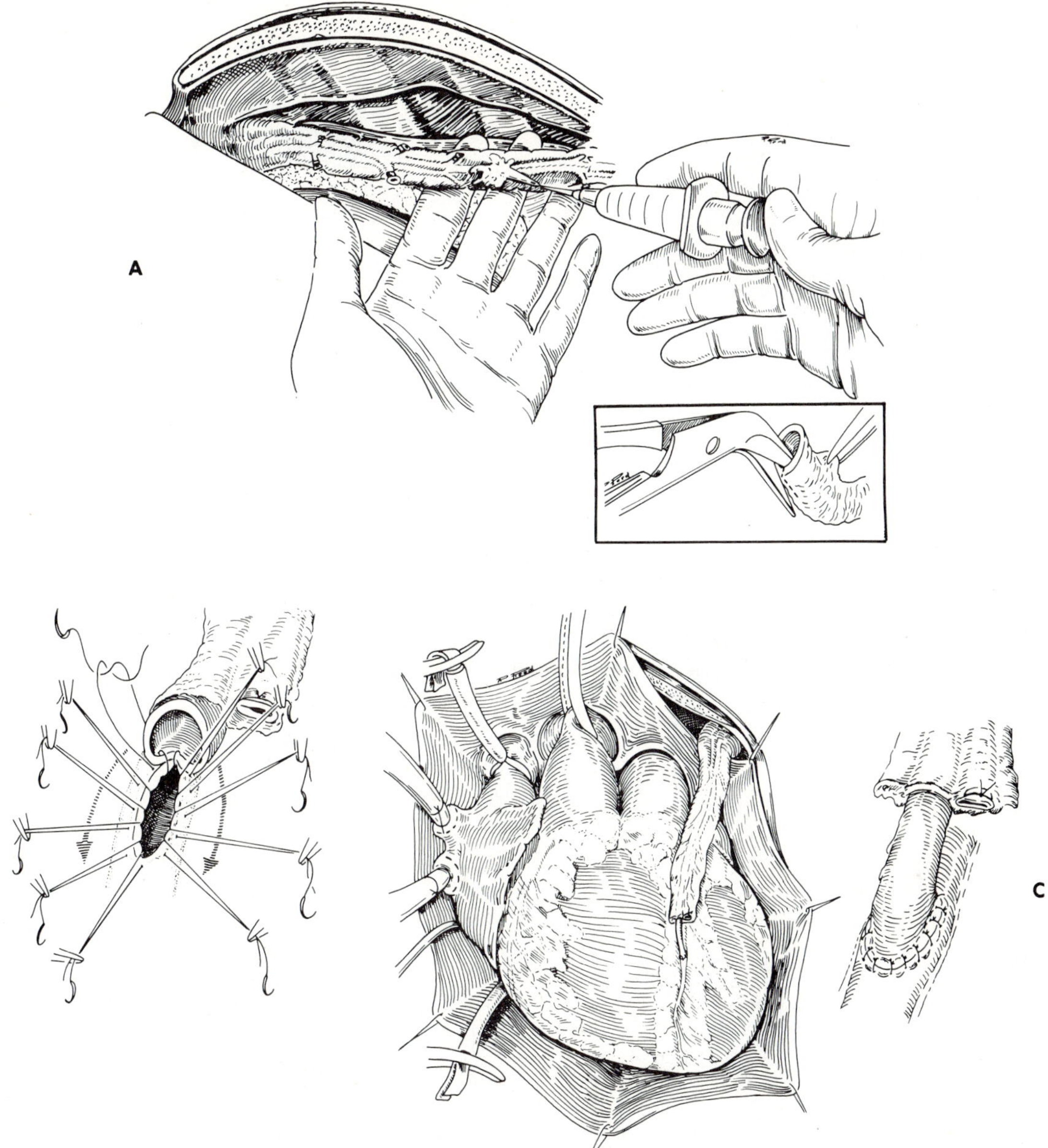

Fig. 18-31. Internal mammary artery–coronary artery anastomosis. **A,** Left IMA is dissected from chest wall as pedicle containing mammary vein. Mobilizing artery in this manner is extremely safe, and side branches are controlled by stainless steel clips. Dilute solution of papaverine is sprayed vigorously into adventitia to effect dilatation of small artery. Pedicle is then wrapped in gauze soaked with papaverine and stored until pump cannulation is performed. *Inset,* Iris scissors are used to divide isolated IMA and slit inferior wall. **B,** End-to-side anastomosis is constructed by interrupted 7-0 silk technique, inserting and tying each suture before next one is placed. This technique allows clear visualization of intimal suture line as grafting progresses. **C,** Artist's conception of left IMA graft to anterior descending branch of left coronary artery. Grafting is performed without any dissection or mobilization of coronary artery. (From Blades, B., editor: Surgical diseases of the chest, ed. 3, St. Louis, 1974, The C.V. Mosby Co.)

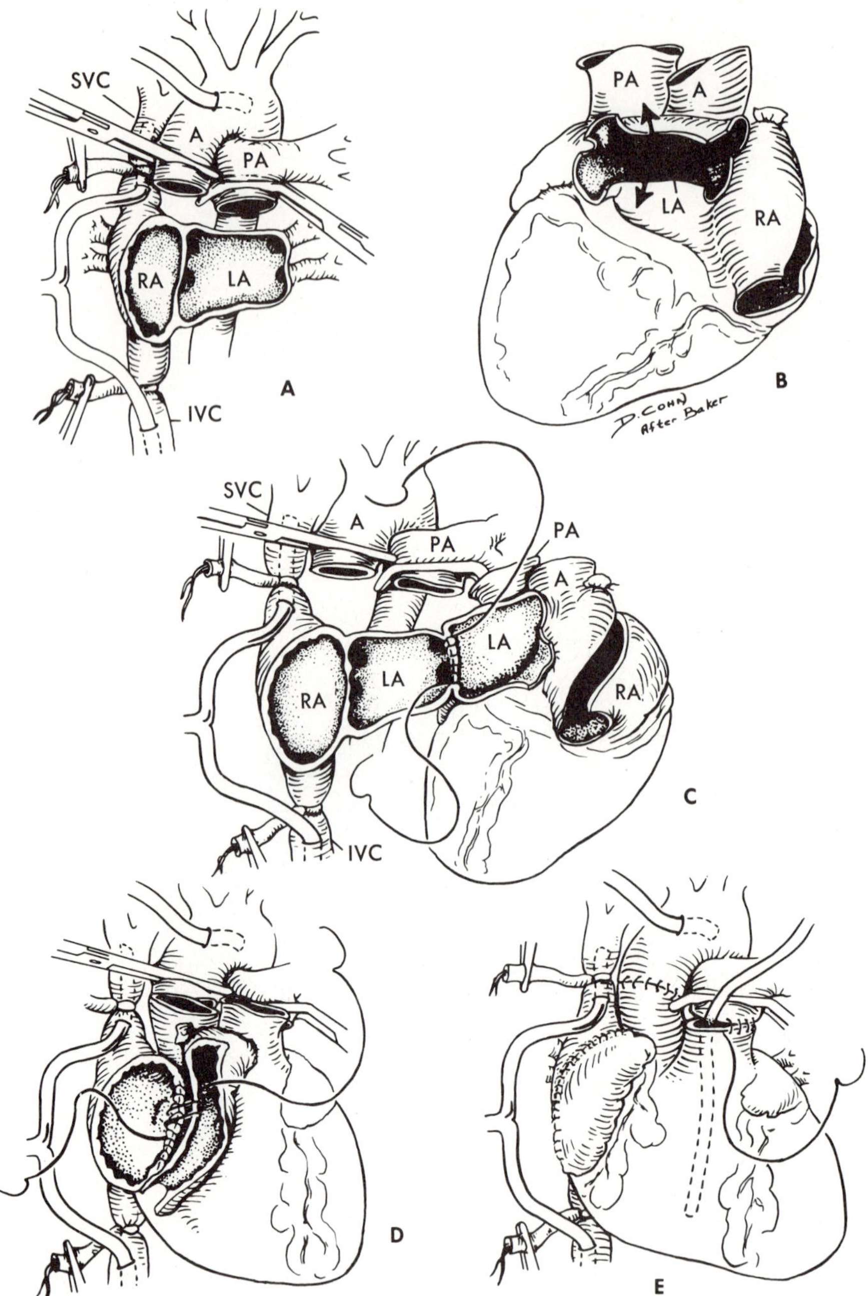

Fig. 18-32. A, Diagram of remaining cuff of recipient heart. Venae cavae and aorta are cannulated in chest to avoid additional incisions, which add to possibility of infection. **B,** Diagram of posterior surface of donor heart. Left atrium is opened through pulmonary veins, and excess removed. Superior vena cava is started on lateral aspect of left atria. **D,** Right atria are then sutured. This technique avoids interatrial tracts. **E,** Aortas are anastomosed first so that coronary circulation can be reestablished. Pulmonary arteries are joined last, and all air is carefully removed from heart. Cardiopulmonary bypass support is weaned off as function is restored. Support with cardiotonic agents is often required temporarily. (From Effler, D.B.: Blades' surgical diseases of the chest, ed. 4, St. Louis, 1978, The C.V. Mosby Co.)

Setup and preparation of the patient. Two individual cardiopulmonary bypass and instrument setups are necessary. The preparation of the operative site and routine draping procedures are carried out as described earlier for open heart procedures.

Operative procedure

Donor heart. Resuscitation of the donor heart is mandatory before proceeding with the recipient. The donor is placed on extracorporeal circulation, as soon after pronouncement of death as possible. The heart is emptied by constricting the venae cavae. The aorta and pulmonary artery are clamped with noncrushing clamps. The venae cavae and pulmonary veins are dissected and transected individually where they enter the atrium. The aorta and pulmonary artery are transected distal to the valves. The donor heart is immediately placed in cold saline solution.

Recipient heart. The recipient is placed on extracorporeal bypass in the usual manner, or peripheral venous cannulation of the venae cavae is achieved by means of the right internal jugular and left common femoral veins. The pulmonary trunk and aorta are dissected immediately above their respective semilunar valves; the atria are incised in such a way as to leave intact portions of the right and left atrial walls and the atrial septum of the recipient. The recipient heart is then removed.

The donor heart is placed in the pericardial well. The interatrial septum and the left and then the right atrial walls are approximated with running cardiovascular sutures. The donor and recipient aortas are similarly joined. Air is removed from the left side of the heart.

The aortic clamp is removed, and a clamp is placed across the donor pulmonary artery. The caval tape is removed, and vigorous ventricular fibrillation of the donor heart commences. Local cooling of the heart is discontinued at this point, and, before the pulmonary artery is sutured, all atrial suture lines are carefully inspected for significant bleeding areas. The pulmonary arteries are united, and the clamp removed. Defibrillation of the ventricles is usually effected by means of a single DC shock. A needle hole is established at the apex of the ascending aorta, so that residual air is expelled. The patient is then removed from extracorporeal bypass after a period of partial bypass. Cannulas are removed from the cavae or the peripheral veins. The incisions are closed as described previously.

REPAIR OF CONGENITAL DEFECTS

Repair of an atrial septal defect

Definition. Under direct vision, closing of a congenital defect in the atrial septum by a simple suture technique or by the insertion of a synthetic prosthetic patch or pericardial patch.

Considerations. An atrial septal defect is a common congenital abnormality, and its classification is based on anatomical location and associated abnormalities (Figs. 18-33 and 18-34).

The *ostium secundum defect* is located in the superior and central portion of the septum. The *ostium primum defect* is located in the lower portion of the atrial septum and is associated with other defects in the atrioventricular canal, usually with a cleft of the mitral valve or occasionally of the tricuspid valve. An accompanying ventricular septal defect may also be present.

An atrial septal defect results in a left-to-right atrial shunt that may be well tolerated in early life if the opening is small. However, if the defect is large or of the ostium primum type, with a marked shunting of blood, the work load of the right side of the heart is increased. The right side of the heart and the pulmonary artery and its branches become enlarged. The vascularity of the lung field is increased, with resulting pulmonary hypertension and subsequent failure of the right side of the heart. At this point the shunt may reverse.

In early life the patient may be asymptomatic. Beginning symptoms may include fatigue, retardation of normal weight gain, and increased susceptibility to respiratory infections. Later symptoms include those of failure of the right side of the heart and cyanosis with a reverse shunt.

A systolic murmur is heard with greatest intensity over the base of the heart.

Setup and preparation of the patient. The patient is placed in the supine position for a median sternotomy or in a right anterior oblique position for an anterolateral thoracotomy.

The instrument setup is as described for basic open heart surgery, with consideration given to the age and size of the patient, plus intracardiac patch material, 2 × 2 inches or larger.

Operative procedure

1. A right anterolateral or median sternotomy incision is performed, and cardiopulmonary bypass begun as described.
2. The right atrium is incised, and the pathological defect determined.
3. The defect is closed with a continuous suture, or a patch of pericardium or prosthetic material may be used. By filling the atrium with blood before the atriotomy is completely closed, air can be expressed from the atrium.

   For the ostium primum defect with a cleft mitral valve, repair of the cleft is accomplished by approximation, using interrupted sutures.
4. Cardiopulmonary bypass is discontinued, and the chest closed as described.

Repair of a ventricular septal defect

Definition. Under direct vision, closing of a congenital defect in the ventricular septum by a simple suture technique or, in most instances, by the insertion of a synthetic prosthetic or pericardial patch (Figs. 18-35 and 18-36).

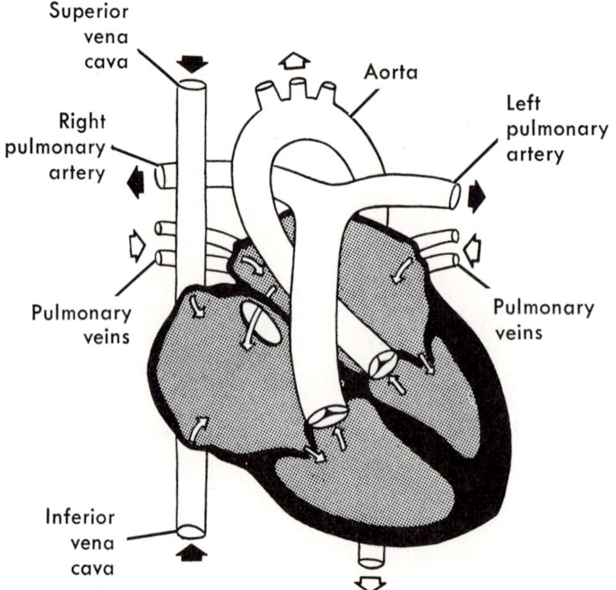

Fig. 18-33. Atrial septal defects. Abnormal opening between right and left atria. Incompetent foramen ovale, high ostium secundum defect, and ostium primum defect usually involve atrioventricular valves. (From Nursing Education Service: General signs and symptoms of congenital heart abnormalities, Columbus, Ohio, Ross Laboratories.)

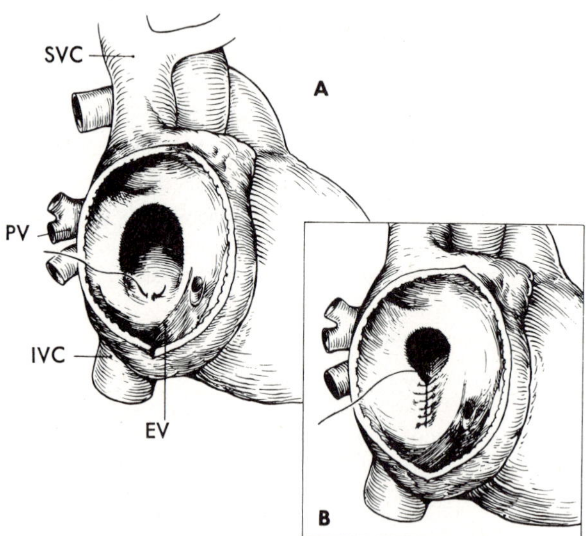

Fig. 18-34. Closure of usual ostium secundum atrial septal defect with simple running stitch. **A,** Suture must be started well to left atrial side at inferior portion of defect, to avoid including eustachian valve (*EV*) if present. If suture is started in eustachian valve, resulting closure will transpose inferior vena cava (*IVC*) to left atrium. *SVC,* Superior vena cava; *PV* pulmonary vein. **B,** Suture line being completed. (From Effler, D.B.: Blades' surgical diseases of the chest, ed. 4, St. Louis, 1978, The C.V. Mosby Co.)

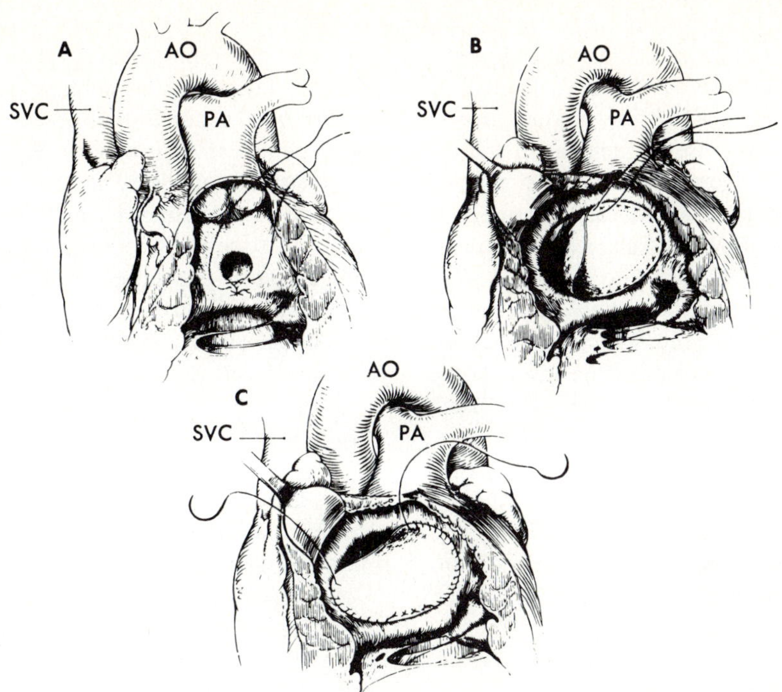

Fig. 18-35. Techniques for closing ventricular septal defects. **A,** Simple interrupted suture may be used if defect is small and has fibrous margins. **B,** Patch closure of ventricular septal defect with interrupted mattress sutures. **C,** Patch closure of ventricular septal defect using interrupted sutures at bottom of defect and continuous suturing technique for remainder of defect. (From Effler, D.B.: Blades' surgical diseases of the chest, ed. 4, St. Louis, 1978, The C.V. Mosby Co.)

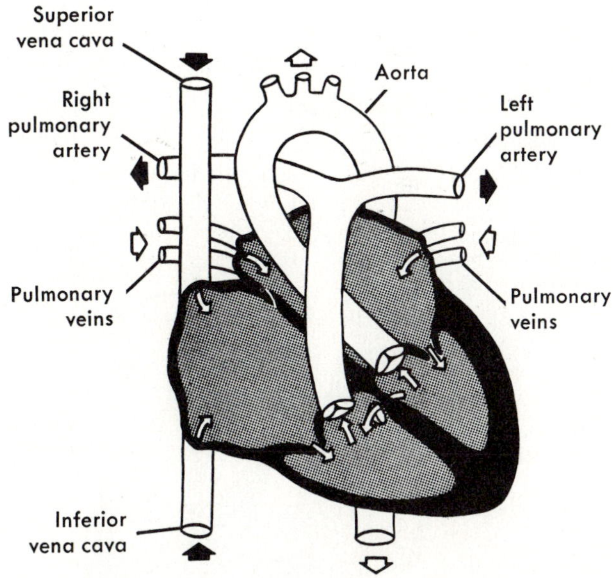

Fig. 18-36. Ventricular septal defects. Abnormal opening between right and left ventricles, which may vary in size and may occur in membranous or muscular portion. (From Nursing Education Service: General signs and symptoms of congenital heart abnormalities, Columbus, Ohio, Ross Laboratories.)

Considerations. One of the most common congenital cardiac anomalies, a ventricular septal defect, if small, is of little physiological importance. The murmur is evident, but the patient is otherwise asymptomatic, and the heart is normal in size. Larger defects with a significant left-to-right shunt, high right ventricular pressure, increased pulmonary blood flow, and enlarged heart are repaired by surgery (Fig. 18-36).

Setup and preparation of the patient. The patient is placed in a supine position. The setup is as described for open heart surgery, with consideration given to the age and the size of the patient, plus intracardiac patch material.

Operative procedure

1. A median sternotomy is performed, and cardiopulmonary bypass begun as described.

2. The right ventricle is opened and the defect is repaired, taking care to avoid damaging branches of the bundle of His.

3. Cardiopulmonary bypass is discontinued, and the sternum closed as described.

Correction of tetralogy of Fallot

General considerations. Tetralogy of Fallot is the most common congenital cardiac anomaly in the cyanotic group. Cyanosis, as seen in the superficial vessels of the skin, is the result of shunting unoxygenated blood into the systemic circulation.

The essential features of this condition are pulmonary stenosis, high ventricular septal defect, and overriding of the septal defect by the aorta, with resulting hypertrophy of the right ventricle—all of which may be subdivided into more complex variations (Fig. 18-37). The *infundibular* form of pulmonary stenosis is a long localized constricture in the pulmonary outflow tract of the right ventricle. It is the most common type of this anomaly. *Valvular stenosis* and infundibular stenosis, however, may occur independently.

Physiologically, in tetralogy of Fallot, blood flow into the lungs decreases as a result of pulmonary obstruction, and a right-to-left shunt of venous blood from the right ventricle to the left ventricle and aorta occurs.

Symptoms of tetralogy are cyanosis, dyspnea, episodes of acute dyspnea, retarded growth, clubbing of extremities, and reduced exercise tolerance. A systolic murmur and secondary polycythemia are usually present. Cardiac catheterization and angiocardiography aid in determining the diagnosis and plan of surgical treatment.

The selection of a *closed* palliative or *open* corrective procedure is based on the age and general condition of the patient and the severity of the pulmonary stenosis.

Shunt for palliation (closed procedure)

Definition. One of several closed palliative procedures designed to divert poorly oxygenated blood from one of the major arteries back through one of the pulmonary arteries to the lungs for reoxygenation, thereby increasing the total blood flow in the pulmonary circulation.

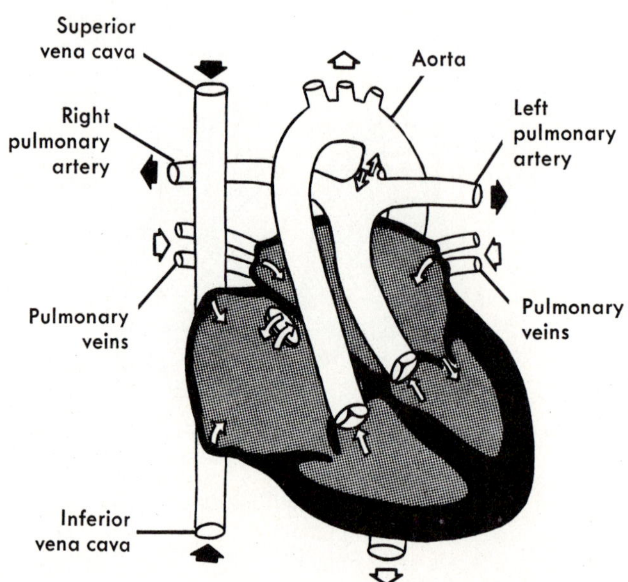

Fig. 18-37. Tetralogy of Fallot is characterized by combination of four defects: pulmonary stenosis, ventricular septal defect, overriding aorta, and hypertrophy of right ventricle. (From Nursing Education Service: General signs and symptoms of congenital heart abnormalities, Columbus, Ohio, Ross Laboratories.)

The *Blalock-Taussig procedure* consists of an end-to-side anastomosis between the proximal end of the subclavian and pulmonary arteries. The procedure is performed on the side opposite the aortic arch. This shunt may be dismantled or ligated if a future operation for full correction is anticipated; however, the shunt has a tendency to reduce in size as the child grows.

The *Potts-Smith procedure* consists of a side-to-side anastomosis directly between the aorta and left pulmonary artery. This procedure may be selected for infants because the size of the anastomosis is not limited by the lumen of the subclavian artery, as it is in the Blalock technique. However, it is more difficult to dismantle if future surgery is anticipated.

The *Waterston procedure* consists of anastomosis of the ascending aorta and the right pulmonary artery. It is the preferred procedure when a systemic-pulmonary artery anastomosis is needed within the first several months of life.

The *Glenn procedure* consists of anastomosis of the superior vena cava to the right pulmonary artery. This operation is employed infrequently in the treatment of tetralogy of Fallot.

Setup and preparation of the patient. The patient is placed in the selected position for the specific procedure. Instruments are as previously described for closed heart surgery, plus the following, with appropriate sizes for infants and children:

2 Potts-Smith aortic occlusion clamps
2 Johns Hopkins modified Potts clamps
2 Hendrin ductus clamps
2 Cooley anastomosis clamps

Operative procedures (Fig. 18-38)

Blalock-Taussig procedure

1. An anterolateral incision is made from the sternal margin to the midaxillary line. The chest cavity is opened and the lung retracted, as previously described.

2. The mediastinal pleura is incised and retracted with a stay suture.

3. The pulmonary artery is dissected from the surrounding tissue, with vascular forceps, dry dissector sponges, and Metzenbaum scissors. As the artery and branches are mobilized, heavy ligatures, moistened umbilical tapes, or fine silicone tubing is placed about them.

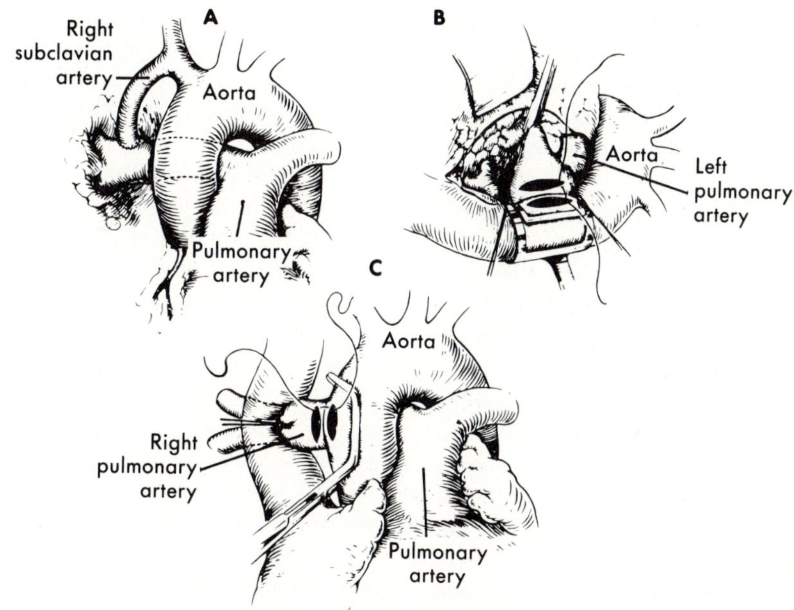

Fig. 18-38. Systemic artery–pulmonary artery shunt operations are designed to increase pulmonary blood flow **A,** Blalock-Taussig operation. Right subclavian artery is dissected free, divided, turned down, and anastomosed to right pulmonary artery, end to side. This operation is accomplished through right lateral thoracotomy. **B,** Potts-Smith anastomosis is primarily of historical interest. This operation, done through left posterolateral thoracotomy, consists of side-to-side anastomosis between descending aorta and left pulmonary artery. **C,** Cooley modification of Waterston anastomosis. Shunt consists of side-to-side anastomosis between ascending aorta and right pulmonary artery. This may be accomplished through pericardium via anterior right thoracotomy. Operation also may be performed, as initially described, by right posterolateral thoracotomy with anastomosis constructed posterior to superior vena cava. (From Effler, D.B.: Blades' surgical diseases of the chest, ed. 4, St. Louis, 1978, The C.V. Mosby Co.)

4. Branches of the vagus nerve are protected and retracted.

5. The subclavian artery is dissected completely from its origin to where it produces the internal mammary and costocervical branches. Its distal end is marked with a silk suture.

6. The subclavian artery is occluded with a vascular clamp, a ligature is placed at the distal segment, and the vessel is divided.

7. The pulmonary artery is occluded temporarily by application of a curved vascular clamp.

8. An incision of sufficient size to accommodate the subclavian artery is made with a no. 11 knife blade and Potts scissors.

9. An end-to-side anastomosis is completed with cardiovascular suture.

10. The clamps are released, and the suture line is inspected for hemostasis.

11. The mediastinal pleura is closed.

12. Closed chest drainage is established, and the chest wound is closed as previously described (Chapter 17).

Potts-Smith procedure. A left posterolateral incision is made in the fourth intercostal space. The pulmonary artery is dissected from its surrounding tissue, and the descending aorta is mobilized. Occluding tapes and Blalock or Potts-Smith clamps are applied. A longitudinal incision is made in each artery, and a side-to-side anastomosis is completed with cardiovascular sutures. The pulmonary artery is released, and the suture line is inspected for hemostasis. The aortic clamps are then removed.

Waterston procedure. A right anterolateral incision is made in the fourth interspace. The pericardium is opened, and the ascending aorta is exposed. The right pulmonary artery is dissected as it passes beneath the ascending aorta. A heavy suture is passed around the right pulmonary artery and is used to temporarily occlude the artery. A curved vascular clamp is placed so that one blade is behind the pulmonary artery and the other occludes a posterolateral portion of the ascending aorta. On closure of the clamp, both the right pulmonary artery and a posterior portion of the ascending aorta are occluded. Parallel incisions are made in both the aorta and the right pulmonary artery. An anastomosis is then made between the ascending aorta and right pulmonary artery.

Glenn procedure. A right anterolateral incision is made in the fourth intercostal space. The pericardium is opened, the right pulmonary artery is dissected, and tapes are placed around the proximal and distal ends of the right pulmonary artery. The right pulmonary artery is clamped with two straight Cooley clamps and divided medial to the vena cava, and its proximal end is oversewn with cardiovascular suture. Then a curved Cooley clamp is placed on the superior vena cava. A circular section is excised from the superior vena cava, and the distal end of the pulmonary artery is anastomosed to the vena cava with cardiovascular suture. The superior vena cava between the anastomosis and the right atrium is ligated, as is the azygos vein.

Open corrective procedure

Definition. Under direct vision, complete repair of the infundibular stenosis or pulmonary valve stenosis and closure of the ventricular septal defect.

Setup and preparation of the patient. The patient is placed on the operating table in a supine position. The setup is as described for open heart surgery, with consideration given to the age and size of the patient. Additional items to be added to the basic open heart setup include the following:

1 Intracardiac patch, 2 × 2 inches
1 Outflow cardiac patch, 2 × 2 inches
1 Felt patch, 4 × 4 inches

Operative procedure

1. A median sternotomy is performed, and cardiopulmonary bypass begun as described.

2. A vertical ventriculotomy over the infundibular area is performed (Fig. 18-39).

3. The ventricular septal defect is identified. Closure requires an intracardiac patch in almost all instances. This can be of a synthetic material or a piece of pericardium.

4. The hypertrophied infundibular muscle is excised, as completely as possible, from the right ventricular outflow tract.

5. Interrupted or continuous cardiovascular sutures are placed in the septum with caution because of the danger of suturing a branch of the neuroconductive system.

6. After closure of the ventricular septal defect, an estimate is made whether the right ventricle can be closed primarily or whether a patch is necessary. If the pulmonic stenosis cannot be relieved adequately by valvulotomy and infundibulectomy, an outflow patch may be needed to enlarge the outflow tract. If the pulmonary artery or valve annulus is quite small, it may be necessary to extend the patch across the valve ring to the proximal portion of the pulmonary artery.

7. Cardiopulmonary bypass is discontinued, and the sternum closed as described.

Operation for tricuspid atresia

Absence of communication between the right atrium and right ventricle is always accompanied by a second defect, an atrial septal defect or a patent foramen ovale, that sustains life. Other abnormalities are also present (Fig. 18-40). The infant displays cyanosis, periods of dyspnea, easy fatigability, and growth retardation. Congestive failure progresses rapidly.

Palliative operations consist of the Blalock-Hanlon procedure, which enlarges the atrial septal defect, or anas-

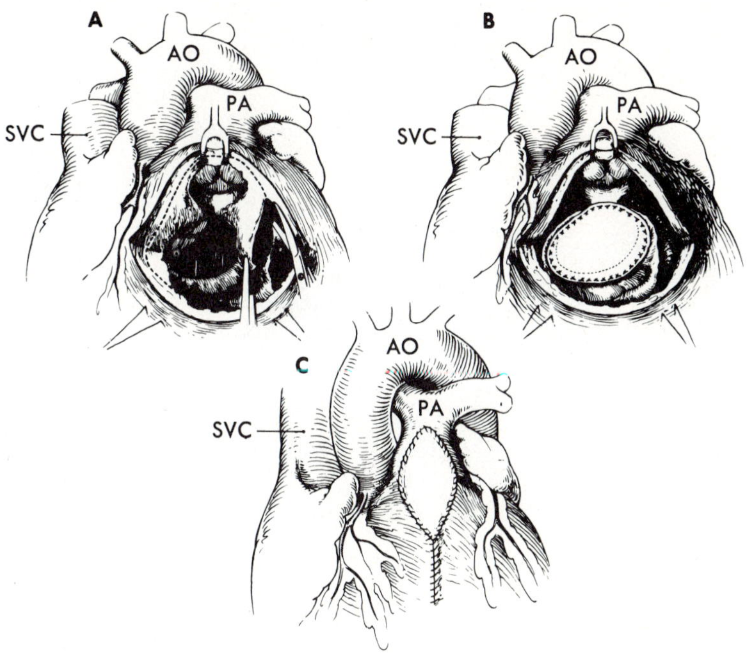

Fig. 18-39. Operation for correction of tetralogy of Fallot. **A,** Infundibulectomy or removal of outflow tract obstruction to right ventricle by sharp dissection. **B,** Closure of ventricular septal defect. **C,** If pulmonary annulus is too narrow, or if infundibulectomy does not open outflow obstruction adequately, patch in outflow tract may be necessary. (From Effler, D.B.: Blades' surgical diseases of the chest, ed. 4, St. Louis, 1978, The C.V. Mosby Co.)

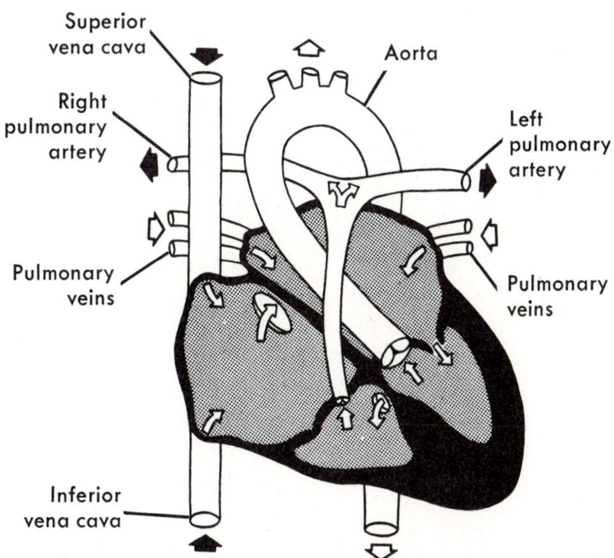

Fig. 18-40. Tricuspid atresia is characterized by small right ventricle, large left ventricle, and diminished pulmonary circulation. Atrial septal or other congenital defect is necessary to sustain life. (From Nursing Education Service: General signs and symptoms of congenital heart abnormalities, Columbus, Ohio, Ross Laboratories.)

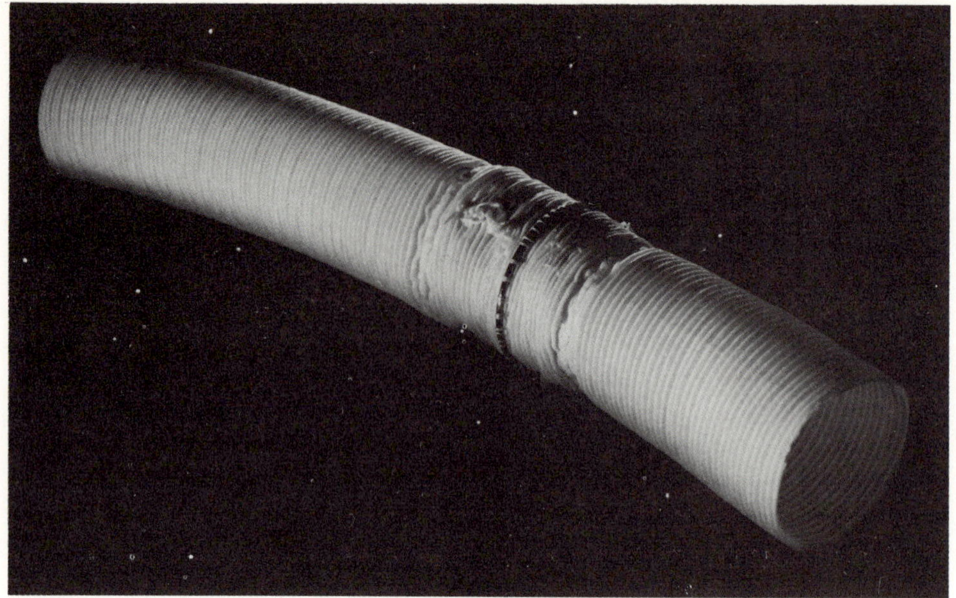

Fig. 18-41. Hancock conduit.

tomotic procedures for shunting the circulation to relieve the cyanosis, including the Blalock-Taussig, Potts-Smith, and Glenn procedures, which have been described previously.

Alternatively, a Fontan procedure may be performed, employing a valved conduit (Fig. 18-41). This allows for redirection of the flow of venous blood from the right atrium to the main pulmonary artery around the atretic tricuspid valve and right ventricle.

Operations for transposition of the great vessels

In this anomaly the aorta arises from the right ventricle and the pulmonary artery from the left ventricle, resulting in reversed circulations (Fig. 18-42). However, to sustain life, there must be a communication between the two sides of the heart or major vessels: a patent foramen ovale, patent ductus arteriosus, atrial septal defect, ventricular septal defect, or partial transposition of the pulmonary veins, which permits oxygenated blood to enter the systemic circulation.

The newborn with this condition is cyanotic at birth and becomes severely incapacitated, with an enlarged heart that rapidly increases in size and progresses to congestive failure.

Corrective procedures for this condition are in the process of refinement and complete evaluation. The Mustard procedure is most commonly performed.

Palliative procedures that tend to improve intracardiac mixing, thereby increasing the oxygen content of the systemic blood, are done to sustain life until the infant has attained sufficient growth to tolerate a long corrective procedure. Palliative procedures include the Blalock-Hanlon and the Rashkind atrial septostomy.

Rashkind atrial septostomy

Definition. Creation of an atrial septal defect to allow mixing of blood.

Considerations. The Rashkind atrial septostomy is performed in the cardiac catheterization laboratory. A balloon-tipped catheter is advanced into the right atrium by way of a peripheral vein and is passed through the foramen ovale into the left atrium. The balloon is then inflated, and the catheter is pulled back into the right atrium, thus creating a large septal defect.

Blalock-Hanlon procedure

Definition. Creation of an opening between the right and left atria at the interatrial groove. Cardiopulmonary bypass is not required.

Setup and preparation of the patient. Similar to shunt operations.

Operative procedure

1. Through a right anterolateral thoracotomy incision, the interatrial groove is exposed.
2. Compression tapes are placed about the right pulmonary artery and the right pulmonary veins.
3. Occlusion of these vessels is completed, and a curved Cooley clamp is applied to include a portion of both the right and left atria.
4. The segment, along with a section of the septum, is excised. The edges of the atrial walls are sutured together. Compression tapes are released.
5. Closure is completed, as previously described.

Mustard procedure

Definition. Under direct vision, the remaining segments of the atrial septum are excised, and a pericardial

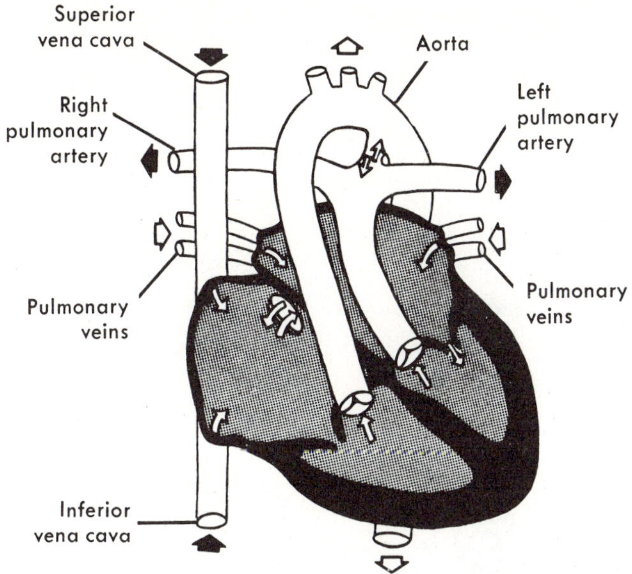

Fig. 18-42. Complete transposition of great vessels produces two separate circulations. Since aorta originates from right ventricle and pulmonary artery from left ventricle, abnormal communication between two chambers must be present to sustain life. (From Nursing Education Service: General signs and symptoms of congenital heart abnormalities, Columbus, Ohio, Ross Laboratories.)

or synthetic patch is sutured in place in the atrial cavities in such a manner that the venous inflow is reversed. This permits the pulmonary venous return to be redirected into the right ventricle and the systemic venous return to be redirected into the left ventricle (Fig. 18-43).

Considerations. Previous creation of an atrial septal defect may serve as a first stage for this procedure. Pericardium or synthetic patch is used as a baffle.

Setup and preparation of the patient. The patient is placed on the operating table in a supine position. The setup is as described for open heart surgery, with consideration given to the age and size of the patient.

Operative procedure

1. A median sternotomy incision is completed as described.
2. A section of pericardium 2 × 3 inches is excised and placed in heparin solution (Fig. 18-43, *A*).
3. Extracorporeal circulation is established as previously described.
4. A curved incision is made in the wall of the right atrium (Fig. 18-43, *B*).
5. The entire atrial septum is excised. The orifice of the coronary sinus is enlarged (Fig. 18-43, *C*).
6. A double-armed suture is placed three fifths of the way along the long margin of the pericardial graft.
7. The pericardial graft or synthetic intracardiac patch is sutured in place, excluding the coronary sinus and the left atrial appendage (Fig. 18-43, *C* and *D*).
8. An additional section of pericardium or synthetic patch is placed in the wall of the right atrium that enlarges the new left atrium.
9. Extracorporeal circulation is discontinued, and closures are completed as previously described.

Open valvulotomy and infundibular resection for pulmonary stenosis

Definition. Separation of the stenosed leaflets under direct vision or resection of the hypertrophied infundibulum.

Setup and preparation of the patient. The patient is placed in the supine position. The basic setup for a sternotomy is used, with consideration given to the age and size of the patient.

Operative procedure

1. A median sternotomy is performed, and the cannulations are made for cardiopulmonary bypass as previously described.

2A. *For open valvulotomy,* the pulmonary artery is opened longitudinally, and the stenotic valve is incised with a scalpel or scissors (Fig. 18-44).

2B. *For infundibular resection,* the outflow tract of the right ventricle is opened, and the resection is performed, as described for tetralogy of Fallot.

Other considerations. Some surgeons use a valved conduit (Fig. 18-41) for the more severe forms of pulmonary stenosis and atresia. The Rastelli procedure involves suturing the conduit to the right ventricle and to the pulmonary artery, thus bypassing the atretic valve.

Closure of patent ductus arteriosus

Definition. Closure of the patent ductus arteriosus, an abnormal communication between the aorta and pulmo-

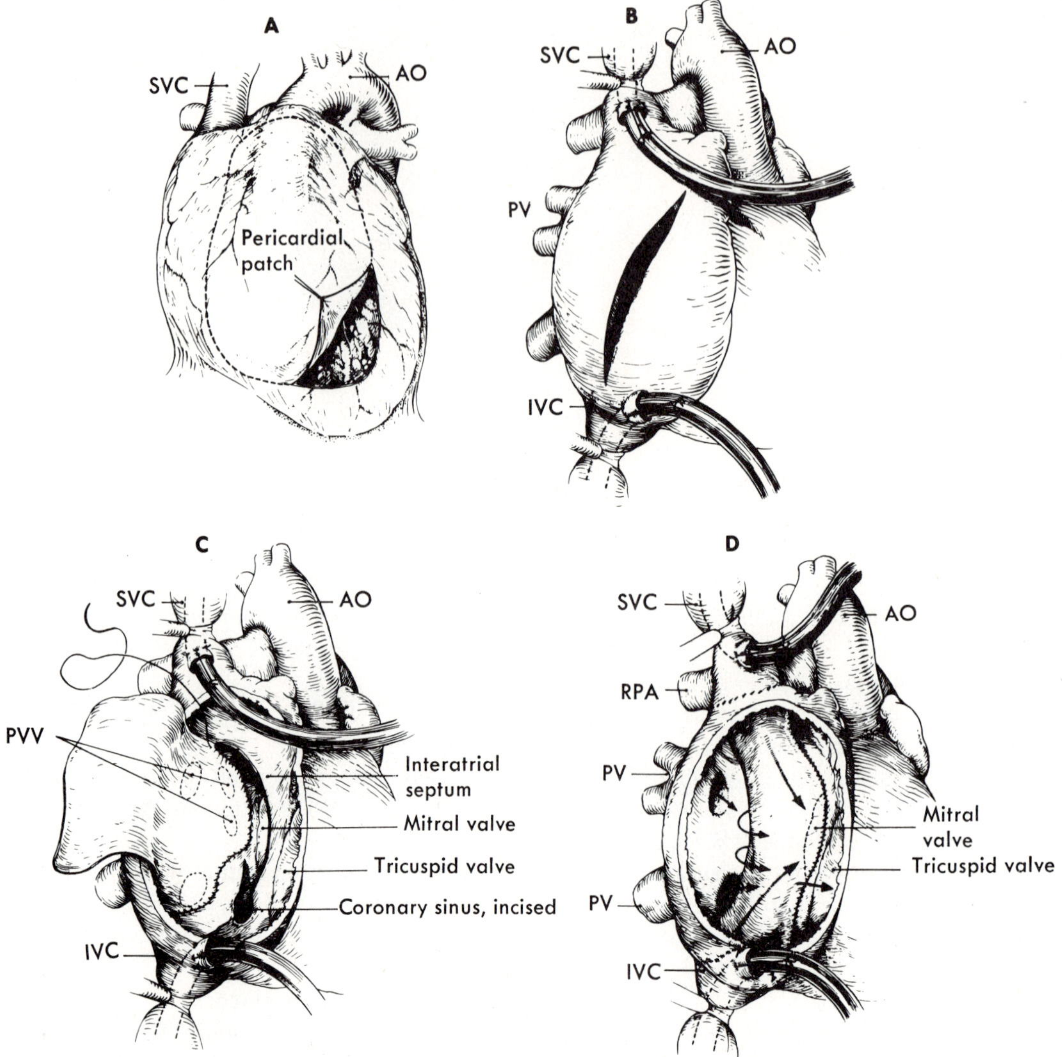

Fig. 18-43. Mustard procedure. **A,** Rectangular patch of pericardium or synthetic material is harvested with its long axis vertically. Length is from diaphragm to reflection onto aorta. Width leaves one comfortably away from phrenic nerves. **B,** Caval cannulas are inserted at junction of venae cavae and right atrium. Superior part of atriotomy goes toward atrial appendage. **C,** Patch is sutured between pulmonary veins and mitral valve, dividing the atrial septal defect in half. Incising the coronary sinus will commit coronary sinus flow into the new systemic venous atrium. **D,** Completed repair. Vena cava flow is now directed to mitral valve, and pulmonary venous blood to tricuspid valve. *SVC,* Superior vena cava; *AO,* aorta; *PV,* pulmonary vein; *IVC,* inferior vena cava; *PVV,* pulmonary veins; *RPA,* right pulmonary artery.

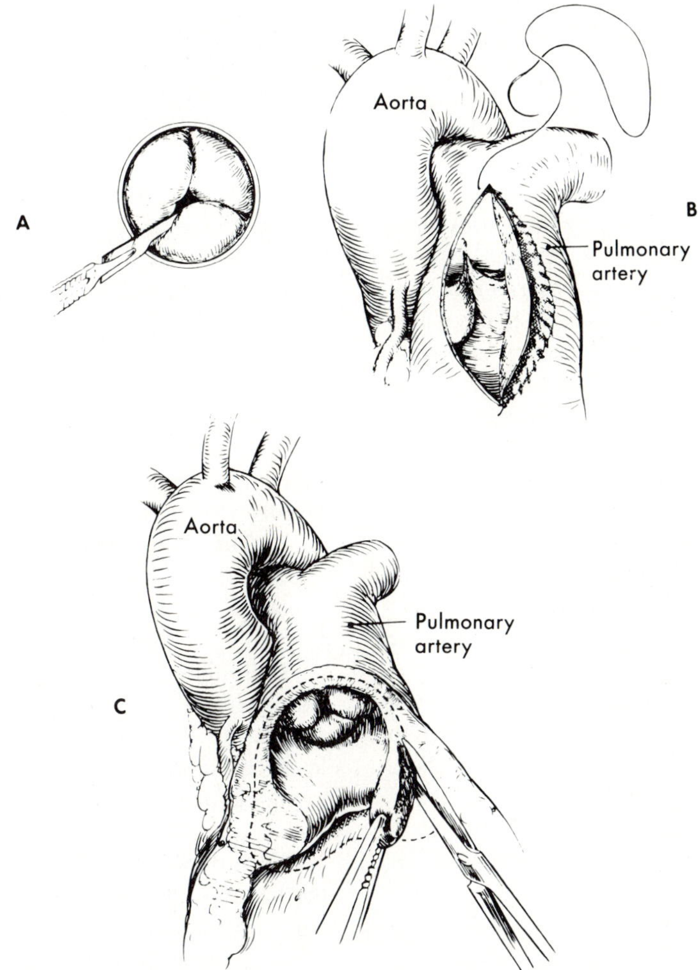

Fig. 18-44. A, Commissurotomy of stenotic valve. Knife is used, and care is taken to incise exactly on commissures. **B,** Diamond-shaped patch being used to enlarge pulmonary outflow tract and pulmonary valve annulus. If vertical pulmonary artery incision is made directly through anterior commissure of valve, the three valve cusps remain intact, and some valve competence is retained. **C,** Excision of obstructing infundibular tissue. (From Effler, D.B.: Blades' surgical disease of the chest, ed. 4, St. Louis, 1978, The C.V. Mosby Co.)

nary artery, by suture ligation or by division of the ductus.

Considerations. The patent ductus arteriosus is an important fetal vascular communication, whereby blood is shunted from the pulmonary artery into the aorta during intrauterine life. During fetal life, the lungs are inactive, and the blood is oxygenated in the placenta. Normally, the muscular coats of the ductus begin to contract soon after birth, with subsequent obliteration of the lumen and cessation of blood flow through the shunt.

When the ductus remains patent after birth (Fig. 18-45), it creates a shunt from the aorta through the ductus into the pulmonary circulation. This increases the work of the heart and causes subsequent enlargement and hypertrophy of the left atrium and ventricle. However, when persistent patency of the ductus is associated with other malformations such as tetralogy of Fallot and extreme stenosis of the pulmonary orifice, it serves as a means of maintaining life. Surgery is not performed if the patent ductus arteriosus is serving in a compensatory capacity.

Many children have few symptoms because of the small size of the shunt. A frequent clinical sign associated with this condition is a harsh, continuous murmur. Since the blood is oxygenated passing through the shunt, there is no cyanosis, clubbing, or reduction in peripheral arterial oxygen saturation. However, growth is retarded in children who have a large ductus. Other symptoms may include dyspnea, frequent upper respiratory infections, palpitation, limited exercise tolerance, and cardiac failure.

Setup and preparation of the patient. For newborn infants, the surgeon and anesthesiologist may elect to perform this procedure in the intensive care nursery bed, since the operation is a short one. Otherwise, the baby will be placed in a right lateral position. The setup is as described, without items for cardiopulmonary bypass, but with special patent ductus clamps.

Generally, a left posterolateral approach is used; in some cases, however, a left anterolateral approach is used.

Operative procedure

1. The incision is carried through the muscles over the fourth interspace. The chest wall is entered through the third or fourth intercostal space, using items as described for thoracotomy (Chapter 17). The wound edges are protected and retracted with a Finochietto rib spreader.

2. The pleura is incised with Metzenbaum scissors, and the left lung is protected and retracted with a moist pack and a malleable retractor.

3. The mediastinal pleura is opened between the phrenic and vagus nerves over the region of the ductus. The pleura is retracted by insertion of stay sutures. The recurrent laryngeal nerve is identified and protected. The aortic arch and pulmonary artery are dissected with fine scissors and dry dissectors. Fine arterial branches are divided and ligated with curved Crile or mosquito hemostats and nonabsorbable ligatures and cardiac suture ligatures.

4. The parietal pleura overlying the ductus is dissected with fine vascular forceps and scissors. Stay sutures are inserted to facilitate retraction (Fig. 18-46).

5. The adventitial layer of the ductus is dissected free. A small portion of the obscure posterior ductus is carefully freed to admit a right-angle clamp. Tapes are passed around the aorta and below the ductus.

6A. *For the suture-ligation method,* two ligatures are placed around the ductus, one near the aorta and the other near the pulmonary artery side, both of which are tied in place. Between these two ligatures, two transfixion sutures are inserted.

6B. *For the division of the ductus method,* the patent ductus clamps are applied as close to the aorta and pulmonary artery as possible. The ductus is divided halfway through and partially sutured with mattress cardiovascular sutures and continued back over the free edge with an over-and-over whip suture. After both openings are sutured, a sponge is held on the area for compression while the patent ductus clamps are removed.

7. The mediastinal pleura is closed with interrupted sutures. The lung is reexpanded, and a chest catheter is inserted for the establishment of closed drainage.

8. The chest wall is closed in layers as previously described, and dressings are applied.

Repair of coarctation of the aorta

Definition. Excision of a constricted segment of the aorta, plus an end-to-end anastomosis—with or without a graft—to reestablish continuity (Fig. 18-47). In some instances, a woven Dacron or PTFE patch may be used to enlarge the aortic diameter at the site of the coarctation.

Considerations. The lesion that narrows or constricts the lumen of the aorta may be classified as *infantile* or *adult.* In the infantile type, the constriction is long and usually located in the aortic arch proximal to the junction of the aorta and ductus arteriosus. The ductus usually remains patent and may be associated with other cardiac defects. In the adult type, the coarctation consists of a constricted area at or just distal to the junction of the aorta and left subclavian artery and the ductus, which is generally closed. This type is compatible with life for a considerable period of time.

Coarctation of the aorta is a fairly common congenital malformation, and the adult patient suffers from hypertension and complains of dyspnea, palpitation, vertigo, headache, epistaxis, and weakness. However, when the aorta is almost obstructed, hypertension is manifested in the upper part of the body with hypotension in the lower extremities. With hypertension above the constriction, the collateral blood supply, which unites the blood vessels of the shoulder, the upper extremities, and the lower ex-

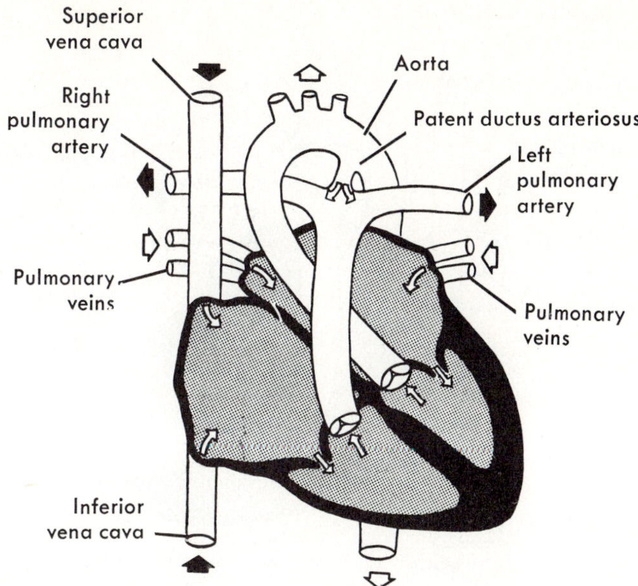

Fig. 18-45. Patent ductus arteriosus. Ductus fails to close after birth. (From Nursing Education Service: General signs and symptoms of congenital heart abnormalities, Columbus, Ohio, Ross Laboratories.)

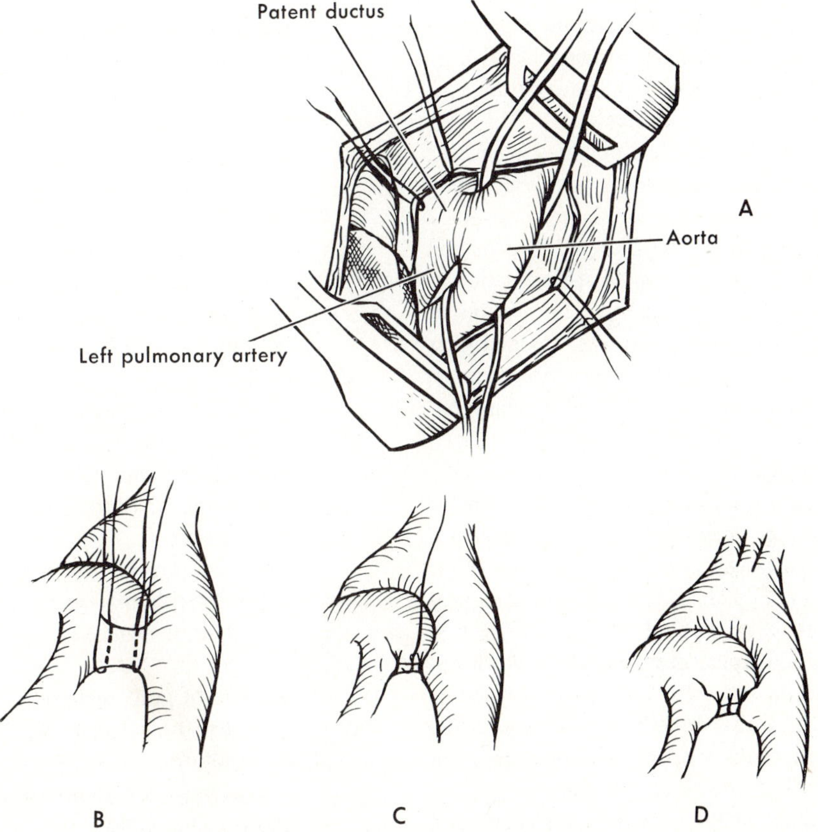

Fig. 18-46. Suture ligation of patent ductus arteriosus. **A,** Potts-Smith aortic clamp and ductus clamp in place. **B,** Ductus arteriosus partially divided. **C,** Closure of ductus arteriosus begun before division completed to permit better control of bleeding should one of clamps slip. **D,** Clamps removed showing completed suture lines.

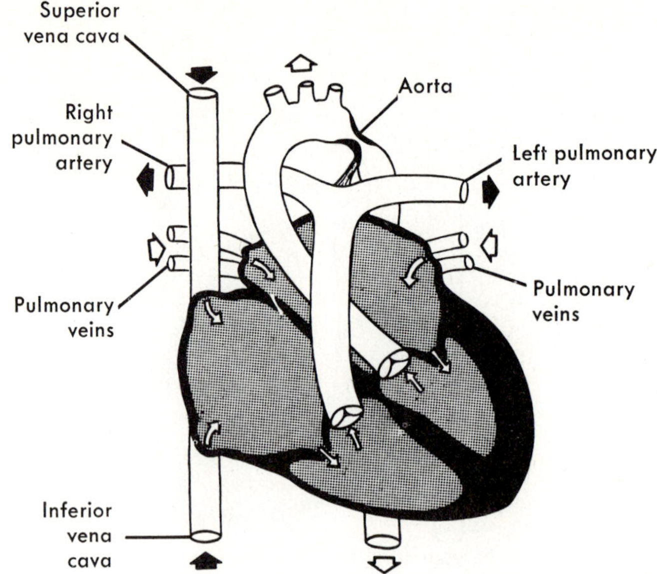

Fig. 18-47. Coarctation of aorta is characterized by narrow aortic lumen and exists as preductal or postductal obstruction, depending on position of obstruction in relation to ductus arteriosus. (From Nursing Education Service: General signs and symptoms of congenital heart abnormalities, Columbus, Ohio, Ross Laboratories.)

tremities, increases markedly. In so doing, the intercostal vessels dilate, allowing their branches to carry blood from the subclavian arteries downward. Occasionally the vessels erode the lower margins of the ribs.

The best results of treatment are obtained when the patient is old enough so that the growth factor regarding the anastomosis is eliminated.

Setup and preparation of the patient. The patient is placed in the right lateral position. Instrumentation is as described for basic cardiac surgery, plus Teflon or Dacron woven or knitted vascular prostheses, assorted sizes (Fig. 18-17), to be used as necessary when primary anastomosis is not possible. Items for cardiopulmonary bypass are not needed.

Operative procedure (Fig. 18-48)

1. A left posterolateral incision is carried through the chest wall with resection of the fourth rib, as described for thoracotomy. As previously stated, the collateral blood vessels are somewhat enlarged, and bleeding may be profuse. Dry sponges are used throughout and weighed to determine accurate blood replacement. A Burford or Finochietto retractor is used.

2. The pleura is incised, and the lung is retracted. The mediastinal pleura is incised over the constricted portion of the aorta, and the edges are sutured to the chest wall.

3. Careful dissection with fine vascular forceps and dry dissectors is continued to mobilize the aorta and the surrounding intercostal vessels. The laryngeal nerve is identified and protected. The ductus arteriosus is ligated and divided between ductus clamps.

4. Resection with graft replacement (Fig. 18-48, *C*)
   a. The curved or angled vascular clamps are applied, and the constricted segment is divided between them. A second set of clamps may be applied above and below, as a safety factor, in fashioning the cuffs for reapproximation.
   b. End-to-end anastomosis is accomplished by means of a continuous, everting mattress technique for the posterior wall and interrupted, everting mattress sutures for the anterior row. If the stricture is long, a synthetic aortic prosthesis is used to bridge the defect.
   c. The clamps are released slowly, the distal one first and then the proximal one. The blood pressure is noted at this time. Removal of clamps is not completed until the blood pressure is stabilized.
5. Patch repair
   a. The curved or angled vascular clamps are applied, and a longitudinal aortotomy is performed with a no. 11 knife blade, a Potts scissors, and vascular forceps.
   b. A piece of graft material is inserted, large enough to widen the aorta, using a continuous cardiovascular suture.
   c. The clamps are removed, one at a time, as described in step 4c.

6. The parietal pleura is closed, leaving a small opening at the lower point. Closed drainage is established, and the chest wall is closed in layers. A dressing is applied.

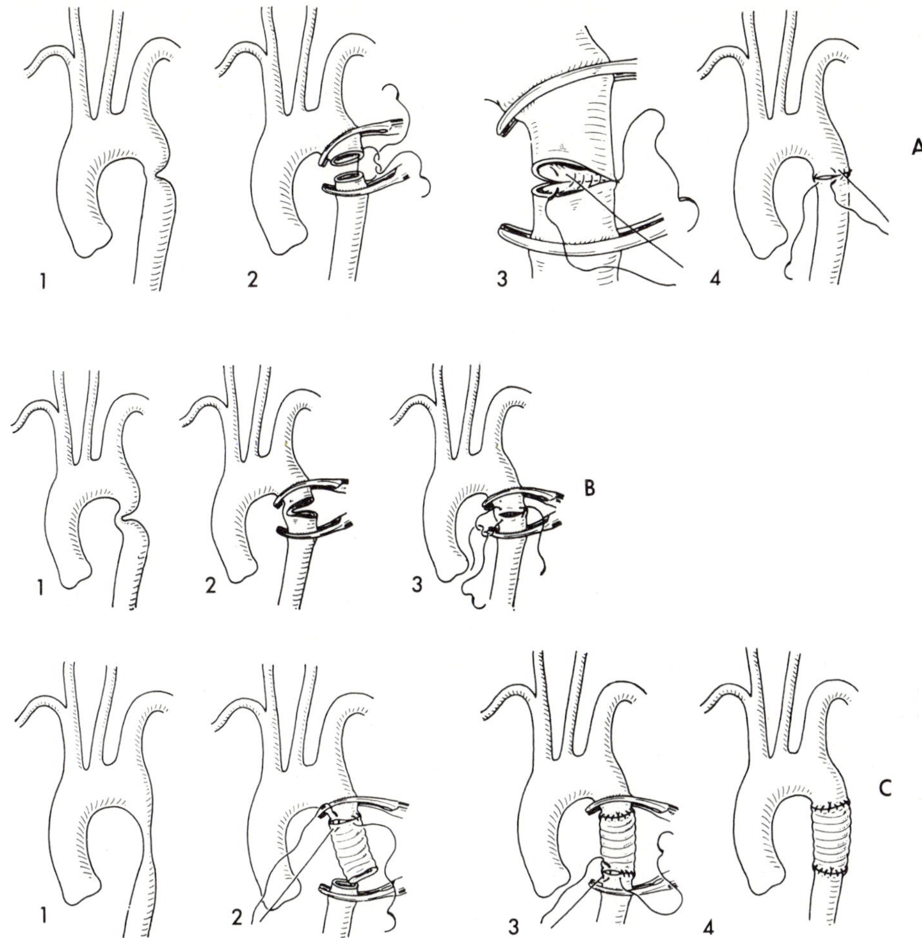

Fig. 18-48. Diagrams showing coarctation of aorta: types with methods of correction. **A,** Short narrow obstruction and steps in end-to-end anastomosis. **B,** Wedge excision with partial anastomosis completed. **C,** Segmental excision with graft replacement. (From Blades, B., editor: Surgical diseases of the chest, ed. 3, St. Louis, 1974, The C.V. Mosby Co.)

Pulmonary artery banding

Definition. Constriction of the pulmonary artery to reduce its diameter, thereby decreasing pulmonary blood flow.

Considerations. The infant with an enlarged heart in intractable failure and a large left-to-right shunt may be treated effectively by a palliative pulmonary artery banding operation. This procedure is designed to reduce the flow of blood through the pulmonary artery to approximately one half to one third of the existing rate. A tape is looped about the artery and secured in place by a simple suture technique. Pressures are measured by direct needle puncture before and after banding. A reduction of the distal pulmonary artery pressure by 50% to 70% is sought. Repair of the interventricular septal defect may be postponed until the child has clinically stabilized and can withstand an open heart procedure. Banding is performed as a palliative procedure for patients who have severe hemodynamic changes from a ventricular septal defect but who are not candidates for total correction.

Setup and preparation of the patient. The patient is placed in the left lateral position, or a median sternotomy may be used. Instruments are as described, plus 8-inch pieces of various width tapes (surgeon's preference), with appropriate sizes for children.

INSERTION OF PERMANENT PACEMAKER

Definition. Permanent implantation of a pulse generator and electrode to initiate ventricular contraction. The most common underlying condition requiring a permanent pacemaker is heart block, in which there is a disturbance of the neuroconductive system (Fig. 18-4). A pacemaker may also be used for the acute forms of heart block that occasionally occur during cardiac surgery.

Considerations. There are two basic methods of placing electrodes for permanent cardiac pacing: transthoracic and transvenous. The transvenous method is preferred because it offers the advantages of not requiring either a major thoracotomy or a general anesthetic and being safer for high-risk patients.

An alternate technique of placing a myocardial electrode may be used. The procedure can be performed under local anesthesia through a subxiphoid incision.

The pulse generator is powered by a mercury-zinc, lithium iodide, nickle-cadmium (rechargeable), or nuclear source (Fig. 18-49, *A*). Several different models are available, but there are basically only two types: asynchronous and demand. The asynchronous model has a fixed rate of pacing, for example, 72 beats per minute, whereas the demand model only fires when the patient's heart rate drops below a preset rate. In addition, unipolar or bipolar systems are used.

A

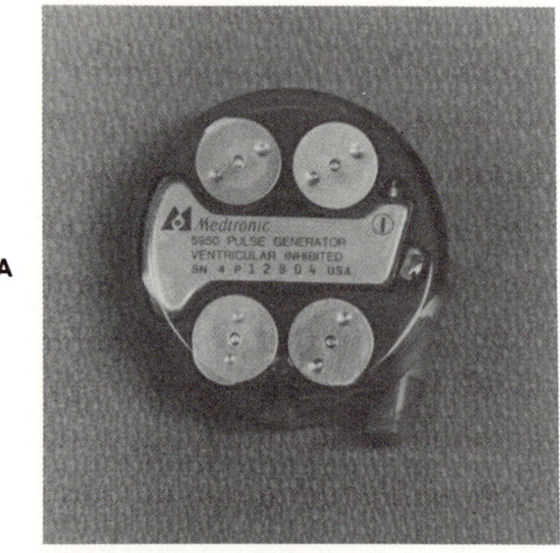

B

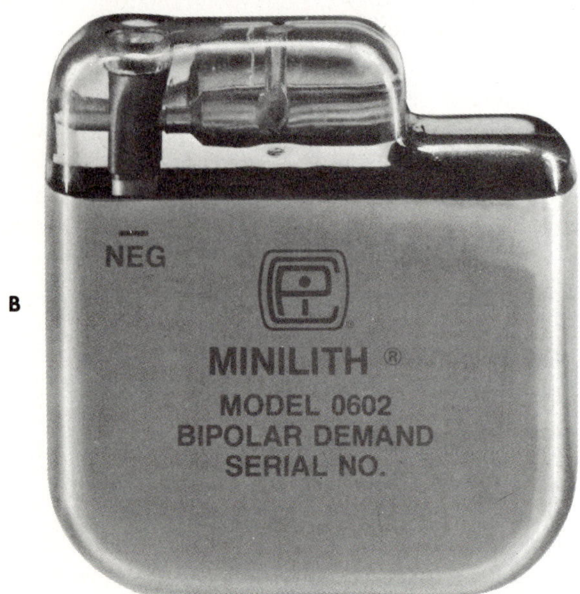

Fig. 18-49. A, Ventricular inhibited pulse generator. **B,** Lithium-powered pulse generator.

There are also two types of electrodes: myocardial (epicardial) and endocardial. The myocardial leads require a thoracotomy because they are placed into the muscle of the heart. This can be accomplished by an anterolateral thoracotomy, which has been the traditional approach, or through the subxiphoid approach.

Recently, lithium-powered pacemakers have come into use (Fig. 18-49, *B*). The advantage of these units is that the life expectancy is 5 to 10 years, as opposed to 2 to 3 years for the mercury-zinc battery-powered models.

Insertion of transvenous (endocardial) pacing electrodes

Setup and preparation of the patient. The patient is placed in the supine position. Continuous electrocardiographic monitoring is essential, so the electrodes must be carefully placed. The patient should be made as comfortable as possible, since this procedure can be lengthy at times and is frequently performed using local and standby anesthesia.

Fluoroscopy is required; thus either a portable image intensifier is needed, or the procedure is done in the special studies section of the radiology department.

A defibrillator and emergency drugs should be available because arrhythmias can occur during catheter insertion.

The majority of these procedures are performed under local anesthesia, but standby for a general anesthetic may be requested.

A minor set of instruments is used, plus the following:

1 Potts vascular scissors
2 Potts vascular forceps
2 Vascular needle holders
1 "Tunneling" instrument, such as a sponge forceps or vaginal packing forceps
Sterile pacemaker and electrodes
External pacemaker (for testing) or a pacing analyzer
Sterile connecting cable

Operative procedure

1. The skin and subcutaneous tissue are infiltrated with a local anesthetic.
2. A cutdown is performed to isolate a jugular or cephalic vein, and the vessel is encircled with heavy sutures or umbilical tapes.
3. A venotomy is performed, usually with a no. 11 scalpel blade, and the pacing electrode is inserted.
4. The electrode is advanced, under direct fluoroscopic vision, into the right atrium, through the tricuspid valve, and into the right ventricle.
5. The surgeon attempts to entrap the tip of the electrode in the *trabeculae carnae* of the right ventricular apex to stabilize it (Fig. 18-50).

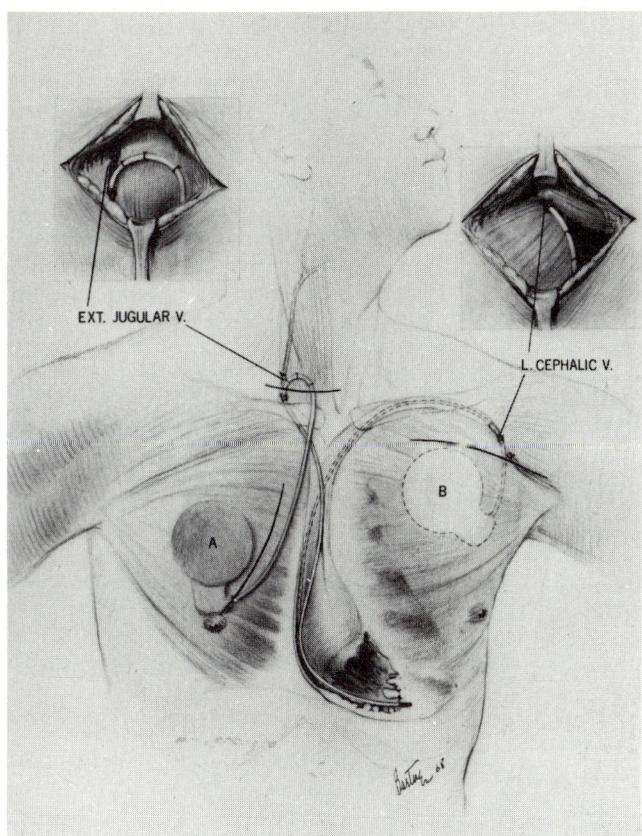

Fig. 18-50. Electrode catheter tip is shown wedged in trabeculae at apex of right ventricle. External jugular approach is shown at left. Strain-relieving loop is in neck. For clarity, cephalic approach is shown on patient's left side, although right cephalic vein is used more often. (From Blades, B., editor: Surgical diseases of the chest, ed. 3, St. Louis, 1974, The C.V. Mosby Co.)

6. The electrode is attached, by appropriate cables, to an external pulse generator or a pacing analyzer for testing.

7. A pocket is created for the implantable pulse generator. The incision is carried down to fascia and a tunnel is formed, subcutaneously with a blunt instrument, to the neck incision.

8. The electrode is brought down through the tunnel and is attached to the pulse generator.

9. The pulse generator is placed in the pocket, and both incisions are irrigated with an antibiotic solution.

10. The incisions are closed with absorbable sutures, subcutaneously, and nonabsorbable sutures on skin.

Insertion of myocardial (epicardial) pacing electrodes

Subxiphoid process approach

Setup and preparation of the patient. As described for placement of endocardial electrodes.

Operative procedure

1. If local anesthesia is used, the subxiphoid process and left, upper quadrant area are infiltrated with the anesthetic.

2. A small, transverse incision is made below the xiphoid process and is carried down to the linea alba. A tunnel is created under the xiphoid process to the pericardium, which is incised to expose the heart.

3. The pacing electrode, mounted on its carrier, is screwed into the ventricular myocardium, and the carrier is removed.

4. The remainder of the procedure is as described for insertion of the endocardial electrode.

Transthoracic approach

Setup and preparation of the patient. Positioning (for anterolateral thoracotomy), nursing considerations, and instrumentation are all as described in Chapter 17.

Operative procedure

1. An anterolateral thoracotomy is performed.

2. The mediastinum is opened with a scissors or scalpel, and an area of myocardium is chosen for placement of the pacing electrodes.

3. The electrode tips are screwed into or are sutured to the myocardium and are attached, by an appropriate cable, to an external pulse generator or pacing analyzer for testing.

4. The pocket and subcutaneous tunnel are created, as described for insertion of the endocardial electrode.

5. A chest drainage catheter is inserted, and the thoracotomy incision is closed.

SUGGESTED READINGS

American Heart Association, Council on Cardiovascular Nursing, and American Nurses' Association, Division on Medical-Surgical Nursing Practice: Standards of cardiovascular nursing practice, Kansas City, Mo., 1975, American Nurses' Association.

Anthony, C.P., and Thibodeau, G.A.: Textbook of anatomy and physiology, ed. 10, St. Louis, 1979, The C.V. Mosby Co.

Ashworth, P.M.: Cardiovascular disorders: patient care, Baltimore, 1973, The Williams & Wilkins Co.

Aspinall, M.J.: Nursing the open-heart surgical patient, New York, 1973, McGraw-Hill Book Co.

Beauchamp, S.P.: Education of the patient and family for cardiovascular surgery, AORN J. **29:**860, 1979.

Berne, R.M., and Levy, M.N.: Cardiovascular physiology, ed. 3, St. Louis, 1977, The C.V. Mosby Co.

Chow, R.K.: Cardiosurgical nursing care, New York, 1976, Springer Publishing Co., Inc.

Cooley, D.A., and Norman, J.C.: Techniques in cardiac surgery, Houston, 1975, Texas Medical Press, Inc.

Effler, D.B., editor: Blade's surgical diseases of the chest, ed. 4, St. Louis, 1978, The C.V. Mosby Co.

Grossman, W., editor: Cardiac catheterization and angiography, Philadelphia, 1980, Lea & Febiger.

Guyton, A.C., and Young, D.B., editors: Cardiovascular physiology, Baltimore, 1979, University Park Press.

Hallman, G.L., and Cooley, D.A.: Surgical treatment of congenital heart disease, ed. 2, Philadelphia, 1975, Lea & Febiger.

Harlan, B., Starr, A., and Harwin, F.M.: Manual of cardiac surgery, New York, 1980, Springer-Verlag, New York, Inc.

King, O.M.: Care of the cardiac surgical patient, St. Louis, 1975, The C.V. Mosby Co.

Lindskog, G.E., Liebow, A.A., and Glenn, W.W.L.: Thoracic and cardiovascular surgery with related physiology, New York, 1975, Appleton-Century-Crofts.

Netter, F.H.: The Ciba collection of medical illustrations, vol. 7, Summit, N.J., 1979, Ciba Pharmaceutical Co.

Reed, C.C., and Clark, D.K.: Cardiopulmonary perfusion, Houston, 1975, Texas Medical Press, Inc.

Reed, E.A.: Intra-aortic balloon pump, AORN J. **23:**995, 1976.

Sabiston, D.C., Jr., and Spencer, F.C.: Gibbon's surgery of the chest, ed. 3, Philadelphia, 1976, W.B. Saunders Co.

Sade, R., Cosgrove, D.M., and Castaneda, A.R.: Infant and child care in cardiac surgery, Chicago, 1977, Yearbook Medical Publishers, Inc.

Seifert, P.C.: An OR nurse's guide to coronary artery bypass, AORN J. **33:**1049, 1981.

Trimiglozzi, B.: Perioperative role in cardiac surgery, AORN J. **29:**856, 1979.

19 Vascular surgery

Vascular surgery is routinely performed in most hospitals today and is no longer limited to larger medical centers. The complexity and diversity of the procedures being performed vary, however. Some are tedious, requiring delicate dissection, and the attentive participation of the nurse is essential.

ANATOMY AND PHYSIOLOGY

Arteries. Arteries are composed of three layers of tissue. The *tunica intima* is the smooth internal endothelial layer that is in contact with the blood, the *tunica media* is the muscular middle portion, and the *tunica adventitia* is the outer layer, composed of connective tissue.

Arteries successively divide into arterioles, which then further subdivide into capillaries, which connect with the venous system. At the capillary level, blood supplies oxygen to body tissues. Arteries can also form *anastomoses* or connections with other arteries. These anastomoses tend to equalize blood distribution and pressure and also to form collateral circulation, when necessary. *Collateral circulation* is important in vascular disease and often provides alternate pathways around occluded vessels.

Vasomotor nerves, which control vascular tone, arise from the sympathetic portion of the autonomic nervous system and are categorized as vasoconstrictor or vasodilator fibers.

Normal arterial function depends on the properties of elasticity and distensibility, which enable the vessels to compensate for changes in blood volume and pressure.

Veins. Veins are thin-walled channels that return the blood to the heart. They are composed of the same three basic layers as arteries, but the tunica media is thin; veins can contract only minimally.

The intimal layer of a vein contains semilunar folds of tissue, or valves. These valves prevent the backflow of blood. Since little pumping pressure from the heart carries across the capillary beds, one-way valves are necessary to overcome the pull of gravity and prevent backflow of blood in the venous system. The negative pressure created by the relaxed right ventricle helps venous return by its sucking effect, and the contraction of visceral and skeletal muscles helps propel venous blood toward the heart.

Capillaries enlarge into venules, which in turn enlarge into successively bigger veins, returning the deoxygenated blood to the heart.

NURSING CONSIDERATIONS

A preoperative assessment is necessary for an adequate understanding of the patient's disease, the patient's response to it, and the proposed surgical procedure.

The patient usually has had arteriograms performed preoperatively, and these should be available in the operating room. If intraoperative arteriograms are anticipated, an appropriate table with additional x-ray materials should be available.

The electrocardiogram and direct arterial lines are used for monitoring purposes. The central venous pressure (CVP) or left atrial pressure (LAP) also may be monitored, depending on the patient's physiological alterations. A general anesthetic is usually administered, and the patient is intubated. Since many patients undergoing vascular surgery have generalized arteriosclerotic disease, the nurse should be alert for cardiac arrhythmias or blood pressure changes.

A urinary catheter should be inserted, especially if the proposed procedure involves the renal arteries or clamping the aorta above the renal arteries or if considerable blood loss is anticipated. The catheter will facilitate the hourly measurement of urine during and after the surgical procedure to assist in the assessment of renal perfusion.

Positioning of the patient undergoing vascular surgery is of particular importance because of restricted circulation distal to the area of arterial obstruction and a generalized state of poor circulation. In addition, the patient's age and medical condition, such as diabetes, can further necessitate the need for attention to positioning. Proper skeletal alignment during surgery will prevent injury to the neuromuscular system. Attention to the skin overlying bony prominences, especially the heels, and the use of proper supports and pads will prevent injury to the patient. For the same reasons, the scrub person should also be cognizant of heavy instruments and drapes resting on the patient's skin and take measures to avoid injury.

Vascular surgery can be lengthy. Attention to the maintenance of the patient's body temperature is important, especially considering the air-conditioned environment of the operating room.

The operating room nurse must be familiar with the location and presence or absence of peripheral pulses. The surgeon may ask the nurse to evaluate the patient's feet for color, temperature, and strength of pedal pulses. This assessment is indicative of tissue perfusion distal to the arterial obstruction. The accomplishment of this nursing activity should be considered during the initial preparation of the patient.

Instrumentation. Vascular instruments are described in Chapter 18, but their uses vary depending on the procedure being performed.

The use of fiberoptic head lights by the surgeon and/or assistants helps illuminate tissues in deep incisions.

The operating room nurse should be familiar with the function and use of an ultrasonic instrument (Doppler). This device detects the change in the frequency of sound as the blood flows through the blood vessels. The sound is amplified through a speaker. The Doppler provides rapid assessment of blood flow and tissue viability when pulses cannot be felt manually.

Sutures. Most vascular sutures are made of synthetic, nonabsorbable materials such as Dacron, polyester, and polypropylene. Occasionally, silk may be used. These sutures are sometimes converted to a monofilament by the impregnation of other synthetics such as Teflon.

Vascular sutures have swaged-on needles of various sizes and are available in sizes 0 to 8-0. The suture may be single-armed or double-armed (that is, a needle on one or both ends). The size and curve of the needle used depend on the vessel and its location.

Prostheses. Arterial prostheses are synthetic, tubular conduits that are designed to replace or bypass diseased vessels. They are available as straight or bifurcated grafts and are usually made of Teflon or Dacron.

Most prostheses are commercially sterilized. If inhospital sterilized, the manufacturer's recommendations should be followed. It is usually not advisable to repeatedly autoclave a prosthesis because the integrity of the fiber may be destroyed. Ethylene oxide, with adequate aeration, is usually recommended.

The Teflon and Dacron grafts are available in either woven or knitted form. Woven grafts do not ordinarily require preclotting, but they tend to fray on cut edges.

Dacron prostheses are available with either the internal or external surface composed of filamental loops called velour. These grafts decrease the potential for bleeding, both initial and delayed, and promote more rapid endothelialization.

Expanded polytetrafluoroethylene (PTFE) is used as an alternative material for vascular prostheses. It is pliable, does not fray, sutures well, and needs no preclotting. Glutaraldehyde-tanned human umbilical vein grafts have also become available as arterial prostheses. This material is available in various lengths and diameters.

Grafts are available in various sizes. The common size used for abdominal procedures is 14 to 22 mm; for the extremities, it is usually 4 to 10 mm.

The graft is prepared before insertion, according to the surgeon's preference. This graft preparation is done to minimize blood loss resulting from seepage through the graft interstices. Sometimes the surgeon prefers to "preclot" the graft with the patient's blood or, after insertion of the graft, to open the occluding clamps individually and momentarily to fill the graft with blood to accomplish the same purpose.

Heparinization. Heparin may be used, locally or systemically, to prevent thrombosis during the operative procedure. When a vessel is completely occluded during the operation, heparin is often injected directly into the distal artery before the clamp is secured. Heparinized saline irrigation also may be used.

The dosage and concentration of heparin in saline solution vary according to the surgeon's preference.

OPERATIONS

Abdominal aortic aneurysmectomy

Definition. Surgical obliteration of the aneurysm, which may or may not include the iliac arteries, with insertion of a synthetic prosthesis to reestablish functional continuity.

Considerations. The majority of abdominal aortic aneurysms begin below the renal arteries and frequently extend to involve the bifurcation and common iliac arteries. Symptoms may be vague or entirely absent until the size of the aneurysm increases sufficiently to produce pressure on surrounding organs. The most reliable physical finding is an abnormal, pulsating, abdominal mass. Severe pain, along with symptoms of hypotension, shock, and distal vascular insufficiency, is usually indicative of rupture or dissection and represents a true emergency condition. The prime surgical consideration when a rupture or dissection occurs is the control of hemorrhage by occluding the aorta proximal to the point of rupture.

Setup and preparation of the patient. The patient is placed in the supine position. The skin is prepared for a midline abdominal incision, and draping is completed to permit access to both groin regions and exploration of femoral arteries (Fig. 19-1).

It is a good idea to mark the pedal pulses before the beginning of the procedure so that they may be located immediately if the surgeon requests a check of the pulses. This assessment of pulses can be done manually or by use of an ultrasonic instrument (Doppler).

The setup includes the basic laparotomy set, plus the following:

Cutting instruments

2 Knife handles, no. 7 with blades nos. 11 and 15
2 Potts-Smith vascular scissors, 1 straight and 1 angled

Holding instruments

4 Potts-Smith tissue forceps, 2 smooth and 2 with teeth
4 DeBakey vascular forceps, 2 long and 2 short

Clamping instruments

4 Angled peripheral vascular clamps
4 Aortic occlusion clamps
3 Satinsky clamps, various sizes
4 DeBakey ring-handled bulldog clamps
4 DeBakey cross-action bulldog clamps

Suturing instruments

4 Needle holders (narrow diamond jaw)

Retractors

2 Kelly retractors, extra large
2 Deaver retractors, extra large
2 Harrington retractors, wide and narrow
2 Weitlaner or Garrett retractors (for extension into the legs)

Accessory items

2 Heparin flushing needles
Crawford-Cooley tunneler
Tissue occlusion clips and applicators (for example, Hemoclips)
Fogarty arterial catheters

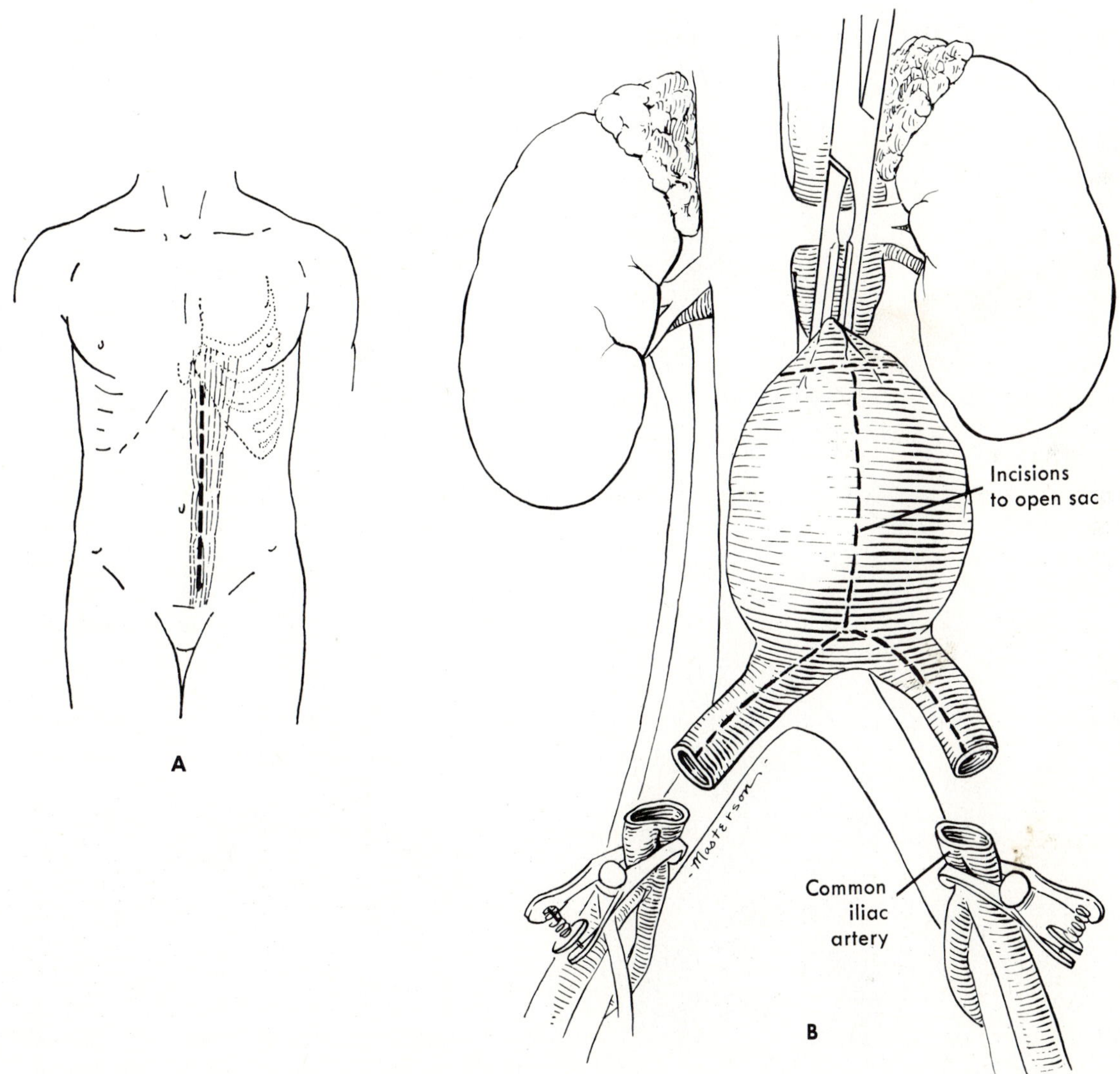

Fig. 19-1. Resection of abdominal aneurysm: end-to-end anastomosis. **A,** Incision. **B,** Sac is opened after obtaining proximal and distal control.

Continued.

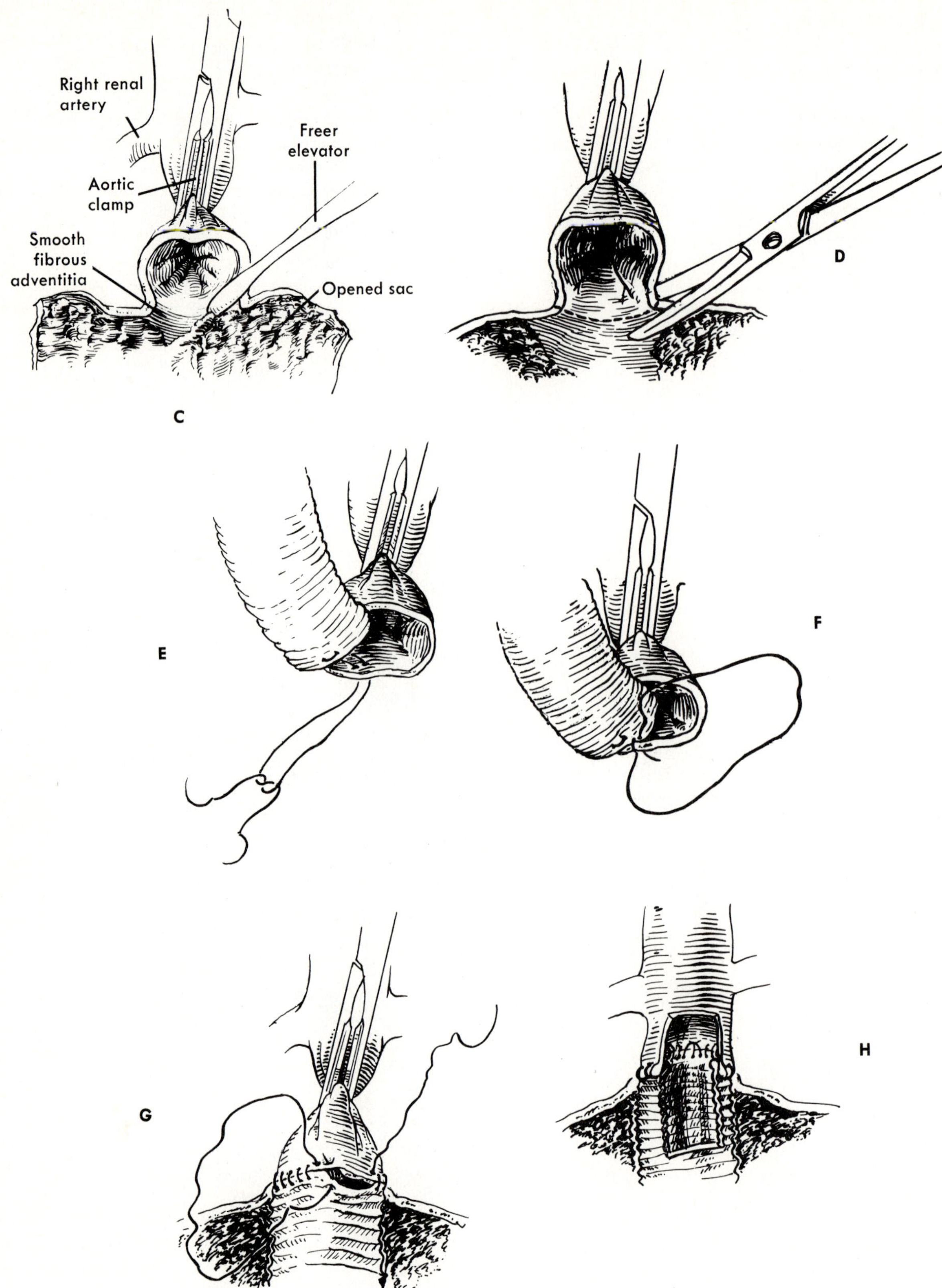

Fig. 19-1, cont'd. C, Endarterectomy at cuff of aorta. **D,** Posterior wall is divided, or, if posterior wall is adherent, anastomosis is performed. **E,** Anastomosis is begun posteriorly. **F,** Sewing over and over from graft to aorta. **G,** Complete anastomosis in front. **H,** Cutaway view.

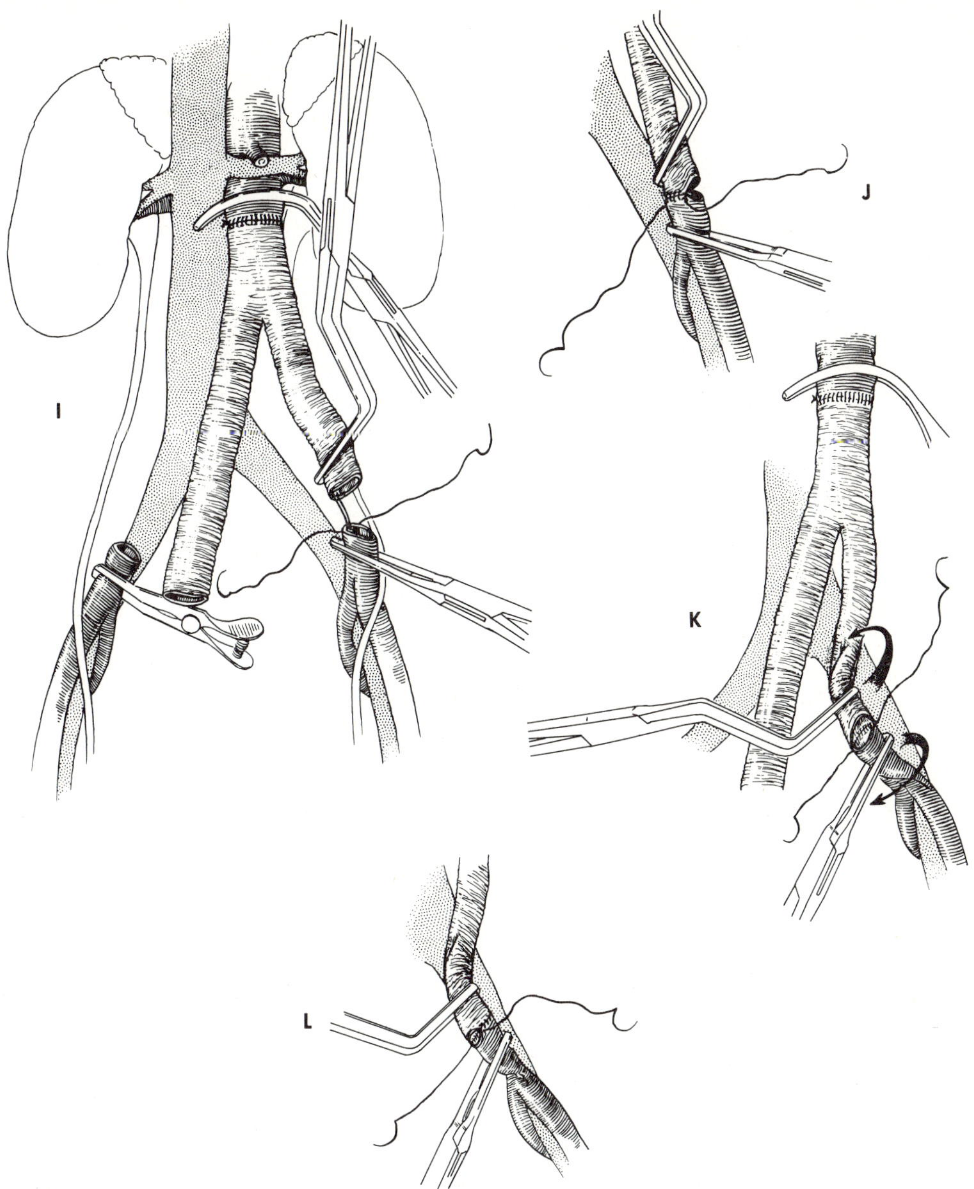

Fig. 19-1, cont'd. I to **L,** First iliac anastomosis: **I,** placement of mattress suture; **J,** medial row; **K,** medial row completed; rotation for lateral row; **L,** lateral row. *Continued.*

Operative procedure

1. The abdomen is opened through a midline incision (Fig. 19-1) from the xiphoid process to the symphysis pubis. Hemostasis is accomplished, and exploration is completed, as described for laparotomy (Chapter 10).

2. Kelly and Deaver retractors are inserted in the wound. If necessary for exposure, a portion of the small bowel can be placed outside the abdomen and covered with moist laparotomy packs or a Lahey bag.

3. The parietal peritoneum is incised over the aorta and extended superiorly to expose the aneurysm and also inferiorly over the bifurcation and beyond the iliac arteries. Metzenbaum scissors, smooth forceps, and hemostats are used.

4. Careful blunt and sharp dissection is continued to expose the aorta above the aneurysm to permit application of moist compression or occlusion tapes (umbilical tape) and loose placement of an aortic clamp. The renal artery and ureters are protected.

5. The iliac vessels and bifurcation are inspected for evidence of small aneurysms, thrombosis, and calcification. Moist tapes are placed about the iliac arteries, and vascular clamps are applied.

6. An aortic clamp such as the Crafoord, Cooley, or Satinsky is applied and closed. Opening of the aneurysm is undertaken with a scalpel or cautery and heavy scissors.

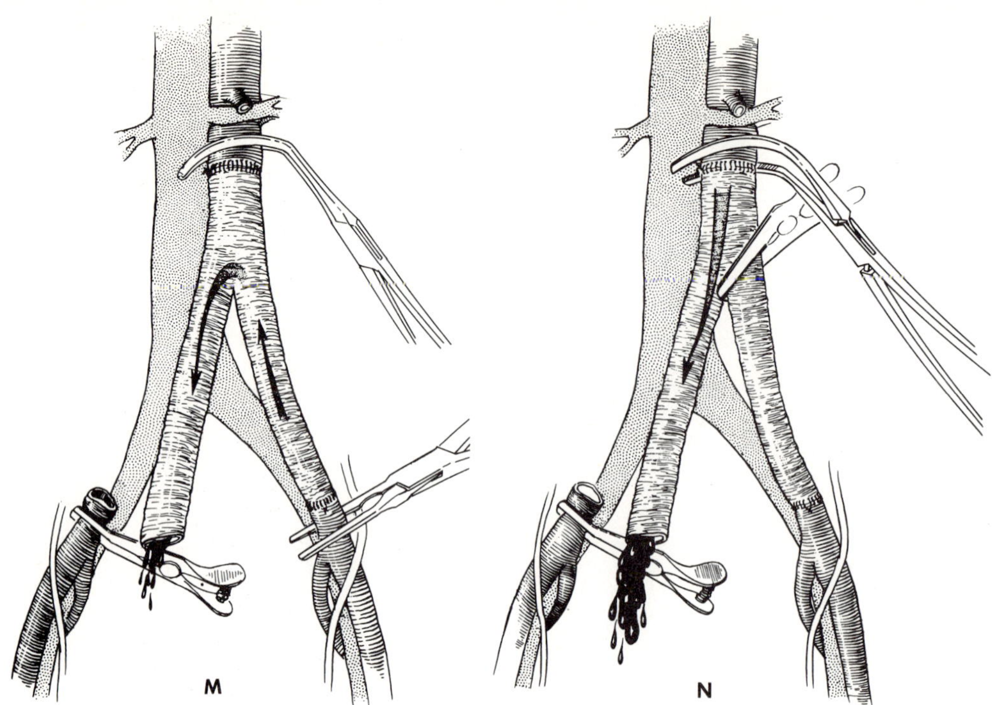

Fig. 19-1, cont'd. M and **N,** Restoration of flow to first leg. **M,** Backflow is checked. **N,** Proximal aorta is flushed. (From Hershey, F.B., and Calman, C.H.: Atlas of vascular surgery, ed. 3, St. Louis, 1973, The C.V. Mosby Co.)

7. The aneurysm is completely opened, and all atheromatous and thrombotic material is removed.

The aneurysm walls may be excised but usually are left in place for eventual reinforcement of the prosthesis. In either case, the posterior aspect of the aorta is left intact.

Bleeding is controlled, especially from the lumbar vessels that enter posteriorly.

8. A bifurcated prosthetic graft of appropriate size is prepared for insertion. Occasionally, if the aneurysm does not involve the aortic bifurcation, a straight tubular graft is used. Preclotting may be accomplished by immersion of the graft in a small quantity of the patient's own blood, as previously described.

9. The aortic cuff is prepared for anastomosis by irrigation with heparinized saline solution and by removal of all fibrotic plaques. One or two vascular sutures (double-armed) are used to accomplish the anastomosis by a through-and-through continuous suture. Additional interrupted sutures may be needed if the anastomosis demonstrates leakage on completion.

10. The distal vessels are opened and inspected for back bleeding, and heparinized saline solution may be injected to prevent clotting.

11. Each limb of the graft is anastomosed to the iliac artery, using a smaller vascular suture and similar technique. After the first side of the anastomosis has been completed, blood is permitted to circulate, and the remaining limb of the graft is clamped gently to prevent both trapping of air and leaking during the last part of the anastomosis. Bleeding is controlled.

12. The parietal peritoneum is closed.

13. The abdominal wound is closed.

Aortoiliac endarterectomy

Definition. Surgical removal of the intraluminal atheromatous obstructive plaques and the restoration of arterial flow to the leg or foot.

Considerations. Aortoiliac endarterectomy is usually accomplished through a vertical arteriotomy with a primary closure. Synthetic patch material of Teflon or Dacron may be used, if necessary, to restore the normal caliber of the artery. The surgeon may choose simply to bypass the obstructed segment, in which case the procedure for abdominal aortic aneurysmectomy would be followed.

Setup and preparation of the patient. As described for abdominal aortic aneurysmectomy, plus endarterectomy instruments or bifurcated and straight tubular synthetic prostheses if endarterectomy is not feasible.

Operative procedure

1. The first five steps of the procedure for aortic aneurysmectomy are followed.

2. An aortic clamp such as the Crafoord or Satinsky is applied, and the arteriotomy is begun. Heparin solution may be injected, and the clamp closed immediately.

3. The arteriotomy incision is completed, and plaques are removed, as shown in Fig. 19-2.

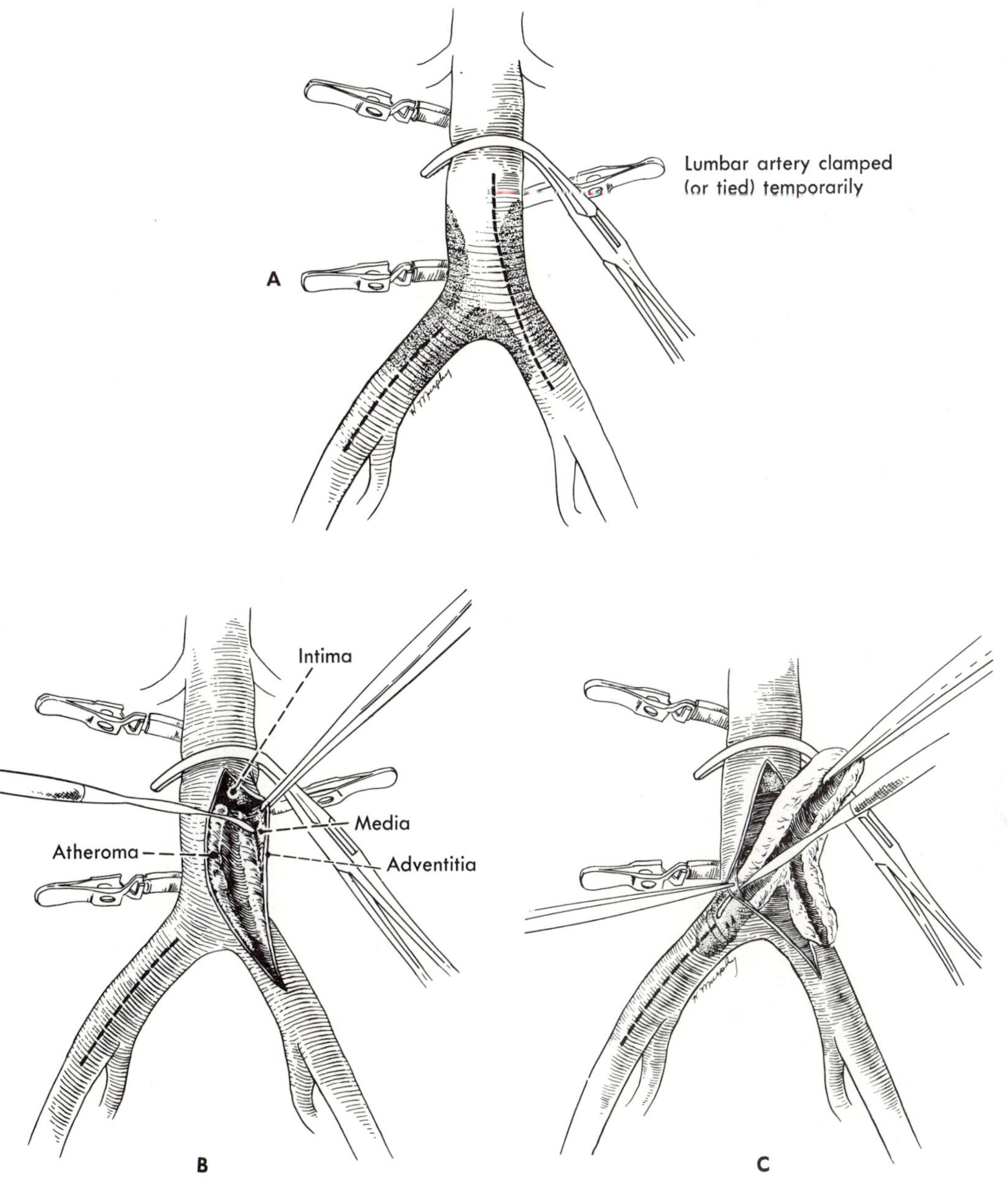

Fig. 19-2. Aortoiliac endarterectomy. **A,** Incisions. **B,** Plane between plaque and media of aorta. **C,** Plaque from other iliac artery from above is freed. *Continued.*

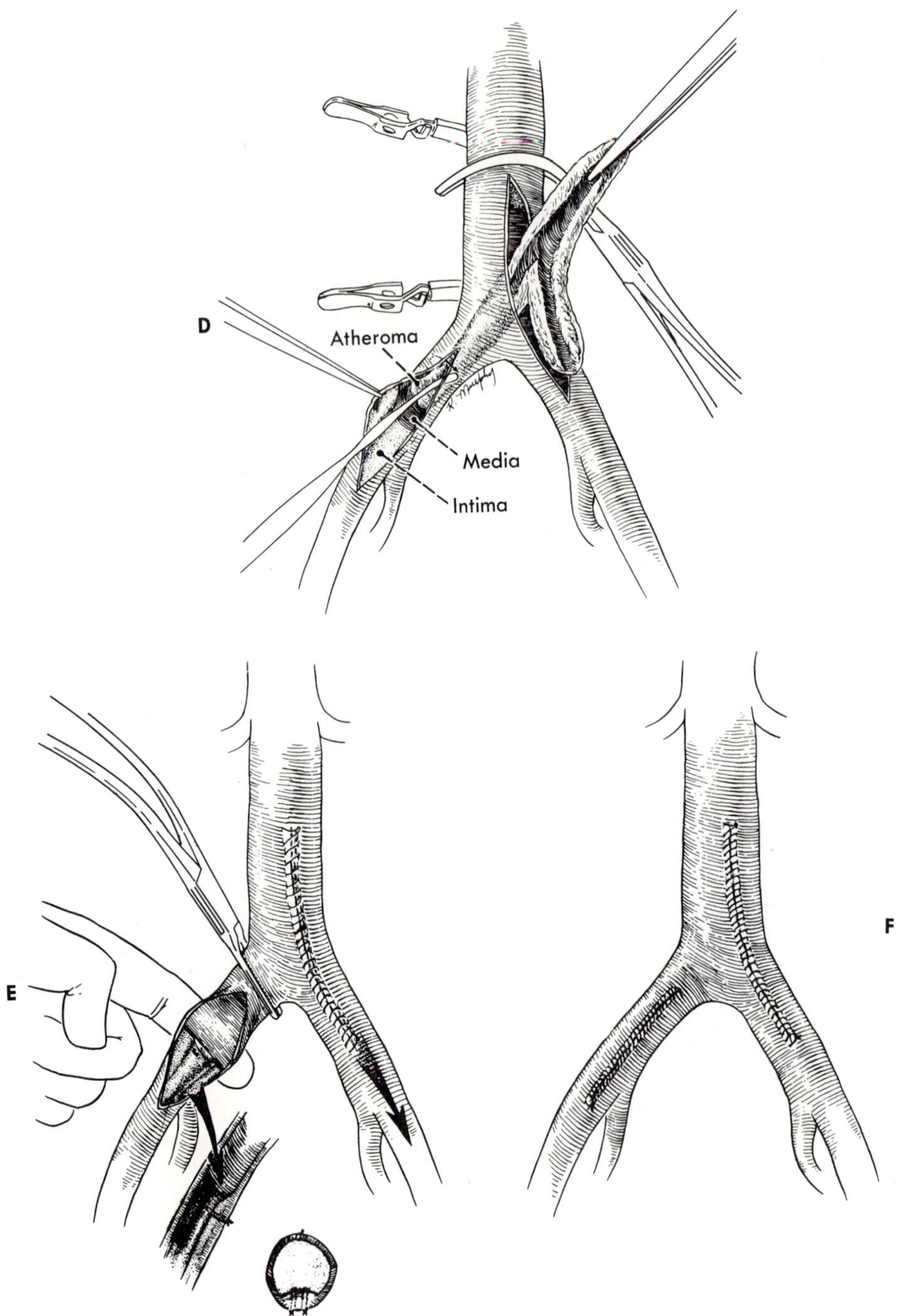

Fig. 19-2, cont'd. D, Plaque is dissected from right iliac artery. **E,** Distal intima is beveled and attached with suture. *Insets,* Side view and cross section. **F,** Arteriotomies sutured. (From Hershey, F.B., and Calman, C.H.: Atlas of vascular surgery, ed. 3, St. Louis, 1973, The C.V. Mosby Co.)

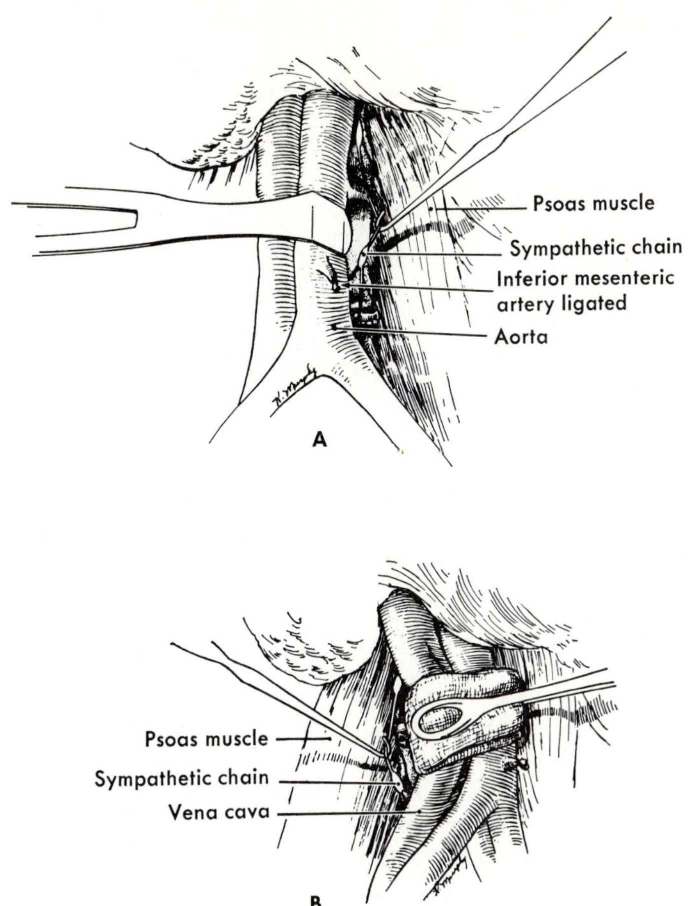

Fig. 19-3. Diagram showing technique of bilateral abdominal sympathectomy. **A,** Left. **B,** Right. (From Hershey, F.B., and Calman, C.H.: Atlas of vascular surgery, ed. 3, St. Louis, 1973, The C.V. Mosby Co.)

4. Arteriotomies are closed with fine, nonabsorbable vascular sutures.

5. A sympathectomy may be performed. The ganglia are identified and grasped with a nerve hook (Fig. 19-3), and occlusion clips are used to clip the nerve. The nerve is then divided with Metzenbaum scissors.

6. The procedure is completed as in steps 12 and 13 for aneurysmectomy.

Femoral-popliteal bypass

Definition. Restoration of blood flow to the leg via a graft bypassing the occluded section of the femoral artery.

Considerations. The bypass may be either a saphenous vein or straight synthetic graft. The patency of the popliteal artery must be demonstrated by angiography for a successful bypass procedure. If popliteal patency is doubtful, exploration of the artery is necessary as the first procedure. Involvement of the popliteal artery may necessitate the exposure and use of the tibial vessels for the lower anastomosis. If this occurs, the procedure could require the use of microvascular instruments and surgical technique.

Setup and preparation of the patient. The patient is placed in a supine position. The thigh is externally rotated and abducted with the knee flexed. Prepping and draping include the entire groin, thigh, and leg below the knee. The instrument setup includes the basic laparotomy and vascular sets plus the following: Gelpi retractors, Garrett or Weitlaner retractors, a Crawford-Cooley tunneler, and supplies and equipment for operative arteriograms.

Operative procedure

Exploration of common femoral artery

1. A vertical incision, extending downward about 6 inches along the medial aspect of the thigh, is made over the femoral artery below the inguinal area, and a Garrett or Weitlaner retractor is inserted.

2. The common femoral artery is located, the sheath of the artery is bluntly dissected in both directions, and the artery is dissected free for complete exposure.

3. Moist umbilical tapes are passed around the common femoral, the superficial femoral, and the deep femoral arteries.

Exploration of upper popliteal artery

1. A vertical incision, extending down just past the patella, is made along the medial aspect of the lower thigh. If the popliteal artery is diseased, an incision below the knee is necessary to expose the tibial vessels.

2. The saphenous vein and nerve are retracted with small retractors.

3. A Weitlaner retractor is used to retract the muscles after blunt dissection or the exploration of the upper and lower artery. However, in exploring the midportion, the gastrocnemius muscle must be divided to expose the artery.

4. The popliteal vein is bluntly dissected from the artery and retracted with either umbilical tape or a small, blunt vein retractor.

5. The popliteal artery is dissected free, the knee is flexed, and moist umbilical tape is passed around it. It may be desirable at this time to perform arteriograms if doubt exists about the popliteal and distal arterial tree.

6. The saphenous vein is exposed by joining the femoral and popliteal incisions the length of the thigh or through multiple short incisions along the medial thigh. If the vein is suitable, the necessary length is resected. If a prosthesis is used, the length and size are determined, and the graft may be preclotted, as previously described.

7. The saphenous vein is prepared for use by carefully ligating side branches with fine silk and dissecting all fibrous bands from the adventitia. Finally, because of venous valves, the vein *must* be reversed so that the end originally in the groin is anastomosed to the popliteal artery.

8. The tunneler is passed beneath the sartorius muscle from the popliteal fossa to the groin.

9. Heparin solution is injected into the common femoral artery, and the vessels are occluded with an angled vascular clamp.

10. An incision is made into the femoral artery with a no. 11 knife blade and extended with a Potts-Smith angulated scissors.

11. The graft is anastomosed to the artery with fine vascular sutures (two single-armed or one double-armed suture).

12. The graft is carefully pulled through the tunnel and positioned to prevent kinks or twists.

13. The knee is flexed, and a vascular clamp is placed on the popliteal artery at the graft site.

14. An incision is made into the popliteal artery as explained for the femoral arteriotomy.

15. The graft is sutured to the popliteal artery, and, before completion, the femoral occluding clamp is momentarily opened to eliminate clots.

16. All occluding clamps are removed, and a check for leaks is made before closure.

17. The incision is closed as described previously.

Arterial embolectomy

Definition. Incision made in the affected artery for removal of thromboembolic material.

Considerations. Emboli may be clot particles, foreign body, air, fat, or a tumor that circulates through the bloodstream and becomes lodged as the vessel decreases in size. More often the direct source is a mural thrombus, associated with cardiac or vascular disease. Pain or numbness distal to the obstruction is the initial symptom, followed by other signs of vascular occlusion, depending on the area affected.

Setup and preparation of the patient. The patient is placed in the supine position, the skin area is prepared, and draping is completed to permit access to the affected area.

The instrument setup includes the basic laparotomy and vascular sets, including Fogarty arterial and irrigating catheters.

Operative procedure

1. The initial incision is completed, and the artery is carefully exposed to permit the application of vascular clamps (Fig. 19-4).

2. An incision is made into the artery with scalpel blade no. 15 or 11. A Fogarty catheter is carefully inserted beyond the point of clot attachment. The balloon is inflated, and the catheter is withdrawn along with detached clot.

3. As backflow is obtained, a vascular clamp is applied below the arteriotomy.

4. The artery may be flushed by injection of heparinized saline solution through a small irrigating catheter.

5. The arterial closure is completed with vascular sutures. The wound closure is accomplished in the usual manner, and dressings are applied.

Carotid endarterectomy

Definition. Removal of an atheroma at the carotid artery bifurcation.

Setup and preparation of the patient. The patient is placed on the operating room table in a supine position with the patient's head supported on a doughnut or head support. A roll may be placed between the scapulas. Instruments used are the basic minor set, with the following vascular instruments as needed:

3 DeBakey arterial clamps
3 DeBakey arterial forceps
4 DeBakey ring-handled bulldog clamps
2 DeBakey cross-action bulldog clamps
1 Potts-Smith vascular scissors
Endarterectomy instruments
Heparin flushing needles

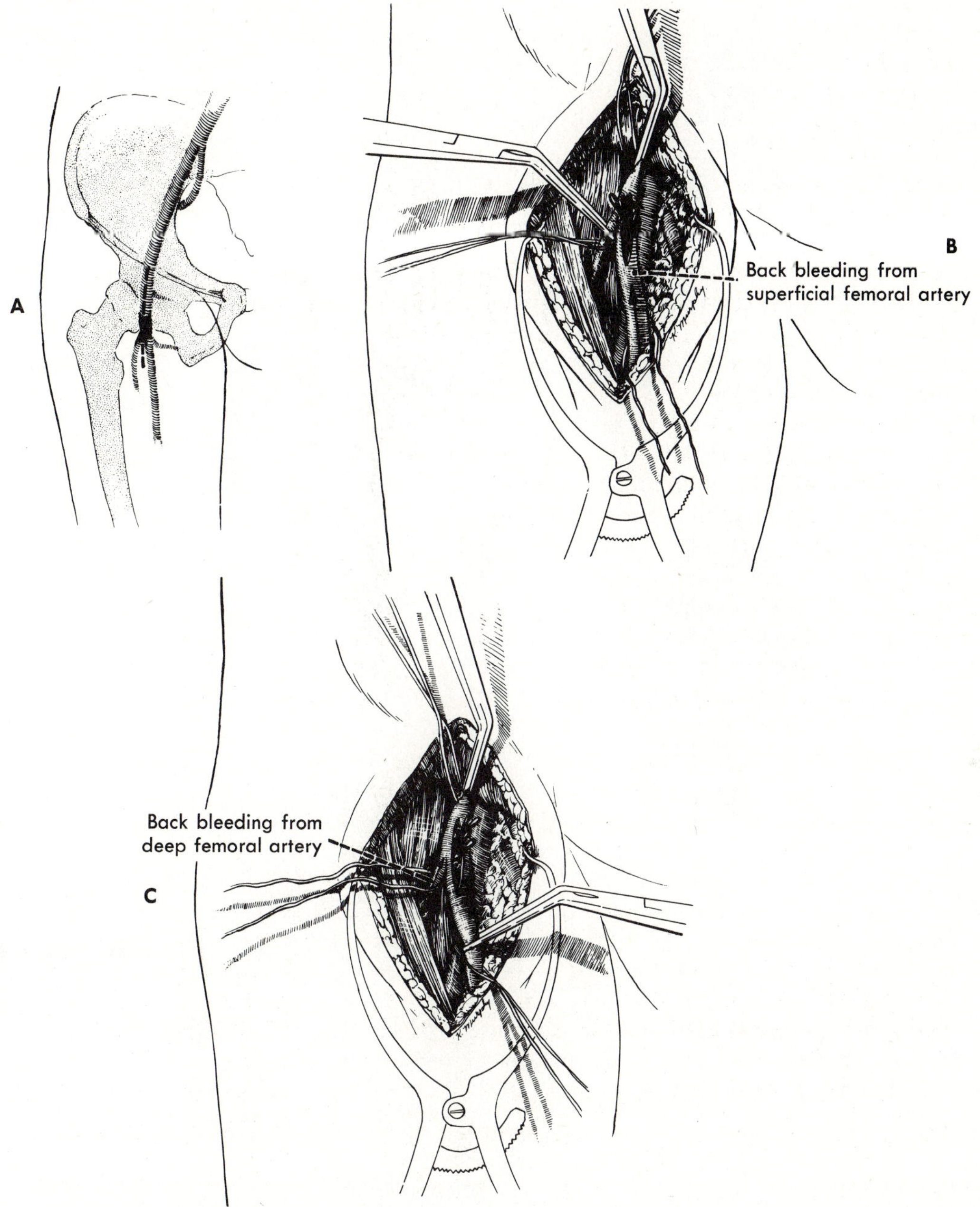

Fig. 19-4. Femoral embolectomy. **A,** Incision. **B,** Backflow from superficial femoral artery is checked. **C,** Backflow from deep femoral artery (profunda femoris) is checked. *Continued.*

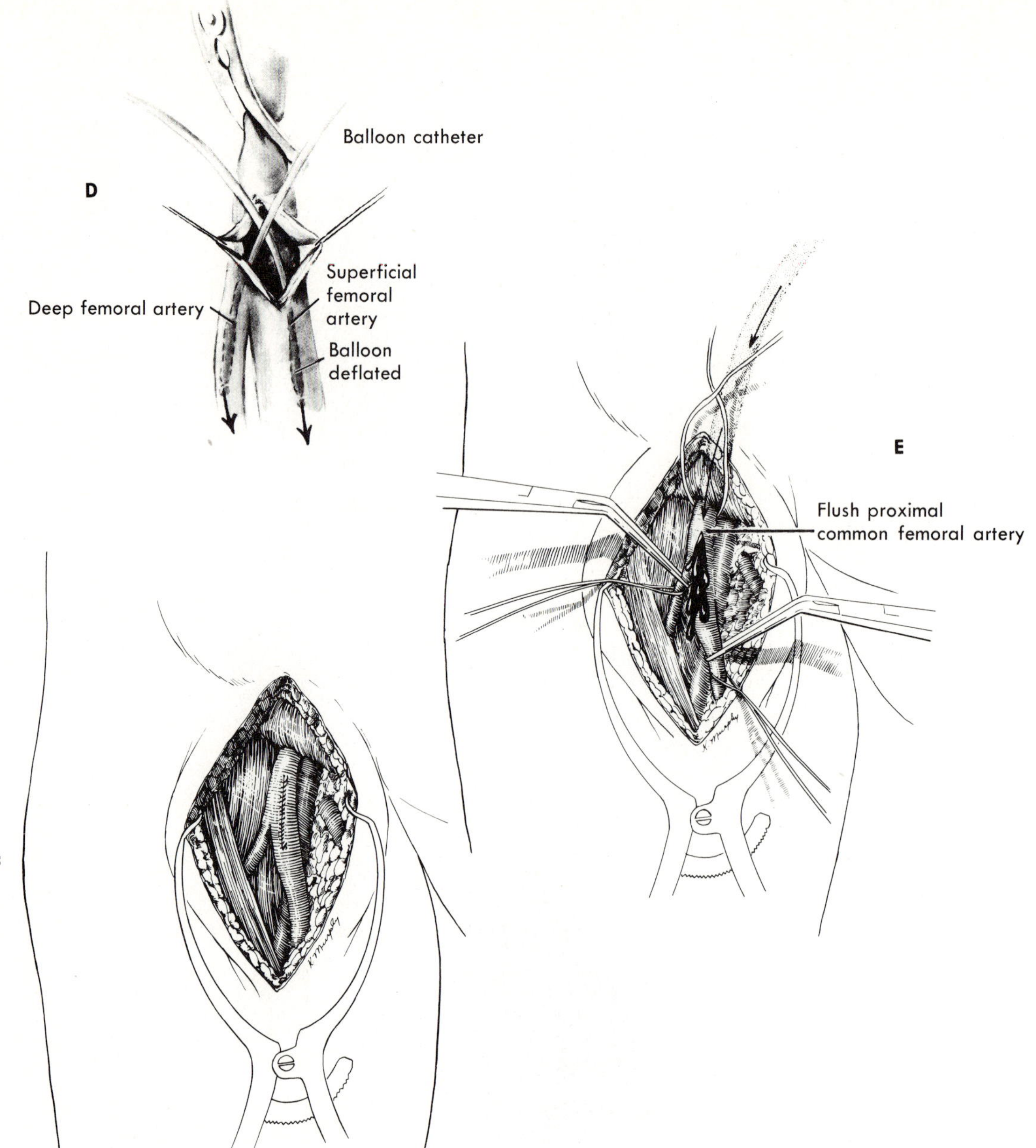

Fig. 19-4, cont'd. D, Balloon catheters are passed into superficial and deep femoral arteries. **E,** Proximal artery is flushed. **F,** Arteriotomy is closed. (From Hershey, F.B., and Calman, C.H.: Atlas of vascular surgery, ed. 3, St. Louis, 1973, The C.V. Mosby Co.)

Operative procedure

1. A longitudinal incision is made over the area of the carotid bifurcation. The Weitlaner self-retaining retractor may be inserted for exposure (Fig. 19-5).

2. With Metzenbaum scissors, the soft tissue is dissected for exposure of the carotid artery and its bifurcation.

3. Blunt dissection with vascular tissue forceps and a small, right-angle clamp is used to dissect and free the carotid artery, including the bifurcated portion. A moistened umbilical tape is passed around the vessel for ease of handling.

4. The external, common, and internal carotid arteries are clamped.

5. With DeBakey tissue forceps and a no. 11 scalpel blade, an arteriotomy is made over the stenotic area. The incision is lengthened with a Potts-Smith angulated scissors to expose the full extent of the occluding plaque.

6. With a blunt dissector, the plaque or plaques are dissected free from the arterial wall. Heparin solution is used as an irrigant to clean the intima.

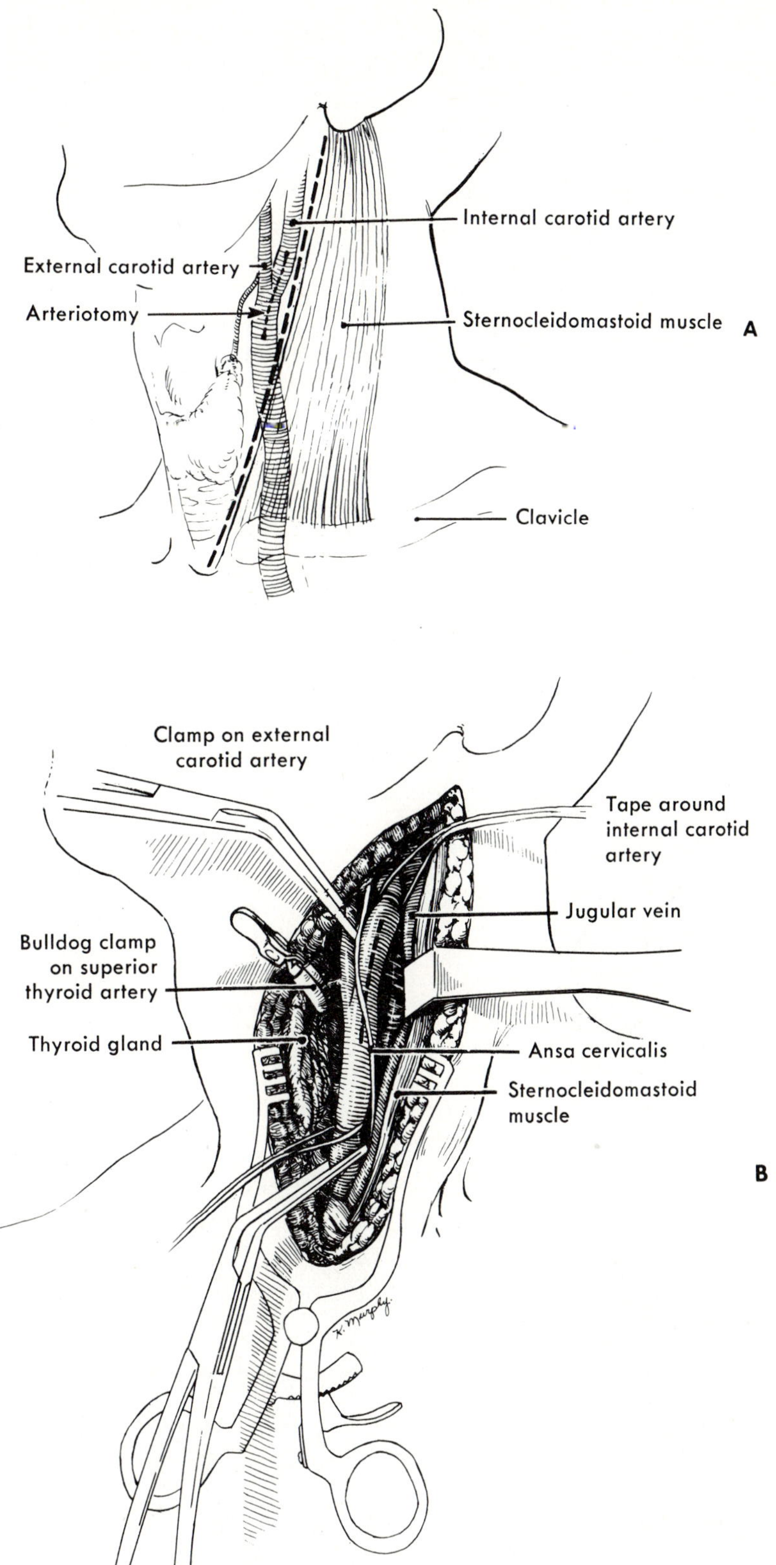

Fig. 19-5. Carotid endarterectomy with patch angioplasty. **A,** Incision. **B,** Exposure of carotid bifurcation. (From Hershey, F.B., and Calman, C.H.: Atlas of vascular surgery, ed. 3, St. Louis, 1973, The C.V. Mosby Co.)

7. Arteriotomy is closed with fine vascular sutures. A synthetic or autogenous patch graft may be used to restore the arterial lumen if it appears to be narrowed.

Before complete closure, blood flow is temporarily restored through the arteries to wash away any free plaques, air, or thrombus. To do this, the occluding clamps are opened and closed individually: first the external artery, then the internal artery, and last the common carotid artery clamps. The closure of the arteriotomy is completed.

8. The occluding clamps are removed from the external and common carotid arteries; the *internal carotid artery clamp is removed last.*

9. Additional interrupted sutures may be needed to control leakage.

10. The wound closure is accomplished in the usual manner, and dressings are applied.

Carotid endarterectomy with temporary bypass

Operative procedure

1. The first five steps as described for carotid endarterectomy are followed.

2. A piece of tubing (polyethylene or silastic) with a suture tied around its center, or a commercially prepared shunt device, is inserted in the common carotid artery and the internal carotid artery to maintain cerebral blood flow and is held in place with tourniquets or ring clamps (Fig. 19-6).

3. The plaque is removed as described for carotid endarterectomy.

4. Before the arteriotomy closure is completed, the ring clamp or tourniquet on the internal carotid artery is released, and the shunt is removed from the internal carotid artery, which is then momentarily reclamped. The shunt is removed from the common carotid artery, and a

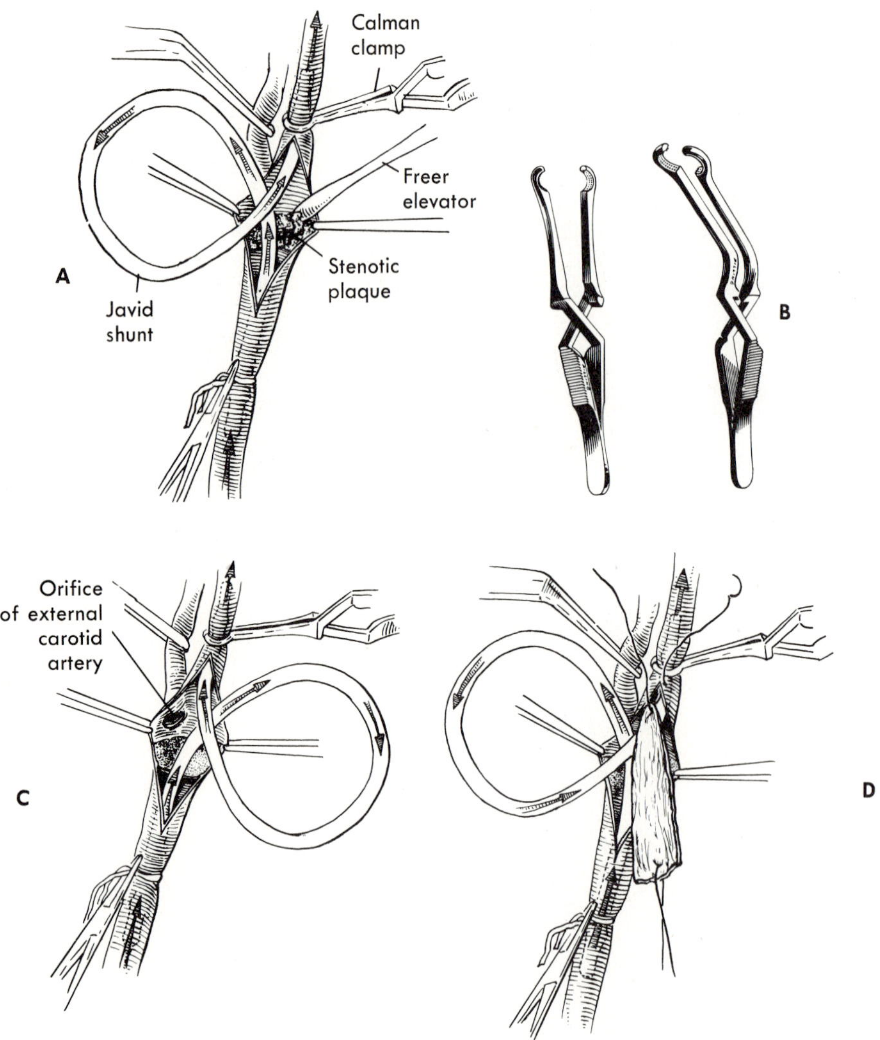

Fig. 19-6. Carotid endarterectomy with internal shunt and patch angioplasty. **A,** Javid shunt in place. Stenotic plaque peeled away. **B,** Calman clamps to hold internal shunts in place. **C,** Shunt rotated for completion of endarterectomy. **D,** Patch angioplasty begun.

partial occlusion clamp, incorporating only the unclosed suture line, is applied. The external carotid occluding clamp is removed, followed by the common carotid artery clamp, and last, the internal carotid artery occluding clamp. This ensures that any minor debris missed will flush harmlessly into the external rather than the internal carotid artery.

5. The closure of the arteriotomy is completed, and the partial occlusion clamp removed.

6. The wound is closed as usual.

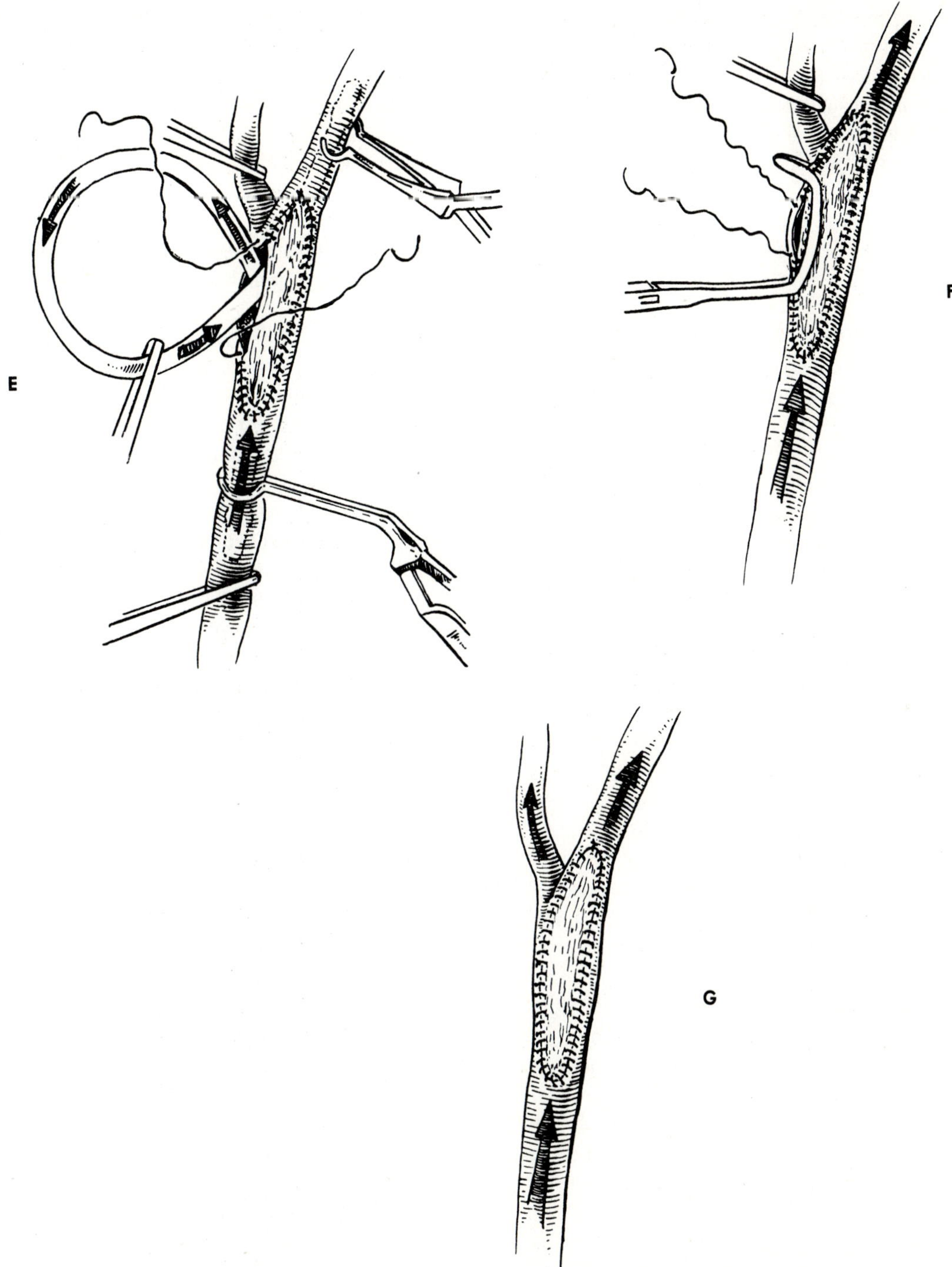

Fig. 19-6, cont'd. E, Shunt being withdrawn from internal carotid artery. **F,** Flow restored to internal carotid artery during completion of patch angioplasty. **G,** Patch angioplasty completed. (From Hershey, F.B., and Calman, C.H.: Atlas of vascular surgery, ed. 3, St. Louis, 1973, The C.V. Mosby Co.)

Shunt operations for portal hypertension

Considerations. Obstruction of the portal system, which may be intrahepatic or extrahepatic, is the direct cause of portal hypertension. Intrahepatic obstruction, which is the more common, may result from cirrhosis or infectious hepatitis. Extrahepatic obstruction, which represents about 15% of the total, may be caused by thrombosis, compression, or congenital abnormalities. The most important indication for surgery is hemorrhage of esophageal or gastric varices. An effective shunt between the hypertensive portal and lower caval circulation produces a fall in portal pressure, with subsequent disappearance of varices and protection against further hemorrhage.

Preoperatively, a portal venogram usually is obtained by percutaneous splenic puncture or the venous phase of mesenteric arteriography.

Portacaval anastomosis

Definition. Through an abdominal incision, an anastomosis is established between the portal vein and the inferior vena cava (Fig. 19-7).

Setup and preparation of the patient. The patient is placed on the operating table in a supine position with a pad under the patient's right side. The instrument setup includes the basic laparotomy and vascular sets, plus the following for measuring portal pressures: a manometer, a three-way stopcock, polyethylene tubing, and a syringe and needles.

Operative procedure

1. The abdominal incision is completed with instruments and materials as previously described. Abdominal exploration is carried out.

2. A jejunal mesenteric vein is isolated and cannulated with polyethylene tubing by a simple cutdown technique, using a no. 11 scalpel blade and fine plastic or vascular scissors, Adson forceps, two curved mosquito hemostats, and silk ligatures. With a three-way stopcock, a spinal manometer is attached to the tubing, and intravenous saline solution is injected into the manometer.

3. The portal pressure is measured and determined by the height of the saline solution meniscus above the right atrium when it comes to rest. Normal limits range from 45 to 150 mm. The abnormal range is from 200 to 600 mm.

4. As the portal vein and inferior vena cava are dissected free, extreme caution is exercised to prevent injury to important surrounding structures, for example, the duodenum, gallbladder, cystic and common bile ducts, and the hepatic artery and its branches.

5. Moist compression tapes are applied to the portal vein and the vena cava, both above and below the prepared sites for anastomosis.

6. Noncrushing vascular clamps are placed on the portal vein. If an end-to-end anastomosis is contemplated, the vein is ligated. If a side-to-side anastomosis is to be established, the vein is incised. Small clots are carefully removed, and the lumen may be irrigated with saline solution.

7. A Satinsky or other suitable partial occluding clamp is placed on the vena cava. An elliptical section of the vessel wall that is secured within the inner aspect of the clamp is excised with vascular scissors. The size of the section removed should correspond to the lumen of the portion of the portal vein that has been prepared for anastomosis.

8. The anastomosis is completed with a continuous vascular suture, fine vascular forceps, and long fine needle holders.

9. The portal pressure is retaken to determine functioning of the shunt.

10. The peritoneum is closed. Closure of the muscle, fascia, and skin is completed. Dressings are applied.

Splenorenal shunt

Definition. Through a left midline or subcostal incision, establishment of an anastomosis between the proximal splenic and the left renal veins (Fig. 19-7).

Setup and preparation of the patient. As described for portacaval shunt.

Operative procedure

1. A midline or subcostal incision is made.

2. The spleen and splenic artery are mobilized, and the pancreas is separated from the splenic pedicle; the phrenocolic ligament is divided.

3. The spleen is removed with angular and curved artery forceps and silk sutures.

4. The renal vein is dissected free, and vascular clamps are applied.

5. An anastomosis of the splenic vein to the left renal vein is carried out in a manner similar to that for the portacaval anastomosis.

6. The wound is closed as described for the portacaval shunt operation.

Distal splenorenal shunt (Warren shunt)

Definition. Anastomosis between the distal end of the splenic vein and the left renal vein (Fig. 19-7).

Setup and preparation of the patient. As described for the splenorenal shunt.

Operative procedure

1. A long transverse or bilateral subcostal incision is made, and a limited abdominal exploration is carried out.

2. The splenic vein lying at the upper border of the pancreas is approached through the lesser omental bursa.

3. The distal end of the pancreas and splenic vein is carefully separated. Multiple fine suture ligatures are required.

4. The gastrocolic ligament is freed from the greater curvature of the stomach, and the gastrocolic vein is ligated.

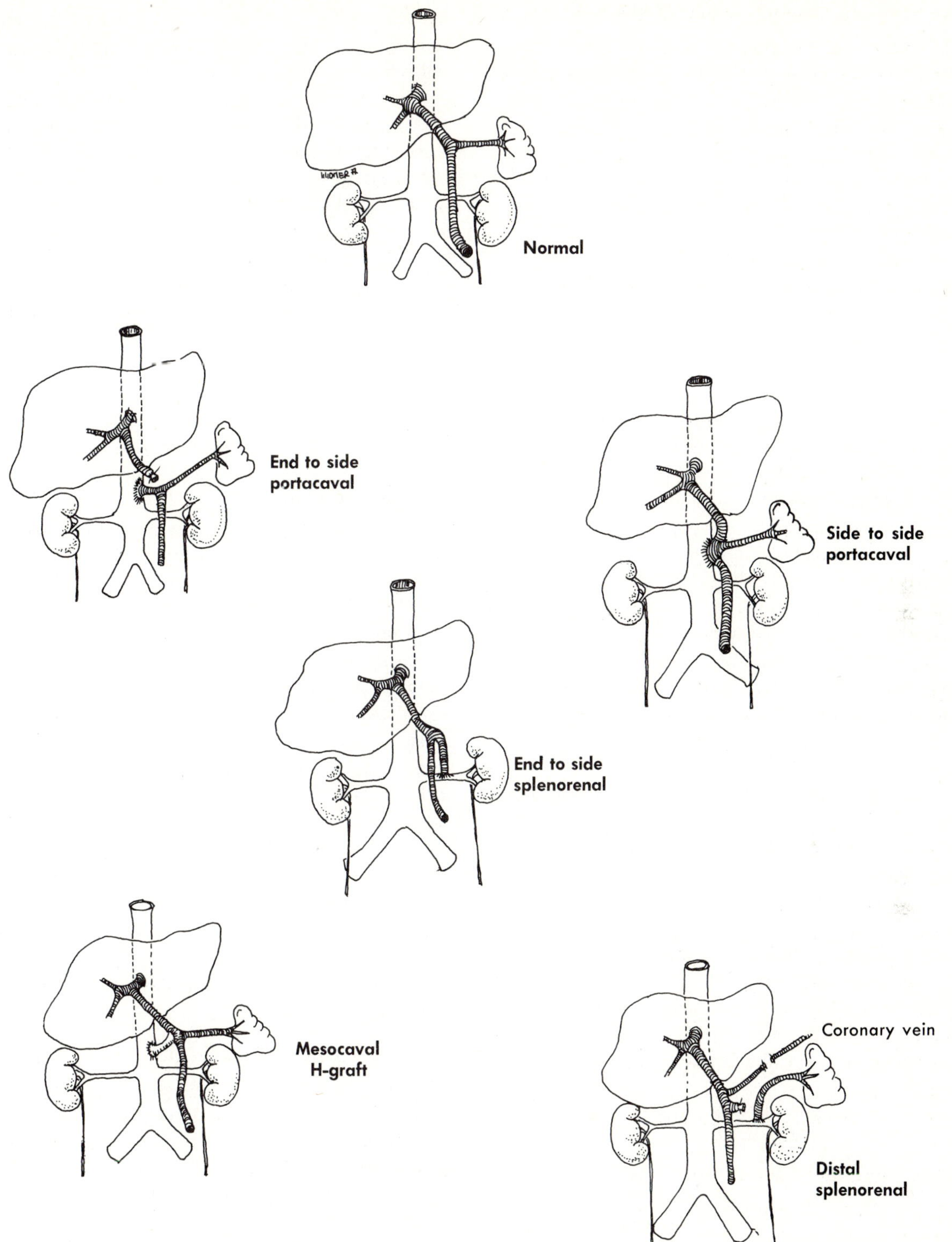

Fig. 19-7. Types of portal-systemic venous shunts used to relieve portal hypertension.

5. The left renal vein is dissected free.

6. The splenic vein is divided near its junction with the mesenteric vein, and the proximal end is closed with a fine continuous vascular suture.

7. The distal (splenic) end of the splenic vein is swung to the renal vein, and an end-to-side anastomosis with a fine vascular suture is accomplished in a manner similar to that for a portacaval anastomosis.

8. The coronary vein is ligated.

9. The wound is closed as described for a portacaval anastomosis.

Mesocaval interposition shunt (Drapanas shunt)

Definition. Placement of a short Dacron prosthetic graft between the superior mesenteric vein and the inferior vena cava (Fig. 19-7).

Setup and preparation of the patient. As described for portacaval shunt.

Operative procedure

1. Incision and pressure measurements are done as in portacaval anastomosis steps 1 to 3.
2. The superior mesenteric vein is identified and isolated through an incision at the base of the transverse mesocolon.
3. The inferior vena cava is approached through the mesenteric reflection of the right colon, and about 4 cm of vein is exposed.
4. A Satinsky clamp is placed partially occluding the vena cava, and an ellipse of vein wall is removed.
5. A short (about 6 to 8 cm) section of an 18- to 20-mm Dacron graft is sutured end to side to the vena cava with a fine vascular suture.
6. The superior mesenteric vein is occluded between vascular clamps, and the graft is sutured end to side to the vein. Appropriate flushing of the graft is carried out before completion of the anastomosis.
7. All vascular clamps are removed, and pressures are again taken, as in portacaval anastomosis.
8. The abdomen is closed as in portacaval anastomosis.

Access procedures

Considerations. Access procedures are performed on patients in chronic renal failure to facilitate hemodialysis. The surgeon may elect to insert a shunting device or to create an arteriovenous fistula.

Arteriovenous shunt

Setup and preparation of the patient. The patient is placed in a supine position with the arms extended on a wide armboard. An arteriovenous shunt is usually done with local or standby anesthesia. A basic minor instrument set is required, plus the following:

4 DeBakey ring-handled bulldog clamps
2 Johns Hopkins bulldog clamps
4 Arteriovenous fistula clamps
2 Vascular forceps
1 Potts-Smith vascular scissors
2 Needle holders
Arteriovenous fistula tunneler
Arterial dilators

Operative procedure

1. After skin cleansing, sterile drapes are applied around the site. A local anesthetic is infiltrated, and a small incision is made over the venous site. Bleeding vessels are clamped and ligated. The vein is dissected free of the fascia, and two heavy silk ties are placed around the vessel and held with clamps. A vascular clamp is applied to the proximal end of the vein, which is then cut and ligated distally.
2. A small incision is made at the selected arterial site after it is infiltrated with local anesthetic. Bleeding vessels are ligated. The artery is exposed and dissected free. Two heavy silk sutures are placed around the artery. A vascular clamp is applied to the proximal end, and the distal end is incised and ligated.
3. Vessel tips are inserted into the open ends of the vein and artery and are tied securely with the heavy silk sutures. A small amount of heparin solution is injected. The selected appliance is then connected to the vessel tips linking the vein and artery. The vascular clamp is removed from the vein, then from the artery, and the shunt has been accomplished.
4. The fascia and skin are closed carefully over the vessel tips and ends of the appliance to prevent twisting or occluding in any way.
5. Sterile dressings are applied and held securely in place with a gauze roller bandage.

Arteriovenous fistula

Considerations. The surgeon may elect to create a direct arteriovenous fistula between the radial artery and the cephalic vein. These vessels would then be used for direct cannulation with large bore needles for hemodialysis. This method is considered to be preferable to an external shunt, which carries a high risk of thrombosis and infection.

Other alternatives are to use a saphenous vein or a prosthetic graft to join the brachial artery and cephalic vein.

Setup and preparation of the patient. Basically the same as for arteriovenous shunt, except that general or regional anesthesia may be used. If a graft is employed a tunneling instrument is required. The anastomosis is done with fine vascular sutures.

Vena cava interruption

Ligation or clipping

Definition. Total or partial occlusion of the vena cava.

Considerations. Ligation or interruption of the vena cava is performed to prevent pulmonary embolism when anticoagulant therapy fails or cannot be initiated. In the female patient, a transabdominal incision may be used to permit ligation of the ovarian veins.

Setup and preparation of the patient. The nursing care and instruments are similar to that required for lumbar sympathectomy (Chapter 24).

Operative procedure

1. Steps 1 and 2 for lumbar sympathectomy are followed.
2. Deep retractors are placed for adequate exposure.
3. The peritoneum and abdominal contents are bluntly

dissected anteriorly, with sponge holders used to expose the vena cava.

4. Deep in the wound, the vena cava is dissected free with sharp and blunt dissecton.

5. With a Mixter forceps, two heavy silk sutures are passed around the vena cava and tied approximately ½ inch above or below the lumbar vein. The vena cava is not cut. A Teflon clip may be used instead of suture ligation. These are available commercially and allow for partial flow of venous blood to reduce vascular congestion in the lower extremities.

6. The incision is closed in layers as described for lumbar sympathectomy.

Umbrella filter

Definition. Partial occlusion of the inferior vena cava with an intravascular umbrella filter, such as a Mobin-Uddin or Kimray-Greenfield, inserted under fluoroscopy with local or standby anesthesia. The Mobin-Uddin device must be inserted through the jugular vein, whereas the Greenfield device offers the option of jugular or femoral vein insertion.

Setup and preparation of the patient. The patient is placed in the supine position with the head turned to the left. Instruments are the same as for arteriovenous shunts. A fluoroscopy unit and equipment are needed as well as the filter setup.

Operative procedure (for insertion of Mobin-Uddin in jugular vein)

1. The filter comes with detailed instructions. These should be read and thoroughly understood before the procedure is begun.

2. The filter is loaded and prepared for use according to these instructions before an incision is made (Fig. 19-8).

3. The incision and approach to the right internal jugular vein are made (Fig. 19-9).

4. The vein is isolated between tapes, and a venotomy is made.

5. The loaded filter is inserted into the vein and threaded under fluoroscopy to the appropriate place in the inferior vena cava.

6. The filter is opened into position, and the stylet removed.

7. The venotomy is closed with a vascular suture.

8. The incision is closed.

High ligation of saphenous veins with or without excision

Definition. Ligation and division of the saphenous trunk with or without subsequent stripping and excision.

Considerations. A series of cup-shaped valves maintains the venous blood flow in a direction toward the heart. Because of disease, the normal functioning of these valves is disturbed, resulting in distention or back pressure. The veins gradually become dilated. Those in the lower extremities are most frequently affected. Dilatation of the saphenous vein produces venous stasis, which may be followed by secondary complications.

The objective of surgical intervention is to interrupt or remove the diseased veins, thus preventing ulceration, secondary edema, pain, and fatigue in the extremity.

Setup and preparation of the patient. The patient is placed on the operating table in a supine position with the legs slightly abducted. Ligation or stripping of the lesser saphenous veins may require placing the patient in the prone position. Drapes are placed to enable flexing and lifting at the knee. Instruments include the basic laparotomy instrument setup (Chapter 10), plus the following:

2 Weitlaner self-retaining retractors
6 Mosquito hemostats, 5½-inches
Vein strippers with various tips available
Elastic bandages

Operative procedure

1. The incision is made in the upper thigh, parallel to the crease in the groin. Bleeding vessels are clamped and ligated.

2. The saphenous vein is identified and isolated. Margins of the wound are separated with a Weitlaner self-retaining retractor.

3. The saphenous vein and branches are doubly ligated with black silk sutures or transfixed, clamped, and divided. The proximal stump is dissected upward to the point at which it enters the femoral vein, where it is carefully religated.

4. If the saphenous vein is to be excised, an incision is made at its distal, pedal portion at the ankle, and the vein is identified, ligated, and divided.

5. A vein stripper is inserted, with the olive tip in place, and is advanced to the proximal end of the vein in the groin, where it is secured with a heavy suture.

6. As the stripper is pulled up the leg, external compression is applied.

7. Tributaries may be ligated through numerous small incisions along the course of the vein.

8. The groin wound is closed in layers with interrupted sutures, and other small incisions are similarly closed. Dressings and circular compression bandages are applied.

Peritoneovenous shunt

Definition. Establishment of a shunt to allow unidirectional flow of fluid from the abdomen through a valve into the venous system, with a resulting increase in intravascular volume and renal perfusion.

Considerations. A peritoneovenous shunt is performed on patients with intractable ascites secondary to cirrhosis or malignancy.

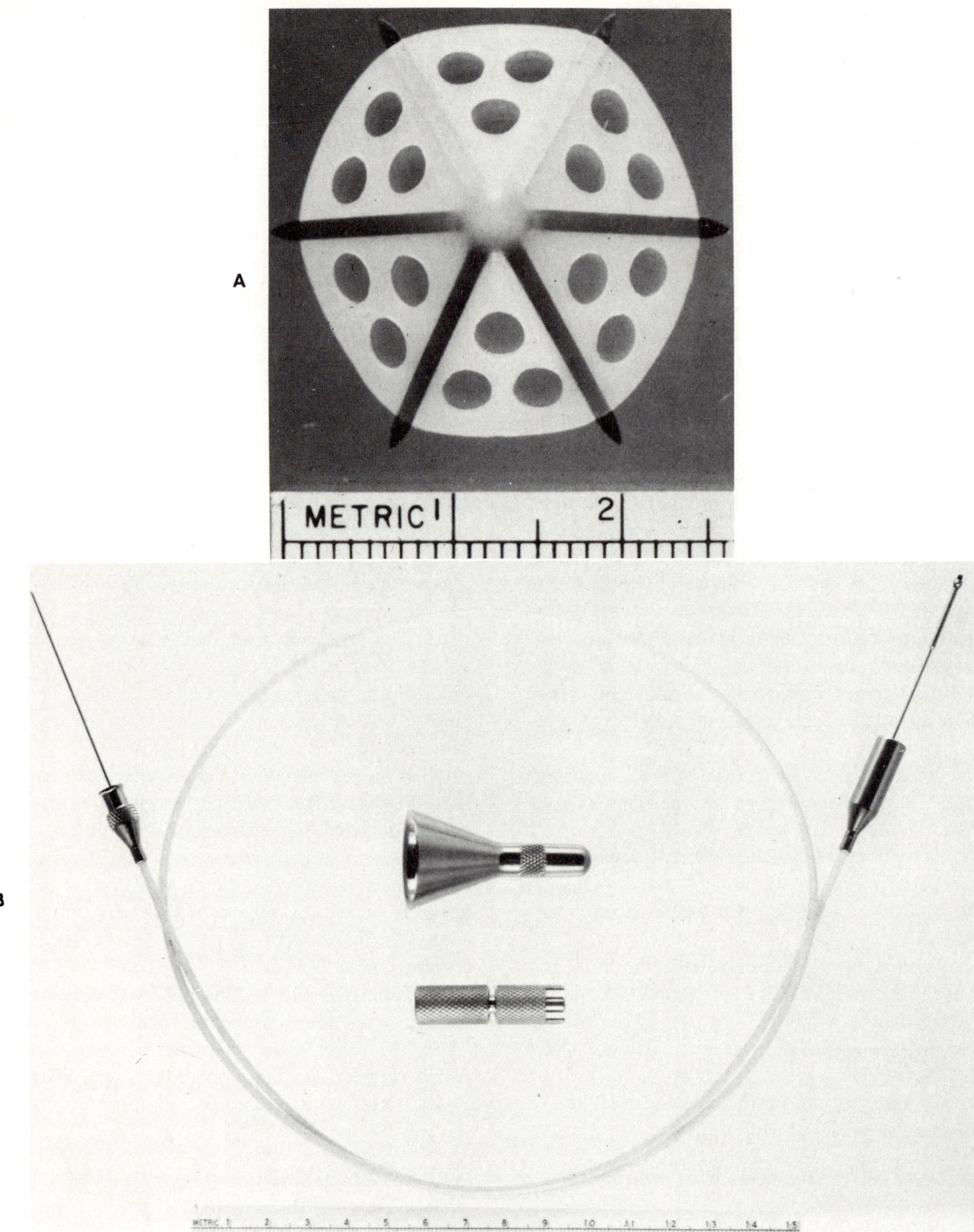

Fig. 19-8. Mobin-Uddin filter. A, Filter. B, Applicator.

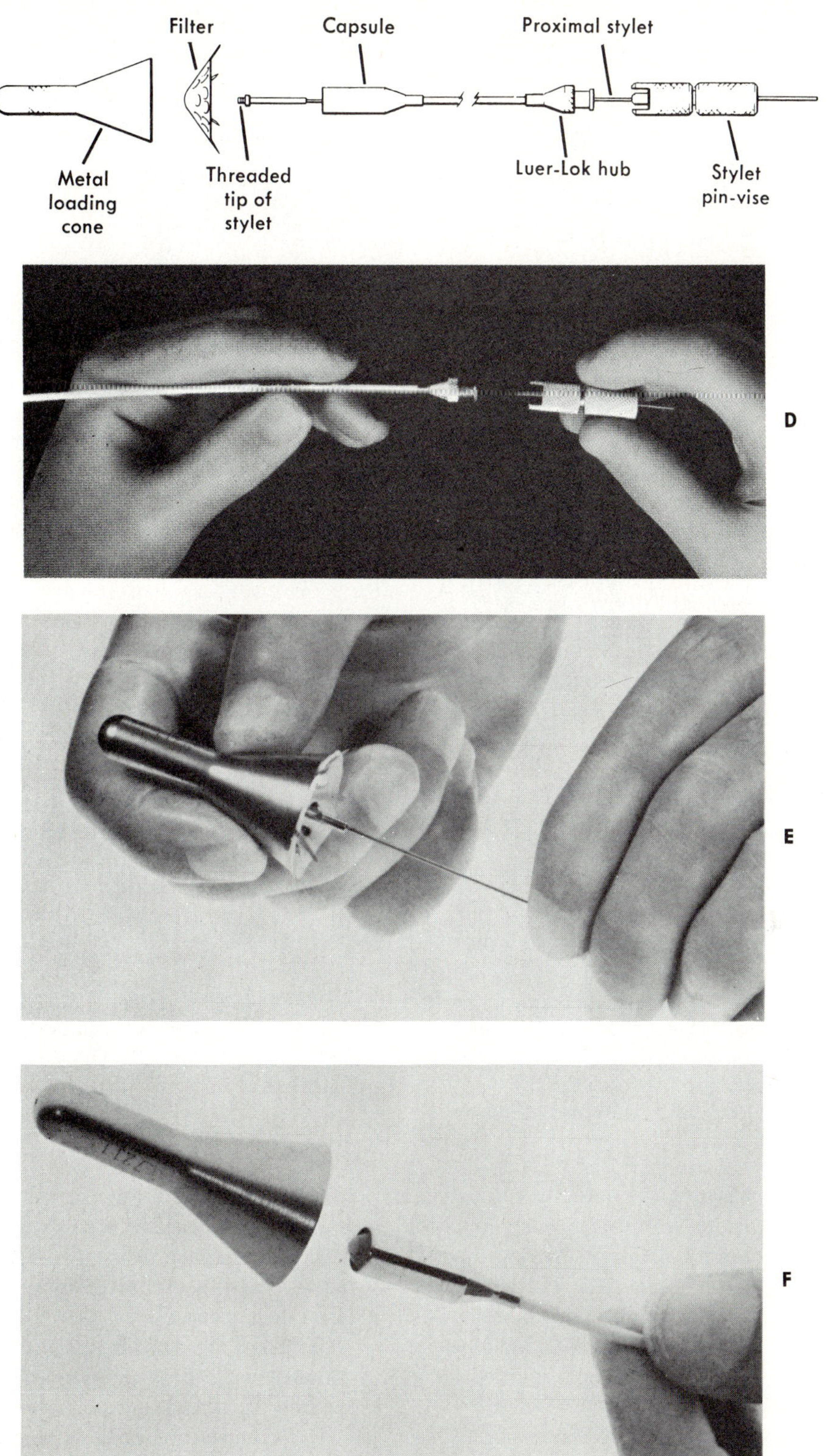

Fig. 19-8, cont'd. C, Diagram of components of applicator. **D,** Luer-Lok hub and stylet pin vise. **E,** Filter advanced into loading cone. **F,** Collapsed filter withdrawn into hollow applicator capsule. (From Hershey, F.B., and Calman, C.H.: Atlas of vascular surgery, ed. 3, St. Louis, 1973, The C.V. Mosby Co.)

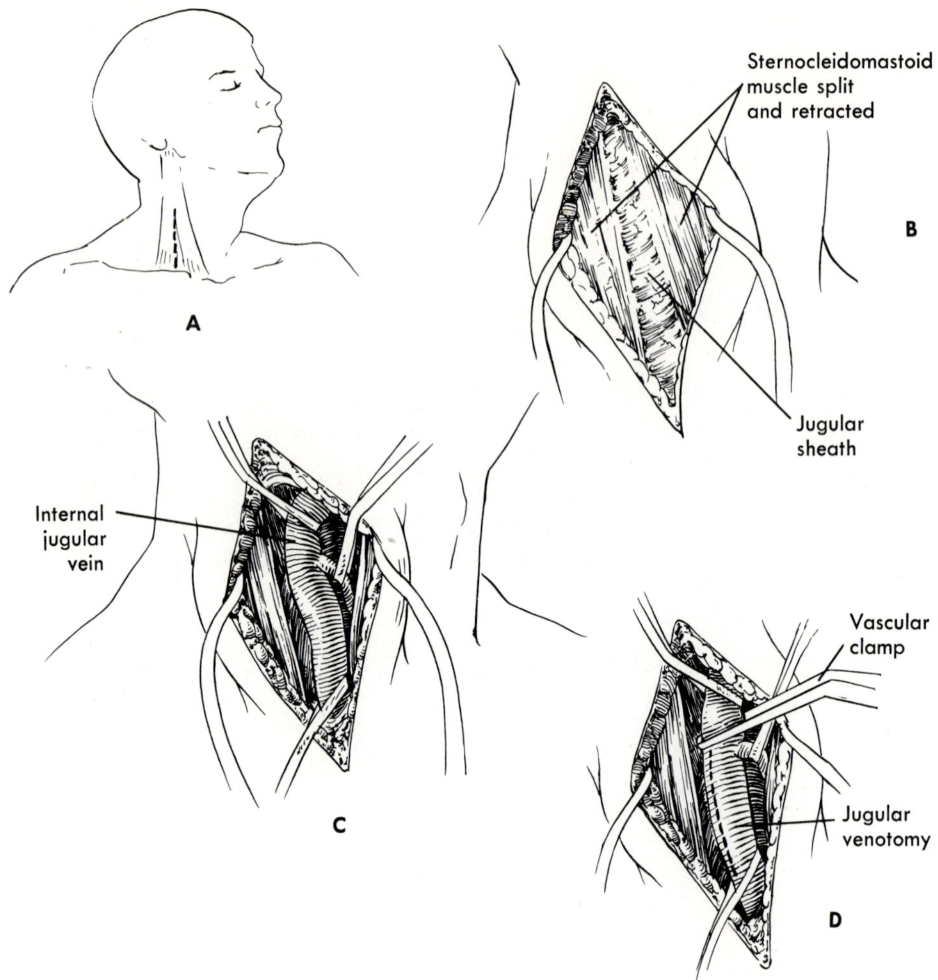

Fig. 19-9. Transjugular venotomy for insertion of Mobin-Uddin filter to interrupt inferior vena cava. **A,** Position of neck and incision. **B,** Sternocleidomastoid muscle split and retracted to reveal jugular sheath. **C,** Internal jugular vein isolated and controlled with tapes. **D,** Jugular venotomy. (From Hershey, F.B., and Calman, C.H.: Atlas of vascular surgery, ed. 3, St. Louis, 1973, The C.V. Mosby Co.)

Setup and preparation of the patient. The patient is placed in a supine position with the shoulders elevated and the head turned toward the left. Preparation and draping include the right side of the neck, clavicular area, anterior thorax, and upper outer quadrant of the abdomen. The instrument setup includes the basic minor setup (Chapter 7), plus the vascular instruments as listed for a carotid endarterectomy.

The shunt is prepared and sterilized according to the manufacturer's instructions.

The procedure can be conducted under local anesthesia with the anesthesiologist monitoring the patient.

Operative procedure

1. A transverse supraclavicular incision is made. Hemostasis is secured. The external or internal jugular vein is exposed and isolated with moist umbilical tapes.
2. A transverse incision is made through the anterior rectus sheath to expose the posterior rectus sheath. Hemostasis is secured.
3. The subcutaneous tunnel is prepared from the abdominal to the neck incision, remaining anterior to the ribs and the clavicle.
4. A tunneler is used to pass the catheter from the abdominal to the neck incision. The outlet tubing of the shunt is ligated to the blunt end of the tunneler with a heavy silk suture.
5. The pointed end of the tunneler is advanced through the superior flap of the abdominal incision, exiting through

the supraclavicular incision. Care is taken to prevent rotational tension of the tubing. All clamps applied to the tubing must be shod with rubber.

6. The tubing is cut flush with the tunneler.

7. Two purse-string sutures of a nonabsorbable vascular material are placed in the posterior rectus sheath and peritoneum. An incision of 1 cm is made through the tissues into the abdomen.

8. The flexible cannula of the shunt is placed into the fluid-filled abdomen. The purse-string sutures are secured around the valve stem to prevent leakage of peritoneal fluid.

9. Valve function is demonstrated by free flow of ascitic fluid through the outlet tubing in the neck.

10. All air bubbles are removed from the outlet tubing, and the tubing is clamped with a rubber shod clamp at the entrance into the supraclavicular incision.

11. A venotomy is made in the jugular vein with a no. 11 scalpel blade. The outlet tubing is advanced into the vein and placed in the superior vena cava.

12. The tubing is secured to the wall of the jugular vein with two encircling nonabsorbable vascular sutures. The cephalic segment of the vein is ligated. Every precaution is taken to prevent air emboli during the venotomy and catheter placement.

13. The rubber-shod clamps are removed from the outlet tubing, and the shunt function is established.

14. The tubing is secured to the fascia and muscle.

15. The neck and abdominal incisions are closed, and the wounds are dressed.

SUGGESTED READINGS

Barker, W.F.: Peripheral vascular disease, ed. 2, Philadelphia, 1975, W.B. Saunders Co.

Beven, E.G.: Carotid endarterectomy, Surg. Clin. North Am. **55:**111, 1975.

Beven, E.G., and Hertzer, N.R.: Construction of arterial venous fistulas for hemodialysis, Surg. Clin. North Am. **55:**1125, 1975.

Bramoweth, E.: Acute aortic dissection, Am. J. Nurs. **80:**2010, 1980.

Butler, S.: Carotid endarterectomy: care in the OR, AORN J. **32:**42, 1980.

Cimochowski, G.E., and others: Greenfield filter vs. Mobin-Uddin umbrella, J. Thorac. Cardiovasc. Surg. **79:**358, 1980.

Cliff, W.J.: Blood vessels, New York, 1976, Cambridge University Press.

Cooley, D., and Wukasch, D.: Techniques in vascular surgery, Philadelphia, 1979, W.B. Saunders Co.

Cranley, J.J., editor: Peripheral venous disease, New York, 1975, Harper & Row, Publishers.

Haimovici, H.: Vascular surgery: principles and techniques, New York, 1976, McGraw-Hill Book Co.

Hermann, R.E.: Shunt operations for portal hypertension, Surg. Clin. North Am. **55:**1073, 1975.

Hessler, K., and Kenny, M.: Using human umbilical vein grafts, AORN J. **33:**862, 1981.

Humphries, A.W.: Technique of bilateral aortofemoral bypass grafting, Surg. Clin. North Am. **55:**1137, 1975.

King, S.: Patient care in vascular surgery, AORN J. **33:**843, 1981.

Long, G.D.: Managing the patient with abdominal aortic aneurysm, Nursing '78 8(8):20, 1978.

Reinhardt, G., and Stanley, M.: Peritoneovenous shunting for ascites, Surg. Gynecol. Obstet. 145:419, 1977.

Rutherford, R.: Vascular surgery, Philadelphia, 1977, W.B. Saunders Co.

Wilson, S., and Owens, M.: Vascular access surgery, Chicago, 1980, Year Book Medical Publishers, Inc.

Wylie, R., Stoney, R., and Ehrenfeld, W.: Manual of vascular surgery, New York, 1980, Springer-Verlag New York, Inc.

20 Orthopedic surgery

Nicholas André first used the word "orthopaedia" in 1741 as the title for a book dealing with the prevention and correction of skeletal deformities in children. The word is derived from the Greek, *orthos* meaning straight, and *paidios* meaning child. Orthopedic surgery has been defined by the American Academy of Orthopaedic Surgeons as "the medical specialty that includes the investigation, preservation, restoration and development of the form and function of the extremity, spine and associated structures by medical, surgical and physical method."

ANATOMY

To be an efficient member of the operating team, the nurse must be aware of the anatomical structures involved in an orthopedic operation. Following is a brief summary of the anatomy of the bones and joints.

The bones of the body form a stable framework that supports the weight of the soft tissues. Diarthrodial joints consist of (1) the ends of the articulating bones that are covered with hyaline cartilage, (2) the supporting ligaments and capsule, and (3) a filmy synovium that forms the inner lining of the joint. Musculotendinous units originate and insert on adjacent bones and pass across the joints. Contraction of the muscle produces motion at the joint and brings about body movements.

Bones are divided into four types, according to their shapes: long, short, flat, and irregular (Fig. 20-1). *Long* bones are present in the limbs and consist of a shaft and two ends; the ends are covered with articular cartilage and provide a surface for articulation and muscle attachment. *Short* bones are present where strength but limited movement is required. *Flat* bones are found in the shoulder and pelvis. *Irregular* bones are found in the skull and vertebral column.

Long bones are divided into three sections: the diaphysis and two epiphyses. The *diaphysis,* or shaft, is the midportion, and each articulating end is an *epiphysis.* Until skeletal maturity, a line of cartilage called the epiphyseal plate separates the epiphyses from the diaphysis.

There are two types of bone tissue: cortical and cancellous bone. *Cortical bone* is the main supporting tissue, the hard bone that forms the shell of all bones. *Cancellous bone* is the soft, spongy bone contained inside cortical bone. Marrow is located in this space. A thin layer of connective tissue called *periosteum* covers all bone.

Shoulder and upper extremity

The *clavicle,* which is a long doubly curved bone, serves as a prop for the shoulder and holds it away from the chest wall. The clavicle rests almost horizontally at the upper and anterior part of the thorax, above the first rib. It articulates medially with the manubrium of the sternum and laterally with the acromion of the scapula and is tethered to the underlying coracoid process of the scapula by the coracoclavicular ligaments.

The *scapula* (shoulder blade) is a flat triangular bone that forms the posterior part of the shoulder girdle lying superior and posterior to the upper chest. The glenoid cavity provides a socket for the humerus, and the acromion process articulates with the clavicle. The scapula is attached to the trunk by muscles.

The *acromioclavicular joint* is the articulating structure (joint) between the outer end of the clavicle and a flattened articular facet situated on the inner border of the acromion.

The *shoulder joint,* a ball-and-socket joint, is formed by the head of the humerus and the glenoid cavity. This joint is surrounded by a loose capsule that allows considerable motion (Figs. 20-2 and 20-3).

The muscles immediately surrounding the shoulder joint are the supraspinous, infraspinous, the teres minor, and the subscapular muscles; together, they are referred to as the rotator cuff. These muscles stabilize the shoulder joint while the entire arm is moved by the powerful deltoid, pectoralis major, teres major, and latissimus dorsi muscles.

The *humerus,* the longest and largest bone of the upper extremity, is composed of a shaft and two ends. The proximal end, or head, has two projections, the greater and lesser tuberosities (Figs. 20-1 and 20-4).

The head articulates with the glenoid cavity of the scapula. The circumference of the articular surface of the humerus is constricted and is termed the *anatomical neck.* The constriction below the tuberosities is called the *surgical neck* and is the site of most fractures. The anatomical neck marks the attachment to the capsule of the shoulder joint.

Text continued on p. 453.

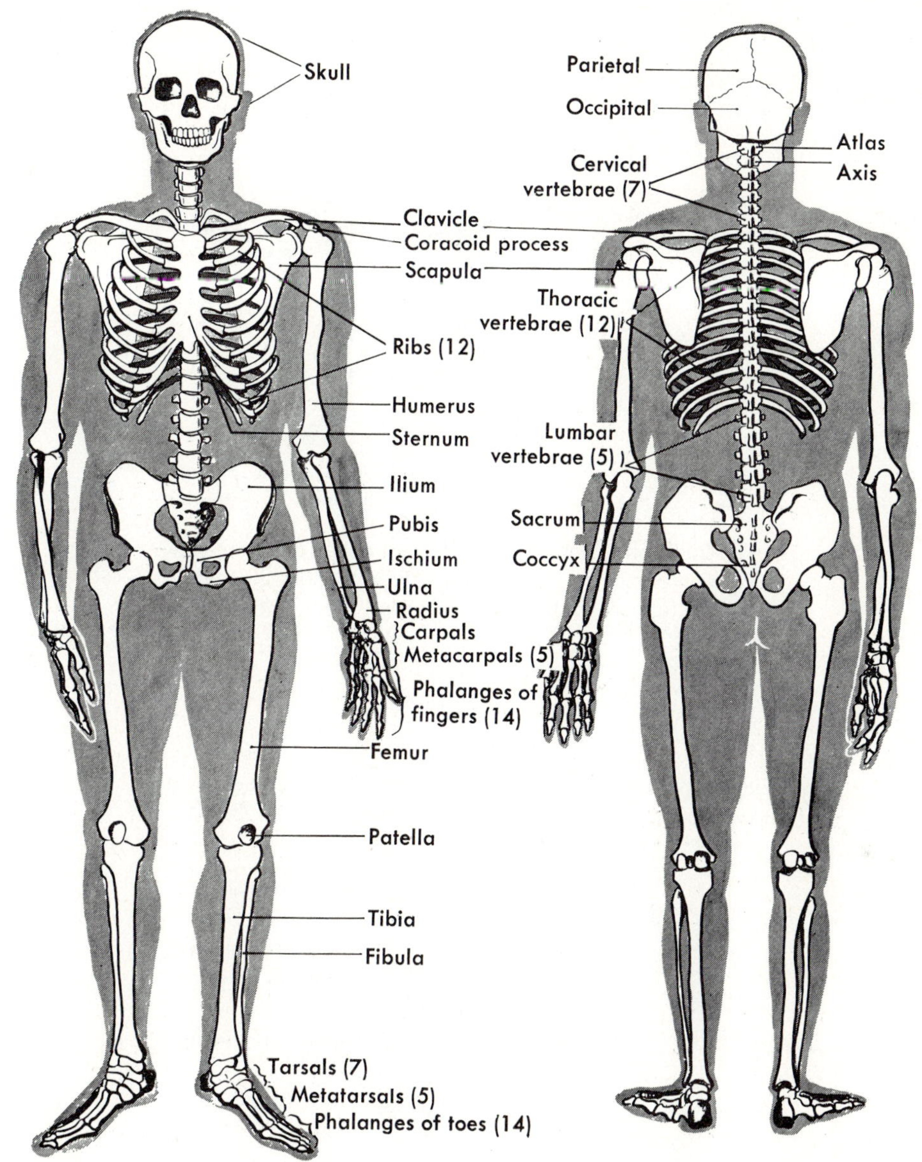

Fig. 20-1. Human skeleton, ventral and dorsal views. Numbers in parentheses indicate number of bones in that unit. In comparison with those of other mammals, the human skeleton is a type of patchwork of primitive and specialized parts. Erect posture brought about by specialized changes in legs and pelvis enabled primitive arrangement of arms and hands (arboreal adaptation of human's ancestors) to be used for manipulation of tools. Development of skull and brain followed as consequence of premium natural selection based on dexterity, better senses, and ability to appraise environment. (Adapted from Hickman, C.P., Hickman, F.M., and Hickman, C.P., Jr.: Integrated principles of zoology, ed. 6, St. Louis, 1979, The C.V. Mosby Co.)

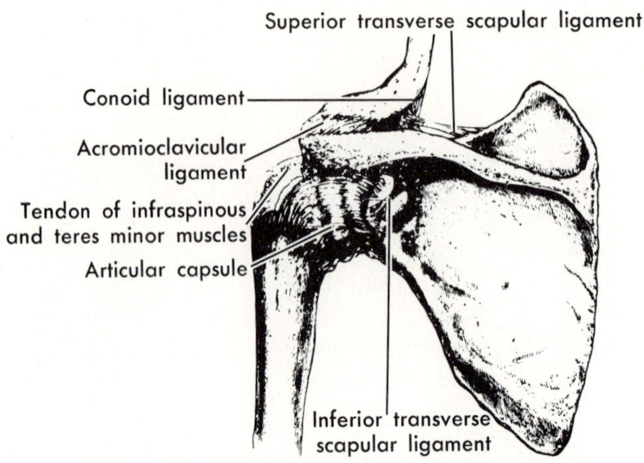

Fig. 20-2. Shoulder joint and related parts: posterior view. Position of clavicle in schematic. (From Anson, B.J., editor: Morris' human anatomy, ed. 12, New York, McGraw-Hill Book Co.)

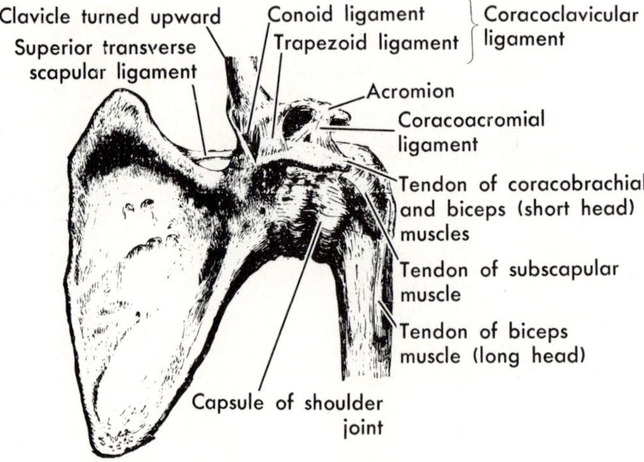

Fig. 20-3. Shoulder joint and related parts: anterior view. Position of clavicle in schematic. (From Anson, B.J., editor: Morris' human anatomy, ed. 12, New York, McGraw-Hill Book Co.)

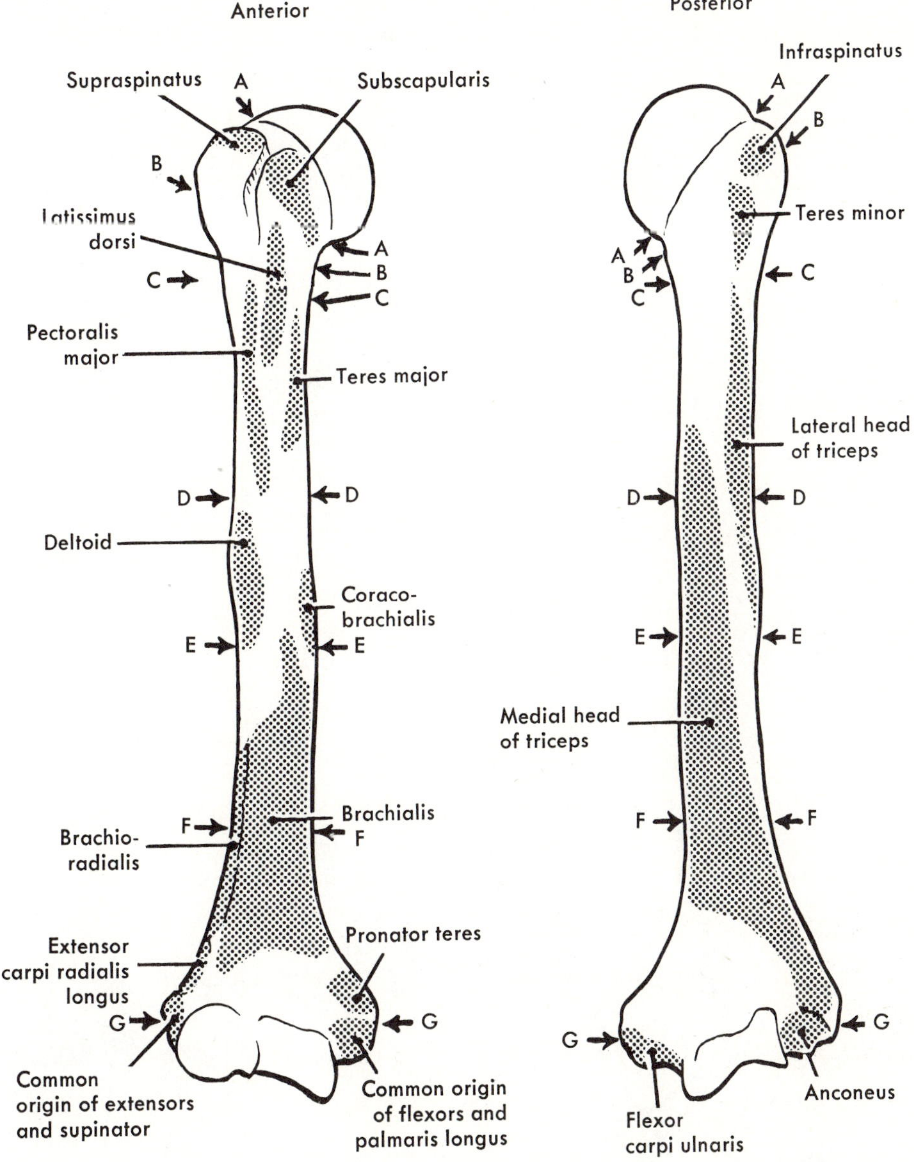

Fig. 20-4. Anterior and posterior views of humerus showing muscle attachments. Arrows *A* to *G* indicate typical locations of fractures. These various fracture sites have different muscle groups asserting pull on fracture fragments; thus fragments assume different characteristic position in each. (From Brantigan, O.C.: Clinical anatomy, New York, McGraw-Hill Book Co.)

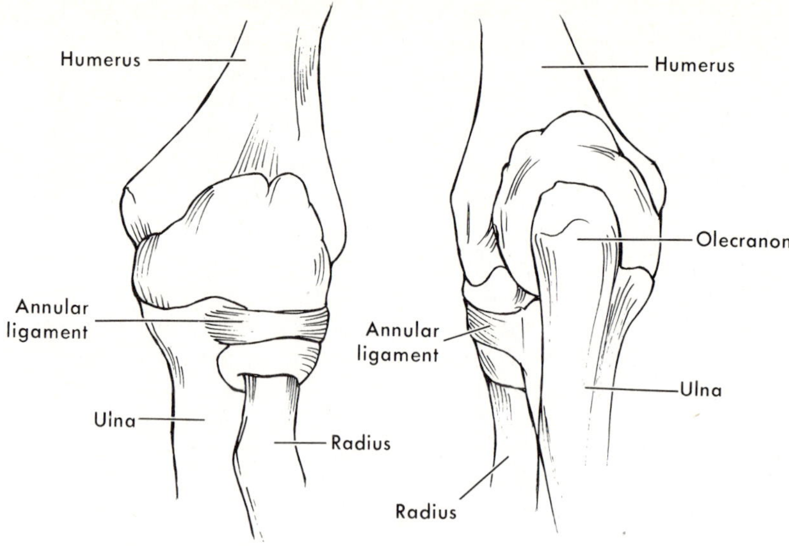

Fig. 20-5. Anatomy of elbow. (Adapted from Gray, H.: Anatomy of the human body, ed. 29, Philadelphia, 1973, Lea & Febiger. [Edited by C.M. Goss.])

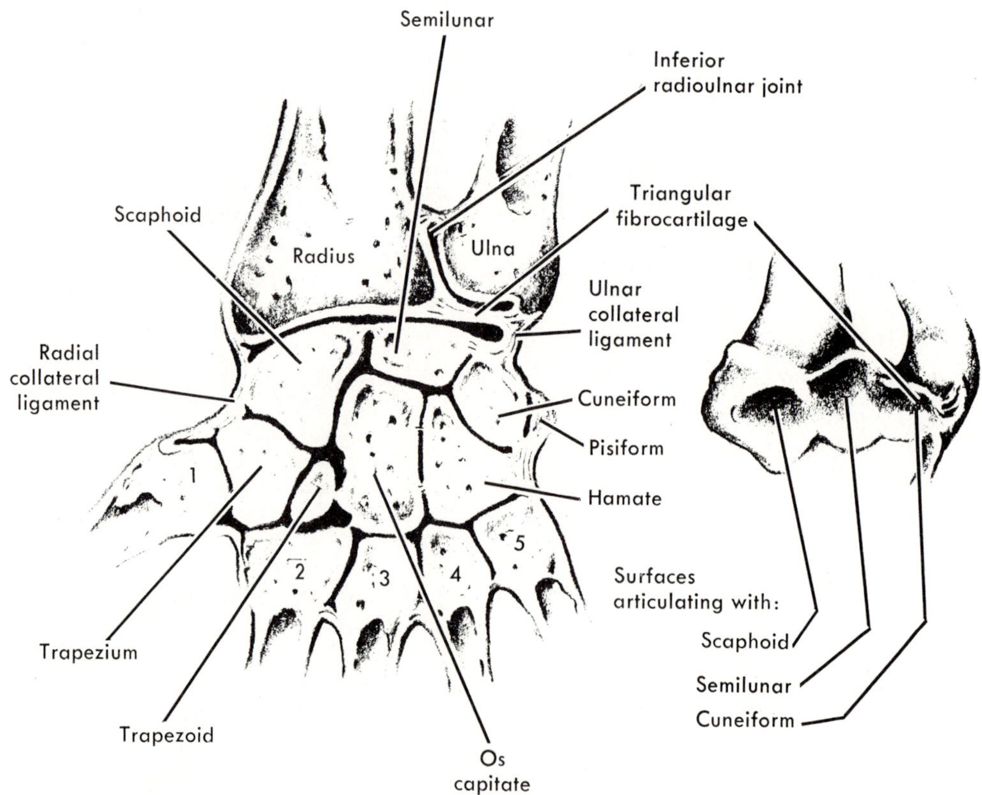

Fig. 20-6. Anatomy of wrist and carpus. (From Moseley, H.F., editor: Textbook of surgery, ed. 3, St. Louis, The C.V. Mosby Co.)

The greater tuberosity is situated at the lateral side of the head. Its upper surface has three impressions where the supraspinous, the infraspinous, and the teres minor tendons insert. This tendinous insertion is known as the *rotator cuff*. The lesser tuberosity is situated in front of the neck and has an impression for the insertion of the tendon of the subscapular muscle. The tuberosities are separated from each other by a deep groove (bicipital groove), in which lies the tendon of the biceps muscle of the arm. The tendon of the pectoralis major inserts on the lateral margin of the bicipital groove, and the latissimus dorsi and teres major insert on the medial margin.

The lower portion of the humerus is flattened and ends below in a broad articular surface, which is divided into two parts by a slight ridge. On either side of the ridge are projections, the lateral and medial condyles. On the lateral condyle, the rounded articular surface is called the *capitellum;* it articulates with the head of the radius. On the medial condyle, the articular surface is termed the *trochlea;* it articulates with the ulna (Fig. 20-5).

The *ulna* is located medial to the radius. The proximal portion of the ulna, the olecranon, articulates with the trochlea of the humerus (Fig. 20-5).

The *radius* rotates around the ulna. At the proximal end is the head, which articulates with the capitellum of the humerus and also the radial notch of the ulna. The tendon of the biceps muscle is attached to the tuberosity just below the radial head. The distal end of the radius is divided into two articular surfaces. The distal surface articulates with the carpal bones of the wrist, while the surface on the medial side articulates with the distal end of the ulna (Fig. 20-6).

Wrist and hand

The skeletal bones of the wrist and hand consist of three distinct parts: (1) the carpals, or wrist bones; (2) the metacarpals, or bones of the palm; and (3) the phalanges, or bones of the digits.

There are eight carpal bones arranged in two rows. The distal row, proceeding from the radial to the ulnar side, includes the trapezium, trapezoid, capitate, and hamate; the proximal row consists of the scaphoid, lunate, triquetrum, and pisiform. Functionally, the scaphoid links the rows as it stabilizes and coordinates the movement of the proximal and distal rows (Fig. 20-7).

Each carpal bone consists of several smooth articular surfaces for contact with the adjacent bones, as well as rough surfaces for the attachment of ligaments. No tendons or muscles are attached to the wrist bones. Consequently, the movement of the carpal bones is dependent on the tendons, which pass across the dorsal and volar surfaces to insert into the metacarpals and phalanges distally.

The five metacarpal bones are situated in the palm. Proximally they articulate with the distal row of carpal bones, and distally the head of each metacarpal articulates with its proper phalanx. The heads of the metacarpals form the knuckles (Fig. 20-7).

The phalanges, called *finger bones,* consist of fourteen bones in each hand, two in the thumb and three in each of the fingers. Each phalanx consists of a shaft and two ends.

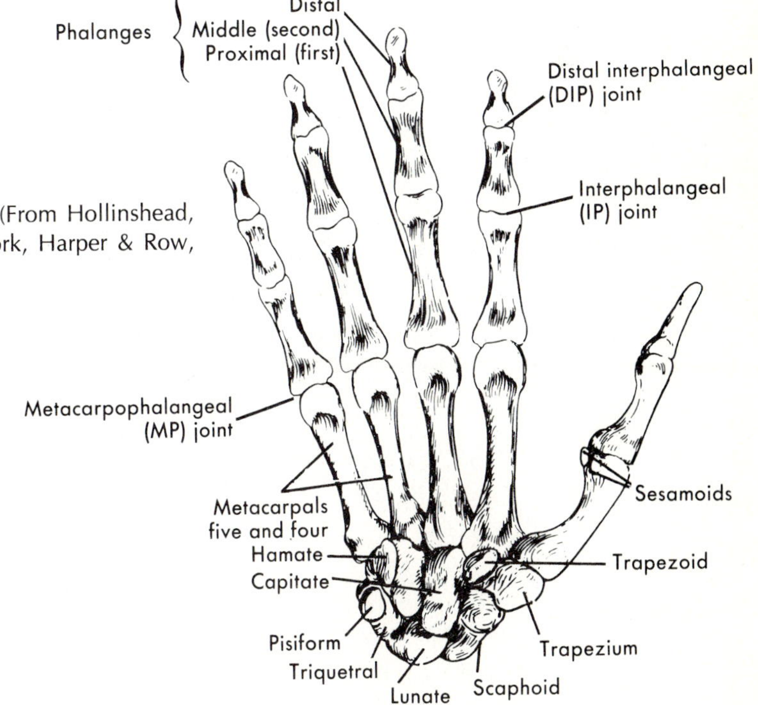

Fig. 20-7. Skeleton of wrist and hand, palmar view. (From Hollinshead, W.H.: Anatomy for surgeons, vol. 3, ed. 2, New York, Harper & Row, Publishers.)

Hip and femur

The *hip joint,* a ball-and-socket joint, is formed by the acetabular portion of the innominate (pelvic) bone and the proximal end of the femur. The hip joint is surrounded by a capsule, ligaments, and muscles (Fig. 20-8).

The acetabulum is a deep, round cavity that holds the head of the femur. The proximal end of the femur consists of the femoral head and neck, the upper portion of the shaft, and the greater and lesser trochanters.

The greater trochanter is a broad process of cancellous bone that protrudes from the outer upper portion of the shaft and projects upward from the junction of the superior border of the neck with the outer surface of the shaft. It serves as a point of insertion for the abductor and short rotator muscles of the hip (Fig. 20-8).

The lesser trochanter is a conical process projecting from the posterior and inferior portion of the base of the neck of the femur at its junction with the shaft. It serves as a point of insertion for the iliopsoas muscle. The lower end of the femur terminates in the two condyles. In front, the condyles are separated from one another by a smooth depression, called the *intercondylar groove,* forming an articulating surface for the patella. Behind, they project slightly, and the space between them forms a deep fossa, the *intercondylar fossa* (Fig. 20-9).

The upper or condylar end of the tibia presents an articular surface corresponding with those of the femoral condyles. The articular surface of the two tibial condyles forms two facets, which are deepened by the semilunar cartilages into fossae for the femoral condyles.

Knee and knee joint

The patella, or *kneecap,* is located anterior to the knee joint in the intercondylar groove of the distal femur. It is a sesamoid bone within the quadriceps tendon. The anterior surface of the patella is united with the patellar tendon (Fig. 20-10). The posterior surface of the patella articulates with the femur.

The knee joint consists of three articular surfaces: two condyle articulations, one between each condyle of the femur and the corresponding meniscus and condyle of the tibia, and a third articulation between the patella and femur. The bones of the knee joint are connected by extraarticular and intraarticular structures. The extraarticular attachments include the capsule, the quadriceps muscle, and two collateral ligaments. The intraarticular ligaments include the two cruciate ligaments and the attachments of the menisci (semilunar cartilages).

The capsule of the knee joint is attached proximally to the femoral condyles, and it is attached distally to the condyles of the tibia and to the upper end of the fibula. The capsule is reinforced—in front by the patellar and quadriceps tendon, on the sides by the medial and lateral collateral ligaments, and posteriorly by the popliteus and gastrocnemius muscles.

The cruciate ligaments, consisting of two fibrous bands, extend from the intercondylar fossa of the femur to attachments in front of and behind the intercondylar surface of the tibia.

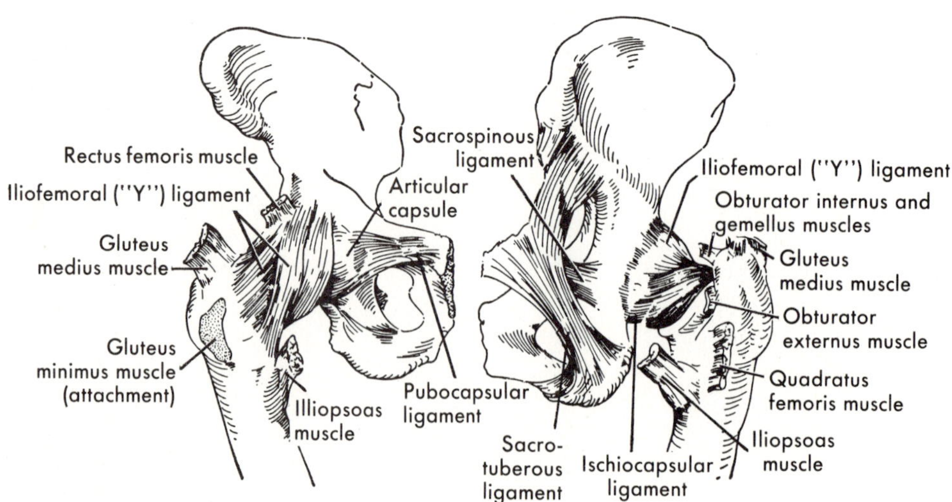

Fig. 20-8. Ligaments and muscles of hip. Anterior and posterior views. (From Howorth, M.B., and others: A textbook of orthopedics, Philadelphia, W.B. Saunders Co.)

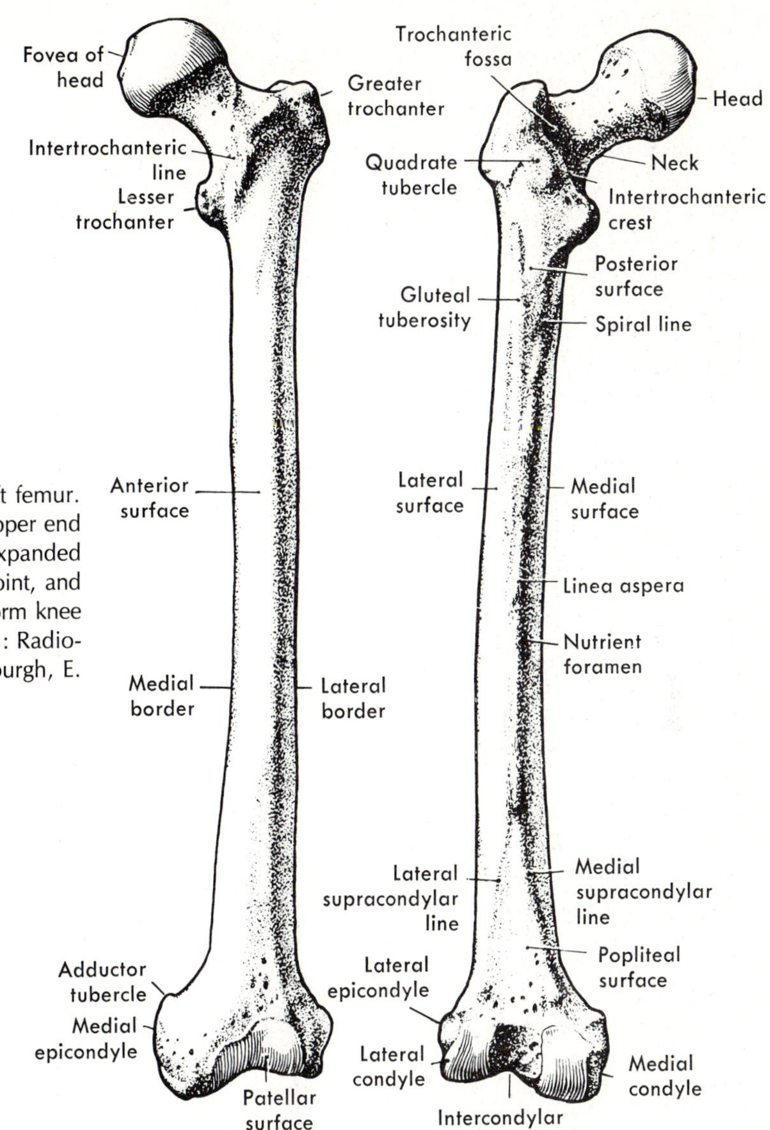

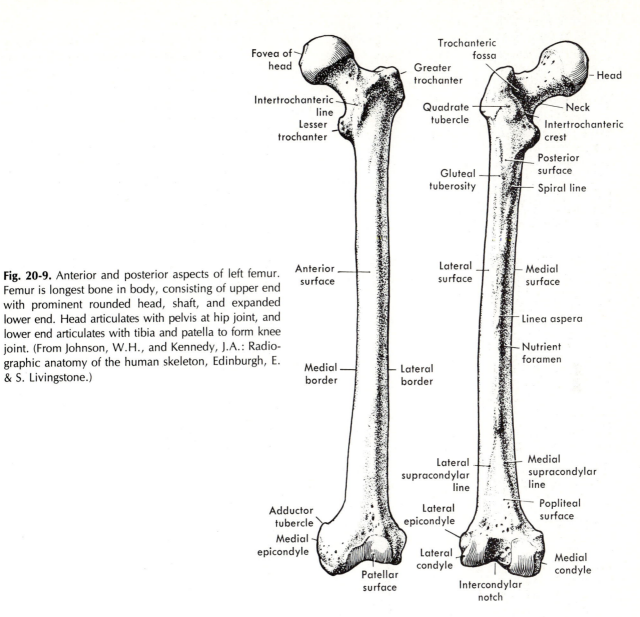

Fig. 20-9. Anterior and posterior aspects of left femur. Femur is longest bone in body, consisting of upper end with prominent rounded head, shaft, and expanded lower end. Head articulates with pelvis at hip joint, and lower end articulates with tibia and patella to form knee joint. (From Johnson, W.H., and Kennedy, J.A.: Radiographic anatomy of the human skeleton, Edinburgh, E. & S. Livingstone.)

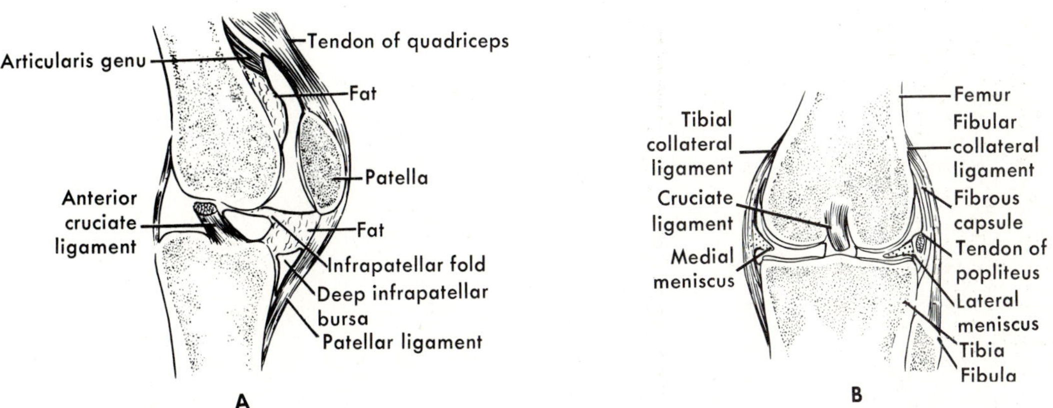

Fig. 20-10. A, Sagittal and, **B,** frontal sections through the knee joint. (From Hollinshead, W.H.: Anatomy for surgeons, vol. 3, ed. 2, New York, Harper & Row, Publishers.)

The semilunar cartilages, known as the *menisci,* are interposed between the condyles of the femur and those of the tibia (Fig. 20-11). Each menisci is attached to the joint capsule. The ends of the cartilages are attached to the tibia in the middle of its upper articular surface.

Synovial membrane lines the capsule of the joint and covers the infrapatellar fat pad, parts of the cruciate ligaments, and portions of the bone.

The portion of the knee joint cavity that extends upward in front of the femur is called the *suprapatellar pouch* or *bursa*.

Ankle and foot

The ankle joint, a hinge joint, is formed by the lower end of the tibia and its malleolus, as well as the malleolus of the fibula. These structures form a mortise for the reception of the upper surface of the talus and its facets (Fig. 20-12).

The bones are connected by ligaments, which spread out from the malleoli to be attached to the calcaneus and navicular bones. The joint is surrounded by a thin capsule.

The *talus* consists of a body, neck, and head. It is an irregular bone that fits into a mortise formed by the malleoli. It articulates with the calcaneus and navicular bones (Fig. 20-13).

The bony framework of the foot comprises seven tarsal bones, five metatarsal bones, and fourteen phalanges.

The calcaneous forms the heel and gives support to the talus (Fig. 20-13). The cuboid bone articulates proximally and posteriorly with the calcaneous and distally with the fourth and fifth metatarsals and the third cuneiform bones.

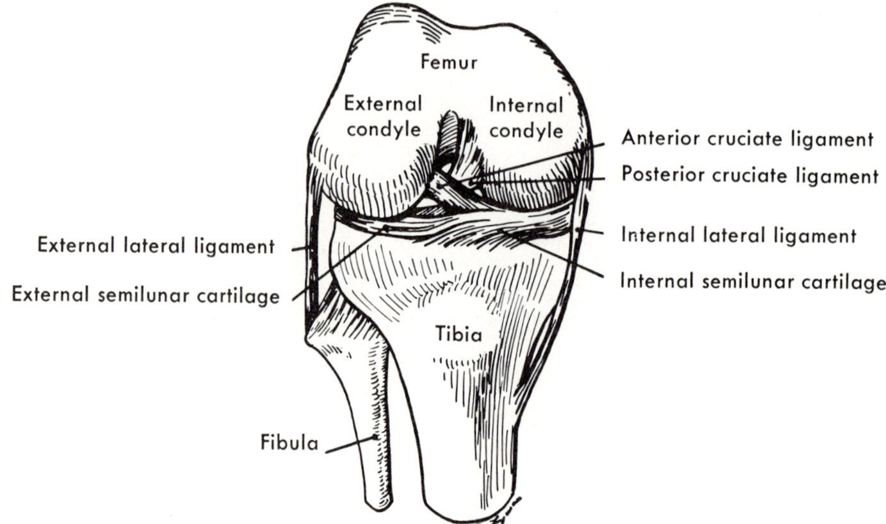

Fig. 20-11. Ligaments of knee joint and semilunar cartilages shown with knee in flexion. (From Larson, C.B., and Gould, M.: Orthopedic nursing, ed. 9, St. Louis, 1978, The C.V. Mosby Co.)

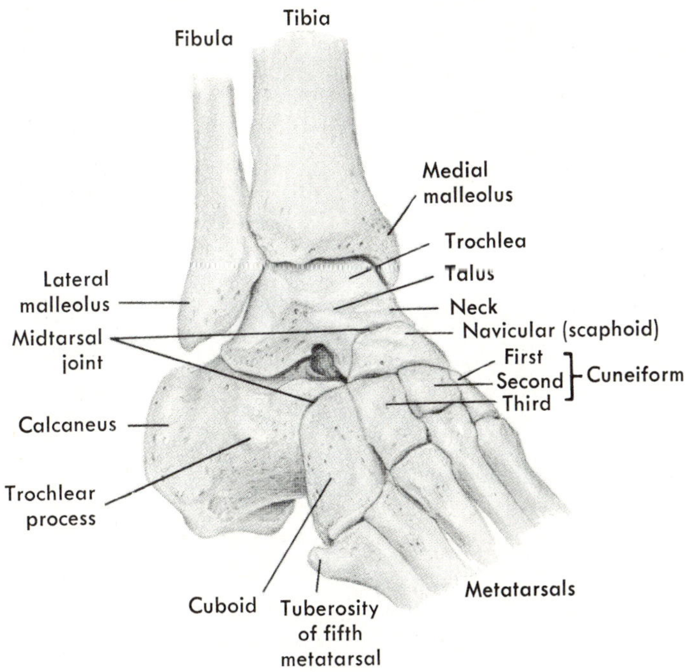

Fig. 20-12. Anatomy of ankle. (Courtesy Zimmer, Inc., Warsaw, Ind.)

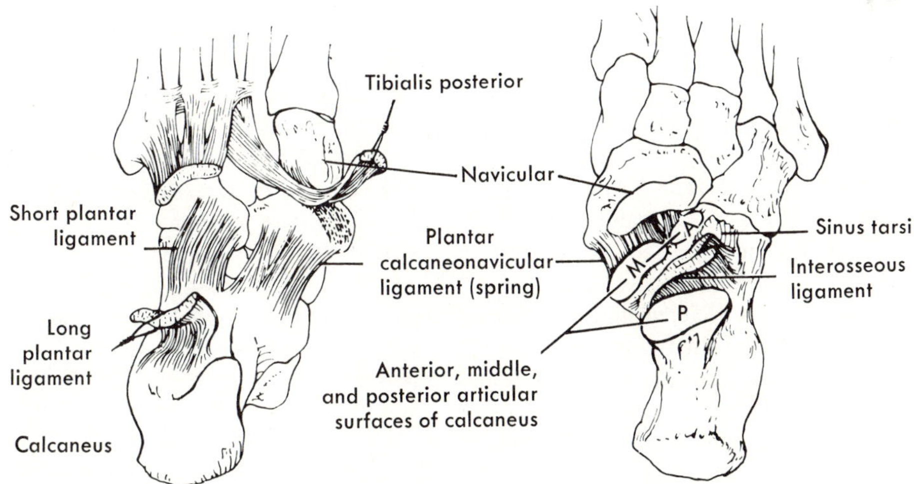

Fig. 20-13. Ligaments of foot. (From DuVries, H.L.: Surgery of the foot, ed. 2, St. Louis, The C.V. Mosby Co.)

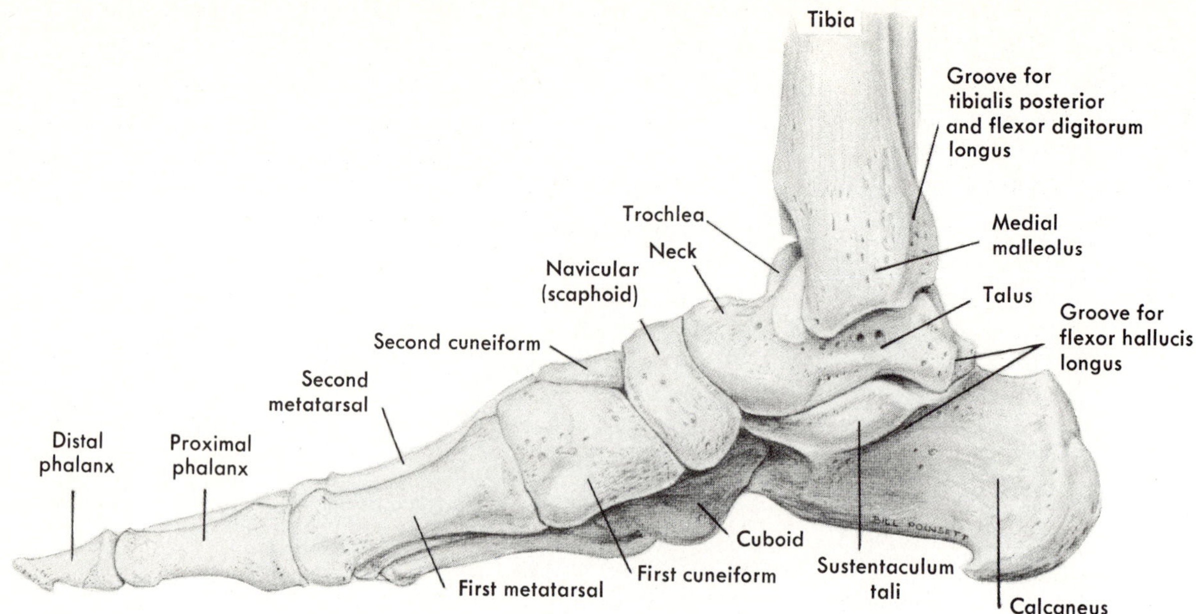

Fig. 20-14. Anatomy of foot. (Courtesy Zimmer, Inc., Warsaw, Ind.)

The navicular bone articulates with the cuneiform bones, which lie side by side in front of the scaphoid. The metatarsal bones articulate proximally with the tarsal bones and distally with the bases of the first phalanges of the corresponding toes. There are two phalanges for the great toe and three for each of the other toes (Fig. 20-14).

NURSING CONSIDERATIONS

Nursing assessment

In the perioperative care of the orthopedic patient, a nursing assessment is done in each phase of care and treatment.

Included in the preoperative assessment are a nursing history and physical examination. In obtaining the history, interview techniques are employed for collecting data. Information specific to orthopedics includes onset of the problem (that is, congenital or developmental), specifics of onset (for example, accident or injury), and functional limitations. Observation skills are needed to perform the physical examination. Appearance of the extremity, range of motion, gait abnormalities, and neurovascular status are noted.

The results of the preoperative assessment are documented. This information will be used throughout the patient's hospital course.

Communication between nursing and surgical personnel is essential for intelligent planning for the orthopedic surgical patient. Information concerning the patient's diagnosis, radiological studies, physical disabilities, surgical approach, position, special equipment, and instruments or supplies needed enables the nurse to plan for the surgical procedure. This preparation can significantly reduce both anesthesia and operating time.

In the operating room, the nurse conducts an assessment while admitting the patient to the surgical suite. Immobilization materials, bandages, and traction equipment are observed. Ascertaining the extremity to be treated with both the patient and chart is imperative. The nurse must know the hazards and precautions, special equipment, and support items needed to position the patient. Before moving the patient, the nurse seeks permission and guidance from the physicians.

Immediately after surgery, the operating room and recovery room nurses assess the condition of the patient. Immobilization techniques are checked, and stabilization is ensured. Special consideration must be given to the neurovascular status of any operative extremity. The affected extremity is usually elevated and checked for warmth, color, sensation, and the presence or absence of pulses.

Preparation of the patient

Considerations. The orthopedic patient requires special handling. The patient with a fractured hip should not be moved from the bed onto a stretcher to be taken to the operating room but should be transported in the bed to avoid unnecessary pain.

Positioning. Proper positioning of the patient on the operating table provides for good body alignment without undue strain or pressure on nerves and muscles, adequate exposure of the operative area, optimum respiratory and

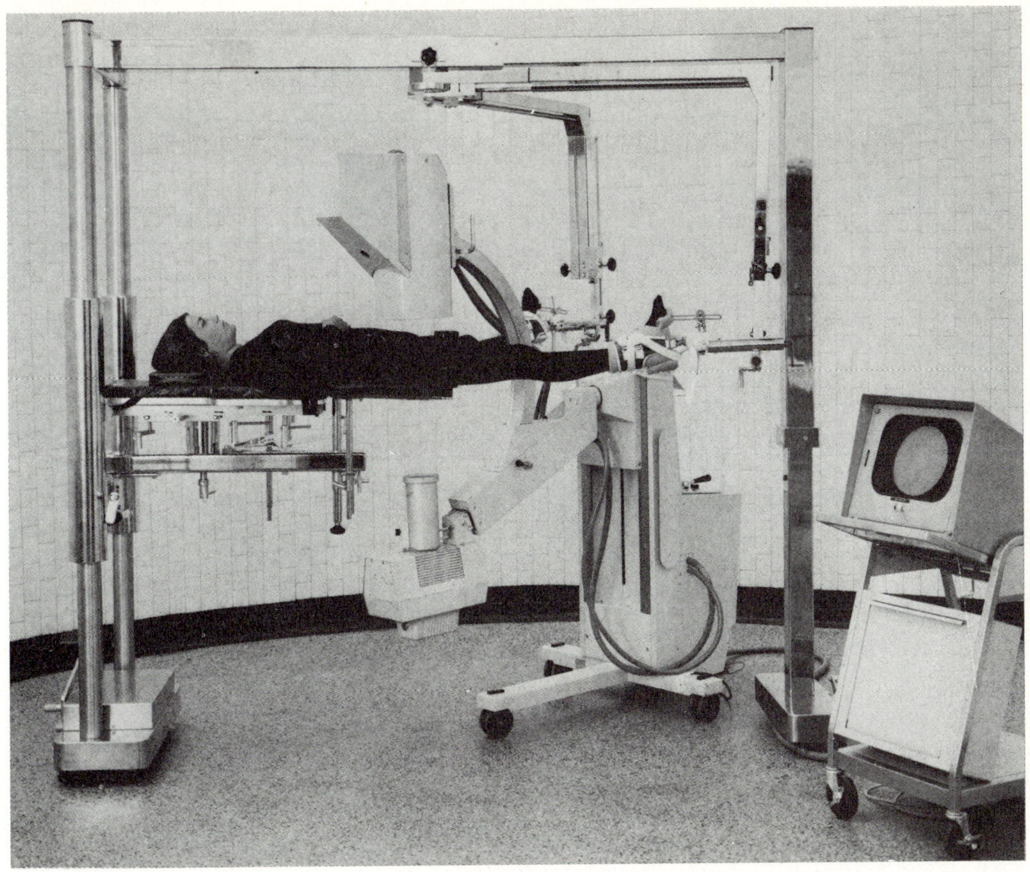

Fig. 20-15. Orthopedic surgical table. (Courtesy Chick Orthopedic, Oakland, Calif.)

circulatory functions, and adequate stabilization of the body.

The surgeon is responsible for supervising the surgical team as they position the patient on the table. The operating room staff should know the meaning of terms such as flexion, extension, abduction, and adduction, which are used in positioning a patient. The nursing assistants should know how to manipulate the operating table and apply the attachments.

The principles of positioning and the different types of positions used in orthopedic surgery are described and illustrated in Chapter 6.

The selection of the position depends on several factors: (1) the type of operation to be performed, (2) the location of the injury or lesion, and (3) the age and physical condition of the patient.

Draping. Application of sterile drapes is the third important step in preparing the patient for the operation. The sterile packs containing sheets, towels, and other drapes should be standardized (Chapter 5). The sterile drapes, towels, and stockinette for operations on the ankle and foot, the knee and midthigh, the hip, the spine, and the upper extremity are described in Chapter 5.

Equipment

Orthopedic operating rooms require a variety of special accessories in addition to routine operating room equipment. Although these vary from hospital to hospital, they serve the same basic purposes.

Orthopedic tables are designed to enable the surgeon to apply traction to a lower extremity while maintaining good alignment and control of the patient. These tables are equipped with radiotranslucent components, trays, and cassette holders to allow x-ray examination of any part of the body. Use of these tables makes it possible to apply a cast to a large body area while properly supporting the patient. The orthopedic surgical table with a full set of equipment is shown in Fig. 20-15. Tables most widely used are the Chick and Stryker.

At times, Wedge frames and Circo-electric beds are used in orthopedics. Wedge frames enable the surgeon to maintain the patient in cervical or halo traction during the procedure, eliminating the need for postoperative transfer. The Circo-electric bed is often employed for postoperative care following spinal procedures. Complete pamphlets with illustrations on each table are available from the manufacturers. A working knowledge of the table before use is very important.

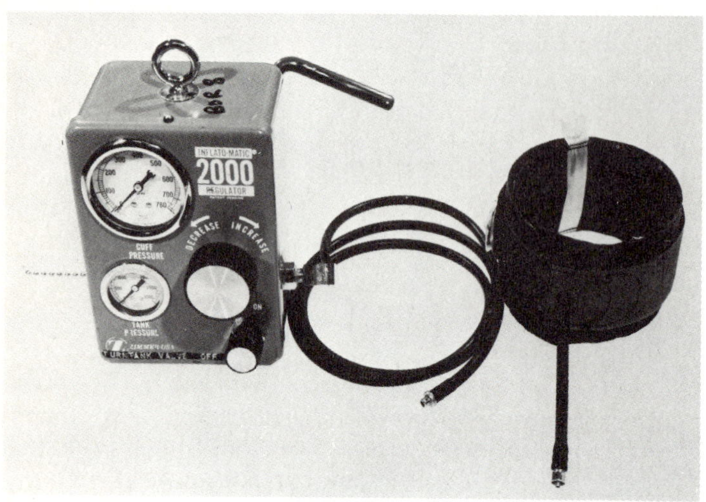

Fig. 20-16. Tourniquet and gauge for unilateral use.

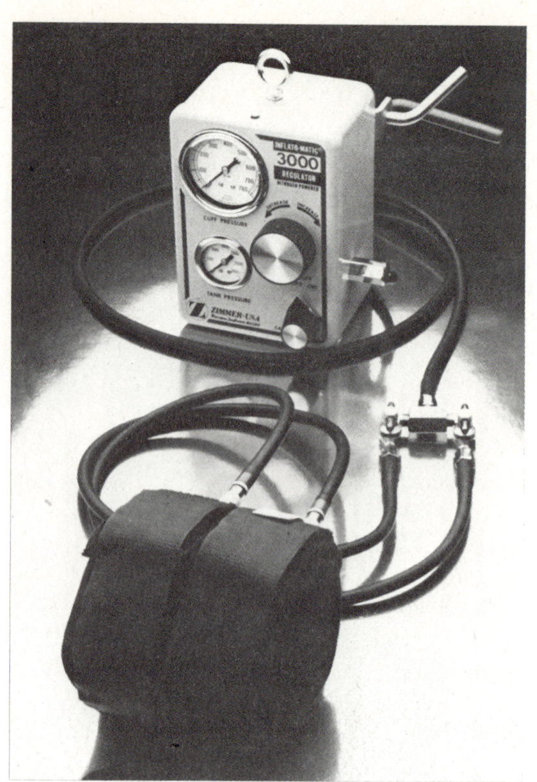

Fig. 20-17. Tourniquet and gauge used for regional anesthesia. (Courtesy Zimmer, Inc., Warsaw, Ind.)

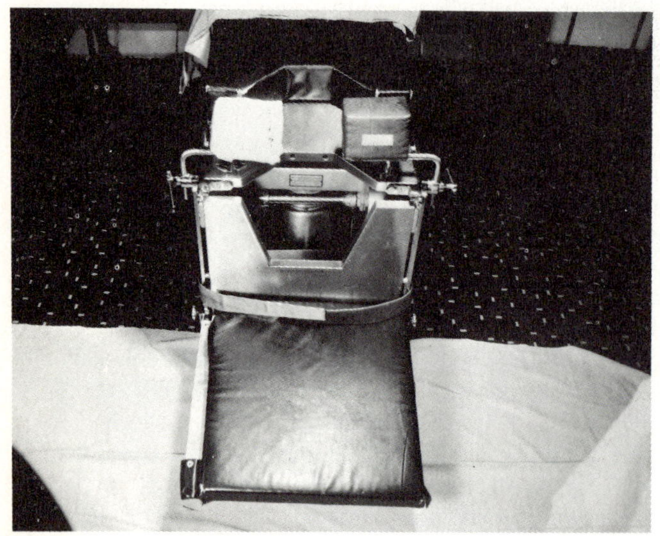

Fig. 20-18. Morgan disc pads.

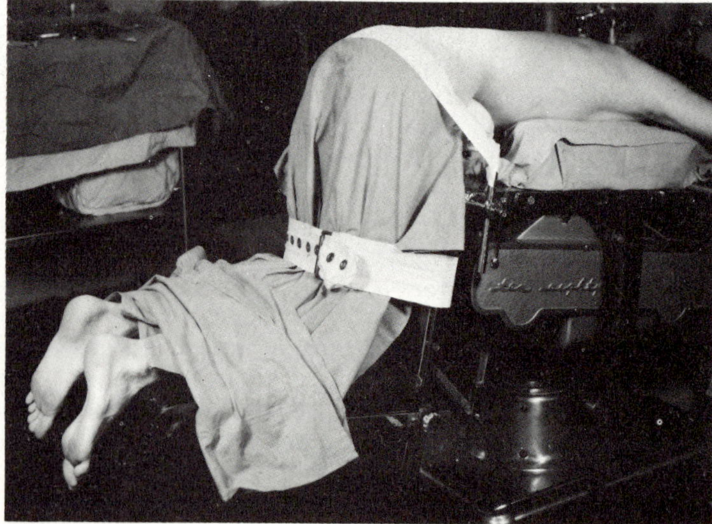

Fig. 20-19. Patient in laminectomy position supported by Morgan disc pads.

Tourniquets are used during most operations on the extremities. They prevent venous oozing but do not totally obstruct the arterial blood supply, thereby leaving the operative field as clear of blood as possible. While elevated, the extremity is wrapped distally to proximally with a 4- or 6-inch Ace wrap or Esmarch rubber bandage to exsanguinate the limb. The tourniquet is then inflated to 250 to 300 mm Hg for an upper limb and 250 to 450 mm Hg for a lower limb (Figs. 20-16 and 20-17). The Esmarch rubber bandages are reusable and should be processed according to hospital procedures.

Tourniquets can be very dangerous if not used properly. The following checks are essential:

1. *Proper application*. Sheet cotton, stockinette, or a tourniquet cover is wrapped smoothly around the limb where the tourniquet will be applied. A tourniquet of sufficient length for the extremity is essential. The ends must overlap at least 2 to 3 inches. The tourniquet must not be placed at the elbow or knee because it will interfere with the superficial neurovascular structures.

2. *Accurate gauge*. Tourniquet paralysis can occur and is usually caused by an inaccurate tourniquet gauge. The accuracy of the gauge must be checked on a regular basis to prevent this complication. Commercial testers are available.

3. *Proper setting*. The original setting is determined by the surgeon and should be checked at intervals by operating room personnel and reported to the surgeon.

4. *Skin preparation*. The cleansing solution must not be allowed to pool under the cuff, since tourniquet burns may result.

5. *Tourniquet time*. Accurate tourniquet time must be recorded and maintained as part of the anesthesia and/or nursing records. The surgeon should be informed of the tourniquet time at hour intervals. Tourniquets are usually released every 2 hours for several minutes. Freon and nitrogen are used most frequently for inflation of tourniquets.

Most orthopedic operations are performed in the supine position. However, to operate on a patient in the prone position, it is necessary to use special devices that permit proper ventilation. Operations on the spine not only require provisions for proper ventilation, but also must allow for flexion at the operative site. Most surgeons favor a particular set of equipment when doing spine operations. Following are some available choices:

1. *Doughnut*. Foam rubber pad about 4 inches thick made in a shape of a slightly oblong doughnut that supports the skeleton but does not compress the viscera
2. *Wilson convex frame*. Provides adjustable flexion of the lumbosacral spine without flexing the operating table
3. *Morgan disc pads*. Flex the patient 90 degrees at the pelvis for maximum exposure of the operative site (Figs. 20-18 and 20-19)
4. *Chest rolls*. Made by rolling and taping two sheets, bath blankets, or large foam pads together; used when flexion is not necessary
5. *Scoliosis frames*. Used for exposure of a large number of vertebrae for spinal fusion

Handling of appliances and instruments

The successful management of an active orthopedic operating room suite depends on the maintenance of adequate inventory levels of standard appliances. Types, styles, and sizes of necessary appliances are usually determined by the operating surgeon, and the number of each depends on the usage. Appropriate companion instruments, such as drivers and extractors, must also be available.

Lot and/or implant serial numbers must be recorded on the patient's chart. An appropriate space should be provided on the operating room record. If one has not been provided or the record is not a permanent part of the patient's chart, it should be recorded in the progress notes.

Many different alloys have been used in orthopedic implants. However, the insertion of implants with different metallic composition must be avoided to prevent galvanic corrosion; internal fixation implants used during an orthopedic procedure should be of the same metal. Screws, for example, should be of the same composition as the metal plate that they fix to the bone. Alloys most frequently used include stainless steel, cobalt-chromium, and titanium-vanadium-aluminum.

It is strongly recommended that no internal fixation devices be reused. Laboratory testing has demonstrated that scratches, abrasions, and the like critically affect the strength of an orthopedic implant. These imperfections are inevitable with use. Bending implants to conform to the contour of the bone should be avoided whenever possible to prevent resultant loss of strength. When bending is necessary, the proper bending press should be used. Once an implant is bent, any attempt to rebend or straighten it should not be allowed. An internal fixation device that has become damaged as a result of improper storage or handling is not usable for similar reasons.

Orthopedic instruments, equipment, and appliances require special care, storage, and handling. All precautions must be taken to prevent the most minute scratches on orthopedic appliances. During sterilization, prostheses and implants are not to be placed in a position in which knocking or bumping might occur. Appropriate sterilizing cases and trays should be used. Implants should be sterilized according to the manufacturer's instructions. Cleaning of instruments frequently presents a problem because of areas that are inaccessible to the cleaning brushes. The most effective cleaning method available is an ultrasonic cleaner.

Instruments and equipment that do not function properly (as a result of dullness, poor adjustment, lack of lubrication, damage, improper fit, or incomplete cleaning) are primary sources of complaints and problems in the operating room. The same instruments and equipment, properly maintained and in good repair, make the operation much easier. The proper maintenance of delicate instruments, such as those used in hand surgery, is particularly important. The operating room nurse is responsible for ensuring such maintenance.

Basic instrument setup

Following are basic instrument sets that should be available in the orthopedic operating room. Additional instruments and appliances are added as needed for specific procedures.

Regular basic set, soft-tissue instruments

Suction tip
Hemostats, straight and curved
Oschner or Kocher forceps
Allis forceps
Towel clamps, large and small
Scissors, straight
Scissors, heavy, curved
Tissue forceps, without teeth
Tissue forceps, with teeth
No. 3 knife handles
Needle holders
Army-Navy retractors
Smooth retractors, assorted
Rake retractors, assorted
Weitlaner retractor

Regular basic set, bone instruments (Fig. 20-20)

Mallet
Periosteal elevators
Gouges
Curettes
Bone-cutting forceps
Osteotomes
Rongeur
Chisels

Small basic set, soft-tissue instruments

Mosquito hemostats, straight and curved
Dissecting scissors, fine
Suture scissors
Suction tip
Tissue forceps, fine
Needle holders
Skin hooks
Retractors, small, smooth
Rakes, small
Towel clamps, small

Air-powered instruments

The use of air-powered surgical instruments in the operating room in recent years has proved to be beneficial to orthopedic surgeons. They eliminate the need for many hand-operated tools, thereby reducing operating time and giving improved results. Fingertip control is available and allows the surgeon to control speed and power instantly. This is especially important in total joint replacement procedures. In using air-powered instruments, it is very important to be aware of the manufacturer's recommended cleaning and lubricating instructions. With proper care, air-powered tools have an indefinite life span (Figs. 20-21 and 20-22).

A

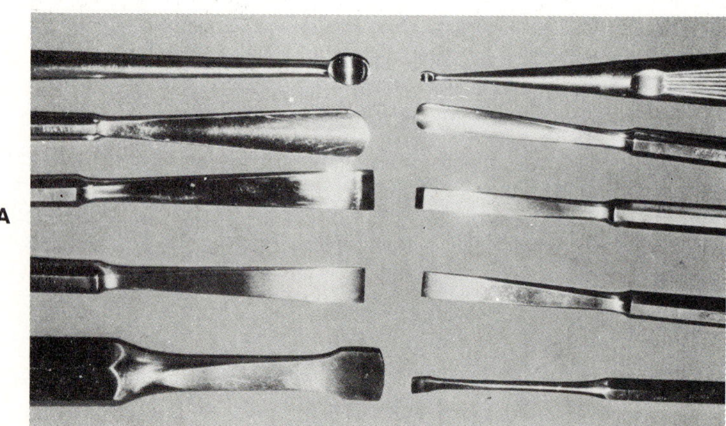

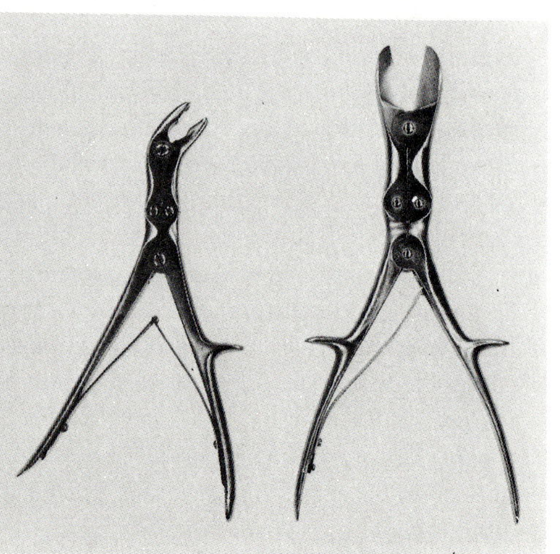

B

Fig. 20-20. A, Regular basic set, bone instruments. **B,** Rongeur and bone cutter.

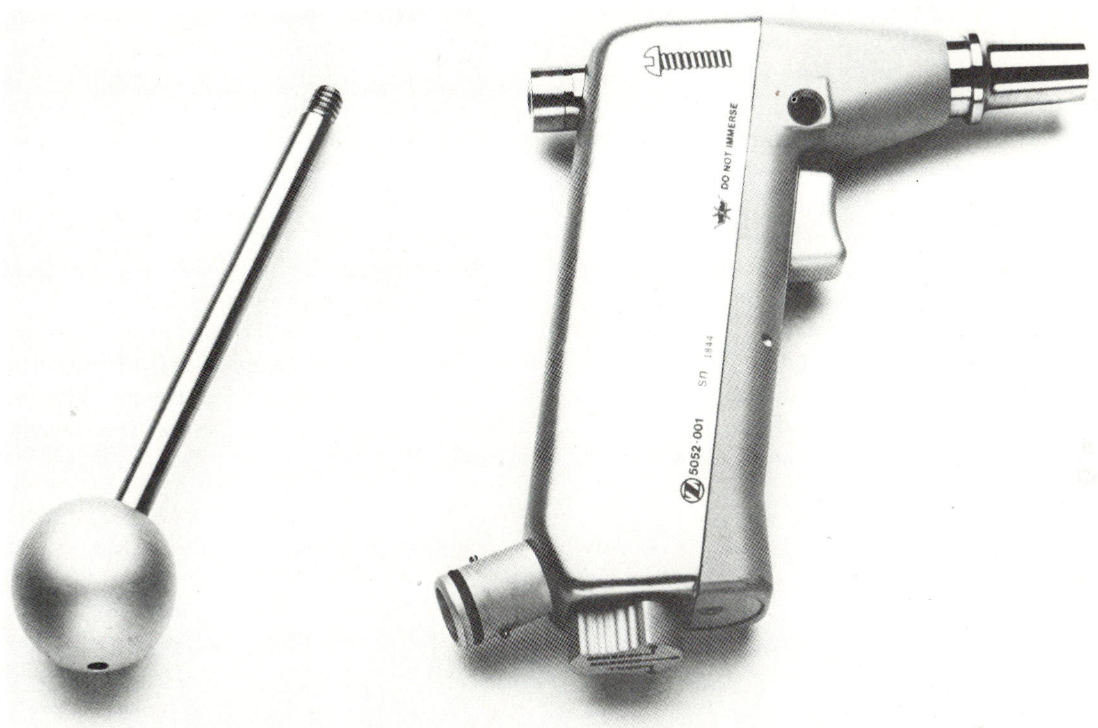

Fig. 20-21. Air-powered equipment. (Courtesy Zimmer, Inc., Warsaw, Ind.)

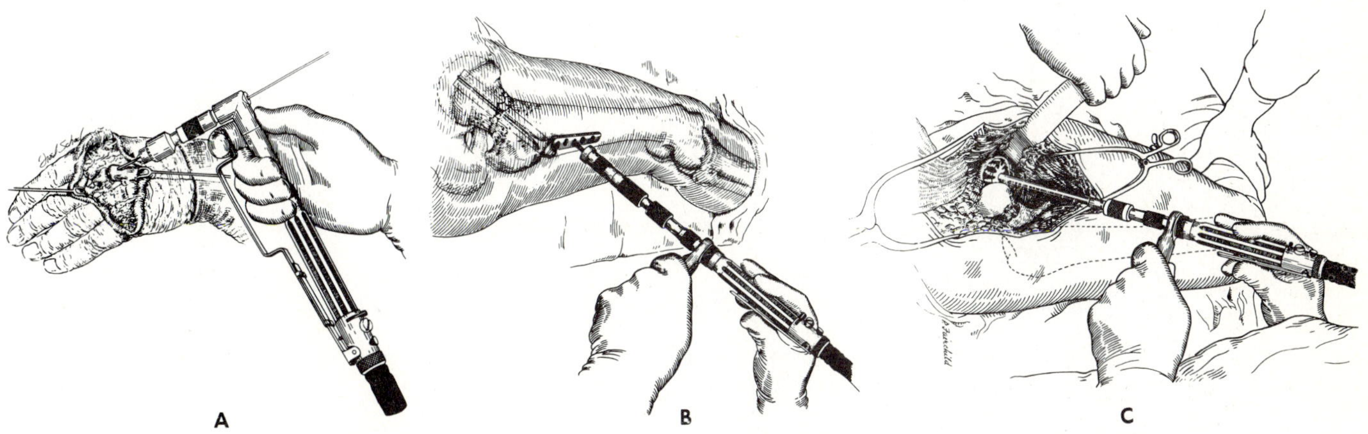

Fig. 20-22. Some uses of air powered drills. **A,** Insertion of threaded or unthreaded wires (using right-angle attachment). **B,** Insertion of screws using fingertip controlled torque in both forward and reserve rotation. **C,** Reaming of acetabulum using cutting power. (From Hall, R.M.: Orthairtome, Warsaw, Ind., Zimmer of Canada, Ltd.; The Fred Schad Co., Inc., Columbus, Ohio.)

FRACTURES AND DISLOCATIONS

A fracture is a break in the continuity of a bone. The care of fractured bones or dislocation of a joint is always complicated because of trauma to the soft tissues, including the muscles, nerves, and blood vessels.

Types of fractures

Fractures are classified into two main groups: closed fractures and compound or open fractures (Fig. 20-23).

Closed (Fig. 20-24, *A*) fractures are those in which there is no communication between the bone fracture and the skin surface. *Incomplete* fractures are those in which the whole thickness of the bone is not broken but is bent or buckled, as in greenstick fractures that occur in children before puberty.

Open (Fig. 20-24, *B*) fractures exist when the break in the bone communicates with a wound in the skin. Since these fractures are contaminated, measures must be carried out to control potential infection.

There are many varieties of fracture architecture, including (1) *transverse* fracture, in which the fracture line runs at a right angle to the longitudinal axis of the bone; (2) *longitudinal* fracture, which runs along the length of the bone; (3) *oblique* fracture and *spiral* fracture, which are similar except for the length; (4) *comminuted* fracture, in which the bone fragments splinter into more than two pieces; (5) *impacted* fracture, in which one fragment is driven into the other end and is relatively fixed in that position; and (6) *pathological* fracture, which may occur when a bone is weakened by disease, thereby permitting a bone to break even with minor trauma (Fig. 20-25).

An *epiphyseal separation* occurs when a fracture passes through or lies within the growth plate of a bone.

An *avulsion fracture* may result from a joint displacement where the ligament or tendon avulses its bony attachment instead of rupturing its fibers. A *dislocation* is a complete displacement of one articular surface of a joint from the other. A *subluxation* is a partial dislocation.

A fracture in the shaft of a long bone is usually described as being in the proximal, middle, or lower third or at the junction of two of these divisions.

A fracture of one of the bony prominences of the end of a long bone is described as a fracture of that prominence by name, for example, a fracture of the olecranon, a fracture of the medial malleolus, or a fracture of the lateral condyle of the femur.

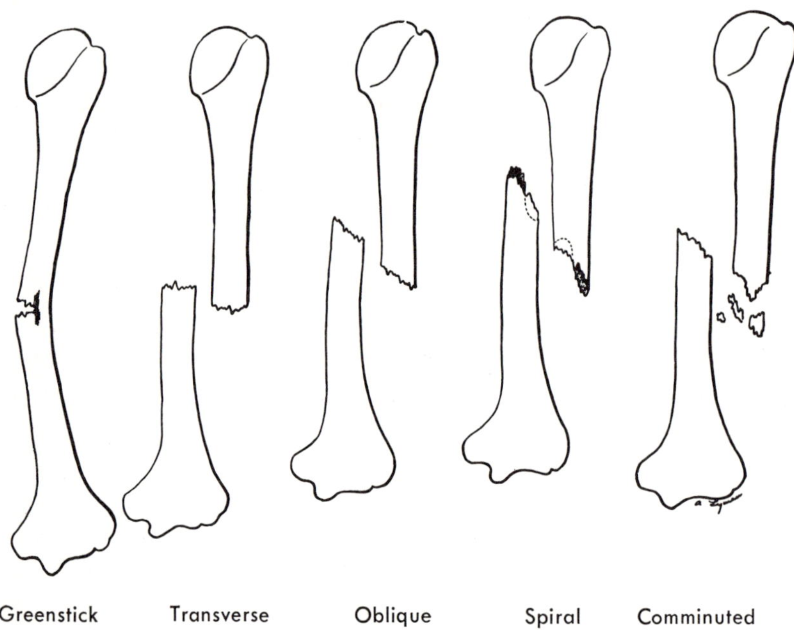

Fig. 20-23. Types of fractures. (From Larson, C.B., and Gould, M.: Orthopedic nursing, ed. 9, St. Louis, 1978, The C.V. Mosby Co.)

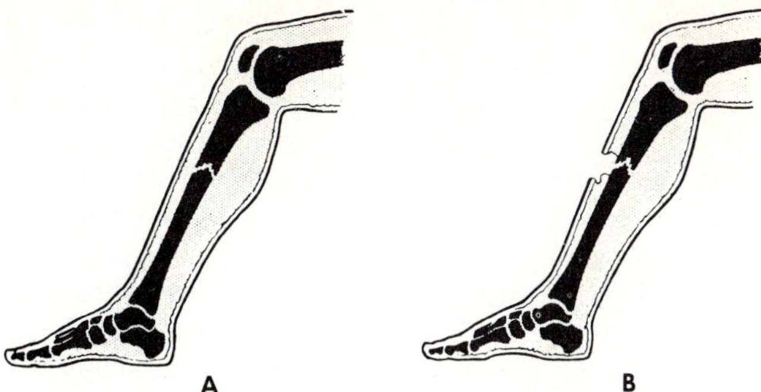

Fig. 20-24. A, Closed, or simple, fracture. No communication between fractured bone and body surface. **B,** Open, or compound, fracture. Wound leading down to site of fracture. Organisms may gain access through wound and infect bone. (From Adams, J.C.: Outline of fractures, ed. 4, Edinburgh, E. & S. Livingstone.)

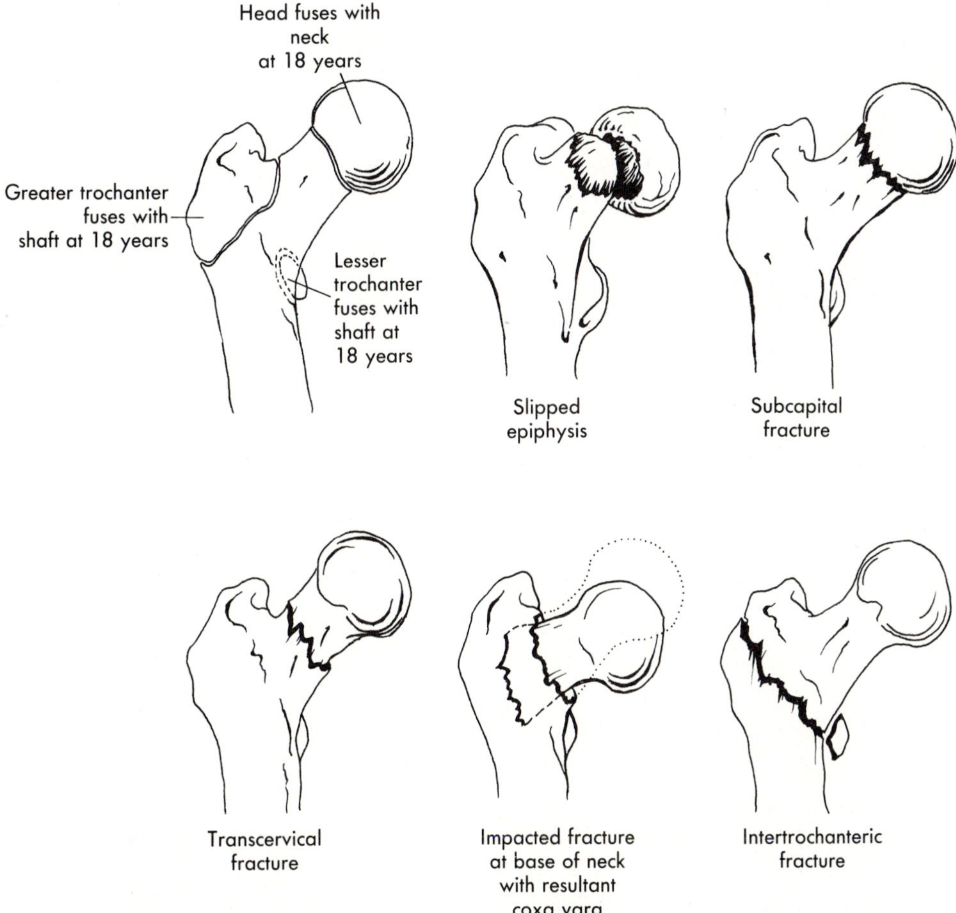

Fig. 20-25. Ossification, slipped epiphysis, and fractures of upper end of femur. (From Moseley, H.F., editor: Textbook of surgery, ed. 3, St. Louis, The C.V. Mosby Co.)

Principles of fracture treatment

The purpose of fracture treatment is to reestablish the length, the shape, and the alignment of the fractured bones or joints and restore their anatomical function to normal or to as near normal as possible.

Fractures of a bone involve two parts: the proximal and the distal fragments. The position of the proximal fragment is controlled by the pull of the attached muscles. For this reason, the distal fragment must be manipulated into the position that is assumed by the proximal fragment. The surgeon selects the method whereby this can be accomplished (Fig. 20-26).

In fractures involving an upper extremity, the surgeon endeavors to preserve mobility because the individual needs a wide range of motion to perform skilled and delicate work. In fractures of a lower extremity, the objectives of surgery are to restore alignment and length and provide stability of the extremity for weight bearing.

In the presence of open fractures involving soft tissues, several associated conditions may arise, including (1) secondary hemorrhage, (2) infection, (3) severe damage to soft tissues, (4) damage to blood vessels and nerves, and (5) Volkmann's contracture.

To accomplish the objectives of surgery, the operating team should keep in mind the following principles: (1) the extremity must be handled gently, (2) the body must have adequate general medical treatment, (3) proper equipment and personnel must be readily available to treat impending or existing shock and to control hemorrhage, (4) aseptic surgical techniques and care must be maintained to control infection, (5) the patient must be positioned properly to provide for adequate circulatory and respiratory functioning, and (6) the comfort of the patient must be considered.

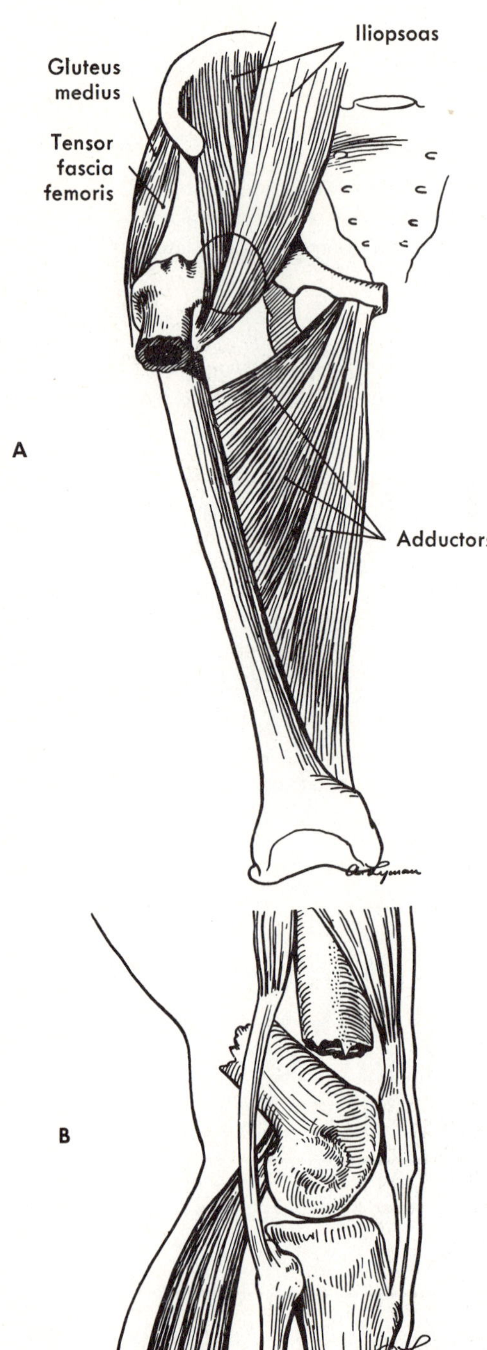

Fig. 20-26. A, Muscle action in subtrochanteric fractures of femur. **B,** Supracondylar fracture of femur (transverse). Note pull exerted by gastrocnemius muscle. (Adapted from Larson, C.B., and Gould, M.: Orthopedic nursing, ed. 9, St. Louis, 1978, The C.V. Mosby Co.)

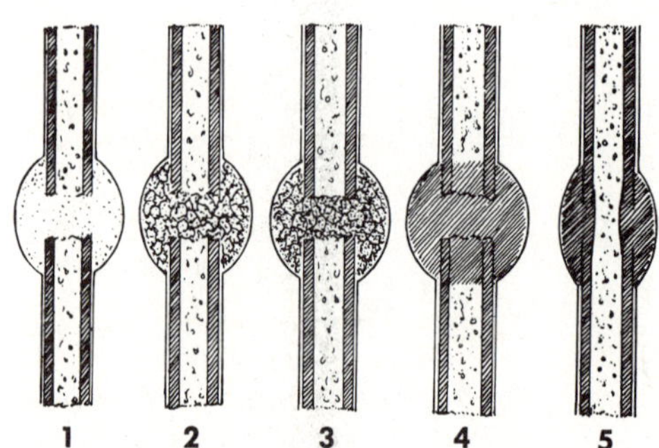

Fig. 20-27. Schematic drawing of the five stages of regeneration of bone. *1,* Hematoma; *2,* granulation; *3,* callus; *4,* consolidation; *5,* remodeling. (From Adams, J.C.: Outline of fracture, including joint injuries, ed. 5, Edinburgh, Churchill Livingstone, Medical Division of Longman Group, Ltd.)

Bone-healing process of fractures

The healing process involves several stages. When a bone is fractured, hemorrhage occurs. The amount of extravasated blood depends on the vascularity of the fracture site. The blood exudate infiltrates the surrounding area, where it forms a clot. The vascular granulation tissue coming from the ends of the bone fragments invades the clot (Fig. 20-27).

After several days, calcium deposits may form in the granulation tissue. These deposits eventually form new bone, known as *callus*. Within the callus, cartilage cells develop a temporary semirigid tissue that helps stabilize the bone fragments (Fig. 20-27). The callus is immature bone that is remodeled by new connective tissue cells (osteoblasts of the periosteum and the inner membrane of the bone cavity). Through this process, mature bone is formed, and the excess callus is reabsorbed (Fig. 20-27).

After several months, depending on the age and physical condition of the individual, the fractured bone becomes firmly united, although the ossification process is not yet completed. Complete union of the fractured bone or joint is determined by means of clinical and radiological examination.

Nonunion of a fracture signifies that the process of healing has ended without producing bony union.

Delayed union signifies that a specific fracture has not healed in the time considered as average for that fracture. The average time for healing of a fracture depends on many factors, and delayed unions must not be considered nonunions until the healing process has ceased without bony union.

Malunion signifies that the fracture has united with deformity sufficient to cause impairment of the function or a significant cosmetic defect.

BASIC TECHNIQUES FOR TREATMENT OF FRACTURES

Closed reduction by manipulation

Whenever possible, fractures are treated by manipulating the fragments into position without incising the skin. If fractures can be treated by this closed method, there is less chance of infection and greater chance for union (healing) of the fracture as long as soft tissue is not caught in the fracture site.

The closed reduction can be performed with (1) infiltration of local anesthetic agent into the fracture site, (2) intravenous regional anesthesia, (3) peripheral or spinal nerve block, or (4) general anesthesia. The choice of anesthesia depends on the site of the fracture and the condition of the patient. After the fracture has been reduced, it is immobilized.

Immobilization by cast

Definition. A form of external mold that places the fractured extremity or joint at rest by immobilizing the joint and both ends of the fractured bone in a rigid casing (Fig. 20-28).

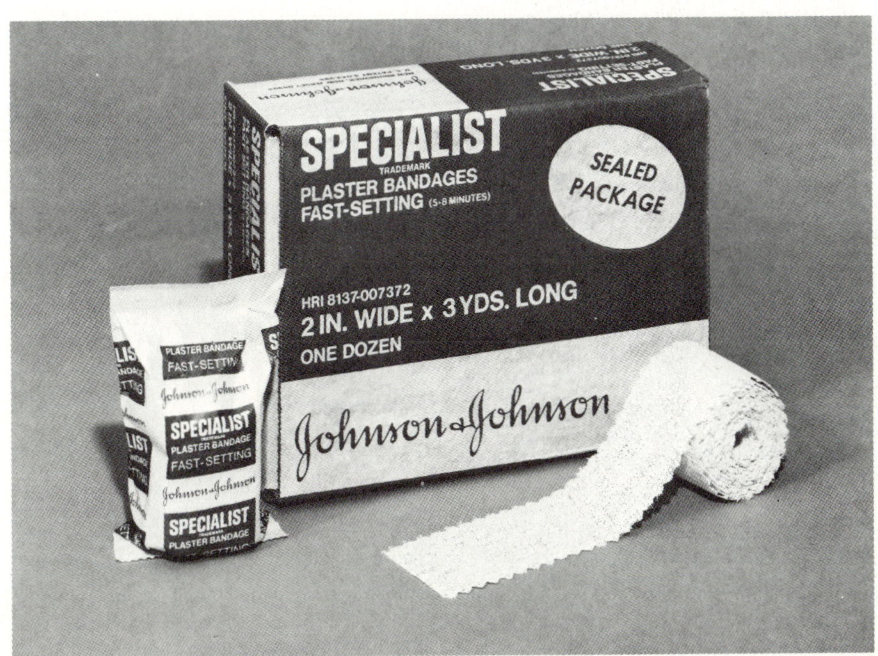

Fig. 20-28. Plaster of Paris casting material. (Courtesy Johnson & Johnson, New Brunswick, N.J.)

Types of casts. A *short leg cast* applied from below the knee to the toes may be used for fractures of the foot and the ankle. A *long leg cast* applied from the groin to the toes may be used to treat fractures of the tibia, fibula, and ankle (Fig. 20-29). A rubber heel or cast shoe may be used with the long leg or short leg cast to allow walking. A *cylinder cast* from the groin to the ankle is used to treat fractures of the patella and to immobilize the knee.

Spica casts are designed to immobilize different parts of the body; for example, a *single hip spica cast* involving the trunk, the affected leg, and foot may be applied to treat a fracture of the femur (Fig. 20-29). A *body jacket cast* encircling the body but not the extremities may be used to treat spinal conditions. A *short arm cast* is applied from below the elbow to the knuckles and is used for wrist fractures. A *long arm cast* is applied from above the elbow to the knuckles and is used to treat fractures of the elbow or the forearm (Fig. 20-29).

The *femoral cast brace* is designed to immobilize a fracture of the femoral shaft without immobilizing the hip joint. It consists of (1) a snug-fitting thigh cast with a specially molded quadrilateral socket at the proximal opening, which controls rotation of the cast brace on the extremity; (2) a short leg walking cast distal to the knee;

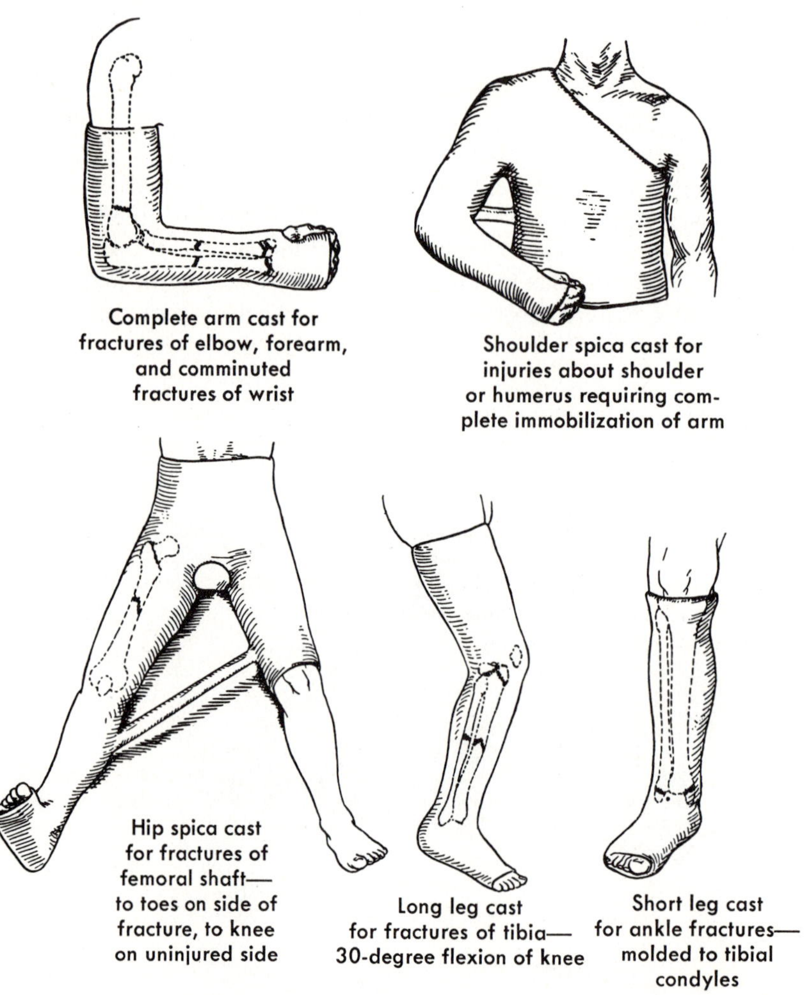

Complete arm cast for fractures of elbow, forearm, and comminuted fractures of wrist
Shoulder spica cast for injuries about shoulder or humerus requiring complete immobilization of arm
Hip spica cast for fractures of femoral shaft—to toes on side of fracture, to knee on uninjured side
Long leg cast for fractures of tibia—30-degree flexion of knee
Short leg cast for ankle fractures—molded to tibial condyles

Fig. 20-29. Several types of plaster casts and some fractures for which they may be indicated. (From Compere, E.L., Banks, S.W., and Compere, C.L.: Pictorial handbook of fracture treatment, ed. 5, Chicago, Year Book Medical Publishers, Inc.)

and (3) hinges at the knee that join the other two components. The hinges allow active knee motion. The cast brace is usually applied after 4 to 6 weeks of skeletal traction when callus formation has been initiated at the fracture site (Fig. 20-30).

Splints are frequently employed in the immediate postoperative period. They do not completely encircle the limb and therefore give some indication as to the degree of swelling and staining.

Casting materials

Synthetic casting materials frequently have a role in the treatment of fractures. They are lightweight, waterproof, and relatively easy to apply. The surgeon's preference will dictate usage. Plaster of Paris is the least expensive material available. It is easily molded and used in patients with acute fractures when maintaining bone alignment is critical. Proper handling of plaster is illustrated in Fig. 20-31.

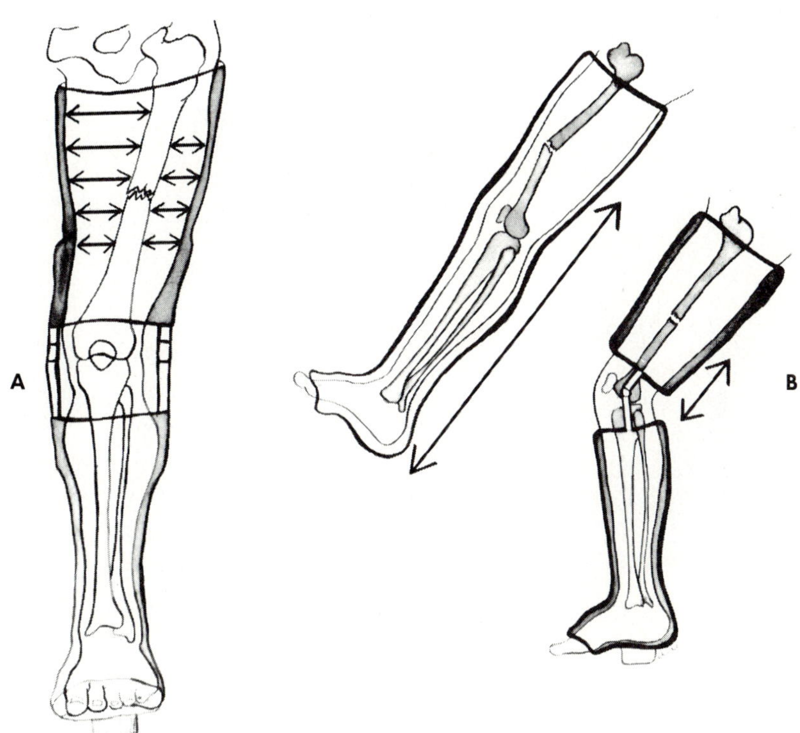

Fig. 20-30. A, Cast brace. **B,** Comparative length of lever arm distal to fracture site, with long-leg cast and with cast-brace. (From Larson, C.B., and Gould, M.: Orthopedic nursing, ed. 9, St. Louis, 1978, The C.V. Mosby Co.)

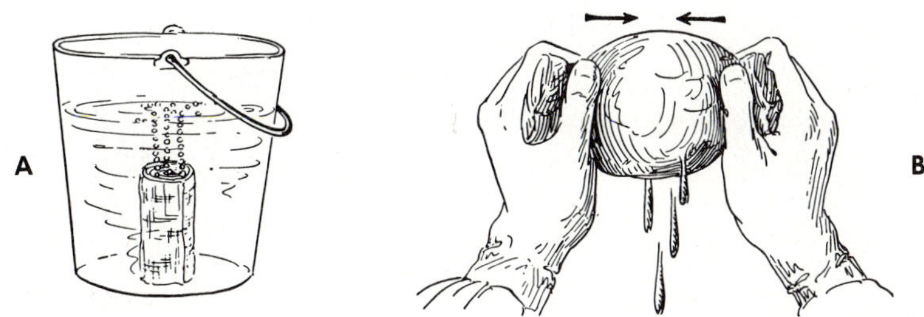

Fig. 20-31. Correct handling of plaster roll. **A,** Roll of plaster placed on end in pail of water. Roll saturated when bubbles cease to appear. **B,** Excess water squeezed (*not* twisted) from plaster roll by pushing both ends toward middle. (From Compere, E.L., Banks, S.W., and Compere, C.L.: Pictorial handbook of fracture treatment, ed. 5, Chicago, Year Book Medical Publishers, Inc.)

In using synthetic casting materials, the manufacturer's instructions are to be followed explicitly. Figs. 20-32 and 20-33 show synthetic casting materials.

Skeletal traction

Definition. Fractures that are difficult to reduce and immobilize in a cast can be treated by applying distal traction to the extremity.

Considerations. The problem with skeletal traction is the long period of confinement in bed, but the incidence of infection and nonunion of the fracture are less with this treatment than with open reduction (Fig. 20-34).

Setup. The following items are sterilized and placed on a sterile table (Fig. 20-35):

Scalpel
Drill and points
Wires or pins, desired type and size
Gauze dressings

Nonsterile times

Traction equipment, desired type

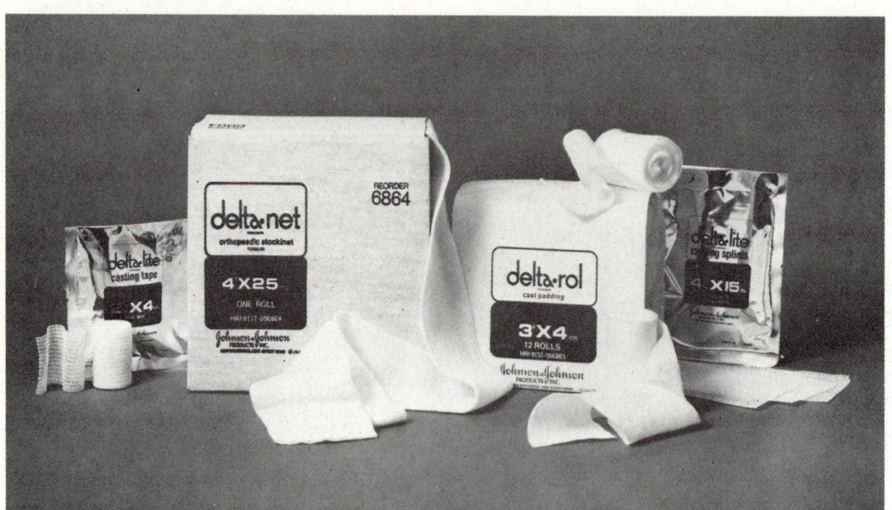

Fig. 20-32. Synthetic casting material supplies. (Courtesy Johnson & Johnson, New Brunswick, N.J.)

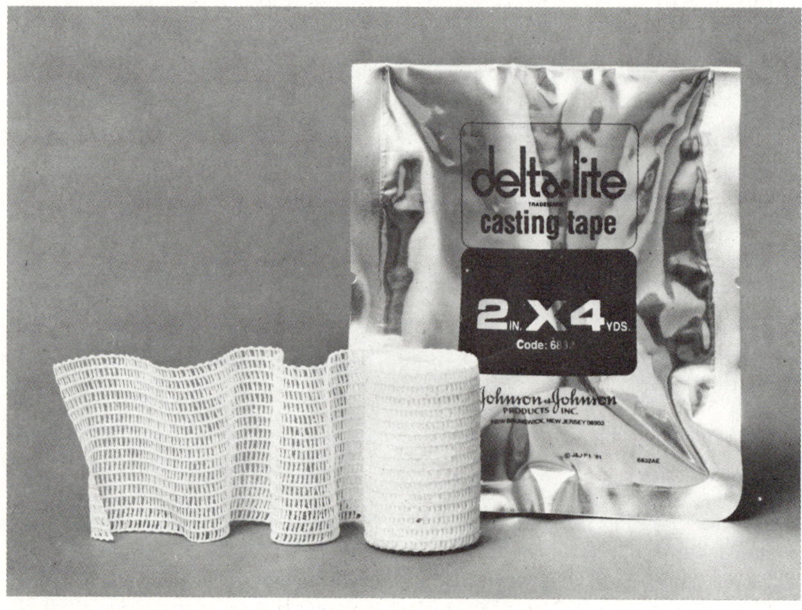

Fig. 20-33. Synthetic casting tape. (Courtesy Johnson & Johnson, New Brunswick, N.J.)

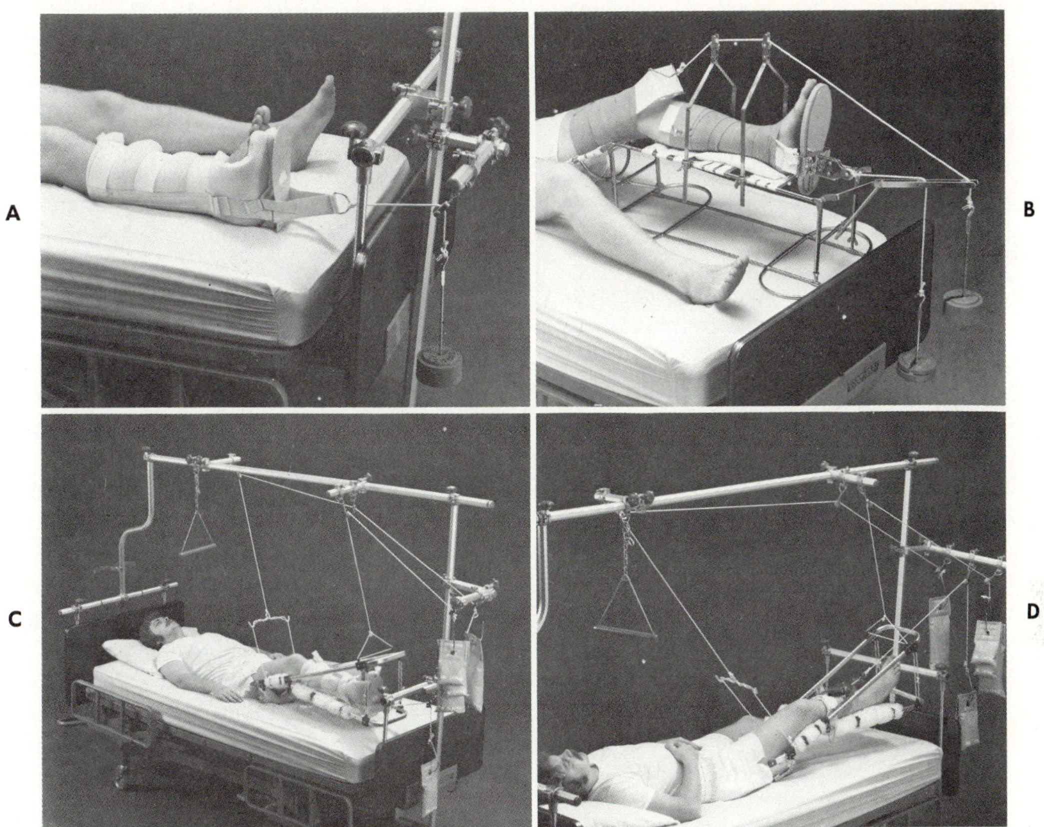

Fig. 20-34. A, Buck's skin traction. **B,** Balanced suspension traction, lower extremity. **C** and **D,** Balanced suspension skeletal traction. (Courtesy Zimmer, Inc., Warsaw, Ind.)

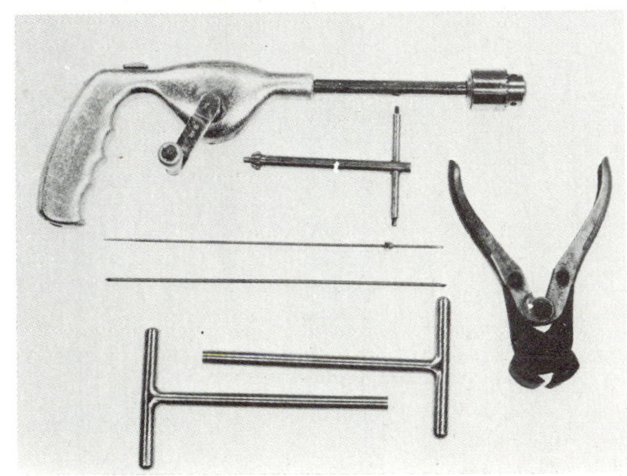

Fig. 20-35. Instruments for insertion of Kirschner wire.

Procedure. A local or general anesthetic may be administered. This procedure may be performed in the plaster room, the emergency room, or the patient's room, depending on the condition of the patient. Aseptic techniques are followed to prevent wound infection.

Under sterile conditions, a pin is passed through the bone distal to the fracture site. A traction bow is attached to the pin and is connected by ropes to weights that pull on the fracture fragments and override the deforming muscle forces, thereby reducing the fracture.

Internal fixation

Definition. Through an open wound, the fracture site is exposed, and the fragments are fixed by pins, nails, intramedullary screws, or plates and screws.

Considerations. Internal fixation is used when satisfactory reduction of a fracture cannot be obtained or maintained by closed methods and when skeletal traction is not indicated (Figs. 20-36 to 20-38). The advantage is that anatomical alignment of the fracture can usually be obtained, and the patient does not have to be confined to bed. However, the incidence of infection and nonunion is increased.

Bone grafting may be used to promote union of fractures at the time of open reduction or to fill cavities and defects in the bone. The type of graft to be used depends on the location of the fracture or defect, the condition of the ends of the fragments, and the preference of the surgeon. Cancellous grafts may be taken from the ilium, olecranon, or distal radius; cortical grafts may be taken from the tibia, fibula, or ribs. The instrumentation for taking a bone graft includes the basic orthopedic sets. Electric or air-powered drills and saws are extremely helpful, if available. A hand drill, drill points, and bone curettes of various sizes are also needed.

A *cancellous bone graft* consists of spongy bone, usually taken from the anterior or posterior crest of the ilium. Exposure of the ilium is relatively easy, since the crest is located subcutaneously. An incision is made along the border of the iliac crest, the muscles on the outer table of the ilium are elevated and retracted. Strips of the iliac crest can be removed with an osteotome parallel to the crest, or a cortical window can be made in the outer table, and cancellous bone chips can be obtained with curettes or gouges.

A *cortical graft* can be taken from the tibia through a curved anteromedial incision. The periosteum is incised and reflected. The size and shape of the graft are outlined with drill holes, and the graft is removed with an osteotome or an oscillating bone saw. The cortical graft is placed across the fracture site and secured.

Setup. The regular bone and soft-tissue sets are used, plus the following: Taylor retractors; a drill, key, and drill points; osteotomes; and a saw, if requested.

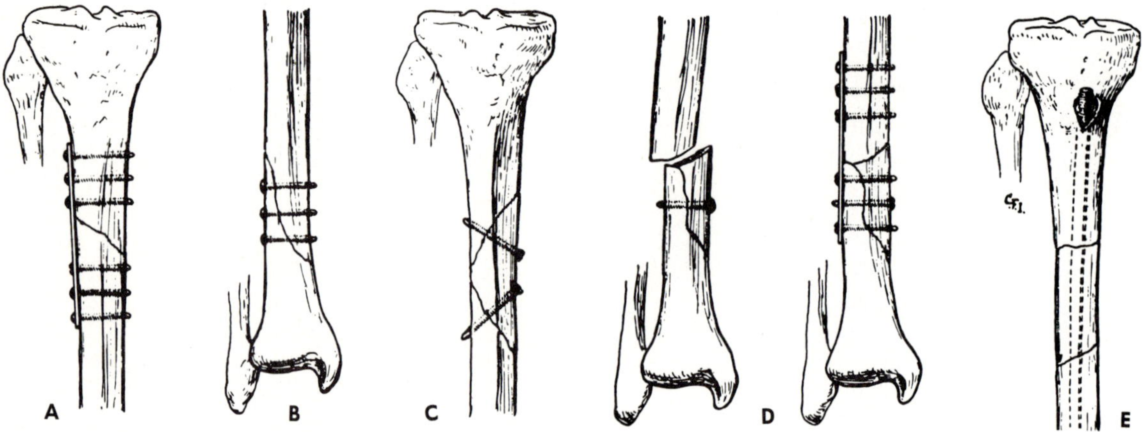

Fig. 20-36. Techniques of internal fixation. **A,** Plate and six screws for transverse or short oblique fracture. **B,** Transfixion screws for long oblique or spiral fractures. **C,** Transfixion screws for long butterfly fragment. **D,** Fixation of fracture with short butterfly fragment. **E,** Medullary fixation. (From Edmonson, A.S., and Crenshaw, A.H., editors: Campbell's operative orthopaedics, ed. 6, St. Louis, 1980, The C.V. Mosby Co.)

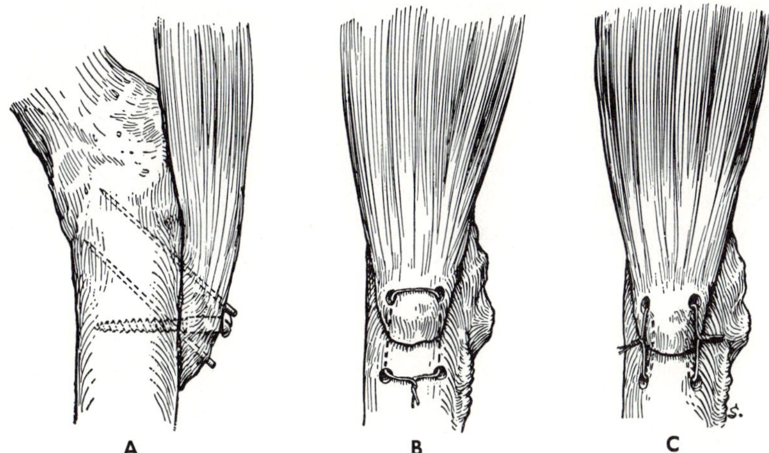

Fig. 20-37. Fixation of osseous attachment of tendon to bone. **A,** Fixation by Vitallium screw or nail. **B,** Fixation by mattress suture of stainless steel wire through holes drilled in bone. **C,** Fixation by wire loops. (From Edmonson, A.S., and Crenshaw, A.H., editors: Campbell's operative orthopaedics, ed. 6, St. Louis, 1980, The C.V. Mosby Co.)

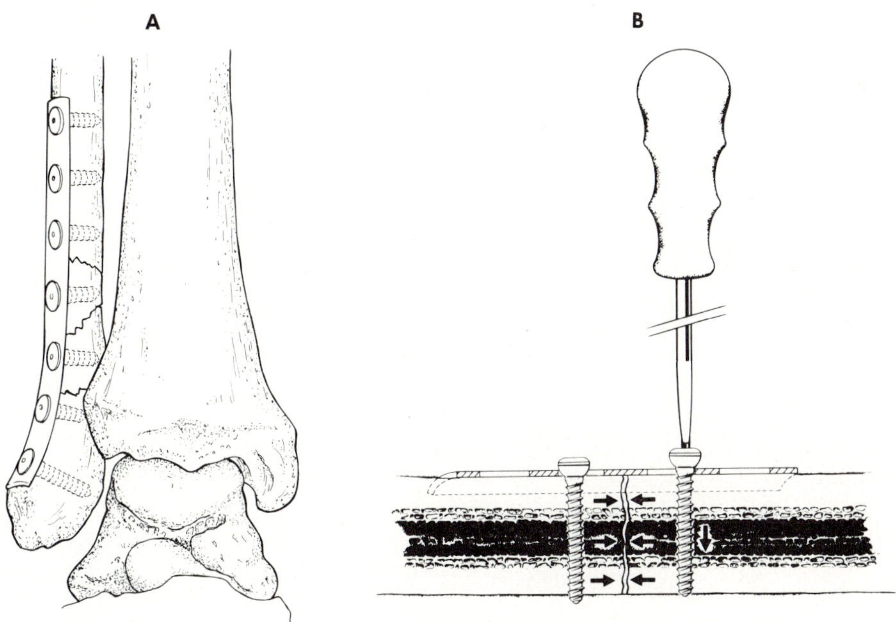

Fig. 20-38. A, Internal fixation of fracture with compression plate and screws. **B,** Forces applied during compression plating. (Courtesy Zimmer, Inc., Warsaw, Ind.)

Electrical stimulation to induce osteogenesis

Definition. Artificially applied electric current that induces or influences osteogenesis. Types include noninvasive, implantable, and percutaneous. The choice of bone stimulator varies according to the patient, pathological condition, and surgeon's preference (Fig. 20-39). Electrical bone stimulation works on the principle that bone, when stressed, produces an electrical charge. The area under compression is electronegative, and the area under tension is electropositive.

Considerations. The bone growth stimulator is used in patients in whom the risk of nonunion is high. This usually includes patients who have undergone previous surgery, who have sustained significant tissue loss, or in whom bone grafting is contraindicated. Once nonunion of a fracture has been established, electrical stimulation may be considered as a treatment alternative. Along with accelerating fracture healing, it has been successfully used in infected nonunions and retards bacterial growth. Some types allow for external monitoring of the current flow.

Setup. A soft-tissue and orthopedic set appropriate to the surgical area. The system is according to the surgeon's preference. *Note:* Instructions and components vary according to type. Special attention should be given to the specifications for autoclaving. The entire surgical team should familiarize themselves with the appropriate technique.

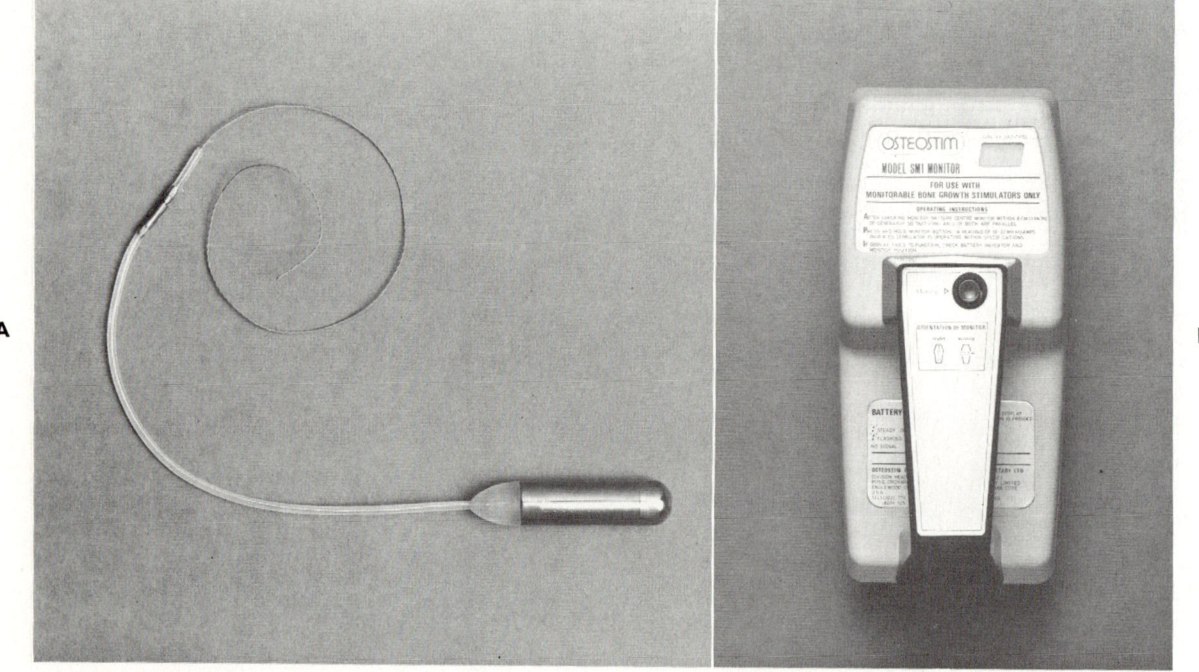

Fig. 20-39. A, Bone growth stimulator cathode and lead. **B,** Monitor for bone growth stimulator. (Courtesy Orthopaedic Division of Telectronics Proprietary, Ltd., Englewood, Colo.)

OPERATIONS ON THE SHOULDER GIRDLE

Acromioclavicular separation

Considerations. Acromioclavicular joint separation is frequently seen in athletes. Not only is the ligamentous support of the acromioclavicular joint disrupted but also the coracoclavicular ligaments that tether the clavicle to the underlying coracoid process of the scapula.

The purpose of surgery in the acute injury patient is to reestablish the proper relationship between the clavicle and the coracoid process. This is done by replacing the coracoclavicular ligament with braided wire, heavy suture, Mersilene tape, or a specially designed (Bosworth) screw. Occasionally, it is also necessary to stabilize the acromioclavicular joint with a smooth pin. Treatment of an old injury involves resection of 1 cm of the distal clavicle to alleviate pain.

Position and incision. The patient is in the supine or semisitting position with a sandbag or folded sheet under the affected shoulder and the head tilted as far as possible to the opposite side. The extremity is draped with stockinette to the midhumeral level, so that it is free to be manipulated. A short curvilinear incision, which also exposes the coracoid process, is made over the distal clavicle.

Setup. The regular bone, small bone, and soft-tissue sets are used, plus the following (Fig. 20-40):

- Bosworth screws
- Screwdriver for Bosworth screws
- Drill and points
- Aneurysm needles (ligature carriers)
- Braided wire
- Pliers, large
- Needle nose pliers
- Wire cutters
- Creggo elevators (Fig. 20-57)

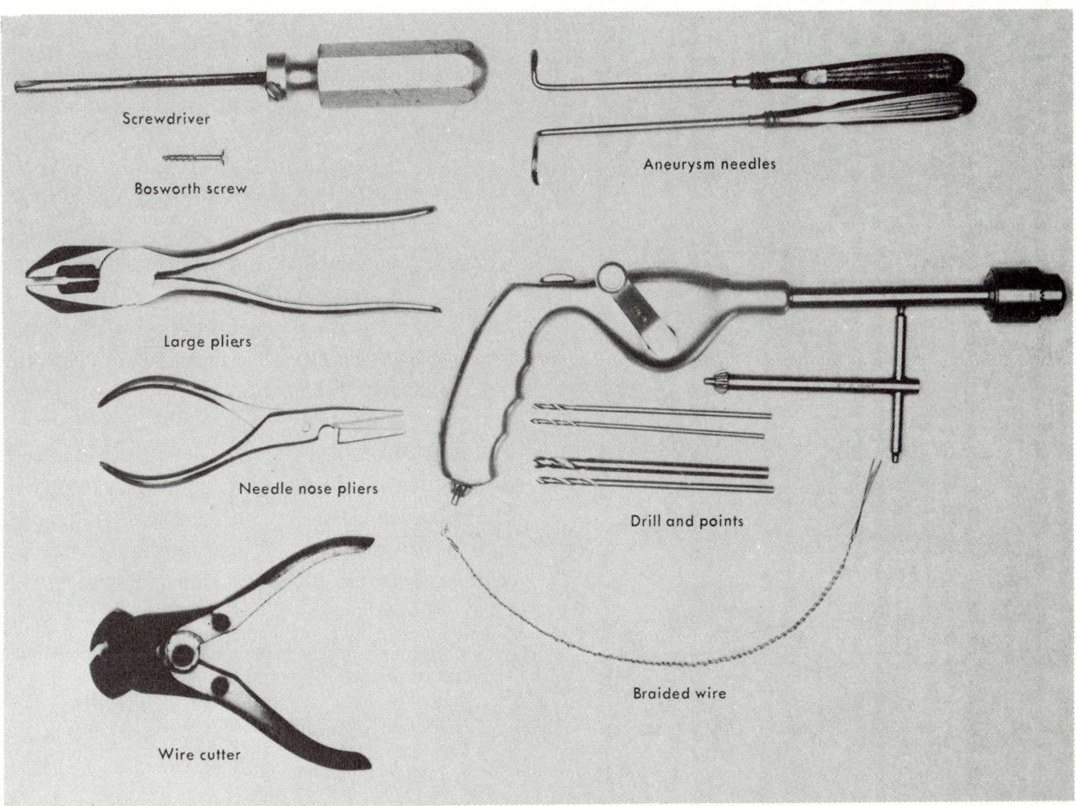

Fig. 20-40. Special instruments for repair of acromioclavicular separation.

Sternoclavicular dislocation

Considerations. Sternoclavicular dislocation usually is treated nonoperatively with immobilizing bandages. In certain severe cases, open reduction may be necessary.

Clavicular fracture

Considerations. Clavicular fracture is usually treated by immobilization in a figure-of-eight splint (Fig. 20-41). When surgery is required, an intramedullary pin is used for internal fixation.

Position and incision. The patient is placed in the supine or semisitting position with a sandbag or folded sheets under the affected shoulder and the head tilted as far as possible to the opposite side. A small incision is made over the distal clavicle if the pinning is to be done without exposing the fracture site. A second incision over the fracture site is occasionally needed to facilitate reduction of the fracture.

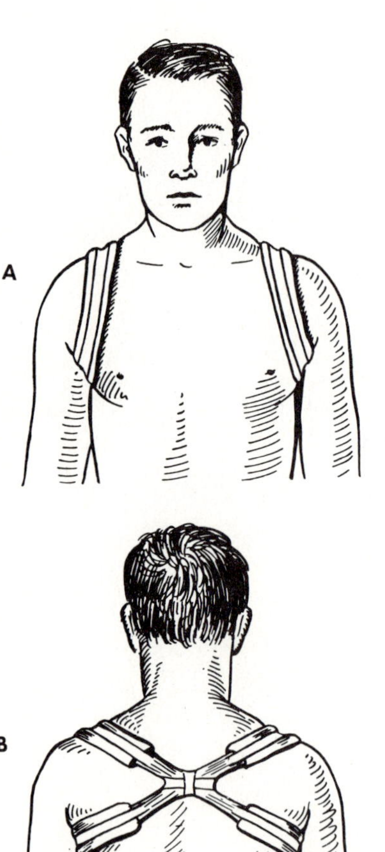

Fig. 20-41. Figure-of-eight dressing. **A,** Front view. **B,** Back view. Felt, bias flannel bandage, and adhesive tape are used. Dressing should be changed every week to 10 days for cleanliness. (From Larson, C.B., and Gould, M.: Orthopedic nursing, ed. 9, St. Louis, 1978, The C.V. Mosby Co.)

Setup. A small bone set and a regular soft-tissue set are required, plus the following:

- Elevators
- Threaded wire, compression plate, or appliance of choice
- Drill and points
- Wire cutters, heavy
- Appliance and accessories of choice

Rotator cuff tear

Definition. Tear occurring through the inserting tendinous fibers of the infraspinous, supraspinous, teres minor, and subscapular muscles on the humerus.

Considerations. Rotator cuff tears frequently follow trauma in patients with weakened tendinous fibers who have degenerative changes within the joint. Patients with this problem are unable to initiate abduction of the shoulder because the stabilizing forces of the ruptured tendons on the humeral head are lost.

Position and incision. The patient is supine or semisitting with a sandbag or folded towel under the affected shoulder. The head is tilted to the opposite side as far as possible. A superior incision that extends both anteriorly and posteriorly is made, and the muscles are detached from the scapula and clavicle.

Setup. Regular bone and soft-tissue sets are required, as well as a drill and drill points, and various shoulder retractors.

Recurrent anterior dislocation of the shoulder

Considerations. The anterior fibers of the shoulder capsule are stretched and weakened as a result of frequent dislocations of the shoulder joint. There are several different methods of repair, but all of the procedures are designed to strengthen the anterior joint capsule. The surgical incision and instruments used for all of the procedures are similar.

Position and incision. The patient is in the supine or semisitting position with a sandbag or folded sheet under the shoulder. The arm is draped free so that the extremity can be manipulated. An anterior curved incision or a longitudinal incision in the anterior axillary fold is made over the shoulder joint.

Setup. A regular soft-tissue set and a regular bone set are required, plus the following:

- Rake retractors, large, smooth
- Bennett retractors
- Drill and points
- Bankart retractors
- Dental drill
- Awls
- Pins with holes
- Aneurysm needles (ligature carriers)

Operative procedure

Bankart procedure. The attenuated anterior capsule is reattached to the rim of the glenoid fossa with heavy sutures, staples, or pullout wires. The glenoid fossa rim is roughened with a chisel to provide a raw surface to which the capsule is attached. A special retractor designed for the Bankart procedure is desirable. Instruments such as an angled drill, a curved awl, or drill points are necessary for making the suture holes in the rim of the glenoid fossa. If the coracoid process is to be removed to obtain better operative exposure, a drill and drill points should be available (Figs. 20-42 and 20-43). Postoperatively, the extremity is immobilized in a sling.

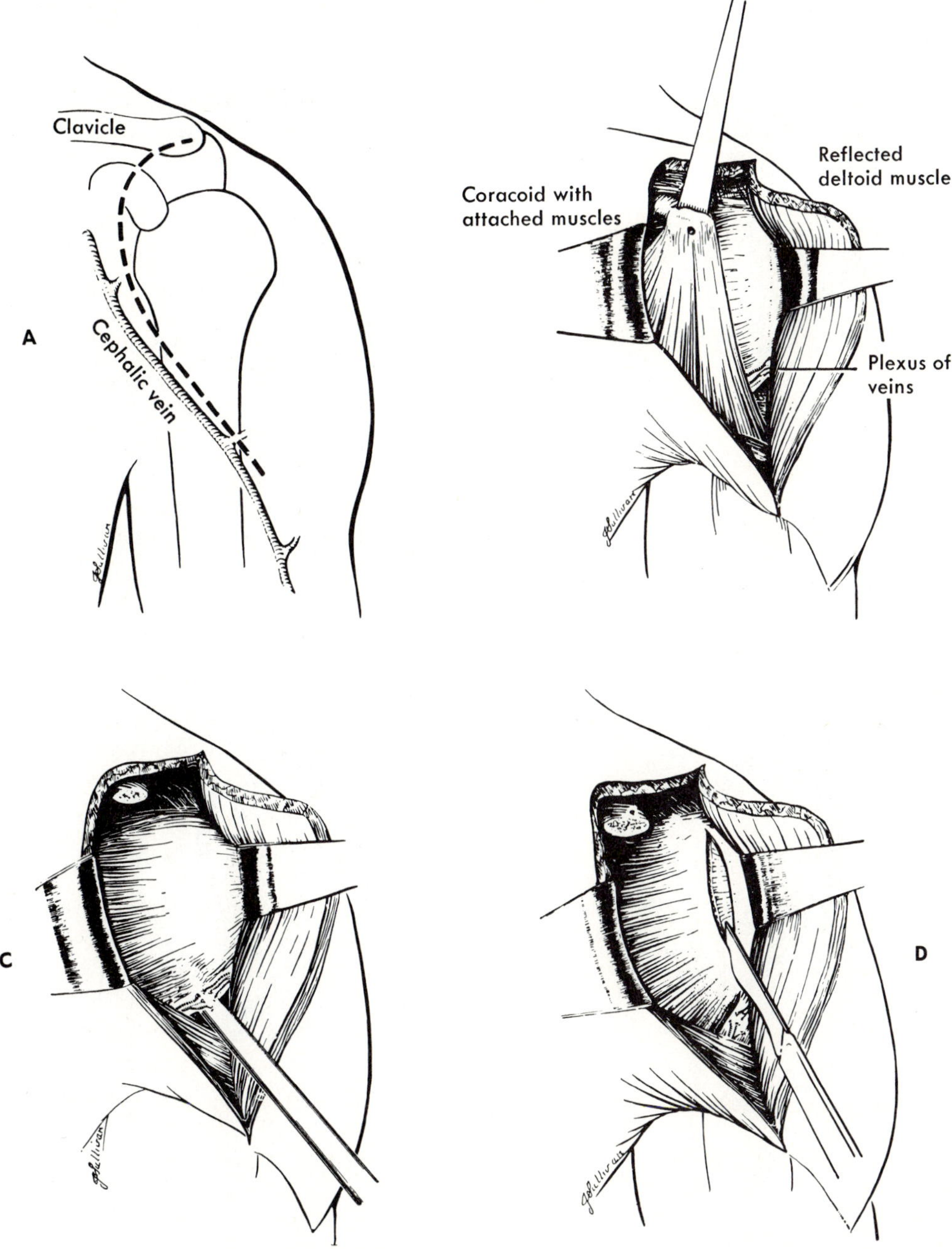

Fig. 20-42. Bankart operation (technique of Cave and Rowe). **A,** Skin incision. **B,** Coracoid divided. **C,** Inferior margin of subscapular tendon identified. **D,** Subscapular tendon divided near lesser tuberosity. **E,** Subscapular tendon retracted medially. **F,** Holes made through rim of glenoid. **G,** Free lateral margin of capsule sutured to rim of glenoid. **H,** Medial margin of capsule lapped over lateral part and sutured in place. (From Edmonson, A.S., and Crenshaw, A.H., editors: Campbell's operative orthopaedics, ed. 6, St. Louis, 1980, The C.V. Mosby Co.)

Continued.

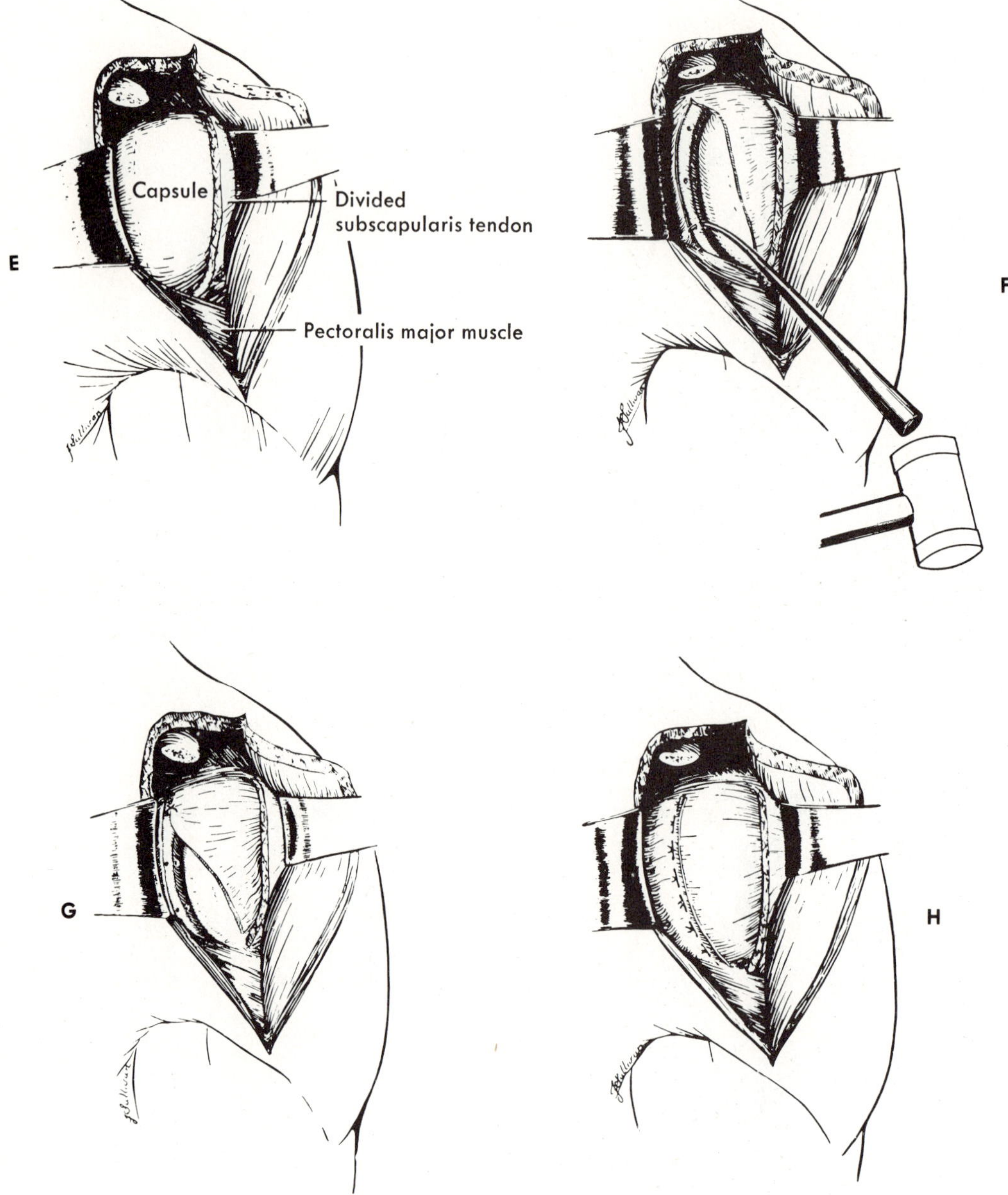

Fig. 20-42, cont'd. For legend see p. 477.

Putti-Platt procedure. The subscapularis tendon and the capsule are detached from the humerus and resutured more laterally on the humeral neck, thereby reducing the laxity of the anterior supporting structures and preventing excess external rotation of the shoulder.

Bristow procedure. The coracoid process, along with the attached muscles, is detached and inserted onto the neck of the glenoid cavity, where it is held with a screw. This stabilizes the anterior joint capsule and prevents recurrent dislocation.

Fracture of the humeral head

Considerations. Comminuted fractures of the humeral head may require open reduction and internal fixation with screws or pins. However, if the fracture is badly comminuted, a prosthetic replacement with the Neer prosthesis (Fig. 20-44) is indicated. Results of this surgery are frequently disappointing, and the operation is used sparingly. Traumatic or degenerative arthritic shoulder joints may be so painful that total shoulder joint replacement is necessary. Again, results are frequently disappointing, and the operation is not often performed. Several total shoulder joint designs are available.

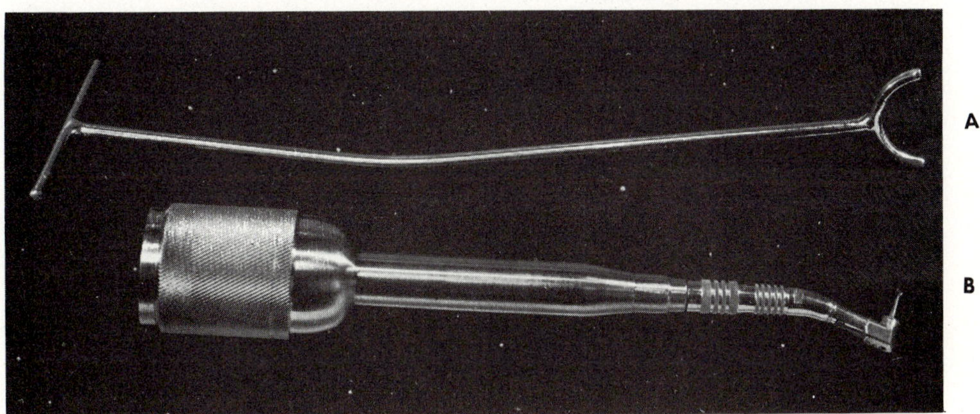

Fig. 20-43. Special instruments for Bankart procedure. **A,** Retractor. **B,** Dental drill designed to fit Luck saw. (From Edmonson, A.S., and Crenshaw, A.H., editors: Campbell's operative orthopaedics, ed. 6, St. Louis, 1980, The C.V. Mosby Co.)

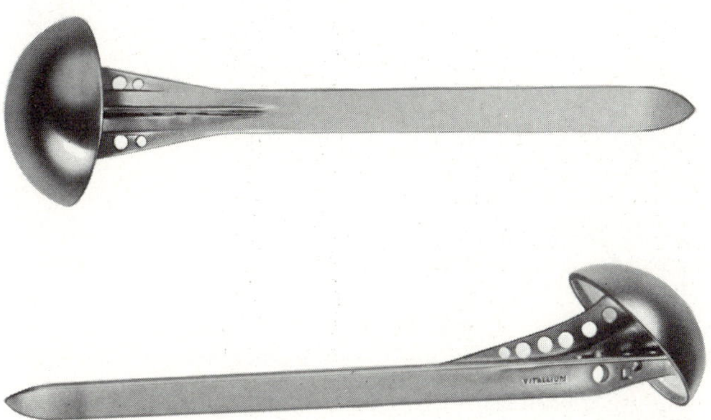

Fig. 20-44. Vitallium Neer shoulder prosthesis. (Courtesy Austenal Co., Division of Vitallium Surgical Appliances, Howe Sound Co., New York, N.Y.)

Position and incision. The patient is placed in the lateral position, and an incision is made superiorly, and can be extended both anteriorly and posteriorly to expose the shoulder joint (Fig. 20-45).

Setup. A regular basic set is used, plus the following:

Bennett retractors
Intramedullary rasp
Intramedullary reamer
Air-powered saw
Drill and drill points
Fixation device of choice

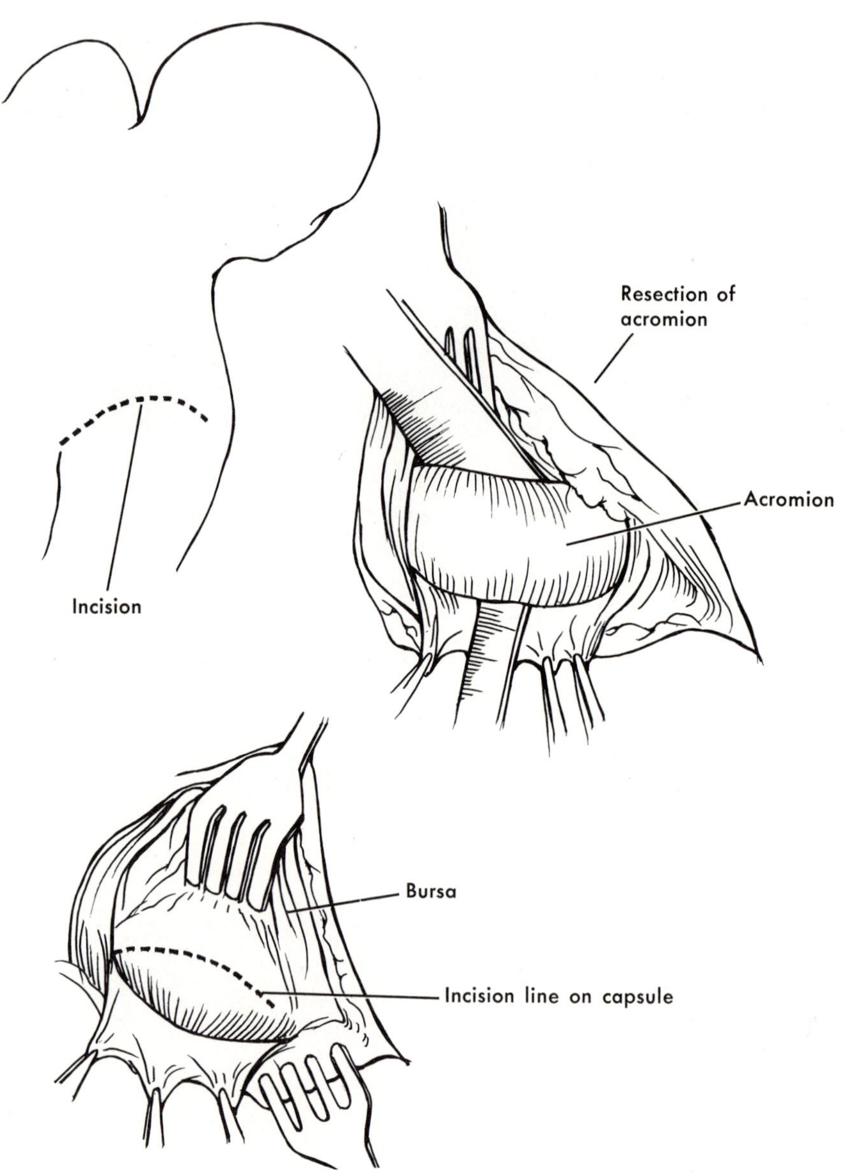

Fig. 20-45. Technique of replacement arthroplasty of shoulder. (From Bateman, L.E.: The shoulder and environs, St. Louis, The C.V. Mosby Co.)

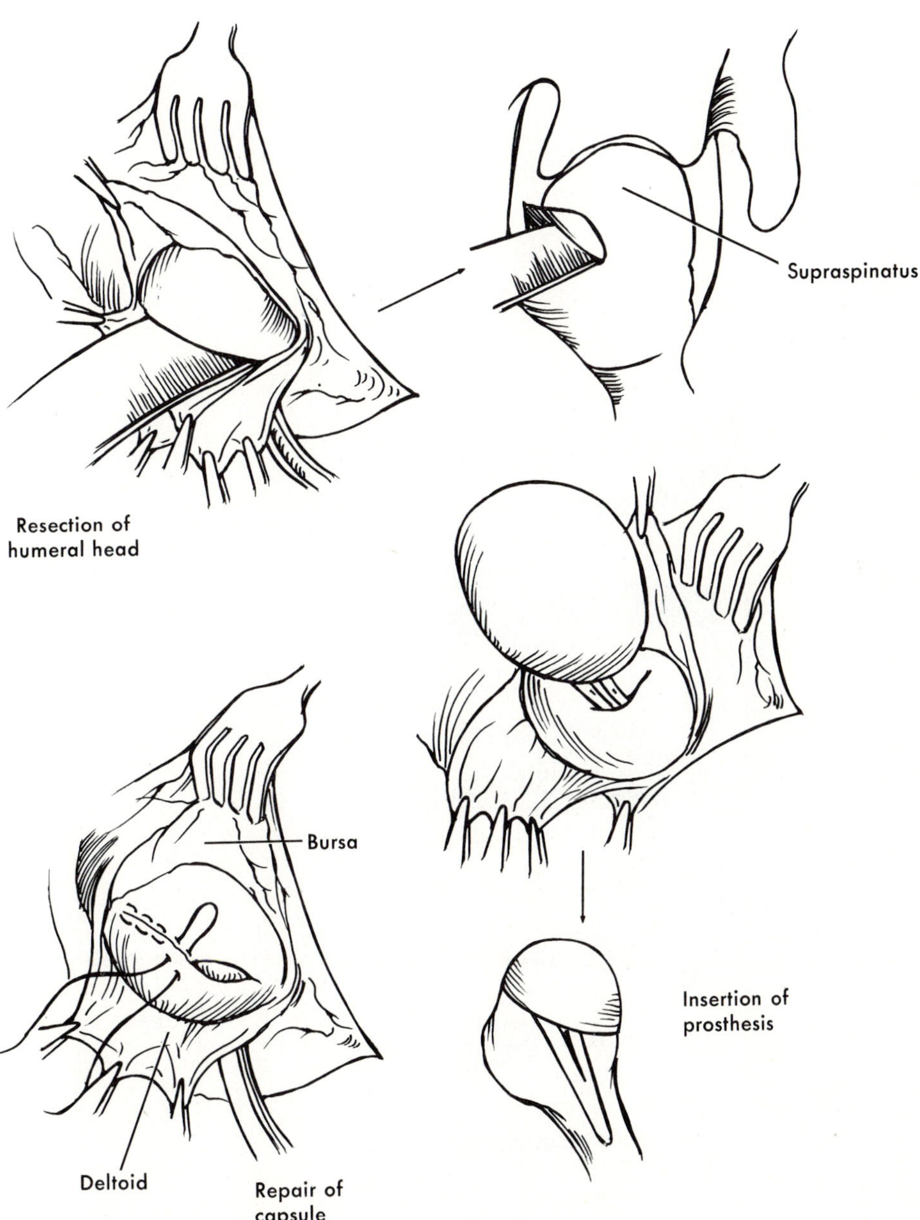

Fig. 20-45, cont'd. For legend see opposite page.

OPERATIONS ON THE HUMERUS, RADIUS, AND ULNA

Fractures of the shaft of the humerus

Considerations. Reduction of the fractured humerus is usually accomplished by closed manipulation and immobilization. When closed reduction is impossible or when nonunion of the fracture has occurred, surgery is indicated. The fracture is reduced and held with Rush rods or a heavy compression plate.

Position and incision. The patient is supine with the extremity prepared and draped from the middle of the chest to below the elbow. The fracture is exposed through a lateral incision.

Setup. Regular soft-tissue and bone sets are required, plus the following (Fig. 20-46):

Bennett retractors	Steinmann pins
Bone holders	Rush rods and awl
Bone hooks	Driver
Drill and points	Extractor
Screwdrivers	Compression set
Plates and screws	

Distal humerus fractures (supracondylar, epicondylar)

Considerations. Distal humerus fractures are particularly difficult to treat by closed methods. Screws, pins, and a variety of different plates can be used for internal fixation. There are circumstances in which it is necessary to transfer the ulnar nerve anteriorly to prevent compression of the nerve.

Position and incision. The patient may be prone with the elbow flexed over a small table, supine with the arm over the chest, or supine with the arm on a hand table. The incision depends on the location of the fracture. A tourniquet is useful during this procedure.

Setup. Regular soft-tissue and bone sets are required, plus the following (Fig. 20-46):

Drill and points	Kirschner wires
Bone holders, medium sized	Rush rods
Steinmann pins	Driver
Wire cutter	Extractor
Y plates and screws	Awl
Screwdrivers	

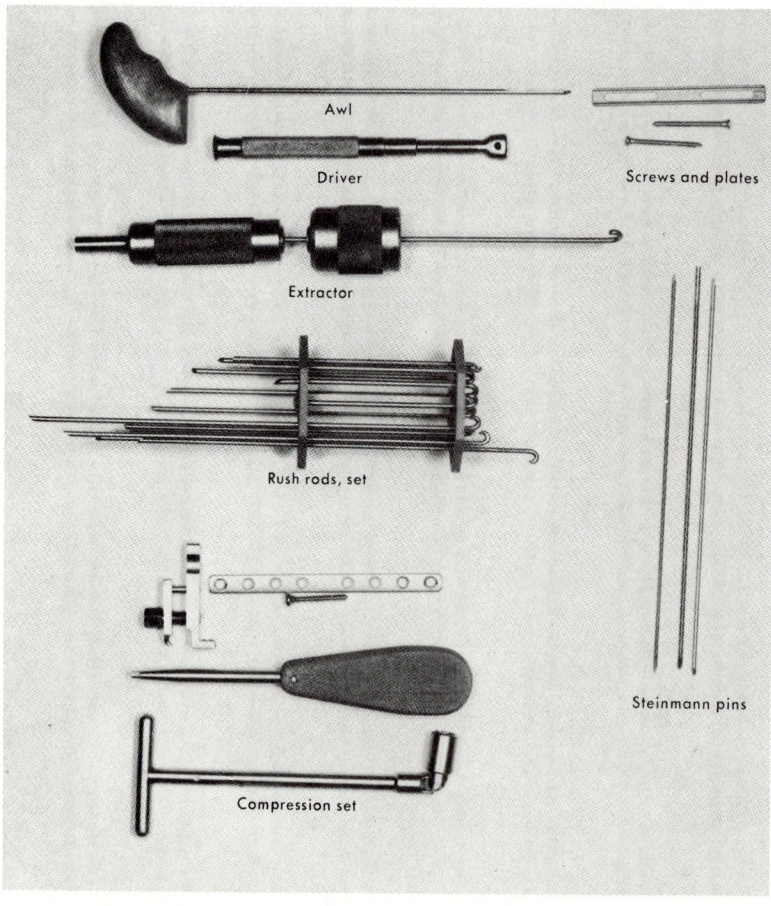

Fig. 20-46. Instruments for open reduction of humeral shaft fracture.

Olecranon fracture

Considerations. If the olecranon fracture fragment is small, it may be excised and the triceps tendon reattached to the ulna shaft. This does not result in loss of stability of the elbow joint. However, larger fragments must be reduced and held with internal fixation. Compression (small fragment) screws (Fig. 20-47), Kirschner wires, Steinmann pins, and figure-of-eight wire may be used (Fig. 20-48).

Setup. Small bone and soft-tissue sets are required, plus the following:

Small fragment compression screws
Drill and points
Elevators
Wire
Steinmann pins
Kirschner wires

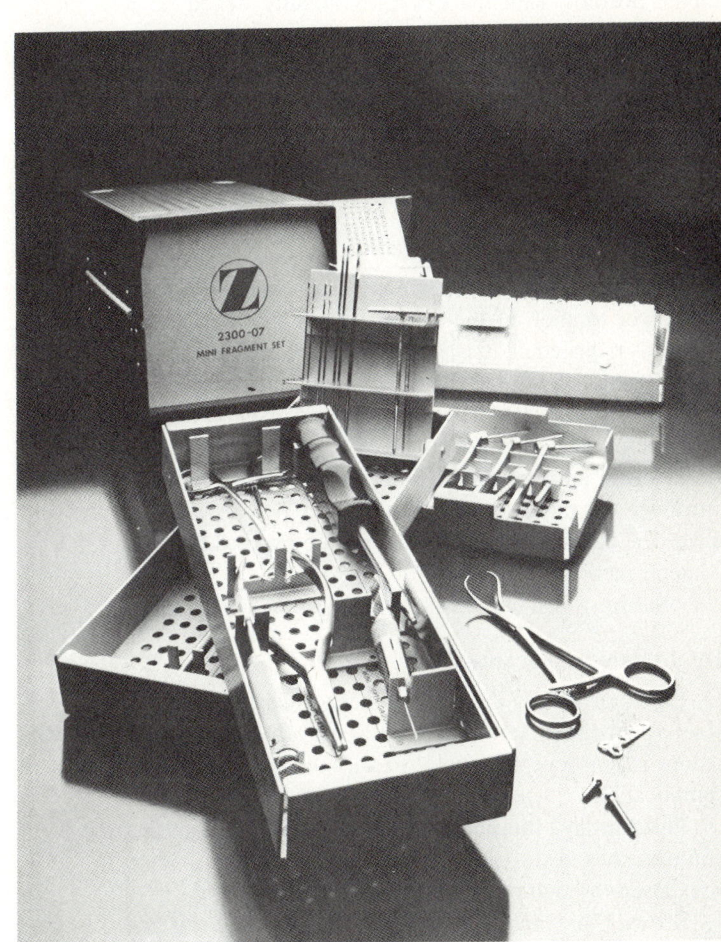

Fig. 20-47. Small (mini) fragment compression set. (Courtesy Zimmer, Inc., Warsaw, Ind.)

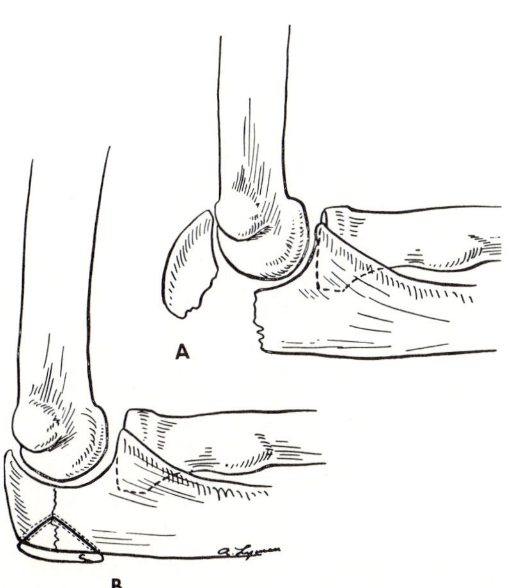

Fig. 20-48. Fracture of olecranon process, which always requires open reduction if fragments are separated. **A,** Fracture. **B,** Wire suture that should be fairly superficial for best results. (From Larson, C.B., and Gould, M.: Orthopedic nursing, ed. 9, St. Louis, 1978, The C.V. Mosby Co.)

Transposition of the ulnar nerve

Considerations. The ulnar nerve is frequently divided or damaged in fractures or wounds of the elbow. Dislocation of the elbow may also cause ulnar nerve damage. Late traumatic neuritis results from stretching of the ulnar nerve caused by an old injury. The hand appears atrophied, and sensory loss is high. In severe cases, a clawhand deformity occurs.

Position and incision. The patient is placed in the supine position with the extremity slightly flexed on a hand table or flexed over the chest. A tourniquet is applied to the upper arm, and the entire arm (fingers to tourniquet) is prepped and draped. An incision is made on the lateral aspect of the elbow near the epicondyle.

Setup. Regular and small soft-tissue sets are required.

Excision of the head of the radius

Considerations. A congruous radial head is essential for proper rotation of the forearm at the elbow. Consequently, in an adult it is necessary to excise the radial head if there is a displaced fracture involving the articular surface (Fig. 20-49). However, the radial head should never be excised in children.

Position and incision. The patient is supine with the arm over the chest or on a hand table. A tourniquet is used. The elbow joint and radial head are exposed through a lateral incision.

Setup. Small soft-tissue and bone sets are required.

Total elbow replacement (Fig. 20-50)

Considerations. Total elbow replacement is done for severe pain and/or loss of motion in the elbow. This procedure is not done frequently because of many potential complications.

Position and incision. The patient is supine with the arm over the chest. A tourniquet is used. The elbow joint is exposed through a lateral incision.

Setup. Small and regular bone and soft-tissue sets are required, plus the following:

Power saw and drill
Total elbow trial prostheses
Total elbow prostheses
Replacement instruments

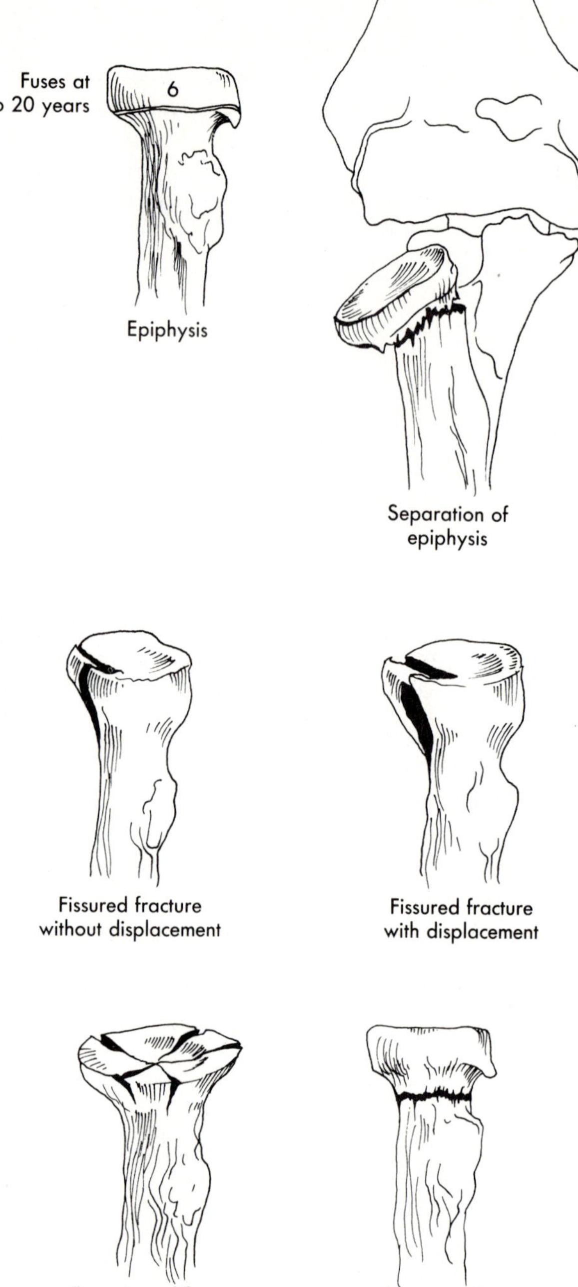

Fig. 20-49. Types of fractures of head and neck of radius. (From Moseley, H.F., editor: Textbook of surgery, ed. 3, St. Louis, The C.V. Mosby Co.)

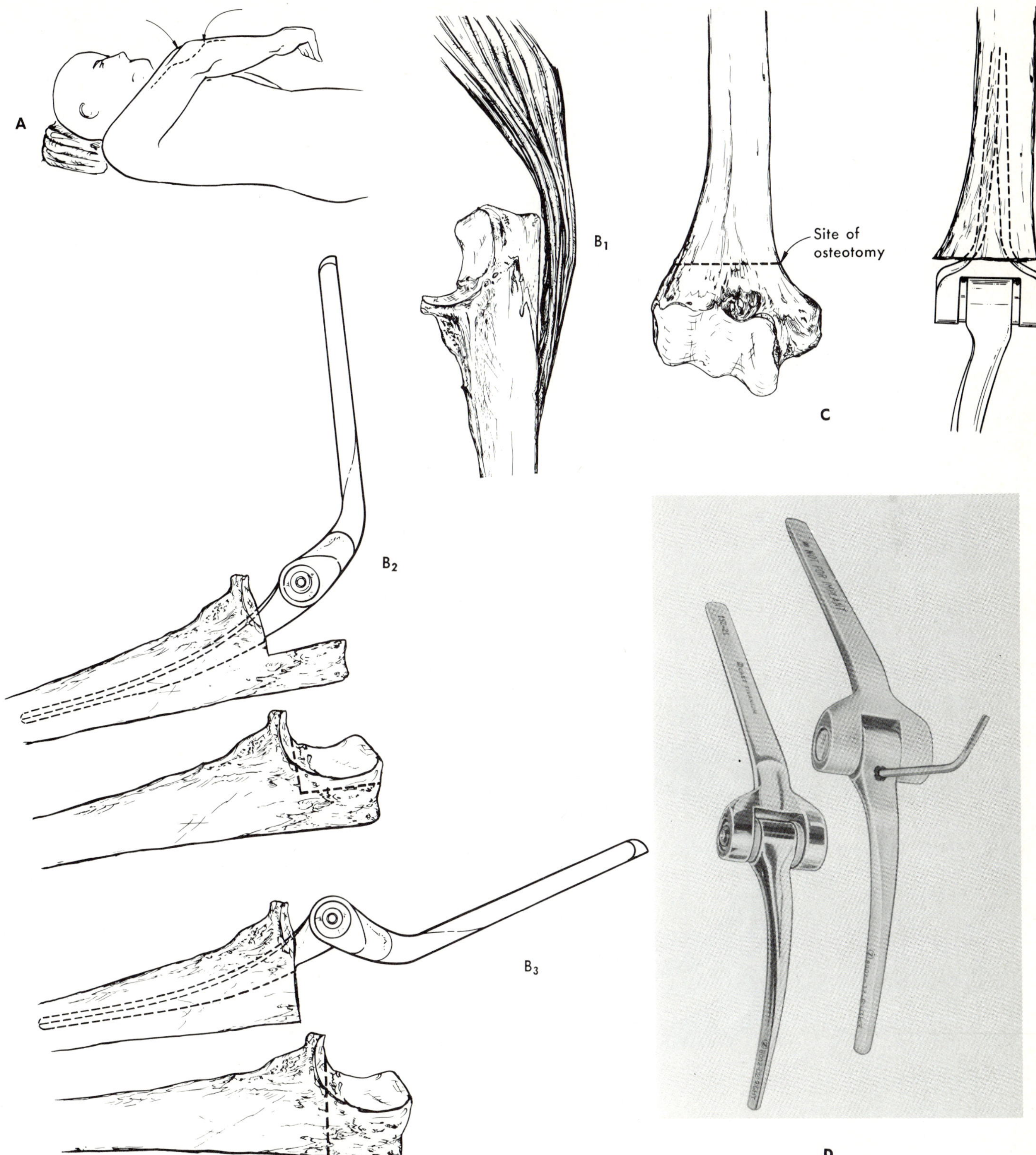

Fig. 20-50. A, Patient position for total elbow replacement procedure. **B_1,** Triceps tendon and periosteum stripped together intact. **B_2,** Bone removal from proximal ulna gives excellent exposure and can include almost entire olecranon and notch. **B_3,** Alternative resection removes articular surfaces while preserving major portion of olecranon. **C,** Bone removal from distal humerus can include both epicondyles to level just proximal to flarin, so as to correctly seat humeral stem. **D,** Total elbow prosthesis. (Courtesy Zimmer, Inc., Warsaw, Ind.)

Fracture of the radius and/or ulna

Considerations. Fractures of the radius and ulna frequently occur in children. As long as there is apposition of the fracture fragments, any angular deformity will be corrected as the child grows, so an operation is not indicated. However, an adult does not correct angular deformities, so anatomical reduction is necessary to permit proper rotation of the forearm. Consequently, open reduction and internal fixation, using intramedullary rods or compression plates, is frequently necessary for displaced fractures of one or both of these bones.

Position and incision. The patient is supine with the arm extended on the hand table. A longitudinal incision is made directly over the fracture(s).

Setup. Regular soft-tissue, regular bone, and small bone sets are used, plus the following:

- Bone holders, small
- Nail set
- Pliers, large
- Pin cutters
- Drill and points
- Rush rods
- Driver
- Extractor
- Rush awl
- Compression set
- Plate and screws

Colles' fracture

Definition. Dorsally angulated fracture of the distal radius.

Considerations. Colles' fracture usually is treated with closed reduction and cast immobilization. If the dorsal cortex is comminuted, the angulation may recur in the cast unless the fracture is held with internal fixation. In this case, Rush pins may be used for fixation.

Position and incision. The patient is in the supine position with the arm extended on a hand table.

Setup. Regular soft-tissue and small bone sets are used, plus a small power drill (Fig. 20-51), Rush pins, a driver, an extractor, and an awl.

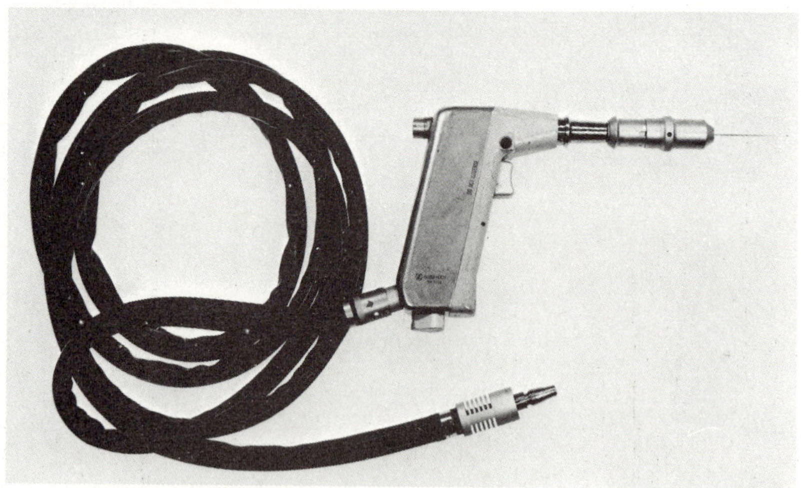

Fig. 20-51. Small power drill.

OPERATIONS ON THE HAND

Certain aspects of hand surgery are covered in Chapter 21. Small power drills are frequently used (Fig. 20-52).

Carpal tunnel release

Considerations. Carpal tunnel syndrome is an entrapment syndrome in which the median nerve becomes compressed at the volar surface of the wrist because of thickened synovium, fractures, or aberrant muscles. This results in numbness and tingling of the fingers and weakness of the intrinsic thumb muscles. The symptoms are usually reversible after the flexor retinaculum is incised, thereby relieving the compressed median nerve.

Position and incision. The patient is in the supine position with the arm on the hand table. A curvilinear, longitudinal volar incision is made from the proximal palm across the wrist joint.

Setup. A small soft-tissue set is required.

Fractures of the carpal bones

Considerations. Most fractures of the carpal bones are treated by closed reduction and immobilization. However, it is occasionally necessary to operate on a fracture because of displacement or nonunion.

Position and incision. The patient is supine with the arm extended on a hand table. Either a longitudinal volar incision or a transverse dorsal incision is made over the scaphoid bone. The fracture can be immobilized with small fragment compression screws or with Kirschner wires. Bone graft from the distal radius or from the olecranon is frequently added.

Setup. Small bone and soft-tissue sets are required, plus the following:

Kirschner wires
Power drill
Bone graft instruments
Small fragment compression set

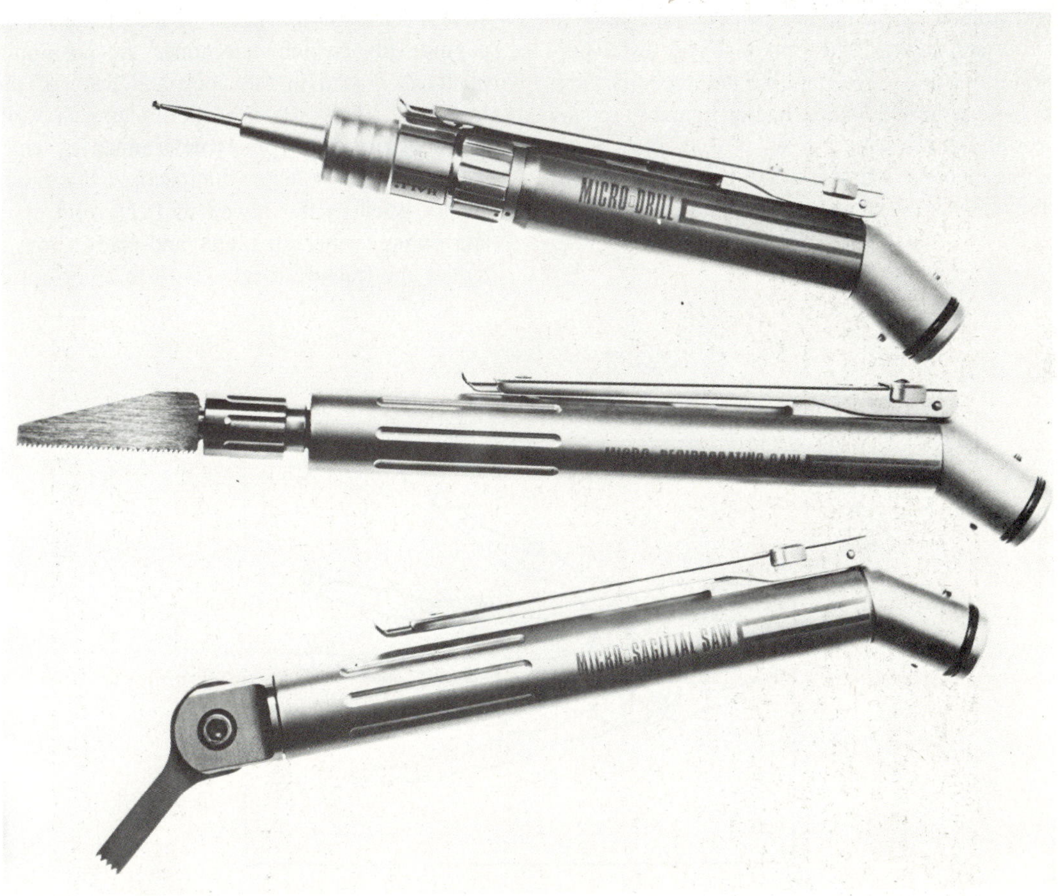

Fig. 20-52. Air-powered microdrill and microsaws. (Courtesy Zimmer, Inc., Warsaw, Ind.)

Excision of ganglia

Considerations. Ganglia are benign out-pouchings of the synovium from the intercarpal joints or tendon sheaths that become filled with synovial fluid. They are usually located on the dorsal surface of the wrist, but can be found on the volar surface also. They appear as firm masses that vary in size. Frequently, ganglia resolve spontaneously, but occasionally they are excised because they cause discomfort or for cosmetic reasons.

Position and incision. The patient is supine with the arm extended on a hand table. A transverse incision is made over each ganglion.

Setup. Small bone and soft-tissue sets are required.

Metacarpal arthroplasty

Considerations. Metacarpal joint replacement is most often performed in patients who have pain or a disabling deformity associated with rheumatoid or degenerative arthritis.

Position and incision. The patient is placed in the supine position with the extremity placed on a hand table. The tourniquet is applied and the entire extremity is prepped and draped. Incisions are made on the dorsum of the appropriate fingers. The proximal and distal portions of the joints are excised, and the intramedullary canals reamed. Appropriate tendon and/or ligament repairs to improve stability are done.

Setup. Small bone and soft-tissue sets are required, plus small reamers and trial and permanent implants (Fig. 20-53).

OPERATIONS ON THE HIP AND FEMUR

Hip fractures

Considerations. Hip fractures include intracapsular femoral neck fractures as well as extracapsular intertrochanteric fractures. Manipulation, reduction, and internal fixation of these fractures are greatly facilitated by a fracture table, which also permits adequate x-ray examination to determine whether the internal fixation implants are properly placed (Fig. 20-25).

Intertrochanteric fractures

Considerations. Intertrochanteric fractures most frequently occur in older people. The fractures usually unite without difficulties. However, since the lower extremity is externally rotated at the fracture site, internal fixation is necessary to prevent malunion. Internal fixation allows patients to get out of bed and helps prevent complications, such as thrombophlebitis, pulmonary emboli, pneumonia, and decubitus ulcers.

Position and incision. The patient is placed in the supine position on the fracture table, and the fracture is reduced by manipulation of the extremity. A lateral incision is made in the region of the greater trochanter, and a guide pin, which determines the position of the implant, is placed in the neck and head of the proximal fragment. The position of the fracture, as well as the position of the guide pin is determined by anteroposterior and lateral views under fluoroscopy. Internal fixation implants, such as the Jewett nail, Deyerle plate and pins, and compression hip plates and screws may be used to reduce the fracture (Figs. 20-54 to 20-56).

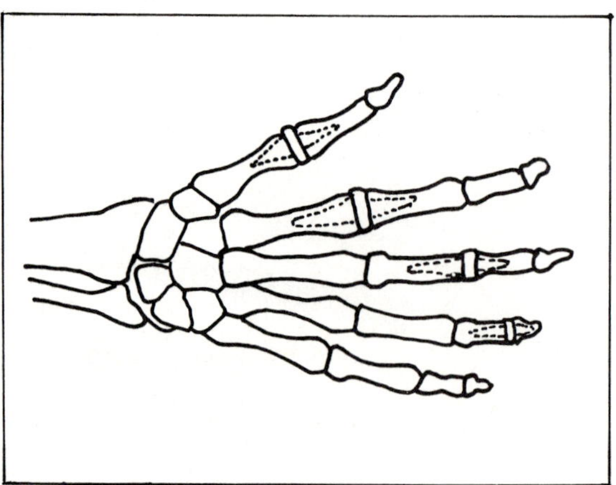

Fig. 20-53. Metacarpal implants, Swanson design. (Courtesy Dow Corning Wright, Arlington, Tenn.)

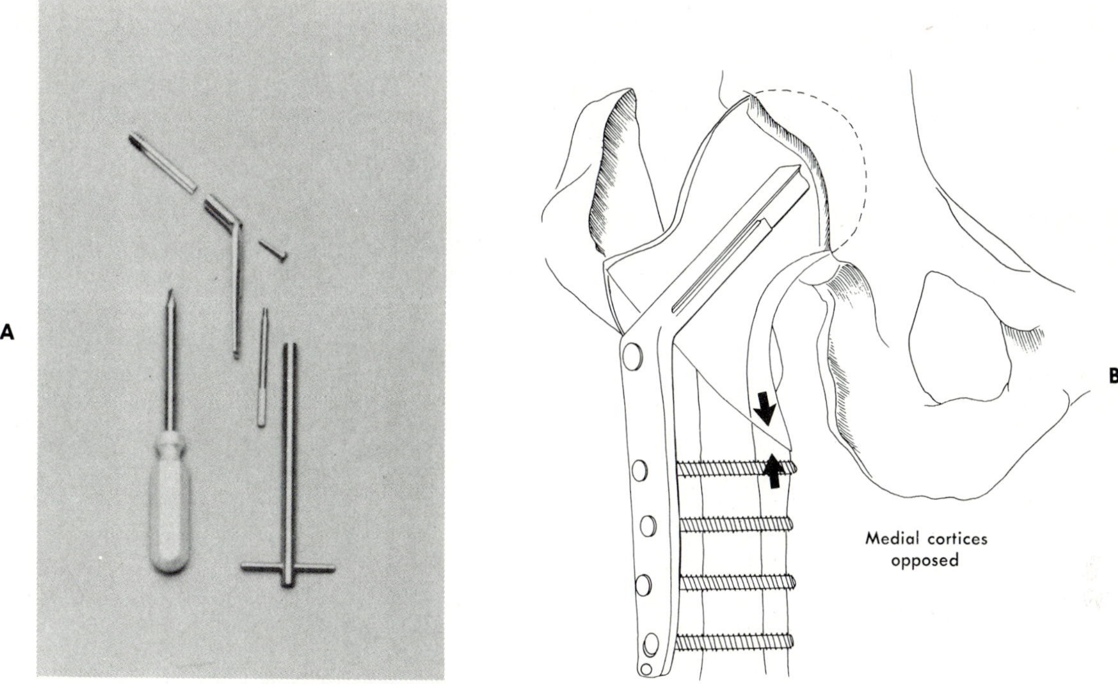

Fig. 20-54. A, Compression hip screw and accessories. **B,** Hip nail. (**A** courtesy Zimmer, Inc., Warsaw, Ind.; **B** from Urist, M.R., editor: Clinical orthopedics and related research, vol. 92, Philadelphia, J.B. Lippincott Co.)

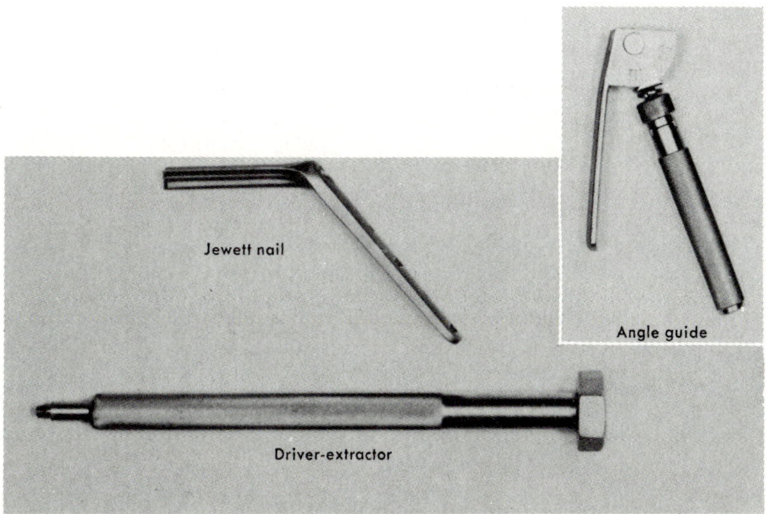

Fig. 20-55. Internal fixation hip device and accessories.

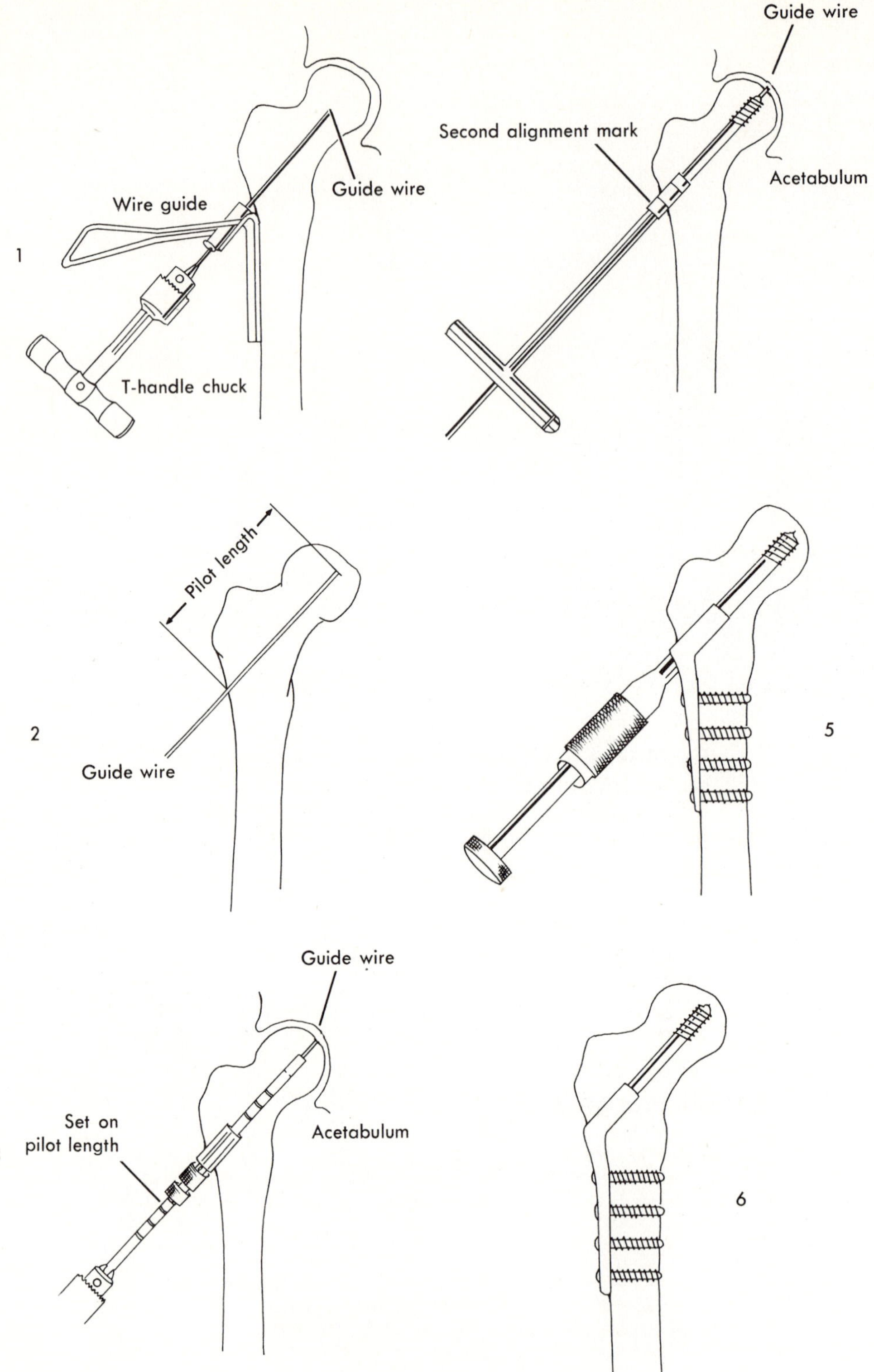

Fig. 20-56. Summary of basic hip fixation technique. (Courtesy Zimmer, Inc., Warsaw, Ind.)

Setup. A regular basic bone set is needed, plus the following (Fig. 20-57):

Hip retractors, assorted
Rake retractors, large
Bone-holding forceps
Bone hooks
Pliers, large
Power drill and points
Angle guide (Fig. 20-55)
Guide wires (Fig. 20-56)
Fixation device of choice with instrumentation
Bone screw set
Depth gauge
Screwdrivers

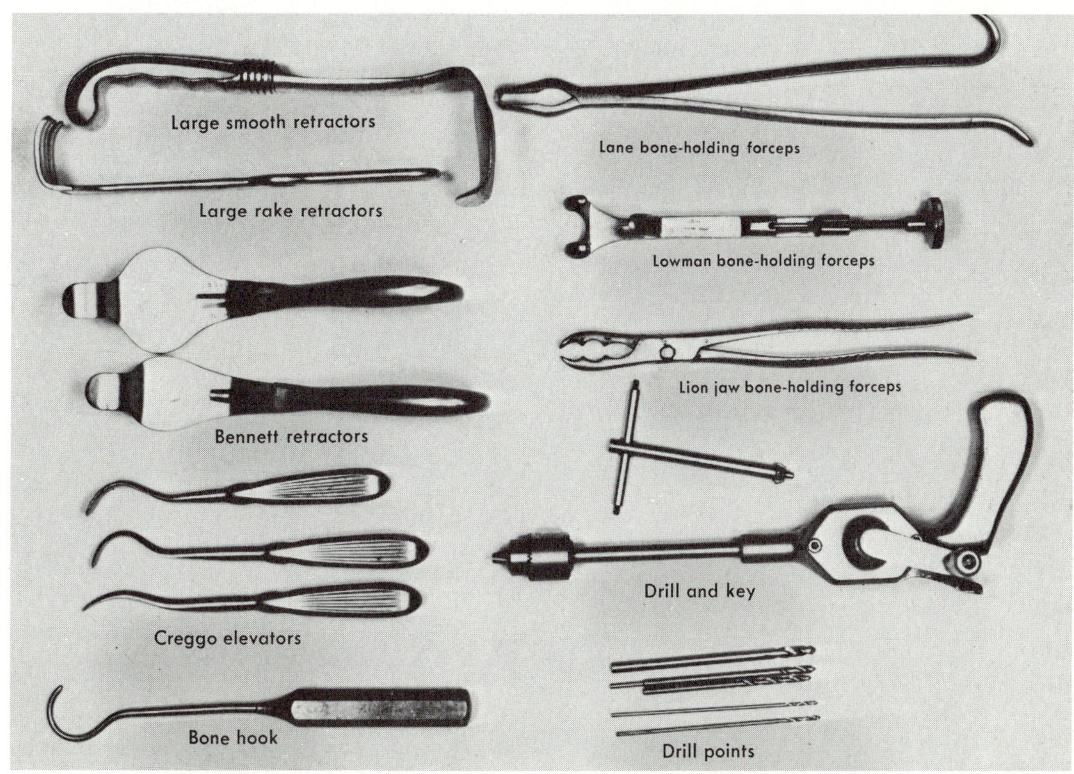

Fig. 20-57. Additional instruments for fixation of intertrochanteric fractures.

Ender nail technique

Considerations. Insertion of Ender nails is performed in patients with minimally displaced or nondisplaced subtrochanteric or intertrochanteric femoral fractures. The nails used are in anteversion. This requires an inventory of both right and left nails. Three to five nails are used on each procedure. The medullary canal should be filled.

Position and incision. The patient is placed on the fracture table, and traction is applied to the extremity. The procedure is performed under fluoroscopy. The incision is made on the medial aspect of the knee.

Setup. Regular bone and soft tissue sets are required, plus an appropriate nail set with instrumentation (Fig. 20-58) and assorted knee retractors.

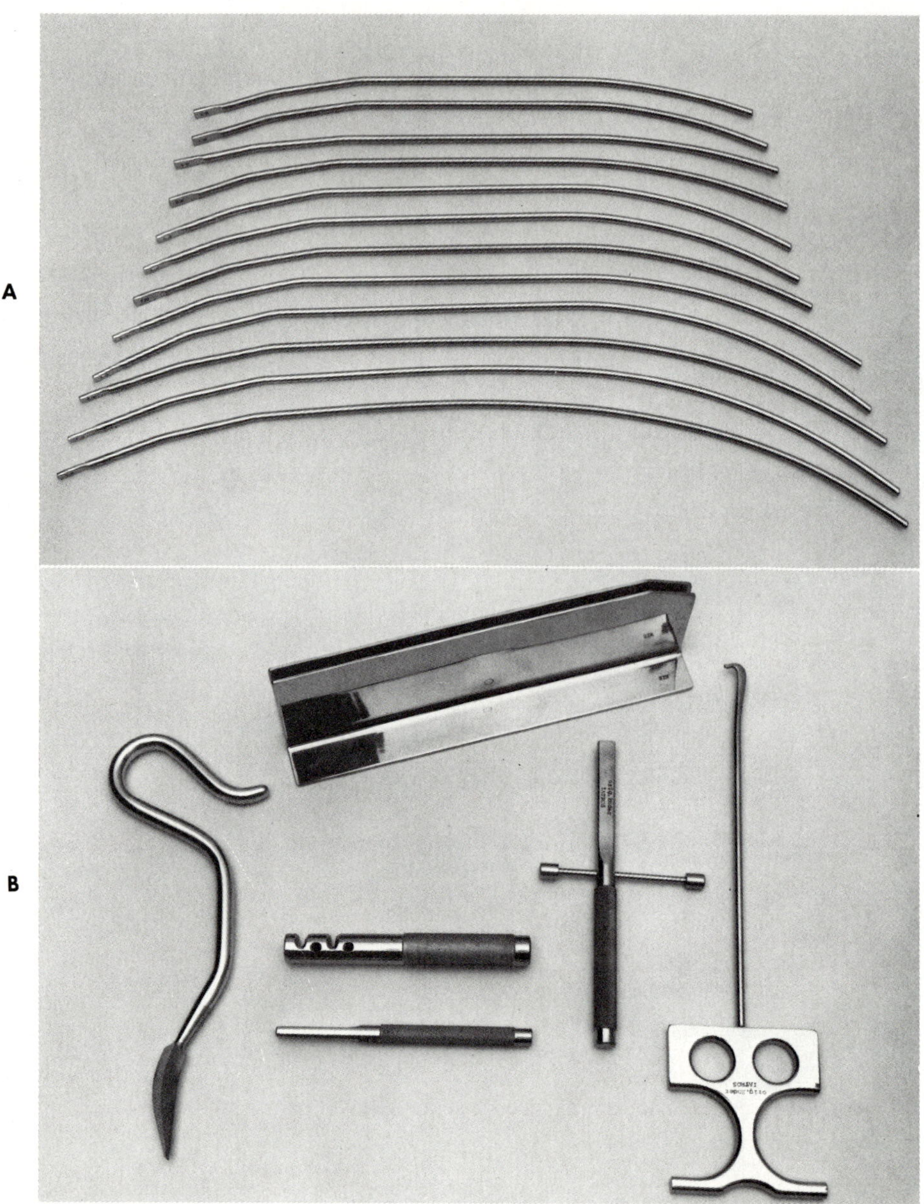

Fig. 20-58. A, Ender nails. **B,** Ender nail instrumentation. (Courtesy Richards Manufacturing Co., Memphis, Tenn.)

Femoral neck fractures
Internal fixation

Considerations. Anatomical reduction is necessary before internal fixation of femoral neck fractures because of the high incidence of associated complications, such as nonunion and aseptic necrosis of the femoral head. Growing children may sustain fractures through the epiphyseal growth plate (slipped capital femoral epiphysis). These injuries are treated by reduction and internal fixation of the femoral head similar to the procedures used in the adult.

Position and incision. The patient is placed on the fracture table, and the fracture is exposed through a lateral incision over the greater trochanter. A guide wire is placed, under fluoroscopy. Multiple pins of various designs, such as Knowles, Hagie, or Deyerle pins, are used (Figs. 20-59 and 20-60).

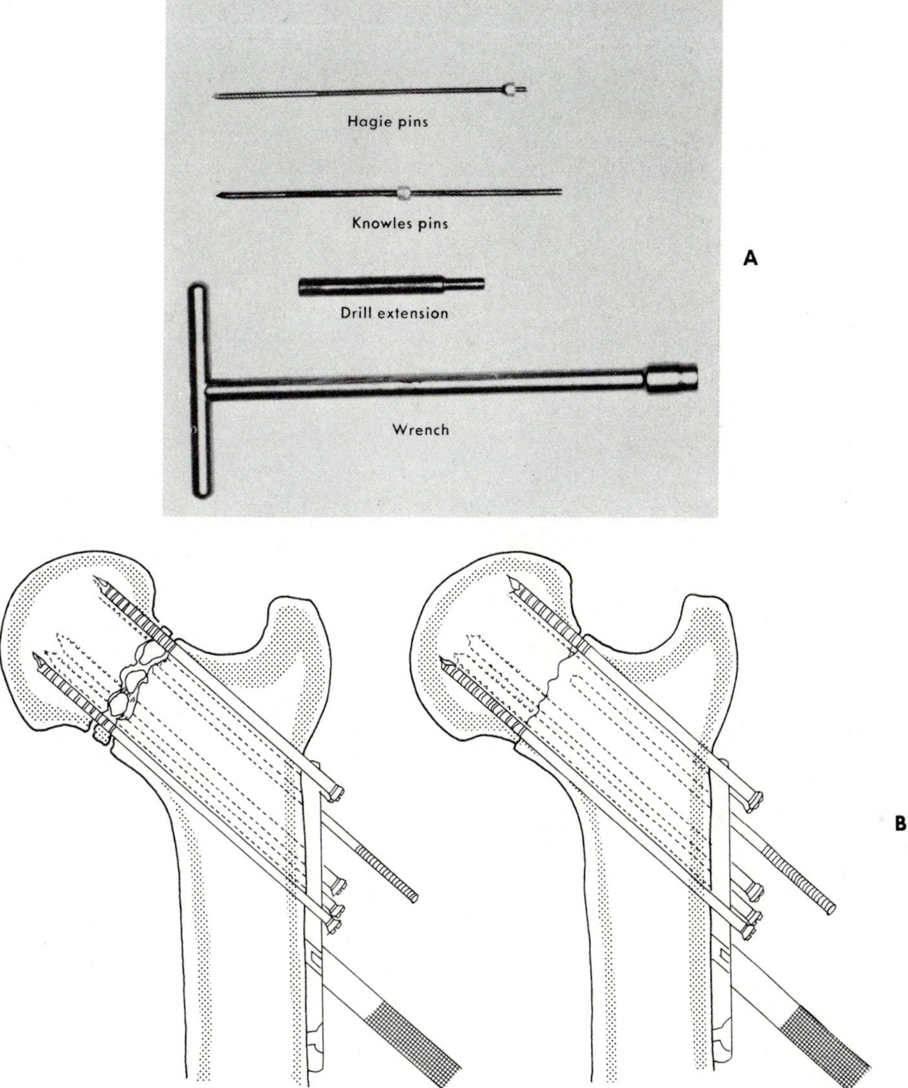

Fig. 20-59. A, Multiple pins for fixation of femoral neck fractures. **B,** Visually controlled impaction with Deyerle pins. After 7 pins have been inserted halfway into the head to prevent loss of reduction, the traction is loosened sufficiently to allow the head to return to its normal position in the acetabulum. (**B** from DePalma, A., editor: Clinical orthopedics and related research, vol. 39, Philadelphia, J.B. Lippincott Co.)

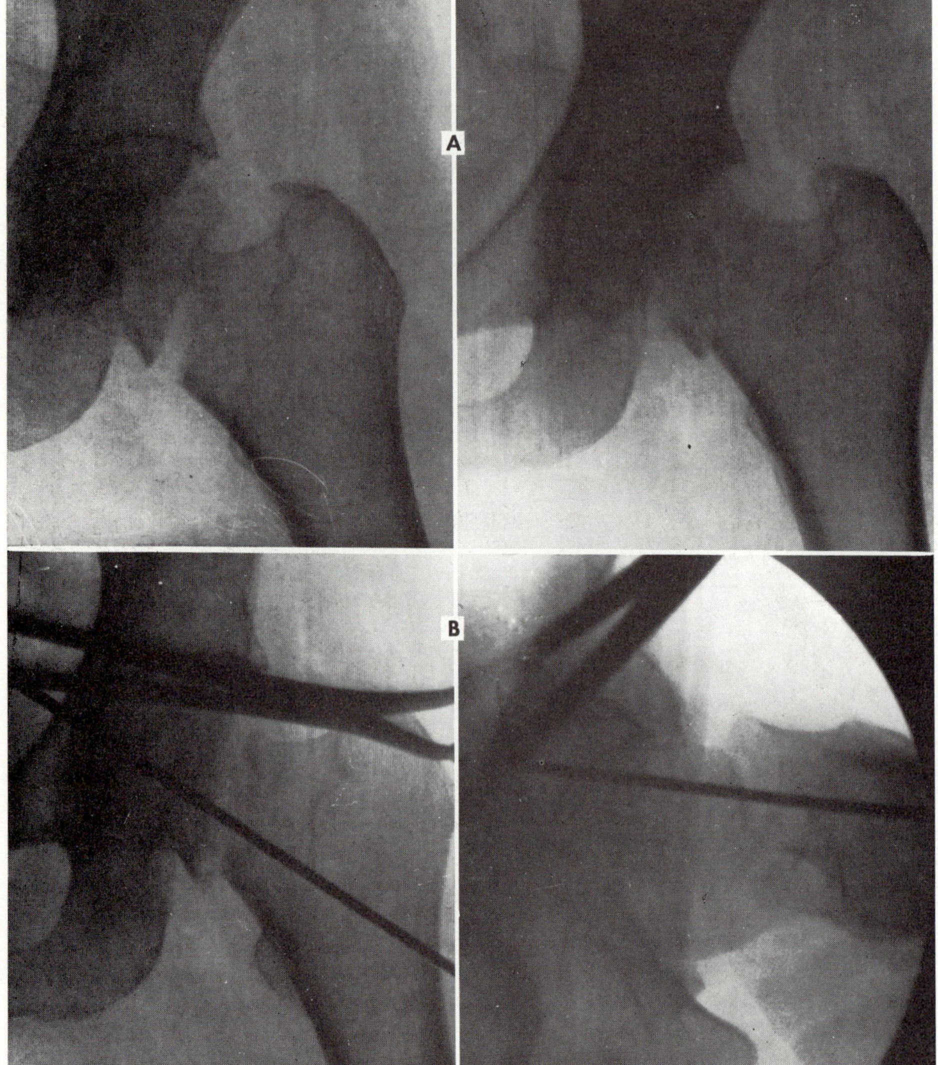

Fig. 20-60. If reduction is unstable, multiple pins are used in preference to compression hip screw, their removal incident to poor position of pins or tilting or displacement of head; this is easier than removal and reinsertion of the hip screw. **A,** Unsatisfactory reduction after first attempt corrected by second maneuvers. Reduction in lateral view (not shown) satisfactory after both attempts. **B,** Guide pin purposely inserted through head into ilium to increase stability. Satisfactory position of pin in anteroposterior view but distraction at fracture. In lateral view, pin is in satisfactory position in neck fragment but engages head in anterior quadrant, tilting it posteriorly. **C,** Fracture has been fixed with four Knowles pins. Usually three pins are preferred. **D,** Fracture has united at 1 year. (From Edmonson, A.S., and Crenshaw, A.H., editors: Campbell's operative orthopaedics, ed. 6, St. Louis, 1980, The C.V. Mosby Co.)

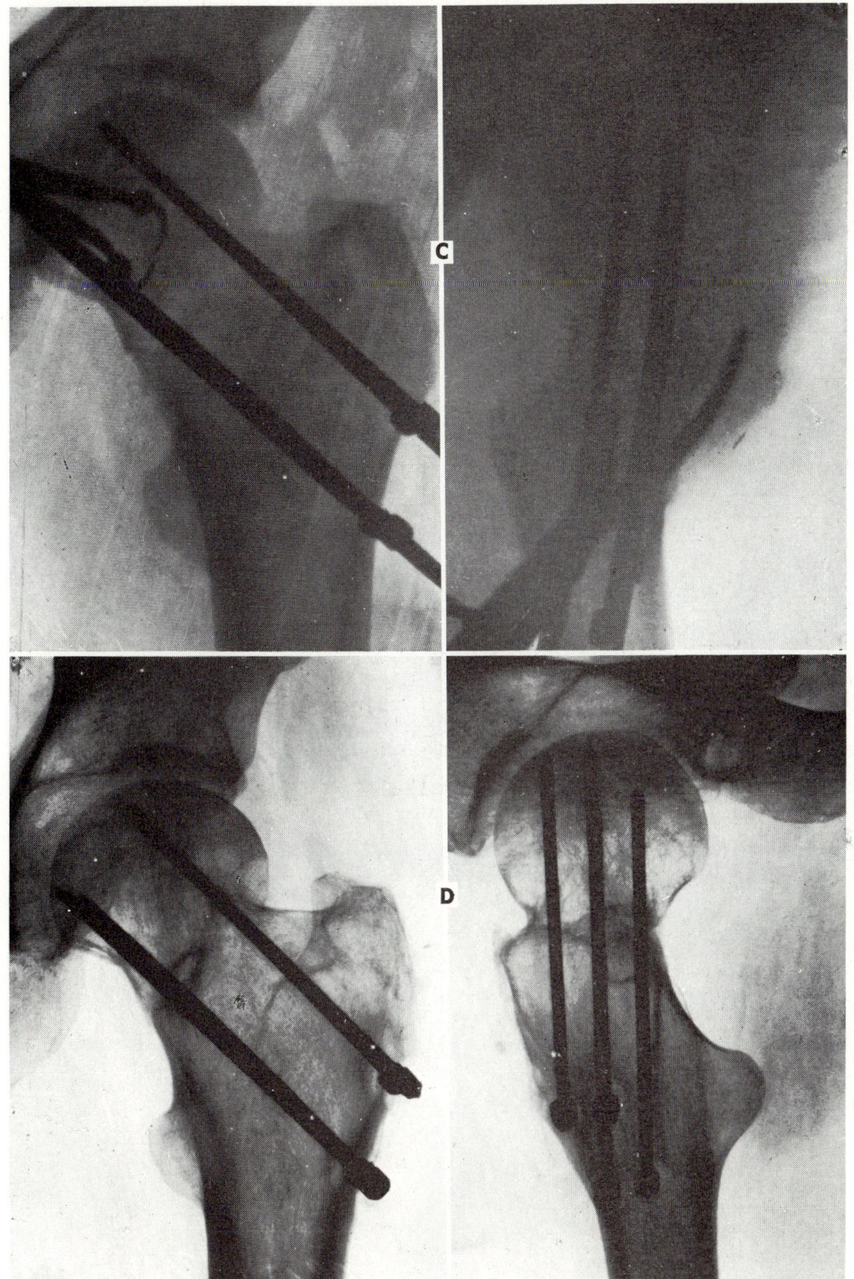

Fig. 20-60, cont'd. For legend see opposite page.

Setup. Regular soft-tissue and bone sets are required, plus the following:

- Hip retractors, assorted
- Rake retractors, large
- Bone-holding forceps
- Bone hooks
- Pliers, large
- Power drill and drill points
- Fixation device of choice, with instrumentation

Femoral head prosthetic replacement

Considerations. If anatomical reduction of a femoral neck fracture cannot be obtained by manipulation in the adult patient, or because of the high incidence of avascular necrosis and nonunion of the fracture, some surgeons prefer to replace the femoral head with an implant. Thompson, Austin-Moore, Bateman, and Mueller are among the many prostheses available (Figs. 20-61 and 20-62).

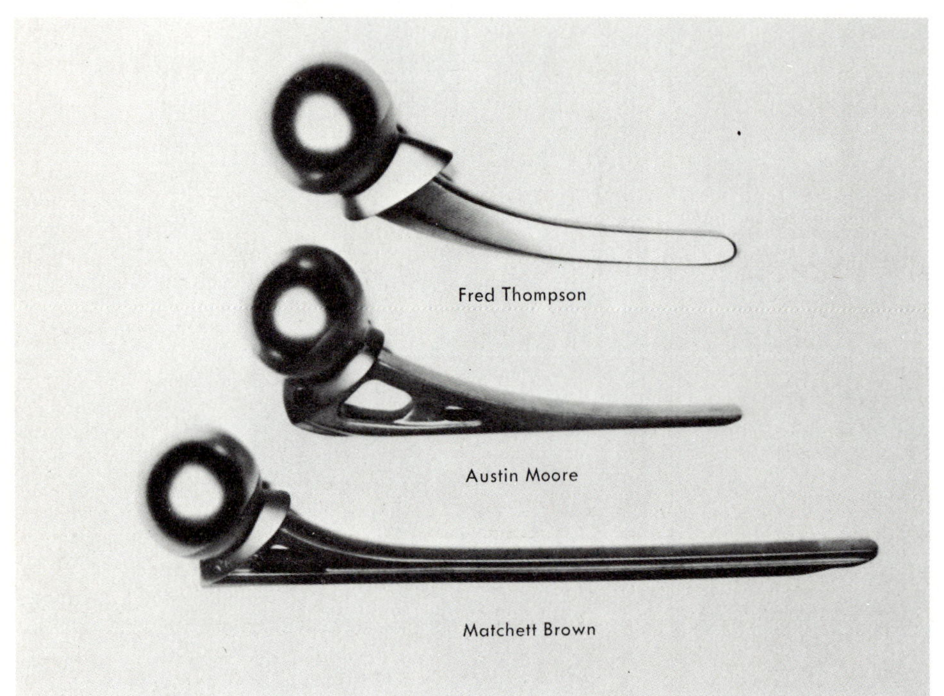

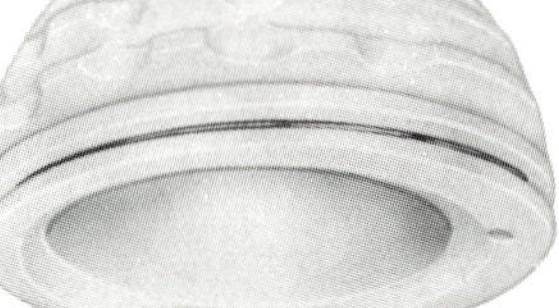

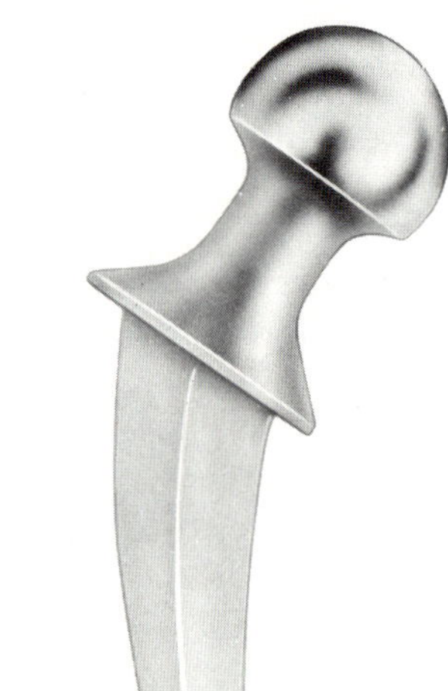

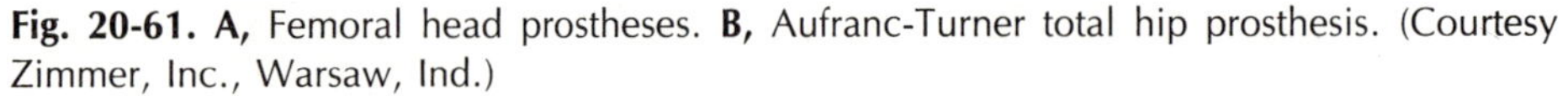
Fig. 20-61. A, Femoral head prostheses. **B,** Aufranc-Turner total hip prosthesis. (Courtesy Zimmer, Inc., Warsaw, Ind.)

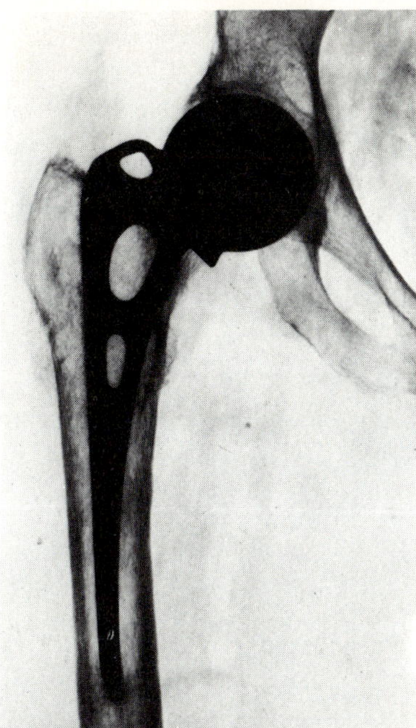

Fig. 20-62. Roentgenograms of hip after replacement arthroplasty with Austin-Moore metal prosthesis in 75-year-old woman who had nonunion of femoral neck fracture and vascular necrosis of femoral head. (From Brashear, H.R., and Raney, R.B.: Shand's handbook of orthopaedic surgery, ed. 9, St. Louis, 1978, The C.V. Mosby Co.)

Position and incision. The patient is placed in the supine position if an anterior approach is used, and in the lateral position if a lateral or posterolateral incision is used (Fig. 20-63). The prep extends from the nipple line to below the knee.

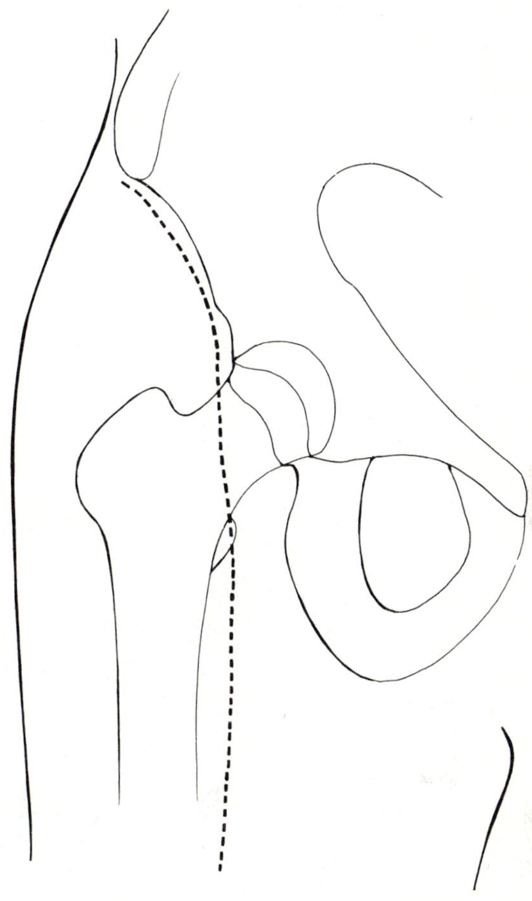

Fig. 20-63. Anterior approach to hip. (Adapted from Nicola, T.: Atlas of orthopaedic exposures, Baltimore, The Williams & Wilkins Co.)

Setup. Regular soft-tissue and bone sets are required, plus the following (Figs. 20-64 to 20-66):

Femoral rasps
Mallet
Driver
Air-powered saw
Femoral head extractor (corkscrew)
Hip gouge
Femoral head caliper
Hip skid
Cement instrumentation (if methyl methacrylate is used)
Prosthesis of choice

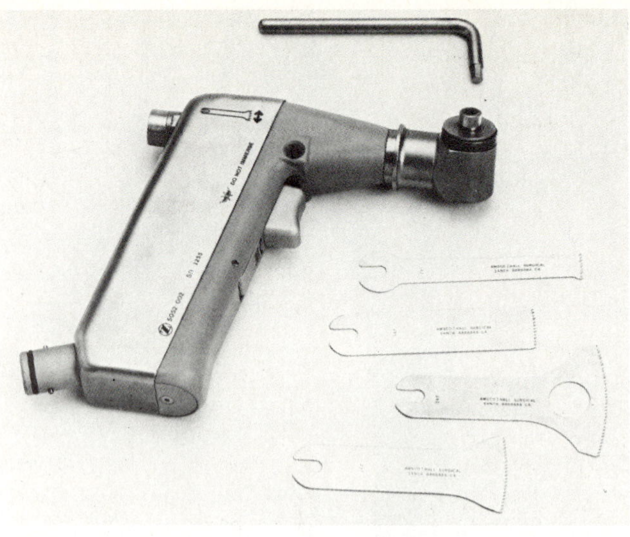

Fig. 20-64. Air-powered saw. (Courtesy Zimmer, Inc., Warsaw, Ind.)

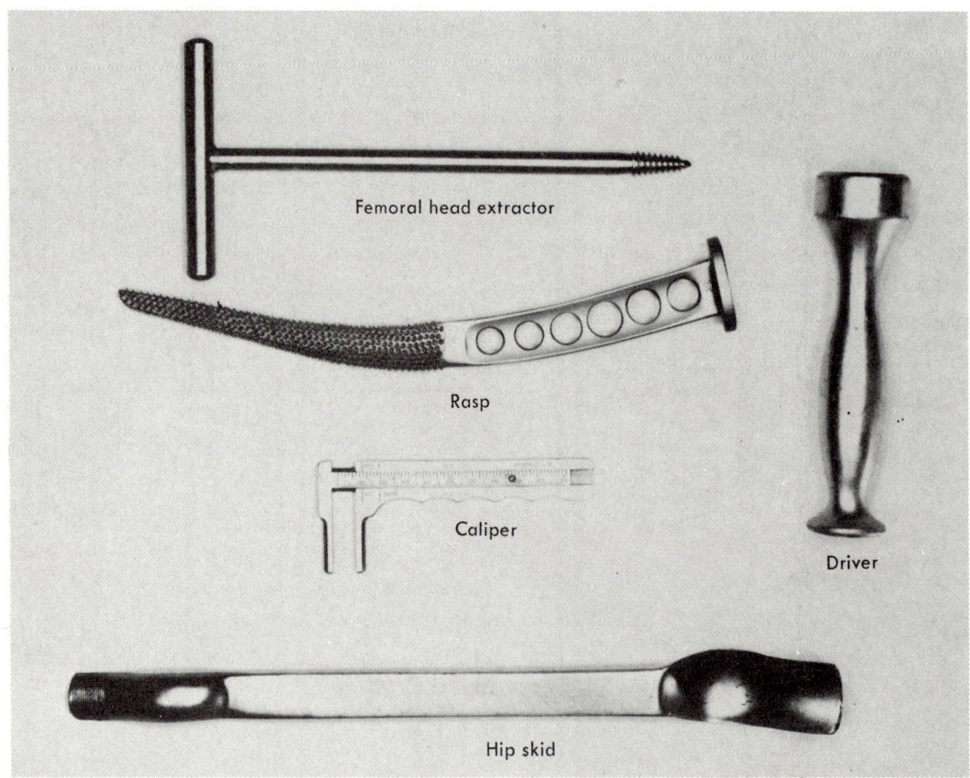

Fig. 20-65. Femoral head prosthetic replacement accessories.

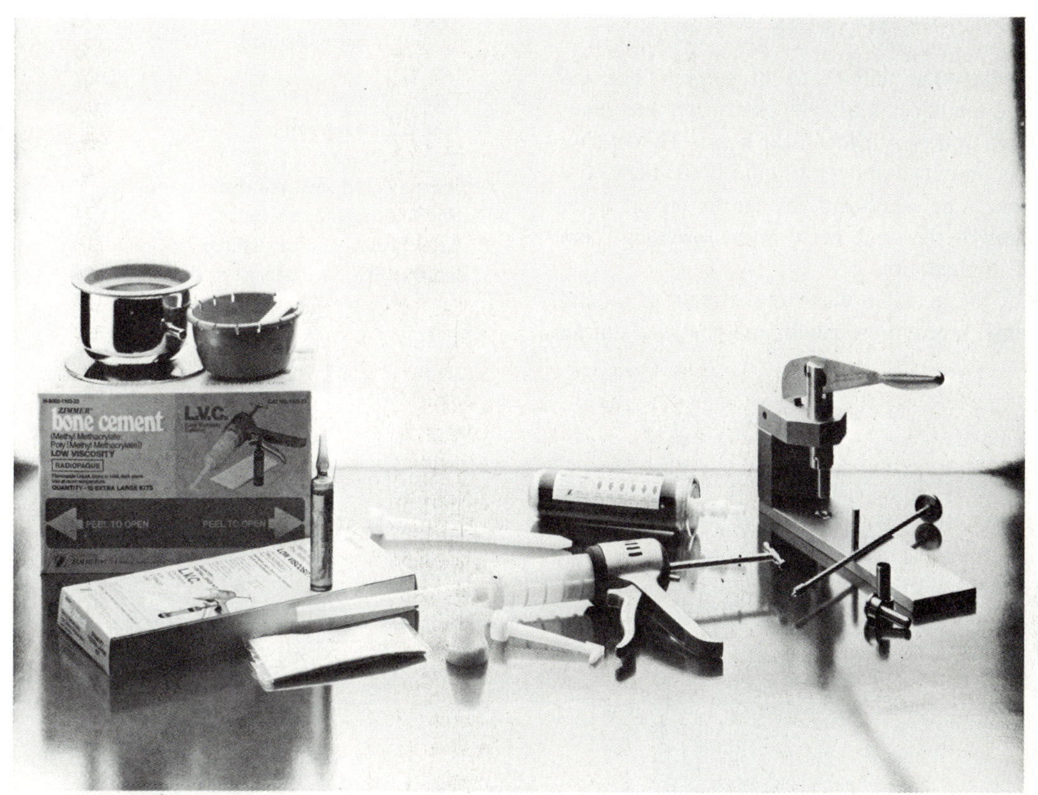

Fig. 20-66. Methyl methacrylate and instrumentation. (Courtesy Zimmer, Inc., Warsaw, Inc.)

Hip reconstruction

Considerations. Hip reconstruction is most commonly indicated in patients with hip pain from rheumatoid arthritis or osteoarthritis.

In the past, reconstructive surgery of the hip consisted of subtrochanteric osteotomy, cup arthroplasty, and prosthetic femoral head replacement. With the development of the total hip arthroplasty, these procedures are rarely done.

In total hip arthroplasty, an acetabular cup, made of high-density polyethylene, and a metal femoral head prosthesis, machined specifically to fit the cup, are held in place with methyl methacrylate. There are numerous total hip implants, such as the Charnley, Charnley-Mueller, Bechtol, and Aufranc-Turner (Figs. 20-67 and 20-68).

Methyl methacrylate adheres to the polyethylene and metal but not to the bone. It fills the cavity and interstices of the bone and forms a mechanical bond. The methyl methacrylate is manufactured as a liquid monomer and a powder polymer. The liquid and powder are mixed under sterile conditions by the scrub nurse in the operating room at the time of implantation.

Because of the possible disastrous effects of wound infection, special precautions usually are observed during total joint replacement, including clean air rooms or exhaust systems, impervious gowns and drapes, antibiotic irrigation solution, and limited movement of personnel in and out of the operating room.

Position and incision. The position and incision are similar to those used for femoral head prosthetic replacement.

Setup. Regular soft-tissue and bone sets are needed, plus the following (Figs. 20-69 to 20-72):

Power acetabular reamers
Hip retractors, assorted
Hip gouges
Rake retractors, large
Methyl methacrylate insertion and mixing devices
Hip skid
Curettes, large, cupped
Driver
Femoral rasp
Hohmann retractors
Cup positioner
Air-powered saw and drill
Femoral head extractor
Trial prostheses (acetabular and femoral)
Trinkle drill, with large drill points

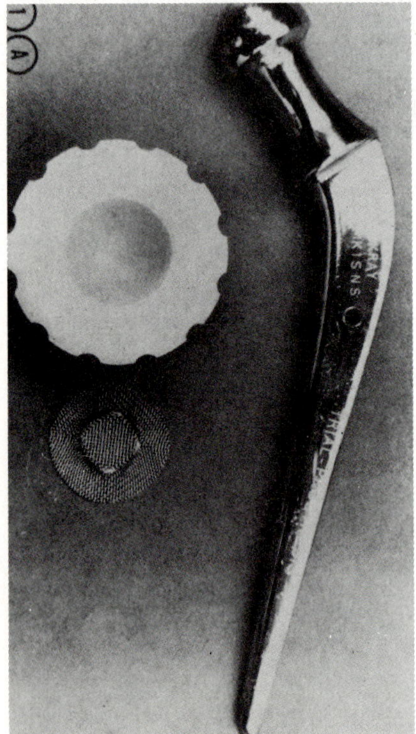

Fig. 20-67. Charnley hip prosthesis and acetabular cup.

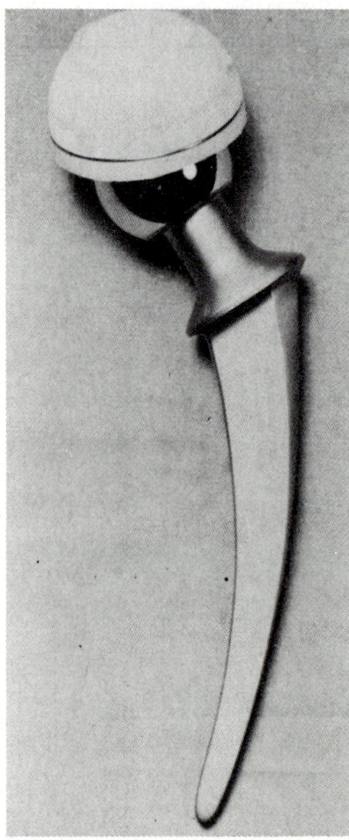

Fig. 20-68. Charnley-Mueller hip prosthesis and acetabular cup.

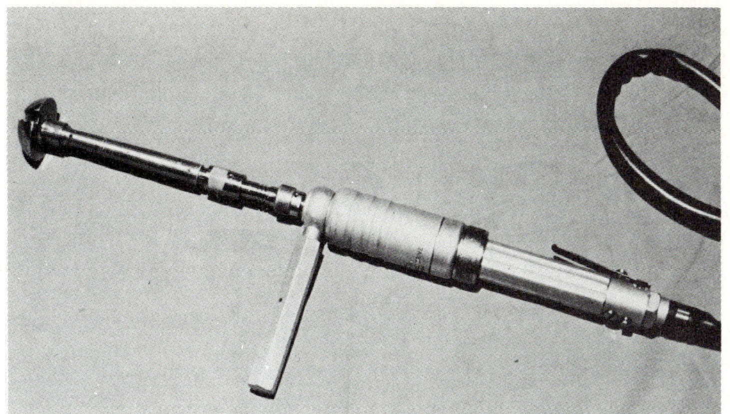

Fig. 20-69. Air-powered acetabular reamer.

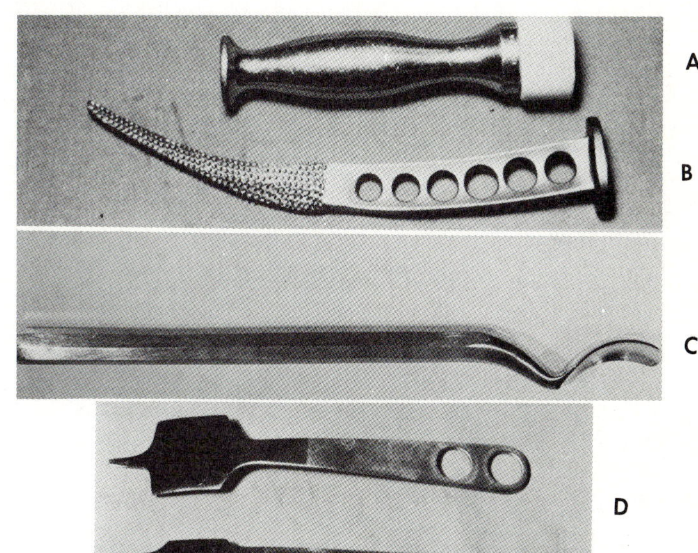

Fig. 20-70. Hip replacement instrumentation. **A,** Teflon-covered driver. **B,** Rasp. **C,** Hip gouge. **D,** Hohmann retractors.

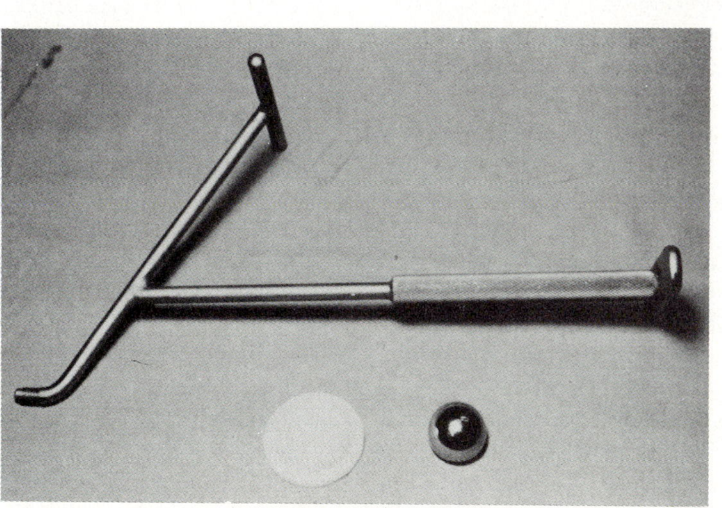

Fig. 20-71. Cup positioner.

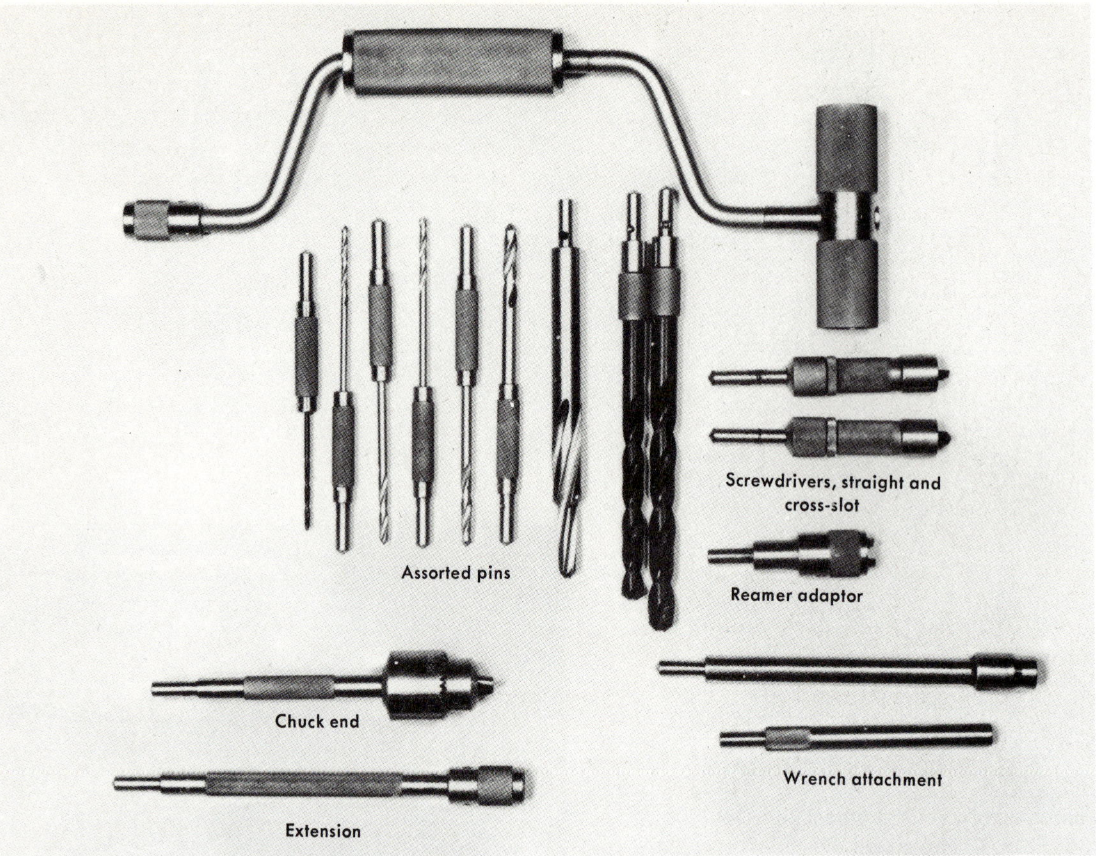

Fig. 20-72. Trinkle drill and large drill bits.

Congenital dislocation of the hip

Considerations. There is much controversy in orthopedic surgery concerning the proper treatment of congenital dislocation of the hip.

Operative procedure. Following are standard operative procedures.

Open reduction. The hip joint is opened, and the soft tissue in the acetabulum is excised. The femoral head can then be reduced into the acetabulum and held by suturing the capsule.

Derotational osteotomy. A derotational osteotomy is performed when there is improper seating of the head in the acetabulum. The femur is placed in internal rotation and is divided. The distal fragment is rotated externally to place the knee and foot straight ahead. In a young child, the osteotomy is frequently performed in the supracondylar region, and the patient is immobilized in a plaster hip spica cast. In an older child, the osteotomy is frequently done in the subtrochanteric region, and the osteotomized fragments are held with an osteotomy blade plate or an intermediate compression screw. Immobilization may not be necessary.

Innominate osteotomy. A complete division of the wing of the ilium is made by an osteotomy from the sciatic notch to the anterior margin of the ilium, superior to the acetabulum. The ilium is then wedged down to increase the depth of the acetabulum by opening the osteotomy site and inserting a bone graft.

Position and incision. The patient is usually in the lateral position for these procedures. An anterior incision is usually made for open reduction, whereas a lateral incision is made for the subtrochanteric osteotomy. The surgeon's preference dictates the incision for an innominate osteotomy.

Setup. Instrumentation varies greatly with the age of the patient, the procedure being done, and the surgeon's preference.

Femoral shaft fractures

Considerations. In children and young adults, femoral shaft fracture is frequently treated with skeletal traction until sufficient callus formation is present at 4 to 6 weeks. At this time the extremity is immobilized in a spica cast or femoral cast brace. It is desirable to avoid prolonged immobilization in older adults because of potential complications, such as decubitus ulcers, pulmonary emboli, atelectasis, and pneumonia. Consequently, open reduction and internal fixation with either an intramedullary nail or compression plate are advocated in older adults.

Position and incision. The patient is placed in the lateral position, and the extremity is prepped and draped from above the iliac crest to the middle of the calf. The fracture is exposed through a lateral incision; a second incision superior to the greater trochanter is necessary if an intramedullary nail is used (Figs. 20-73 and 20-74).

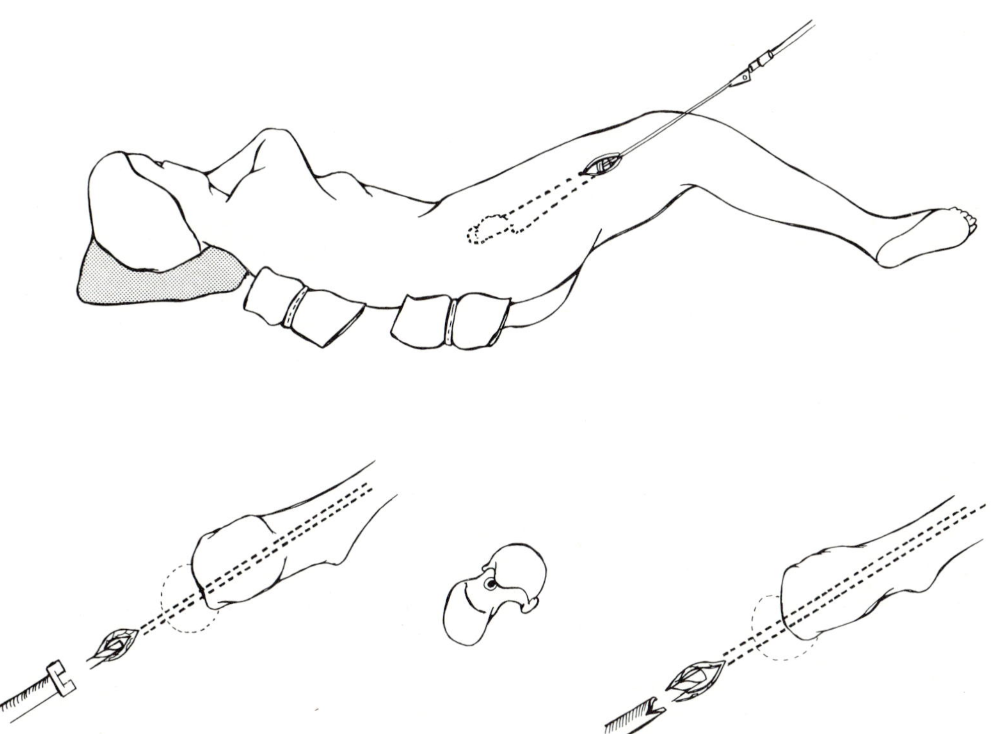

Fig. 20-73. Details of insertion of intramedullary nail. Guide pins emerge through small incision in upper outer quadrant and buttock. Trochanteric reamer placed over guide pin and holes drilled in correct alignment with medullary canal. Küntscher nail inserted into proximal femoral fragment over guide pin. When nail has been driven down to level of fracture site, guide pin is removed and fracture reduced. Nail is then driven correct distance in distal fragment. (From Smith, H.: Radiology **61**:194.)

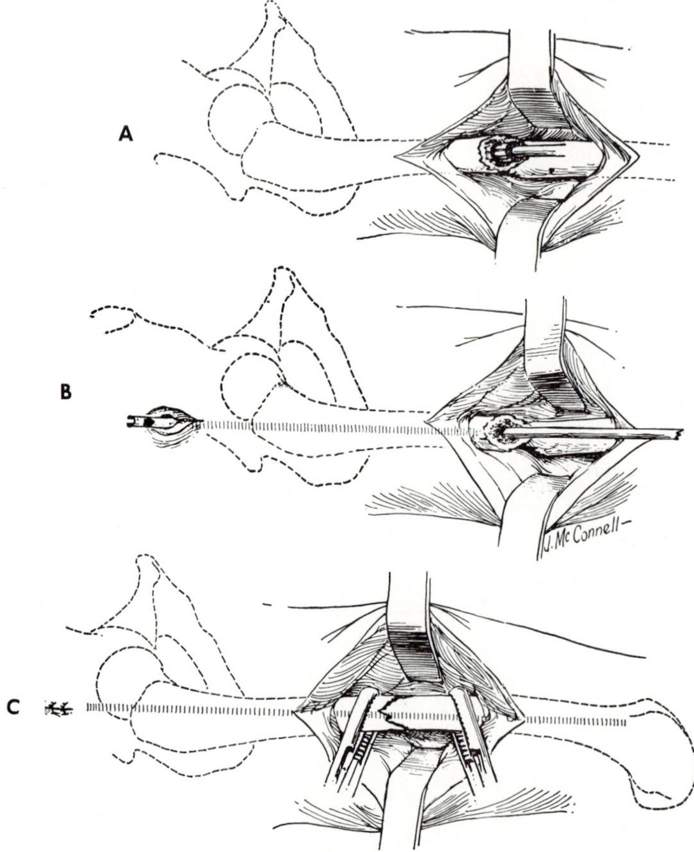

Fig. 20-74. Introduction of intramedullary rod into femur by retrograde method. Fracture is exposed through lateral incision. **A,** Stainless steel rod of correct size and length is driven upward through medullary canal of proximal fragment so that rod pierces cortex of neck just medial to greater trochanter. **B,** Skin incision is made over end of rod where it presents on gluteal region so that is can emerge far enough for other end of rod to be introduced into distal fragment. **C,** After fracture is reduced, rod is drawn into distal fragment at level corresponding to patella. Reamer is used to enlarge canal if it is too small to accept rod or if it is obstructed by bone. (From Compere, E.L., Banks, S.W., and Compere, C.L.: Pictorial handbook of fracture treatment, ed. 5, Chicago, Year Book Medical Publishers, Inc.)

Intramedullary nailing

Considerations. Several intramedullary nails are available, including the Küntscher and Lottes (Fig. 20-75). After the fracture has been exposed and the femoral canal reamed to appropriate size, either the nail or a guide wire is driven retrogradely up the proximal fragment to emerge out the greater trochanter through the second incision. The fracture is reduced, and the nail is driven across the fracture into the distal fragment.

Setup. Regular bone and soft-tissue sets are required, plus the following:

Hip retractors, assorted
Rake retractors
Richardson retractors
Bone-holding forceps, large
Intramedullary reamers
Drivers
Extractors
Set of nails of choice (Lottes or Küntscher)

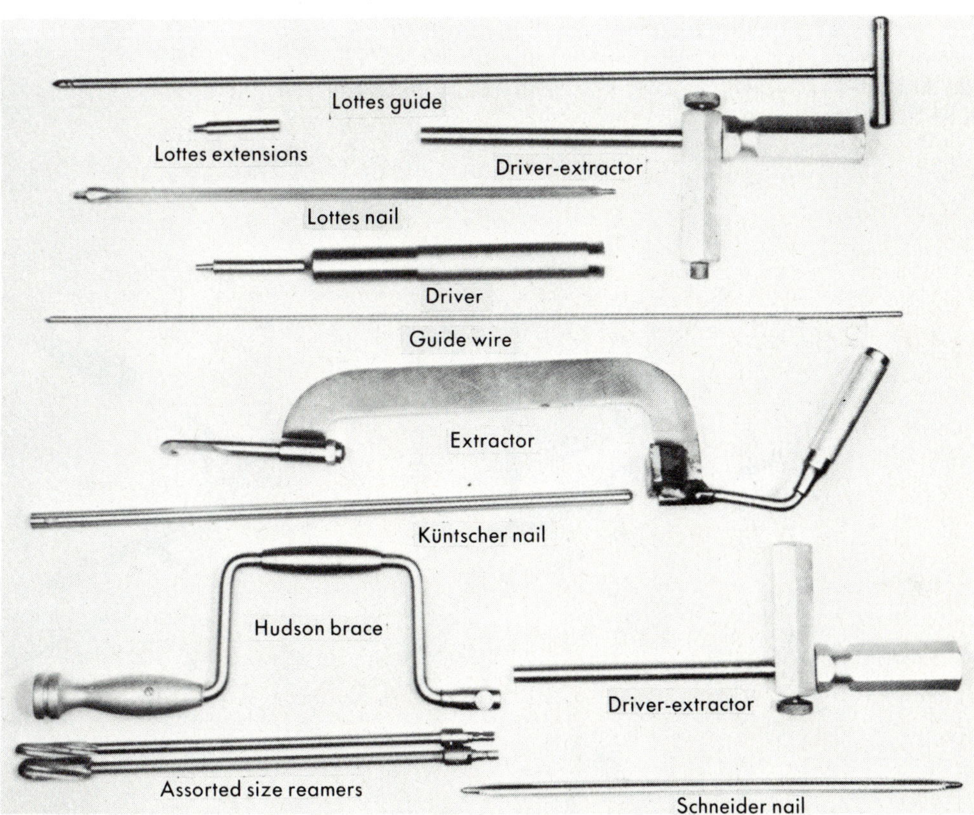

Fig. 20-75. Intramedullary nails for fixation of femoral shaft fractures.

Compression plating

Considerations. Occasionally surgeons prefer to fix a fracture internally with compression plates.

Position and incision. The fracture is exposed and reduced through a lateral incision. A large compression plate with a minimum of three holes above and three holes below the fracture is necessary. A single compression plate is applied on the lateral surface of the femur; if two plates are used, they are at 90-degree angles to each other, laterally and superiorly (Fig. 20-76).

Setup. Regular bone and soft-tissue sets are required, plus the following:

Hip retractors, assorted
Rake retractors, large
Richardson retractors, large
Bone-holding forceps, large
Compression set (Fig. 20-77)
Air-powered drill

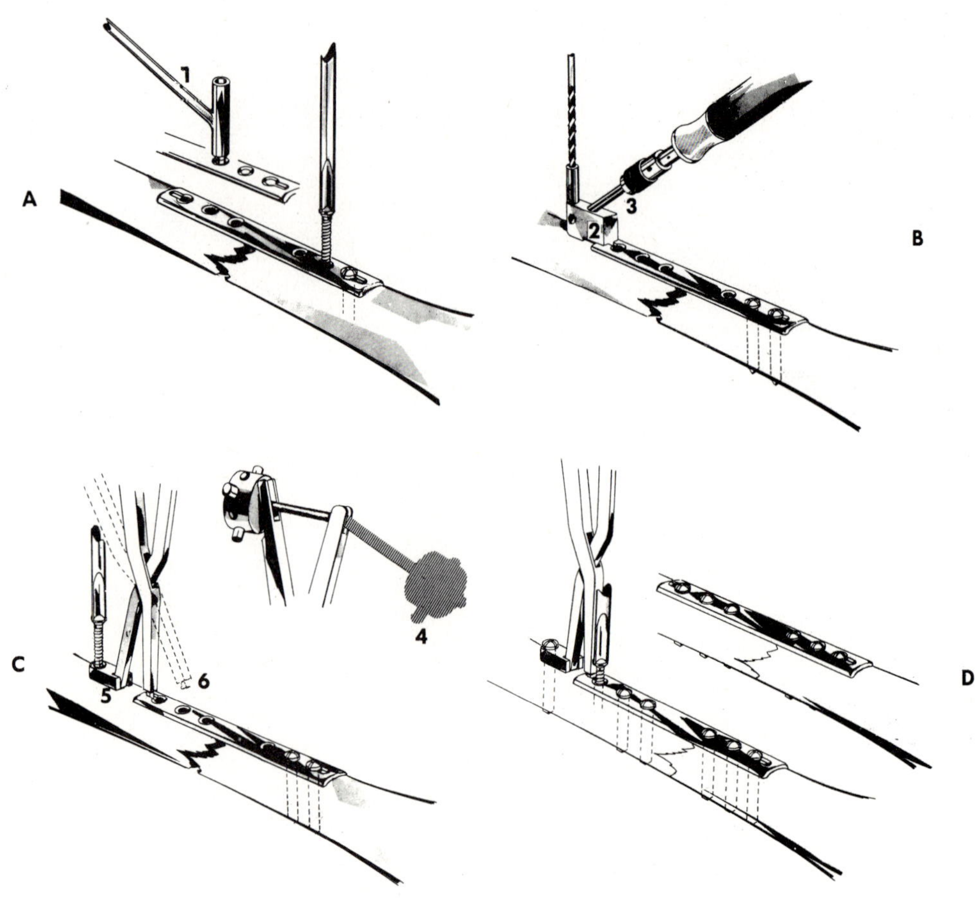

Fig. 20-76. Compression plating of fractures. (Courtesy Zimmer, Inc., Warsaw, Inc.)

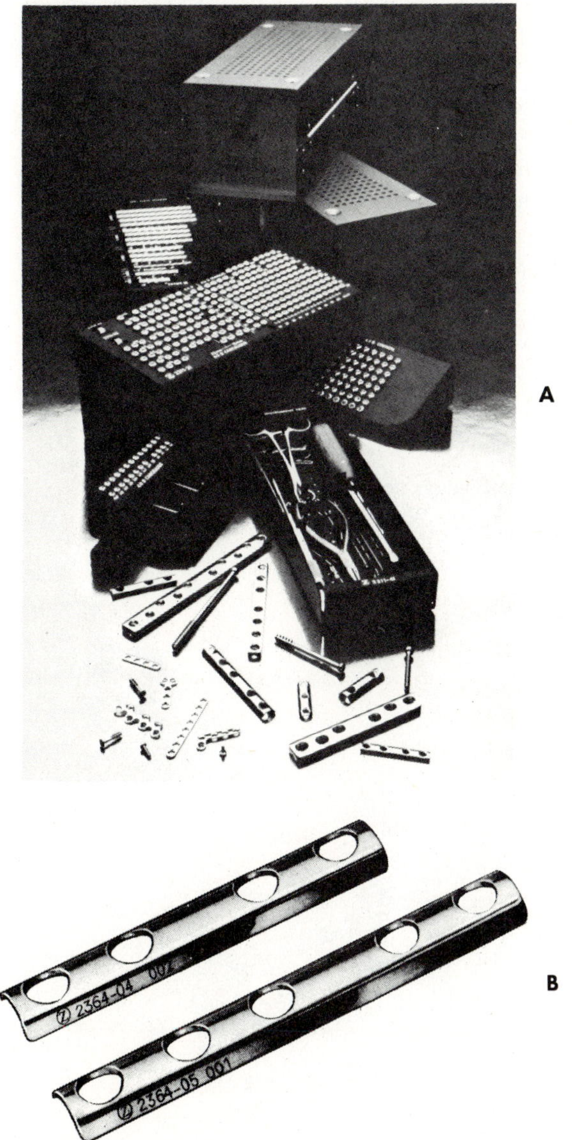

Fig. 20-77. A, Standard plate and screw set, European compression technique. **B,** Semitubular compression plates. (Courtesy Zimmer, Inc., Warsaw, Ind.)

External fixation

Considerations. Because of the increased chance of infection in patients with an open fracture, external fixation is often the preferred treatment. External fixation offers stabilization of the fracture along with direct visualization of the wound. In fractures with a substantial amount of soft-tissue damage, rigid immobilization is mandatory. Advantages of external fixation include the ability to care for the wound, the absence of plaster, and the performance of range-of-motion exercises on proximal and distal joints. Subsequent surgical procedures such as skin grafts may be performed as needed.

Principles

1. The fixation pins are inserted by hand. This keeps bone necrosis to a minimum, thereby eliminating loose pins.
2. The pin guide is used to ensure parallel placement.
3. Compression is applied whenever possible to aid in union.

Setup. Regular bone and soft-tissue sets are required, plus the following:

Curettes
Irrigation basin and syringe
Bone-holding forceps
Hand drill, drill points, and key
Large pin cutters
Fixation device of choice with instrumentation, for example, the Anderson, Hoffman (Fig. 20-78), Wagner, and Vidal-Adrey

OPERATIONS ON THE KNEE AND TIBIA

Position and incision. Most operations on the knee are performed in the supine position with the knee prepped and draped from the groin to the middle of the calf or including the entire foot. It is occasionally necessary for the surgeon to operate with the foot of the operating table dropped and the knee flexed to 90 degrees. Consequently, it is important to position the patient so that the knee is at a "break" in the table; then the lower leg can be flexed at the knee during the operation, if necessary. One of many possible incisions is used for surgery of the knee joint (Fig. 20-79).

Setup. A basic set of specifically designed instruments must be available for all operations involving the knee joint (Fig. 20-80).

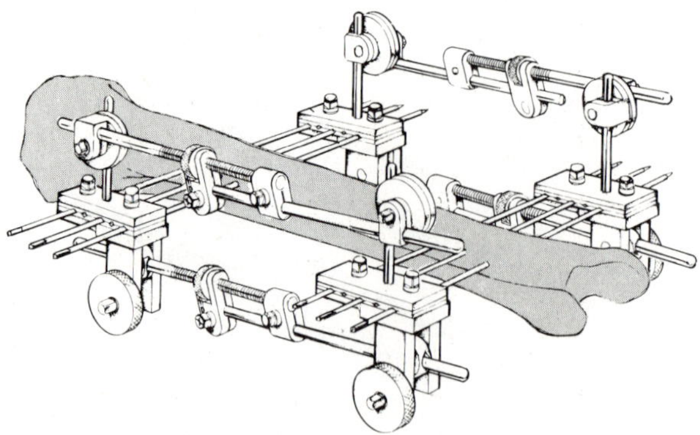

Fig. 20-78. Hoffman external fixation device. (Courtesy Zimmer, Inc., Warsaw, Inc.)

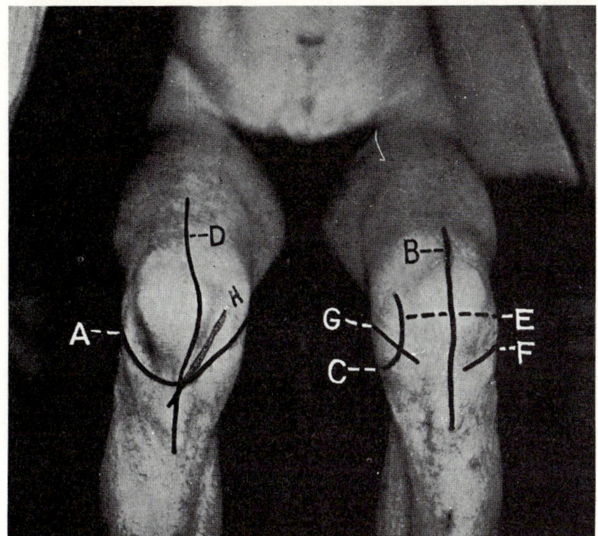

Fig. 20-79. Various incisions for operations on knee joint. (From Conwell, H.E., and Reynolds, F.C.: Key and Conwell's management of fractures, dislocations, and sprains, ed. 7, St. Louis, The C.V. Mosby Co.)

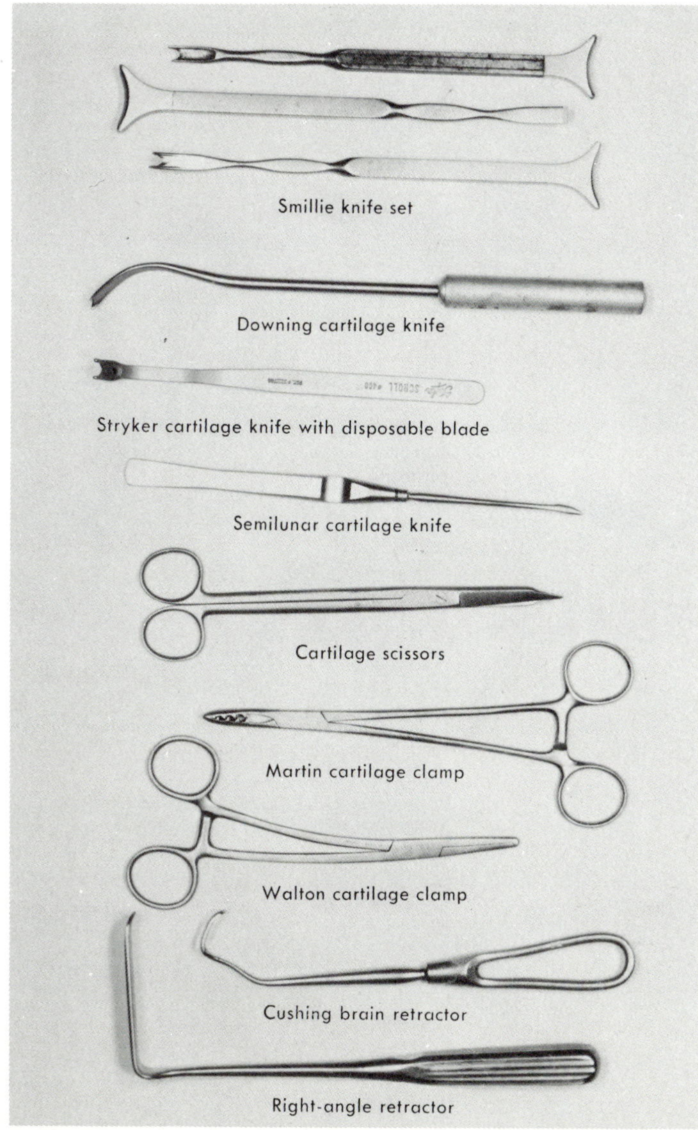

Fig. 20-80. Specifically designed instruments necessary for all knee operations.

Femoral condyle and tibial plateau fractures

Considerations. It is important to anatomically align the articular surfaces of the distal femur and proximal tibia to provide joint stability and to decrease the chance of subsequent posttraumatic arthritis. In a markedly comminuted fracture, alignment can best be obtained with a distal tibial traction pin and early range of motion. However, the surgeon may attempt to restore the articular surfaces by reducing the larger bone fragments and holding them with various metal implants: 95-degree osteotomy blade plates are often used with compression techniques. Central depression fracture of the tibial plateau frequently requires elevation of the articular surface through a ''window'' in the anterior tibia, which is then packed with bone graft to give additional support (Fig. 20-81).

Setup. Regular soft-tissue and bone sets are used, plus the following:

Knee retractors
Drills and drill points
Compression screw set
Threaded wires
Curettes
Osteotomes
Condyle plates (assorted) and threaded wires and pins with or without washers

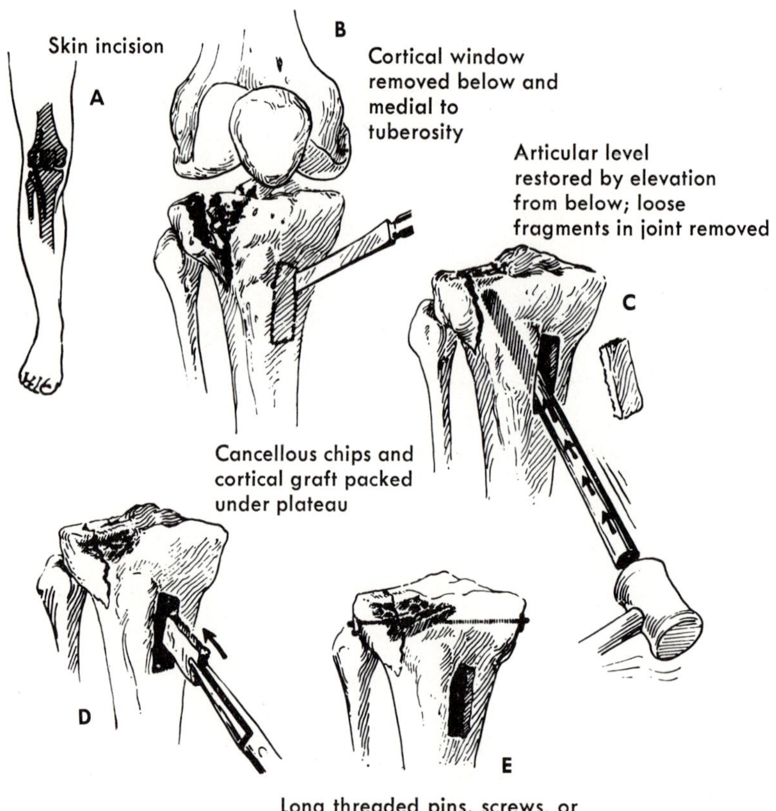

Fig. 20-81. Surgical restoration of lateral articular surface of knee. (From Compere, E.L., Banks, S.W., and Compere, C.L.: Pictorial handbook of fracture treatment, ed. 5, Chicago, Year Book Medical Publishers, Inc.)

Patellectomy and reduction of fractured patella

Considerations. It is possible to excise a portion of the patella (for comminuted fracture) or the entire patella (for painful degenerative arthritis) without significantly affecting the function of the knee joint. Removal of the entire patella may result in relative lengthening of the knee extensor mechanism, so it becomes necessary to imbricate the quadriceps tendon to prevent a lag in knee extension at the time of operation. If the fracture consists of two large fragments that can be anatomically reduced, fixation is accomplished with a circumferential wire (Fig. 20-82). Postoperatively, the knee is immobilized in a cylinder cast or knee immobilizer, allowing full weight-bearing.

In case of mild chondromalacia of the patella, the softened and frayed articular cartilage can be shaved or excised, and range-of-motion exercises are begun early in the postoperative period.

Setup. Regular bone and soft-tissue sets, knee instruments, a drill and drill points, and heavy wire are required.

Patella reconstruction

Considerations. Teenagers with a shallow femoral condylar groove and a patella proximal to the normal anatomical position may have recurrent lateral dislocation of the patella. If the condition persists, chondromalacia may occur. Numerous operations have been designed to realign the knee extensor mechanism. All of the operations include incising the lateral quadriceps tendon and shifting the insertion of the patellar tendon medially.

Setup. Regular bone and soft-tissue sets, knee instruments, a drill and drill points, and a screw rack are required.

Collateral or cruciate ligament tears

Considerations. The stability of the knee depends on the integrity of the cruciate and collateral ligaments. If any of these supporting structures is damaged, an unstable knee is likely unless properly repaired. Injuries to these supporting structures do not usually occur as isolated injuries. More frequently, several of these ligaments are injured at the same time. As an example, common injuries referred to as the "terrible triad" include a torn anterior cruciate ligament, torn medial meniscus, and torn medial collateral ligament.

Examination under anesthesia is required for complete evaluation of a ligamentous injury. The knee demonstrates grave disability with major ligamentous disruption. The collateral ligaments reinforce the knee capsule medially and laterally. They resist varus and valgus stresses on the knee. The cruciates control anteroposterior stability. Along with the ligaments, the muscle groups serve to stabilize the joint and control movement. Because muscle strength is the first line of defense for the knee, damage is repaired to protect the ligaments. For optimum function of the joint, damaged structures should be reconstructed as closely as possible to the original anatomy. If left untreated, osteoarthritis will develop. Procedures may vary from a capsular tightening to a partial intraarticular transfer of a ligament. Nonabsorbable sutures, wires, and staples are frequently used.

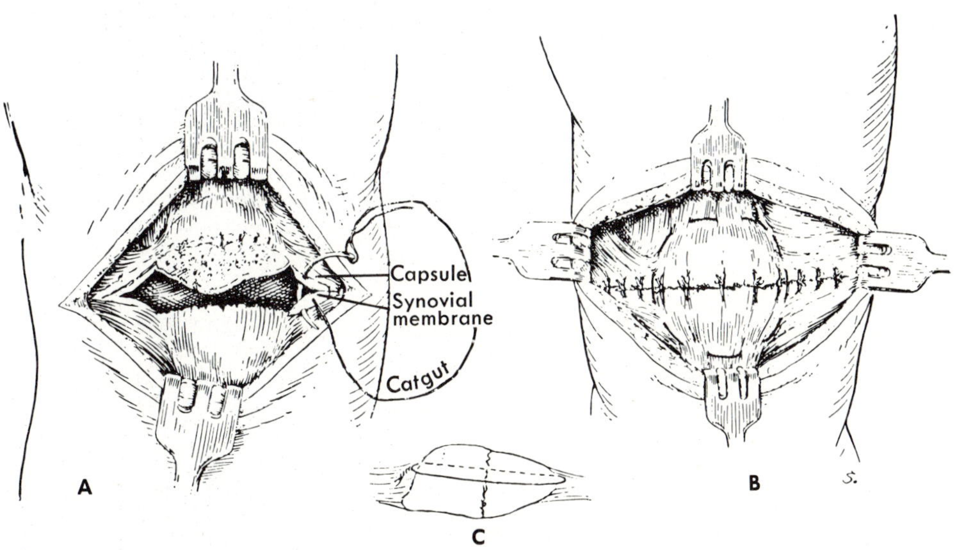

Fig. 20-82. Open reduction of fracture of patella. Fixation of fragments by circumferential wire loop. Lateral tears in capsule and synovial membrane repaired with catgut. (From Edmonson, A.S. and Crenshaw, A.H., editors: Campbell's operative orthopaedics, ed. 6, St. Louis, 1980, The C.V. Mosby Co.)

Position and incision. The patient is placed in the supine position. The extremity is prepped and draped for a routine knee procedure. Incisions vary depending on the area to be reconstructed (Fig. 20-79). One of the following will be used:

- Medial parapatellar
- Lateral parapatellar
- Posteromedial
- Posterolateral
- S-shaped
- Anteromedial
- Anterolateral

Setup. Regular bone and soft-tissue sets, knee instruments, drill and drill points, wire passer, and hook are required. The following supplies may be requested by the surgeon:

- Kirschner wires
- Polyethylene buttons
- Nonabsorbable suture
- Staples
- Driver
- Extractor

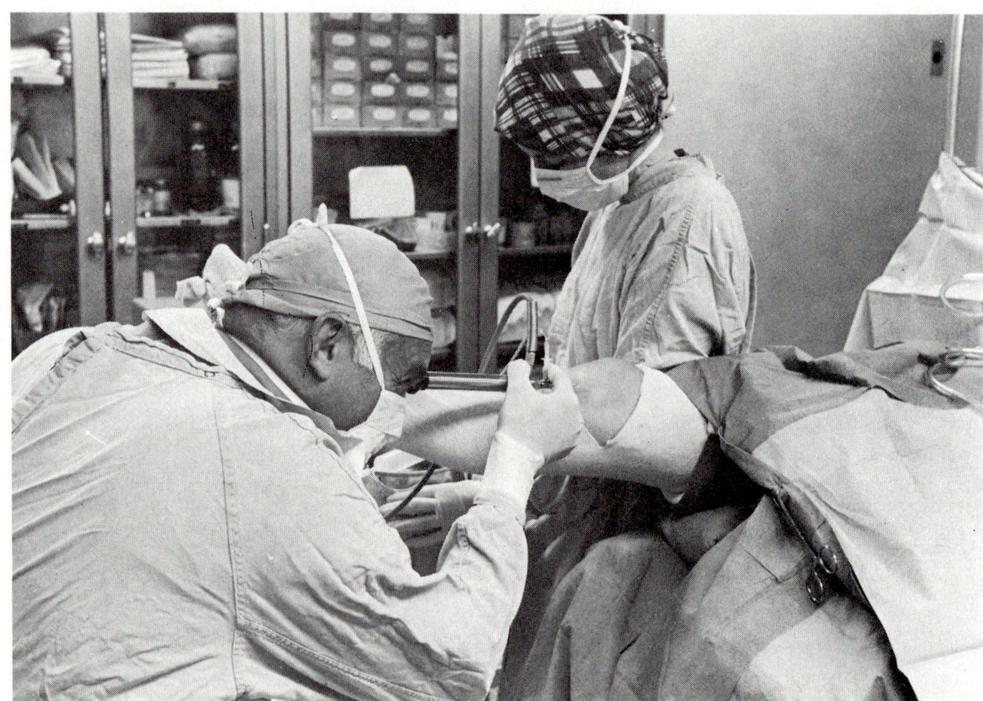

Fig. 20-83. Arthroscopy of knee. After entry has been confirmed and saline has distended joint, suprapatellar pouch and patellar area may be visualized. (From Johnson L.L.: Diagnostic and surgical arthroscopy: the knee and other joints, ed. 2, St. Louis, 1981, The C.V. Mosby Co.)

Arthroscopy (Figs. 20-83 to 20-88)

Considerations. Learning the art of arthroscopy is an enormous task; it requires superb technical skills. Through a small-diameter endoscope inserted into the knee joint, visualization of the intraarticular structures and cleansing of the joint is possible. Two categories of patients are candidates for arthroscopy: patients whose diagnosis cannot be determined by history, physical examination or arthrogram—the findings were insufficient to warrant surgical exploration—and patients who show an intraarticular abnormality or ligamentous injury. Arthroscopy may be performed before an anticipated arthrotomy. Frequently, surgical treatment is modified following the findings of the arthroscopic examination.

Setup. If subsequent arthrotomy is to be performed, two sterile setups are required. A second draping and prepping are necessary after arthroscopy. Following is the equipment needed for an arthroscopy:

Scalpel
Hemostats
Suture scissors
Towel clamp
Needle holder
Syringes
Large-bore needle
Basin for normal saline
2 Pieces rubber tubing
Metal stopcock
Normal saline (IV drip, 2000 ml)
Irrigation tubing
Arthroscope according to surgeon's preference (small-diameter scopes usually preferred)
Light source, with high-intensity setting
Light cables, with thermal-resistant covering
Cannulas for scope, irrigation, and suction

Care and handling of arthroscopic equipment. Ethylene oxide sterilization is recommended because steam sterilization is known to cause deterioration of arthroscopes. Proper ethylene oxide sterilization usually takes 3 to 7 hours, plus aeration time. Most equipment used with the scopes is steam sterilizable.

Although sterilization is optimum and should be encouraged, liquid disinfection according to the manufacturer's instructions is often performed. ''Cold sterilization'' (disinfection) with an activated glutaraldehyde solution has become the standard of practice among some established arthroscopists.

The fiberoptic cords used in the surgery should never be kinked or twisted. Gradual deterioration occurs in the cables: fibers in the cable break, and light cannot be transmitted. When stored, the cords should be loosely coiled or hung.

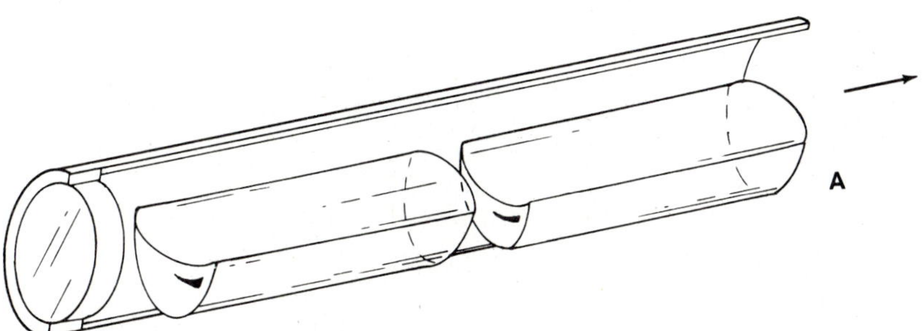

Fig. 20-84. A, Rod-lens system is series of glass cylinders separated by small areas of air, or reverse of thin-lens system. (From Johnson, L.L.: Diagnostic and surgical arthroscopy: the knee and other joints, ed. 2, St. Louis, 1981, The C.V. Mosby Co.) *Continued.*

Fig. 20-84, cont'd. B, Storz telescope, with sheath, obturators, and bridge. **C,** Storz 70-degree inclined view rod-lens telescope, with cannula and sharp and blunt obturators. This telescope is used in viewing posterior compartment. **D,** Dyonics rod-lens system, with insertion instrumentation. **E,** *Left to right,* 4-mm diameter Dyonics rod-lens endoscope; 2.2-mm Needlescope seen in end view; 1.7-mm Needlescope; No. 18 needle, shown for relative size comparison.

B

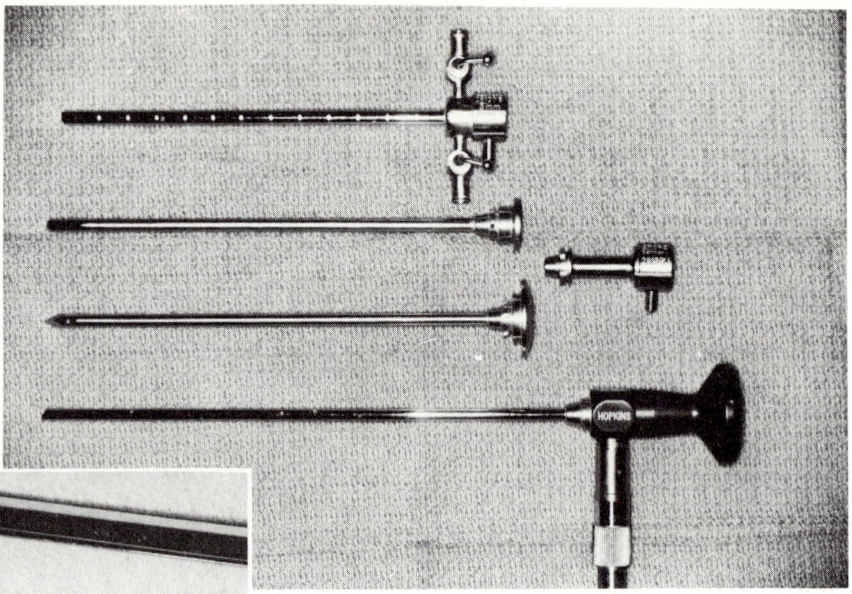

C

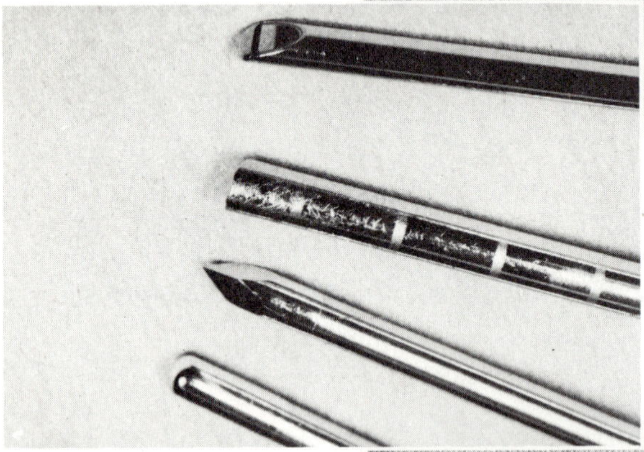

D

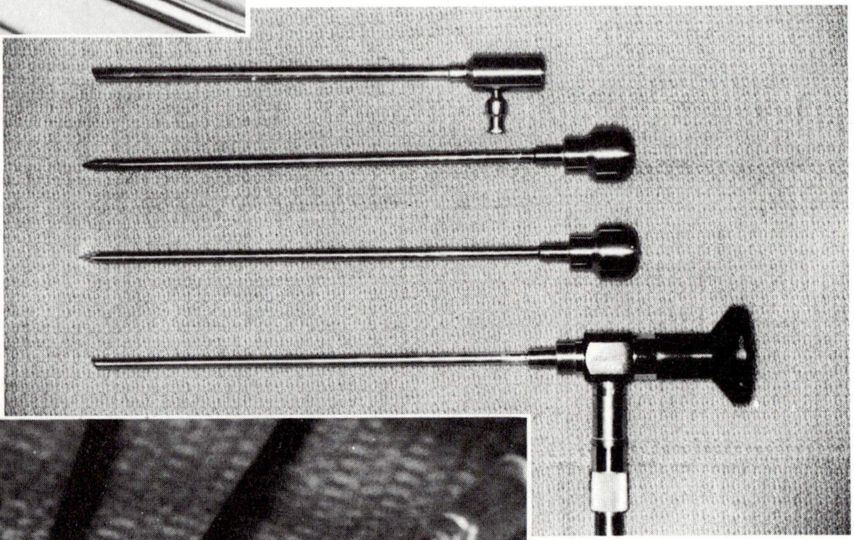

E

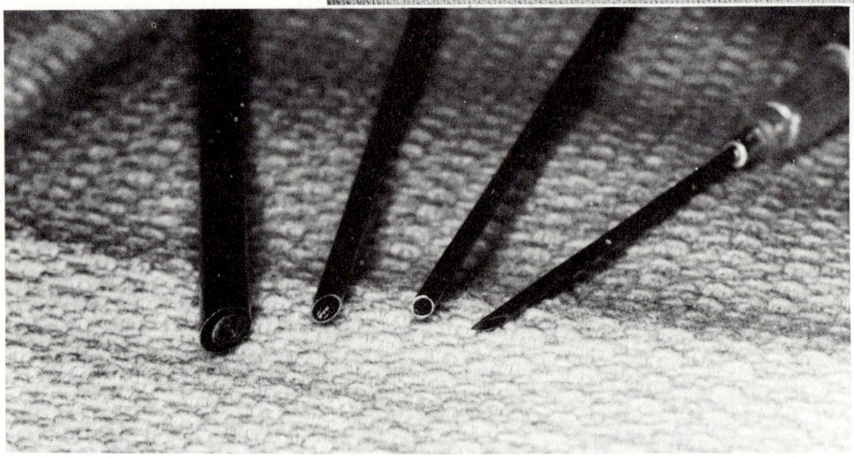

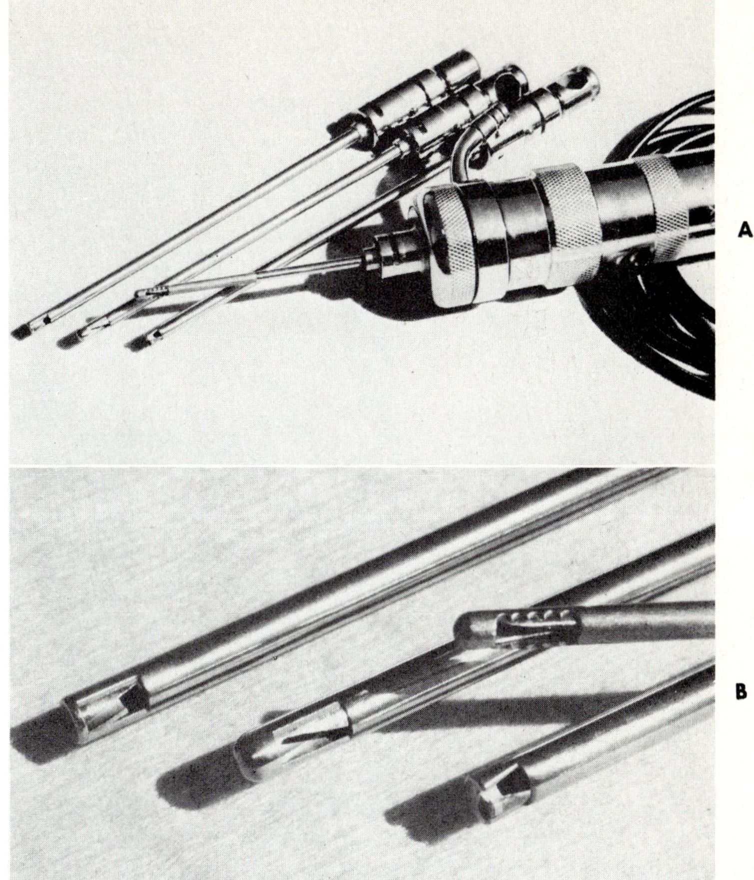

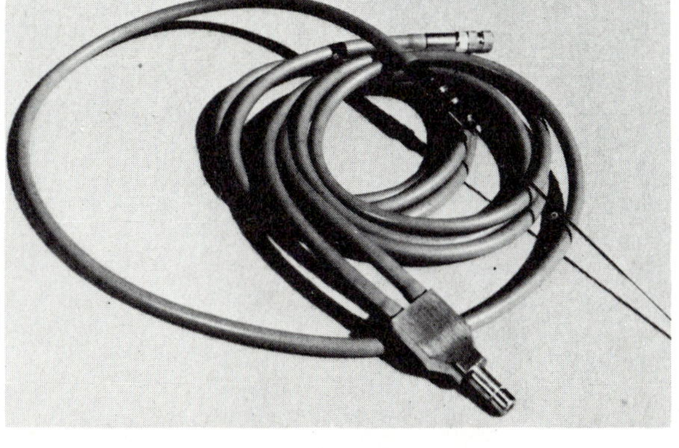

Fig. 20-85. Bifurcated cable. (From Johnson, L.L.: Diagnostic and surgical arthroscopy: the knee and other joints, ed. 2, St. Louis, 1981, The C.V. Mosby Co.)

Fig. 20-86. A, Intra-articular Shaver. **B,** Close-up of cannulas. (From Johnson, L.L.: Diagnostic and surgical arthroscopy: the knee and other joints, ed. 2, St. Louis, 1981, The C.V. Mosby Co.)

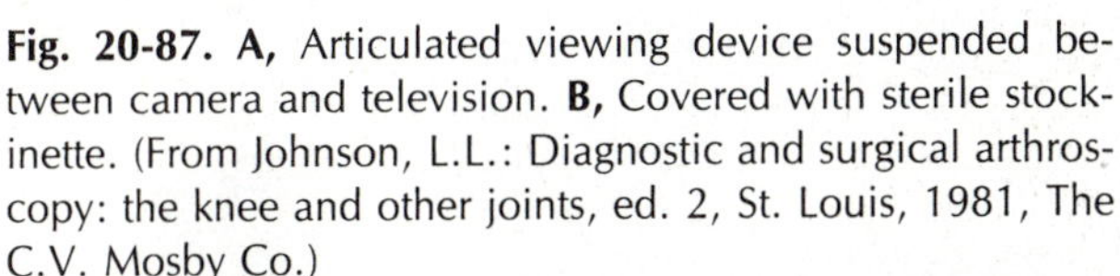

Fig. 20-87. A, Articulated viewing device suspended between camera and television. **B,** Covered with sterile stockinette. (From Johnson, L.L.: Diagnostic and surgical arthroscopy: the knee and other joints, ed. 2, St. Louis, 1981, The C.V. Mosby Co.)

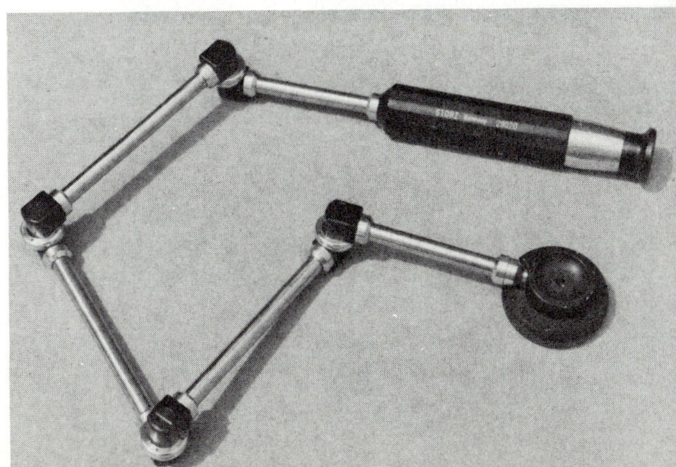

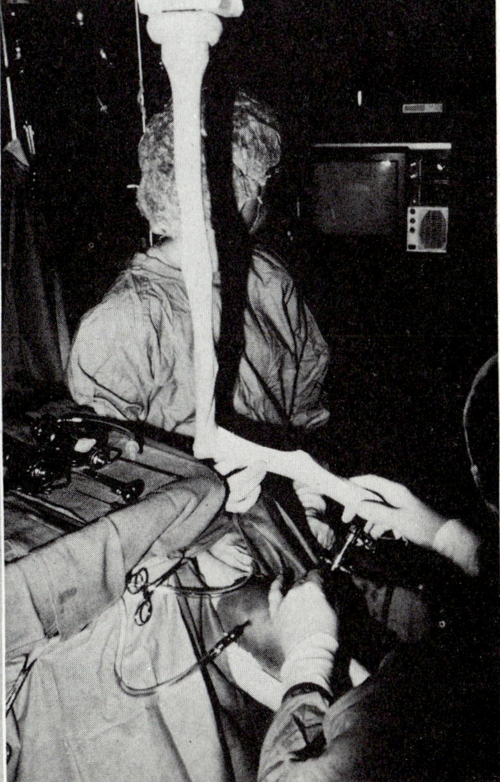

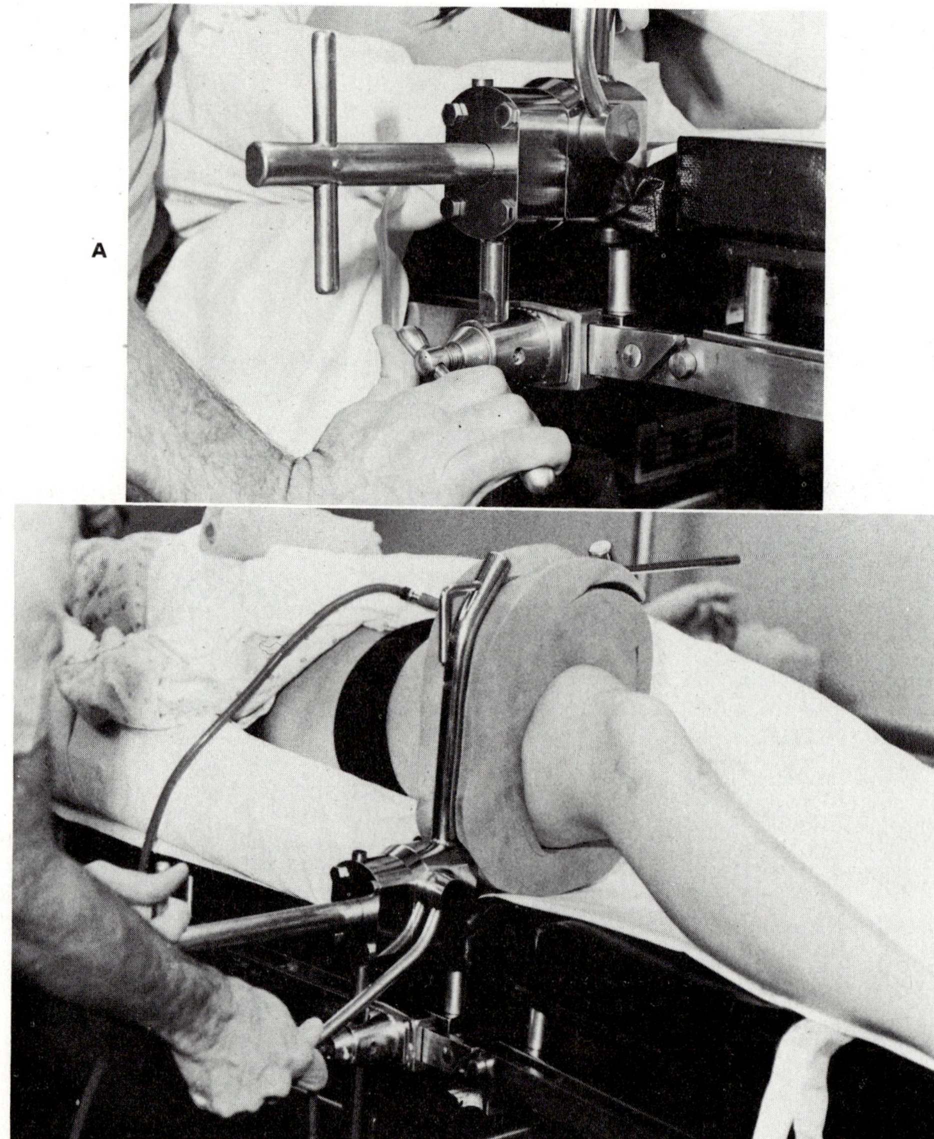

Fig. 20-88. A, Clark stirrup accessory, which attaches Surgical Assistant to standard operating table. **B,** Surgical Assistant is secured to patient manually and with pumping of cam action lever. (From Johnson, L.L.: Diagnostic and surgical arthroscopy: the knee and other joints, ed. 2, St. Louis, The C.V. Mosby Co.)

Arthroscopic surgery

Considerations. The following arthroscopic surgical procedures may be performed:

- Synovial biopsy
- Excision, loose body
- Resection of plicae
- Shaving of patella
- Meniscectomy
- Chondroplasty
- Synovectomy
- Repair of osteochondritis dissecans

Setup. Minor set and arthroscopy equipment is required, plus the following:

- Forceps: pituitary, grasping, and biopsy
- Intraarticular power instrumentation: cutter, shaver, and trimmer
- Articulated telescopic viewing device (teaching arm)
- Television camera

The articulating viewing device is the link between the ocular eyepiece of the arthroscope and the suspended television camera. The viewing device may not undergo sterilization. It is covered with a sterile stockinette or transparent drape. The television camera allows freedom of both hands, which benefits personnel.

Position. For positioning the patient, a standard operating room table with a foot drop is needed. The bed should have a Clark attachment in place. A positioning device called a "surgical assistant" is used. It consists of a steel frame with a foam insert and crossbar. This device serves to hold the thigh securely.

• • •

Procedures may be recorded on videocassette tapes for instruction and research.

Emphasis on preoperative organization and planning is stressed. All procedures are done in a similar manner, and members of the team acquaint themselves with each step. It is beneficial to have the same surgical team whenever possible.

Arthrotomy and meniscectomy

Considerations. A tear in the meniscus is the most common injury of the knee requiring surgery (Fig. 20-89). An injured meniscus will not heal and must be excised. If left untreated, an injured meniscus alters the gait pattern of the knee and may result in degenerative changes of the articular cartilage and permanent damage. Although both menisci can sustain tears, the medial meniscus is injured much more frequently than the lateral meniscus.

Setup. Regular bone and soft-tissue sets, knee instruments, and a nerve hook are required.

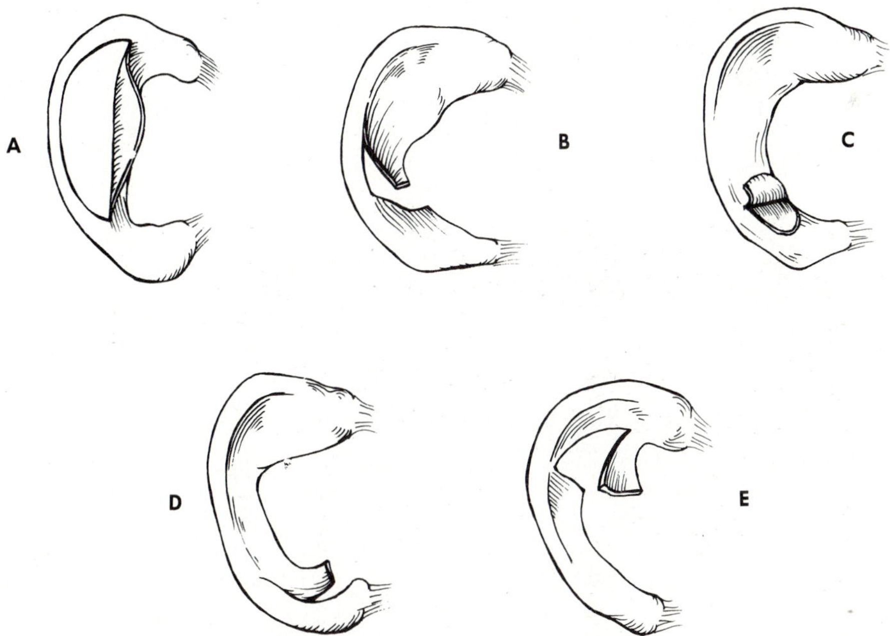

Fig. 20-89. Meniscal cartilage injury. **A,** Longitudinal splitting (bucket-handle type). **B,** Tear of middle third. **C,** Tear of anterior tip. **D,** Longitudinal splitting of anterior third. **E,** Tear of posterior third. (Adapted from Brashear, H.R., and Raney, B.R.: Shand's handbook of orthopaedic surgery, ed. 9, St. Louis, 1978, The C.V. Mosby Co.)

Synovectomy of the knee

Considerations. Proliferative synovitis of the knee as seen in rheumatoid arthritis, pigmented villonodular synovitis, and synovial chondromatosis may produce pain as well as ligamentous and articular cartilage destruction. Early in the disease process, synovectomy can relieve the pain and probably prevent further damage if the cartilage and ligamentous structures have not yet been affected by the disease process. However, late in the disease process, reconstructive surgery such as total knee joint replacement is necessary in addition to synovectomy.

Setup. Regular bone and soft-tissue sets and knee instruments are required.

Popliteal (Baker's) cyst excision

Definition. Removal of a cyst from the popliteal fossa.

Considerations. The cysts are frequently painful and can become very large, especially when associated with rheumatoid arthritis. Whereas cysts in the popliteal fossa occur without a precipitating cause in children, in adults they are frequently indicative of an intraarticular disease process, such as rheumatoid arthritis, or a torn medial meniscus. Consequently, it may be necessary to expose the knee joint and correct the intraarticular condition at the same time a cyst is removed.

Position and incision. In contrast to other operative procedures on the knee, the patient is placed in the prone position with chest rolls under the thorax during surgery. A curvilinear incision is made over the cyst.

Setup. Regular bone and soft-tissue sets are required.

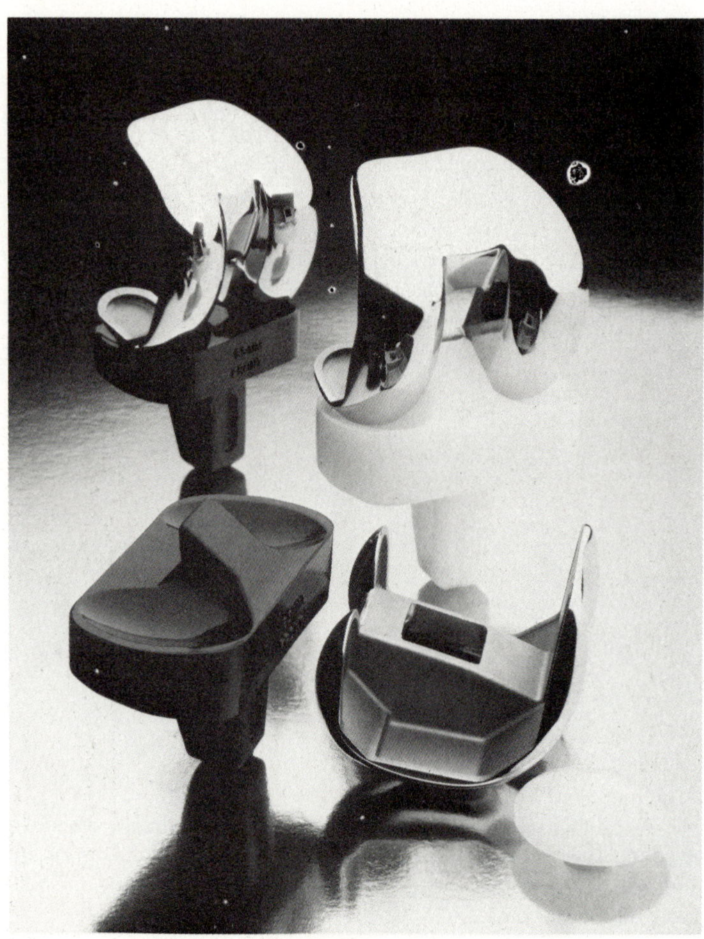

Fig. 20-90. Geometric total knee replacement. (Courtesy Zimmer, Inc., Warsaw, Ind.)

Total knee joint replacement arthroplasty

Considerations. Patients with degenerative arthritis or rheumatoid arthritis of the knee complain of pain and instability. Total knee joint replacement arthroplasty has been successful in relieving pain and providing a stable knee.

Many models are available, but basically only two types of knee joint replacement designs exist. The non-hinge type is similar to the total hip replacement in that a stainless steel distal femoral component articulates with a high-density polyethylene tibial component. The femoral and tibial components are fixed to the bone with methyl methacrylate. The polycentric, geometric, total condylar, and modular are among the many models of this type available (Fig. 20-90). The second design is the hinge type of total knee prosthesis. A metallic implant in the distal femoral shaft is fixed to another metallic implant in the proximal tibial shaft by a bolt, thereby forming a hinge. The components are again held in the bone with methyl methacrylate. This hinge type of prosthesis is used when there is marked instability of the knee with destroyed supporting ligaments. The Walldius and offset hinges are among the available models (Fig. 20-91).

Setup. Regular bone and soft-tissue sets are required, plus the following:

Knee instruments
Power drill and drill points
Power saw
Rakes, retractors, large
Nerve hooks
Duval elevators
Pituitary rongeurs
Ruler
Instruments for inserting implant of choice
Curettes, large, cupped
Methyl methacrylate insertion and mixing devices
Trial prostheses

Often during total knee arthroplasty, patellectomy and placement of a "patellar button" is performed. Surgical preference and technique determine the need.

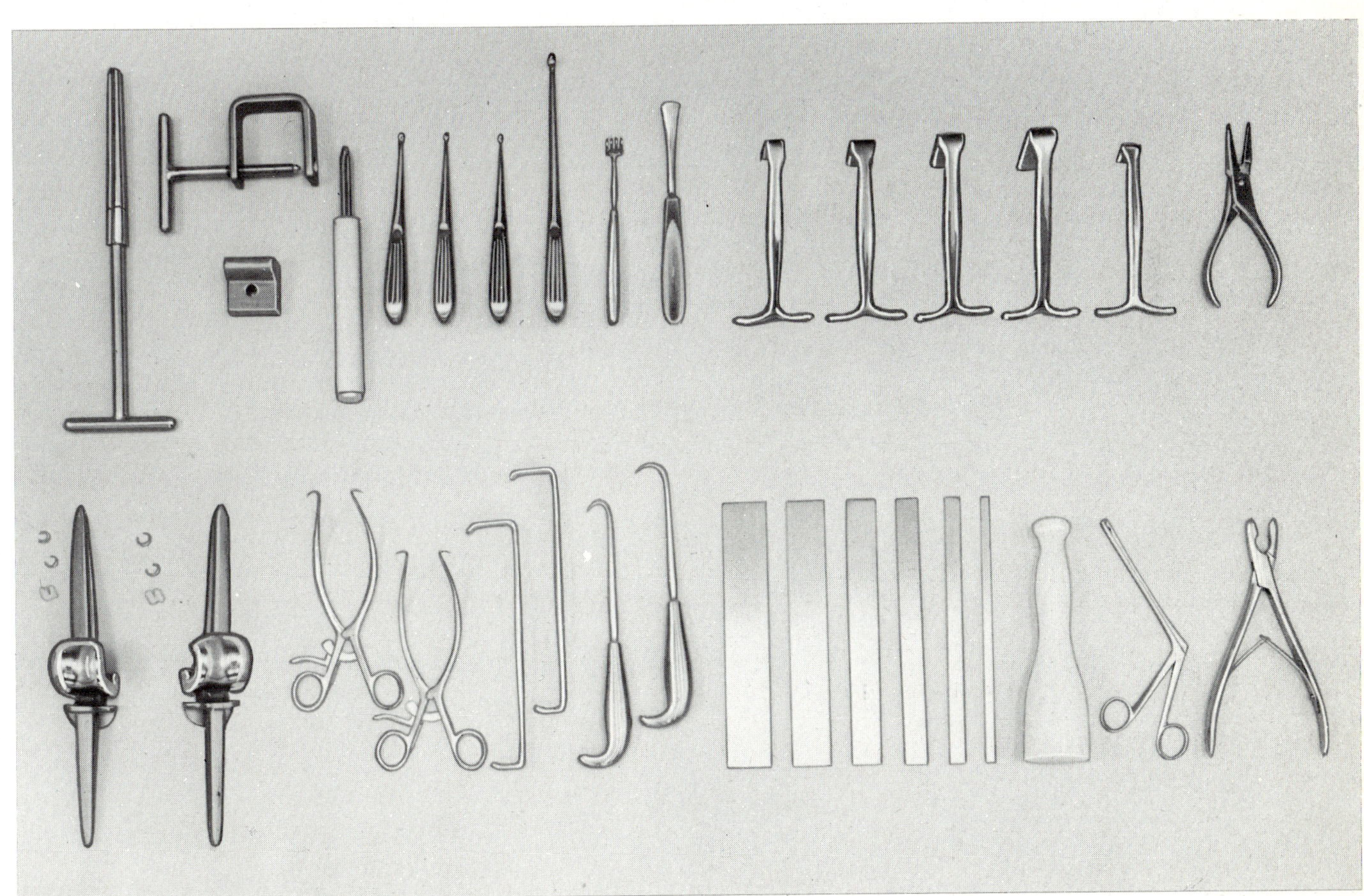

Fig. 20-91. Offset hinge total knee and instruments. (Courtesy Zimmer, Inc., Warsaw, Ind.)

Fractures of the tibial shaft

Considerations. Fractures of the tibial shaft are usually treated by closed reduction and plaster casting, since excellent healing is obtained without significant nonunion or infection. When surgery is necessary, screws, compression plates, and intramedullary nails should be available (Fig. 20-92).

Position and incision. The patient is supine with the incision made directly over the fracture. In the case of closed nailing, a small incision is made at the proximal tibia, and the nail is passed across the fracture site under fluoroscopy without exposing the fracture site.

Setup. Regular bone and soft-tissue sets are required, plus bone holders, and instruments for inserting the appliance of choice.

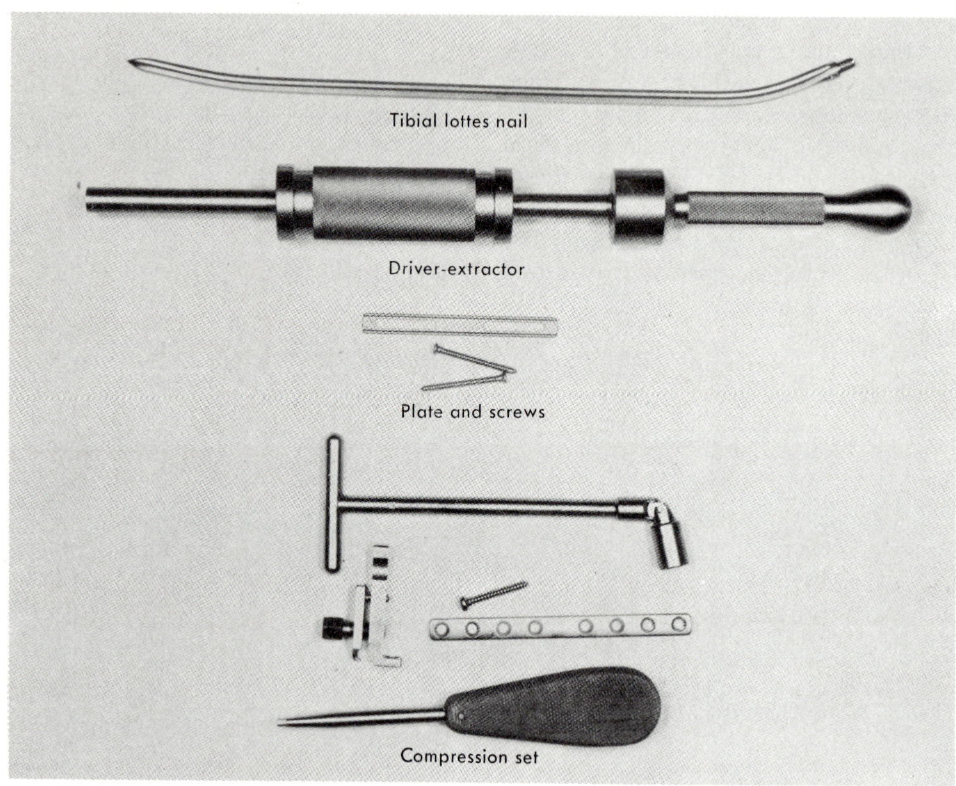

Fig. 20-92. Implant and instrumentation for fixation of tibial shaft fracture.

OPERATIONS ON THE ANKLE AND FOOT

Ankle fractures

Definition. Ankle fractures include fractures of the medial malleolus (tibia), lateral malleolus (fibula), and posterior malleolus (posterior aspect of the articular surface of the distal tibia). The terms malleolar, bimalleolar and trimalleolar are used depending on the number of fractures involved.

Considerations. Since medial malleolar and posterior malleolar fractures involve the distal weight-bearing articular surface of the tibia, open reduction and anatomical alignment are necessary. Displaced fractures are treated with open reduction and internal fixation. Screws or pins are usually used (Fig. 20-93). The lateral malleolus is important for lateral and rotational stability of the joint, and open reduction with internal fixation, using Steinmann pins or Rush rods, is frequently necessary. Postoperatively, a long leg cast is used for immobilization. Anatomical reduction is accomplished to prevent degenerative joint disease.

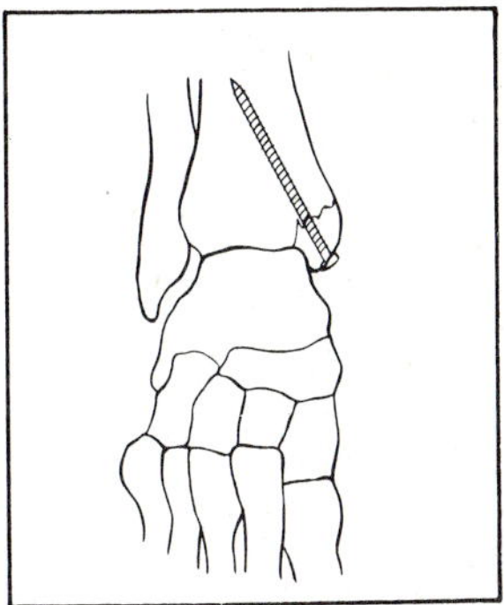

Fig. 20-93. Reduction of medial malleolar fracture with insertion of screw. (Courtesy Zimmer, Inc., Warsaw, Ind.)

Position and incision. Incisions are made directly over the fracture (Figs. 20-94 and 20-95). The patient is in the supine position for most malleolar fractures.

Setup. Small bone and soft-tissue sets are required, plus the following:

- Kirschner wires
- Steinmann pins
- Rush rods
- Driver
- Awl
- Drill and drill points
- Compression set, small fragment

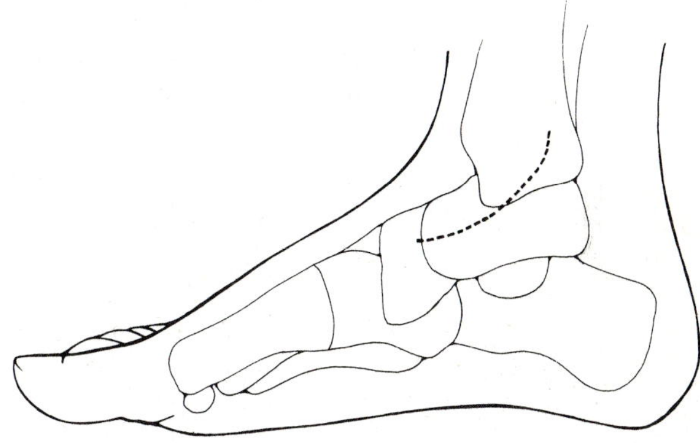

Fig. 20-94. Medial approach to ankle. (Adapted from Nicola, T.: Atlas of orthopaedic exposures, Baltimore, The Williams & Wilkins Co.)

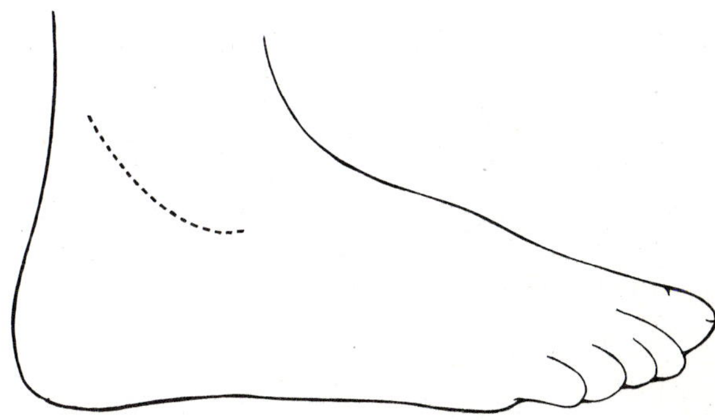

Fig. 20-95. Lateral approach to ankle. (Adapted from Nicola, T.: Atlas of orthopaedic exposures, Baltimore, The Williams & Wilkins Co.)

Triple arthrodesis

Considerations. It is necessary to fuse the talocalcaneal (subtalar), talonavicular, and calcaneocuboid joints in patients with marked inversion or eversion deformities of the foot. Such deformities occur in clubfoot, poliomyelitis, and rheumatoid arthritis. Occasionally, this operation is necessary for patients with pain resulting from degenerative or traumatic arthritis. This triple fusion does not interfere with flexion and extension of the foot at the ankle joint (Fig. 20-96).

Positon and incision. The patient is placed in the supine position, and an oblique incision is made laterally over the sinus tarsi.

Setup. Small bone and small soft-tissue sets and regular bone and regular soft-tissue sets are required, plus bone-graft instruments, Steinmann pins, staples, and a small vertebral spreader.

Total ankle joint replacement

Considerations. Since flexion and extension of the ankle joint are of great importance to weight-bearing and ambulation, all efforts should be made to maintain this motion (Fig. 20-97). Total ankle joint replacement with high-density polyethylene and metal components has been developed (Figs. 20-98 and 20-99).

Position and incision. The patient is placed in a supine position, and a longitudinal incision is made over the anterior ankle joint.

Setup. Small bone and soft-tissue sets are required, plus the following:

Air-powered saw, small
Air-powered drill, small
Air-powered bur set
Total ankle joint-replacement instruments
Trial prostheses
Methyl methacrylate and instrumentation

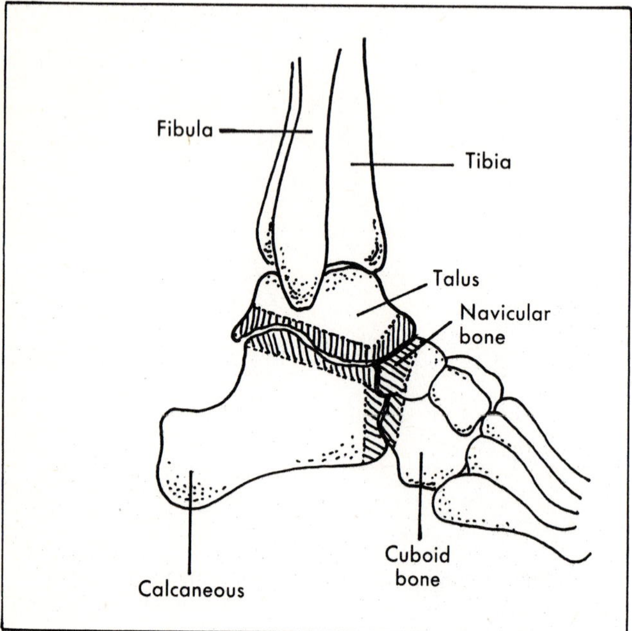

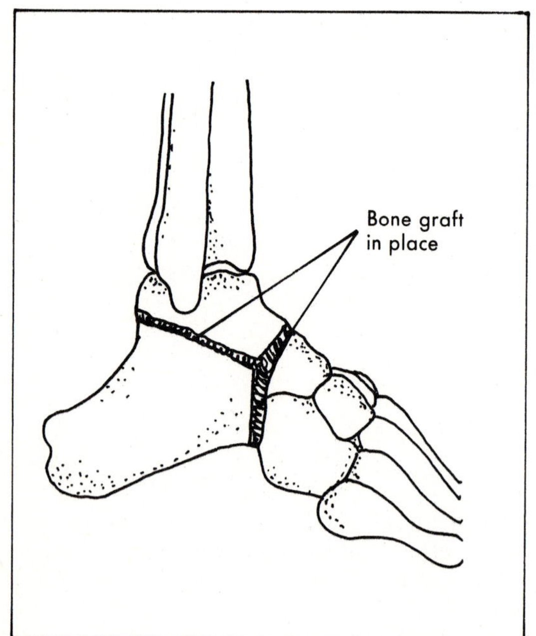

Fig. 20-96. Lateral views of joint fusion—triple arthrodesis. *Shading,* Area of bone to be resected. (From Brantley, P., and Analla, M.: The nurse and orthopedic surgery, Rutherford, N.J., 1980, Howmedica, Inc.)

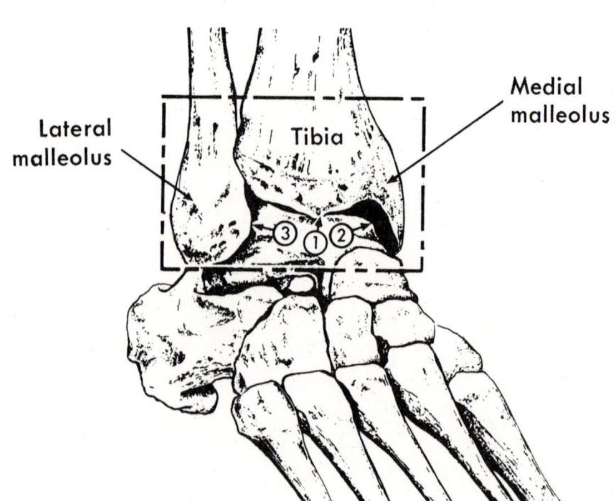

Fig. 20-97. Ankle joint. (Courtesy Zimmer, Inc., Warsaw, Ind.)

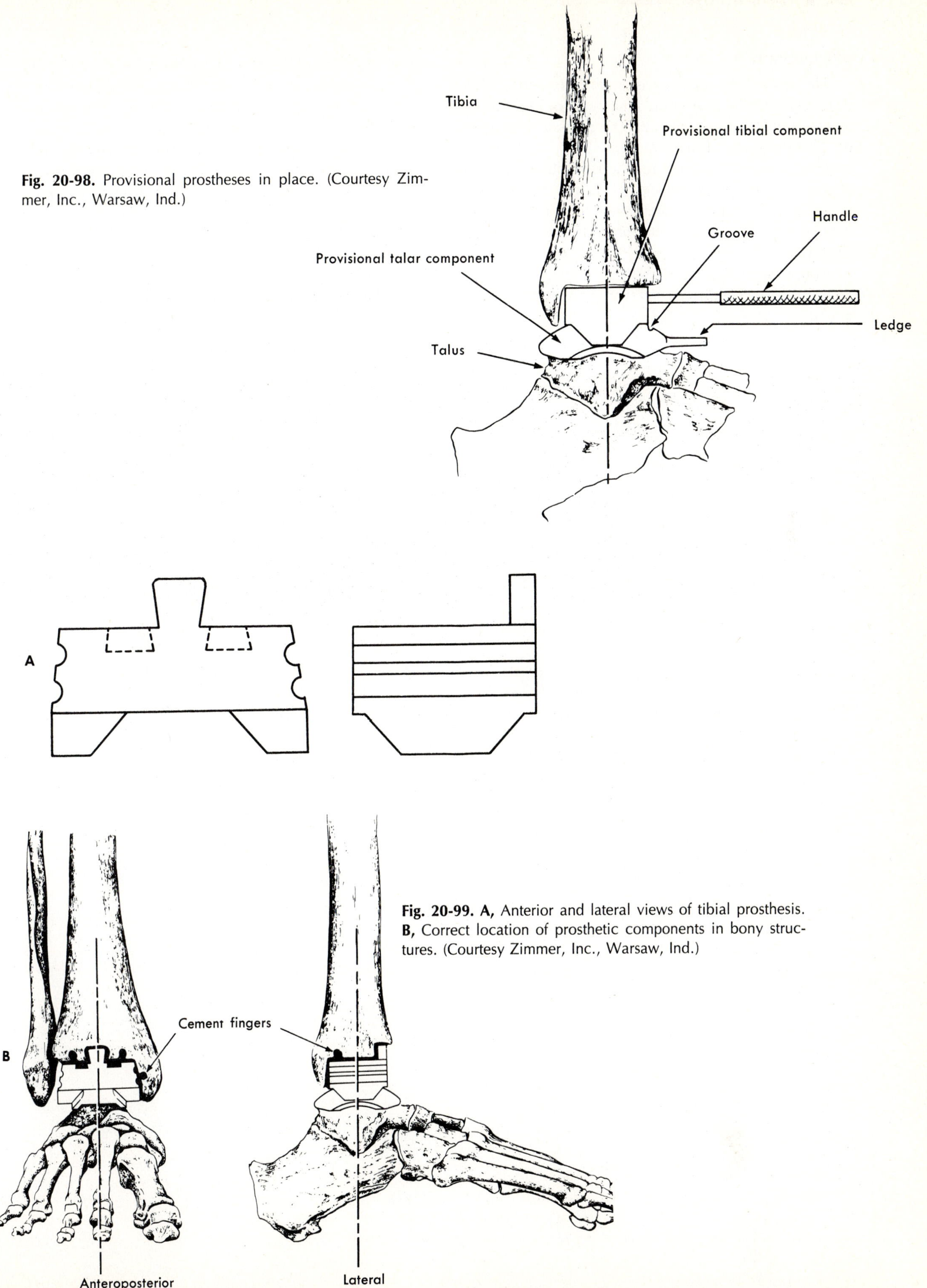

Fig. 20-98. Provisional prostheses in place. (Courtesy Zimmer, Inc., Warsaw, Ind.)

Fig. 20-99. A, Anterior and lateral views of tibial prosthesis. **B,** Correct location of prosthetic components in bony structures. (Courtesy Zimmer, Inc., Warsaw, Ind.)

Bunionectomy

Considerations. A bunion is a soft-tissue and/or bony mass at the medial side of the first metatarsal head. It is associated with a valgus (Fig. 20-100) position of the great toe. When painful it should be excised.

A variety of operations are available; all of them remove the exostosis and attempt to realign the great toe by removal of bone, transfer of tendons, osteotomy of the first metatarsal shaft, or appropriate imbrication of soft tissue.

Setup. Small bone and soft-tissue sets, a drill and drill points, a minidriver, and Kirschner wires are required.

Hammer-toe deformity

Considerations. A hammer-toe flexion deformity develops at the proximal interphalangeal joint of four lateral toes. This deformity causes painful calluses on the dorsal joints of the four lateral toes, as the cocked-up digits rub against the shoes. The deformity is treated by incising the long extensor tendon to the toes and fusing the middle joint. A smooth Kirschner wire is frequently used to stabilize the fusion and position the toe properly during the postoperative period.

Setup. Small bone and soft-tissue sets, Kirschner wires, and a microdrill or minidriver are needed.

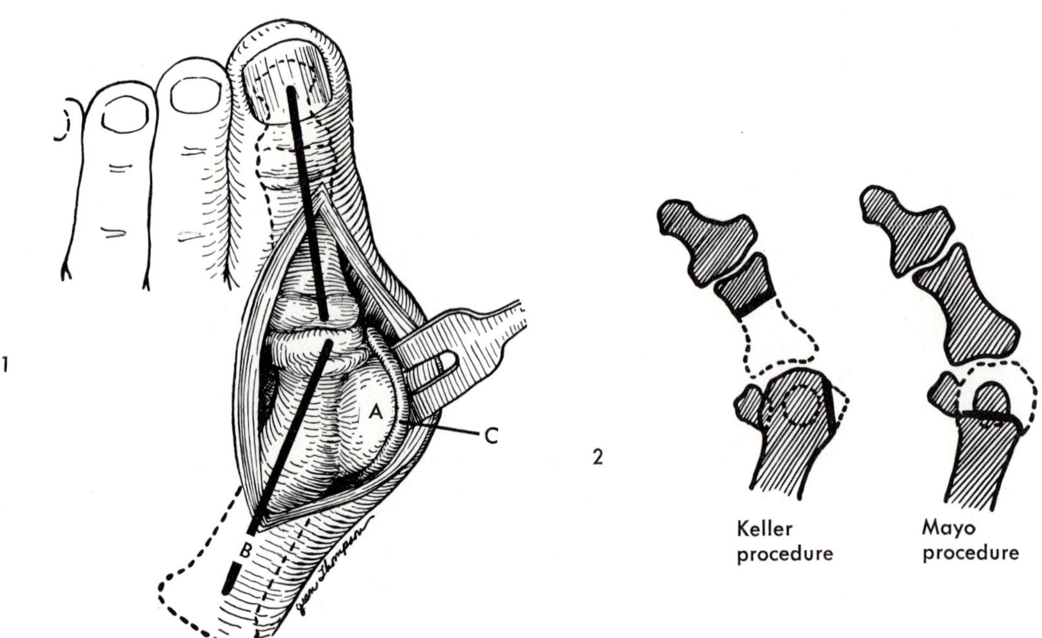

Fig. 20-100. 1, Bunion: *A,* exostosis of metatarsal head; *B,* hallux valgus deformity; *C,* overlying bursa. **2,** Operations for hallux valgus. (From Richards, V.: Surgery for general practice, St. Louis, The C.V. Mosby Co.)

Metatarsal head resection

Considerations. Patients with rheumatoid arthritis frequently have dorsally dislocated toes and prominent and painful metatarsal heads on the plantar surface of the feet. Excision of all the metatarsal heads frequently relieves the pain and corrects an associated bunion deformity.

Position and incision. The patient is placed in a supine position, and the heads of the metatarsals are excised through a transverse plantar incision.

Setup. Small bone and soft-tissue sets, Kirschner wires, and a microdrill or minidriver are needed.

Metatarsal arthroplasty

Considerations. Silastic implantation is indicated in the treatment of deformities associated with rheumatoid arthritis, hallux valgus, and a painful or unstable joint.

Position and incision. The patient is placed in the supine position. A tourniquet is applied, and the entire extremity is prepped and draped. The incision is made over the appropriate joints. Resection of the proximal phalanx with removal of exostosis of the metatarsal head is carried out. The medullary canal is reamed, and the implant seated.

Setup. Small bone and soft-tissue sets are required, plus the following:

Drill, key, and drill points
Trial and permanent implants (Fig. 20-101)

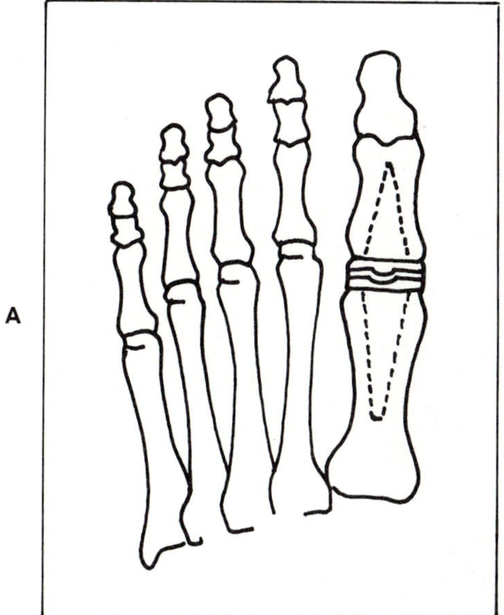

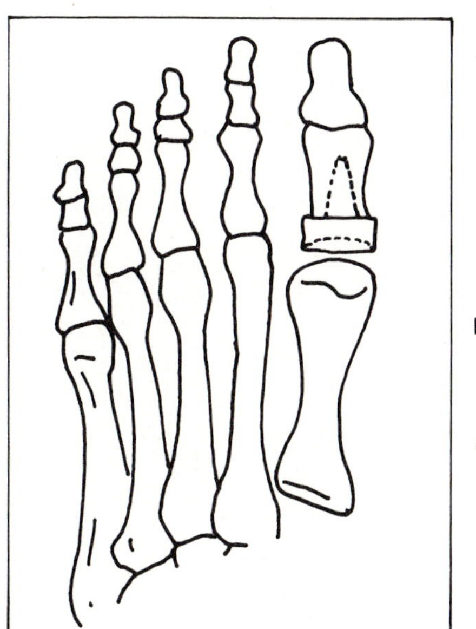

Fig. 20-101. A, Metatarsal implant, Swanson design. **B,** Great toe implant, Swanson design. (Courtesy Dow Corning Wright, Arlington, Tenn.)

OPERATIONS ON THE SPINAL COLUMN

Surgery of the spine is covered in Chapter 24, except for the treatment of scoliosis.

Treatment of scoliosis

Definition. Correction of scoliosis (Fig. 20-102) by fusion of the vertebral bodies involved in the curve.

Posterior spinal fusion with Harrington instrumentation

Considerations. Posterior spinal fusion is most frequently performed in teenagers, while the curve is still relatively flexible.

Harrington rods are internal splints that help maintain the spine as straight as possible until the vertebral body fusion has become solid. The Harrington method of treatment of scoliosis involves placing distraction rods on the concave side of the curve and compression rods on the convex side. The distraction rods are anchored to hooks fixed to the transverse processes of the vertebrae above and below the curve on the concave side. On the convex side of the curve, three to eight hooks are inserted in the transverse processes of the vertebrae and pulled together with a threaded rod. In this way the scoliotic deformity can be corrected as much as the flexibility of the spine allows.

The posterior elements of the vertebrae are denuded of soft tissue, and bone graft is added. Considerable blood is lost in this extensive operative procedure, and an accurate record of loss must be maintained. After surgery the patient is placed in an immobilizing jacket.

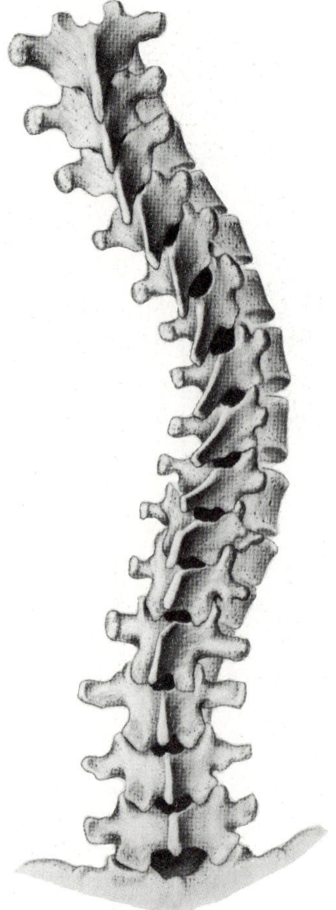

Fig. 20-102. Scoliosis deformity. (Courtesy Zimmer, Inc., Warsaw, Ind.)

Position and incision. The patient is placed in the prone position with rolls under the chest and abdomen to facilitate respiration. A straight midline incision is made in the back. Because of the amount of bleeding, the skin and subcutaneous tissues are often infiltrated with a vasoconstricting solution, such as epinephrine.

Setup. Harrington rod instruments include the following (Fig. 20-103):

1. *Distraction rods.* Relatively heavy rods, ratcheted on one end
2. *Compression rods.* Somewhat flexible threaded rods with nuts designed to maintain the force against each of the separate hooks used with the compression rod
3. *Distraction and compression hooks.* Several varieties of these anchor the distraction and compression rods to the vertebrae
4. *Hook clamps.* Hold the hooks during insertion and manipulation
5. *Rod clamps.* Hold and stabilize the rod as corrective forces are applied with the spreader
6. *Spreader.* Advances the ratchets through the hooks
7. *Drivers.* Drive the various hooks into the prepared area of the vertebrae
8. *Wrench.* Turns the nuts on the compression rod
9. *Outrigger.* Designed to temporarily apply distracting forces during the operation but is out of the operative field; replaced by the distraction rod after the vertebrae have been prepared to receive the bone graft
10. *Heavy wire or washer.* Placed between the distraction hook in the last ratchet on the rod to prevent slippage
11. *Large pin cutter.* Especially designed cutter to cut large pins but provided with a small end, so that it will fit in the wound

A separate instrument table is used for the Harrington rod equipment.

An x-ray cassette is placed under the patient before the procedure begins, so that an x-ray film can be taken during the operation to accurately identify the vertebrae to be fused.

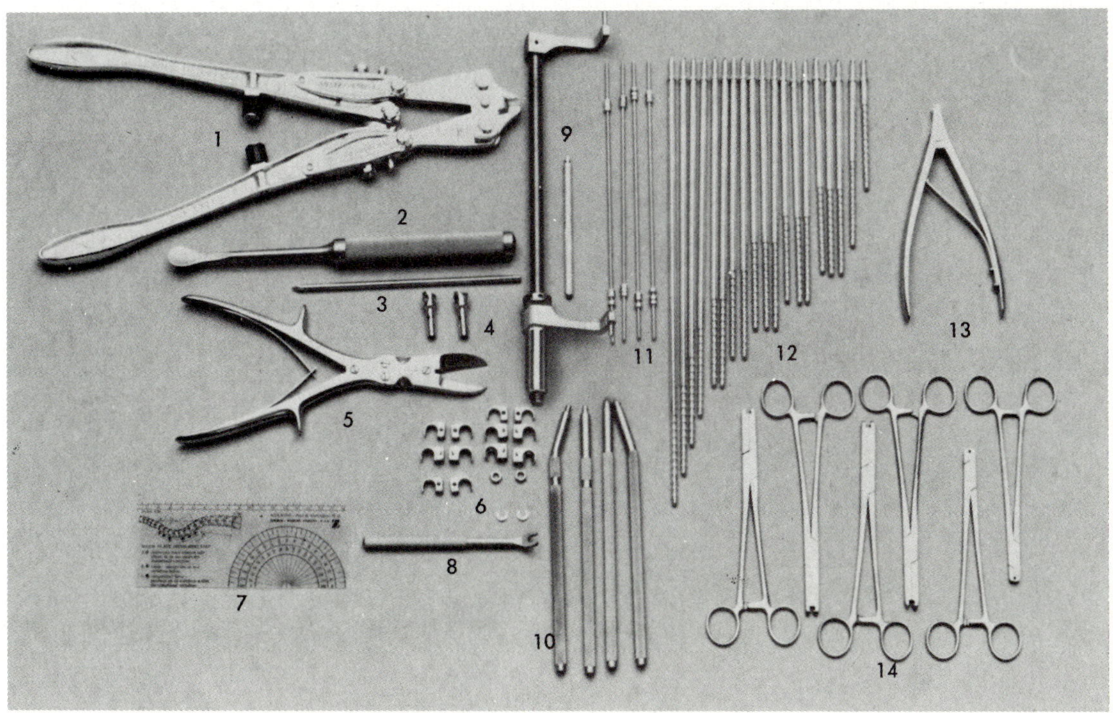

Fig. 20-103. Harrington rod instruments. *1,* Pin cutter; *2,* Harrington special elevator; *3,* Steinmann pin; *4,* sacral rod, nut, and eyelet; *5,* large bone cutter; *6,* hooks for distraction rod; *7,* protractor; *8,* flat wrench; *9,* outrigger distraction unit; *10,* drivers; *11,* compression rod assembly; *12,* distraction rods; *13,* spreader; *14,* hook clamp.

Anterior spinal fusion with Dwyer instrumentation

Considerations. Anterior spinal fusion is most frequently performed in patients with idiopathic thoracolumbar scoliosis and lordosis. Patients with congenital anomalies of the spine are also candidates.

Intervertebral discs are removed, and autologous bone from a rib graft is used. Dwyer instrumentation is frequently used, and consists of a titanium cable threaded through a series of screws and staples. The cable is placed on the convex side of the curve. As the cable is tightened, the curve is straightened.

Position and incision. The patient is placed in the lateral decubitis or chest position with the convex side of the curve superior. An intercostal incision is made, and a rib is excised. The rib is used for the bone graft.

Setup. Routine thoracotomy and spinal instrumentation is required, plus Dwyer instrumentation (Fig. 20-104):

Cables
Staples
Screws
Beads
Crimper
Cable tightener
Staple inserter
Staple driver
Screwdriver

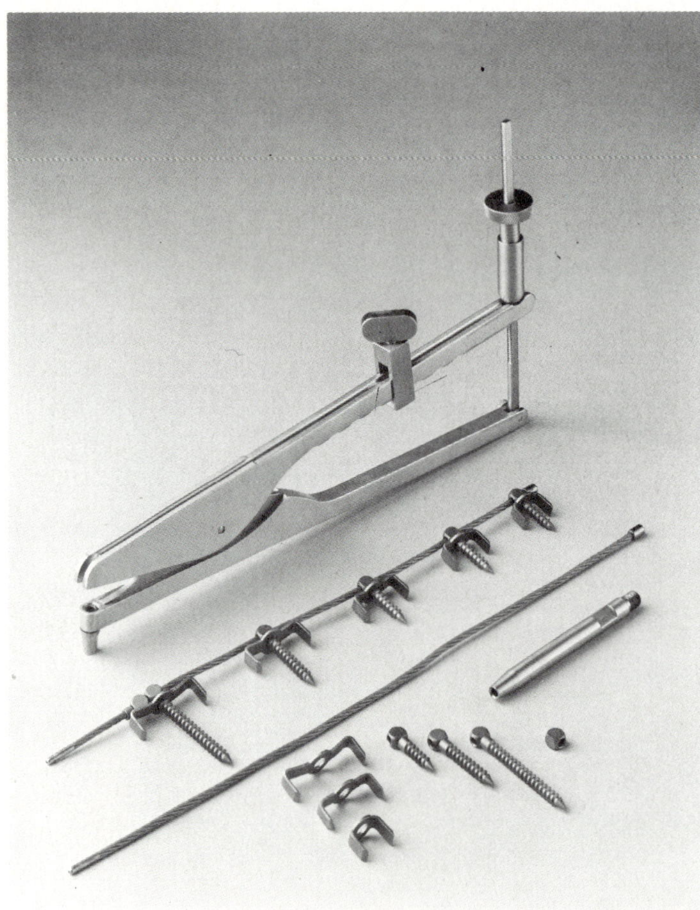

Fig. 20-104. Dwyer instrumentation. (Courtesy Zimmer, Inc., Warsaw, Ind.)

SUGGESTED READINGS

Bassett, C.A.L., Mitchell, S.N., and Gaston, S.R.: Treatment of ununited tibial diaphyseal fractures with pulsing electromagnetic fields, J. Bone Joint Surg. **63-A:**511, 1981.

Blauvelt, C.T., and Nelson, F.R.T.: A manual of orthopaedic terminology, ed. 2, St. Louis, 1981, The C.V. Mosby Co.

Brantley, P., and Analla, M.: The nurse and orthopedic surgery, Rutherford, N.J., 1980, Howmedica, Inc.

Brashear, H.R., and Raney, R.B.: Shand's handbook of orthopaedic surgery, ed. 9, St. Louis, 1978, The C.V. Mosby Co.

Brown, C.: Continuity of care for the orthopedic patient, AORN J. **31:**1128, 1980.

Brown, C.: The child undergoing anterior spinal surgery, Orthop. Nurs. **1:**33, 1982.

Brunner, N.A.: Orthopedic nursing: a programmed approach, ed. 4, St. Louis, 1983, The C.V. Mosby Co.

Deyerle, W.M., Crossland, S., and Sullivan, H.G.: Methylmethacrylate: uses and complications, AORN J. **29:**696, 1979.

Donahoo, C.A., and Dimon, J.H.: Orthopedic nursing, Boston, 1977, Little, Brown & Co.

Donahoo, C.A., and Spickler, L., editors: Core curriculum of orthopedic nursing, Atlanta, 1980, Orthopedic Nurses Association.

Driscoll, J.: Criteria for selecting arthroscopes, AORN J. **27:**831, 1978.

Edmonson, A.S., and Crenshaw, A.H., editors: Campbell's operative orthopaedics, ed. 6, St. Louis, 1980, The C.V. Mosby Co.

Electrical stimulation: an alternative to bone grafting, Englewood, Colo., 1980, Telectronics Orthopedic Division of Telectronic Proprietary, Ltd.

Ellison, A.E.: Distal iliotibial-band transfer for anterolateral rotatory instability of the knee, J. Bone Joint Surg. **61-A:**330, 1979.

Fowler, P.J.: The classification and early diagnosis of knee joint instability, Clin. Orthop. **147:**15, March-April 1980.

Gallagher, L.L.: Shoulder arthroplasty, Nursing '80 **10**(7):46, 1980.

Grana, W.A., and Pons, S.: Arthroscopy to diagnose knee disorders, AORN J. **27:**823, 1978.

Grana, W.A., and Randel, R.L.: Roger Anderson device for distal radius fractures, AORN J. **28:**1036, 1978.

Hay B.K., and Karas, C.B.: External fixation: option for fractures, AORN J. **34:**417,1981.

Hilt, N.E., and Cogburn, S.B.: Manual of orthopedics, St. Louis, 1980, The C.V. Mosby Co.

Johnson, L.L.: Diagnostic and surgical arthroscopy: the knee and other joints, ed. 2, St. Louis, 1981, The C.V. Mosby Co.

Johnson, R.J.: Care of orthopedic equipment, AORN J. **27:**44, 1978.

Kane, W.J.: A technique for insertion of the totally implantable bone growth stimulator, Englewood, Colo., 1979, Telectronics Orthopedic Division of Telectronic Proprietary, Ltd.

Krempen, J.F., Silver, R.A., and Sotelo, A.: The use of the Vidal-Adrey external fixation system. 1. The treatment of open fractures, Clin. Orthop. **140:**111, May 1979.

Larson, C.B., and Gould, M.: Orthopedic Nursing, ed. 9, St. Louis, 1978, The C.V. Mosby Co.

Larson R.L.: Combined instabilities of the knee, Clin. Orthop. **147:**68, March-April 1980.

Lombardo, S.J., and others: The modified Bristow procedure for recurrent dislocation of the shoulder, J. Bone Joint Surg. **58-A:**256, 1976.

Lovell, W.W., and Winter, R.B., editors: Pediatric orthopedics, Philadelphia, 1978, J.B. Lippincott Co.

Olerud, S.: Treatment of femoral fractures with Ender nails (letter), Clin. Orthop. **142:**262, July-Aug. 1979.

Paterson, D.C., Lewis, G.N., and Cass, C.A.: Treatment of delayed union and nonunion with an implanted direct current stimulator, Clin. Orthop. **148:**117, May 1980.

Roaf, R., and Hopkinson, L.J.: Textbook of orthopedic nursing, ed. 3, Oxford, England, 1980, Blackwell Scientific Publications, Ltd.

Robb, S.: Bunion surgery, Am. J. Nurs. **74:**2181, 1974.

Salter, R.B.: Textbook of disorders and injuries of the musculoskeletal system, Baltimore, 1970, The Williams & Wilkins Co.

Shibe, J.C.: Joint implants for arthritis, AORN J. **24:**442, 1976.

Thompson, V.R.: Injuries and the athlete, Point of View **13:**4, 1976.

Tobiason, S.J.: The arthritis patient comes to surgery, AORN J. **32:**608, 1980.

Volz, R.G., and Jones, A.B.: Upper extremity total joint replacement, AORN J. **28:**843, 1978.

21 Reconstructive plastic surgery

The word plastic is derived from the Greek *plastikos,* which means to mold or give form. Plastic surgery therefore deals with the healing and restoration of patients with injury, disfigurement, or scarring resulting from trauma, disease, or birth defects. As increasing emphasis is placed on the *quality of life,* restoration of normal function and normal appearance are the goals of the plastic surgeon. These goals are achieved by combining fundamental surgical techniques with an active imagination. Meticulous attention to detail is necessary because the results of plastic surgery are often highly visible.

Plastic surgery is not limited to a single anatomical or biological system; it encompasses all areas of the body. Only the anatomy and physiology of the hand are discussed in detail in this chapter because other anatomical areas are described elsewhere in this book.

A wide variety of operations are a standard part of operating room procedure in plastic and reconstructive surgery. The advancement of microsurgical techniques has expanded the repertoire of the surgeon to perform sophisticated procedures in replantation of limbs, digits, free flaps, and the like to restore and retain functional use of esthetic configuration. Breast augmentation, reconstruction, and reduction are included in this chapter, as well as free flap technique of jejunal tissue transfer for the reconstruction of the esophagus. Recession and advancement of the mandible and maxilla and treatment of hypertelorism and Crouzon's disease are also included to demonstrate the role of the surgeon, nurse, and specialty team members in successful accomplishment of these procedures.

The esthetic problems, varieties of congenital and acquired deformities, and diversity of operative techniques combined with psychological responses of patients offer unique learning experiences and challenges for providing perioperative nursing care.

NURSING CONSIDERATIONS

It is important for the nurse and all personnel coming in contact with the plastic surgery patient to be sympathetic to that patient's need for seeking help. Preoperative and postoperative patient visits by operating room nurses provide a sound basis for better understanding of the patient and his or her particular problem.

Most operations require that the operative site and adjacent areas be cleansed the night before surgery. This treatment is ordered by the physician. Special attention is given to fingernails, for patients undergoing hand surgery; to hair, for operations of the face, head, or neck; and to oral hygiene, for operations in or near the mouth.

Anesthesia. Many operations in plastic surgery are done under local, topical, or regional anesthesia administered by the surgeon. A registered nurse or anesthesiologist should be in attendance for these procedures. A blood-pressure cuff and cardiac-monitor leads are applied to the patient, and infusion equipment, emergency drugs, and resuscitation equipment should be available before the local, topical, or regional anesthetic is administered. All drugs that are to be used should be clearly labeled, including those placed on the sterile Mayo stand.

Drugs most frequently used for local anesthesia are 0.5%, 1%, or 2% lidocaine, plain or in combination with epinephrine 1:100,000 or 1:200,000. Epinephrine is a vasoconstrictor that decreases bleeding from the operative site and prolongs the effect of the local anesthetic agent. Drugs most frequently used for topical anesthesia are 4% cocaine and 2% tetracaine. Lidocaine *without* epinephrine is used for regional anesthesia, including digital nerve blocks. Because of its vasoconstrictive action, epinephrine is usually not used in surgery on an extremity, since it might result in necrosis.

Diazepam (Valium) and meperidine (Demerol), as well as other sedatives, narcotics, or hypnotics, are often given intravenously in small increments during a prolonged operative procedure under local anesthesia.

Adverse reactions to these medications consist primarily of possible cardiovascular and respiratory depression and/or arrest, cardiac arrhythmias, and convulsions. Hence there is a need for resuscitation equipment and emergency drugs in the operating room.

Positioning and draping. The operating table must be positioned so that remaining space in the room can comfortably accommodate anesthetic equipment, the scrub nurse and instrument tables, and any special equipment that is to be used, such as a hand table or drills. The patient is positioned so that all operative sites are well exposed.

Skin preparation is discussed in Chapter 5. Most plastic surgeons prefer an iodine-alcohol mixture, povidone-iodine solution, or hexachlorophene.

Correct draping procedure depends on the location of the operative site or sites. The most frequently used draping techniques in plastic surgery are the "head drape" and the "hand drape." The latter can also be applied to other upper or lower extremity procedures. The advantage of these techniques is that each allows maximum mobility of the head or extremity.

The *head drape* consists of the following (Fig. 21-1):

1. One barrier sheet folded in half and one towel are placed beneath the patient's head with the towel uppermost. The folded half sheet covers the operating table or headrest. The towel is brought around the patient's head on each side to cover all hair, leaving the entire face (which has been prepped) exposed, and is secured with two small towel clamps.

2. Two towels are placed diagonally across the neck just under the chin and are secured to each other in the middle over the neck and on each side to the towel around the head with a total of three small towel clamps.

3. A full sheet is placed to cover the patient from neck to feet.

Before proceeding with the "hand drape," a pneumatic tourniquet is applied to the upper arm over padding. The patient is supine on the operating table, with the affected arm extended and supported on a hand table. While an assistant on the other side of the operating table holds the arm with both hands around the tourniquet, the skin preparation solution is applied from fingertips to tourniquet.

The following comprises the *hand drape* (Fig. 21-2):

1. Two folded barrier sheets cover the hand table. The first sheet covers the end of the hand table. The second sheet is placed with a folded edge on top, nearest the patient (thus forming a cuff), and lies directly beneath the tourniquet.

2. Double-thickness, 4-inch stockinette is used to cover the extremity, and the edge is rolled over the tourniquet.

3. The upper arm and upper half of the body are covered by a folded sheet, with the folded edge placed across the part of the stockinette that covers the tourniquet.

4. A small towel clamp that grasps the edge of the folded top sheet, the stockinette, and the edge of the cuff of the bottom sheet is placed on each side of the arm. This excludes the tourniquet from the sterile field.

5. The remainder of the body is covered with one or two additional sheets.

Dressings. Dressings are often an essential part of the operative procedure in plastic surgery and may determine the ultimate outcome of the operation. Dressings are usually applied while the patient is still anesthetized. In general, the dressing should accomplish immobilization of the affected part and even pressure over the wound, allowing for drainage and comfort. A pressure dressing is essential in the elimination of dead space and the prevention of hematoma formation. In some instances, instead of using a pressure dressing, the same result can be achieved by use of catheters or drains placed beneath the operative site and connected to negative-pressure suction devices, such as a Hemovac or Jackson-Pratt apparatus.

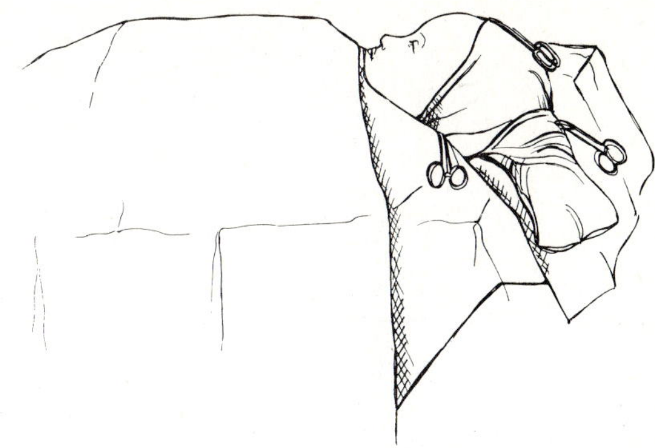

Fig. 21-1. Head drape.

The operating room nurse is responsible for having the following general dressing supplies available in sterile form:

- Nonadherent gauze, such as Adaptic, Xeroform, or Scarlet Red
- Petrolatum gauze, ½ inch (for nasal packing)
- Telfa
- Gauze, fine mesh
- Gauze dressing sponges
- Abdominal pads
- Mechanic's waste
- Acrylic fiber
- Cotton sheets and balls
- Kling and Kerlix gauze rolls
- Steri-strips
- Tape: adhesive, paper, or silk

Alloplastic materials. Autogenous tissue has always been considered the best implantation material and is used wherever feasible, in preference to synthetic material. In certain instances, however, use of alloplastic (synthetic) materials is indicated.

Silicone is presently the most frequently used alloplastic material in plastic surgery. The advantages of medical grade silicone are heat and time stability, versatility, nonadherence, minimal tissue reaction, and lack of attack or alteration by the body. Various forms of medical grade silicone are available: silicone rubber (Silastic), silicone sponge, silicone sheeting, and silicone blocks. Some of these may be carved into various shapes and sizes. A variety of preformed silicone prostheses (Fig. 21-3) are available for surgical implantation: nose, chin, ear, breast, testicular, and penile implants for contour restoration; silicone rods for formation of tendon sheaths before tendon grafting; and bone and joint implants for resection arthroplasty in hand surgery (Fig. 21-4).

Most silicone products are supplied in sterile form by manufacturers. However, they may be resterilized a number of times without any change in physical properties.

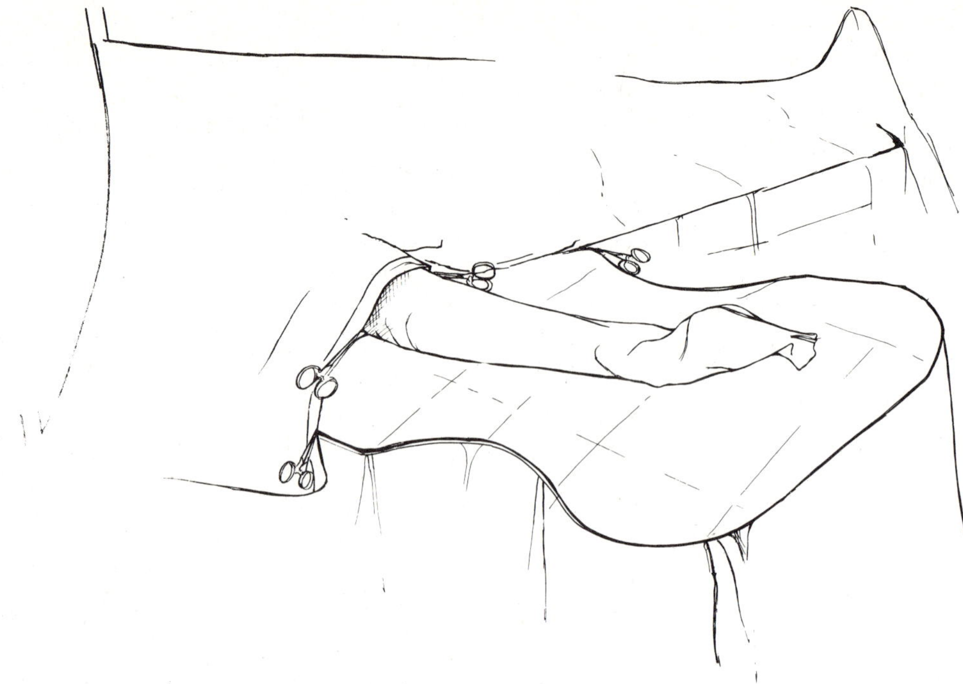

Fig. 21-2. Hand drape.

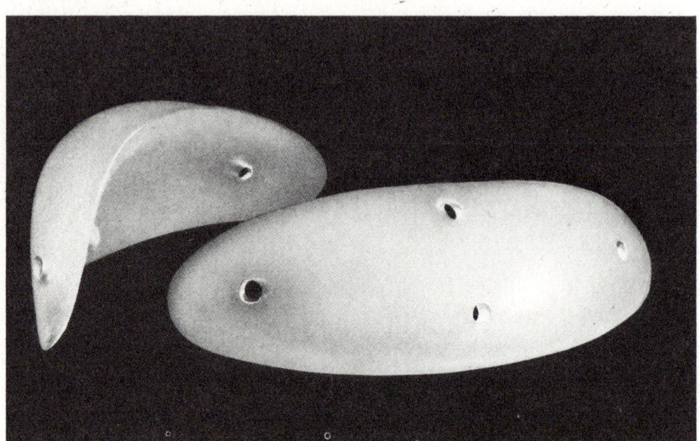

Fig. 21-3. Preformed silicone chin implants. (Courtesy McGhan Medical/3M, St. Paul, Minn.)

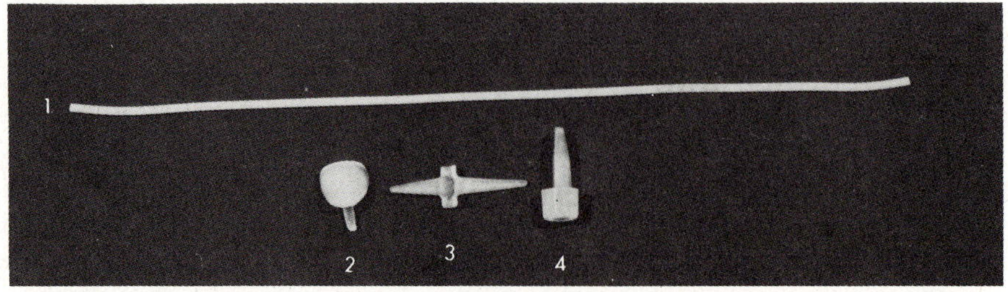

Fig. 21-4. Silicone rubber implants for hand surgery. *1,* Tendon rod; *2,* carpal lunate; *3,* Swanson finger joint prosthesis; *4,* carpal trapezium.

Special mechanical devices. Many special mechanical devices are used in plastic surgery. The operating room nurse must be familiar with the operation and proper safety regulations of all equipment used. Manufacturers' instructions for proper sterilization techniques and for special care after use must be followed. Each piece of equipment must be kept in working order. The following types of mechanical devices are used in plastic surgery.

Dermatomes. Used for removing split-thickness skin grafts from donor sites, dermatomes are of three basic types—knife, drum type, and motor driven:

1. *Knife dermatomes*
   a. *Ferris-Smith* (Fig. 21-5). Grafts obtained in "freehand" manner; sterile blades supplied by manufacturer
   b. *Humby.* Has adjustable roller to control thickness of graft
2. *Drum-type dermatomes.* Operate on principle of fixing outer surface of skin to half of a metal drum, then moving rotating blade back and forth close to surface of drum to obtain split-thickness skin graft
   a. *Reese* (Fig. 21-6). Tape containing adhesive is fixed to drum; dermatome cement is applied to skin in thin layer and allowed to dry for 3 minutes; distance between blade and drum (thickness of graft) is adjusted by inserting shim (0.008 to 0.034 inch) adjacent to blade in carrying arm; sterile dermatome tapes, cement, and blades available from manufacturer
   b. *Padgett-Hood* (Fig. 21-7). Grafts available in three sizes: baby model (3 × 8 inch), standard model (4 × 8 inch), and giant size (4 × 16 inch); cement applied to skin and directly to drum or used with dermatome tape; calibrated dial on dermatome can be adjusted to between 0.005 and 0.05 inch for desired level between knife blade and drum; sterile dermatome tapes, cement, and blades available from manufacturer
3. *Motor-driven dermatomes.* Graft obtained with knife blade that moves back and forth like blade of hair cutter; power supplied by electricity or compressed gas; long sterile cable serves as drive shaft and runs between dermatome and its power source; motor activated by foot pedal or hand control
   a. *Brown* (Fig. 21-8). Available with electrical or pneumatic power source; thickness of graft adjusted by one or two calibrated knobs on dermatome (in thousandths of an inch); sterile blades supplied by manufacturer; may be gas or steam sterilized
   b. *Castroviejo* (Fig. 21-9). Used primarily for cutting small mucosal grafts from inner sur-

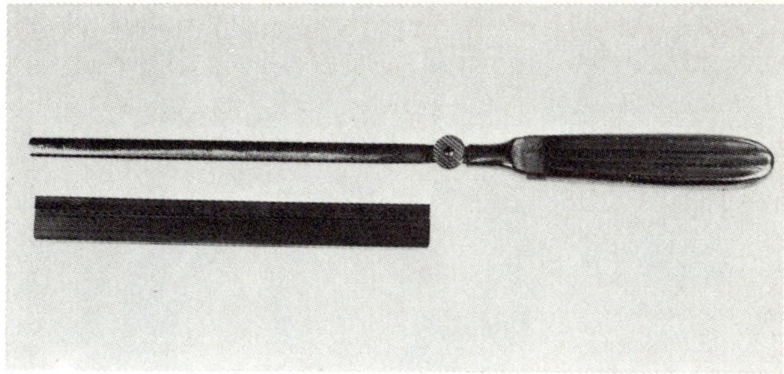

Fig. 21-5. Ferris-Smith knife dermatome handle and blade (straight razor).

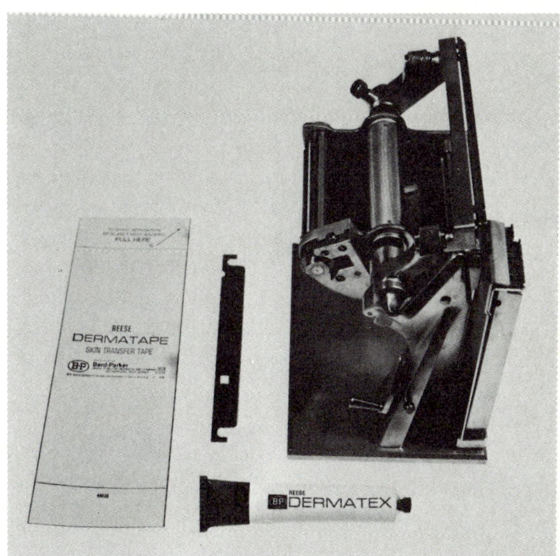

Fig. 21-6. Reese dermatome on stand, with tape, blade, and glue; shims are stored at lower right of dermatome stand.

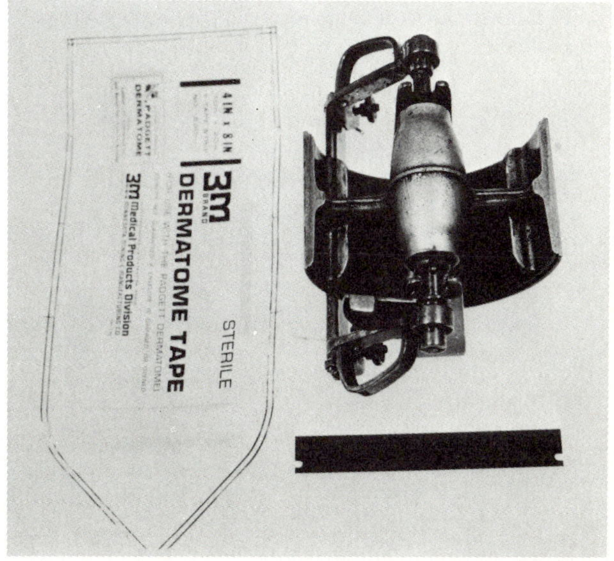

Fig. 21-7. Padgett-Hood dermatome with tape and blade.

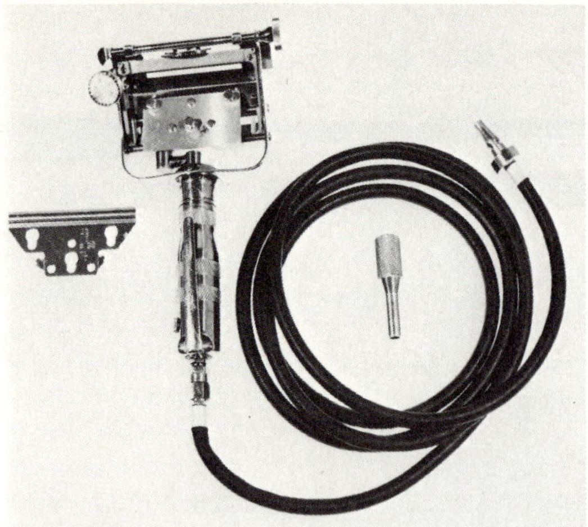

Fig. 21-8. Brown air dermatome and hose assembly with blade and chuck for securing blade.

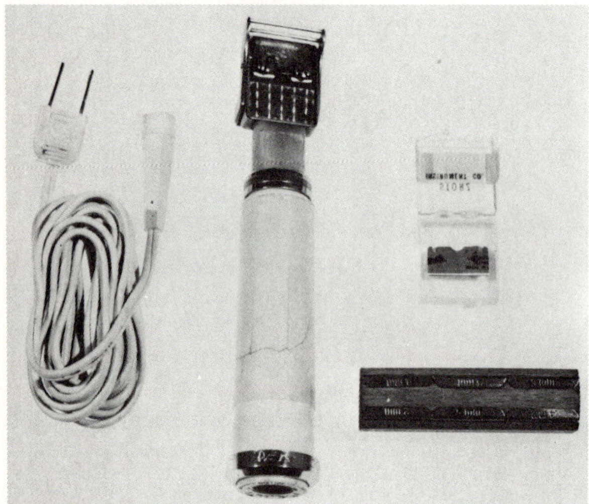

Fig. 21-9. Castroviejo dermatome with electric cord, blades, and guards.

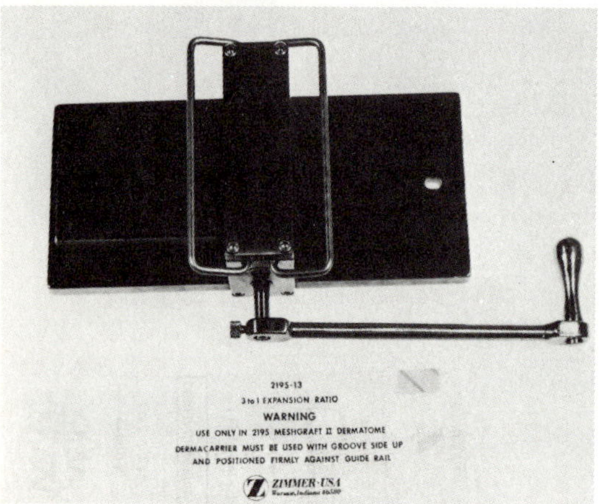

Fig. 21-10. Zimmer mesh graft II dermatome and carrier with 3:1 skin expansion ratio.

face of lips and cheeks; thickness of graft measured in millimeters rather than thousandths of an inch; blades and dermatome should be gas sterilized

4. *Skin meshers* (Fig. 21-10). Several types available, each designed to produce multiple uniform slits in a skin graft, approximately 0.05 inch apart, which allow for expansion of graft and multiple apertures in graft for drainage; graft placed on carrier and passed through mesher; sterile carriers for mesher supplied by manufacturer, usually in several sizes, which determine expansion ratio of skin graft (3:1 and 10:1 ratios most commonly used)

Insertion of the knife blade and guards or shims with any dermatome is done by the surgeon. It is also the surgeon's responsible to remove the knife blade after obtaining a graft, before any instrument-cleaning procedures are begun by operating room personnel. The blade is replaced in the original wrapper for identification before disposal.

Stryker pneumatic-powered instruments (Fig. 21-11). The power source is inert, nonflammable, and explosion-free compressed gas. The motor is activated by a foot pedal. The various attachments may be gas or steam sterilized (*not* immersed in liquid); the following attachments are used in plastic surgery:

Kirschner wire driver and bone drill
Oscillating bone saw
Reciprocating saw
Roto osteotome, straight
Derma-Tattoo (used with reciprocating saw handpiece)
Dermabrader

Hall II air drill (Fig. 21-12). The Hall II air drill is pneumatic powered; the motor is activated by a pedal on a handpiece. Burs and drill points of varied sizes are available for precision cutting and shaping of bone or for drilling holes in bone for wire-passing. The drill may be steam or gas sterilized (*not* immersed in liquid).

Luck-Bishop bone saw (Fig. 21-13). The electric motor is activated by a variable speed foot switch. A twist drill attachment is used for insertion of Kirschner wires in treatment of facial fractures. The Luck-Bishop bone saw may be steam or gas sterilized (*not* immersed in liquid).

Bipolar coagulation unit. Described in Chapter 24.

Fiberoptic instruments (Fig. 21-14). Light source is described in Chapter 17. Attachments used in plastic surgery include a head light for rhinoplasties, augmentation mammoplasties, and other procedures; a mammary retractor for augmentation mammoplasties; a rhytidectomy retractor; a Dingman mouth gag attachment for cleft palate repairs.

Pneumatic tourniquet with inflatable cuff (Chapter 20). This tourniquet is used with most hand surgery procedures as well as other upper and lower extremity operations.

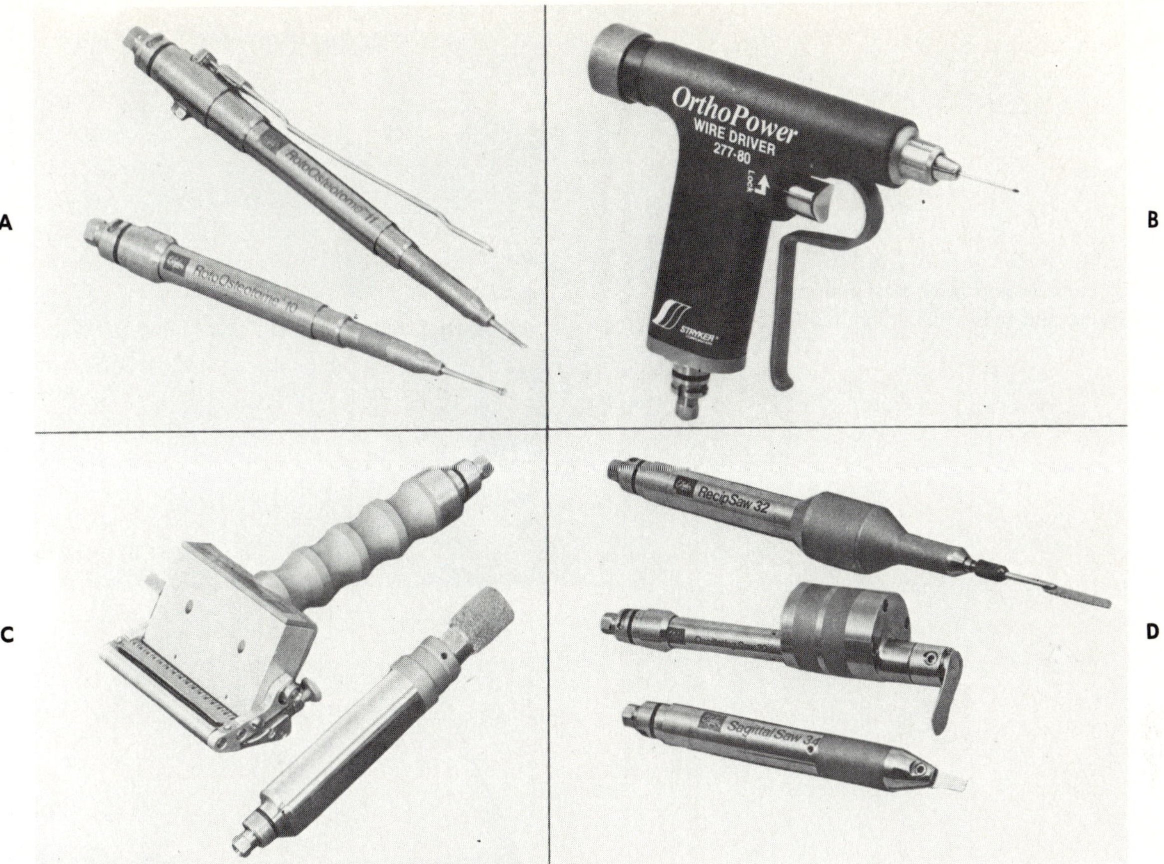

Fig. 21-11. Pneumatic-powered instruments. **A,** Osteotomes. **B,** Kirschner wire driver. **C,** Dermatome and dermabrader. **D,** Power saws.

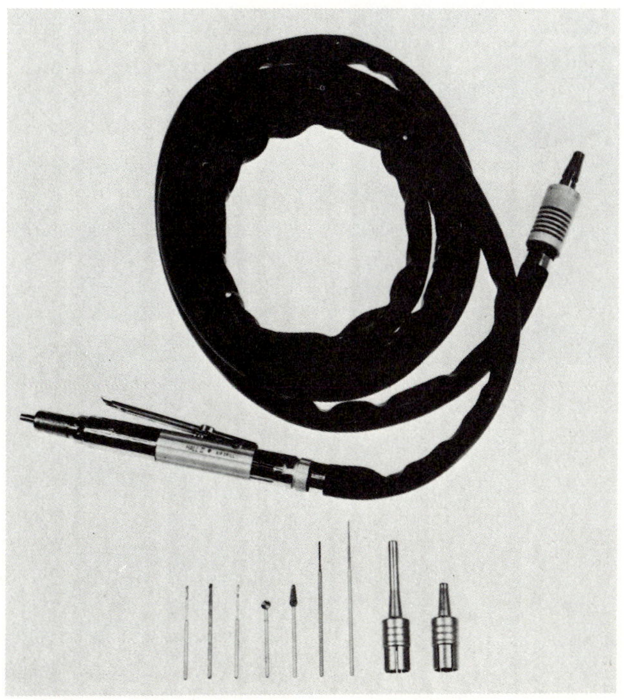

Fig. 21-12. Hall II air drill and hose assembly with assorted burs and long and medium bur guards.

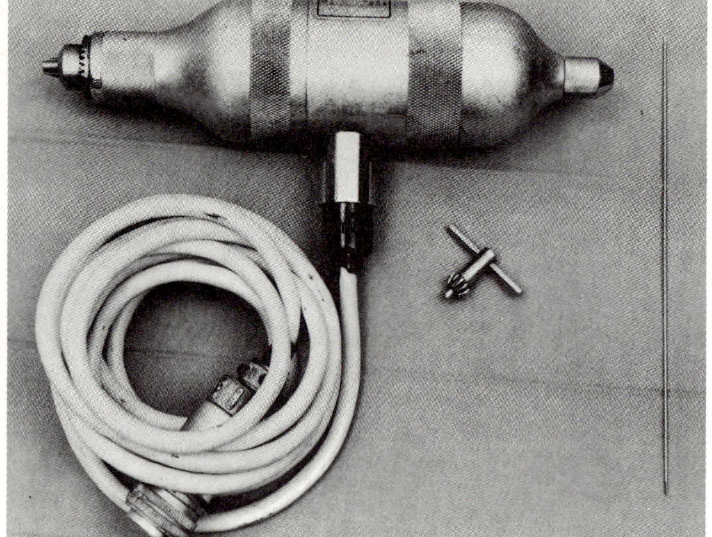

Fig. 21-13. Luck-Bishop bone saw with motor unit, cord assembly, and twist drill attachment.

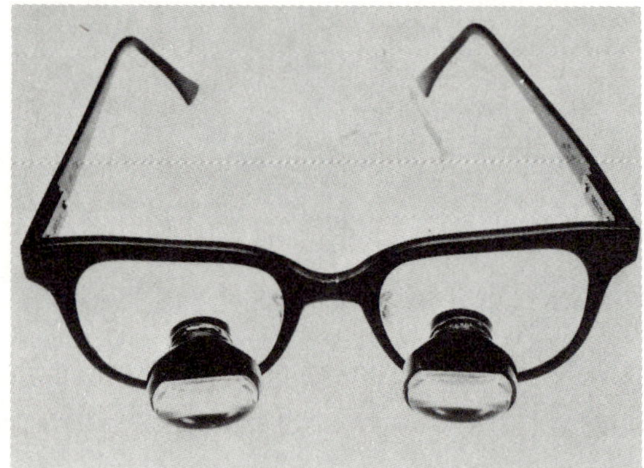

Fig. 21-15. Loupes—used for magnification.

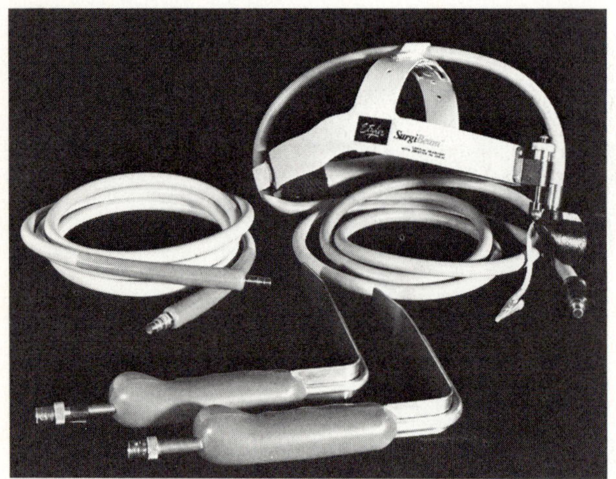

Fig. 21-14. Fiberoptic equipment: head light, mammary retractors, and cord for power supply.

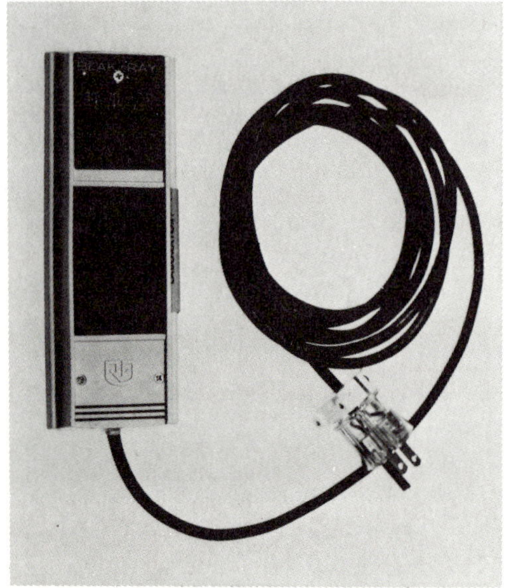

Fig. 21-16. Woods lamp and cord assembly.

Loupes (Fig. 21-15). Loupes are magnifying lenses used for microvascular surgery and nerve repair.

Operating microscope. Described in Chapter 22.

Woods lamp (Fig. 21-16). The Woods lamp is an ultraviolet light used in determining viability of skin flaps in darkened room after intravenous injection of 20 ml of 5% sodium fluorescein.

BASIC INSTRUMENT SETUP

Basic instrument sets. Three types of sterile basic instrument trays are kept available in the plastic surgery operating room. With modification by addition of instruments for specific operations, these trays suffice for all plastic surgery operations:

PLASTIC LOCAL INSTRUMENT SET (Fig. 21-17)

Cutting instruments

2 Bard-Parker knife handles, no. 3, 4 inches
1 Stevens tenotomy scissors, curved
2 Iris scissors, 1 curved and 1 straight
1 Metzenbaum scissors, curved, 5¼ inches
1 Brown dissecting scissors, curved, 5¾ inches

Holding instruments

1 Sponge forceps, straight, 7 inches
10 Towel clamps, 3 inches
2 Adson tissue forceps, 2 × 1–inch teeth
1 Adson dressing forceps
2 Brown-Adson tissue forceps
1 Dressing forceps, 5 inches
1 Bayonet dressing forceps, 5 inches
2 Skin hooks, single
2 Skin hooks, double, 10 mm

Clamping instruments

12 Mosquito hemostats, curved, 5¼ inches
6 Mosquito hemostats, straight, 5 inches

Exposing instruments

2 S-shaped retractors
2 Senn-Kanavel retractors

Suturing instruments

2 Brown needle holders, 6¾ inches
2 Webster needle holders

Accessory items

1 Joseph periosteal elevator
1 Freer septal elevator
2 Frazier-Ferguson suction tips, nos. 7 and 9
1 Anthony suction tip
1 Ruler
1 Bowl, small
1 Luer-Lok syringe, 5 ml
2 Needles, 25 and 22 gauge
2 Medicine cups

BASIC PLASTIC INSTRUMENT SET (Fig. 21-18)

Cutting instruments

3 Bard-Parker knife handles, no. 3, 4 inches
1 Bard-Parker knife handle, no. 3, 8⅜ inches
1 Stevens tenotomy scissors, curved
1 Iris scissors, straight
1 Metzenbaum scissors, curved, 5¼ inches
1 Mayo scissors, straight, 6 inches
1 Wire suture scissors, 4¾ inches

Holding instruments

1 Sponge forceps, straight, 7 inches
10 Towel clamps, 3 inches
4 Towel clamps, 5¼ inches
2 Adson tissue forceps, 2 × 1–inch teeth
1 Adson dressing forceps
2 Brown-Adson tissue forceps
1 Dressing forceps, 5 inches
1 Tissue forceps with teeth, 5 inches
2 Bayonet dressing forceps, 5 and 7 inches
4 Allis clamps, 6 inches
2 Skin hooks, single
2 Skin hooks, double, 10 mm

Clamping instruments

24 Mosquito hemostats, curved, 5¼ inches
12 Halsted forceps with teeth, straight, 5 inches
4 Ochsner clamps, 6½ inches
4 Kelly hemostats, curved, 5½ inches

Exposing instruments

2 S-shaped retractors
2 Senn-Kanavel retractors
2 Cushing vein retractors
2 Army-Navy retractors
2 Rake retractors, four blunt prongs
5 Ribbon malleable retractors, assorted widths (4 to 7 inches)
6 Richardson retractors, assorted
2 Weider tongue depressors, 1 large and 1 small

Suturing instruments

2 Webster heedle holders
2 Brown needle holders, 6¾ inches
2 Mayo-Hegar needle holders, 8 inches

Accessory items

1 Joseph periosteal elevator
1 Freer septal elevator
1 Ruler
1 Silver probe, 6 inches
2 Nasal specula, 1 short and 1 long
2 Bite blocks, 1 large and 1 small
1 Jaw hook
2 Anthony suction tips
3 Frazier-Ferguson suction tips, nos. 7, 9, and 11
1 Yankauer suction tip

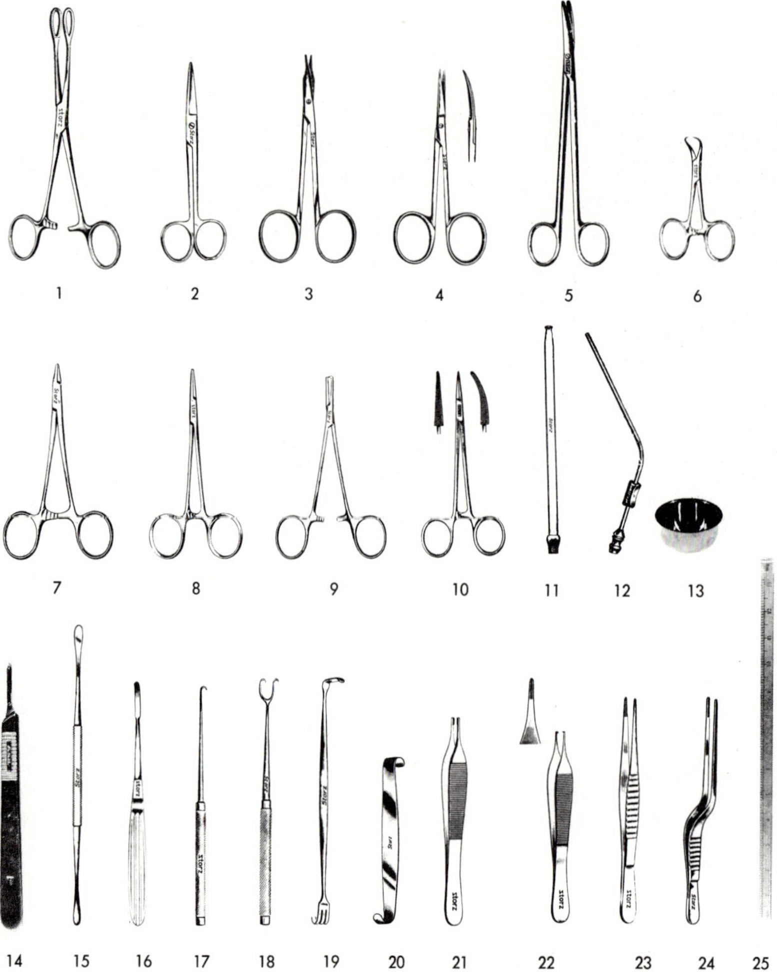

Fig. 21-17. Plastic local instrument set. *1,* Sponge forceps; *2,* Brown dissecting scissors; *3,* Stevens tenotomy scissors; *4,* straight and curved iris scissors; *5,* Metzenbaum scissors; *6,* towel clamp; *7,* Brown needle holder; *8,* Webster needle holder; *9,* straight mosquito hemostat with teeth; *10,* straight and curved mosquito hemostats; *11,* Anthony suction tip; *12,* Frazier-Ferguson suction tip; *13,* small bowl; *14,* Bard-Parker knife handle no. 3; *15,* Freer septal elevator; *16,* Joseph periosteal elevator; *17,* single skin hook; *18,* double skin hook; *19,* Senn-Kanavel retractor; *20,* S-shaped retractor; *21,* Brown-Adson tissue forceps; *22,* Adson tissue and dressing forceps; *23,* dressing forceps; *24,* bayonet dressing forceps; *25,* ruler.

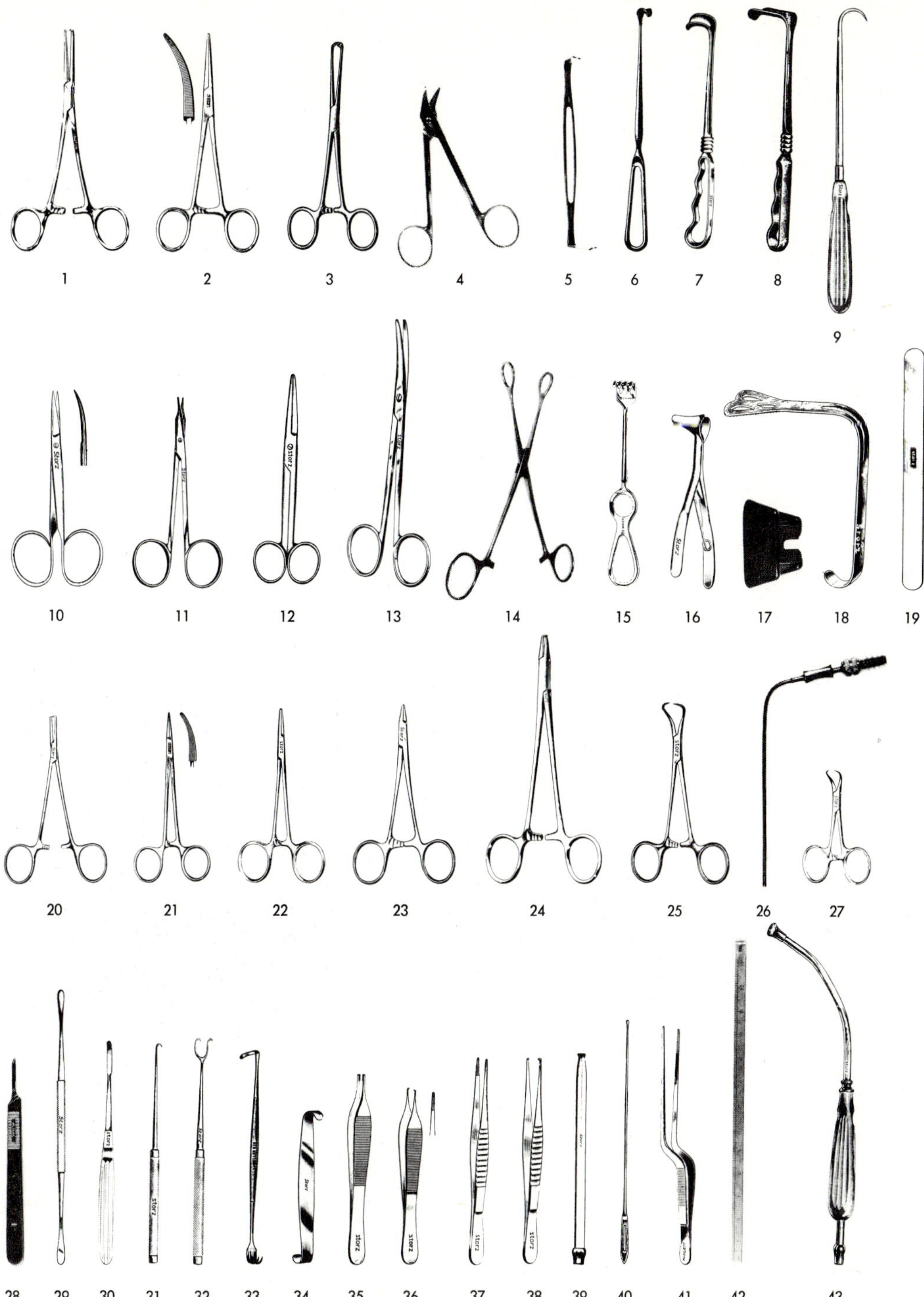

Fig. 21-18. Basic plastic instrument set. *1,* Ochsner clamp; *2,* straight and curved Kelly hemostats; *3,* Allis clamps; *4,* wire suture scissors, *5,* Army-Navy retractor; *6,* Cushing vein retractor; *7* and *8,* Richardson retractors; *9,* jaw hook; *10,* straight and curved iris scissors; *11,* Stevens tenotomy scissors; *12,* straight Mayo scissors; *13,* curved Metzenbaum scissors; *14,* sponge forceps; *15,* rake retractor with blunt prongs; *16,* nasal speculum; *17,* bite block; *18,* Weider tongue depressor; *19,* ribbon malleable retractor; *20,* Halsted forceps with teeth; *21,* straight and curved mosquito hemostats; *22,* Webster needle holder; *23,* Brown needle holder; *24,* Mayo-Hegar needle holder; *25,* large towel clamp; *26,* Frazier-Ferguson suction tip; *27,* small towel clamp; *28,* Bard-Parker knife handle no. 3; *29,* Freer septal elevator; *30,* Joseph periosteal elevator; *31,* single skin hook; *32,* double skin hook; *33,* Senn-Kanavel retractor; *34,* S-shaped retractor; *35,* Brown-Adson tissue forceps; *36,* Adson tissue and dressing forceps; *37,* dressing forceps; *38,* tissue forceps with teeth; *39,* Anthony suction tip; *40,* silver probe; *41,* bayonet dressing forceps; *42,* ruler; *43,* Yankauer suction tip.

PLASTIC HAND INSTRUMENT SET (Fig. 21-19)

Cutting instruments

3 Bard-Parker knife handles, no. 3, 4 inches
1 Stevens tenotomy scissors, curved
1 Metzenbaum scissors, curved, 5¼ inches
1 Iris scissors, straight
1 Mayo scissors, straight, 6 inches
2 Bone-cutting forceps, 1 angular and 1 straight, 7 inches
1 Wire suture scissors, 4¾ inches

Holding instruments

2 Sponge forceps, straight, 7 inches
2 Towel clamps, 5¼ inches
10 Towel clamps, 3 inches
2 Adson tissue forceps, 2 × 1–inch teeth
2 Adson dressing forceps
2 Brown-Adson tissue forceps
1 Tissue forceps with teeth, 5 inches
2 Allis clamps, 6 inches
2 Skin hooks, single
2 Skin hooks, double, 10 mm

Clamping instruments

6 Hartmann mosquito hemostats, curved
12 Mosquito hemostats, curved, 5¼ inches
2 Mosquito hemostats, straight, 5¼ inches
2 Kelly hemostats, curved, 5½ inches
2 Ochsner clamps, 6½ inches

Exposing instruments

6 Senn-Kanavel retractors
2 S-shaped retractors
2 Cushing vein retractors
2 Army-Navy retractors
2 Rake retractors, four blunt prongs

Suturing instruments

3 Webster needle holders

Accessory items

1 Joseph periosteal elevator
1 Freer septal elevator
1 Ruler
1 Bunnell hand drill
2 Needle-nose pliers, 6¼ inches
2 Frazier-Ferguson suction tips, nos. 7 and 9
2 Ruskin rongeurs, 1 large and 1 small
1 Lempert rongeur
1 Set Kirschner wires
1 Kirschner wire cutter
Curettes, assorted

Special supplies. In addition to the basic instrument sets, the following sterile supplies are available at all times and are added to instrument sets for nearly all procedures:

Marking pen
Epinephrine 1:200,000 for injection
X-ray film, unexposed (for pattern making)
Bard-Parker knife blades, no. 15
Cautery

OPERATIONS

Replacement of lost tissue

Free skin graft

Definition. Segment of epidermis and dermis that is completely separated from its blood supply at the donor site before being transplanted to another area of the body—the recipient site.

Considerations. A *split-thickness* (or *partial-thickness*) skin graft contains epidermis and only a portion of the dermis of the donor site. A *full-thickness* skin graft contains epidermis and all of the dermis from the donor site (Fig. 21-20). The donor site for a split-thickness skin graft heals by regeneration of epithelium from dermal elements that remain intact. Therefore only a dressing is placed over this donor site. Since no dermal elements remain when a full-thickness skin graft is taken, this donor site will not heal spontaneously. It will heal only if another layer of skin is placed over it—either by suturing the wound edges of the donor site together or applying another skin graft over it. A scar remains at the donor site of a skin graft. Therefore donor sites that are covered by clothing are generally chosen.

The "take," or survival, of a free skin graft depends on revascularization of the graft by ingrowth of blood vessels from the recipient bed. It is therefore necessary to prevent accumulation of material between the graft and the recipient site that increases the distance through which new blood vessels must grow; that is, hematoma or wound exudate. A stent or tie-over dressing is often placed over a skin graft (Fig. 21-21). This exerts even pressure, assuring good contact between graft and recipient site. It also eliminates potential shearing forces at the graft–recipient site interface, which might disrupt new blood vessels that are growing into the graft.

Setup and preparation of the patient. A plastic local instrument set is required, plus a dermatome of choice, marking pen, and unexposed x-ray film.

The patient is positioned so that both donor and recipient sites are well exposed. Both areas are prepared and draped to maintain adequate exposure and mobility, as required.

Operative procedure

1. The recipient site is prepared as necessary. This may involve excision of a benign or malignant skin tumor, debridement of an open wound, or release of a scar contracture.

2. When feasible, a pattern of the recipient site is made with unexposed x-ray film. This pattern is transferred to the donor site and outlined with a marking pen.

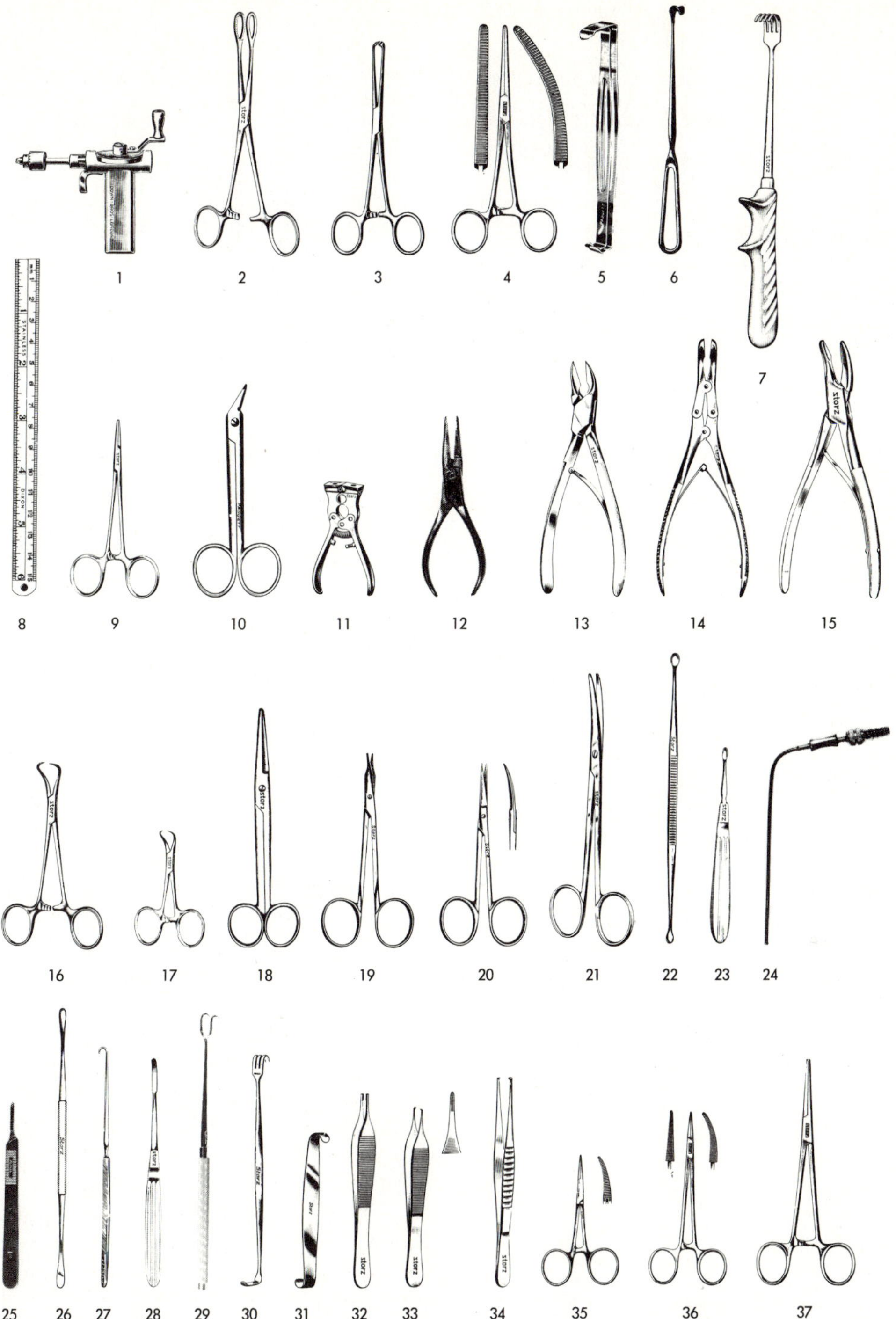

Fig. 21-19. Plastic hand instrument set. *1,* Bunnell hand drill; *2,* sponge forceps; *3,* Allis clamp; *4,* straight and curved Kelly hemostats; *5,* Army-Navy retractor; *6,* Cushing vein retractor; *7,* rake retractor with blunt prongs; *8,* ruler; *9,* Webster needle holder, *10,* wire suture scissors; *11,* Kirschner wire cutter; *12,* needle-nose pliers; *13,* bone-cutting forceps; *14,* Ruskin rongeur; *15,* Lempert rongeur; *16,* large towel clamp; *17,* small towel clamp; *18,* straight Mayo scissors; *19,* Stevens tenotomy scissors; *20,* straight and curved iris scissors; *21,* curved Metzenbaum scissors; *22* and *23,* curettes; *24,* Frazier-Ferguson suction tip; *25,* Bard-Parker knife handle no. 3; *26,* Freer septal elevator; *27,* single skin hook; *28,* Joseph periosteal elevator; *29,* double skin hook; *30,* Senn-Kanavel retractor; *31,* S-shaped retractor; *32,* Brown-Adson tissue forceps; *33,* Adson tissue and dressing forceps; *34,* tissue forceps with teeth; *35,* straight and curved Hartmann mosquito hemostats; *36,* straight and curved mosquito hemostats; *37,* Ochsner clamp.

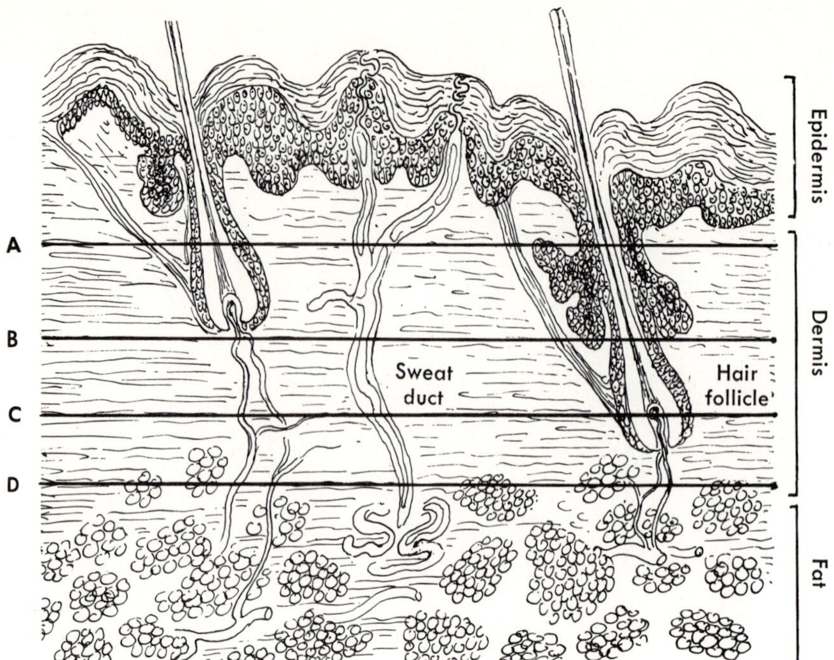

Fig. 21-20. Layers of skin. Level *A* corresponds to a superficial or thin split-thickness graft and level *D* to a full-thickness graft, with levels *B* and *C* representing intermediate-thickness split grafts. (From Wood-Smith, D., and Porowski, P.C., editors: Nursing care of the plastic surgery patient, St. Louis, The C.V. Mosby Co.)

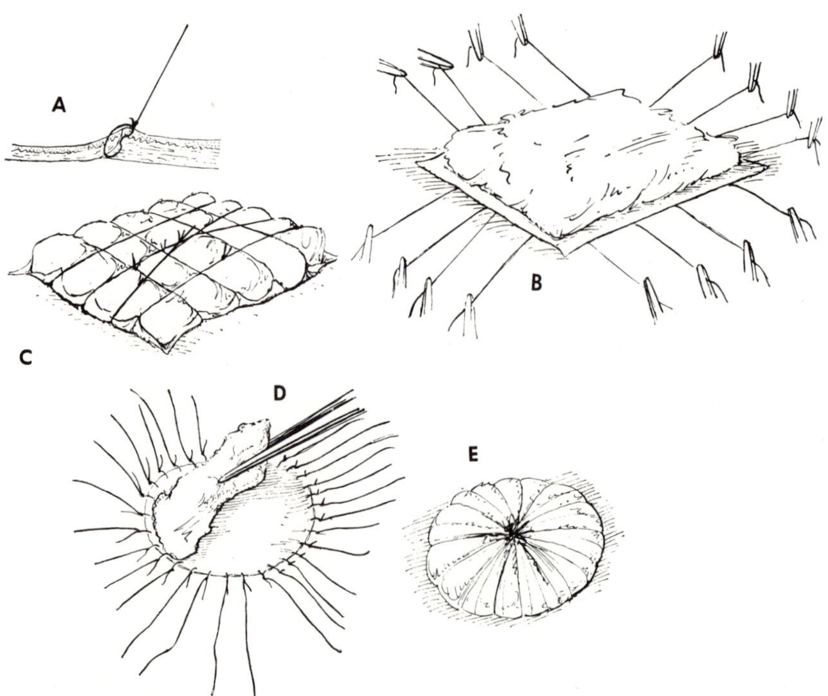

Fig. 21-21. A, Method of fixation of skin graft to edges of wound. **B,** Nonadherent dressing is applied over skin graft, and on this a generous pad of acrylic fiber. **C,** Long ends of suture are tied over fiber to produce area of pressure between graft and base. **D,** Similar dressing is applied to circular graft. **E,** Long suture ends are tied over circular graft (often called "stent" dressing). (From Wood-Smith, D., and Porowski, P.C., editors: Nursing care of the plastic surgery patient, St. Louis, The C.V. Mosby Co.)

3. The edges of the donor site are sutured together. Fat adherent to the graft is trimmed. The graft is applied to the recipient site, usually sutured at the edges, and these sutures are left long to tie over a stent dressing (Fig. 21-21). Blood clots beneath the graft are removed by saline irrigation before the dressing is applied.

4. Split-thickness grafts are obtained with a dermatome. Additional skin preparation of the donor site may be requested by the surgeon, such as mineral oil for use with Brown or Weck dermatomes.

5. Moist sponges are first applied to donor sites to aid hemostasis. These are replaced by the surgeon's choice of dressing, such as fine mesh gauze or nonadherent gauze.

6. If the graft is to be meshed, it is now applied to specifically supplied carriers for use with certain skin meshers.

7. A graft that is not immediately applied to the recipient site dries quickly, particularly a meshed graft. Therefore grafts should be kept in moist gauze sponges that are secured to the Mayo stand with a towel clamp to prevent inadvertent loss of the graft. Meshed skin should not be removed from its carrier until it is applied directly to the recipient site.

8. Whether applied as a sheet or meshed, split-thickness grafts may or may not be sutured. Nonadherent gauze is usually applied as the first dressing layer over a graft. Moist dressings should be applied to all meshed grafts to prevent desiccation and loss of the graft.

Flap

Definition. Tissue that is completely detached from its donor site and transferred to the recipient site, where microvascular anastomoses of at least one artery and two veins (between flap and recipient site) provide the means of continued viability of flap tissue.

Considerations. Because flaps carry their own blood supply, they are usually used to cover recipient sites that have poor vascularity. They are useful for padding bony prominences. They may be used in situations where it is necessary to operate through the wound at a later date to repair underlying structures. Flaps containing skin and subcutaneous tissue retain more properties of normal skin and shrink less than do skin grafts. Therefore they are often used to repair defects of the face. Flaps, however, have some disadvantages, such as bulky appearance, failure to match tissue of the recipient site in texture or color, ability to carry hair into non-hair-bearing areas, and possibility of requiring multiple operations and prolonged hospitalization.

Flaps may be classified as *direct flaps,* which are applied at the same time they are raised, and *delayed flaps,* which are raised in stages to improve the blood supply before permanent application to the recipient site. Flaps may also be classified as *local flaps,* which contain tissue adjacent to the recipient site, and *distant flaps,* which contain tissue at a distance from the recipient site. Local and distant flaps may be transferred as direct or delayed flaps. In addition, distant flaps are sometimes transferred to the recipient site by an intermediate site, or "carrier," when donor and recipient sites are far removed from one another, that is, transfer of a flap from the trunk to the lower leg, using the wrist as an intermediate carrier.

Setup and preparation of the patient. A basic plastic instrument set is required, plus the following:

Cautery
Clamping instruments, extra
Dermatome of choice
Marking pen
X-ray film, unexposed

Positioning, preparation, and draping of the patient are carried out to maintain adequate exposure and mobility of both the flap donor and recipient sites.

Operative procedure

1. The recipient site is prepared in the same manner as for a skin graft.

2. When feasible, a pattern of the recipient site is made and transferred to the donor area.

3. The flap is incised, elevated, and transferred to the recipient site. The edges of the flap are sutured to the periphery of the recipient site.

4. The flap donor site is repaired by approximating the skin edges directly or by covering the defect with a skin graft or another flap.

5. Drains are usually placed under flaps.

6. Dressings are applied with particular attention given to immobilization of the flap. This may require stockinette, padding, and/or plaster of Paris.

7. When a pedicle flap is divided, the surgeon may want to check the adequacy of circulation within the flap. This can be done by placing rubber-shod clamps across the base of the pedicle and injecting 20 ml of 5% sodium fluorescein intravenously. After all lights in the operating room are turned off, a Woods lamp is held over the flap to determine the presence or absence of fluorescence within the flap.

Composite graft

Definition. Compound tissues that are completely separated from the blood supply of the donor site and transplanted to another area of the body.

Considerations. The survival of a composite graft depends on ingrowth of new blood vessels from the recipient site around the periphery of the graft. Therefore composite grafts are usually small, so that no portion of the graft is greater than 1 cm from its periphery. Examples of compound tissues used as composite grafts are (1) a segment of external ear, composed of skin, subcutaneous tissue, and cartilage, which is used to reconstruct defects of the alar rim of the nose, and (2) hair transplants, composed of skin, fat, and hair follicles, which are used to treat male-pattern baldness.

Setup and preparation of the patient. A plastic local instrument set is required, plus the following:

Marking pen
X-ray film, unexposed
Nasal specula, when indicated
Nasal packing, when indicated
Brown nasal splint, when indicated

Positioning, preparation, and draping of the patient are such that adequate exposure of both donor and recipient sites is maintained.

Operative procedure

1. The recipient site is prepared by excising tissue, such as a scar or a benign or malignant skin lesion.
2. When feasible, a pattern of the recipient site is made and transferred to the donor site.
3. The donor site is closed by approximating its skin edges or may be left unsutured (such as in hair transplant donor sites).
4. Meanwhile, the composite graft is kept in a moist sponge, until it is sutured to the edges of the recipient site.
5. Dressings of choice are applied to the composite graft and donor site.

Free tissue transfer

Definition. Single-stage reconstruction with a free jejunal transfer in patients requiring removal of the entire hypopharynx, cervical esophagus, and neck dissection for carcinoma.

Considerations. Reconstructive problems in patients undergoing laryngectomy and upper cervical esophagectomy can be adequately solved by free jejunal transfer. Modern microsurgical techniques greatly improve the success rate. Free jejunal transfers have proved beneficial:

1. In patients with massive resections of the laryngopharynx when resection may extend into the oropharynx or even the lower nasopharynx and encompass a large portion of the cervical esophagus
2. In patients with radiation failure in whom laryngopharyngoesophagectomy is required
3. In patients with secondary reconstruction of the hypopharynx or cervical esophagus in whom other methods have failed because of flap necrosis or radiation
4. In patients in whom primary pharyngoesophageal closure of radiation has resulted in hypopharyngeal stricture unresponsive to dilatation
5. In isolated cases in which a large area of oral lining is lost

Setup and preparation of the patient. The patient is positioned, prepped, and draped for laryngectomy with the abdomen exposed. The abdomen is covered with sterile towels during laryngectomy. When laryngectomy is completed, all instruments and drapes are discarded after the wound has been covered with sterile towels. The patient is again prepped and draped for the free tissue graft.

Standard plastic surgery instruments are used, plus abdominal instruments for the graft and microsurgical and vascular instruments for the graft anastomosis. The operating microscope or loupes may be used for preparation of the graft and graft placement.

Operative procedure. A two-term approach is used. Neck dissection is carried out, at which time donor vessels are identified and preserved. The abdomen is opened, and the ligament of Treitz located. A suitable segment is identified in the first 2 feet of jejunum with a single dominant vascular pedicle. The segment with its pedicle is resected, and bowel continuity reestablished. The abdomen is closed as the microsurgeon prepares the bowel vessel for anastomosis. The donor-recipient vessels in the neck are prepared, using the miscroscope. The proximal bowel anastomosis is made, followed by the vascular anastomosis. When the microvascular clamps are removed, pulsation of the mesenteric vessels and peristalsis should begin. The distal bowel anastomosis is then done. The neck is closed, leaving a small Silastic window over the jejunal segment to allow for close, postoperative observation of the transplant.

Breast reconstruction with latissimus dorsi flap

Definition. Single-stage reconstruction of the breast after mastectomy using a latissimus dorsi myocutaneous island flap.

Considerations. The breast is the leading site of cancer in women. Since breast cancer is the number one killer of women in the United States, mastectomy is the preferred treatment. In recent years use of a latissimus dorsi myocutaneous island flap has made reconstruction possible in one surgical procedure. The goal of reconstruction is to return the woman, as nearly as possible, to her premastectomy state. Change in body image is one of the most difficult psychological aspects of having a breast removed.

Breast reconstruction can be done as early as 6 weeks after a mastectomy, although 3 to 4 months to allow for adequate healing of the surgery site is not unusual. Chemotherapy or radiation therapy may delay reconstruction for a year or more.

Contraindications for having breast reconstruction include very large invasive tumors, extensive chest wall or axillary metastasis, and extensive disease involving other body systems.

Setup and preparation of the patient. The skin island and area of dissection for the latissimus dorsi flap are drawn on the patient's back before prepping and draping (Fig. 21-22).

The patient is placed in a lateral position with the arm on the operative side placed on a sling support. Pressure points are protected by the use of pillows and sheet rolls. The patient is prepped and draped, exposing the affected breast area and muscle.

Standard plastic instruments are used, plus long Metzenbaum scissors, long DeBakey forceps, Freeman areolar markers, lighted breast retractors, and a second electrocautery unit.

Two surgical teams work simultaneously, one freeing the muscle flap and the other preparing the recipient site.

Operative procedure. Initially, the island of skin is incised transversely across the back. The muscle is then freed from the overlying skin by undermining so that part or all of the muscle may be mobilized. The skin island and the muscle are then tunneled through the axilla to the chest wall. The insertion of the muscle on the humerus and accompanying blood vessels are left undisturbed. The latissimus dorsi muscle fills the space left by the missing pectoralis muscle. The island of skin is oriented to the recipient site, and both are sutured into place. A silicone implant is placed under the muscle before suturing to reconstruct the breast mound (Fig. 21-23). The wound is drained by suction drain catheters (Fig. 21-24).

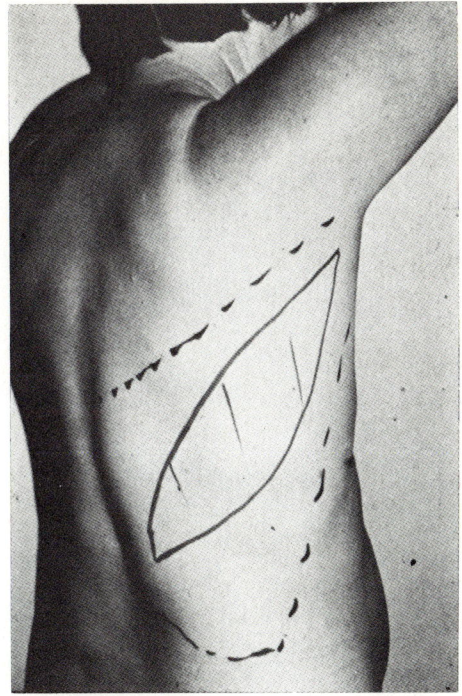

Fig. 21-22. Skin island and dissection for latissimus flap. Flap has been outlined on patient before surgical preparation.

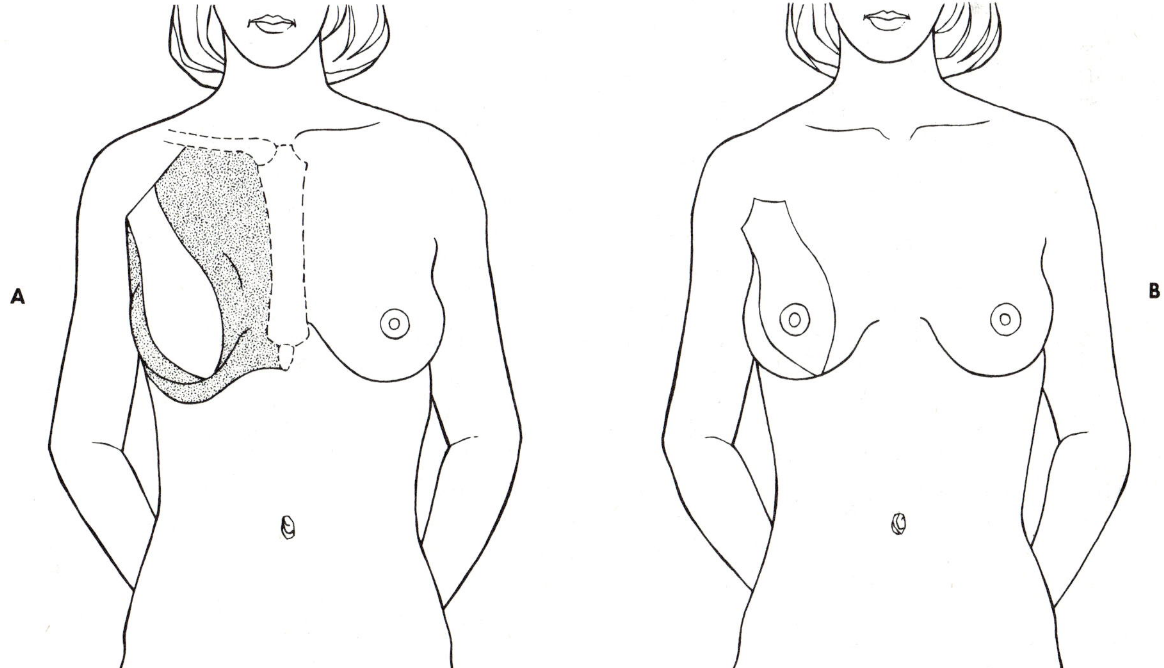

Fig. 21-23. A, Orientation of muscle and skin island over mastectomy site. **B,** Skin and muscle flap in place with silicone prosthesis beneath.

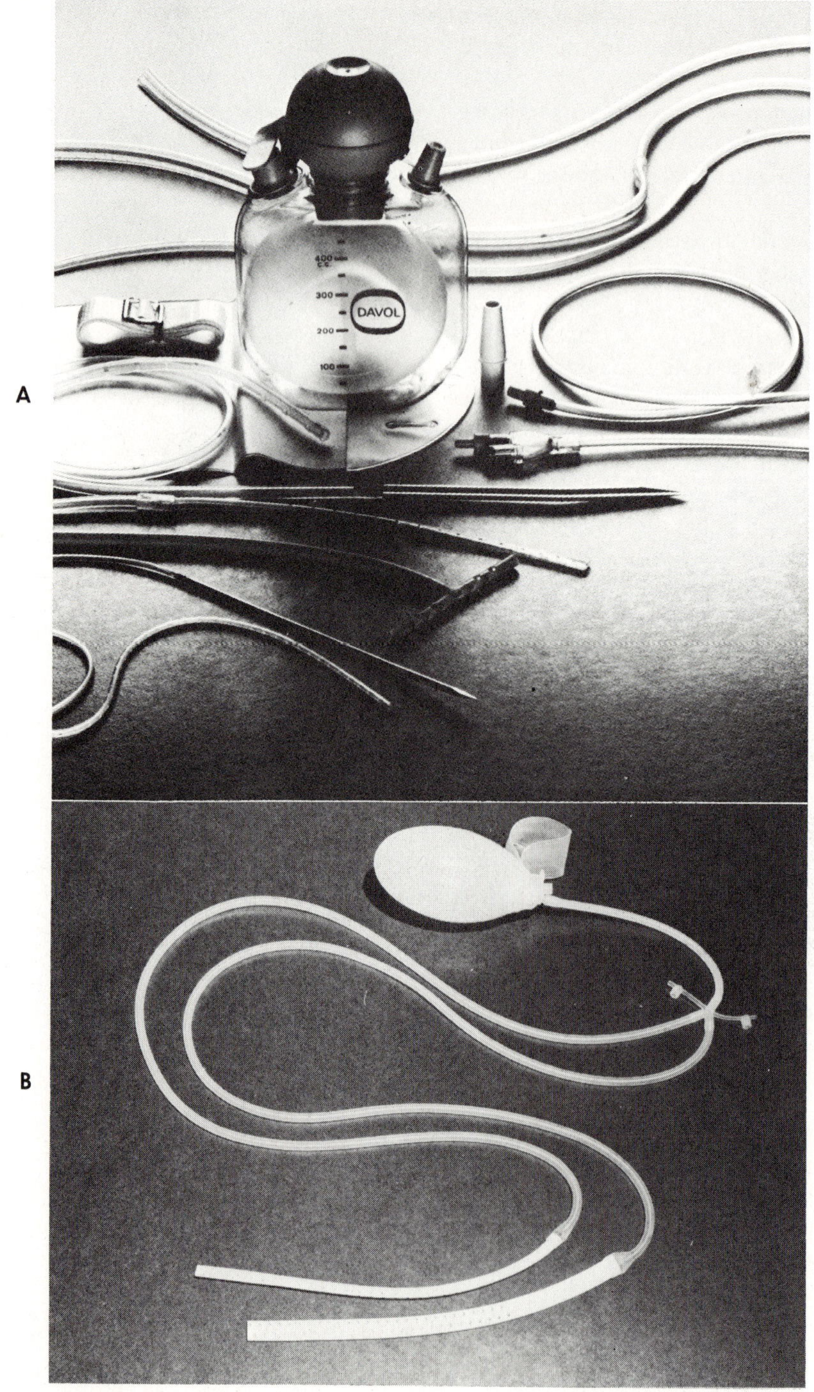

Fig. 21-24. A, Davol drain system. **B,** Heyer-Schulte (Jackson-Pratt) suction drain system. (**A** courtesy Davol, Inc., Cranston, R.I.; **B** provided by American Heyer-Schulte Corp., Goleta, Calif.)

The nipple-areola complex may also be reconstructed by sharing the nipple on the unaffected side or by using groin or auricular tissue. This can be done at the time of reconstruction or at a later date as a minor procedure under local anesthesia (Fig. 21-25).

Augmentation mammoplasty

Definition. Insertion of a silicone breast prosthesis to enlarge or form the breast mound.

Considerations. Breast augmentation is done for hypomastia, to correct breast asymmetry, and to recreate the breast after mastectomy. Formation of a fibrous capsule after insertion of a silicone prosthesis is one of the associated problems. Postoperative exercises aid in reducing capsule formation. Placing the implant under the pectoralis muscle also contributes to softness (Fig. 21-26).

Setup and preparation of the patient. Standard plastic surgery instruments are used, plus lighted fiberoptic retractors. The breast implants are packaged in sterile containers from the manufacturer and given to the scrub nurse when breast size is determined (Fig. 21-27). The patient is placed in a supine position with the arms extended on armboards to approximately 60 degrees. Prepping and draping are carried out in the routine manner to expose the operative site.

Operative procedure. Augmentation mammoplasty is done through areolar, inframammary, or axillary inci-

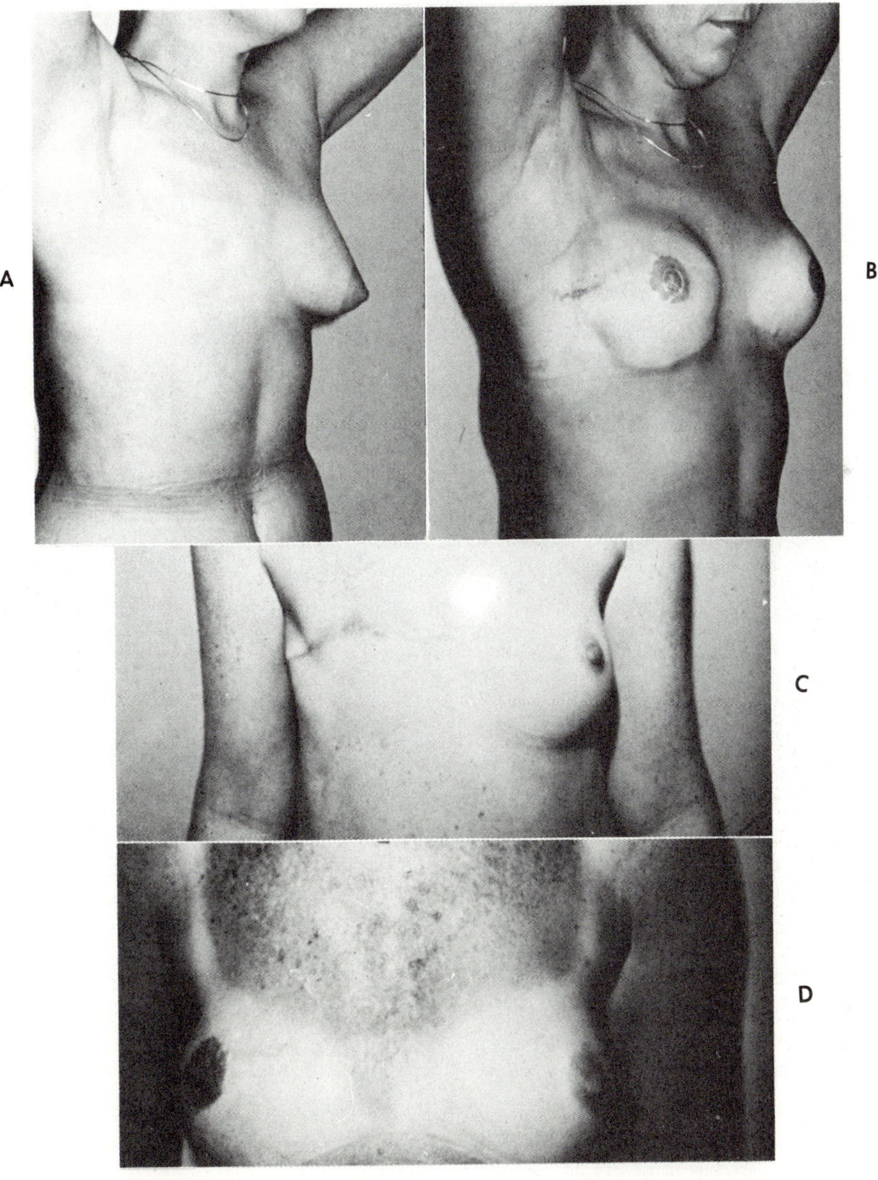

Fig. 21-25. **A** and **C,** Before and, **B** and **D,** after breast reconstruction.

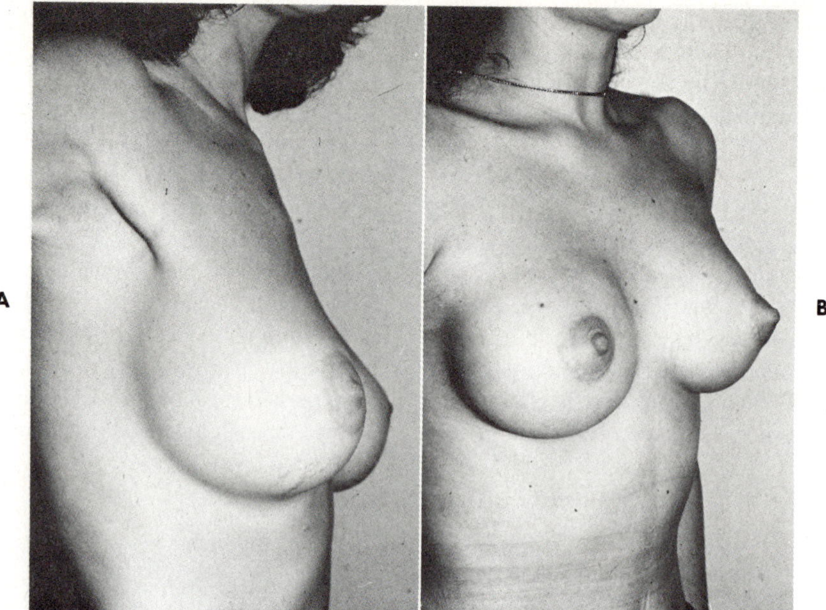

Fig. 21-26. A, Augmentation mammoplasty implant under muscle. B, Implant under breast tissue.

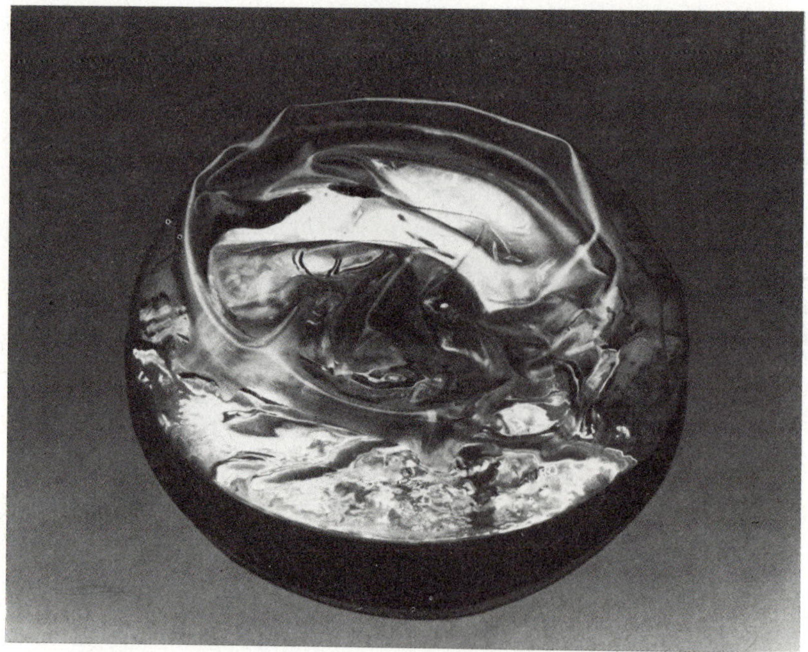

Fig. 21-27. McGhan double-lumen round mammary implant. (Courtesy McGhan Medical/3M, St. Paul, Minn.)

sions. The tissue is elevated, either the breast tissue from the underlying muscle or the pectoralis muscle from the chest wall. A pocket is dissected, and the implant placed in the pocket. Electrosurgical coagulation or suture ligatures may be used to achieve hemostasis. The pocket may be irrigated with an antibiotic solution before placement of the implant. The wound is closed in layers and a light gauze dressing applied. A bra or an Ace wrap may be used for support.

Reduction mammoplasty

Definition. Excision of excessive breast tissue and its overlying skin with reconstruction of breast contour, size, shape, and symmetry (Fig. 21-28).

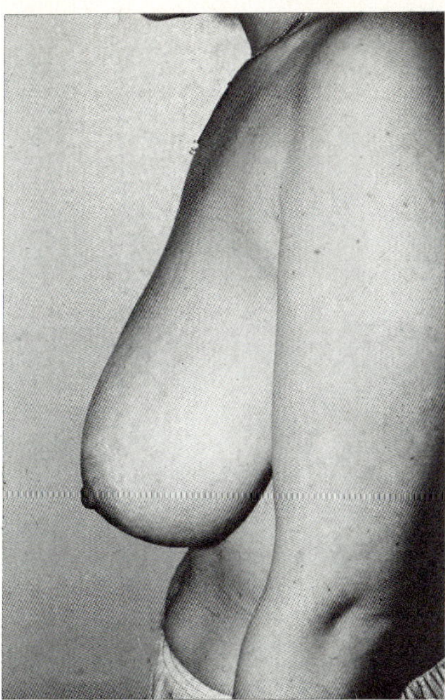

Fig. 21-28. Patient with pendulous breast before reduction mammoplasty.

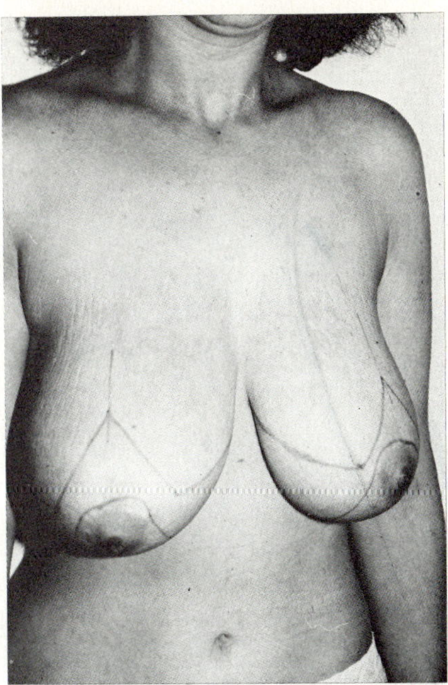

Fig. 21-29. Area of excision marked before surgery.

Considerations. Reduction of the amount of breast tissue may be indicated for the patient with ptosis, disproportion of breast size and body build, or back pain related to posture and the weight of large breasts and obesity. Reduction mammoplasty may be desirable on the unaffected breast following reconstruction of a previous mastectomy site.

Setup and preparation of the patient. Regular plastic surgery instruments are used, plus a Freeman areola marker ("cookie cutter"), a skin stapler, an electrocautery unit, and a marking pen.

The patient is placed in sitting position with arms angled out on armboards. Standard prepping and draping are done.

Operative procedure

1. The skin to be excised, as well as the new site for the nipple, is marked (Fig. 21-29).
2. The skin between the new nipple site is incised and removed, the nipple remaining attached to the underlying breast tissue.
3. The redundant segment of breast tissue inferior to the nipple is excised through an inverted-T incision. Tissue from each breast is measured and kept separately.
4. The nipple and adjacent tissue are mobilized and sutured in place.
5. The medial and lateral skin edges are approximated in a vertical suture line inferior to the nipple.
6. The inframammary elliptical incision is trimmed and closed transversely (Fig. 21-30). Suction drainage catheters may be placed. The wound is dressed.

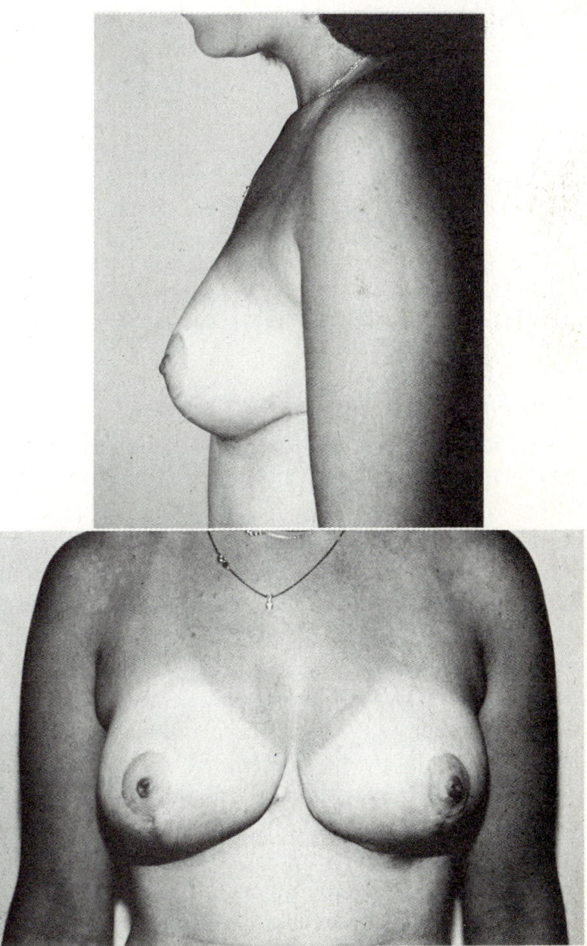

Fig. 21-30. Postoperative reduction mammoplasty.

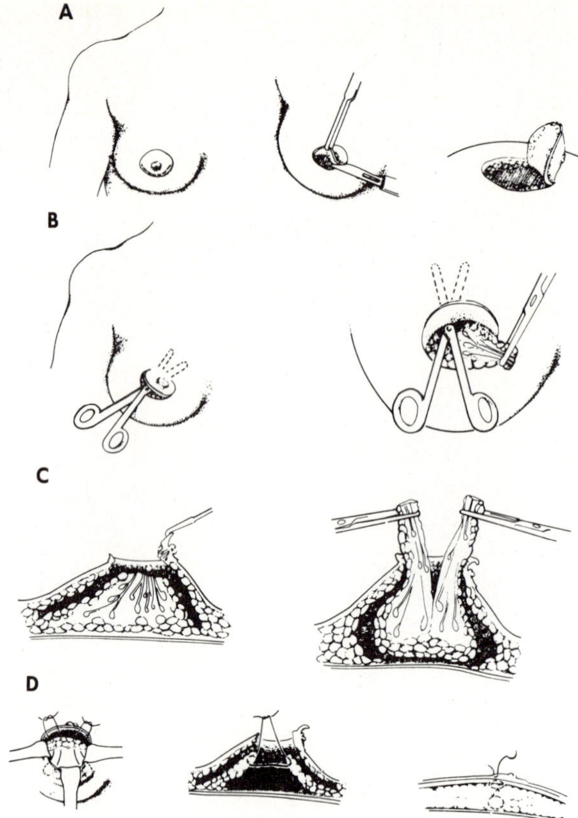

Fig. 21-31. A, Classical intraareolar incision allows access to subjacent fibrofatty breast tissue. **B,** All involved breast tissue is dissected free by careful undermining through intraareolar incision. **C,** Breast tissue is totally removed either as single mass or in sections, depending on size. **D,** Reconstruction is accomplished by adjacent rotation flaps and layered closure to prevent depression in area of resection. (Redrawn from Webster, J.P.: Ann. Surg. **124:**557; from Masters, F.W., and Lewis, J.R.: Symposium on aesthetic surgery of the face, eyelid, and breast, vol. IV, St. Louis, 1972, The C.V. Mosby Co.)

Esthetic reduction of the male breast

Definition. Removal of all subareolar fibroglandular tissue and surgical reconstruction of the resultant defect.

Considerations. Gynecomastia is a relatively common pathological lesion that consists of bilateral or unilateral enlargement of the male breast. It occurs primarily during puberty or after the age of 40, and, although it may be produced by a variety of diseases, it is usually related to excessive hormone production or alterations in hormonal balance. It may also be seen in elderly men after estrogen therapy for carcinoma of the prostate gland.

Setup and preparation of the patient. The patient may be positioned as for a simple mastectomy or in a semi-Fowler position, according to the surgeon's preference. Supplies and equipment needed will be the same as for a simple mastectomy, plus one plastic surgery set.

Operative procedure (Fig. 21-31)

1. An intraareolar incision is made around the inferior half of the areola (Fig. 21-31, A). Through this incision, the fibrous and ductal attachments of the underlying glandular tissue to the nipple are divided. A cuff of fatty tissue is left attached to the underlying nipple surface to protect the blood supply (Fig. 21-31, *B*).
2. With the nipple elevated on the fat-based pedicle, the breast tissue mass is gently dissected (Fig. 21-31, *C*). It is usually necessary to carry the dissection to the pectoral fascia to remove the entire mass.
3. The breast tissue mass is removed through the intraareolar incision. This may be done as one mass, or, if the tissue mass is too large, the mobilized breast tissue can be removed in sections.
4. Hemostasis is carefully controlled by use of ligatures or electrocautery. Adjacent fibrofatty pedicles are mobilized to minimize distortion of the nipple or an obvious depression of the chest wall.
5. When all subcutaneous tissue has been mobilized, a three-layer closure is carried out (Fig. 21-31, *D*). A small rubber drain may be inserted to prevent hematoma formation. A firm pressure dressing is applied.

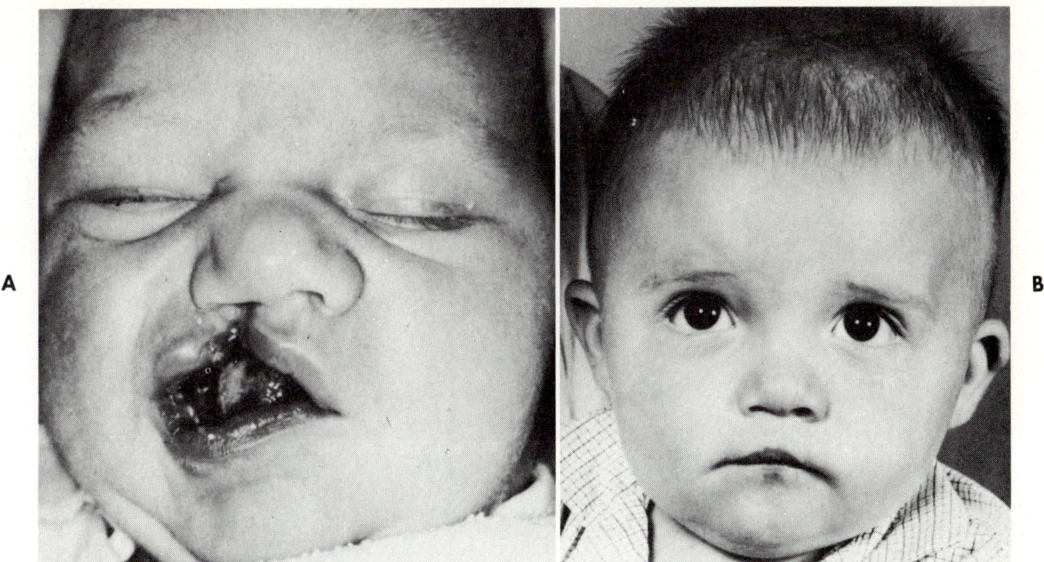

Fig. 21-32. A, Infant with complete unilateral cleft of lip. **B,** Repair, 1 year later.

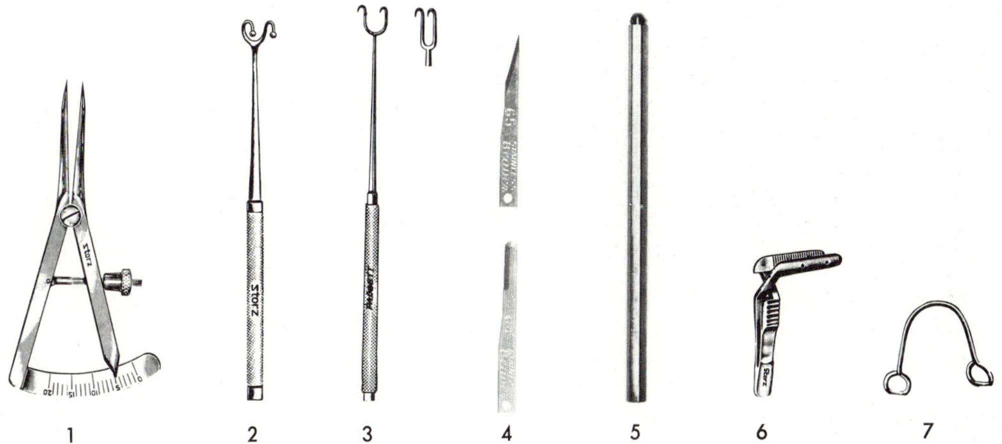

Fig. 21-33. Special instruments for cleft lip repair. *1,* Caliper; *2,* Fomon retractor; *3,* 10-mm and 5-mm double skin hooks; *4,* Beaver scalpel blades nos. 64 and 65; *5,* Beaver scalpel handle; *6,* Brown lip clamp; *7,* Logan's bow.

Correction of congenital deformities

Cleft lip repair

Considerations. The normal upper lip is composed of skin, underlying orbicularis oris muscle, and mucosa. Two skin ridges near the midline outline the central philtrum of the lip. The vermilion (red portion of the lip) peaks at the philtral ridge on each side and gently curves downward as it reaches the midline to form the Cupid's bow. A deficiency in tissue (skin, muscle, and mucosa) along one or both sides of the upper lip, or rarely in the midline, results in a cleft at the site of this deficiency. The deficiency of tissue present with a cleft lip results in distortion of the Cupid's bow, absence of one or both philtral ridges, and distortion of the lower portion of the nose. Cleft lip is usually associated with a notch or cleft of the underlying alveolus and a cleft of the palate.

Cleft lip repair is most often performed when the infant is about 3 months of age. Lip repair is directed toward rearrangement of existing tissues to approximate the normal lip as closely as possible (Fig. 21-32). Some consideration may also be given to correcting the nasal deformity at the time of cleft lip repair.

Setup and preparation of the patient. A plastic local instrument set is required, plus the following special instruments (Fig. 21-33):

2 Brown lip clamps
2 Calipers
1 Fomon retractor
2 Skin hooks, double, 5 mm
Beaver scalpel handles and blades
Logan's bow
2 Bard-Parker knife blades, no. 11
1 Needle, 25 gauge, on straight hemostat
2 Cotton-tipped applicator sticks
1 Tongue depressor, disposable
Marking pen
Methylene blue
Epinephrine 1:200,000 (for injection)

The patient is placed in the supine position, with the head at the edge of one end of the operating table. The head drape is used. The surgeon may stand or sit at the patient's side or just above the patient's head during the operation.

Operative procedure. Many types of cleft lip repair are in common use, one of which is illustrated in Fig. 21-34. The following steps are applicable to all lip repairs:

1. Normal landmarks are identified and marked or tattooed. Precise measurements, using calipers and a ruler, are made so that corresponding points can be marked along the cleft.
2. The lip may be infiltrated with epinephrine 1:200,000, or lip clamps may be used to aid hemostasis.
3. Incisions are made along the markings for the repair.
4. The abnormal musculature is dissected.
5. Additional dissection along the maxilla and nose may be performed.
6. Closure is done in three layers: muscle, skin, and mucosa.
7. A Logan's bow is applied to the cheeks with tape strips.

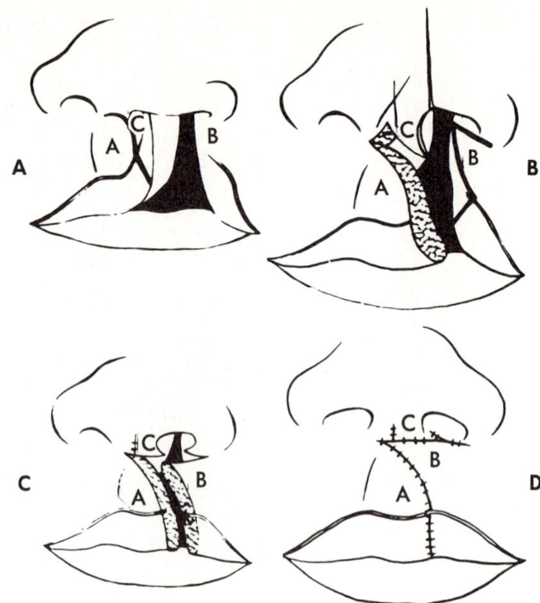

Fig. 21-34. Rotation-advancement method to correct complete unilateral cleft of lip. **A,** Rotation incision marked so that Cupid's bow-dimple component *A* will rotate down into normal position; flap C will advance into columella and then form nostril sill. **B,** Flap *A* has dropped down, flap C has advanced into columella, and flap *B* has been marked. **C,** Flap *B* is being advanced into rotation gap; white skin roll flap is interdigitated at mucocutaneous junction line. **D,** Scar is maneuvered into strategic position where it is hidden at nasal base and floor and philtrum column and interdigitated at mucocutaneous junction. (From Millard, D.R.: In Grabb, W.C., and Smith, J.W., editors: Plastic surgery: a concise guide to clinical practice, Boston, Little, Brown & Co.)

Cleft palate repair

Considerations. The palate is made up of the bony or hard palate anteriorly and the soft palate posteriorly. The alveolus borders the hard palate. A separation or cleft of the palate occurs in the midline and may involve only the soft palate or both hard and soft palates. The alveolus may be cleft on one or both sides.

The major function of the soft palate is to aid in the production of normal speech sounds. An intact hard palate is necessary to prevent escape of air through the nose during speech and to prevent the egress of liquid and food from the nose.

Cleft palate repair is usually performed when a child is from 12 to 18 months old. The various operations used to achieve surgical closure of the palate all employ tissue adjacent to the cleft (in the form of flaps) and shift it centrally to close the defect.

Setup and preparation of the patient. A basic plastic instrument set is required, plus the following special instruments (Fig. 21-35):

Dingman mouth gag with assorted blades
1 Blair palate hook
2 Palate knives
1 Blair palate elevator, L-shaped
2 Burlisher clamps, curved
2 Crile-Wood needle holders, 6 inches
2 Fomon lower lateral scissors, 1 short and 1 long
2 Cushing tissue forceps, 7 inches
2 Cushing dressing forceps, 7 inches
1 Brown forceps, 6 inches
12 Cottonoids with strings, 1 × 1 inch
Epinephrine 1:200,000 (for injection)
Marking pen
Bipolar cautery
Volumetric suction bottle

The patient is placed in the supine position, with the head at the edge of one end of the operating table. The head drape is used. Many surgeons sit just above the pa-

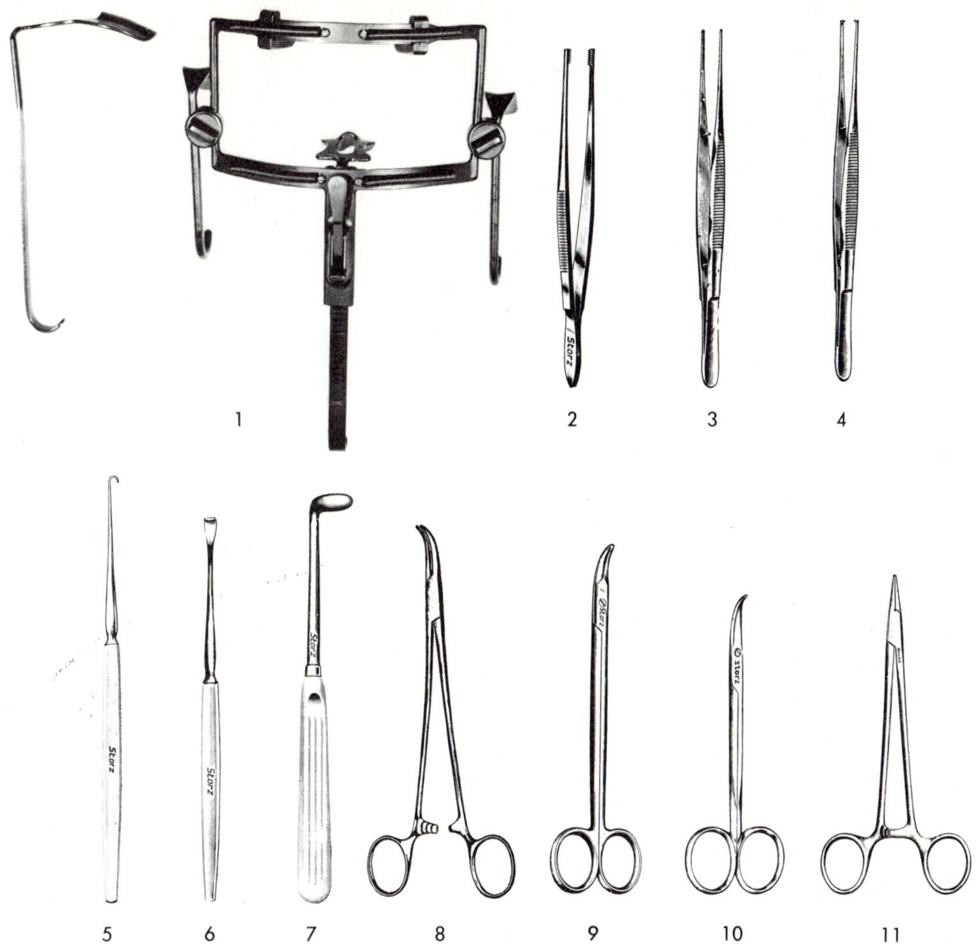

Fig. 21-35. Special instruments for cleft palate repair. *a*, Dingman mouth gag with assorted blades; *2*, Brown forceps; *3*, Cushing dressing forceps; *4*, Cushing tissue forceps; *5*, Blair palate hook; *6*, palate knife; *7*, Blair L-shaped palate elevator; *8*, curved Burlisher clamp; *9*, long Fomon lower lateral scissors; *10*, short Fomon lower lateral scissors; *11*, Crile-Wood needle holder.

tient's head and cradle the head on their lap (with the patient's neck hyperextended).

Operative procedure. One of the most frequently used cleft palate repairs is illustrated in Fig. 21-36. The following steps are common to all palate repairs:

1. The Dingman mouth gag is inserted. Maintenance of the position of the endotracheal tube is crucial at this point.
2. The outlines of the palatal flaps are marked.
3. The palate is injected with epinephrine 1:200,000 for hemostasis.
4. The flaps are incised and elevated.
5. Closure is in three layers: nasal mucosa, muscle, and palatal mucosa.
6. A large horizontal mattress traction suture is placed through the body of the tongue. If the patient experiences upper airway obstruction after extubation, traction is placed on this suture to pull the tongue forward, rather than inserting an airway that might harm the palate repair.

Pharyngeal flap

Definition. Tissue taken from the posterior pharyngeal wall and used to add tissue to a deficient soft palate.

Considerations. When abnormal speech (velopharyngeal insufficiency) results despite a cleft palate repair, a secondary surgical procedure may be necessary to improve speech. Typical "cleft palate speech" is characterized primarily by an excess of air escaping through the nose during speech. This hypernasality often results from insufficient bulk and/or movement of the muscles of the soft palate. To decrease or eliminate this problem, tissue from the pharynx, in the form of a pharyngeal flap, is added to the soft palate. This flap also reduces the size of the opening between the oropharynx and nasopharynx,

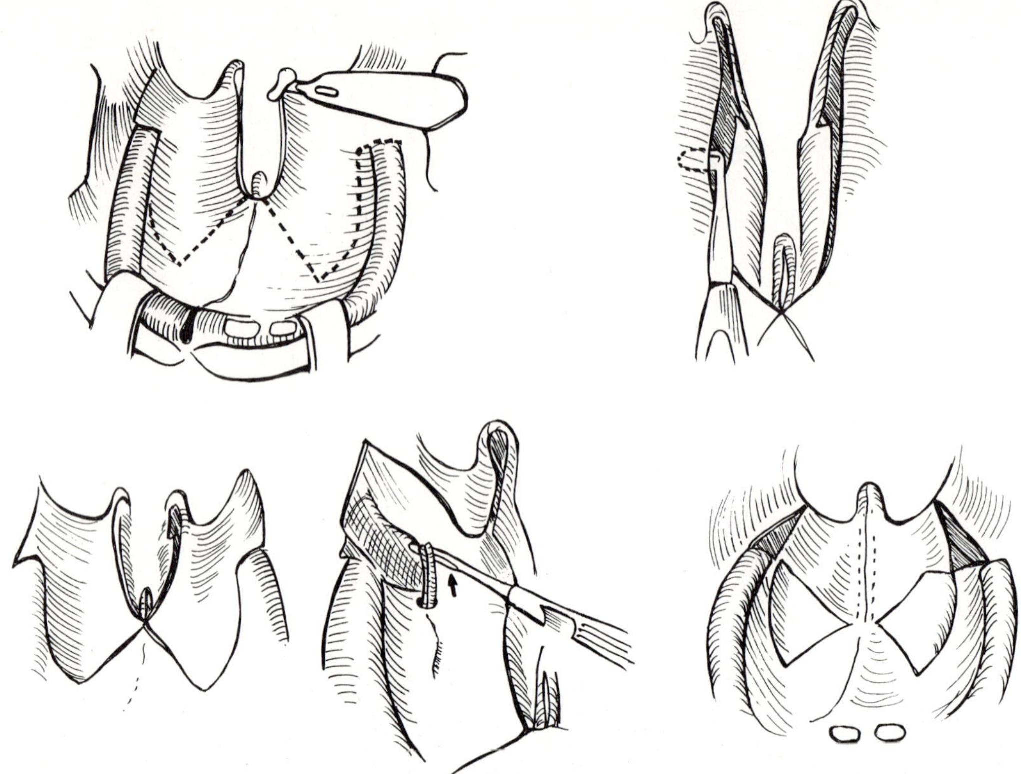

Fig. 21-36. Closure of cleft of soft palate by V-Y (Wardill-Kilner) palatoplasty. A V-shaped incision is made on oral side of palate; mucoperiosteal flaps are elevated on oral and nasal sides, with preservation of blood vessels; Y-shaped closure (in three layers) closes cleft and lengthens palate. (Redrawn from Randall, P.: In Grabb, W.C., and Smith, J.W., editors: Plastic surgery: a concise guide to clinical practice, Boston, Little, Brown & Co.)

thus decreasing or eliminating the nasal escape of air during speech.

A pharyngeal flap repair may be done at any age, but most are done before the patient is 14 years old. A pharyngeal flap also may be a part of primary cleft palate repair.

Setup and preparation of the patient. The same instruments are needed as for cleft palate repair, plus two no. 14 Fr red rubber catheters.

Positioning and draping of the patient are as described for cleft palate repair.

Operative procedure

1. The Dingman mouth gag is inserted.
2. The palate and posterior wall of the pharynx are injected with epinephrine 1:200,000 for hemostasis.
3. The palate is incised, and the pharyngeal flap is incised and elevated.
4. The pharyngeal wall donor site may be sutured or left open.
5. The pharyngeal flap is sutured to the palate, and the palate is closed.
6. A traction suture is placed through the body of the tongue.

Ear reconstruction for microtia

Considerations. Microtia refers to congenital total or subtotal absence of the external ear. The technique of ear reconstruction for microtia described here also may be applied to traumatic defects of the external ear. The external ear is a complex structure composed of numerous fine details. Its basic framework is cartilage with a thin layer of subcutaneous tissue and skin covering the cartilage. It is difficult to reproduce the fine detail of the normal ear. The general principles of ear reconstruction include placing a framework (carved costal cartilage) in a subcutaneous tissue pocket and, later, lifting this away from the side of the head. This requires several individual operations, or stages, to complete. Since the external ear has attained virtually full growth by age 6 years, ear reconstruction is usually started at age 4 years and completed by the time the child begins school.

Setup and preparation of the patient. A plastic local instrument set is required, plus calipers, a marking pen, and epinephrine 1:200,000 for injection.

If the operation includes obtaining an autogenous costal cartilage graft, the following separate setup is required in addition to a plastic local instrument set:

2 Bard-Parker knife blades, no. 10
1 Key periosteal elevator
1 Duckbill rongeur
1 Rib shears, small
1 Alexander costal periostome
1 Teflon cutting board
Bipolar cautery
X-ray film, unexposed

The patient is placed in the supine position on the operating table. The head drape is used, leaving both ears and postauricular areas well exposed. The lower costal cartilages on one side are also prepared and draped if a cartilage graft is to be used.

Operative procedure

1. During the first-stage operation, the ear remnants are excised or repositioned, as indicated.

2. Simultaneously, or during a second-stage operation, a costal cartilage graft (which must be carved to resemble the normal auricular cartilage framework) or a preformed silicone ear implant is placed in a subcutaneous pocket along the side of the head.

3. Several months later, the ear framework in its subcutaneous pocket is elevated from the side of the head and, a split-thickness skin graft is used to cover the retroauricular defect.

4. Subsequent stages include various adjustments, often using split-thickness or full-thickness skin grafts, to make the ear appear more normal.

Otoplasty

Definition. Correction of a congenital deformity in which the ear protrudes abnormally from the side of the head.

Considerations. This deformity is generally the result of an absent or insufficiently pronounced antihelical fold of the external ear. The various methods of otoplasty attempt correction by creating an antihelical fold, which "pins" the ear back against the side of the head (Fig. 21-37). Protruding ears may be unilateral or bilateral. Otoplasty is usually performed on children just before they start school. It is also performed on adults, in which case either general or local anesthesia may be used.

Setup and preparation of the patient. A plastic local instrument set is needed, plus the following:

Calipers
Milliner's needles
Cotton-tipped applicator sticks
Methylene blue
Dingman oto rader
Marking pen
Epinephrine 1:200,000 for injection

The patient is placed in the supine position on the operating table, and a head drape is used, leaving both ears well exposed. The patient's head is turned with the affected ear up and with the lower ear well padded to avoid pressure injury.

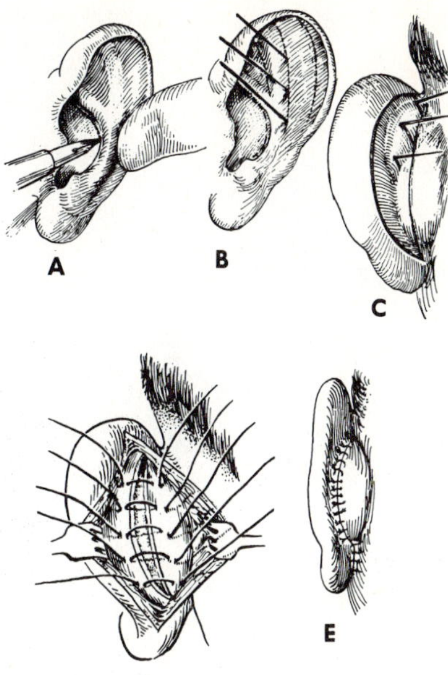

Fig. 21-37. Otoplasty for correction of protruding ears. **A,** Antihelix defined by applying pressure to ear. **B,** Position of antihelical fold marked by passing milliner's needles through ear. **C,** Needle points visible along posterior surface of ear with ellipse of skin to be excised marked. **D,** Section of ear cartilage incised and scored or excised with sutures placed to hold cartilage back. **E,** Posterior ear incision sutured. (Redrawn from Wood-Smith, D., and Porowski, P.C., editors: Nursing care of the plastic surgery patient, St. Louis, The C.V. Mosby Co.; and Converse, J.M., editor: Reconstructive plastic surgery, vol. 3, Philadelphia, W.B. Saunders Co.)

Operative procedure

1. The antihelical fold is created by bending the external ear backward. The position of the antihelical fold is marked by placing approximately six milliner's needles through the ear from anterior to posterior, applying methylene blue to the tip of the needles, and withdrawing them.

2. An ellipse of skin is excised from the posterior surface of the ear after it has been infiltrated with epinephrine 1:200,000 for hemostasis.

3. The ear cartilage is usually incised near the antihelical fold, and the anterior surface of the cartilage is scored to allow it to bend backward.

4. Sutures are usually placed to hold the cartilage in its new position.

5. The skin incision is closed.

6. A bulky dressing exerting moderate compression on the ears is applied. Cotton is usually placed behind the ear to avoid pressing the posterior ear surface against the side of the head.

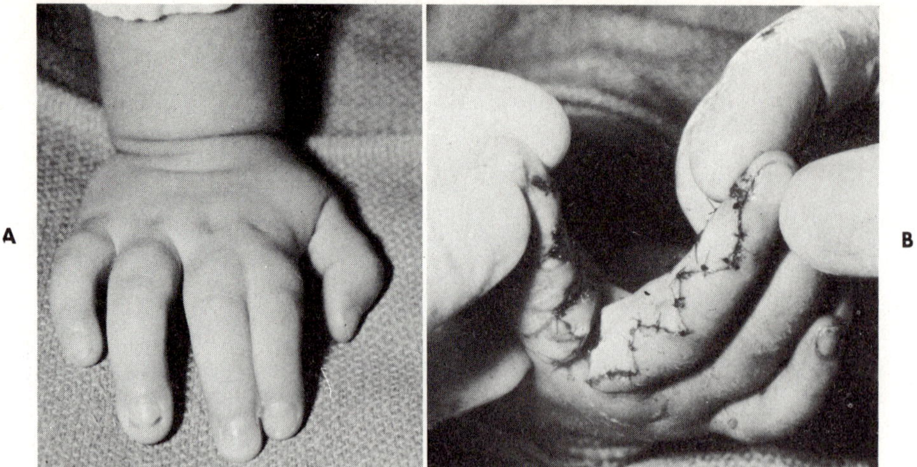

Fig. 21-38. A, Syndactyly involving index and long fingers. **B,** Skin web separated; triangular flaps and skin grafts visible along sides of both fingers.

Repair of syndactyly

Considerations. Syndactyly refers to webbing of the digits of the hand or feet. The most common form of syndactyly is symmetrical webbing in two otherwise normal hands. It may, however, be associated with other abnormalities in the hand, such as extra fingers (polydactyly) or bony abnormalities. In syndactyly with normal digits, a web of skin joins adjacent fingers; each finger, however, has its own tendons, vessels, nerves, and bony phalanges. Although the skin web may appear loose, a deficiency in skin is always present when surgical separation is undertaken. Plans for taking a skin graft (usually full thickness) should always be made (Fig. 21-38). Surgical separation of syndactyly is performed at any time after the age of approximately 12 months.

Toe syndactyly is less often treated surgically than finger syndactyly, since proper function of the foot does not necessitate fine movements of individual toes. Although the setup and description that follow are for the repair of finger syndactyly, they can also be applied to the repair of toe syndactyly.

Setup and preparation of the patient. A plastic local instrument set is required, plus a marking pen, unexposed x-ray film, a pediatric pneumatic tourniquet, and an Esmarch bandage.

The patient is placed in the supine position on the operating table with the affected arm extended on a hand table. A pediatric pneumatic tourniquet is used. A hand drape is used, and both inguinal areas are prepped and draped (donor sites for full-thickness skin grafts).

Operative procedure

1. Skin incisions are marked, and the tourniquet is inflated.
2. The skin is incised, and small flaps at the sides of fingers and in the web are elevated.
3. After these flaps have been sutured into position, patterns of areas of absent skin on sides of fingers are made and transferred to the skin-graft donor site.
4. The skin graft is taken, and the donor-site wound is dealt with appropriately.
5. Skin grafts are sutured to fingers.
6. Stent dressings are placed over the skin grafts. The entire hand is immobilized in a bulky dressing (see hand surgery section) or in a long-arm plaster cast.

Hypospadias repair

Considerations. Hypospadias is a congenital anomaly in which the urethra ends on the ventral surface of the penile shaft or in the perineum. This is usually accompanied by a downward curvature of the penis, called *chordee,* especially during erection.

The goal of hypospadias repair is to allow for a normal urinary stream and for normal sexual function. This requires excision of the scar tissue that causes the chordee and construction of a urethra that extends to the distal end of the penis (Chapter 15). Hypospadias repair is usually performed between the ages of 1 and 2 years, so that psychosocial problems can be prevented.

Construction of a new urethra requires the addition of new tissue along the ventral surface of the penis. Most patients with hypospadias have not been circumcised. This is advantageous because the prepuce can be used to provide the extra tissue that is needed (usually in flap form). Some methods of hypospadias repair make use of free skin grafts.

More than 150 different operations have been described for the correction of hypospadias. The advances in the state of the art of hypospadias repair over the past decade have led to a one-stage procedure usually with the technique of Horton and Devine. The Hodgson technique

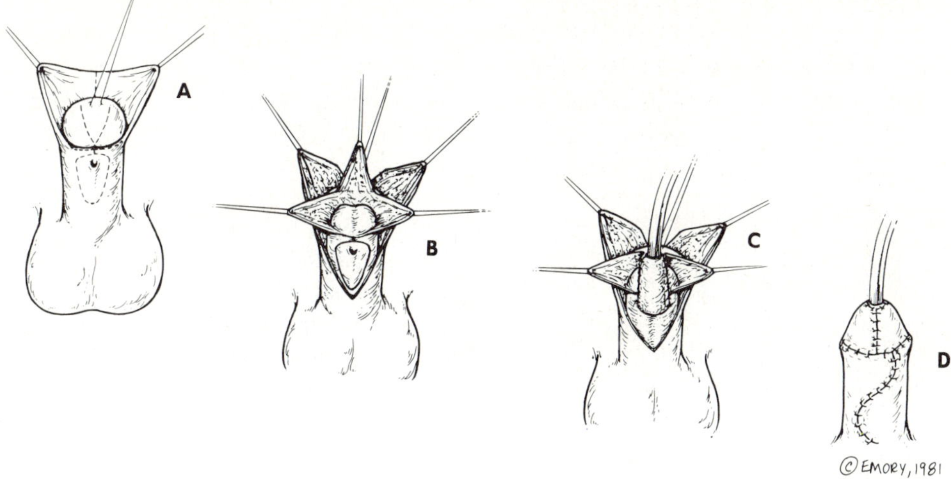

Fig. 21-39. Horton-Devine repair of hypospadias. **A,** Incisions from meatus to coronal sulcus. **B,** Triangular flap is elevated, and lateral wings of glans are freed. **C,** Urethral meatus is outlined and elevated. **D,** Functional and cosmetic closure is completed with small feeding tube or Foley catheter in place. (Courtesy Emory University School of Medicine, Atlanta, Ga.)

is an alternative for repair of the defect, depending on the choice of the surgeon and characteristics of the patient's deformity. It employs the establishment of an island of tissue from which a tube may be constructed to connect the urethra through an acceptable cosmetic channel to the tip of the penis. A transurethral plastic stent remains in place postoperatively for 7 days. Although the Hodgson method is a popular approach to repair of hypospadias, the Horton-Devine repair will be detailed here. The suggested readings at the end of the chapter include references for specific variations and alternatives for the one- or mutliple-stage repair and the rationale for selecting each technique.

Setup and preparation of the patient. Instrumentation includes a plastic local instrument set, plus urethral sounds, nos. 8 to 22 Fr; red rubber urethral catheters, nos. 8 to 22 Fr, with a guide or stylet; a small feeding tube; a lubricant for the catheter and sounds; and a bipolar cautery.

The patient is placed in the supine position on the operating table, with a folded sheet beneath the buttocks to elevate the hips slightly and with legs stabilized in a frog-leg position. The perineum is scrubbed with soap and water and is towel dried, followed by an application of the routine skin preparation.

Operative procedure. The Horton-Devine repair (Fig. 21-39) consists of the following steps:

1. Lidocaine with 1:200,000 epinephrine is injected for hemostatic purposes.
2. Incisions are made into the shaft and fibrous tissue beginning at the meatus and continuing to the coronal sulcus and encircling the glans penis. The chordee (scar tissue) is resected.
3. The dissection continues beneath the glans, a triangular flap is elevated, and lateral wings of the glans are freed with sharp dissection.
4. On the ventral surface of the penis a long penile flap, based distally on the urethral meatus, is outlined and elevated.
5. The glans flap is used to form the roof of the urethra using nos. 5-0 and 6-0 Dexon sutures.
6. The retrograde portion of the flap is flipped forward to form the ventral surface of the urethra, using multiple interrupted sutures to complete the reconstruction of the glans.
7. The lateral wings are now brought around the neourethra and are sutured together at the midline.
8. The ventral skin deficit is closed with preputial flaps.
9. A small feeding tube or indwelling Foley catheter is left in place for 3 days after surgery.
10. Postoperative edema is controlled with a compression dressing of Elastoplast, which is placed snugly but not tightly around the shaft of the penis.

The two-stage operation described by Byars yields reproducible results and is therefore described here.

First stage (Fig. 21-40, *A*)

1. An indwelling catheter is placed into the bladder through the existing urethral meatus.
2. A traction suture is placed through the glans penis.
3. The chordee (scar tissue) is excised from the urethral opening to the tip of the glans.
4. The prepuce is incised in the dorsal midline, creating two folded flaps.
5. Both preputial flaps are unfolded and rotated ventrally to cover the defect between the meatus and tip of the glans left by excision of the chordee.

6. The flaps are sutured in place with the ends of the sutures left long.

7. A dressing of nonadherent gauze and acrylic fiber is placed over the flaps, and the long ends of the sutures are tied over it. The entire penile shaft is then encased with inch-wide strips of Elastoplast.

8. The catheter is taped to the patient's thigh, and open drainage is maintained by placing the end of the catheter within two folded abdominal pads held in place at the thigh by ties.

Second stage (Fig. 21-40, *B*)

1. A French catheter with a stylet in the lumen is inserted into the bladder through the existing meatus.

2. The stylet is rotated to permit palpation of its tip in the perineum; an incision is made over the prominence into the urethra.

3. The distal (flared) end of the catheter is pulled out through the perineal urethrostomy and sutured in place.

4. A traction suture is placed through the glans penis.

5. A rectangular area surrounding the urethral defect is incised from the meatus to the tip of the glans. This tissue is tubed by suturing the edges together, thus forming the new urethra. The surrounding skin edges are undermined and sutured together over the new urethral tube.

6. The penile shaft is dressed with gauze and inch-wide Elastoplast strips.

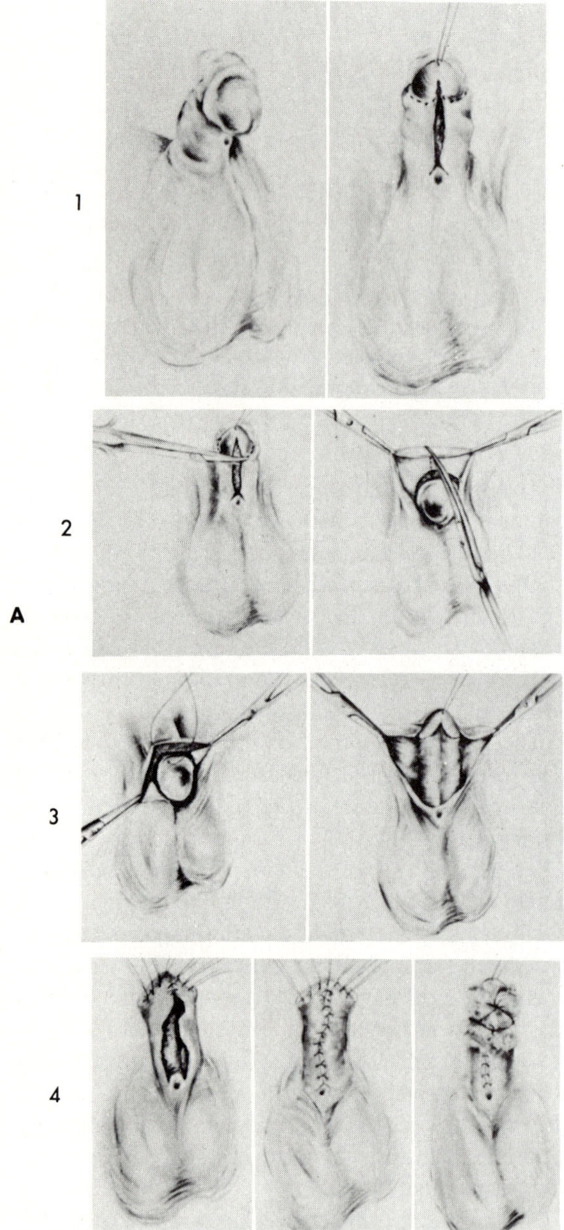

Fig. 21-40. Byars hypospadias repair. **A,** First stage. *1,* Midpenile shaft hypospadias with chordee at left; traction suture through glans and initial incision of first stage at right. *2,* Preputial incision at left; dorsal slit incision at right. *3,* Preputial flaps developed, and midline suture placed dorsally to stabilize known points at left; ventral surface presents large raw area where scar has been excised to straighten penis at right. *4,* Preputial flaps sutured over ventral penile shaft raw surface, and tie-over dressing placed over flaps. (From Byars, L.T.: Surg. Gynecol. Obstet. **92:**149.)

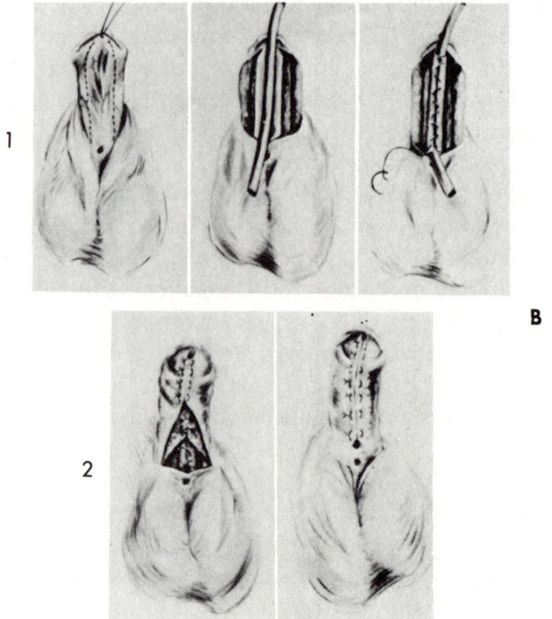

Fig. 21-40, cont'd. B, Second stage (perineal urethrostomy has been done). *1,* Rectangular incision from meatus to tip of glans; sides of this flap are elevated and inverted to form new urethral tube. *2,* Closure of subcutaneous tissue and skin in multiple tiers over new urethral tube. Operation depicted here was done in three stages; it is now done in two stages with new urethral tube and existing meatus connected at time of second-stage repair. (From Byars, L.T.: Surg. Gynecol. Obstet. **92:**149.)

7. Catheter drainage is the same as step 8 of the first-stage operation.

The major complication of these procedures is urethrocutaneous fistulas, which may require further surgery or heal spontaneously. Of note in the one-stage technique is the use of the Gittes and McLaughlin manner of injection to induce penile erection, thus indicating the degree of success of the removal of the constricting chordee.

Orbital-craniofacial surgery

Considerations. A number of congenital anomalies involve the orbital-craniofacial skeleton. These include (1) hypertelorism (Fig. 21-41), in which the distance between the orbits is increased; (2) Crouzon's disease (Fig. 21-42), which includes premature closure of the cranial sutures, resulting in an abnormally shaped skull, exophthalmos and hypertelorism, parrot's beak nose, and maxillary hypoplasia; and (3) Apert's syndrome, which includes the same craniofacial deformities as Crouzon's disease plus syndactyly or other hand anomalies. Recent advances in plastic surgery make surgical correction of some of these deformities possible.

Binocular vision is normal in humans. It involves the coordinated use of both eyes to obtain a single mental impression of objects. Binocular vision is usually absent in the craniofacial anomalies because of the increased distance between the orbits. The purpose of orbital-craniofacial surgery is to provide the patient with binocular vision, by moving the orbits closer together, and to provide the patient with a more acceptable appearance, by moving the bones of the orbital-craniofacial skeleton into a more normal position. Correction of the deformity seen in Crouzon's disease and Apert's syndrome involves a surgically created Le Fort III maxillary fracture.

Although an extracranial approach may be used, an intracranial approach is used in most cases; therefore a neurosurgeon as well as a plastic surgeon performs these operations through a bifrontal (coronal) craniotomy approach. A tracheostomy may be done before the start of the procedure. Bone grafts are necessary to augment areas of bone deficit, which result from movement of the craniofacial skeleton.

These operations are usually performed on children. They are very extensive procedures, often lasting 12 to 14 hours. Blood loss is considerable. Postoperative complications, such as cerebral edema or meningitis, can be formidable. The operating room nurse must pay particular attention to the following important details: (1) insertion of a Foley catheter into the patient's bladder before the operation is started, (2) positioning of the patient on the operating table so that all bony prominences are well padded, and (3) availability of accurate means for measuring blood loss (usually a volumetric suction bottle and scales for weighing sponges).

Setup and preparation of the patient. A basic plastic instrument set, craniectomy instruments and supplies (Chapter 24), and tracheostomy instruments and supplies (Chapter 22) are required, plus the following:

Hall II air drill
Stryker oscillating and reciprocating bone saws
6 Osteotomes, assorted sizes, straight and curved
1 Mallet
3 Curettes, assorted
3 Rongeurs, assorted
2 Calipers
1 Brown fascia needle
1 Set coil arch bars
2 Rowe maxillary forceps
2 Polyethylene buttons
2 Foam rubber pads, small
Volumetric suction bottle
Marking pen

A separate setup is necessary for obtaining the bone graft. It includes a plastic hand instrument set, plus the following:

1 Weitlaner retractor
3 Curettes, assorted
6 Osteotomes, assorted
1 Mallet
Hall II air drill
Teflon cutting board

The patient is positioned, prepped, and draped as described for a bifrontal craniotomy (Chapter 24). The entire face is left exposed, however, and may temporarily be covered with a plastic drape until the portion of the operation requiring access to the face is reached. The bone-graft donor site is also prepped and draped so that both iliac crests and the lower ribs are exposed.

Operative procedure

1. Tracheostomy, if required, is performed first, followed by application of arch bars, when indicated (as in Crouzon's disease and Apert's syndrome).

2. The bifrontal craniotomy/craniectomy is performed.

3. Orbital osteotomies into the anterior cranial fossa are performed bilaterally.

4. Bilateral conjunctival (lower eyelid) and labiogingival sulcus incisions (for Crouzon's disease and Apert's syndrome) are made for other orbital and for maxillary osteotomies.

5. The bones of the orbital-craniofacial region are now moved, based on measurement of the intercanthal distance (in hypertelorism) and/or occlusion of the teeth (in Crouzon's disease and Apert's syndrome).

6. Bone grafts are obtained from the iliac crest and/or lower ribs.

7. Bone grafts are fixed in place with interosseous wires and by means of intermaxillary fixation applied to arch bars (for Crouzon's disease and Apert's syndrome) (Fig. 21-43).

8. The craniotomy, conjunctival, intraoral, and bone-graft donor-site incisions are closed.

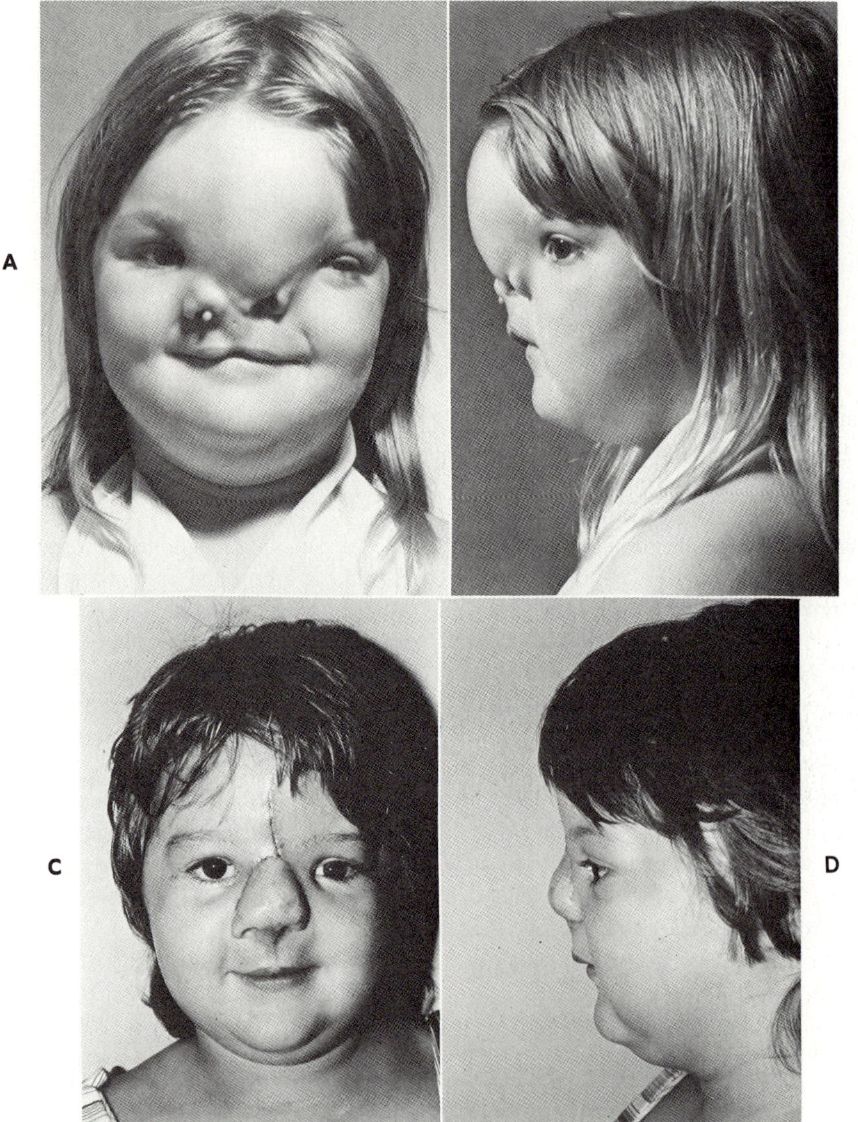

Fig. 21-41. Hypertelorism. **A** and **B,** Before surgery, front and side views. **C** and **D,** After surgery, front and side views. (Courtesy Emory University School of Medicine, Atlanta, Ga.)

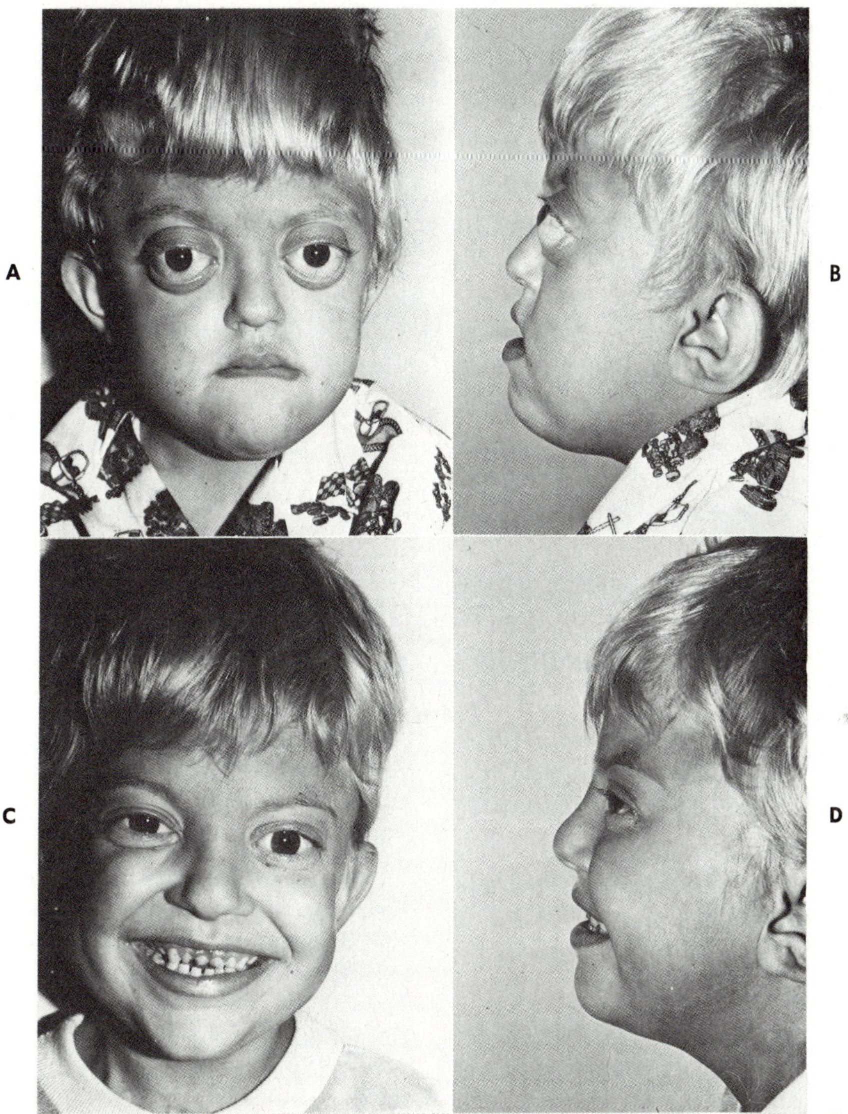

Fig. 21-42. Crouzon's disease. **A** and **B,** Before surgery, front and side views. **C** and **D,** After surgery, front and side views. (Courtesy Emory University School of Medicine, Atlanta, Ga.)

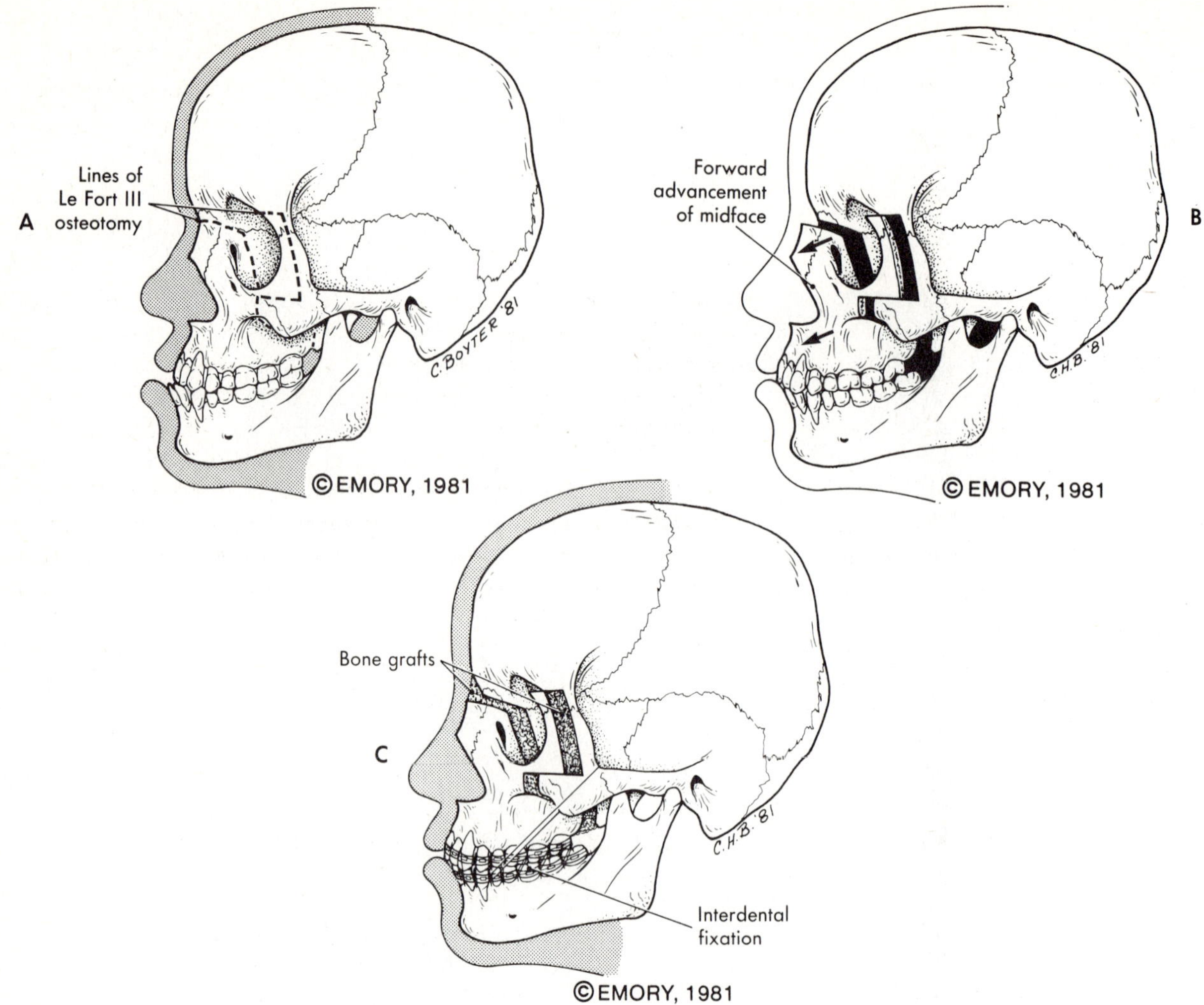

Fig. 21-43. Steps in surgical correction of Crouzon's disease deformities. (Courtesy Emory University School of Medicine, Atlanta, Ga.)

Surgery for maxillofacial trauma

Reduction of nasal fracture

Definition. Usually a closed procedure performed by digital and instrumental manipulation. Rarely, an open reduction with interosseous wire fixation of nasal bone fragments is necessary.

Considerations. A nasal fracture may involve a fracture of the nasal bones and/or cartilage (including the septum). Closed reduction of a nasal fracture is most often performed under local and topical anesthesia.

Setup and preparation of the patient. A plastic local instrument set is required, plus the following:

2 Nasal specula, 1 short and 1 long
1 Asch forceps or rubber-shod Kelly forceps
4 Metal applicator sticks and wisps of cotton
1 Brown nasal splint
Nasal packing of choice
Local and topical anesthetic agents of choice

The patient is placed in the supine position on the operating table. An intravenous infusion is started and a blood pressure cuff is applied. The head drape is used.

Operative procedure

1. Topical anesthesia for the nasal mucosa and nerve-block anesthesia around the nose are administered.
2. The Asch forceps is introduced intranasally to elevate the bony fragments, while with digital pressure, the surgeon's other hand molds the bones into position.
3. The nasal septum is inspected and realigned with the Asch forceps, if necessary.
4. Bilateral anterior nasal packs are placed.
5. Half-inch tape strips are applied over the skin of the nose, followed by application of the nasal splint and a nasal drip pad.

Reduction of mandibular fractures

Definition. Correction of malocclusion, a condition resulting from a fracture of the mandible (lower jaw) wherein the biting (occlusal) surfaces of the teeth do not meet properly.

Considerations. The purpose of treatment for a mandibular fracture is to restore the patient's preinjury dental occlusion. With some types of fractures, a closed reduction with immobilization by means of intermaxillary fixation is sufficient for treatment. With a majority of mandibular fractures, however, it is necessary to perform an open reduction with internal wire fixation, plus supplemental intermaxillary fixation to achieve adequate immobilization for healing.

Intermaxillary fixation is most often accomplished by applying arch bars to the maxillary and mandibular teeth. No. 25 stainless steel wires are placed around the necks of the teeth and are ligated around the arch bars to hold the latter in place. Latex bands are attached to the tongs on the maxillary and mandibular arch bars to fix the teeth in occlusion (Fig. 21-44). If the patient is edentulous, arch bars are attached to dentures or specially fabricated dental splints. The dentures or splints are held in place by means of wires placed around the mandible (for the mandibular arch bar) and through the nasal spine and around the zygomatic arches (for the maxillary arch bar).

Setup and preparation of the patient. A basic plastic instrument set, plus the following instruments and supplies, are needed for an open reduction of a fractured mandible:

1 Hall II air drill
2 Dingman bone-holding forceps (Fig. 21-45)
1 Concept nerve stimulator
Stainless steel wires, nos. 25, 26, and 28
1 Marking pen
1 Electrocautery
Epinephrine 1:200,000 for injection

For the application of arch bars or other types of interdental wiring techniques, a separate Mayo table setup with the following instruments and supplies is required:

1 Coil arch bars and Latex bands
1 Stainless steel wire, no. 25 or 26
2 Mayo-Hegar needle holders, 8 inches
1 Wire suture scissors, 4¾ inches
2 Weider tongue depressors, large and small
1 Yankauer suction tip
1 Freer septal elevator
6 Mosquito hemostats, curved, 5¼ inches
1 Brown fascia needle (if dentures or splints are used)
1 Penrose drain, small

If arch bars are applied before the open reduction is performed, this latter setup must be kept completely separate from the instruments used for the open reduction. Since the mouth is a contaminated area, a complete change of gowns, gloves, and drapes is necessary after the intraoral procedure.

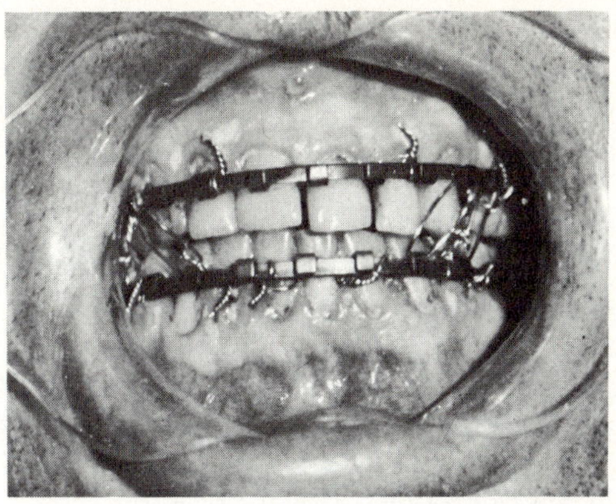

Fig. 21-44. Teeth in occlusion with arch bars in place. Tong on arch bars will accept latex bands, which maintain occlusion for several weeks (wires around tongs are shown).

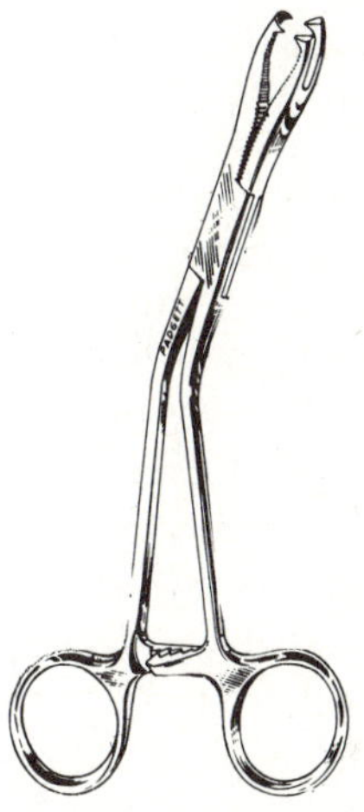

Fig. 21-45. Dingman bone-holding forceps used in reduction of mandibular fractures.

The patient is placed in the supine position on the operating table. The head drape is used.

Operative procedure

1. Arch bars may be applied before or after the open reduction.

2. A line inferior and parallel to the lower border of the mandible at the fracture site is marked, and the area is infiltrated with epinephrine 1:200,000 for hemostasis.

3. The incision is made so that the inferior border of the mandible is exposed. The nerve stimulator may be used to aid in identification of the marginal mandibular branch of the facial nerve in fractures of the posterior body and angle of the mandible.

4. The fracture is reduced by manipulation. Holes are drilled into the mandible on each side of the fracture line with the Hall II air drill, while an assistant holds the reduction of the fracture with the aid of Dingman bone-holding forceps.

5. Stainless steel wire is inserted through the holes and twisted tightly to secure the fracture fragments in anatomical alignment.

6. A small Penrose drain is usually placed in the wound, and the wound is closed in layers (periosteum, platysma muscle, and skin).

7. The Latex bands may be applied to the arch bars at this time, but more frequently are applied later, after the patient is fully awake and reactive.

8. A moderate compression dressing is applied to cover the submandibular wound and drain.

Reduction of maxillary fractures

Definition. Restoration of dental occlusion and correction of the facial deformity caused by a fracture of the maxilla, or upper jaw, which constitutes the middle third of the face. Maxillary fractures are usually classified as follows: (1) Le Fort I, or transverse maxillary fracture; (2) Le Fort II, or pyramidal maxillary fracture; (3) Le Fort III, or craniofacial disjunction, which includes fractures of both zygomas and the nose.

Considerations. A maxillary fracture produces malocclusion, as does a mandibular fracture. In addition, depending on the severity of the fracture, it also may produce considerable deformity of the middle of the face, usually perceived as a flattening or "smashed-in" appearance of the middle of the face.

Closed reduction with intermaxillary fixation suffices for treatment of Le Fort I and some Le Fort II fractures. The more severe Le Fort II and all Le Fort III fractures require open reduction in addition to intermaxillary fixation.

Setup and preparation of the patient. The basic plastic instrument set is required, plus the following:

Hall II air drill
Stainless steel wires, nos. 25, 26, and 28
Rowe maxillary forceps, right and left
Brown fascia needle
Polyethylene buttons
Small foam rubber pad
Marking pen
Electrocautery
Epinephrine 1:200,000 for injection

A separate Mayo table setup for the application of arch bars is required, as described for reduction of mandibular fractures.

The patient is placed in the supine position on the operating table. The head drape is used.

Operative procedure. Arch bars are applied before or after the open reduction, or they may be the only mode of treatment in closed reduction. In addition to ligating the maxillary arch bar to the teeth, it must also be suspended from stable bones superior to the fractured maxilla (which is unstable). In Le Fort I fractures, suspension may be around both zygomatic arches via passage of percutaneous wires. In Le Fort II and III fractures, suspension wires are placed through holes drilled bilaterally in the zygomatic process of the frontal bone. This requires incisions in both lateral eyebrow areas. The following description pertains to open reduction of Le Fort II and III fractures:

1. After injection of epinephrine 1:200,000 for hemostasis, bilateral incisions are made to expose the infraorbital rims and frontozygomatic suture lines.

2. The Rowe maxillary forceps are applied intranasally and intraorally to disimpact and reduce the maxilla.

3. Holes are drilled into bone on each side of fracture lines along the infraorbital rim (and frontozygomatic area for Le Fort III fractures, after reducing the zygomatic fractures).

4. Stainless steel wires are passed through these holes and twisted down tightly to maintain the reduction.

5. Suspension wires are passed from the eyebrow incisions, behind the zygomatic arches, into the mouth with the Brown fascia needle. A pullout wire is looped through each suspension wire within the eyebrow incision, brought out through the skin near the hairline, and tied down over a polyethylene button and foam rubber padding.

6. Incisions are closed.

7. When indicated, reduction of the nasal fracture is performed at this time.

Reduction of zygomatic fractures

Definition. Correction of fractures of the zygoma (the cheek, or malar, bone). The two most common types of zygomatic fractures are depressed fractures of the arch and separation at or near the zygomaticofrontal, zygomaticomaxillary, and zygomaticotemporal suture lines, which constitutes a *trimalar* fracture.

Considerations. Although fractures of the zygoma can interfere with the ability to open and close the mouth properly, their chief consequence is a flattening of the cheek on the involved side, which results from a depressed trimalar or zygomatic arch fracture. Treatment is directed toward elevating the depressed fracture and maintaining the reduction. Closed reduction is the procedure used for treatment of zygomatic arch fractures, while most trimalar fractures are reduced by means of open reduction with internal fixation.

Setup and preparation of the patient. A plastic local instrument set, a Suraci zygoma hook-elevator, and a jaw hook are required for a closed reduction. A basic plastic instrument set, plus the following instruments and supplies, are required for an open reduction:

Hall II air drill
Stainless steel wires, nos. 26, 28, and 30
1 Suraci zygoma hook-elevator
1 Jaw hook

1 Kerrison rongeur
2 Blair retractors
Luck-Bishop drill with assorted set of Kirschner wires and sterile cork (optional)
Bipolar cautery
Marking pen
Epinephrine 1:200,000 for injection

The patient is placed in the supine position on the operating table. The head drape is used.

Operative procedure. Closed reduction is performed by elevating the depressed fracture with a percutaneous bone hook. Stabilization of a trimalar fracture may then be achieved by drilling with the Luck-Bishop drill and inserting a transantral Kirschner wire from the fractured side to the normal side.

The technique of open reduction of a trimalar fracture is as follows:

1. Incisions are marked along the lateral eyebrow and lower eyelid over the zygomaticofrontal suture line and zygomaticomaxillary suture line (infraorbital rim) fractures, respectively.
2. After injection with epinephrine 1:200,000 for hemostasis, incisions are made down to bone, and fracture lines are identified and exposed.
3. The depressed zygoma is elevated with a Kelly clamp or periosteal elevator placed behind the body of the zygoma through the lateral eyebrow incision. Bone hooks placed percutaneously or at the fracture sites may be used instead.
4. Holes are drilled in bone on each side of the fracture lines. Stainless steel wires are passed through the holes and twisted down tightly to maintain the reduction. (Reduction and stabilization of two of the three fractures is sufficient.)
5. An alternate method of stabilization of the fractures is interosseous wiring of the zygomaticofrontal fracture and placement of a transantral Kirschner wire.
6. Incisions are closed.
7. An eye-patch dressing may be applied.

Reduction of orbital-floor fractures

Considerations. The orbital floor is the eggshell-thin bone on which the eye and periorbital tissues rest. It separates the orbit from the maxillary antrum. Orbital-floor fractures usually occur in combination with fractures of the infraorbital rim (maxillary and zygomatic fractures). An isolated depressed orbital-floor fracture with an intact infraorbital rim is called a "blowout" fracture.

Symptoms of orbital-floor fractures are diplopia and/or enophthalmos. Diplopia is caused by entrapment of periorbital fat and/or extraocular muscles in the fracture line, which restricts movement of the eyeball. Enophthalmos usually results from a fracture extensive enough to allow herniation of periorbital fat into the maxillary antrum, which gives the eye a sunken appearance. Treatment is directed toward relief of these symptoms.

Because the orbital floor is so thin, comminuted fractures occur frequently and segments of bone may be irretrievably lost into the maxillary antrum. If the floor cannot be reconstructed by elevating the bony fragments, its integrity must be restored with an implant (cartilage graft, bone graft, or alloplastic material).

Setup and preparation of the patient. A basic plastic instrument set is required, plus the following:

2 Blair retractors
Hall II air drill
Alloplastic material of choice (Teflon or Silastic sheet) (Fig. 21-46)
Marking pen
Bipolar cautery
Epinephrine 1:200,000 for injection

In addition, instruments and supplies listed for reduction of maxillary and zygomatic fractures may also be needed, since orbital-floor fractures often occur in combination with these fractures.

The patient is placed in the supine position on the operating table. The head drape is used.

Operative procedure

1. A lower eyelid incision is marked and the eyelid injected with epinephrine 1:200,000 for hemostasis and incised down to the infraorbital rim.
2. Periosteum is elevated from the infraorbital rim and orbital floor.
3. The fracture is identified, and any entrapped periorbital tissues are reduced by gentle traction.
4. Continuity of the orbital floor is reestablished by reducing the fracture, replacing any bone chips if possible, or inserting an autogenous graft or alloplastic implant.
5. The orbital floor implant is secured anteriorly to the infraorbital rim with a suture after a hole has been drilled in the bone.
6. The incision is closed in one layer (skin).
7. An eye-patch dressing may be applied.

Elective orthognathic surgery

Considerations. A large number of patients are afflicted with either acquired or congenital facial defects that affect the maxilla and/or mandible. The condition of many of these patients can be improved dramatically with orthodontic care; however, many also require surgical rearrangement of the maxilla or mandible.

Psychosocial and functional deficits are related to abnormalities of the maxilla and mandible. Surgical correction of these defects can improve the quality of life for these patients. Surgery is usually delayed until an adequate number of permanent teeth are in place for postoperative immobilization. Proper preoperative planning is of great importance to these patients.

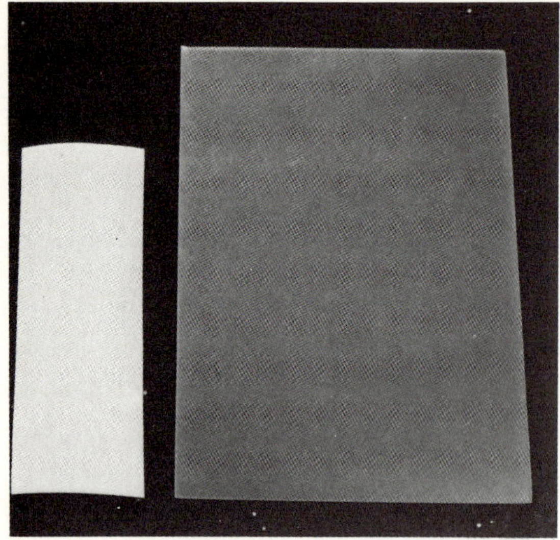

Fig. 21-46. Sheets of alloplastic implant material: *left,* Teflon; *right,* Silastic. Small segments are cut to fit for reconstruction of fractured orbital floor.

Setup and preparation of the patient. As described for craniofacial surgery.

Operative procedure

1. Arch bars are applied for postoperative immobilization.
2. Exposure is accomplished through intraoral incisions.
3. The maxilla or mandible is cut as indicated by the preoperative workup.
4. Bone is advanced or set back to a predetermined position.
5. Bones are wired in place with grafts in defects as needed.

Surgery for acute burns

Definition. Reestablishment of an intact skin barrier after injury to the skin. A majority of burns result from exposure to high temperatures, which injures the skin. Thermal skin injury may be caused by flame, scald, or direct contact with a hot object. Similar destruction of skin can result from contact with chemicals such as acid or alkali or contact with an electrical current. The latter, however, often involves extensive destruction of underlying tissue in addition to skin.

Considerations. Intact skin provides protection against the environment for all underlying tissues and organs. It aids in heat regulation, prevents water loss, and is the major barrier against bacterial invasion. The greater the degree of injury to the skin, as expressed in percent of total body surface burned and the depth of the burn, the more severe is the injury. Burn patients are therefore some of the most severely ill patients brought to the operating room.

Partial-thickness (first- and second-degree) burns heal by regeneration of skin from dermal elements that remain intact. Full-thickness (third degree) burns require skin grafting to heal, since no dermal elements remain intact. Both partial- and full-thickness burns may require debridement of necrotic tissue (eschar) before healing can occur by skin regeneration or grafting.

The essentials of skin grafting are discussed in the section on free skin grafts. This section therefore deals only with the procedure for debridement of burn wounds.

Setup and preparation of the patient. A basic plastic instrument set is required, plus a knife dermatome, an electrocautery, a pneumatic tourniquet for isolated extremity burns, and a topical antibacterial agent of choice.

Since most burn wounds become infected within a few days, burns are contaminated, and appropriate operating room procedures are followed.

Most burn patients arrive in the operating room with dressings covering their wounds. These are removed after the patient has been anesthetized, to minimize pain and loss of body heat through the open burn wounds. The temperature in the operating room should be elevated above normal levels if extensive burn areas are to be exposed.

Operative procedure

1A. Nonviable tissue is excised down to underlying muscle fascia, using a scalpel.

1B. An alternate method is tangential excision of the burn wound, which is performed with a knife dermatome. This type of excision is usually carried down only to subcutaneous fat, rather than to fascia.

2. Hemostasis is obtained with the electrocautery.

3. Dressings saturated with the topical antibacterial agent of choice are applied.

Although skin grafting may be done at the time of wound debridement, it is usually performed several days later in burns that are extensive.

Esthetic surgery

Rhinoplasty

Definition. Operative procedure wherein the nose is reshaped and its size reduced. A procedure to alter the nasal septum, *septoplasty* or *submucous resection* (SMR), often accompanies rhinoplasty.

Considerations. Deformities of the external nose and nasal septum may be congenital or secondary to previous trauma. The goal of rhinoplasty is to improve the appearance of the external nose. This is accomplished by reshaping the underlying framework of the nose (Fig. 21-47), which allows the overlying skin and subcutaneous tissue to redrape over the new framework. Reshaping the nasal skeleton usually includes rasping down of a dorsal hump, partial excision of the lateral and alar cartilages, shortening of the septum, and osteotomy of the nasal bones.

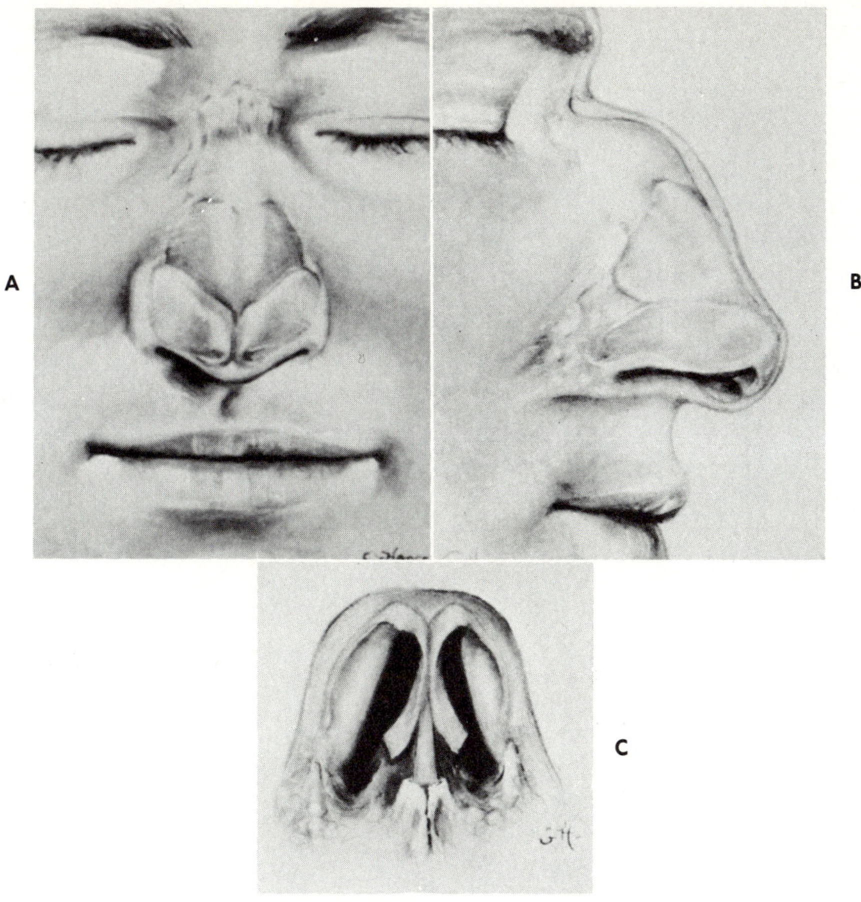

Fig. 21-47. Skeleton of abnormal nose with soft tissues superimposed. (From Brown, J.B., and McDowell, F.: Plastic surgery of the nose, ed. 2, Springfield, Ill., Charles C Thomas, Publisher.)

The goal of SMR is to improve the nasal airway by resecting a segment of septal cartilage. Septoplasty reshapes the existing septal cartilage; it may aid in altering the appearance of the nose or in improving the airway.

Rhinoplasty is performed through incisions made inside the nose; it therefore leaves no visible scars. Rarely, small external incisions at the alar bases and near the nasal bridge are also used to narrow the nose.

Setup and preparation of the patient. A plastic local instrument set is required, plus the following special instruments (Fig. 21-48):

3 Nasal specula, assorted lengths
4 Metal applicator sticks and wisps of cotton
1 Aufricht nasal retractor
1 Fomon retractor
3 Pituitary rongeurs, assorted sizes, straight and upturned
1 Nasal scissors, angled
1 Kazanjian nasal forceps
1 Fomon lower lateral scissors
2 Joseph button-end knives, straight and angular
1 Ballenger swivel knife, straight
2 Joseph saws, 1 right and 1 left
2 Chisels, 2 mm and 4 mm
1 Cinelli double-guarded osteotome, straight
2 Guarded chisels, straight, right and left
1 Mallet
1 Brown nasal rasp (upward stroke)
1 Maltz nasal rasp (downward stroke)
1 Diamond rasp (optional)
Fomon rasp
Silver osteotomes
1 Nasal septum forceps (for SMR)
Brown nasal splint
Nasal packing
Anesthetic agents of choice, local and topical
Fiberoptic light source and head light (optional)
Atomizer (optional)

A separate local anesthetic tray should contain the following:

Bayonet forceps
Sponges
Local anesthetic
Syringe, 10 ml
Needle, 26 gauge
Cotton or gauze (for packing)

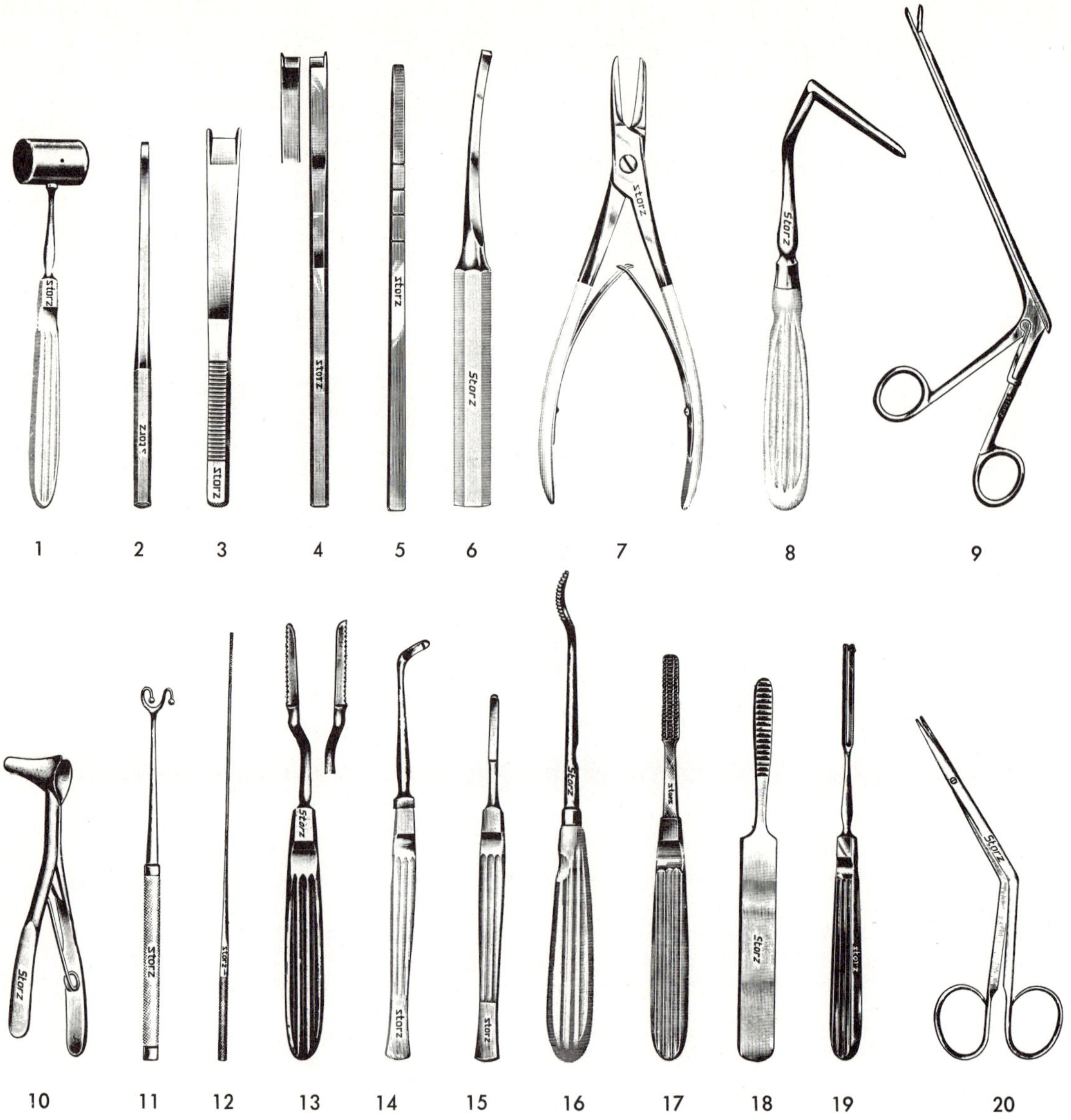

Fig. 21-48. Special instruments for rhinoplasty. *1,* Mallet; *2,* 2-mm chisel; *3,* Cinelli double-guarded osteotome; *4,* right and left straight-guarded chisels; *5,* 4-mm chisel; *6,* Blair chisel; *7,* Kazanjian nasal forceps; *8,* Aufricht nasal retractor; *9,* pituitary rongeur; *10,* nasal speculum; *11,* Fomon retractor; *12,* metal applicator stick; *13,* right and left Joseph saws; *14,* Joseph angular button-end knife; *15,* Joseph straight button-end knife; *16,* Aufricht rasp; *17,* Maltz nasal rasp; 18, Brown nasal rasp; *19,* Ballenger straight swivel knife; *20,* angled nasal scissors; *21,* Fomon rasps; *22,* silver osteotomes.

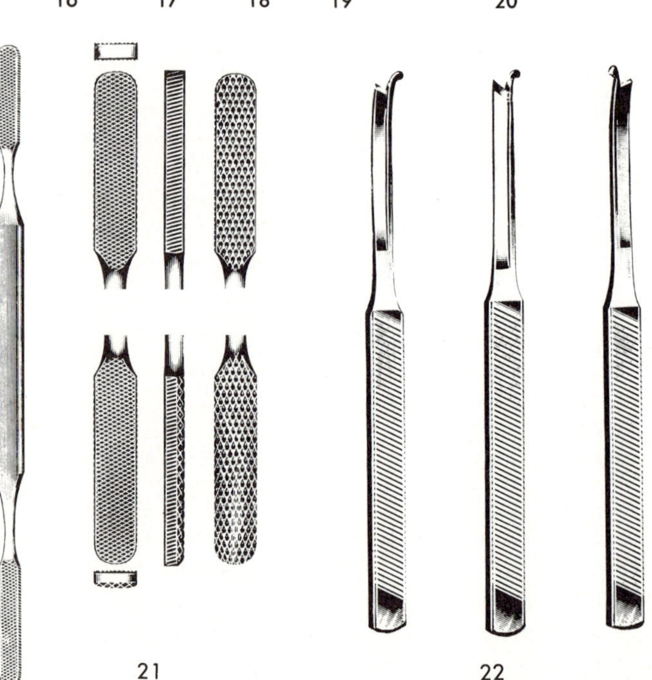

From this tray (before scrubbing) the surgeon can do the preliminary nasal preparation, inject the local anesthetic, and pack the nose with gauze or cotton soaked in 4% cocaine solution. With this procedure the local anesthesia can take effect while the surgeon is scrubbing. (Rhinoplasty is almost always performed using local anesthesia.) Intravenous fluids are started, and a blood-pressure cuff and leads to a cardiac monitor are placed.

The patient is placed in the supine position on the operating table. The head drape is used. The surgeon may use a head light while performing the operation.

Operative procedure

1. Local and topical anesthetics are administered by the surgeon. The topical anesthetic is applied with applicator sticks or an atomizer.
2. Intranasal incisions are made, and the skin and soft tissues of the nose are elevated from the underlying nasal bones and cartilage.
3. The tip of the nose is reshaped by excising portions of the alar and lateral cartilages on each side.
4. The nasal dorsum (hump) is reduced by removing portions of bone and septum.
5. The nasal bridge is narrowed by means of medial and lateral osteotomies of the nasal bones.
6. The intranasal incisions are sutured.
7. Bilateral anterior nasal packs are inserted, and a nasal splint and drip pad (moustache dressing) applied.

If an SMR is performed at the time of rhinoplasty, it usually immediately precedes step 2. Septoplasty may be performed at any time during the operative procedure.

Blepharoplasty

Definition. Removal of loose skin and protruding periorbital fat of the upper and lower eyelids.

Considerations. The aging process causes a sagging or relaxation of eyelid skin and the orbital septum. As the latter becomes weaker, it allows periorbital fat to bulge. These changes are perceived as baggy eyelids, which give the patient a chronically tired appearance. The goal of blepharoplasty is to improve the patient's appearance. The upper eyelid skin can be so redundant that it encroaches on the patient's field of vision and causes a decrease in the visual field. Blepharoplasty is often performed with a rhytidectomy.

Setup and preparation of the patient. A plastic local instrument set is required, as well as two Blair retractors, a bipolar cautery, a marking pen, and a local anesthetic.

Blepharoplasty is usually performed under local anesthesia. Intravenous fluids are started, and a blood-pressure cuff and leads to a cardiac monitor are applied.

The patient is placed in the supine position on the operating table. The head drape is used.

Operative procedure (Fig. 21-49)

1. The local anesthetic is injected after the incisions have been marked bilaterally.
2. An ellipse of excess skin is excised from the upper eyelids.
3. After incising or removing a strip of the orbicularis oculi muscle and orbital septum, protruding periorbital fat is excised.
4. The upper-eyelid incisions are sutured in one layer.
5. The lower-eyelid incisions are made close to the ciliary margin.
6. A skin flap or skin-muscle flap is elevated away from the orbicularis oculi muscle.
7. Protruding periorbital fat is excised from beneath the obicularis muscle.
8. The skin flaps are draped over the lower eyelids, and any excess skin is excised. Removal of too much skin for the lower eyelid can cause an ectropion.
9. The lower eyelid incisions are sutured in one layer.
10. Finely crushed ice in all-gauze 4 × 4 pads is applied to the eyes.

Rhytidectomy

Definition. Excision of redundant or loose skin of the face and upper neck (also called a facelift).

Considerations. As the aging process progresses, the skin of the face and neck becomes loose and redundant. This is particularly noticeable in the "jowl" areas and just beneath the chin. A rhytidectomy is designed to improve the patient's appearance by removing some of this excess skin and sometimes the excess fat of the neck. Rather than excising the redundant skin directly, incisions adjacent to or within hairlines are used so that scars are virtually indiscernible.

Setup and preparation of the patient. A basic plastic instrument set is required, plus the following:

1 Castanares facelift scissors (Fig. 21-50)
2 Deaver retractors, 1 inch
2 Army-Navy retractors
2 Cushing tissue forceps, 7 inches
2 Brown-Adson forceps
2 Cushing dressing forceps, 7 inches
6 Burlisher clamps, curved
Rhytidectomy retractor
Double hooks
Metzenbaum scissors, long
Marking pen
Bipolar cautery
Fiberoptic light source
Local anesthetic agent of choice
Skin stapler

A rhytidectomy is usually performed with local anesthesia. Intravenous fluids are started, and a blood-pressure cuff and cardiac monitor leads applied. The patient is placed in the supine position on the operating table. The head drape is used. Minimal or no hair is shaved.

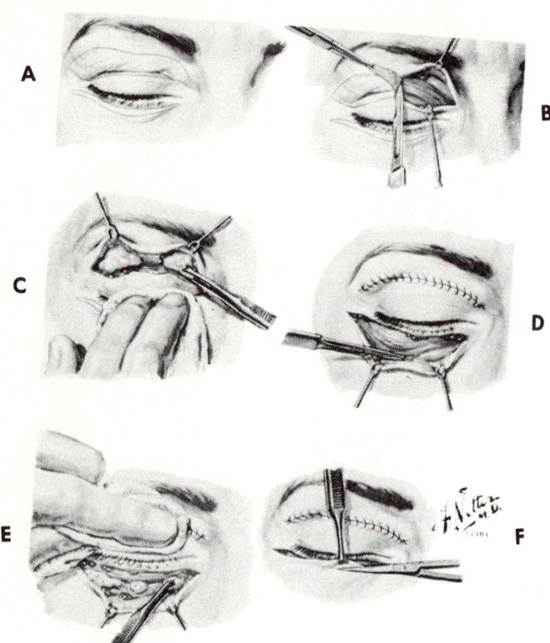

Fig. 21-49. Blepharoplasty for baggy eyelids. **A,** Areas of proposed skin excision marked with methylene blue or marking pen. **B,** Strip of skin excised from upper lid; fat pad shining through orbital fascia and orbicular muscle of eye. **C,** Orbital fascia opened in two places (medially and laterally). Pressure on eyeball causes fat pads to bulge. They are teased out meticulously. **D,** Upper lid incision sutured with continuous no. 6-0 silk. Orbicular muscle fibers are separated from skin. **E,** Orbital fascia opened; fat pads bulge because of digital pressure and are teased out meticulously. **F,** Skin tailored to fit and sutured. (Copyright CIBA-GEIGY CORPORATION. Reproduced with permission from CLINICAL SYMPOSIA, illustrated by Frank H. Netter, M.D. All rights reserved.)

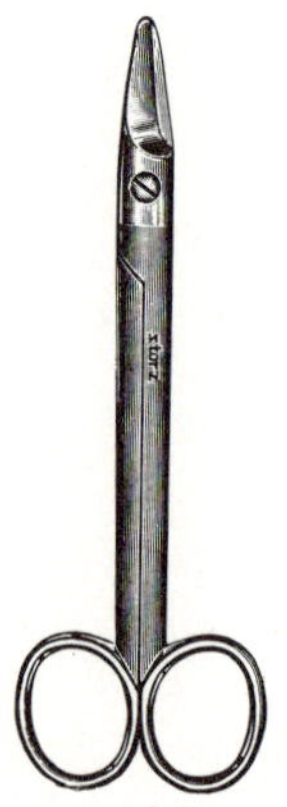

Fig. 21-50. Castanares facelift scissors.

Operative procedure (Figs. 21-51 and 21-52)

1. Bilateral incisions are marked—from the temporal scalp, in front of the ear in a natural skin wrinkle line, around the earlobe, onto the posterior surface of the ear, and into the occipital scalp.
2. The incisions, both temples, cheeks, upper neck, and the submental area are injected with the local anesthetic agent.
3. After the incisions are made, large flaps of skin and subcutaneous tissue are elevated from the face and upper third of the neck, meeting in the midline in the submental area.
4. The edges of the flaps are grasped with Allis clamps, and superior and posterior traction is placed on the flaps. If there is excess fat in the neck, it is sometimes excised. The submental incision is used to give better access to the central neck to remove fat. To obtain a tighter and perhaps longer lift the deeper tissues and platysma muscles can be sutured in a separate layer.
5. Excess skin at the flap edges is excised, which pulls the tissue in the previously redundant areas tight.
6. Drains, if used, are inserted.
7. Incisions are closed in one or two layers. Sometimes skin staples are used on the scalp.
8. A moderate compression dressing is applied.

Dermabrasion

Definition. Sanding, or planing, of the skin, used primarily to smooth scars and surface irregularities of the skin.

Consideration. Dermabrasion is most commonly performed to improve the appearance of facial scars, especially the irregular scars resulting from acne vulgaris. It may also be used for the removal of acute, traumatic foreign-body tattoos. It is less successfully used for removal of professional body tattoos and to smooth fine wrinkle lines of the face.

The goal in treating irregular surfaces with dermabrasion is to sand or plane down the high points or elevations so that the low ones appear less deep. Dermabrasion removes epidermis and a portion of the dermis of the skin. Healing occurs from residual dermal elements, as in partial-thickness burns or split-thickness skin-graft donor sites.

Setup and preparation of the patient. Instrumentation includes a plastic local instrument set, a Stryker dermabrader, and a marking pen.

The operation may be performed under general or local anesthesia. The patient is positioned and draped so that the area to be dermabraded is well exposed.

Operative procedure

1. The bases of pitted scars and depressions are marked.
2. The skin is planed with the Stryker dermabrader.
3. A single layer of the dressing of choice is applied to the dermabraded area.

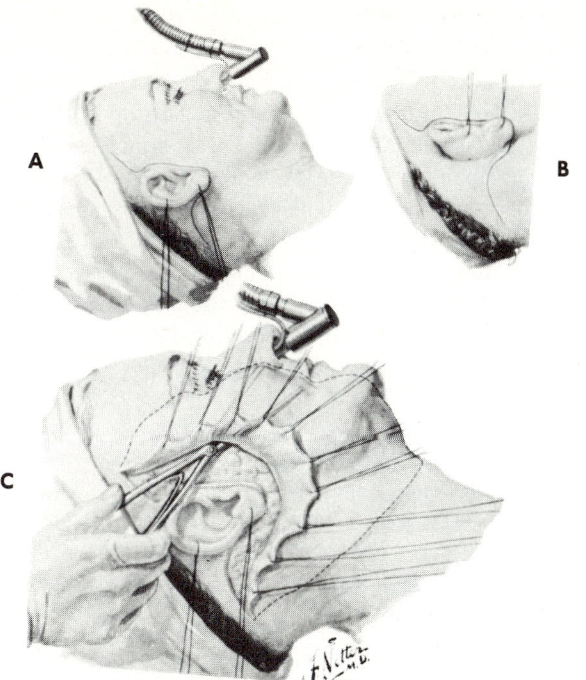

Fig. 21-51. Rhytidectomy: line of incision and undermining. A, Traction sutures of no. 4-0 silk placed in auricle; temporal incision curved posteriorly to better support upward pull. B, Incision carried under earlobe, then curved posteriorly upward and then caudad toward midline. C, Skin undermined almost to nasolabial fold, to area of mental foramen, and to midline of neck as far down as thyroid cartilage. Care is taken to avoid injury to submandibular branches of facial nerve and facial artery. (Copyright CIBA-GEIGY CORPORATION. Reproduced with permission from CLINICAL SYMPOSIA, illustrated by Frank H. Netter, M.D. All rights reserved.)

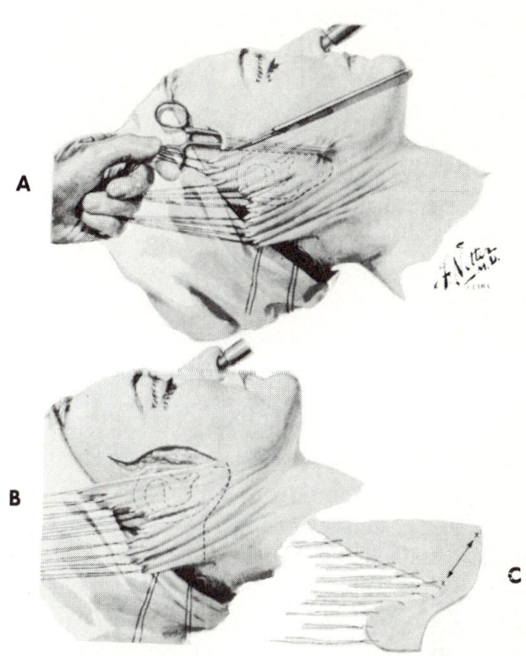

Fig. 21-52. Rhytidectomy: removal of superfluous skin. A, Skin drawn upward to proper degree of tension and incision made along posterior margin of clamp. B, Incision continued upward around posterior margin of auricle and then backward to excise skin specimen. C, Specimen: distance *x* to *x′* usually measures 1 to 2 inches. (Copyright CIBA-GEIGY CORPORATION. Reproduced with permission from CLINICAL SYMPOSIA, illustrated by Frank H. Netter, M.D. All rights reserved.)

Scar revision

Definition. Rearranging or reshaping of an existing scar by means of a scar revision procedure, so that the scar is not as noticeable. It is impossible to completely eradicate a scar.

Considerations. The simplest form of scar revision is excision of an existing scar and simple resuturing of the wound. This may improve scars that are wide.

The Z-plasty is the most widely used method of scar revision. It breaks up linear scars, rearranging them so that the central member of the Z lies in the same direction as a natural skin line. Scars that are parallel to skin lines are less noticeable than scars that are perpendicular to skin lines. A contracted scar line also can be lengthened to a limited extent with a Z-plasty.

Setup and preparation of the patient. A plastic local instrument set and a marking pen are required.

The operation may be performed under local or general anesthesia. The patient is positioned, prepped, and draped so that the scar that is to be revised is well exposed.

Operative procedure

1. The scar and pattern for the planned revision are marked and incised.
2. The scar is excised.
3. The skin is sutured.
4. Dressings may or may not be applied.

Abdominoplasty

Definition. Excision of loose or redundant abdominal skin, plus the subcutaneous fat immediately beneath this skin, and repair of any muscle laxity.

Considerations. Abdominoplasty is particularly useful in improving the appearance (and to a certain extent, function) of persons who have lost a great deal of weight. Patients who have undergone an intestinal bypass operation for the treatment of morbid obesity are often candidates for abdominal lipectomy. Obesity produces distention and stretching of the skin of the abdomen. Although weight loss reduces the volume of the underlying fat, it does not produce concomitant reduction in the excess surface area of the overlying skin, resulting from destruction or insufficiency of elastic fibers in the skin. The stretched skin remains as an apron that hangs from the lower abdomen, sometimes as far as the knees. The rectus abdominus fascia is also stretched in obese patients, and weight loss does not restore its integrity. Abdominoplasty is therefore often accompanied by some type of fascial plication procedure.

Abdominoplasty is usually performed to remove stretch marks and redundant skin and fat of the lower abdomen, which occur after multiple pregnancies. It also repairs any laxity of the rectus muscle.

Setup and preparation of the patient. A basic plastic instrument set is required, as well as extra clamping instruments, an electrocautery, and a marking pen.

The patient is placed in the supine position, with slight flexion at the hips. Draping is such that the entire abdomen, lower costal margins, upper thighs, and both anterior iliac spines are exposed.

Operative procedure

1. A low, transverse abdominal incision across both inguinal areas laterally and the superior border of the mons pubis in the midline is marked and incised down to fascia.
2. A large flap of skin and subcutaneous tissue is elevated away from the fascia of the anterior abdominal wall.
3. The umbilicus is left in its normal position.
4. The abdominal flap is elevated further until the xiphoid process of the sternum and the lower costal margins are reached.
5. If diastasis of the rectus abdominus fascia is present, plication is performed from the xiphoid process to the mons pubis.
6. The flap of abdominal skin and subcutaneous tissue is pulled inferiorly, and excess tissue is excised.
7. A small incision is made in the midline of the flap to accommodate the umbilicus, which is then sutured peripherally to the flap.
8. Drains may or may not be used, followed by closure of the lower abdominal incision in two layers.
9. The patient is placed in the hospital bed in high Fowler's position.

Miscellaneous operations

Pressure sores

Definition. Pressure sores result from prolonged compression of soft tissues overlying bony prominences. *Decubitus ulcer* defines a type of pressure sore that is produced while the patient is lying down.

Considerations. Prolonged pressure causes thrombosis of small blood vessels and anoxia of soft tissues, with eventual necrosis. A person with normal sensation perceives discomfort in an area of prolonged or excessive pressure and changes position before irreversible soft-tissue damage occurs. Pressure sores, therefore, occur in patients who lack normal sensation, such as paraplegics, or in patients who are too ill or weak to change their positions, even though they are uncomfortable.

The most common sites for the occurrence of pressure sores are over the sacrum, the greater trochanter, and the ischial tuberosity. The basic principles of the surgical repair of pressure sores are excision of the ulcer and underlying bony prominence, followed by adequate soft-tissue coverage of the area (usually a local flap with a skin graft used to cover the flap donor site).

Setup and preparation of the patient. A basic plastic instrument set is required, plus the following:

Osteotomes, assorted sizes, straight and curved
Mallet
Gigli saw and handle
Curettes, assorted
Key periosteal elevator
Duckbill rongeur
Bone wax
Dermatome of choice
Electrocautery
Marking pen

The patient is positioned and draped so that the pressure sore, adjacent flap donor site, and a skin graft donor site are well exposed.

Operative procedure

1. The area to be excised and the local flap are outlined.
2. The ulcer is excised along with the underlying bony prominence.
3. Large suction catheters are placed into the defect left by excision of the ulcer and beneath the flap.
4. The flap is sutured in place.
5. A split-thickness skin graft is usually used to resurface the flap donor site.
6. A stent dressing is placed over the skin graft, and gauze dressings or a plastic spray dressing are applied over the suture lines.

HAND SURGERY

Plastic surgery of the hand is directed toward restoration of function. It deals with the treatment of acute injuries, as well as reconstruction in established deformities. A systemic surgical approach for the restoration of hand function includes (1) replacement of lost tissue covering; (2) restoration of bony architecture; (3) repair of severed nerves; (4) restoration of the motor unit, either by tendon repair, tendon graft, or tendon transfer; and (5) replantation of severed digits.

Functional anatomy

The functional unit in hand surgery consists of the hand, digits, wrist, and forearm. Each of these structures has a *radial* and an *ulnar* side, as determined by its position in relation to the radius and ulna of the forearm,

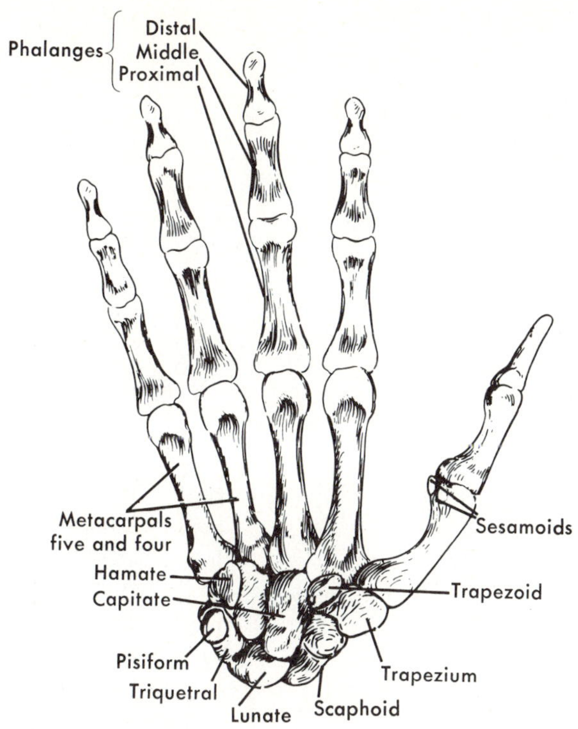

Fig. 21-53. Skeleton of wrist and hand, palmar view. (From Hollinshead, W.H.: Anatomy for surgeons, vol. 3, The back and limb, ed. 2, New York, 1969, Harper & Row, Publishers.)

rather than a lateral and medial side. Each also has a *dorsal* and *volar,* or *palmar,* surface. To avoid confusion, the digits of the hand are referred to as the thumb and the index, long, ring, and little fingers.

The skeletal framework of the hand and wrist consists of three distinct parts: (1) the metacarpals, or bones of the hand; (2) the phalanges, or bones of the digits; and (3) the carpals, or bones of the wrist (Fig. 21-53). The five metacarpals articulate distally with the proximal phalanges of each digit at the metacarpophalangeal (MP) joints. The two bones of the thumb are the proximal phalanx and the distal phalanx, which articulate at the interphalangeal (IP) joint. Each of the four fingers contains three bones: a proximal phalanx, a middle phalanx, and a distal phalanx. Each finger therefore has three joints: (1) the metacarpophalangeal joint, (2) the proximal interphalangeal (PIP) joint between the proximal and middle phalanges, and (3) the distal interphalangeal (DIP) joint between the middle and distal phalanges.

The carpus (wrist) consists of eight bones arranged in two rows. The proximal row includes the scaphoid (navicular), lunate, triquetrum, and pisiform. The distal row includes the trapezium (greater multangular), trapezoid (lesser multangular), capitate, and hamate. The metacarpals articulate proximally with the distal row of carpal bones. The proximal row of carpal bones articulates with the radius and ulna of the forearm.

Motion of the thumb and fingers is achieved through the action of muscles intrinsic and extrinsic to the hand. The intrinsic muscles are those whose muscle bellies lie within the hand: (1) the interosseous and lumbrical muscles of the hand, which flex the MP joints while extending the PIP and DIP joints and permit spreading and approximation of the fingers; (2) the muscles of the thenar eminence, which aid in adduction, abduction, flexion, and opposition of the thumb; and (3) the muscles of the hypothenar eminence, which aid in abduction, flexion, and opposition of the little finger.

The extrinsic muscles are so called because the muscle bellies are located in the forearm while the tendons pass into the hand, dorsally beneath the extensor retinaculum (Fig. 21-54) and volarly beneath the flexor retinaculum (Fig. 21-55) at the wrist, to insert on the phalanges of the thumb and fingers. The dorsal group consists of the extensor tendons, which extend the finger MP joints and the thumb MP and IP joints. The volar group consists of the flexor tendons, one for the thumb and two to each finger. The paired finger flexors are the superficial (sublimis) flexor tendons, which flex the PIP joints, and the deep (profundus) flexor tendons, which flex the DIP joints. In addition to the finger and thumb flexors and extensors, other muscles of the forearm have tendinous insertions that work to abduct the thumb and flex and extend the wrist.

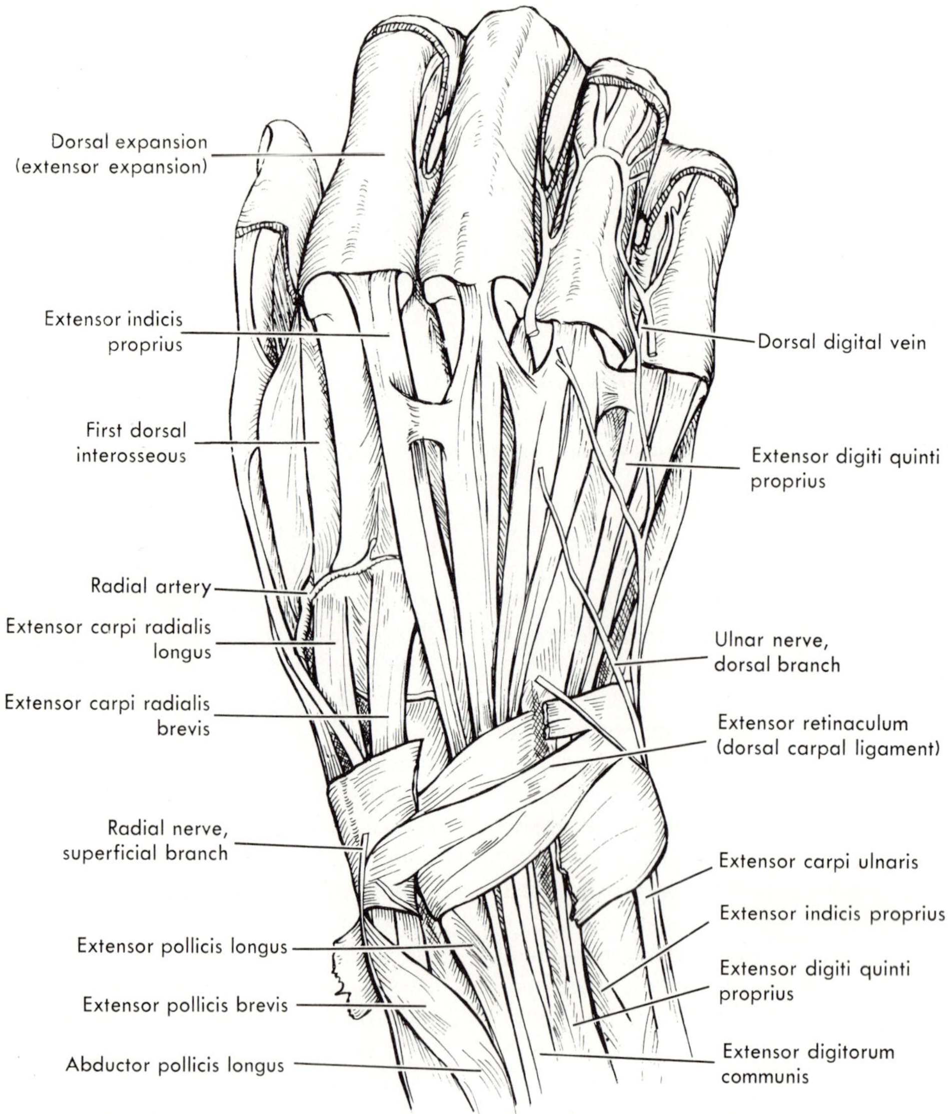

Fig. 21-54. Dorsum of hand and wrist; finger and long thumb extensor tendons pass under extensor retinaculum at wrist. (Reproduced by permission. From J.C.B. Grant's atlas of anatomy, 6th ed., copyright © 1972, The Williams and Wilkins Co.)

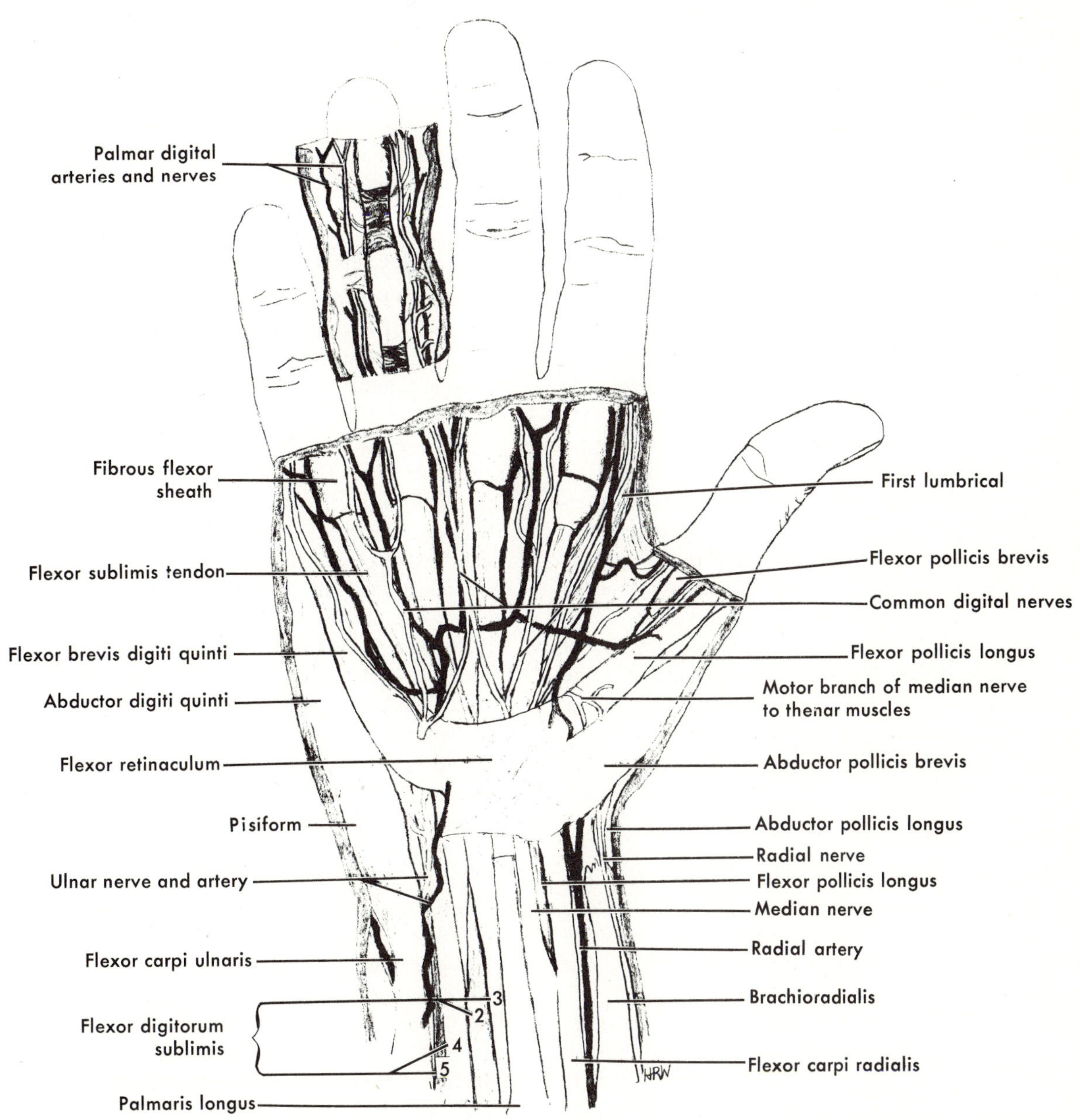

Fig. 21-55. Volar (palmar) surface of hand and wrist; median nerve, finger, and long thumb flexor tendons pass beneath flexor retinaculum (transverse carpal ligament) at wrist. (Courtesy Heather R. Weeks, The Jewish Hospital School of Nursing, St. Louis, Mo.)

Although hand movements are achieved by the action of various muscles and their tendons, muscle function depends on adequate innervation of the muscle belly. The motor nerves of the hand are (1) the radial nerve to the extensors, (2) the median nerve to a majority of the flexor tendons and a few intrinsic muscles, and (3) the ulnar nerve to a majority of the intrinsic muscles and the remaining flexors.

Sensation in the hand is provided by the same three nerves: (1) the radial nerve supplies the dorsal radial hand and fingers; (2) the median nerve, the volar (palmar) radial hand and digits (thumb, index, long, and radial side of the ring finger); and (3) the ulnar nerve, the remaining dorsal and volar ulnar hand and fingers. As the terminal sensory branches of the median and ulnar nerves enter the thumb and fingers, they are called digital nerves (Fig. 21-55).

The principal blood supply for the hand is from the radial and ulnar arteries that form a superficial and deep palmar arch in the hand, giving off terminal branches to both sides of each digit, called digital arteries after they enter the fingers and thumb (Fig. 21-55). A rich network of dorsal veins serves to return blood from the hand.

A minimum of skin and subcutaneous tissue covers the dorsum of the hand and digits. The skin covering the volar (palmar) surface is anchored to underlying fascia in areas of skin folds. Because of these fascial attachments, the skin and subcutaneous fat pads of the volar (palmar) surface do not move about during flexion and grasping of an object. The palmar fascia is a thick fibrous structure overlying the blood vessels, tendons, and nerves in the palm of the hand, to which skin is anchored, principally at the palmar skin creases. The palmar fascia sends extensions into each digit.

Special equipment

Pneumatic tourniquet (see also Chapter 20). Because it renders the operative field relatively bloodless, a tourniquet is almost essential in dealing with the complex, delicate, and vital structures within the hand. The tourniquet should be the pneumatic type, inflated with compressed gas, the pressure of which can be determined with an accurate gauge. Each tourniquet must be checked at regular intervals against a mercury manometer to maintain the accuracy of its gauge. The tourniquet can be a dangerous instrument when not in good working order and when improperly used.

The arm cuff of the tourniquet should be smooth and broad so that pressure is distributed evenly over a wide area. It should be placed as far proximally on the arm as possible, where a greater amount of soft tissue provides padding for underlying nerves and blood vessels as they are compressed against bone when pressure is applied. There should be no kinking of the tubing between the cuff and gas-regulating mechanism. To prevent a chemical burn, antimicrobial solutions used for skin preparation should not be allowed to run beneath the tourniquet cuff.

The arm is exsanguinated by progressively wrapping the arm from fingertips to tourniquet cuff (distal to proximal) with an Esmarch rubber bandage. The tourniquet is quickly inflated, to prevent filling of superficial veins before occlusion of the arterial blood flow. The Esmarch bandage is removed after inflation of the tourniquet cuff. The amount of pressure used to inflate the tourniquet depends on the size of the extremity and the patient's age and systolic blood pressure.

Tourniquet time should be kept to a minimum. Times of inflation and deflation should be recorded. After completion of the surgical maneuver that required use of the tourniquet, deflation of the cuff should be accompanied by total removal of the tourniquet from the arm. If the cuff is left on the arm after being deflated, it may cause some obstruction to the return of venous blood, which is perceived as increased bleeding at the operative site.

Boyes-Parker hand operating table (Fig. 21-56). The hand table is used for most hand operations. Adjustable legs allow fitting to any standard operating table level. The legs also provide maximum stability of the operative field. The surgeon and assistants sit during the operation. A stainless steel pan with drain and plug may be placed in the hand table to facilitate irrigation of wounds.

Stryker SurgiLav (Fig. 21-57). The SurgiLav is a sterile disposable system for lavage and debridement of tissue. It provides a pulsating jet stream of fluid when attached to a standard solution bag or bottle. Sterile disposable handpieces and tubing assemblies are available from the manufacturer, as well as several different types of irrigation tips and splash shields.

Intravenous regional anesthesia

Intravenous regional anesthesia (Chapter 9) is often used for hand operations and may be administered by the surgeon or an anesthesiologist. A pneumatic tourniquet with a double cuff plus dual control valves and tubing (Fig. 21-58) is used. A butterfly needle is inserted into a vein of the affected extremity and secured with tape. The position of the needle within the vein is assured by irrigating with sterile saline solution in a 10-ml syringe, which is left attached to the tubing of the butterfly needle. An Esmarch bandage is used to exsanguinate the extremity, and the proximal cuff of the tourniquet is inflated. After removal of the Esmarch bandage, 0.5% lidocaine is injected intravenously through the butterfly needle (usual dosage is 3 mg/kg of body weight, not exceeding a total dose of 250 mg). The butterfly needle is removed, and pressure is applied at the venipuncture site for several minutes. Preparation and draping of the patient usually follow.

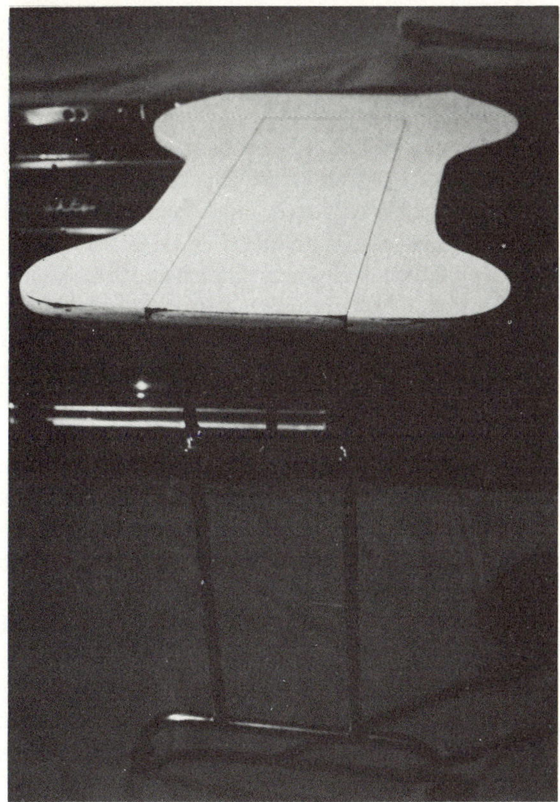

Fig. 21-56. Boyes-Parker hand operating table. Central segment slides out so stainless steel pan can be inserted during wound irrigation.

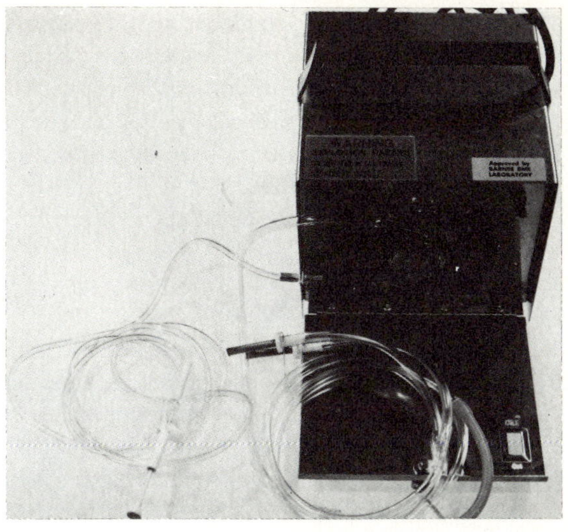

Fig. 21-57. Stryker SurgiLav for wound irrigation in hand surgery. Wheel at back of assembly is shown with tubing at bottom, which leads to solution bag or bottle; tubing at left delivers pulsatile flow of solution through multiple orifice irrigation tip shown here.

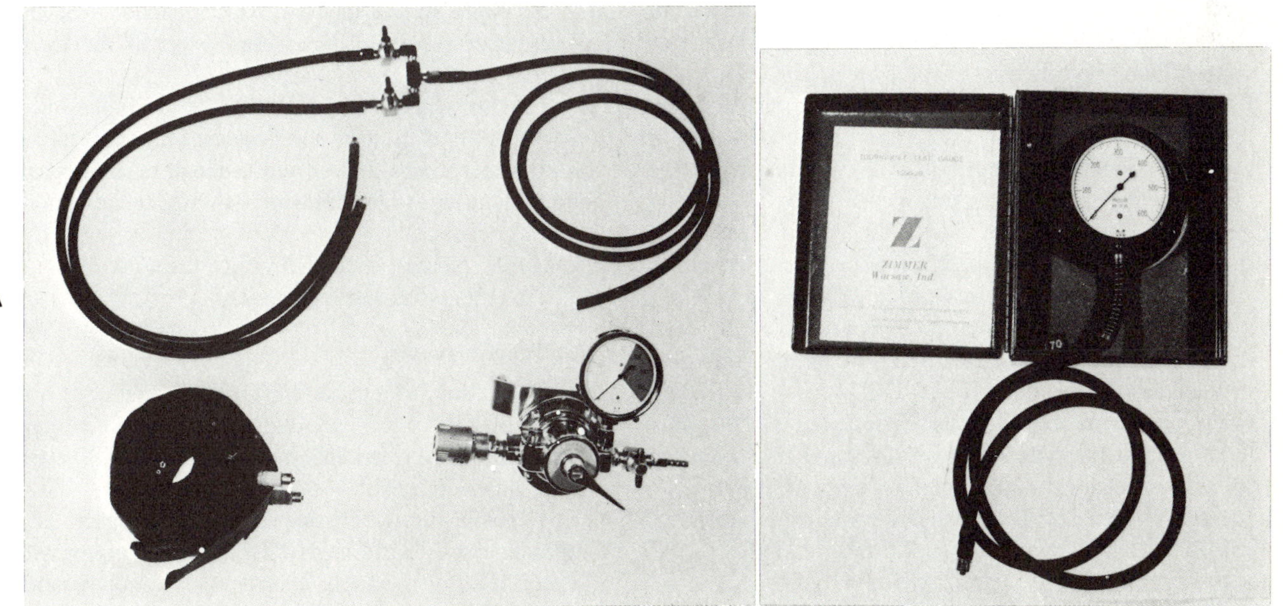

Fig. 21-58. Dual tourniquet cuff set for use with regional intravenous anesthesia. **A,** Dual cuff, dual control valves with tubing, and tourniquet pressure gauge (in mm Hg). **B,** Tourniquet test gauge.

The advantage of a tourniquet with a double cuff is as follows: The patient usually experiences moderate to severe tourniquet pain approximately 30 minutes after the procedure starts. When this occurs, the distal cuff may be inflated. The distal cuff lies over an anesthetized area of the arm, and the patient's discomfort should be reduced. After inflation of the distal cuff, the proximal cuff is deflated.

Dressings and immobilization

Basic conditions for good wound healing after hand surgery are immobilization and elevation. Adequate immobilization achieves support and splinting, to protect against both active and passive motion. With most hand operations, because of many closely related movements, it is usually necessary to immobilize the entire hand, fingers, wrist, and distal two thirds of the forearm. This immobilization is often maintained for 3 or 4 weeks after surgery. Application of the means of immobilization must therefore be performed with care, while the patient is still anesthetized. Although plaster of Paris may be used to achieve immobilization, many surgeons prefer a soft, bulky hand dressing. Steps in the application of a hand dressing are as follows:

1. An assistant supports the hand, which is elevated by flexing the elbow and resting it on the hand table.
2. Nonadherent gauze is applied over incisions.
3. Gauze dressing sponges in thin layers are placed between the fingers to prevent maceration. These sponges must be of uniform thickness from proximal to distal to prevent pressure on digital blood vessels.
4. A thicker layer of gauze is placed between the thumb and index finger to prevent an adduction contracture of the thumb. In addition to abduction, the thumb is also rotated into opposition as the dressing is applied.
5. Mechanic's waste or acrylic fiber is placed in the palm of the hand for bulk, so that it can support the PIP and DIP joints of the fingers in extension. It may also be added to the thumb-index finger web space to maintain thumb abduction.
6. Folded abdominal pads are placed vertically across the dorsal and volar surfaces of the wrist for support.
7. Two Kling gauze rolls are wrapped around the hand and forearm so that the MP joints are in approximately 90 degrees flexion, the PIP and DIP joints are extended, the thumb is in abduction and opposition, and the wrist is in neutral position. All fingertips must be exposed to permit inspection for determining viability.
8. Inch-wide strips of adhesive tape are applied vertically over the dressing (to avoid constricting bands).

Operations

Treatment of fractures

Considerations. Fractures within the scope of hand surgery may involve the phalanges in the fingers, the metacarpals in the hand, and/or the carpals in the wrist. The basis for treatment of any fracture is reduction of the fracture and immobilization until healing occurs.

Reduction of a fracture may be closed or open. Closed reduction is performed by manipulating the fracture fragments beneath intact skin and subcutaneous tissue. X-ray studies verify the reduction. Open reduction is performed by making an incision, visualizing the fracture site, and then manipulating the fragments under direct vision. X-ray films are usually also obtained after open reduction.

Immobilization of a fracture may be external or internal. External methods include splinting and/or casting. Internal immobilization in hand fractures is usually accomplished by inserting Kirschner wires (Fig. 21-59). This may be the sole method by which a reduction can be stabilized. It has the additional advantage of allowing motion in a maximum number of hand joints while immobilizing only the injured part, thus preventing unnecessary joint stiffness.

Setup and preparation of the patient. A plastic hand instrument set, a Stryker Kirschner-wire driver, an Esmarch bandage, and a marking pen are required.

The patient is placed in the supine position on the operating table with the arm extended on a hand table. The hand drape is used.

Operative procedure (open reduction, internal fixation)

1. The incision is marked.
2. The pneumatic tourniquet is inflated.
3. The incision is made, and the fracture is exposed.
4. The fracture is reduced by manipulating the fragments digitally or instrumentally under direct vision.
5. While an assistant holds the reduction, Kirschner wires are driven into bone, usually across the fracture site.
6. After x-ray films are obtained to verify the fracture reduction, the Kirschner wires are cut off so that the ends are buried beneath skin or with a short segment protruding through skin. This segment is twisted down with needle-nose pliers.
7. The incision is sutured in one layer (skin).
8. A hand dressing is applied.

Tendon repair

Definition. When continuity of a tendon is interrupted by avulsion or laceration, a specific active movement of one or more joints of the hand is lost. The treatment is tendon repair.

Considerations. Primary flexor or extensor tendon repair is usually performed at the time of injury or within several days of the acute injury. When adequate tendon length is present on each side of the laceration, repair is performed by suturing the tendon ends together (Fig. 21-60). When the laceration is near the bony insertion of the tendon, the distal tendon segment is too short to permit

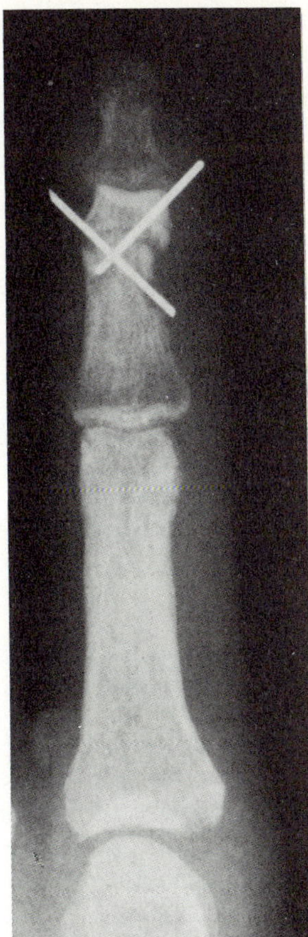

Fig. 21-59. Radiograph shows fracture of middle phalanx of index finger following open reduction, with internal fixation by means of crossed Kirschner wires across fracture site.

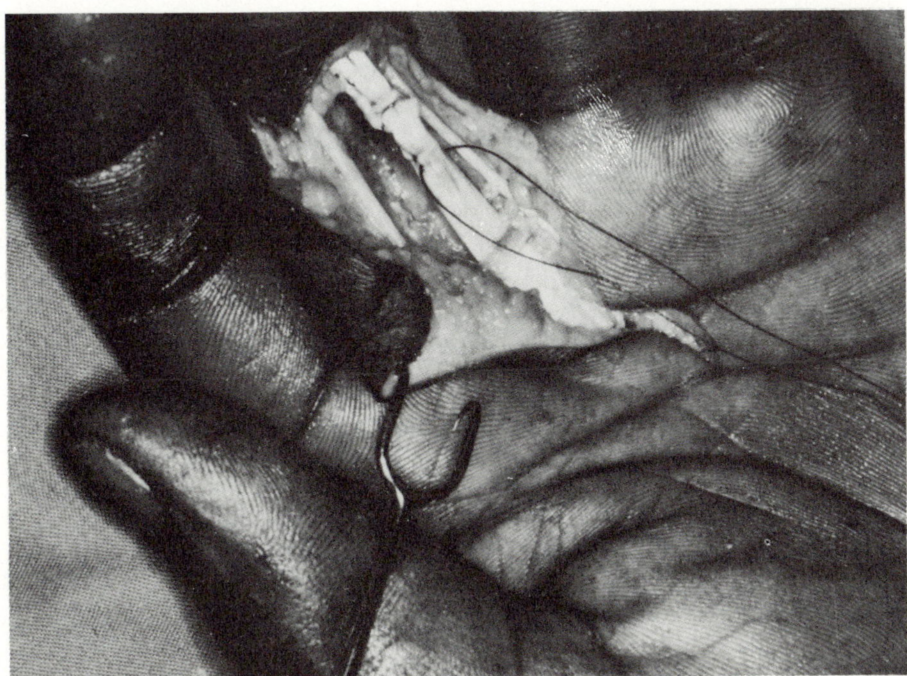

Fig. 21-60. Primary repair of flexor profundus tendon of long finger in distal palm.

adequate purchase for a suture. In this case, tendon repair is performed by reinserting the proximal end of the tendon into bone.

Setup and preparation of the patient. A plastic hand instrument set, an Esmarch bandage, a marking pen, and no. 3-0 or 4-0, double-armed, nonabsorbable suture are required.

The patient is placed in the supine position on the operating table, with the arm extended on a hand table. The hand drape is used.

Operative procedure

1. The skin laceration is usually enlarged to permit adequate exposure of the tendon laceration, after first marking the skin extensions for the laceration and inflating the tourniquet.
2. An additional incision in the hand and/or wrist may be necessary to identify the retracted proximal tendon end.
3. The tendon is repaired by placing a no. 4-0 or 5-0, double-armed, nonabsorbable suture through the tendon ends and approximating the ends. A pullout suture may or may not be placed through the tendon suture.
4. If the repair involves reinsertion of the tendon into bone, a small bone flap is raised, a straight Keith needle is drilled through the bone with the hand drill, and the suture ends from the tendon are passed through the bone and are tied down over foam-rubber padding and a polyethylene button.
5. Incisions are closed in one layer.
6. A hand dressing is applied.

Flexor tendon graft

Definition. Graft used to restore function when the original tendon is incapable of so doing because of a large gap between ends of a lacerated tendon or because of a failed primary tendon repair. Although extensor tendon grafts are possible, the vast majority of free tendon grafts are flexor profundus and flexor pollicis longus tendon grafts.

Considerations. A gap large enough to preclude approximation by direct suture of the tendon ends results from loss of a segment of tendon at the time of injury or from shortening of the proximal tendon end if too long a time has elapsed since the original injury. A failed primary tendon repair is usually caused by scar tissue that inhibits adequate tendon gliding. Tendon gliding must be sufficient to produce appropriate joint movement when the muscle belly of the tendon contracts. If a great deal of scar tissue is present in the tendon bed, a free tendon graft also may fail to glide sufficiently to produce adequate joint movement. In this case, a silicone rod may be inserted into the tendon bed. The scar tissue that forms around the rod creates a pseudosheath through which a tendon graft is placed 6 to 8 weeks later. The pseudosheath often permits better tendon gliding.

The most commonly used donor tendon for a free graft is the palmaris longus tendon in the wrist and forearm. The plantaris tendon in the leg is also frequently used. Toe extensor tendons are used less commonly.

Setup and preparation of the patient. A plastic hand instrument set is required, plus the following special instruments (Fig. 21-61):

1 Brand tendon stripper
1 Sanders-Brown fascia needle
1 Silver probe, 9 inches
1 Hegar dilator, no. 6, with hole
1 Freer septal elevator with hole
1 Keith needle, straight
1 Polyethylene button
1 Foam rubber pad, small
1 No. 4 Lane needle, cutting and taper points
1 Goniometer
1 Esmarch bandage
Marking pen
Double-armed nonabsorbable suture, no. 3-0 or 4-0
Silicone tendon rod, 3 mm (optional)

The patient is placed in the supine position on the operating table, with the arm extended on a hand table. The hand drape is used. If the plantaris tendon or a toe extensor tendon is to be used as the donor tendon, the lower extremity also must be prepped and draped. Use of a pneumatic tourniquet on the leg is optional.

Operative procedure

1. After marking incisions and inflating the pneumatic tourniquet, a distal incision is made to expose the insertion of the flexor profundus tendon into the distal phalanx, and a proximal incision is made in the hand and/or wrist.
2. Scar tissue in the tendon bed is excised.
3. If the flexor tendon bed is not deemed suitable for a tendon graft, a 3-mm silicone rod is inserted and sutured distally to the profundus tendon remnant attached to the distal phalanx (Fig. 21-62).
4. If the tendon bed is suitable or a silicone rod has previously been inserted, a free tendon graft is obtained with the Brand tendon stripper.
5. Approximation of the proximal tendon end and graft is performed in the palm or wrist.
6. The graft is threaded through the tendon bed to the distal phalanx (Fig. 21-63), where it is inserted as described in step 4 of tendon repair, after the tension of the graft has been carefully adjusted.
7. The incisions are closed in one layer.
8. A hand dressing is applied.

Peripheral nerve repair and grafting

Definition. Nerve repair by direct approximation or by means of a nerve graft, for interruption of the continuity of a nerve in the hand, wrist, or forearm, which causes loss of sensation and/or motor function.

Fig. 21-61. Special instruments for flexor tendon graft. *1,* Freer septal elevator (with hole); *2,* Sanders-Brown fascia needle; *3,* silver probe; *4,* no. 6 Hegar dilator (with hole); *5,* Keith needle; *6,* foam rubber; *7,* polyethylene button; *8,* Brand tendon stripper.

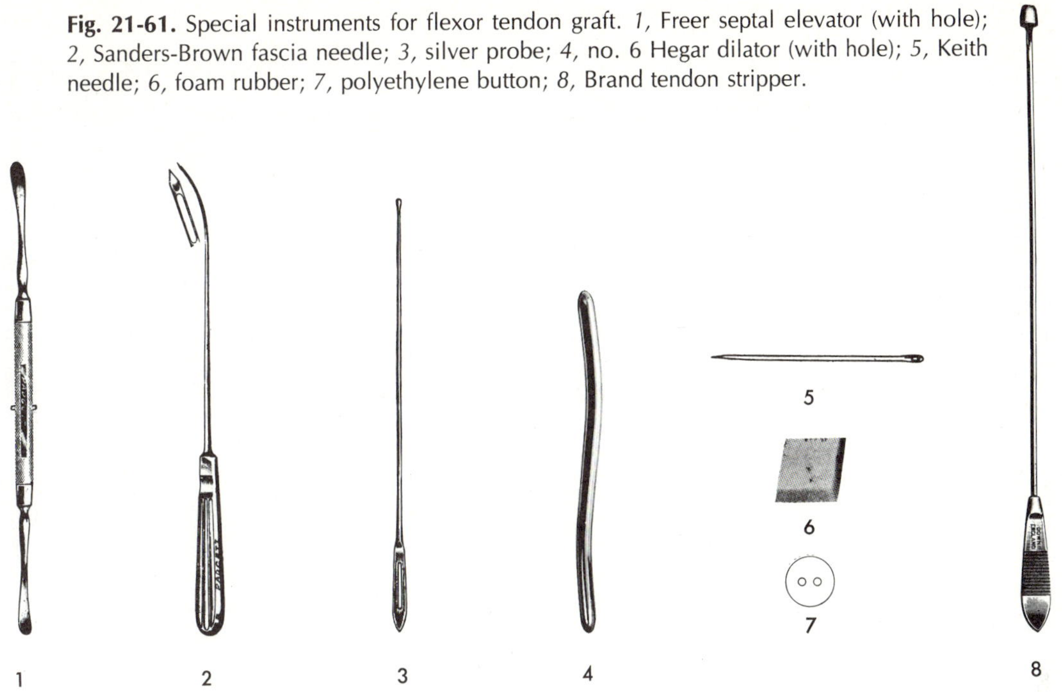

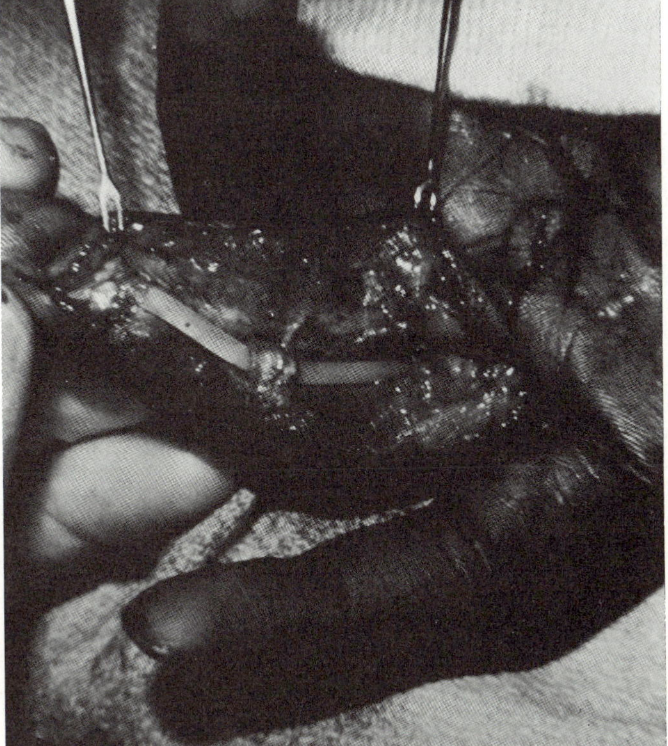

Fig. 21-62. Tendon prosthesis of silicone rubber placed into profundus tendon bed of long finger in preparation for flexor tendon grafting.

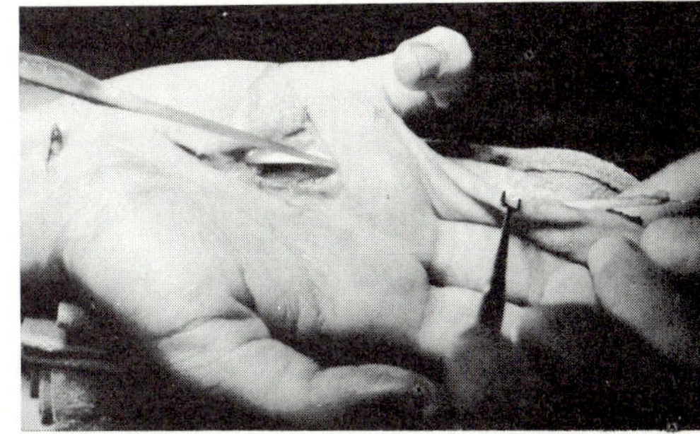

Fig. 21-63. Flexor tendon graft being threaded through profundus tendon bed of ring finger from palm to distal phalanx. Palmaris longus tendon has been obtained with Brand tendon stripper through small wrist incision.

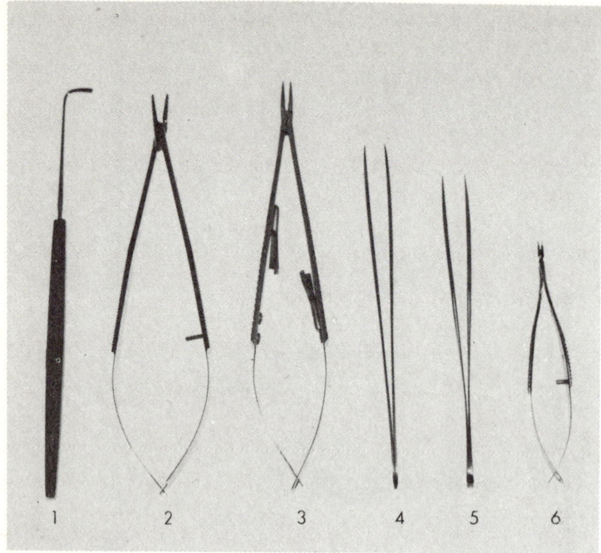

Fig. 21-64. Special instruments for nerve repair and grafting. *1,* von Graefe muscle hook; *2,* Castroviejo needle holder without lock; *3,* Castroviejo needle holder with lock; *4* and *5,* jeweler's forceps; *6,* Castroviejo-Vannas scissors.

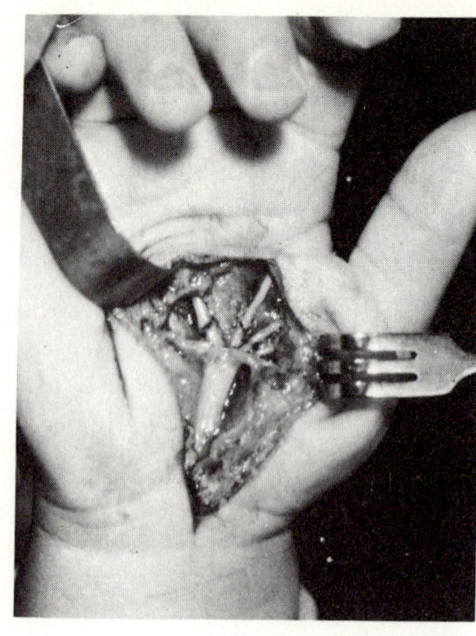

Fig. 21-65. Severed branches of median nerve have been reapproximated with fine sutures.

Setup and preparation of the patient. A plastic hand instrument set is required, plus the following special instruments (Fig. 21-64):

1 Jeweler's forceps
1 Castroviejo-Vannas scissors, curved
2 Castroviejo needle holders, straight, with and without lock
Nerve hook (von Graefe muscle hook)
Razor blade
Nerve stimulator
Esmarch bandage
Marking pen
Loupes or microscope

The patient is placed in the supine position on the operating table, with the arm extended on a hand table. The hand drape is used. If a nerve graft is to be used, the lower extremity is also prepped and draped. Use of a pneumatic tourniquet on the leg is optional.

Operative procedure

1. After incisions are marked and the tourniquet is inflated, the proximal and distal nerve ends are exposed.

2. Devitalized nerve tissue or scar at the severed nerve ends is resected sharply with a razor blade, back to normal nerve tissue, where individual nerve bundles can be visualized.

3. With the aid of loupes or the operating microscope, individual nerve bundles are each approximated (Fig. 21-65) with a fine, nonabsorbable suture (usually no. 7-0 to 10-0 nylon).

4. If a nerve graft is used, it is obtained through a series of short transverse incisions or one long vertical incision along the posterolateral aspect of the leg. Approximation of the nerve bundles between the graft and proximal and distal nerve ends is performed as in step 3.

5. The incisions are sutured.

6. A hand dressing is applied so that tension at the site of repair is prevented.

Implant arthroplasty

Definition. Excision of the joint surfaces to achieve motion in joints that are stiff as a result of destruction of their articular surfaces. Insertion of an implant may accompany an arthroplasty.

Considerations. Destruction of the cartilage that forms the articular surface of a joint results in stiffness and pain during movement of the joint. Traumatic arthritis and rheumatoid arthritis are the most common causes of destruction of articular joint surfaces. Excision of the diseased joint surface affords relief of pain and improves joint motion. Insertion of an implant is an adjunct to resection arthroplasty. The implant serves as a dynamic joint spacer, not a joint prosthesis.

The most commonly used implants in hand surgery are flexible implants made of silicone rubber (Silastic). Flexible implants available for arthroplasty within the scope of hand surgery are finger joints (for MP and PIP joints), wrist joint, carpal trapezium, lunate, and navicular (scaphoid).

Setup and preparation of the patient. A plastic hand instrument set is required, plus the following:

Stryker oscillating bone saw
Hall II drill with Swanson burs
Alloplastic implant of choice (Fig. 21-4)
Esmarch bandage
Marking pen

The patient is placed in the supine position on the operating table, with the arm extended on a hand table. The hand drape is used.

Operative procedure

1. The involved joint is exposed through an appropriate incision after the incision is marked and the pneumatic tourniquet is inflated.

2. In finger-joint resection arthroplasty, the joint surfaces are excised together with comprehensive soft-tissue release of the joint capsule. In resection arthroplasty of a carpal bone, the involved bone is completely excised.

3. In finger-joint arthroplasty, the medullary canals of the two adjacent bones are reamed with the Hall II drill with Swanson burs. In carpal bone implant resection arthroplasty, holes are reamed in one appropriate adjacent bone.

4. The two stems of a finger or wrist-joint implant or the single stem of a carpal-bone implant are seated in adjacent bones.

5. Soft tissues of the joint capsule (ligaments, tendons) are repaired.

6. The skin incisions are closed.

7. A hand dressing is applied.

Palmar fasciectomy

Definition. Partial or total excision of the palmar fascia, employed for Dupuytren's contracture.

Considerations. Dupuytren's contracture is a progressive disease, involving the palmar fascia and the digital extensions of the palmar fascia. It usually begins with a small nodular thickening in the palm, most frequently in line with the ring finger. With progression of the disease, additional nodules appear, usually with skin adherent to them. Subsequent contracted longitudinal bands of palmar fascia may appear beneath the skin. When the digital extensions of the palmar fascia become involved in the disease process, flexion contractures of the finger MP and PIP joints result.

The cause of Dupuytren's contracture is unknown. One or both hands may be involved. The disease may also be present in the foot in the form of nodules and cords involving the plantar fascia. It does not result in contracture of the toes, however, because the plantar fascia has no digital (toe) extensions.

Surgery is the preferred treatment for Dupuytren's contracture, preferably at an early stage in the disease, before irreparable joint damage occurs as the result of prolonged fixed flexion contracture. Surgical procedures include fasciotomy (simple division of contracted bands) or partial or total excision of the palmar fascia. In long-standing disease with irreversible joint changes, amputation of the finger may be the only treatment possible.

Setup and preparation of the patient. A plastic hand instrument set is required, plus an Esmarch bandage and a marking pen.

The patient is placed in the supine position on the operating table, with the arm extended on a hand table. The hand drape is used.

Operative procedure (Fig. 21-66)

1. Incisions are marked, often with several Z-plasties to lengthen the involved skin of the finger and palm (as for scar revision).

2. The tourniquet is inflated.

3. After incisions are made, flaps of skin and subcutaneous tissue are carefully elevated to preserve their blood supply, exposing the fibrotic palmar fascia and its digital extensions.

4. Part or all of the palmar fascia and digital extensions are excised.

5. The tourniquet is usually released before skin closure, so hemostasis can be obtained.

6. Incisions are sutured. A shortage of skin is sometimes noted at this point, in which case coverage by means of a full-thickness skin graft is required.

7. If skin grafts are used, they are stented, and then a hand dressing is applied.

Carpal tunnel release

Definition. Incision or excision of the transverse carpal ligament, with or without synovectomy, to relieve the symptom complex produced by compression of the median nerve within the carpal canal at the wrist.

Considerations. The carpal tunnel is located along the volar surface of the wrist. Its rigid boundaries consist of carpal bones along three sides and the transverse carpal ligament along the fourth (volar) side. The median nerve, superficial and deep finger flexors, and the long thumb flexor tendon all pass through the carpal tunnel before entering the hand (see Fig. 21-55). Any condition that decreases the size of the canal, such as fracture of a carpal bone, or increases its volume, such as the hypertrophic synovitis of rheumatoid arthritis, may cause pressure on the median nerve with resultant symptoms of carpal tunnel syndrome. However, in a majority of cases the cause of carpal tunnel syndrome is unknown.

The symptoms of median nerve compression at the wrist are usually pain and paresthesia in the thumb, the index finger, the long finger, and the radial half of the ring finger. Long-standing median nerve compression may result in hand weakness and thenar muscle atrophy. The condition may be unilateral or bilateral.

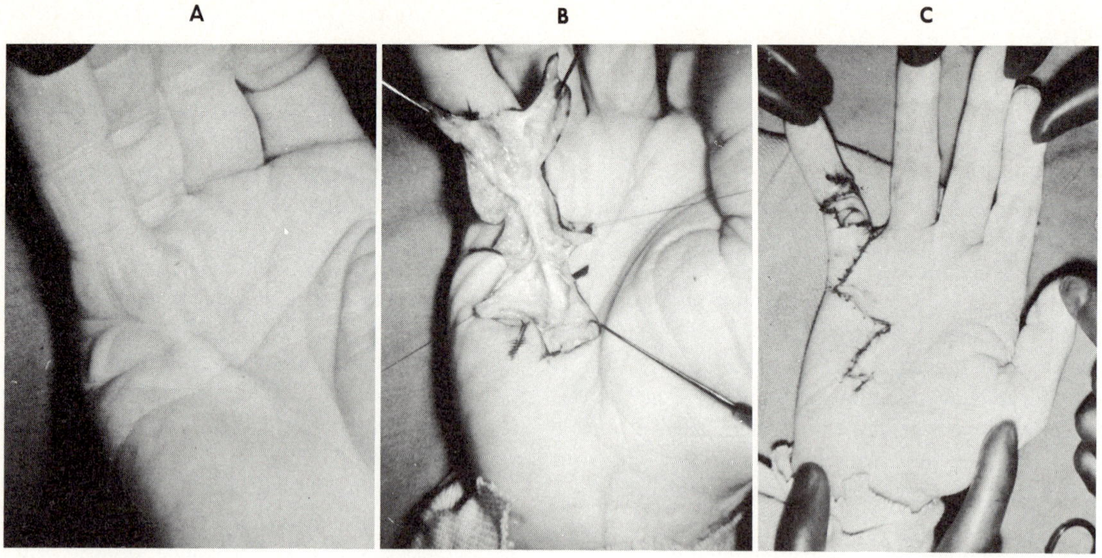

Fig. 21-66. Dupuytren's contracture involving palmar fascia and its digital extensions into little finger. **A,** Cord and nodules in palm with mild flexion contracture of little finger. **B,** Contracted band of palmar fascia exposed. **C,** Wound closure with multiple Z-plasties to lengthen contracted skin.

Setup and preparation of the patient. A plastic hand instrument set, is required, plus an Esmarch bandage and a marking pen.

The patient is placed in the supine position on the operating table, with the arm extended on a hand table. The hand drape is used. The operation may be performed under general, axillary block, or intravenous regional anesthesia.

Operative procedure

1. After appropriate skin marking and inflation of the pneumatic tourniquet, an incision is made across the volar wrist surface and base of the palm, to adequately expose the transverse carpal ligament.
2. The transverse carpal ligament is incised along its entire length. A segment of it may be excised.
3. Synovectomy of structures within the carpal canal may or may not be performed.
4. The incision is closed in one layer.
5. A hand dressing is applied.

Microsurgery

Definition. Relatively new art of operating with the aid of an operating microscope, which has applications in various surgical subspecialties. In plastic surgery, microsurgery serves as a method for transplantation or salvage of composite tissues by means of microneurovascular anastomosis and repair.

Considerations. The most common plastic surgery operation requiring microsurgical techniques is replantation of amputated parts (usually digits). Digital replants are done under the following conditions: (1) an attempt should always be made to replant the thumb; (2) with loss of multiple fingers, an attempt should be made to replant at least one of the fingers; (3) single-digit replants of an amputated finger are done only in females for cosmetic reasons and in children in whom a better functional result can be expected; and (4) occasionally a microsurgical transfer of the great toe to the hand is indicated to replace a lost thumb.

The success of digital replantation primarily depends on microsurgical repair of one digital artery and two digital veins. Replantation of an amputated part is ideally performed within 4 to 6 hours after injury, but success has been reported up to 24 hours after injury, if the amputated part has been cooled. The success of replantation also depends in part on the type of injury causing the amputation; that is, greater success is achieved with the guillotine type of amputation than in avulsion or crush injuries. Most centers performing replantations now report an 80% to 90% viability rate with replantation of guillotine amputations as far distally as the distal phalanx of the finger.

The ultimate aim of replantation is the restitution of function beyond that provided by a prosthesis. Function primarily depends on the quality of recovered sensation, and this is accomplished by means of digital nerve repair using microsurgical techniques. Skin coverage, freedom from pain, and the ability to position the part are also

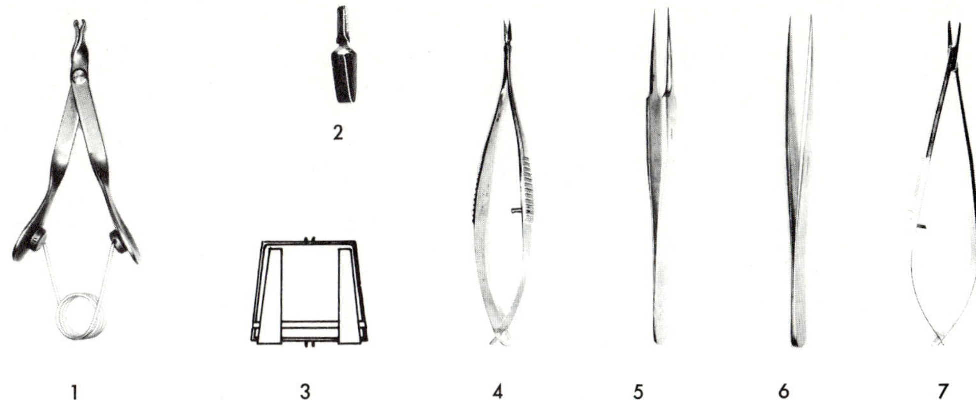

Fig. 21-67. Special instruments for microsurgery. *1,* Microvessel clip applying forceps; *2,* microvessel clips; *3,* Acland double clamps with frame; *4,* Barraquer needle holder; *5* and *6,* jeweler's forceps; *7,* Castroviejo-Vannas scissors.

important considerations in the return of function.

Setup and preparation of the patient. A plastic hand instrument set is required, plus the following special instruments (Fig. 21-67):

Jeweler's forceps, nos. 2, 3C, and 5
Barraquer needle holder, curved
Castroviejo-Vannas scissors, curved
Microvessel clips, assorted
Microvessel clip applying forceps
Approximating clamp, double
Stryker Kirschner-wire driver
Operating microscope
Bipolar cautery
Heparin, 100 units/ml
Lidocaine 1%

For digital replantation, two teams usually operate simultaneously. One team prepares the amputated part, often starting before the patient arrives in the operating room. The patient is placed in the supine position on the operating table, with the affected arm extended on a hand table. A pneumatic tourniquet is placed on the upper arm, and a hand drape is used.

Operative procedure

1. Bone ends are shortened to eliminate any tension on the vascular anastomoses to be done later; the bone is stabilized by means of internal fixation with Kirschner wires.

2. Flexor and extensor tendon repairs are usually performed next.

3. The digital nerves are repaired with the aid of loupes or the operating microscope.

4. With microsurgical instruments and techniques, two digital veins are repaired, followed by repair of one digital artery. If ischemic time is prolonged, digital-vessel repair may precede repair of tendons and nerves.

5. The skin is sutured.

6. A bulky supportive hand dressing is applied.

SUGGESTED READINGS

Bostwick, J., III: Breast reconstruction: a comprehensive approach, Clin. Plast. Surg. **6:**143, 1979.

Bostwick, J., Vasconez, L.O., and Jurkiewicz, M.J.: Breast reconstruction after a radical mastectomy, Plast Reconstr. Surg. **61:**682, 1978.

Burt, B., and Bostwick, J.: Nipple-areola reconstruction with auricular tissues, Plast. Reconstr. Surg. **60:**353, 1977.

Byars, L.T.: A technique for consistently satisfactory repair of hypospadias, Surg. Gynecol. Obstet. **100:**184, 1955.

Chang, W.H.: Fundamentals of plastic and reconstructive surgery, Baltimore, 1980, The Williams & Wilkins Co.

Chouinard, F., and others: Vigilant nursing care after reconstructive microsurgery, Nursing '79 **9**(6):18, 1979.

Converse, J.M., editor: Reconstructive plastic surgery: principles and procedures in corrective reconstruction and transplantation, ed. 2, Philadelphia, 1977, W.B. Saunders Co.

Gittes, R.F., and McLaughlin, A.P., III: Injection technique to induce penile erection, Urology **4:**473, 1974.

Grabb, W.C., and Smith, J.W., editors: Plastic surgery: a concise guide to clinical practice, ed. 3, Boston, 1973, Little, Brown & Co.

Grazer, F.M., and Klingbeil, R., editors: Body image: a surgical perspective, St. Louis, 1980, The C.V. Mosby Co.

Hester, R., and others: Reconstruction of cervical esophagus, hypopharynx and oral cavity using free jejunal transfer, Am. J. Surg. **487,** 1980.

Hodgson, N.B.: A one stage hypospadias repair, J. Urol. **104:**281, 1970.

Hollinshead, W.H.: Anatomy for surgeons, vol. 3, ed. 2, New York, 1969, Harper & Row, Publishers.

Horton, C.E.: Plastic and reconstructive surgery of the genital area, Boston, 1980, Little, Brown & Co.

Mathes, S.J., and Nahai, F.: Clinical atlas of muscle and musculocutaneous flaps, St. Louis, 1979, The C.V. Mosby Co.

Mauldin, B.: Breast reconstruction after mastectomy, AORN J. **32:**612, 1980.

Milford, L.: The hand, ed. 2, St. Louis, 1982, The C.V. Mosby Co.

Rees, T.D.: Aesthetic plastic surgery, Philadelphia, 1980, W.B. Saunders Co.

Sheen, J.H.: Aesthetic rhinoplasty, St. Louis, 1978, The C.V. Mosby Co.

Tessier, P., and others, editors: Symposium on plastic surgery in the orbital region, vol. 12, St. Louis, 1976, The C.V. Mosby Co.

Wood-Smith, D., and Porowski, P.C., editors: Nursing care of the plastic surgery patient, St. Louis, 1967, The C.V. Mosby Co.

Woodward, J.R., and Cleveland, R.: Application of Horton-Devine principles to the repair of hypospadias, J. Urol. **127:**1155, 1982.

22 Ear, nose, and throat surgery

■ Ear

The Latin word *audire* means to hear; thus the word auditory refers to the sense of hearing. The physical nature of sound pertains to the pressure waves and moving molecules, whereas the sensations humans feel lie in the ears, nerves, and brain. The study of the ear and its diseases is known as otology, derived from the Greek word *otos,* meaning ear.

The ear is a complex mechanism that receives sound waves, discriminates their frequencies, and then transmits this auditory information to the central nervous system. When a person falls asleep, the sense of hearing is the last of the senses to disappear, and when a person awakens, it is the first sense to return. In humans, the ear has an additional function in relation to the maintenance of body equilibrium.

ANATOMY AND PHYSIOLOGY

Ear

The ear is comprised of three distinct divisions: the external ear (pinna, or auricle), the middle ear, and the inner ear (Fig. 22-1). The middle and inner ear structures are situated in the temporal bone cavity.

External ear. The external ear consists of an *auricle,* or *pinna,* and an external *auditory meatus* (a tube that ends at the tympanic membrane, or drum, Fig. 22-2). The auricle is almost lacking in function and is motionless in humans. It is covered with skin and consists of a plate of elastic cartilage and some subcutaneous tissue, which form elevations and depressions. The skin on the outer side (front) of the auricle adheres tightly to the underlying cartilage, whereas that on the posterior (back) surface is looser (Fig. 22-2). For this reason a skin graft is frequently taken from the posterior surface, thus resulting in less gross deformity and scarring.

The external ear has an abundant blood and lymphatic supply. The nerve supply to the external ear is primarily derived from the trigeminal nerve (fifth cranial) and from the cervical nerves. A branch of the vagus nerve (tenth cranial) enters the posterior part of the ear canal. There is a good neural anastomosis between the external ear and middle ear (Fig. 22-1).

The external auditory canal collects sound waves and serves as a protector and a pressure amplifier. This canal is a twisting passageway about half an inch long, directed inward and forward, lying between the concha and the tympanic membrane (Fig. 22-3). It terminates medially in a sulcus (depression) of the tympanic membrane. The walls of the outer third of the canal are fibrocartilaginous; those of the inner two thirds are bony. When the physician inspects the eardrum, the cartilaginous portion of the canal is straightened by drawing the auricle upward and backward with an aural speculum. Lying within the cartilaginous portion of the auricle are fine hairs, sebaceous glands, and special glands that produce cerumen. The tympanic membrane, or eardrum, is the so-called closing membrane. It stretches across the deepest part of the ear canal, thereby serving as a partition between the external canal and the tympanic cavity (Fig. 22-1).

Tympanic membrane. The *tympanic membrane* is composed of three layers: the external layer, which is continuous with the epidermal lining of the meatus; the middle fibrous layer; and the inner layer, which is a continuation of the mucous membrane of the middle ear. The small upper portion of the tympanic membrane is known as Shrapnell's membrane or the pars flaccida (Fig. 22-3). The larger, vibrating part of the tympanic membrane, which has a fibrous layer, is called the *pars tensa* (Fig. 22-3). The fibers of the tympanic membrane at its margins form a thickened incomplete band called the *annulus.* It fits into the bony tympanic sulcus. The annulus breaks superiorly between the anterior and lateral ligaments of the malleus.

Middle ear. The middle ear is a narrow, irregular, oblong, air-conditioning cavity located in the tympanic portion of the temporal bone, which is directly behind the eardrum. In this air-filled space are three very small bones, or ossicles: the malleus, incus, and stapes (Figs. 22-1 and 22-4), as well as the facial nerve (seventh cranial), which controls movements of the face, and the chorda tympani nerve, which provides taste for most of the anterior portion of the tongue (Fig. 22-5). The temporal lobe of the brain and its meninges are in association with the middle ear and mastoid (Fig. 22-5). This cavity communicates anteriorly, via the eustachian tube, with the nasopharynx and posteriorly, via the aditus, with the mastoid process. The middle ear is lined with mucous membrane, which extends into the eustachian tube (Figs. 22-1 and 22-5).

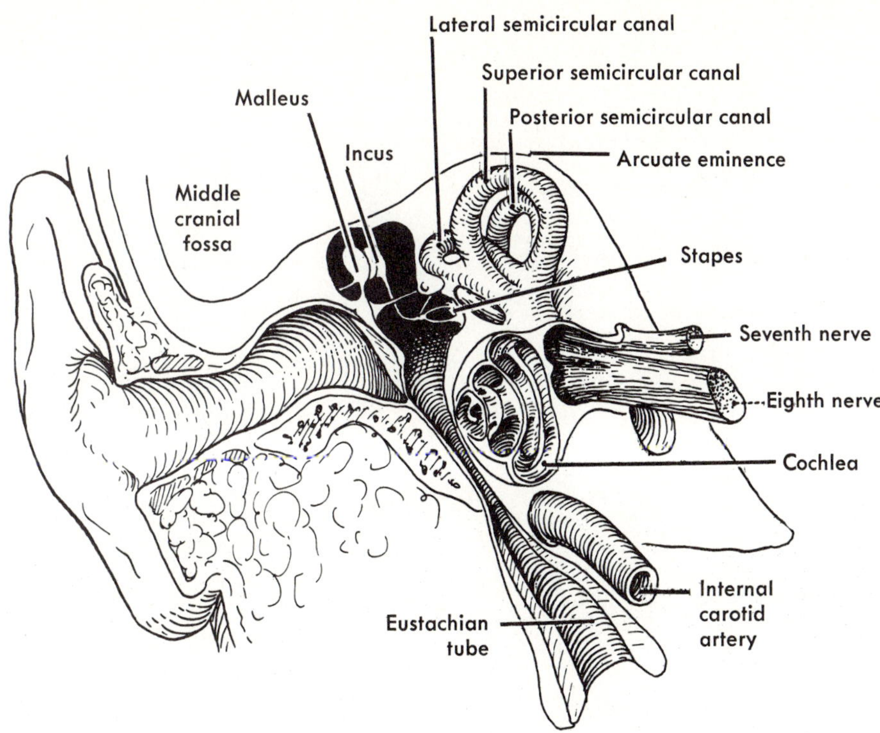

Fig. 22-1. Schematic drawing of external ear, middle ear, and inner ear. It is not possible to show all structures in a single plane; therefore there are distortions from actual anatomy in this schema. (From DeWeese, D.D., and Saunders, W.H.: Textbook of otolaryngology, ed. 3, St. Louis, The C.V. Mosby Co.)

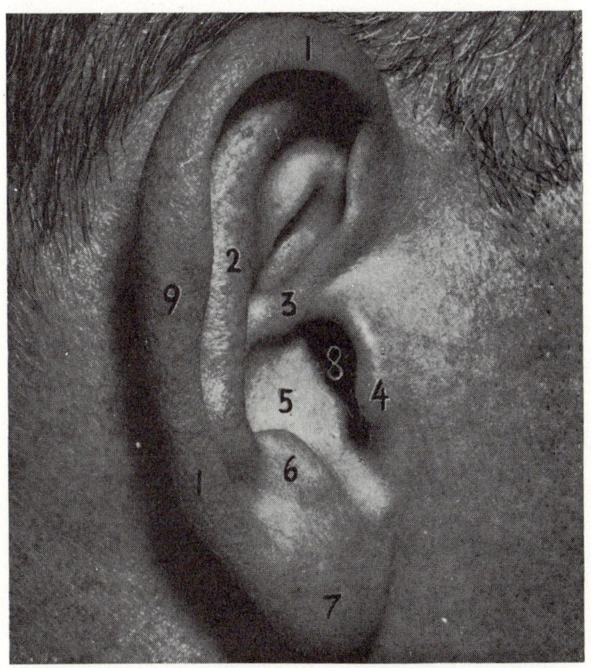

Fig. 22-2. Auricle. *1,* Helix; *2,* antihelix; *3,* crus of helix; *4,* tragus; *5,* concha; *6,* antitragus; *7,* lobule; *8,* external auditory meatus; *9,* Darwin's tubercle. (From DeWeese, D.D., and Saunders, W.H.: Textbook of otolaryngology, ed. 6, St. Louis, 1982, The C.V. Mosby Co.)

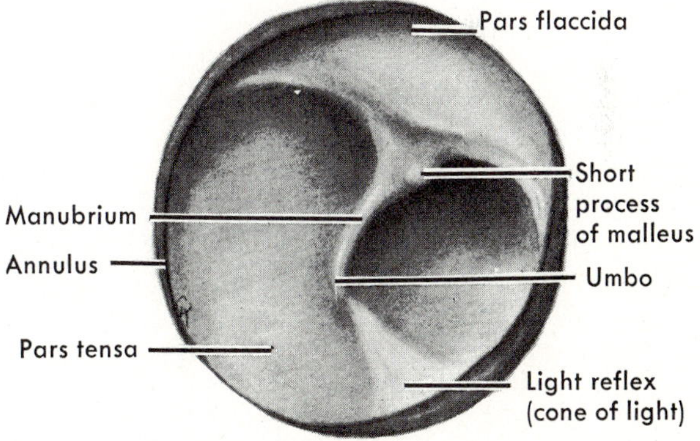

Fig. 22-3. Landmarks of right tympanic membrane. Size of pars flaccida is exaggerated in this drawing. (From DeWeese, D.D., and Saunders, W.H.: Textbook of otolaryngology, ed. 6, St. Louis, 1982, The C.V. Mosby Co.)

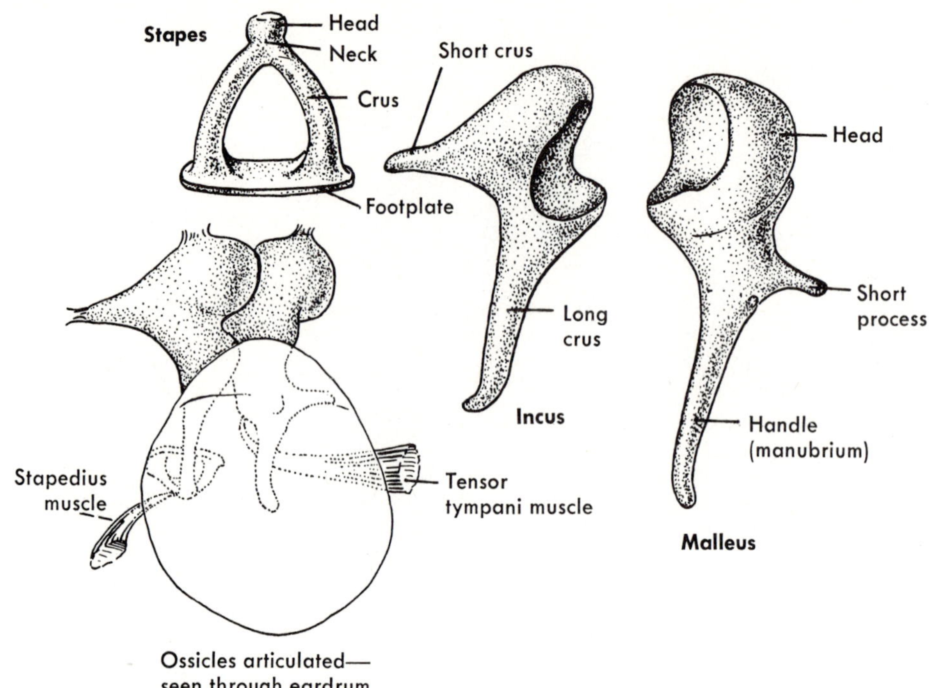

Fig. 22-4. Drawing of right ear showing articulated ossicles of middle ear. (From DeWeese, D.D., and Saunders, W.H.: Textbook of otolaryngology, ed. 6, St. Louis, 1982, The C.V. Mosby Co.)

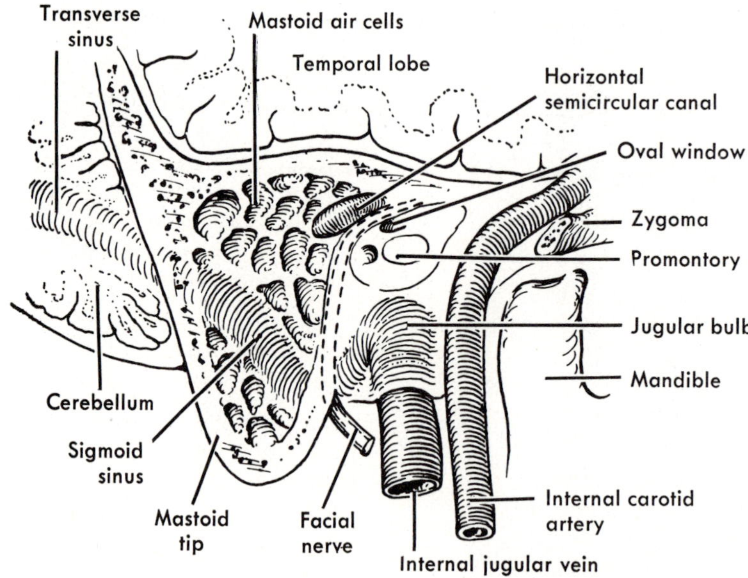

Fig. 22-5. Composite drawing of right ear showing relationship between middle ear, mastoid, and surrounding structures. (From DeWeese, D.D., and Saunders, W.H.: Textbook of otolaryngology, ed. 6, St. Louis, 1982, The C.V. Mosby Co.)

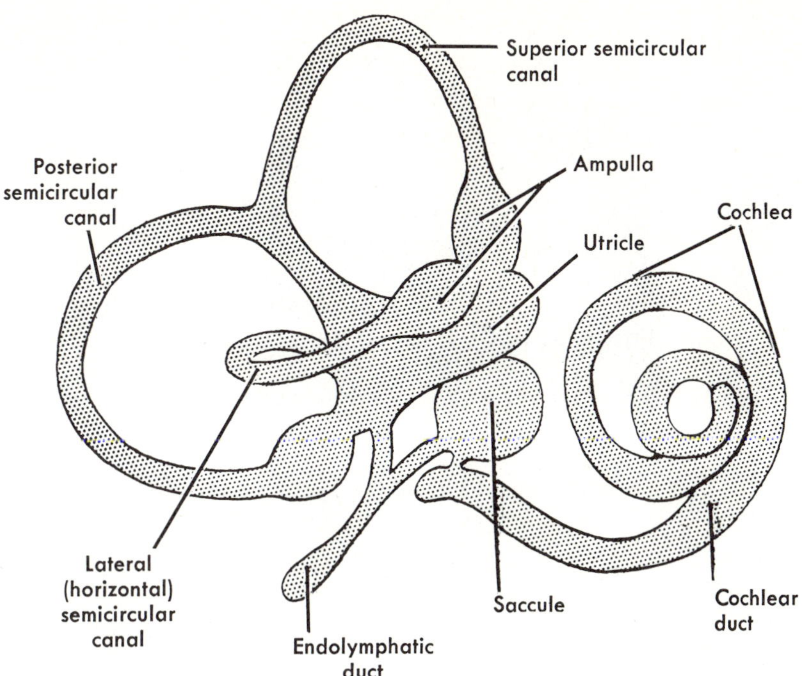

Fig. 22-6. Membranous endolymphatic system of right ear, lateral view. Endolymph of cochlea and labyrinth is continuous. Bony capsule of internal ear surrounds endolymphatic system and is separated from it by perilymphatic space. (From DeWeese, D.D., and Saunders, W.H.: Textbook of otolaryngology, ed. 3, St. Louis, The C.V. Mosby Co.)

The middle ear cavity is separated from the inner ear by the former's medial or inner wall. There is a promontory on the medial wall that marks the first turn of the cochlea in the internal ear (Fig. 22-6). Above and slightly behind the promontory is an opening, called the *oval window* to which the stapes is connected (Figs. 22-1 and 22-5). Below the promontory, covered by mucous membrane, is the round window.

The auditory ossicles in the middle ear cavity form a chain that conducts sound from the eardrum across the middle ear to the oval window, the opening in the inner ear (Fig. 22-5). The *malleus,* resembling a hammer, consists of a head, neck, handle, and long and short processes (Fig. 22-4). The handle and short process of the malleus are attached to the eardrum by very small muscles and join the second bone, the *incus*. Resembling an anvil, the incus consists of a body and long and short processes. The long crus of the incus is in contact with the third and innermost bone, the *stapes* (Fig. 22-4). Resembling a stirrup, the stapes consists of a head, neck, anterior and posterior crura, and footplate that fits in the oval window (Fig. 22-4). The tensor tympani muscle and stapedius muscle and their ligaments connect the ossicles. The ligaments and muscles attached to the ossicles are essential to their proper functioning. For example, the tensor tympani muscle acts to draw the drum inward to increase tension of the drum, whereas the stapedius muscle acts to draw the stapes away from the oval window to lessen tension of the drum. The middle ear and mastoid process are supplied with blood from the branches of the internal maxillary artery, a branch of the external carotid system. Important vascular channels are closely associated with the middle ear (Fig. 22-5). It has an abundant neural anastomosis.

Difficulties in hearing airborne sound may be corrected by a hearing aid, but proper bone conduction is essential to hearing one's own voice. When a bony growth is present in the ossicular chain, the ligaments and bones are unable to move mechanically as intended and thus interfere with the passage of sound waves to the inner ear.

Inner ear. The inner ear is a complex structure located in the petrous or rock-like, portion of the temporal bone. It has two distinct parts, each with specific functions that are delicately coordinated. One part (cochlea) is concerned with the special sense of hearing, and the other part (vestibular labyrinth) with the maintenance of equilibrium (Fig. 22-6). The two major parts of the inner ear—the cochlea and the vestibular labyrinth—have various compartments.

The bony cochlea and vestibular labyrinth lie in the petrous portion of the temporal bone (Fig. 22-5). In the small channels of these two structures are two distinct fluids: the perilymph and endolymph. The perilymph, lying in the bony canals, surrounds the membranous inner ear, thus serving as a protective cushion to the end organ re-

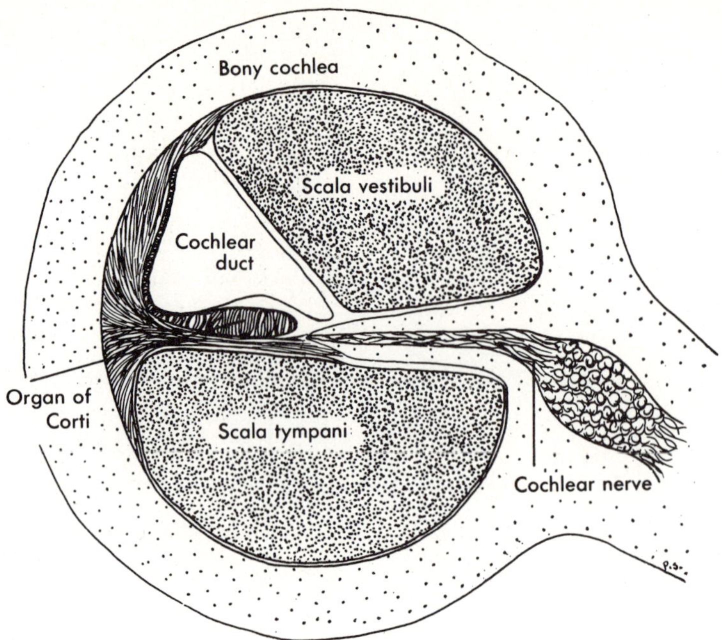

Fig. 22-7. Diagram of cross section of cochlea. (From DeWeese, D.D., and Saunders, W.H.: Textbook of otolaryngology, ed. 3, St. Louis, The C.V. Mosby Co.)

ceptors for hearing. The perilymph is continuous with the subarachnoid space and its cerebrospinal fluid through the aqueduct of the cochlea (cochlear duct). The endolymph, which is contained in a fragile membranous tube, bathes and nourishes the sensory cells and their supporting structures. The endolymph in the cochlea and labyrinth is contained in a continuous closed system with no ducts (Fig. 22-6).

Cochlea. The *cochlea* is a tubular formation that winds as a spiral around a central part, called the *modiolus*. Within the cochlea are three compartments (Fig. 22-7): the scala vestibuli, which is associated with the oval window; the scala tympani, which is associated with the round window; and the cochlear duct. The scala vestibuli and scala tympani rest in perilymph, whereas the cochlear duct contains endolymph.

On the vestibular surface of the basilar membrane of the cochlea is the delicate neural end organ for hearing, called the *organ of Corti*. From its neuroepithelium project thousands of fragile *hair cells* that are set in motion by the sound waves on entrance into the cochlea (Fig. 22-7). The organ of Corti extends along the entire length of the cochlea, except at the apex of the modiolus (helicotrema), where the scala tympani and scala vestibuli join.

The cochlea transmits sound waves to the auditory nerve and also acts as a microphone through which the mechanical energy of vibrations is converted into electrochemical impulses, probably by means of the hair cells of the organ of Corti.

The inner ear is connected with the brain through the eighth cranial (acoustic) nerve, which enters the temporal cortex of the cerebrum, where the impulses are interpreted as meaningful sound. This connecting fiber system (transverse gyri of Heschl) is located on both sides of the brain.

Vestibular labyrinth. The *vestibular labyrinth* of the inner ear is composed of the utricle, saccule, and three semicircular canals (Fig. 22-6) known as the lateral, superior, and posterior canals. In each ear, the canals are arranged at right angles to one another so that any movement of the head affects one or more of the semicircular canals. For example, when the head is in an erect position, the lateral (horizontal) canal is not quite horizontal. When a patient is turned quickly on the operating table, a current is set up in the endolymph by the neural cells in the vestibular labyrinth, thereby resulting in vertigo. Each canal is enlarged at a point near the utricle. This enlargement is called the *ampulla* of the canal, in which resides the specialized neuroepithelium (end organ of equilibrium).

The utricle of the vestibular labyrinth is concerned with static equilibrium and regulation of the sense of position in space. Stimulation of the utricle results in compensatory eye positions. The neural fibers from the utricle and semicircular canals join to form the vestibular portion of the eighth cranial nerve.

The blood supply of the internal ear is derived from the internal auditory branch of the basilar artery and the stylomastoid branch of the posterior auricular artery. The internal auditory artery enters the internal meatus and divides into the cochlea and vestibular labyrinth branches. The veins from the cochlea and labyrinth unite at the bottom of the semicircular canals to form the internal auditory veins.

Temporal bone

The temporal bone is composed of five separate parts, which are joined by suture lines (Fig. 22-5). Only the tympanic and petrous portions contain structures directly related to hearing. The *squamous* portion is a large piece of bone that is frequently pneumatized (Fig. 22-24). On its external surface is a groove for the middle temporal artery; on its internal surface are grooves for the middle meningeal vessels.

The *mastoid* portion of the temporal bone lies behind and below the squamous portion, attached to the sternocleidomastoid and digastric muscles. The internal surface of the mastoid process is in close association with important intracranial structures and with those of the middle ear (Fig. 22-5). The interior of the mastoid process is composed of a cortex that covers a system of intercommunicating air cells. The mastoid antrum is the largest of these air cells and connects directly with the middle ear through the aditus. The air cells are lines with a thin mucous membrane that is continuous with that of the middle ear.

The *petrous* portion of the temporal bone fuses with the base of the skull and contains the structures of the inner ear, including the sensory end organs of hearing and equilibrium. In the petrous portion are openings for the trigeminal ganglion, facial and auditory nerves, and internal auditory artery.

The *zygomatic* portion of the temporal bone extends anteriorly and joins the zygoma or malar bone of the cheek.

The *tympanic* portion of the temporal bone contains the middle ear and forms part of the ear canal.

Hearing loss

The amplitude of the air waves that strike the tympanic membrane determines the loudness or intensity of the sound.

In dealing with hearing loss, the loudness is measured in decibels (db). It is a logarithmic method of dealing with large numbers: the decibel is a ratio, not an absolute value; it compares the relationship between two sound intensities and the smallest perceptible change in loudness that the human ear can hear. Hearing loss is expressed by recording auditory acuity for each frequency in decibels.

• • •

The physiology of hearing may be summarized as follows:

1. The sound waves collect in the auricle.
2. The vibrating air waves pass into the external canal and hit the eardrum.
3. The ossicles, arranged in a lever system, respond to the vibration, thus amplifying the sound. First the malleus moves, and then this movement is transmitted to the incus, which in turn transmits it to the stapes.
4. The small footplate of the stapes delivers the sound to the inner ear by rocking the oval window.
5. Sound pressure, delivered through the oval window into the cochlea, agitates the perilymph and endolymph.
6. Relief of pressure is provided by shielding of the round window from sound.
7. The receptors of hearing (hair cells) are distorted.
8. Mechanical sound is transformed into electrochemical impulse.
9. These impulses are sent by way of the acoustic nerve to the temporal cortex of the brain, where they are interpreted as meaningful sound.

NURSING CONSIDERATIONS

Antibiotics, the operating microscope, delicate instrumentation, and ongoing improvement in implantable prosthetic devices coupled with better understanding of the anatomy and physiology of the ear enable the otological surgeon to perform procedures not only to improve hearing in a patient, but also to more carefully and fully control diseases of the mastoid.

New concepts and procedures are being introduced, and older procedures are constantly being refined. Surgical treatment for sensorineural hearing loss, or Ménière's disease, can be offered to patients who are afflicted by an intolerable tinnitus or vertigo that is severe enough to be disabling. Surgical treatments aimed at correcting hearing losses resulting from conduction apparatus abnormalities include stapedectomy and stapes replacement procedures.

Preoperative assessment

The preoperative assessment of the patient undergoing otological surgery should include all elements of an assessment done for any other type of surgery: chart review, conferring with appropriate unit personnel who are responsible for the care of the patient, and, of prime importance, the patient interview. Chart review should include close attention to patient allergies, expecially if drug related, since many otological procedures are performed under local anesthesia. Any antibiotic sensitivities should also be carefully noted. Physical limitations such as arthritis and back or neck problems should be observed to provide for optimum patient comfort during the surgical procedure. The operating room nurse should be able to answer patient questions related to the procedure in a clear and concise manner.

Patient teaching should include the following:

1. The patient should be advised to shampoo his hair as a part of the preoperative preparation because shampooing is not permitted for a period of 10 days to 2 weeks after surgery. The ear canal must be kept dry during this time. The patient should also be told that some hair may be shaved from around the ear depending on the procedure that is to be done. This may cause some concern for the black patient, since hair regrowth in these patients may be slow.

2. The patient should be cautioned not to lie on the operated ear for the first 24 hours after surgery. The head of the bed should be elevated during this period.

3. The patient should be told that there may be some vertigo for a day or so after surgery. If this occurs, the patient should request nursing assistance to get out of bed. Moving slowly and smoothly may help alleviate these unpleasant sensations. If the symptoms persist or are severe, antimotion drugs may be necessary.

4. The patient should be cautioned against deep coughing or nose-blowing. If sneezing is unavoidable, both the nose and mouth should be kept open. These points are important and should be reinforced; strict adherence may prevent a graft or prosthesis from being dislodged.

5. The patient should be made aware that hearing may be somewhat diminished during the immediate postoperative period. It should be reinforced that this is a temporary condition and that the hearing will improve gradually over a period of time.

6. The patient should be reminded about not going swimming or diving during the first weeks after surgery. In addition, the patient should be reminded not to drive during the first postoperative week. Air travel is also not advised during the first postoperative week; after that, it may be allowed only on a commercial airliner.

7. If the patient develops an upper respiratory infection or any other change in physical status, the physician should be contacted immediately.

8. Other special preoperative instructions may be needed depending on the individual physical condition or special requests of the operating surgeon. It should be understood by nursing personnel that the surgeon will usually discuss these points with the patient when the decision for surgery is made. Nursing personnel can discuss the principles with the patient and clarify any questions that the patient may have.

Intraoperative care

Duties of the circulating nurse

A smooth intraoperative phase is dependent on good preoperative preparation and assessment of the patient and proper application of information gained from the assessment process. If the patient has neck or back problems caused by arthritis or other conditions, special paddings and/or supports can be readied before the day of surgery, thereby allowing the circulating nurse more time to devote to the patient on arrival in the operating room.

Drug allergies can also be handled more effectively if known before the day of surgery. Appropriate alternatives should be available in accord with the surgeon's choice.

The circulating nurse should be capable of providing appropriate care for the awake patient. This care begins as soon as the patient enters the surgical suite. Depending on departmental policy, an intravenous infusion may be started to provide the patient with fluids during surgery and to provide a pathway for additional medications.

The circulating nurse should have the necessary equipment ready for monitoring the patient during surgery. This includes a cardiac monitor, blood pressure apparatus, oxygen setup, suction equipment, and emergency drugs.

The surgeon may begin the local anesthetic administration in a holding area or even in the operating room proper before the surgical preparation begins. With this in mind, the circulating nurse must assist in starting the procedure as efficiently as possible and at the same time observe the patient for signs of any reaction to the local anesthetics if administered or injected prior to the surgical preparation. Some of these signs are restlessness, apprehension, skin pallor, sweating, palpitations (if epinephrine is added to the local anesthetic), tremors, weakness, and in some instances fainting or any other adverse reaction by the patient. As with other patient complications, these should be reported to the surgeon immediately.

Because of preoperative sedation, the patient's visual and hearing perception may be altered somewhat. It is the responsibility of the circulating nurse to provide a quiet atmosphere during the surgery; a gentle reminder to those in the room to speak quietly and a sign posted on the outside of the operating room door indicating that a local anesthetic has been administered to the patient is helpful. In some instances, a radio playing softly in the background may be soothing to the patient. If departmental policy permits radios to be used in the operating room, they must be inspected and approved for use by appropriate electrical safety personnel. For infection control purposes, radios should be kept within the surgical suite.

During the course of surgery, the circulating nurse or a monitor nurse should continually monitor vital signs, the rate of fluid infusion, and the patient's general condition. If the patient becomes restless, the nurse should try to make the patient more comfortable. Often, just seeing the nurse is enough to reassure the patient. If the patient becomes extremely restless and uncooperative, it may be necessary for the surgeon to order additional medication for the patient. This should be done in accordance with departmental standards, and the patient should be observed closely for any adverse reactions.

Duties of the scrub nurse

During the course of surgery the scrub nurse can be of great assistance to the surgeon. The nurse must be familiar with the procedure being done, the instrumentation needed, and the care of the instruments during and after surgery. Because many of these procedures are done in semidarkness with the only illumination coming from the microscope light, an x-ray view box, or perhaps a small spotlight over the back table, the nurse must keep the Mayo stand in absolute order to be able to find the various fine-tipped instruments in the darkened operating room. The fine needle suction tips must be constantly flushed to be kept free of debris.

Preparation of the patient

For most otological procedures, the hair is removed and skin shaved at least 1½ inches from the site of the proposed incision. The hair is removed mainly from the area above the ear for an endaural approach and from behind the ear for a postauricular approach. Petrolatum may be rubbed into the hair along the hairline and then the hair brushed away from the operative field.

A solution of mild soap and water, a hexachlorophene soap (Hexagerm, Hibiclens, or pHisoHex) and water, or a povidone-iodine preparation is used to cleanse the exposed auricle and the periauricular skin. The meatus is cleansed with the aid of cotton applicators. A small amount of acetone or other type of skin degreaser may be applied around the ear to remove some of the soap fats and allow a disposable drape to adhere more securely to the skin.

Positioning

Quietness and immobility of the patient are most important in otological surgery. In some procedures, such as myringotomy under local anesthesia, an attendant should hold the patient's head firmly in position. For other operations (stapedectomy), the patient's head may be immobilized and supported in a padded headpiece attached to the operating table. Several available commercial foam headrests may be used, such as the Shea headrest. The comfort of the patient and proper body alignment are most important, especially in long procedures, such as tympanoplasty. Principles of positioning are discussed in Chapter 6.

The patient is placed on the operating table in a dorsal recumbent position, head resting on a firm pad or brace and turned to the side, with the affected ear uppermost. The upper extremities should rest alongside the body and be secured physiologically by a restraint sheet. The arms and body of an infant may be wrapped in a mummy type of sheet. To relieve pressure on nerves and to support muscles, firm padding of suitable shape and size should be used. In some cases the surgeon may prefer the patient to be in the prone position with a headpiece or firm pad.

For effective visualization, the head of the patient is turned with the affected ear uppermost; the surgeon stands or sits at the head of the patient. With inclined oculars, the surgeon looks directly ahead to visualize the post-canal wall. The entire operating table is tilted laterally 20 degrees to bring the external canal into proper position.

Draping

A standard ear pack is used. For major otological procedures, the towels and sheets are placed on the patient as follows.

Three towels, folded lengthwise, are placed around the operative site. The first towel is placed horizontally above the ear; the second towel is placed diagonally on the outer prepared skin area, surrounding the ear; and the third towel is placed vertically in front of the meatus, thereby creating a triangular operative field around the affected ear. A disposable, antistatic, adhesive small-aperture drape may be applied either over or under the draped towels or the fenestrated sheet.

A folded fenestrated sheet is unfolded over the patient and table, with the operative site in view through the opening.

The draped tables with sterile instruments and the operating microscope are positioned around the patient. For example, if the operation involves the left ear and is being done under general anesthesia, the sterile instrument tables are placed near the left side of the operating table. If the operation is under local anesthesia, the instrument tables are placed across the patient (Fig. 22-13). The scrub nurse usually sits or stands near the instrument table and passes the instruments in such a manner that the surgeon does not have to turn away from the operating microscope.

INSTRUMENTS AND SUPPLIES (Figs. 22-8 to 22-14)

Endaural mastoidectomy instruments

The endaural mastoidectomy setup includes the major ear pack, a head drape, a basin set, a skin prep set, operating table appliances, and the following instruments:

2 Lancet knives
1 Lempert flap knife
1 Myringotomy knife, curved
2 No. 3 knife handles with no. 15 blades
2 Dental picks, nos. 11 and 12
2 Dental picks, curved
2 Scissors, small, curved; 1 sharp and 1 blunt
1 Scissors, small, straight, sharp
1 House-Tragus hook
2 Mayo scissors, 1 straight and 1 curved
1 Endaural speculum
3 Walsh hand retractors, assorted
6 Endaural curettes, nos. 5-0 through 1
1 Olivecrona rongeur
1 Malleus nipper
1 Periosteal elevator, heavy
1 Periosteal elevator, light
2 Metal applicators
1 Bur holder with assorted cutting burs
2 Fine tissue forceps with and without teeth
2 Heavy tissue forceps with and without teeth
1 Bayonet tissue forceps

1 Adson tissue forceps
2 Needle holders
3 Mosquito forceps, straight, 5 inches
6 Mosquito forceps, curved, 5 inches
4 Towel clamps
1 Allis clamp, 6 inches
1 Rochester-Pean forceps, curved, 6¼ inches
1 Crile forceps, curved, 5½ inches
2 Self-retaining retractors with and without teeth
2 Wullstein-Weitlaner retractors
1 Littauer ear forceps
Endaural specula, assorted sizes
Ferguson-Frazier suction tubes, assorted sizes
2 Baron suction tubes, nos. 5 and 7 Fr

Accessory items

2 Irrigating bulbs, large, and plastic tips
1 Sana-Lok control syringe, 10 ml
1 Suction tubing
1 Tube antibiotic ointment
1 Gauze pack
1 Closure suture (silk no. 3-0 swaged to a cutting needle)
1 Jordan-Day or ototome drill set
1 Electrosurgical unit
1 Operating microscope with sterile cover (Figs. 22-13 and 22-14)
1 Head light

Text continued on p. 599.

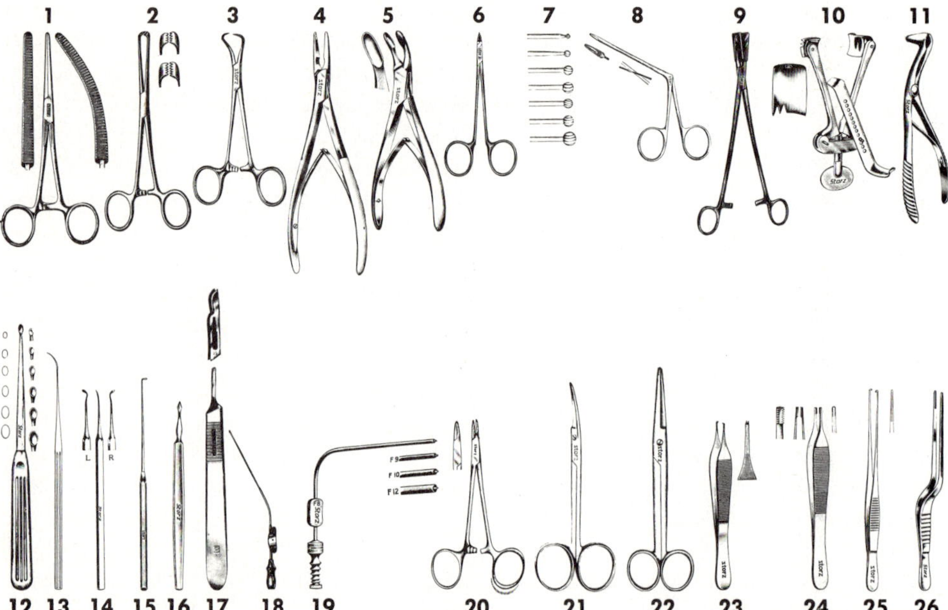

Fig. 22-8. Mastoidectomy instruments. *1,* Rochester-Pean forceps; *2,* Allis forceps; *3,* towel clamps; *4,* Lempert rongeur; *5,* Hartmann rongeur; *6,* malleus nipper; *7,* assorted dental burs; *8,* Littauer ear forceps; *9,* Proud fascia crusher; *10,* House endaural retractor; *11,* endaural speculum; *12,* assorted endaural curettes; *13,* straight pick; *14,* picks, right and left curved; *15,* incus hook; *16,* lancet knife; *17,* knife handle and no. 15 blade; *18,* ear suction tube; *19,* assorted Ferguson-Frazier suction tubes; *20,* Crile-Wood needle holder; *21,* Mayo scissors, curved; *22,* Mayo scissors, straight; *23,* Adson forceps; *24,* Brown-Adson forceps; *25,* Walsh dressing forceps, with and without teeth; *26,* nasal dressing forceps. (Courtesy Storz Instrument Co., St. Louis.)

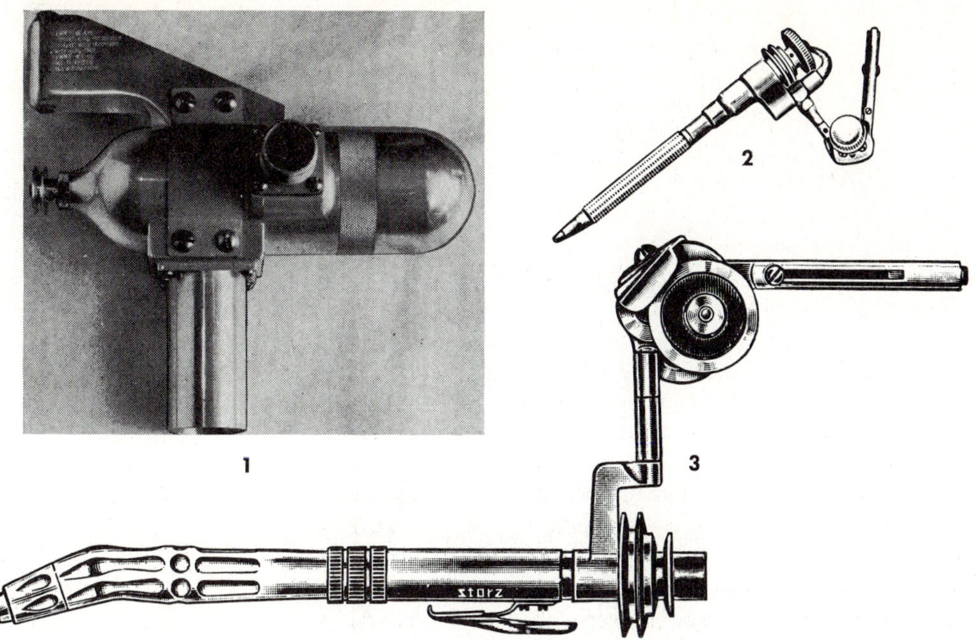

Fig. 22-9. Drills for ear operation. *1,* Storz Jordan-Day motor; *2,* Chayes handpiece; *3,* Wullstein handpiece for use with Jordan-Day motor. (Courtesy Storz Instrument Co., St. Louis.)

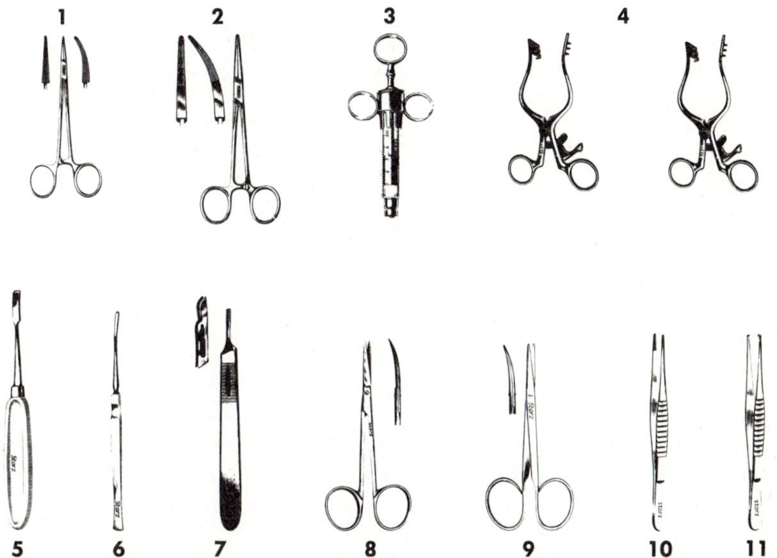

Fig. 22-10. Mastoidectomy instruments, continued. *1,* Mosquito hemostat; *2,* Crile hemostat; *3,* Sana-Lok syringe; *4,* Wullstein-Weitlaner retractors; *5,* Lempert elevator, heavy; *6,* Lempert elevator, angled; *7,* knife handle and no. 15 blade; *8,* small eye scissors, straight and curved; *9,* blunt scissors, straight and curved; *10,* dressing forceps without teeth; *11,* dressing forceps with teeth. (Courtesy Storz Instrument Co., St. Louis.)

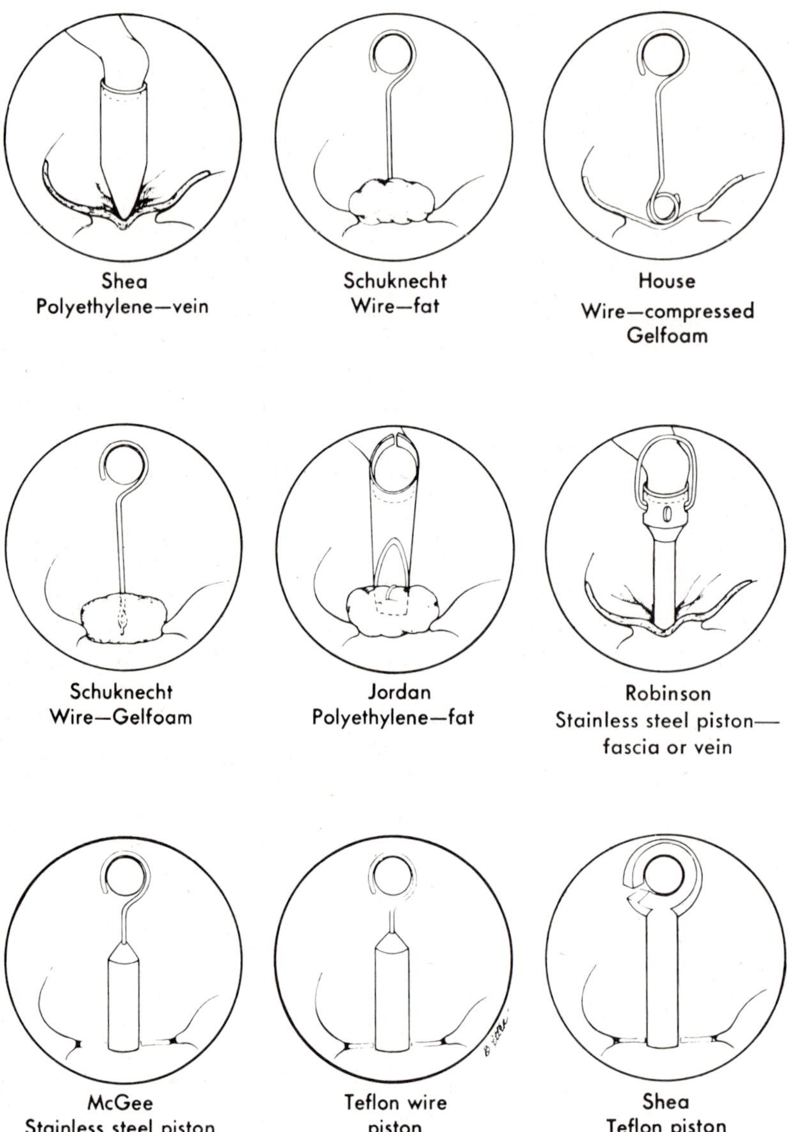

Fig. 22-11. Examples of more commonly used ear prostheses shown immediately after being implanted. Grafts will gradually thin out and become continuous with mucoperiosteum in ear. (From Saunders, W.H., and others: Nursing care in eye, ear, nose, and throat disorders, ed. 4, St. Louis, 1979, The C.V. Mosby Co.)

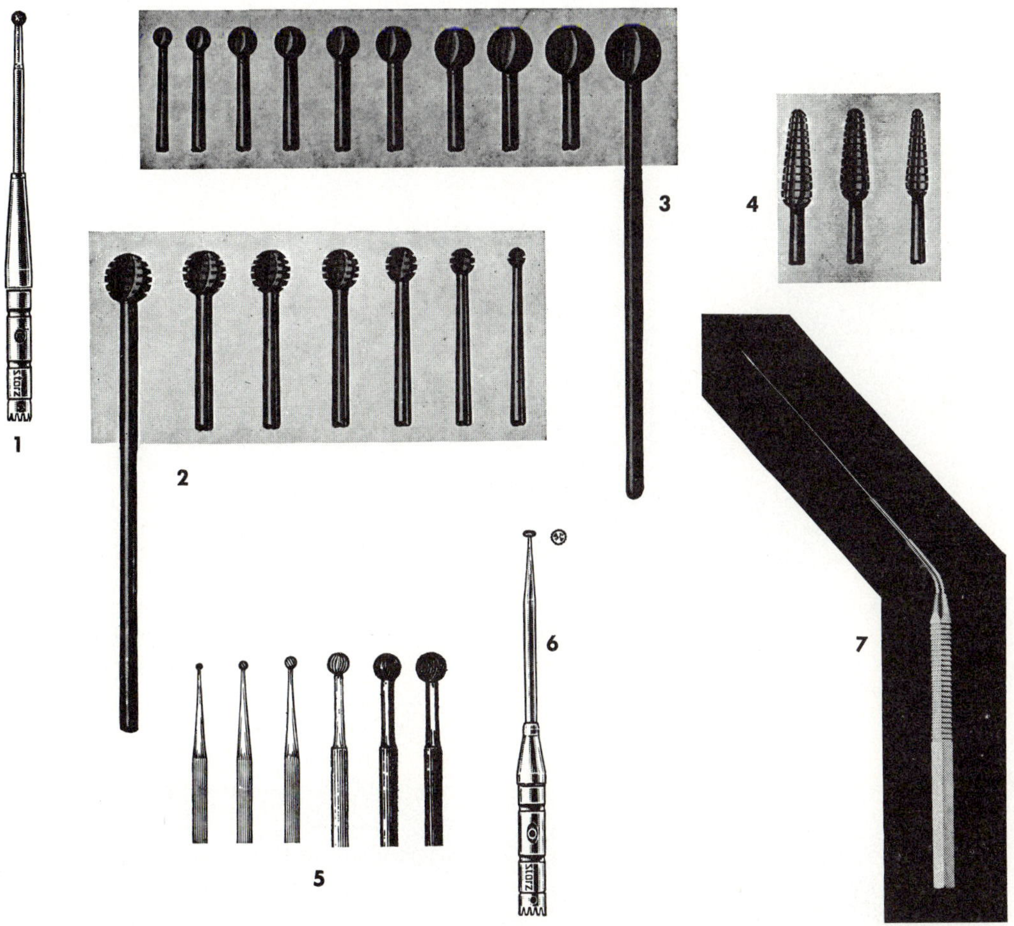

Fig. 22-12. Instruments for operations on middle and inner ear. *1,* Wullstein diamond bur, available in various sizes; *2,* crosscut burs, sizes 6 to 2 mm; *3,* cutting round burs, sizes 2.3 to 8 mm; *4,* perforating burs, various sizes; *5,* polishing burs, various sizes; *6,* Hough-Wullstein crurotomy saw bur; *7,* Goodhill strut introducer. (Courtesy Storz Instrument Co., St. Louis.)

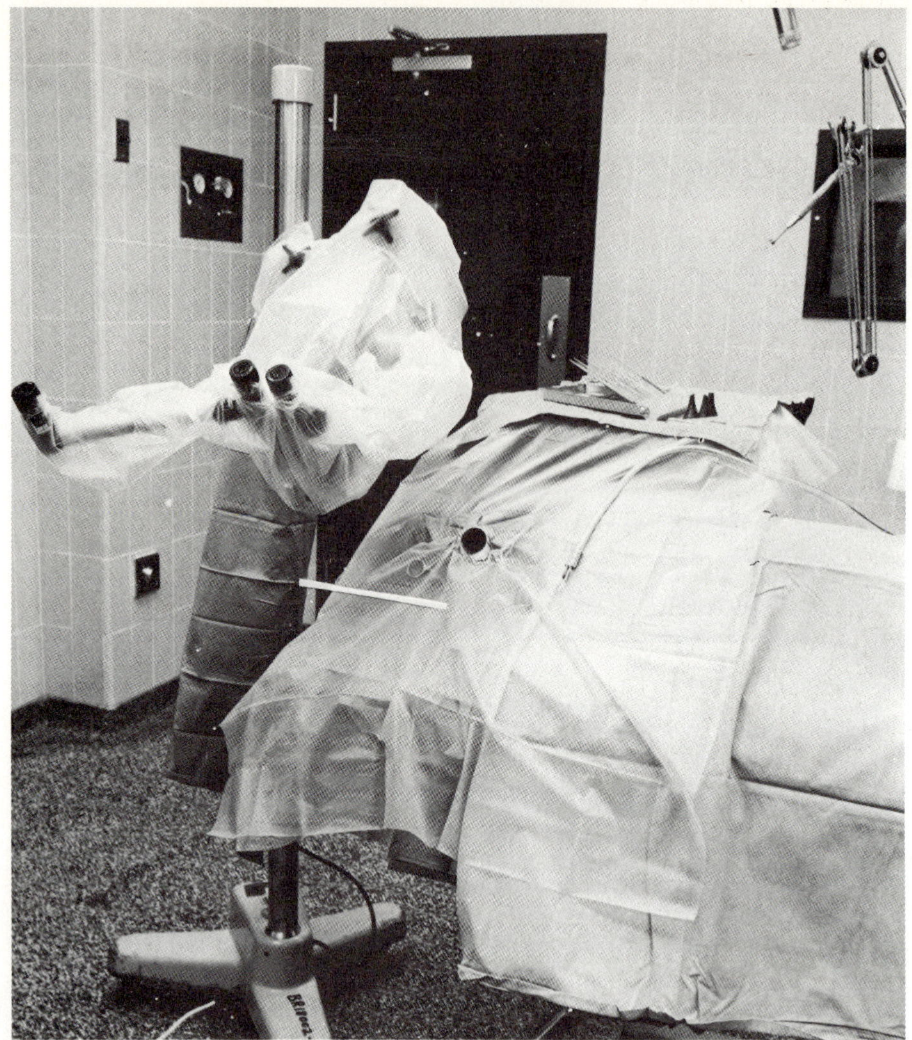

Fig. 22-13. Draped microscope and Mayo stand are shown in place over patient in preparation for stapedectomy. Suction and tubing and Jordan-Day drill are assembled in position ready for use. Instruments are in tray, and aural speculum is in place. Microscope is draped with sterile disposable cover.

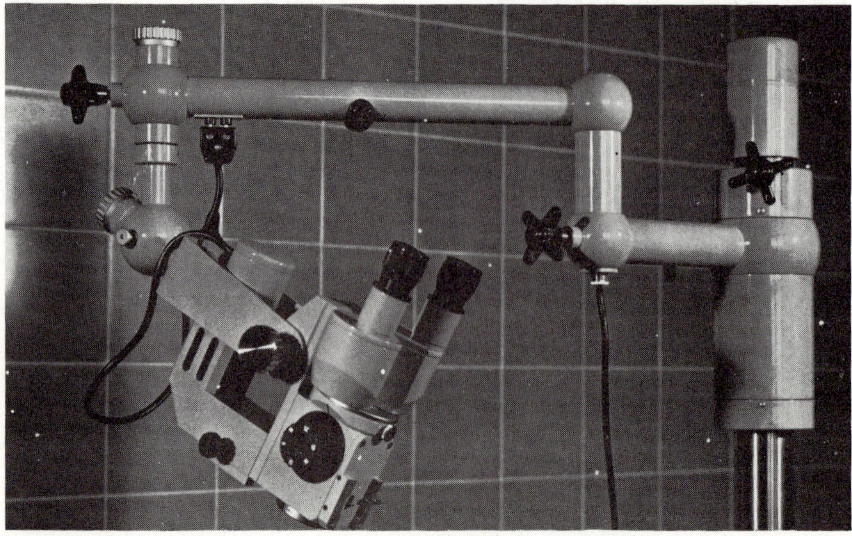

Fig. 22-14. Operating microscope used during stapes mobilization, fenestration, and tympanoplasty procedures. Lens system allows magnification change from 6 to 40 times without change in distance between microscope and ear. (From DeWeese, D.D., and Saunders, W.H.: Textbook of otolaryngology, ed. 6, St. Louis, 1982, The C.V Mosby Co.)

Stapedectomy and mobilization instrument setup (Figs. 22-15 and 22-16)

The items include a head drape pack and basin set, a skin-cleansing preparation set, an operating table side extension, a local anesthesia set, and the following instruments:

1 Guilford-Wright flap knife
1 Myringotomy knife, curved
1 Walsh crurotomy knife
1 House elevator
1 House strut guide
1 Walsh footplate chisel
1 Hough pick, 45-degree angle
1 Hough pick, straight
1 House curette
1 House pick, 1 mm, 90-degree angle
1 Walsh footplate pick, 90-degree angle
1 Walsh footplate pick, 30-degree angle
1 Walsh pick, curved up
1 Shea oblique pick
1 Shea fenestra hook, 25-degree angle
1 Crimper forceps
2 House strut forceps
2 Fine serrated ear forceps
1 Littauer ear forceps
2 Bellucci scissors, left and right
1 Knife handle no. 3 with no. 15 blade
1 Straight scissors, small, sharp
2 House suction tubing adapters
6 Rosen suction tubes, assorted
2 Baron suction tubes, nos. 5 and 7 Fr
1 Suction tubing
4 House strut calipers
1 Tuning fork
6 Ear specula, assorted sizes
1 Bulb syringe, small
1 Shea speculum holder
8 Towel clamps, 3 inches
1 Needle, 28 gauge × 1½ inches
1 Sana-Lok control syringe, 5 ml
Prosthesis of choice
1 Microscope with sterile cover
1 Drill with assorted burs
1 Wire bending die
1 Ruler
1 Schuknecht wire cutter
Steel wire, 28 gauge

For graft harvest

1 Plastic instrument set
1 Minor drape pack
1 Eye sheet
1 Local anesthesia set

Care and handling

Each piece of equipment must be kept in working order. The basic principles of care, handling, and sterilization of instruments are discussed in Chapter 5. Delicate instruments should be handled on an individual basis. To prevent damage, they should not be put into a large basin of cleaning solution and allowed to come into contact with each other. They should be washed, rinsed, and dried individually. A soft bristled toothbrush can be used to clean the instruments, and care should be used to prevent damage to the tips of the instruments. Fine, delicate instruments for tympanoplasty and stapedectomy procedures should be kept in a special rack type of instrument tray. This type of metal tray provides for the separation of instruments from each other, thereby protecting them from damage and facilitating easy handling during surgery. The instruments should be arranged in the rack from left to right or from right to left, in the order of use.

Operating microscope. Proper illumination of the operative site is provided by means of the microscope that illuminates and magnifies the small delicate anatomical structures encountered in otological surgery. Several kinds of operating microscopes (Figs. 22-13 and 22-14) are available, with different attachments. For operations through an ear speculum, the microscope provides direct light and permits the surgeon to work effectively at a distance, using selected magnification of 6, 10, 16, 25, or 40 times.

The microscope is draped with a sterile cover (Fig. 22-13). The surgeon adjusts the microscope before it is draped for surgery and manipulates it during the procedure.

Several types of operating microscopes are available for otological surgery. The microscope may either be a floor type or a ceiling-mounted model. Numerous types of heads are available for the microscope along with teaching attachments for observers to view the surgery. The lens, type of head used, and eyepiece angulation are selected by the surgeon.

The lenses used in the microscope come in various powers and are interchangeable for various powers of magnification. Before lenses are put into the microscope, they should be checked carefully to be sure that they are free of lint, dust, fingerprints, and soil. There are several methods of cleaning the lenses:

1. *For lint.* The lint can be blown off with a rubber bulb syringe, or the lens can be wiped with a special lens cleaning paper or with a clean, dry, soft brush.

2. *For fingerprints.* A lens cleaner should be used for this. Alcohol or Freon solutions should not be used because they are solvents and in time will dissolve the cement holding the lens in place. Over a period of time, the lens may also become cloudy as a result of using these solutions.

The stand of the microscope can be wiped with a cloth and a germicidal solution. The wheels should be kept free of pieces of suture and other debris to prevent problems of mobility of the scope, causing it to tip over and fall if the wheels do not turn properly. It is advisable for two people to move the mobile microscope to prevent it from

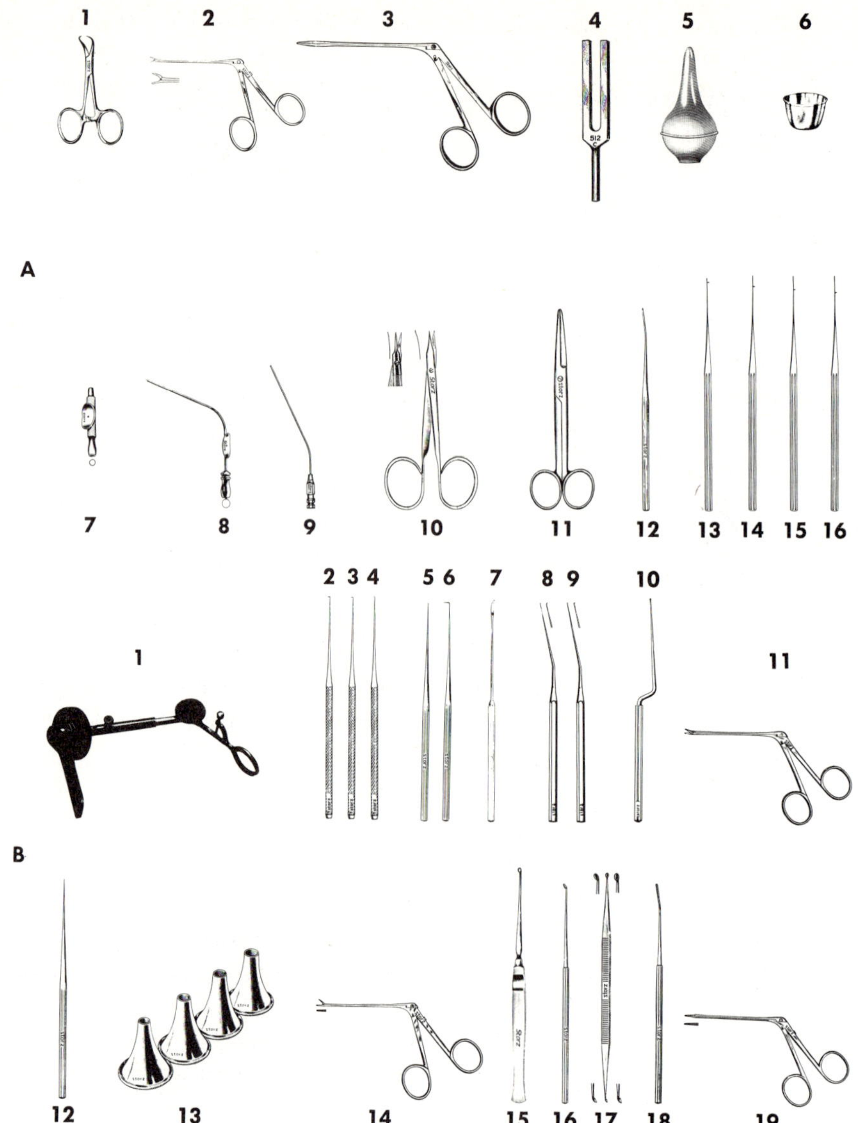

Fig. 22-15. Stapedectomy instruments. **A,** *1,* Towel clamp; *2,* McGee wire closure forceps; *3,* Noyes ear forceps; *4,* tuning fork; *5,* ear syringe; *6,* basin; *7,* suction adapter; *8,* Baron ear suction; *9,* Rosen suction tube; *10,* scissors, small sharp-pointed; *11,* Mayo scissors, straight; *12,* House strut guide; *13* to *16,* House strut calipers. **B,** *1,* Shea speculum holder; *2,* Shea fenestra hook, 90-degree; *3,* Shea fenestra hook, 25-degree, short; *4,* Shea pick; *5* and *6,* House picks; *7,* myringotomy knife; *8,* Hough pick, 45-degree; *9,* Hough pick, 90-degree; *10,* Walsh footplate chisel; *11,* Bellucci scissors; *12,* House straight pick; *13,* assorted ear specula; *14,* House alligator forceps; *15,* Lempert flap knife; *16,* House lancet knife; *17,* House curette; *18,* House elevator; *19,* House alligator and crimper forceps. (Courtesy Storz Instrument Co., St. Louis.)

tipping, which could severely damage the scope and possibly injure operating room personnel. Before moving the scope, the knobs on both the arm and column should be tightened and the arm folded as closely as possible to the column, so that the arm does not swing around, causing possible damage during moving.

The microscope has several electrical connections, which should be checked before use for their integrity and proper fit. If connections are loose and wires frayed, the microscope should not be used until these conditions are corrected.

An extra microscope bulb should be available in case the lamp in the scope burns out during the procedure. The bulb may be changed easily without contaminating

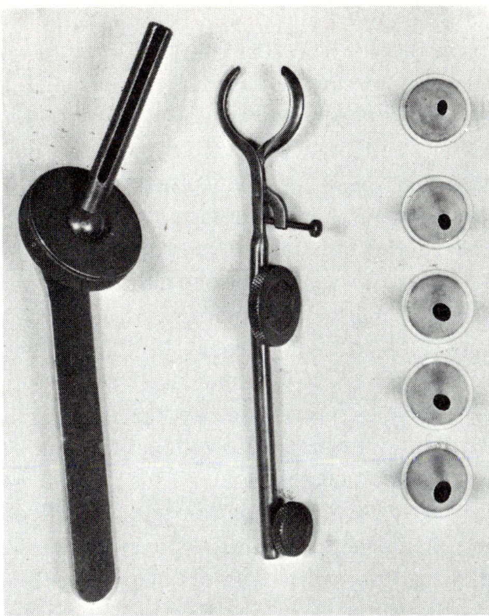

Fig. 22-16. Shea speculum holder.

the scope: the nurse (1) disconnects the scope, protecting the fingers in some manner to prevent burns, since these bulbs become very hot during use; (2) reaches under the cover, removes the bulb housing and bulb, twists the old bulb out, replaces it with a new bulb, and replaces the housing; and (3) reconnects the scope and aids in repositioning it, if necessary. This procedure takes a very short time; however, if the anticipated procedure is to be lengthy, it may be advisable to change the bulb before the procedure starts as a precautionary measure.

Care should be taken when removing the drapes from the microscope so as not to discard the eyepieces with the drapes or to drop them on the floor. Eyepieces have been either lost or damaged in this manner, necessitating costly repair or replacement.

When the microscope is not in use, it should be kept in a storage area that is away from traffic, free of dust, and properly ventilated. Ideally, a set of eyepieces should be left in the scope to prevent the scope from getting dusty on the inside. The microscope may also be covered with either a sheet or a plastic bag.

Specula. Varying sizes of specula are needed to fit the different sizes and shapes of the ear canals encountered.

Needles and syringes for local injection. Local anesthesia is preferred for some operations and is given by block injection (Chapter 9).

For stapes surgery, the initial local anesthetic such as a solution of lidocaine with epinephrine is injected, using a 28-gauge, 1½-inch needle attached to a 5-ml, double-ringed Sana-Lok syringe. For the secondary injection, a heavier-gauged needle (26-gauge, 1½-inch) is generally used.

Knives. For myringotomy, a sharp knife in perfect condition is needed. After one use, the myringotomy knife should be resharpened. Prepackaged, sterile, disposable myringotomy sets are available from several manufacturers and are now being widely used. They are relatively inexpensive and provide good instrumentation for the surgeon. For stapes surgery, the circumferential knives with blades facing to the right and others to the left are designed for various purposes: (1) to make the primary incision, (2) to elevate the periosteum, (3) to enucleate the fibrous annulus, (4) to separate the incudostapedial joint, and (5) to dissect or resect the scar tissue or the stapedial tendon.

Scissors. Mayo scissors, curved and straight, are used for the radical mastoidectomy approach. Delicate scissors with angular blades (Bellucci type) are used in middle ear operations to incise and divide the stapedial tendon or incise this tendon and scar tissue bands (Figs. 22-8, 22-10, and 22-15, *B*).

Drills and burs. Electric or air-driven dental drills or ototomes and burs are used to remove bone (Fig. 22-12). Cortical and hard cellular bone may be removed by means of an electric drill with a rotating type of bur. For stapes procedures, several microburs are needed. Both cutting and diamond types of burs are used. These burs may be attached to an angular Wullstein handpiece driven by a cable-driven engine (Fig. 22-9). Many surgeons are now using an air-driven dental type of drill because the speed can be regulated by lowering the pressure on the tank gauge or at the wall hookup.

A mini-Stryker or Hall micro-ototome drill fitted with either the straight or angled handpiece may be the drill of choice in this circumstance. A complete selection of bits, from round cutting burs to diamond polishing burs (Fig. 22-17), should be available. During surgery, the surgeon holds the handpiece in the same manner as a pen and uses the sides of the bur as the cutting edge. A soft toothbrush or similar brush may be sterilized and used by the scrub nurse to keep the burs clean and free of bone bits during the procedure. At the end of the procedure, the burs should be thoroughly cleaned and inspected for nicks or other damage and discarded, if necessary.

Rongeurs, periosteal elevators, and dissectors (Figs. 22-8 and 22-10). To remove overhanging cortical bone, a Kerrison type of rongeur may be desired. To remove the thin bony plate, meatal wall, or bridge, a delicate narrow rongeur may be preferred. Fine dissectors of many variations are available.

For radical mastoidectomy or tympanoplasty procedures, fine narrow-angle periosteal elevators and dissectors are needed to free the periosteum from the bone (Fig. 22-10).

For stapes surgery, very fine hooks of 45-degree, 90-degree, and 180-degree angles are essential dissecting tools (Fig. 22-15, *B*).

Bone curettes. Various types of bone curettes are used to remove soft bone or substance on the dura, on the sinus wall, or in the vicinity of the facial nerve. Curettes must be sharp.

For stapes surgery, strong shank curettes are needed to remove the annulus and posterior canal wall bone or bridge. Right and left curettes, each with large and small cups, are also needed (Fig. 22-15, *B*).

Dissecting forceps. In radical mastoidectomy and tympanoplasty, several types of grasping and cutting alligator forceps are needed for manipulation within the canal and the middle ear (Fig. 22-8).

Stapes strut introducer, malleable probes, and needles (Fig. 22-15). The malleable fine probes are used to determine the mobility of a footplate fragment, palpate other areas within the middle ear, or palpate the position of the facial nerve. The sharp needle probe is used to manipulate fragments of the tympanic membrane. The strut introducer is used to open the collar of the articulated Silastic strut so that it may encircle and grasp the short process and create an effective articulated incus-strut union.

Suction tubes. For mastoidectomy and tympanoplasty procedures, several patent suction cannulas are needed. Adequate suctioning must be available at all times.

For stapes surgery, the tips of the suction apparatus must be available in three gauges—18, 22, and 24—and equipped with cutoffs to vary the degree of suction (Fig. 22-15, *A*). These fine needle suction tips must be flushed frequently during the procedure with either saline or sterile water to prevent clogging.

Cauterization and coagulation tips. In radical mastoidectomy, tympanoplasty, and stapes procedures, electrocoagulation is desired to control oozing. In stapes sur-

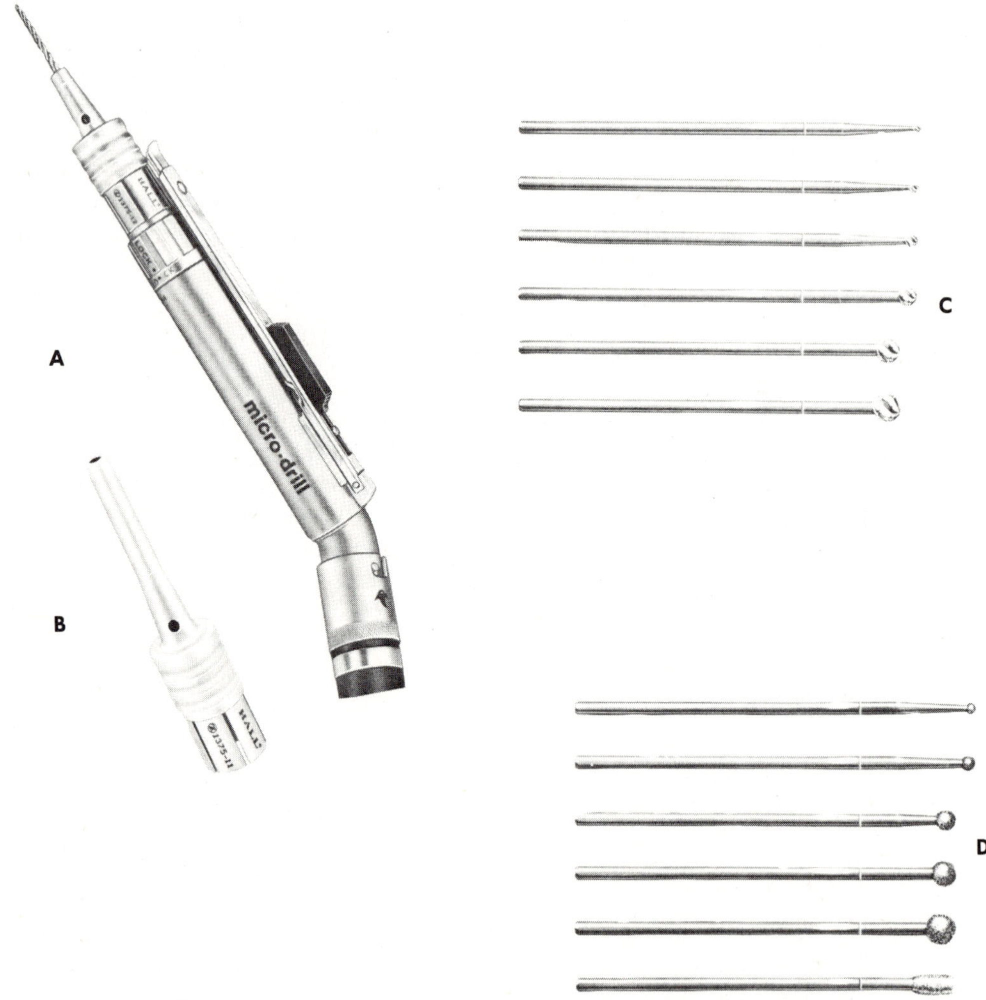

Fig. 22-17. Hall micro-ototome. **A,** Angled handpiece. **B,** Long bur guard. **C** and **D,** Sampling of various, **C,** cutting and, **D,** polishing burs used during middle ear surgery. (Courtesy Zimmer, Inc., Warsaw, Ind.)

gery, an insulated suction tube may be used to cauterize small bleeding vessels at the margin of the incision. This tube is attached to the active electrode of a delicate coagulating machine. The objective is to control oozing and prevent blood from entering the middle ear during suctioning.

Continuous irrigation equipment. Irrigation of the operative field is done frequently with sterile warm saline or Ringer's solution, suctioning apparatus, and bulb syringes to prevent clogging of the bur and to remove bone dust in areas where osteogenesis is to be avoided.

Synthetic materials to control bleeding. Absorbable gelatin sponge (Gelfoam) plugs or pledgets may be placed against the bone. Bone wax may be used in some cases; however, since it is a foreign body, absorbable substances are preferred.

Anesthesia. Ear procedures in children are done with general anesthesia; adults may receive local or general anesthetics. For procedures such as endaural radical mastoidectomy and tympanoplasty, a general anesthetic with endotracheal intubation is used. A local block anesthetic such as lidocaine with epinephrine or occasionally a general anesthetic may be administered for stapes surgery.

OPERATIONS

Incisional approaches

The endaural (vertical) incision frequently is used for temporal operations, except for simple mastoidectomy. The first incision extends from the superior meatal wall, and the second extends directly upward to a point between the meatus and the upper edge of the auricle, where the two incisions join (Fig. 22-18).

The high posterior incision may be used in operations on infants or young children. The incision is placed at a higher posterior level than is the endaural incision, thereby preventing possible damage to the facial nerve.

The postaural incision may be used to expose the mastoid process. If follows the curve of the postaural fold, beginning at the upper attachment of the auricle and continuing behind the postaural fold downward to the tip of the mastoid process (Fig. 22-18).

For stapes surgery, a circumferential incision is made in the posterior half of the canal, starting at the inferior aspect of the annulus and ending posterior to the short process of the malleus.

For myringotomy, a circumferential (posteroinferior) incision is made. It provides for wide drainage and removal of pus or fluid under pressure from the middle ear (Fig. 22-19).

Myringotomy

Definition. Incision of the tympanic membrane under direct vision.

Considerations. Myringotomy is done to treat acute otitis media, in the presence of an exudate, or, more commonly now, for the presence of fluid in the middle ear that produces a hearing loss. The patient has severe pain. There is a bulging of the membrane (Figs. 22-20 and 22-21). By releasing the pus or fluid, hearing is restored, and the infection controlled. Frequently, tubes are inserted through the tympanic membrane.

Setup and preparation of the patient. Positioning, prepping, and draping of the patient are as described previously. The instrument setup includes the following:

1 Myringotomy knife
2 Aural applicators, metal
1 Hartmann aural forceps, delicate type
  Aural specula, assorted sizes
1 Culture tube
1 Square cotton, absorbent
1 Suction set
1 Minor ear drape pack
3 Buck ear curettes

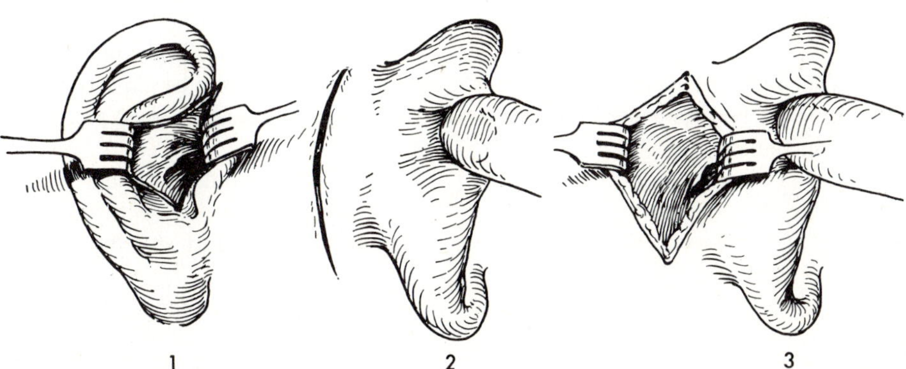

Fig. 22-18. Mastoidectomy incisions. **1,** Endaural. **2,** Postaural. **3,** Postaural incision open. (From DeWeese, D.D., and Saunders, W.H.: Textbook of otolaryngology, ed. 6, St. Louis, 1982, The C.V. Mosby Co.)

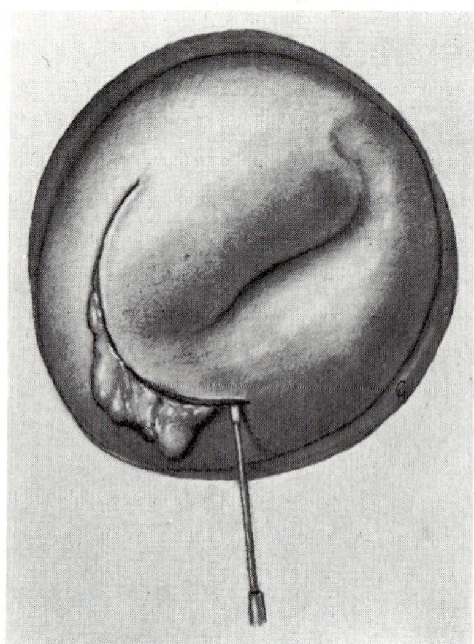

Fig. 22-19. Circumferential incision provides for visibility of eardrum without damage to ossicles and for removal of pus or fluid from middle ear. (From DeWeese, D.D., and Saunders, W.H.: Textbook of otolaryngology, ed. 6, St. Louis, 1982, The C.V. Mosby Co.)

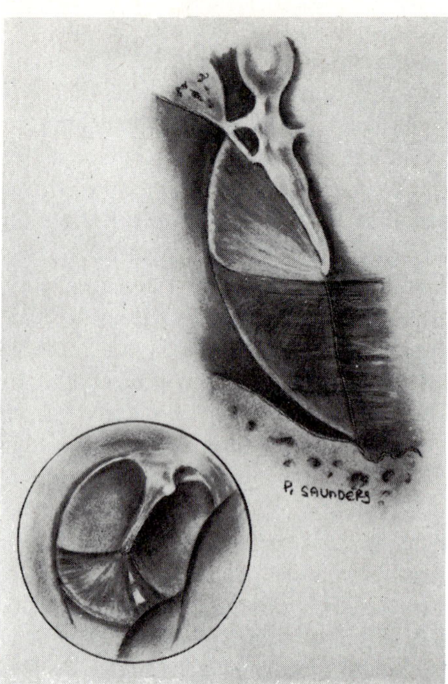

Fig. 22-20. Air-fluid level behind tympanic membrane. *Inset,* Typical appearance of retracted drumhead and meniscus. (From DeWeese, D.D., and Saunders, W.H.: Textbook of otolaryngology, ed. 6, St. Louis, 1982, The C.V. Mosby Co.)

Several disposable myringotomy kits are available. They are relatively inexpensive and afford a more expedient procedure.

Operative procedure

1. Through microscopic visualization, the aural speculum is inserted in the canal; with a sharp myringotomy knife, a small curved incision is made in the posteroinferior quadrant or the pars tensa, and the thickened membrane is cut.
2. A culture is taken to determine the type of organisms present.
3. Pus and fluid are suctioned out.
4. A prosthesis is usually put into place (Fig. 22-22, *A* and *B*).

Several types of disposable myringotomy tubes are available for implanting in the tympanic membrane to facilitate drainage of the middle ear (Fig. 22-22, *C*).

Radical mastoidectomy (Figs. 22-23 and 22-24)

Definition. Removal of the mastoid air cells and the tympanic membrane, thereby converting the middle ear and mastoid process into a single cavity, and removal of any remaining portions of the tympanic membrane, the malleus, and the incus while preserving the stapes and the facial nerve.

Considerations. A radical mastoidectomy is done to treat chronic otitis media when it has involved the mastoid air cells. A cholesteatoma, which is a mass of dead skin, may be associated with chronic otitis media. In this condition, skin from the external auditory canal has grown into the middle ear, where it acts as a foreign body producing erosion and more serious complications. A cholesteatoma should be surgically removed.

Although now seldom done, a radical mastoidectomy is of benefit to patients who have had chronic mastoid infections along with chronic otitis media. It does not affect hearing in the sense that hearing will be lost because hearing is already diminished when the operation is performed. However, if the stapes and cochlea are intact, acceptable hearing can be attained with the use of a hearing aid. Because of the presence of chronic infection, the facial nerve may be exposed, thereby leaving it prey to injury, which is the most serious complication of this procedure.

Radical mastoidectomy may also be done to provide adequate exposure in the treatment of facial nerve decompression to drain an extradural abscess in the bony labyrinth.

Facial nerve damage is always a possibility with this procedure. If the facial nerve has been damaged, the patient will be able to wrinkle only half of the forehead and close only one eye, and the mouth will pull to the unaffected side when an attempt to smile or show the teeth is made.

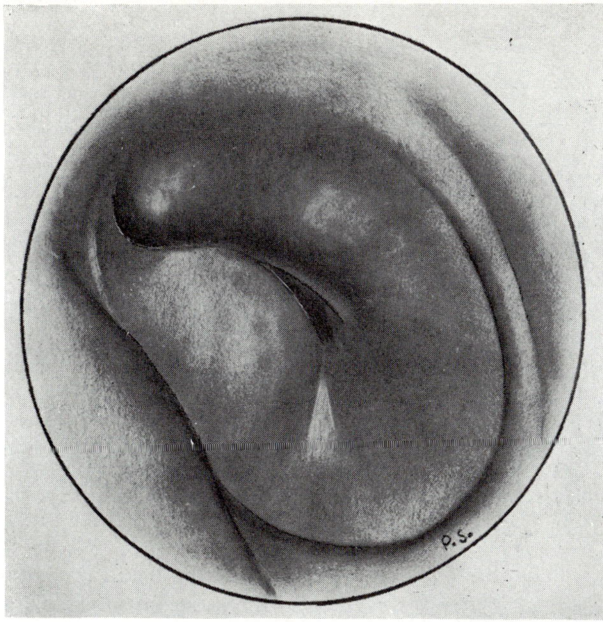

Fig. 22-21. In purulent otitis media, pus under pressure pushes eardrum outward, thus resulting in bulging tympanic membrane. (From DeWeese, D.D., and Saunders, W.H.: Textbook of otolaryngology, ed. 6, St. Louis, 1982, The C.V. Mosby Co.)

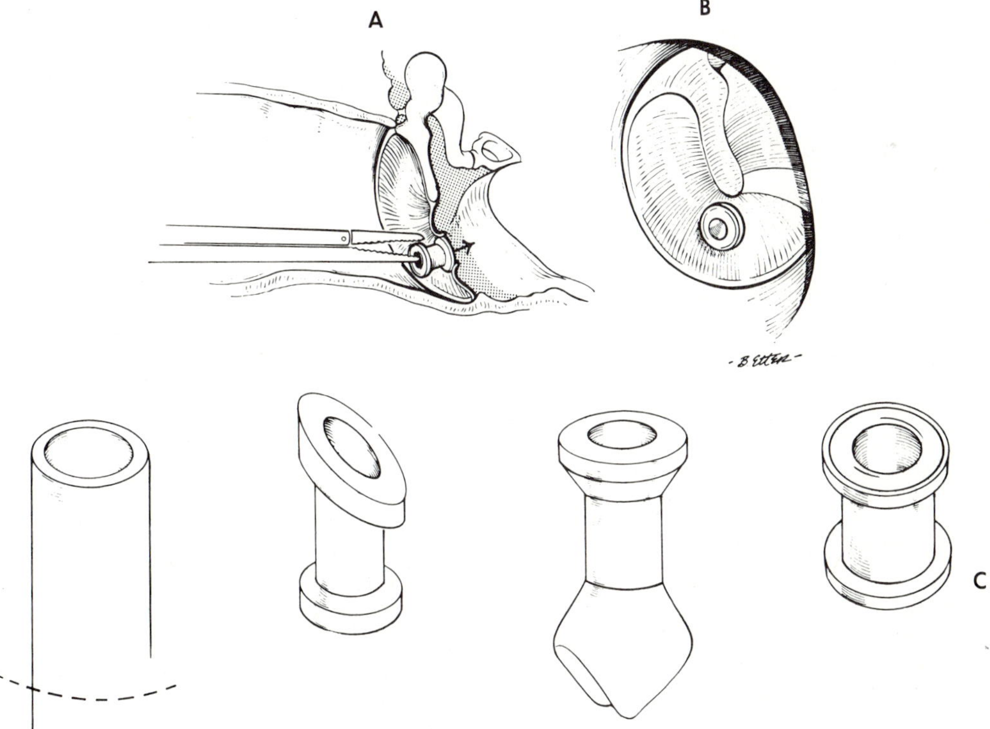

Fig. 22-22. A, Illustration of tube (placed on end of alligator forceps) being inserted into tympanic membrane. B, Tube in place. C, Several types of plastic tubes that may be inserted into tympanic membrane. Purpose of tubes is to aerate middle ear and reduce need for adenoidectomy. (From Saunders, W.H., and others: Nursing care in eye, ear, nose, and throat disorders, ed. 4, St. Louis, 1979, The C.V. Mosby Co.)

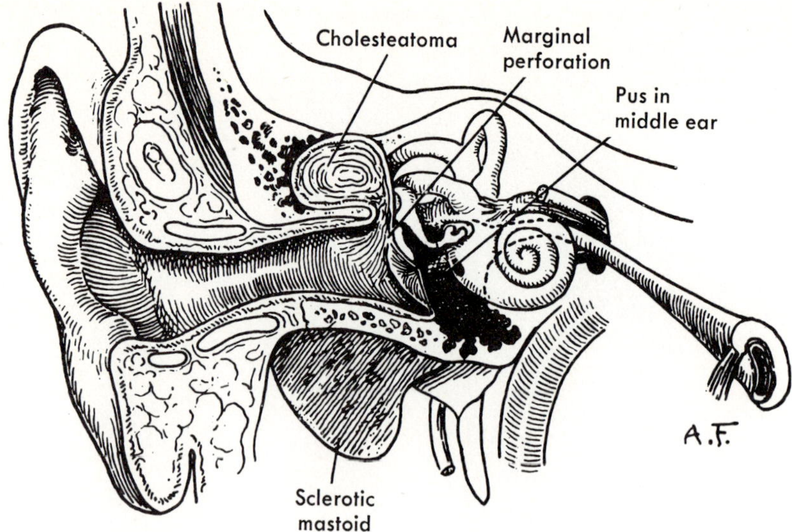

Fig. 22-23. Cholesteatoma of middle ear is mass of epidermoid cells arranged in concentric layers, intermingled with cholesterin crystals. Squamous epithelium grows through tympanic perforation to form pouch, which finally lines middle ear cavity and adjacent mastoid cells. Center of pouch tends to become necrotic and houses infectious bacteria. These lesions increase in size slowly at margins of tympanic membrane. (From Davis, H., and Fowler, E.P. In Davis, H., and Silverman, S.R., editors: Hearing and deafness, rev. ed., New York, Holt, Rinehart & Winston, Inc.)

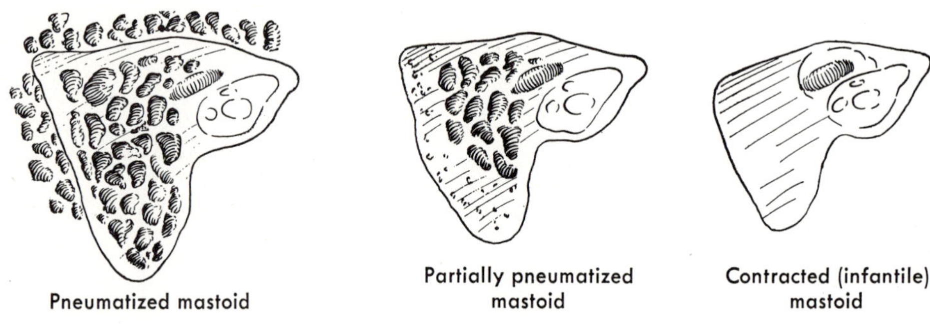

Fig. 22-24. Types of mastoid pneumatization. Otitis media in infancy or early childhood can arrest normal pneumatization at any stage. (From DeWeese, D.D., and Saunders, W.H.: Textbook of otolaryngology, ed. 6, St. Louis, 1982, The C.V. Mosby Co.)

Setup and preparation of the patient. The patient is placed in a supine position. Since this can be a lengthy procedure, the patient should be made as comfortable as possible by the use of small pillows or pads.

Skin preparation, draping techniques, and placement of the sterile instrument tables and other equipment follows the basic otological setup as described earlier in this chapter.

Operative procedure

1. An endaural or postaural incision is made, and bleeding vessels are clamped and ligated. With a second knife, the periosteum is incised and freed to form a flap. The wound is retracted with a self-retaining retractor (Fig. 22-10).

2. The meatal flap is cut, exposing the mastoid area by means of a circumferential knife, narrow periosteal elevator, and curved scissors.

3. The mastoid antrum is exposed. By means of round cutting burs attached to an electric or air drill, the bone of the outer cortex is removed. The osseous meatal walls are removed with rongeurs or burs. The wound is irrigated and suctioned. Cotton pledgets are used for sponging the operative site.

4. The thin bridge of bone between the meatus and antrum is removed with angular dissectors and fine curettes.

5. The tympanic membrane, malleus, incus, and mucoperiosteal lining of the middle-ear cavity are ex-

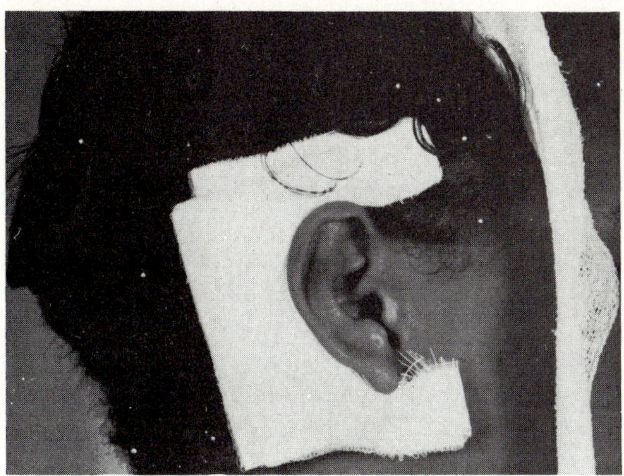

Fig. 22-25. Head dressing after mastoidectomy. Space directly behind ear is padded because ear, if pressed lightly against skull, becomes painful. Gauze strip of bandage will later be used to tie together several windings of gauze. (From Saunders, W.H., and others: Nursing care in eye, ear, nose, and throat disorders, ed. 4, St. Louis, 1979, The C.V. Mosby Co.)

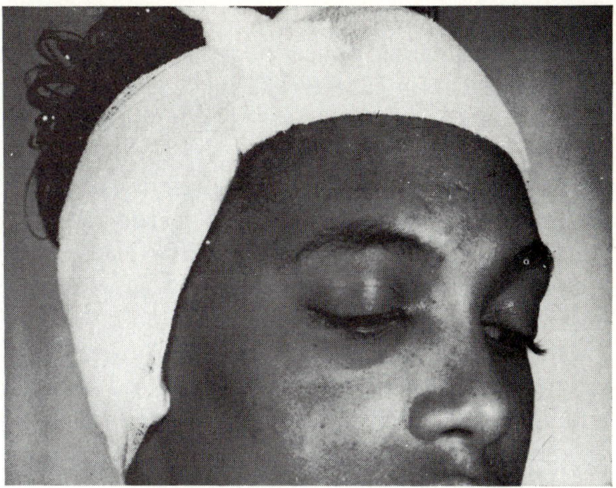

Fig. 22-26. Head dressing after completion of mastoidectomy. Several fluffed 8 × 4–inch dressings are placed over ear to absorb drainage before gauze is wrapped about head. Dressing is placed high enough so that it does not fall over eyes. Dressings should actually be over hair, not across forehead. (From Saunders, W.H., and others: Nursing care in eye, ear, nose, and throat disorders, ed. 4, St. Louis, 1979, The C.V. Mosby Co.)

cised by means of stapes instruments, as for a stapes operation.

6. The tympanic cavity is cleaned. The wound is closed with sutures. A musculoplasty may be done by taking a strip of temporalis muscle from above the ear and placing it in the mastoid cavity. In time, the skin grows over the muscle.

7. The mastoid cavity is usually packed with a strip of ½ × 8–inch gauze packing that has been impregnated with petrolatum or an antibiotic ointment. The wound is closed.

8. The ear dressing is applied, including a shaped ear pad (Fig. 22-25). Fluffed 8 × 4–inch gauze sponges are placed around and behind the affected ear, and then flat compresses over the affected ear. A gauze bandage is applied to hold the dressings in place and prevent pressure (Fig. 22-26).

Simple mastoidectomy

Definition. Removal of the air cells of the mastoid process without disturbing the contents of the middle ear (Fig. 22-24).

Considerations. Simple mastoidectomy may be done occasionally to treat acute empyema of the mastoid process. However, because of the effectiveness of antibiotics, this procedure is almost obsolete. Simple mastoidectomy is still the procedure of choice in the presence of complications following acute mastoiditis. The nursing care of the patient is the same as that of the radical mastoidectomy patient. The patient should be told to expect some dizziness, nausea and perhaps vomiting, and a certain amount of drainage after surgery.

Setup and preparation of the patient. As described for radical mastoidectomy, but omitting the stapes instruments.

Operative procedure. A postaural or endaural incision is made. The steps of the procedure are followed as described for radical mastoidectomy. A drain may be inserted.

Modified radical mastoidectomy (atticoantrotomy)

Definition. Simple mastoidectomy, plus the removal of the bony posterior external auditory canal wall. This exposes the mastoid cavity to the external auditory canal for drainage. The middle ear is not disturbed.

Considerations. A modified radical mastoidectomy may be done in the presence of a small tympanic perforation or in the presence of an attic and mastoid-antrum disease but does not involve the middle ear. It may also be done as a preliminary surgical exposure for a fenestration operation.

Setup and preparation of the patient. As previously described for radical mastoidectomy, but omitting the stapes instruments.

Operative procedure. As described for radical mastoidectomy, steps 1 through 4 and 6 and 7. The middle ear structures and drum are preserved. The eardrum is left attached to the skin of the external auditory canal posteriorly. Both are used to seal the middle ear from the mastoid cavity.

Tympanoplasty

Definition. Group of operations selected to restore or improve hearing in patients with middle ear or the conductive type of hearing loss, resulting from chronic otitis media.

Considerations. Conductive deafness is caused by an obstruction in the external canal or middle ear, which impedes the passage of sound waves to the inner ear. The action of the round window and oval window has been reviewed previously.

The objectives of tympanoplasty are to restore two functions of the middle ear: the areal ratio and sound protection for the round window. The objective of the skin graft laid across the middle ear, touching the stapes and leaving an air pocket about the round window, is to improve hearing. The sound waves are transmitted through the graft to the stapes and the oval window. The sound waves striking the graft covering associated with the round window are reflected backward, thereby providing sound protection.

Types of procedures (Fig. 22-27; Table 3). Many procedures are now in the developmental stage. Various methods and materials are being introduced as a means of constructing a closed, air-contained middle-ear cavity and restoring a sound-pressure transformer action.

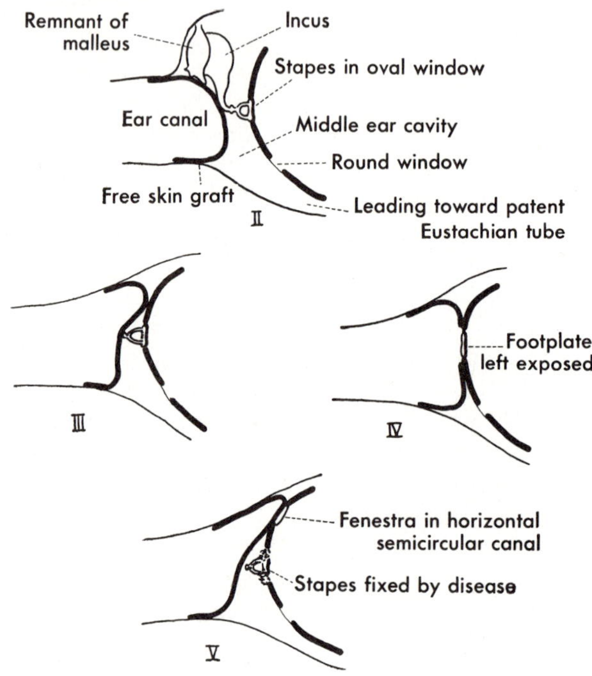

Fig. 22-27. Tympanoplasty types II, III, IV, and V. (From DeWeese, D.D., and Saunders, W.H.: Textbook of otolaryngology, ed. 5, St. Louis, 1977, The C.V. Mosby Co.)

Table 3. Tympanoplastic procedures

Type	Damage to middle ear	Methods of repair
I	Perforated tympanic membrane with normal ossicular chain	Closure of perforation; type I same as myringoplasty
II	Perforation of tympanic membrane with erosion of malleus	Closure with graft against incus or remains of malleus
III	Destruction of tympanic membrane and ossicular chain *but with* intact and mobile stapes	Graft contacts normal stapes; also gives sound protection for round window
IV	Similar to type III but with head, neck, and crura of stapes missing; footplate mobile	Mobile footplate left exposed; air pocket between round window and graft provides sound protection for round window
V	Similar to type IV plus *fixed* footplate	Fenestra in horizontal semicircular canal; graft seals off middle ear to give sound protection for round window

From DeWeese, D.D., and Saunders, W.H.: Textbook of otolaryngology, ed. 6, St. Louis, 1982, The C.V. Mosby Co.

In tympanoplasty types I, II, and III, fresh tissue—either a vein or a piece of perichondrium, fascia, or skin from the inner third of the external auditory canal—is used to repair the tympanic membrane and close off a pocket of air in front of the round window. In some cases, a new areal ratio is created if there is a sufficient ossicular chain present.

Tympanoplasty types IV and V provide only sound protection for the round window, since the areal ratio cannot be restored. In tympanoplasty type IV, a new opening into the inner ear is established by placing a graft over the fenestra in the lateral canal (fenestration operation).

Tympanoplasty type I (myringoplasty)

Definition. Reconstruction of the tympanic membrane by means of a sliding graft fashioned from the inner part of the ear or by means of a fascial graft taken from the temporalis muscle behind the ear.

Considerations. The nursing care given to these patients follows the same pattern as for other types of otological surgery. Depending on the type of tympanoplasty to be performed, the patient may be given a general or a local anesthetic. Postoperatively, there may be some dizziness and nausea. If the dizziness is severe, the patient may exhibit a jerking movement of the eyes (nystagmus), which results from stimulation of the labyrinth during surgery.

Setup and preparation of the patient. The setup as listed previously includes instruments for modified radical mastoidectomy and for stapedectomy and vein graft.

Positioning, skin prepping, and draping of the patient have been described earlier in this chapter under the general instructions for otological surgery.

Operative procedures. Many different incisional approaches are used; however, an endaural approach is commonly preferred.

Wullstein technique

1. The ear speculum is introduced, and then the microscope is brought into place. An endaural incision is made either within the meatus, as for stapes mobilization, or extended upward from the meatus by means of a knife, sharp curettes, and fine cupped forceps.

2. The tympanic membrane is entered, and a modified radical mastoidectomy may be done, depending on the extent of the disease.

3. The antrum is inspected, and a stapedial fossa tympanotomy is accomplished by means of burs, dissectors, suction, and forceps.

4. The graft is taken. The middle ear is reconstructed by placing the graft in position with smooth forceps, fine knives, and moist cotton pledgets. Small pledgets of Gelfoam or a similar substance may be inserted to lightly hold the graft in position. A cotton ball is used to occlude the outer meatus.

5. The wound is closed witth no. 4-0 silk sutures, and a mastoid dressing is applied (Figs. 22-25 and 22-26).

Austin-Shea technique

1. A segment of vein may be taken from the antecubital fossa or forearm, and excessive connective tissue is trimmed from the adventitial surface. The vein graft is split or thinned, cut, converted into a quadrilateral graft, and stored in a sponge saturated with normal saline or Ringer's solution, until needed. Fascia from the temporalis muscle is an excellent choice for graft material. Some surgeons prefer that the graft be put into a small press (Fig. 22-8) to be flattened and thinned, making it easier to handle.

2. The ear speculum is inserted, and an endaural incision is made. Tympanotomy is performed.

3. The ossicular chain or remnants are mobilized; diseased bone may be removed with stapes instruments.

4A. Diseased mastoid cells are cleared. The middle ear is reconstructed by means of a vein graft, resulting in closure of the perforated membrane.

4B. Reconstruction of the middle ear may be done by other methods, depending on the condition of the structures encountered. A prosthetic substitution may be used that becomes a strut from malleus to footplate, from incus to footplate, or from membrane to footplate, or the tympanic remnant and graft may be used to secure sound protection of the round window.

5. Bleeding is controlled, the skin flap and drum replaced to original position, and the incision closed with no. 4-0 silk sutures. Antibiotic solution is instilled in the ear. A mastoid dressing is applied.

Fenestration operation

Definition. Reconstruction of the outer and middle parts of the ear by means of a new drum or skin flap or creation of a new window into the internal ear mechanism by a newly established drum or skin flap; also partial mastoidectomy.

Considerations. The Lempert endaural fenestration operation is done to restore hearing in persons who have had bilateral conduction deafness because of otosclerosis of the tympanic membrane and ossicles (Fig. 22-28).

Otosclerosis is the most common cause of conductive hearing loss in people from 15 to 50 years of age. It is a hereditary defect of unknown cause, is more common in women than in men, and is not common in blacks.

In otosclerosis, the normal bone is absorbed and replaced by otosclerotic bone, which is vascular. It grows into the bony labyrinth, thus causing progressive fixation of the footplate of the stapes.

The objective of surgery is to restore the mechanical aspects of the middle ear and the external canal.

The objective of fenestration is to create a new permanent window through which sound waves can enter the inner ear when the oval window is fixed.

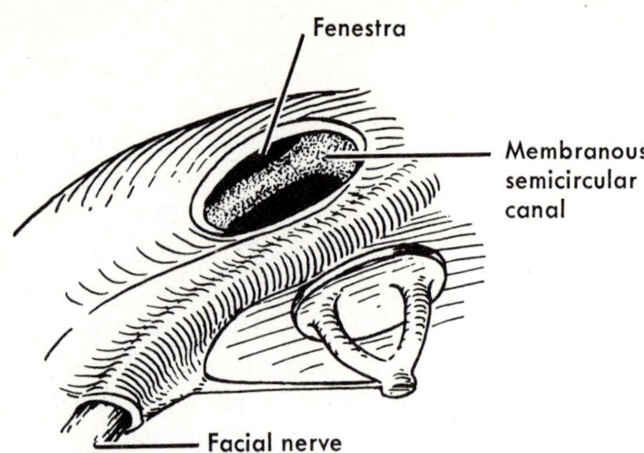

Fig. 22-28. Fenestration operation. Fenestra made in horizontal semicircular canal for otosclerosis. Incus is removed. Fenestra is ready to be covered by flap fashioned from eardrum and skin of external auditory canal. (From DeWeese, D.D., and Saunders, W.H.: Textbook of otolaryngology, ed. 6, St. Louis, 1982, The C.V. Mosby Co.)

Setup and preparation of the patient. As described for endaural mastoidectomy and stapes surgery.

Operative procedure

1. An endaural incision is made inside the ear by means of an ear speculum, microscope, and small knife.

2. A modified radical mastoidectomy is done. The bridge is reduced, incus removed, and head of malleus amputated by means of electric drill with burs attached, Rosen knives, and Bellucci scissors. The ampulla and lateral semicircular canals are identified. The operative field is irrigated with warm normal saline solution.

3. A fenestra is created by using diamond burs, working through the microscope. The membranous labyrinth is left exposed by a thin dome or cupola of endosteal bone, which is removed. The edges of the fenestra are trimmed with fine picks.

4. A pedicle flap is made from the skin and periosteum of the superior and posterior canal walls.

5. Endosteum and bone dust are removed by fine excavators. The graft is laid over the fenestra (Fig. 22-28). The cavity may be lined by pledgets of synthetic sponge.

6. The endaural incision is closed with fine silk sutures. The meatal opening is lightly packed with gauze saturated with an antibiotic solution. Mastoid dressing is applied (Figs. 22-25 and 22-26).

Stapedectomy

Definition. Removal of the stapes (the head, neck, and crura) and reestablishment of linkage between the incus and oval window by interposition of a vein graft, polyethylene tube, or other prosthetic material (Fig. 22-11).

Considerations. Stapes surgery is done to restore hearing in patients with conductive deafness caused by otosclerotic stapedial ankylosis, which causes a gradually progressive hearing loss.

If the stapes is fixed in the oval window, the stapes is either freed (stapes mobilization) or removed and replaced with an artificial bone (stapedectomy).

Hearing is generally restored while the patient is in the operating room. The hearing will diminish as the ear is packed and dressed. There may be bleeding in the middle and external ear that impedes the hearing until the clot dries and cracks and once again allows the sound waves to enter into the ear.

Setup and preparation of the patient. As described for stapes surgery, plus graft set (Figs. 22-12 to 22-16).

Operative procedure (Fig. 22-29)

1. With the aid of a microscope, knife, and suction needles, an incision is made in the posterior half of the osseous meatal wall about 5 mm from the annulus. The posterior flap, consisting of skin and periosteum, is dissected from the bone with a large circumferential knife and wet cottonoid pledgets or applicators. The elevation is carried medially until the posterior margin of the annular sulcus is reached, using narrow or duckbill elevators, modified Kos or angular Rosen elevators, or right or left Shea elevators.

2. The delicate middle ear mucosa is separated, and the tympanic membrane is folded forward on itself to expose the contents of the middle ear, using delicate periosteal elevators. With a microscope, the middle ear is inspected for patency of the round window. The posterior superior bony canal rim is removed with a small, round, flat knife (Rosen, Shea, or Goodhill), spud, and curettes above the exit of the chorda tympani nerve to provide for exposure of the incudostapedial joint. The incus, the incudostapedial joint, and the head of the stapes are palpated, using Rosen picks or a Derlacki mobilizer.

3. The crura are fractured from the footplate, and the stapes superstructure is removed (Fig. 22-30).

4. Fragments of the footplate are removed. The opening into the vestibule is covered with a graft. The prosthesis is articulated with the long process of the incus by means of stapes forceps. Blood is gently suctioned from the tympanic cavity, and the tympanic membrane is replaced in its original position.

5. On completion of the lysis or the prosthetic procedure, audiometric status is determined by lightly striking a 256-cycle magnesium tuning fork. All blood is gently suctioned from the tympanic cavity, and the operative wound is closed. The tympanic membrane–posterior skin flap is gently replaced in position with Rosen or Shea picks and House alligator forceps.

6. The extraneous blood is suctioned from the canal. Part of the incision is covered with several Gelfoam sponges moistened in epinephrine solution to keep the meatal skin in position and prevent bleeding into the middle ear. In some cases, several saline-soaked strips of rayon are placed over the skin incision area to line the bony external auditory canal.

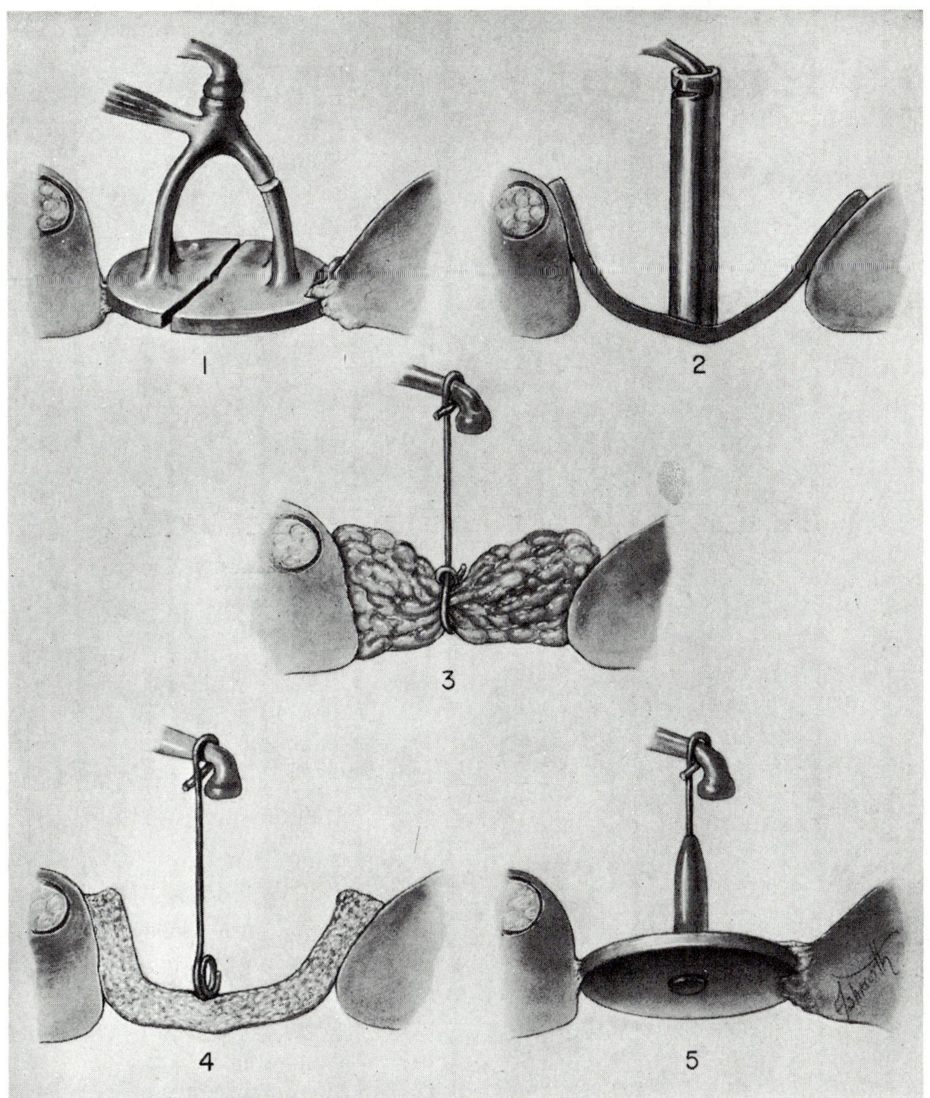

Fig. 22-29. Techniques of stapedectomy. **1,** Partial stapedectomy by cutting anterior crus and bisecting footplate. Posterior crus and remaining footplate are mobile (Hough procedure). **2,** Stapes removed and replaced with vein graft. Polyethylene strut provides continuity (Shea procedures). **3,** Wire-fat prosthesis replacing stapes (Schuknecht procedures). **4,** Oval window covered with Gelfoam. Preformed wire placed on Gelfoam (House procedure). **5,** Footplate not removed. Footplate drilled and preformed wire-Teflon piston placed through hole in footplate (Shea and Guilford procedures). Otosclerotic fixation of anterior footplate margin is shown in **1** and **5.** (From DeWeese, D.D., and Saunders, W.H.: Textbook of otolaryngology, ed. 5, St. Louis, The C.V. Mosby Co.)

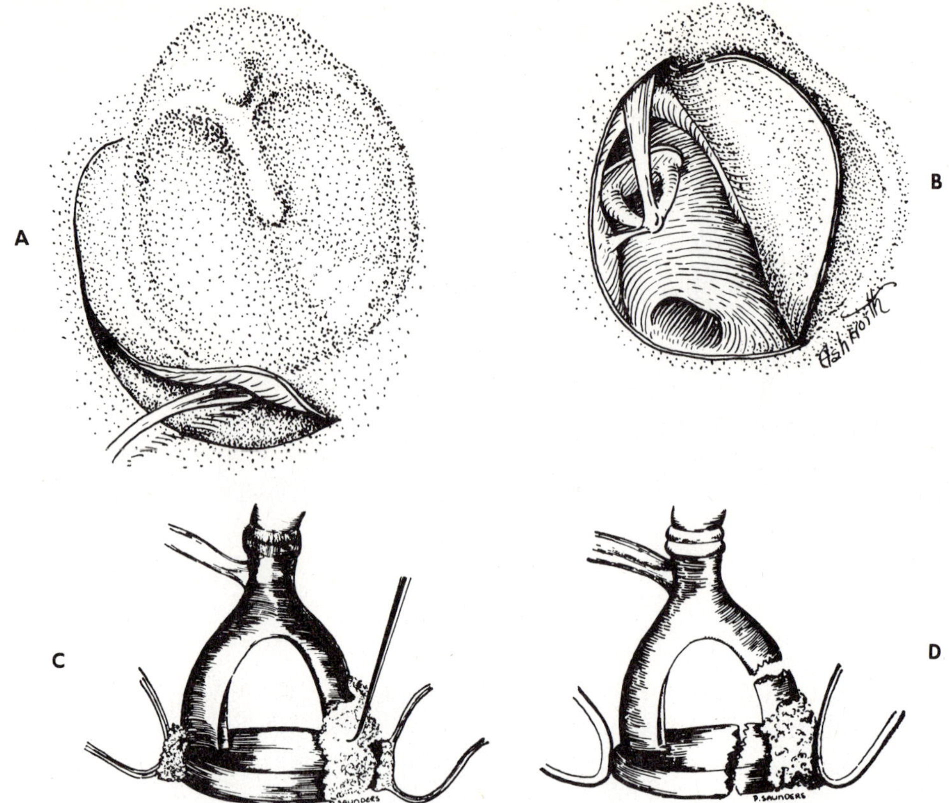

Fig. 22-30. Stapes mobilization. **A,** Incision in posterior ear canal wall. **B,** Operative field seen through aural speculum. **C,** Fracturing through otosclerotic focus. Earlier, surgeons applied pressure only to incus or head of stapes. **D,** Anterior crurotomy technique—otosclerotic focus is bypassed. (From DeWeese, D.D., and Saunders, W.H.: Textbook of otolaryngology, ed. 6, St. Louis, 1982, The C.V. Mosby Co.)

Stapes mobilization

Definition. Creation of an opening into the vestibule of the labyrinth and reestablishment of a functioning linkage between the incus and the inner ear (Fig. 22-30).

Considerations. This procedure involves remobilization of the entire middle ear mechanism. The term *stapediolysis* means removal or lysis of bony or fibrous adhesions around the stapes. Patients with conductive hearing loss resulting from fixation of the stapes are selected for stapes mobilization.

Setup and preparation of the patient. As described for stapes surgery.

Operative procedure. The major steps and items used are similar to those for stapedectomy (Fig. 22-30). The stapes is freed from the hardened otosclerotic membrane by means of fine probes, dissectors, and picks. The auditory canal is packed, and mastoid dressing applied.

Labyrinthectomy

Definition. Opening of the labyrinth to destroy the inner ear.

Considerations. Labyrinthectomy is done to relieve the medically uncontrollable symptoms of unilateral Ménière's disease or to prevent the intracranial spread of infection from the labyrinth.

Setup and preparation of the patient. As described for tympanoplasty.

Operative procedures. These are dependent on the type of approach used. The transmeatal approach is performed as a stapedectomy. After the stapes is removed, the inner ear is suctioned to remove the membranous labyrinth. The round and oval windows are combined by the use of a bur to make a single large window. In the transmastoid approach a modified radical mastoidectomy is performed. The stapes is removed, the inner ear is suctioned to remove the membranous labyrinth, and the semicircular canals are opened.

■ Nose

Surgery of the nose is performed to treat external injuries and malformations and provide for effective function of the respiratory system (Fig. 22-31).

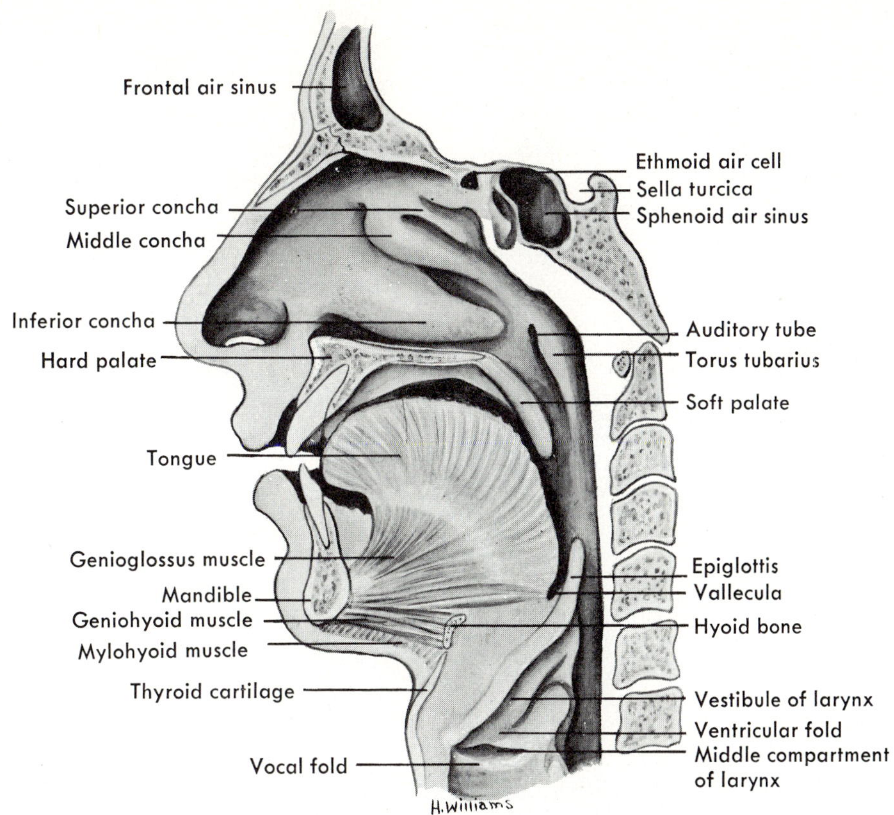

Fig. 22-31. Sagittal section of face and neck. (From Francis, C.C., and Martin, A.H.: Introduction to human anatomy, ed. 7, St. Louis, 1975, The C.V. Mosby Co.)

ANATOMY AND PHYSIOLOGY

The nose is divided into the prominent external portion and the internal portion known as the nasal cavity. The chief purpose of the nose is the preparation of air for use in the lungs.

The *external* nose projects from the face. The upper portion of the external nose is formed by the nasal bones and the frontal process of the maxillae, and the lower portion is formed by a group of nasal cartilages and connective tissue covered with skin (Fig. 22-32). The nostrils and the tip of the nose are shaped by the major alar cartilages. The nares are separated by the columella, which is formed by the lower margin of the septal cartilage, the medial parts of the major alar cartilages, and the anterior nasal spine, all of which are covered by skin.

The nasal septum is composed of three structures: the nasal cartilage, the vomer bone, and the perpendicular plate of the ethmoid bone. The septum is covered by mucous membrane on either side. The deviated or fractured septum may be repaired surgically by mobilization of the fracture or removal of the deformed cartilage or bone.

The *internal* portion, or nasal cavity, is divided by the nasal septum into two parts at its midline. The nasal cavity communicates with the outside by its external openings, call the *nares*. The nares open into the nasopharynx through the choanae. The nasal cavity is also associated with each ear by means of the eustachian tube and with the paranasal air sinuses (frontal, maxillary, ethmoidal, and sphenoidal) through their respective orifices (meatuses). The nasal cavity also communicates with the conjunctiva through the nasal duct. The nasal cavity is separated from the lingual cavity by the hard and soft palates (Fig. 22-33) and from the cranial cavity by the ethmoid bone. The nasal cavity is held together by periosteal covering and by perichondrium, which extends over the cartilages.

The *turbinate bones* of the nasal structure are arranged one above the other, separated by grooves, or meatuses. These act as drainage passages of the accessory sinuses and are known as the sphenoethmoidal recesses and the superior, middle, and inferior meatuses, respectively (Fig. 22-33).

The nasal sinuses serve as air spaces and communicate with the nasal cavity through the meatuses. Anteriorly, on each side of the skull, the frontal sinus, the anterior ethmoidal sinus, and the maxillary sinus (antrum of Highmore) drain into the middle meatus; posteriorly, the ethmoidal and the sphenoidal sinus drain into the superior meatus and the sphenoethmoidal recess. A passageway for the flow of air is provided by the irregular air spaces present between these structures. Because of their shape, the air is forced to flow in thin air waves.

The sensory nerve supply of the nasal cavity is derived from the trigeminal nerve.

The nose and sinuses receive their blood supply (Fig. 22-34) from the branches of the internal maxillary artery. There are masses of communicating veins below the epithelial layer of the turbinate bones, and the veins lying just beneath the skin anastomose freely. Dilatation of the superficial veins may cause the turbinate bones to swell, whereas contraction of these vessels may cause the bones to shrink.

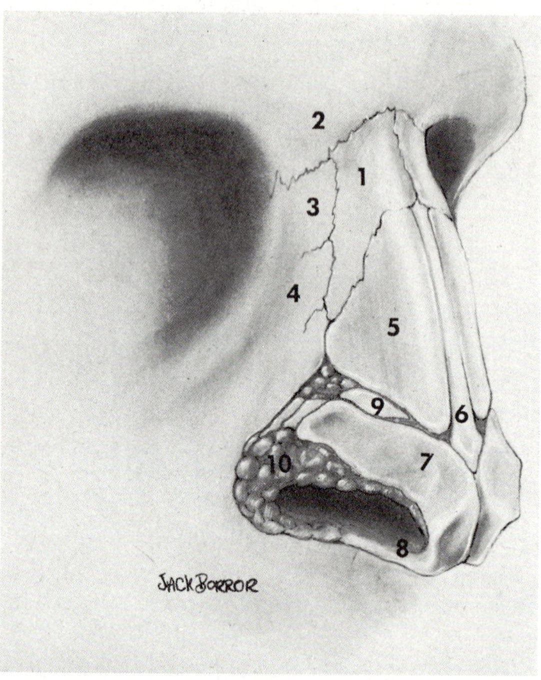

Fig. 22-32. Nasal bony framework. *1,* Nasal bone; *2,* frontal bone; *3,* lacrimal bone; *4,* maxillary bone; *5,* upper lateral cartilage; *6,* nasal septum; *7,* lower lateral cartilage, lateral crus; *8,* lower lateral cartilage, medial crus; *9,* sesamoid cartilage; *10,* fibrofatty tissue. (From Saunders, W.H., and others: Nursing care in eye, ear, nose, and throat disorders, ed. 4, St. Louis, 1979, The C.V. Mosby Co.)

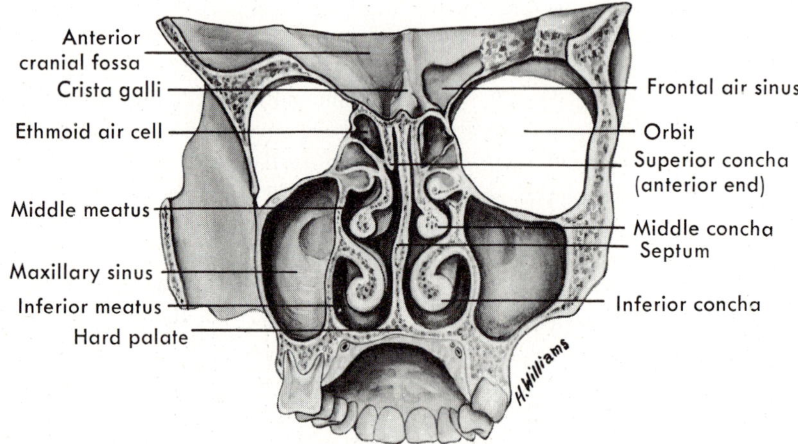

Fig. 22-33. Vertical section through nose. Plane of section passes slightly obliquely through left first molar tooth and behind second right premolar tooth. Posterior wall of right frontal sinus removed. (From Francis, C.C., and Martin, A.H.: Introduction to human anatomy, ed. 7, St. Louis, 1975, The C.V. Mosby Co.)

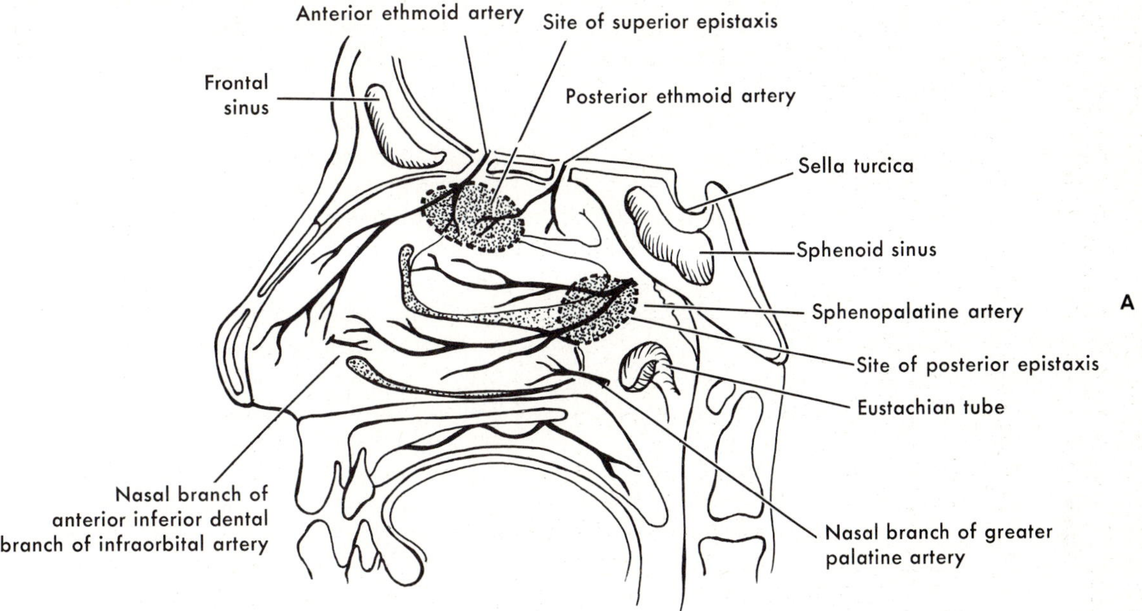

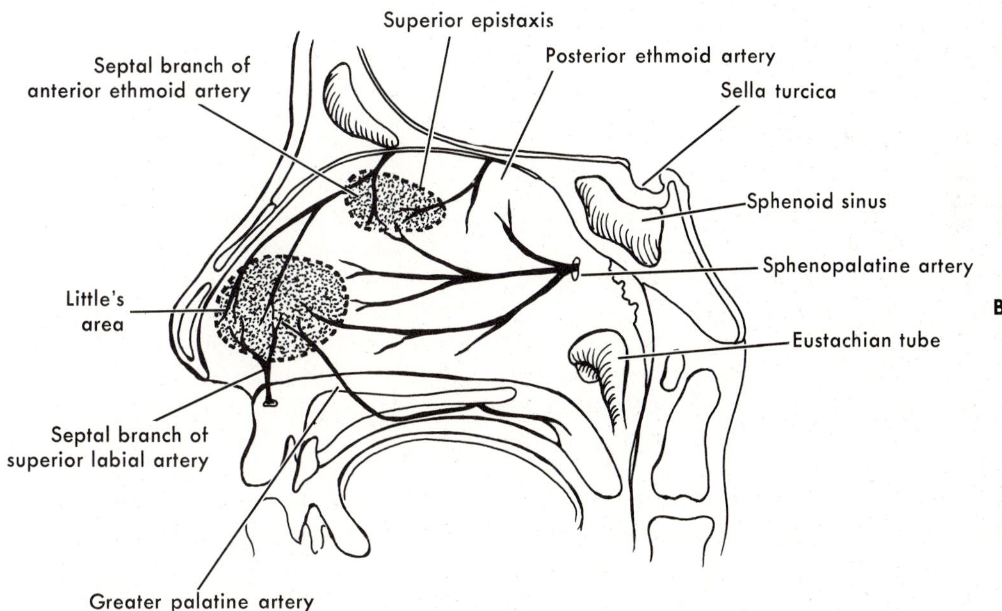

Fig. 22-34. A, Blood supply of lateral nasal wall. **B,** Arteries of nasal septum. (Adapted from Ryan, R.E., and others: Synopsis of ear, nose, and throat diseases, ed. 3, St. Louis, 1970, The C.V. Mosby Co.)

NURSING CONSIDERATIONS

Since nasal surgery is usually done under a local anesthetic, close attention should be paid during preoperative assessment to allergies and drug reactions or sensitivities, especially if related to the administration of local anesthetics. Questions about previous dental experiences involving this type of anesthesia and the patient's tolerance to it can provide a clue to how the patient will react to the anesthetic agents.

Cardiac status should be noted, since many surgeons use epinephrine as an additive to the local anesthetic. The epinephrine acts as a vasoconstrictor and reduces the blood loss during surgery but may also contribute to cardiac arrhythmias. Any respiratory conditions, such as asthma, should be noted. Physical limitations of the patient can determine additional aspects that should be included in the intraoperative care of the patient.

Several principles of nursing care are basic to all types of nasal surgery. The following information should be given to the patient:

1. Some discomfort may occur during the initial administration of a local anesthetic. If the surgeon uses a topical anesthetic as the first phase of anesthesia, the patient may find the packing uncomfortable or may have the urge to sneeze. This will disappear as the anesthetic takes effect. There may be some momentary discomfort from the needle and perhaps a burning sensation as the anesthetic is injected. If the surgeon uses epinephrine with the local agent, the resulting weak, quivery feeling and the increased heart rate are effects of the epinephrine and will disappear after a few minutes. The patient's cardiac status should be noted at this time.

2. Certain procedures may be performed on entry to the operating room or holding area in accordance with the individual operating room's policies, for example, insertion of intravenous lines, application of monitoring devices, and oxygen administration.

3. During the surgical procedure, the patient will feel the surgeon working and may feel pressure at some point, but *no* pain should be felt. The patient should let the surgeon know if any discomfort is felt during the procedure, and more anesthetic can be given.

4. After surgery, the head of the bed will be elevated to facilitate both breathing and drainage.

5. A nasal pack probably will be inserted, and there may be some difficulty in swallowing. When the patient attempts to swallow, a sucking action occurs in the throat because the packing does not allow air passage through the nose, thereby creating a partial vacuum.

6. Frequent oral hygiene will be offered and encouraged because of the postoperative mouth breathing.

7. Some bruising and swelling can be expected after surgery. It should be emphasized that this will gradually subside.

8. Forceful nose-blowing must be avoided for a time to prevent movement of the newly arranged nasal structures.

9. The sense of smell will be diminished for a time after surgery, but will gradually return.

10. Some numbness may be noticed postoperatively, but this too will gradually disappear.

11. A moderate amount of discomfort should be expected after surgery; medication will be ordered for this.

12. There is a procedure for changing the "moustache" dressing that will be in place postoperatively to absorb any drainage.

Preparation of the operating room includes checking the availability and functional capability of suction, the surgeon's head light, emergency drugs, oxygen administration equipment, and the cardiac monitor.

Preoperative preparations. Before the patient arrives, the operating table may be made into a reclining chair by use of a footpiece and pillows placed to protect the feet from pressure and to relieve strain on vessels and tendons of the lower extremities. The reclining chair is adjusted to meet the physical characteristics and comfort of the patient. The table is raised or lowered to accommodate the surgeon. In some cases the surgeon may request that the patient be placed on the table in a dorsal recumbent (supine) position.

In some cases, the hair of the nostrils may be clipped with fine, curved scissors. Sterile mineral oil drops or an antibiotic ointment may be put into the eyes of the patient to protect them from the prep solutions. The face is scrubbed with a mild soap and water. Prepping and draping of the patient is usually done before injection of the local anesthetic. However, the surgeon may request the topical anesthetic to be placed on the prep table so that the nose may be topically anesthetized for a period before the injections of anesthetic are started. This allows the topical anesthetic to take effect earlier and is more comfortable for the patient. Some surgeons may also request that the local anesthetic be placed on the prep table so that it can be injected before the skin is prepared. The circulating or monitor nurse should observe any changes in the vital signs of the patient. When cocaine or another similar narcotic agent is used, a thiopental (Pentothal) sodium setup and oxygen equipment should be in the room. The amount of the agents used for both the topical and the local anesthetics and any additions to the local, such as epinephrine, should be recorded on the appropriate chart.

Draping. The patient is draped with sterile towels and sheets as follows:

1. A small sheet with two towels on top of it is placed over the head of the table and under the head of the patient ("head drape").

2. The uppermost towel is brought around the head, including the hairline.

3. The ends of the uppermost towel are secured with a towel forceps, and the free ends tucked under the patient's head.

4. A large sheet is draped over the patient, bringing its upper end up to the chin.

5. Moist gauze pads are placed over the patient's eyes to protect them from possible injury by instruments and from nasal drainage.

INSTRUMENTS AND SUPPLIES

Sterile instruments, supplies, and other items include the following:

Local anesthesia setup

Cocaine 10% (topical)
Lidocaine 1% or 2% (usually with epinephrine 1:100,000)
Luer-Lok syringes, 5 and 10 ml
Needles: 25 gauge, ½ inch, and 27 gauge, 1½ inches
Cotton applicator sticks
Bayonet tissue forceps
Cotton balls, ½ × 3–inch cottonoid sponges, or other packing material

Supplies

1 ENT drape pack
1 Tube petrolatum gauze packing, ½ inch wide
3 Medication cups, labeled
1 Basin set
Gloves
1 Gown pack
1 Skin prep set

Cutting instruments (Figs. 22-35 and 22-36)

1 Myles septum-cutting forceps
1 Knife handle no. 3 with no. 15 blade
2 Ballenger swivel knives
1 Freer septum knife, rounded blade
1 Septum forceps
1 Kerrison septum punch forceps
1 Luc nasal cutting forceps, curved sideways
1 Freer septum chisel
2 Douglas nasal snares with wires
1 Freer dissecting elevator
1 Ballenger nasal gouge
1 Pierce submucous dissector, double-ended, right or left

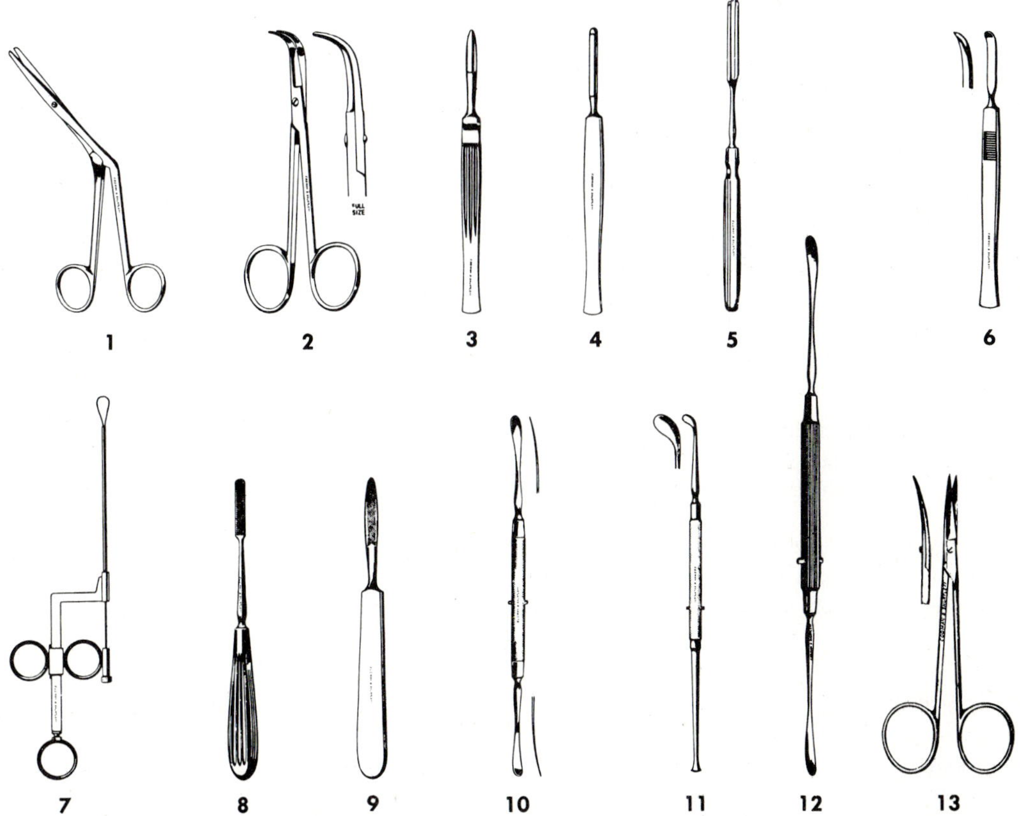

Fig. 22-35. Cutting instruments for operations on external nose and nasal cavity. *1,* Nasal scissors, angled; *2,* Fomon upper lateral scissors; *3,* cartilage knife, beveled blade; *4,* cartilage knife, straight; *5,* cartilage knife, swivel blade; *6,* cartilage nasal knife, curved; *7,* nasal snare; *8,* nasal rasp, narrow; *9,* nasal rasp; *10,* double-ended elevator; *11,* golf stick elevator-dissector; *12,* Freer dissecting elevator; *13,* iris scissors, straight and curved. (Courtesy Codman & Shurtleff, Inc., Randolph, Mass.)

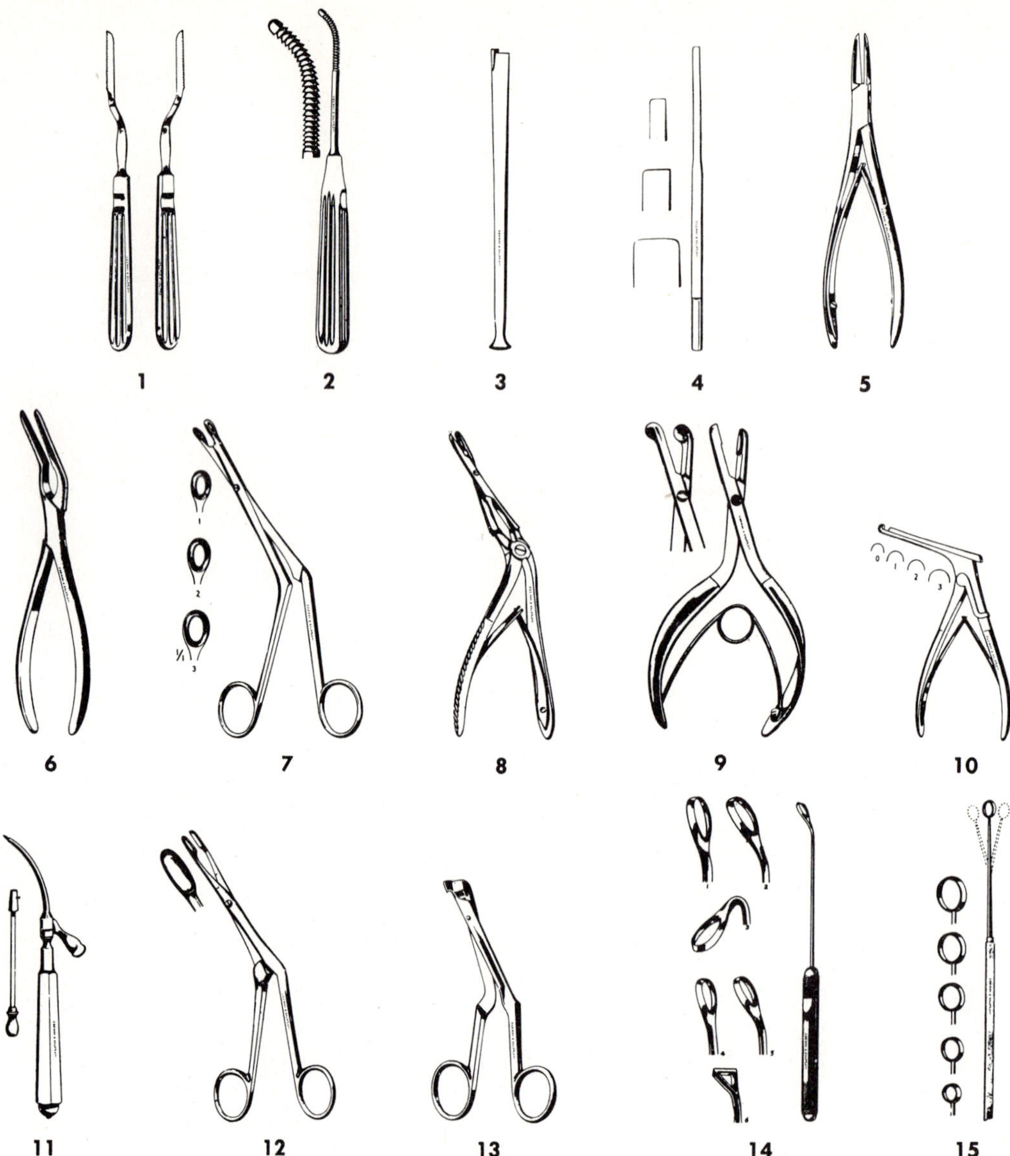

Fig. 22-36. Cutting instruments for operations on external nose and nasal cavity, continued. *1,* Freer nasal saws, right and left; *2,* reamer; *3,* nasal chisel with guard; *4,* osteotome, narrow widths; *5,* nasal bone cutter; *6,* Asch septum forceps; *7,* Bruening septum forceps; *8,* double-action nasal rongeur; *9,* McCoy septum forceps; *10,* Kerrison punch; *11,* antrum trocar and stylet; *12,* septum-cutting forceps; *13,* septal ridge–cutting forceps; *14,* Coakley ethmoidal sinus curettes; *15,* Myles antrum ring curettes. (Courtesy Codman & Shurtleff, Inc., Randolph, Mass.)

Holding and clamping instruments (Figs. 22-37 and 22-38)

1 Dandy nerve hook
3 Towel clamps
2 Kelly forceps, straight
1 Mayo hemostat, curved
1 Adson bayonet forceps
1 Adson tissue forceps
1 Tissue forceps

Exposing instruments (Fig. 22-39)

1 Nasal self-retaining wire speculum
Retractors, assorted sizes
2 Killian nasal specula

Suturing items (Chapter 7)

1 Needle holder, small
1 Septal suture, as desired, and taper point needle

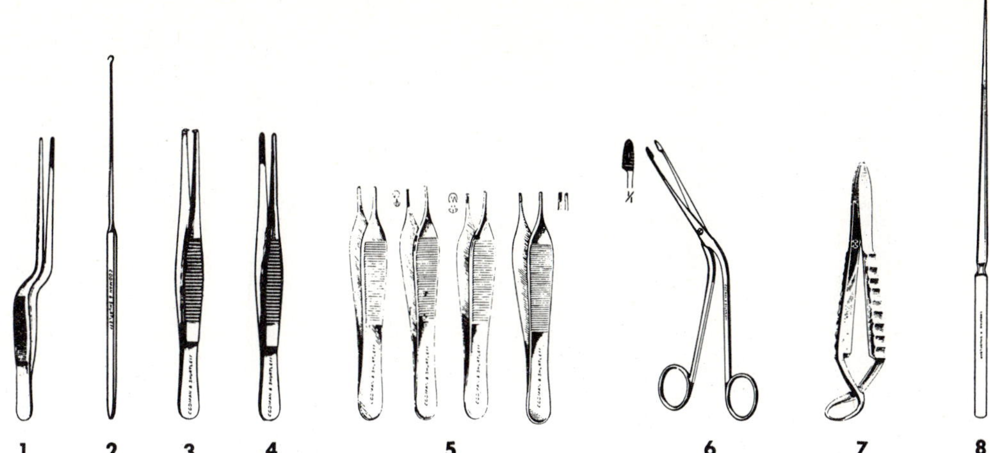

Fig. 22-37. Holding instruments for operations on external nose and nasal cavity. *1,* Adson bayonet dressing forceps; *2,* single hooks; *3,* Adson tissue forceps; *4,* dressing forceps; *5,* Adson dural forceps; *6,* Hartmann forceps; *7,* Jones towel clamps; *8,* Dandy nerve hook. (Courtesy Codman & Shurtleff, Inc., Randolph, Mass.)

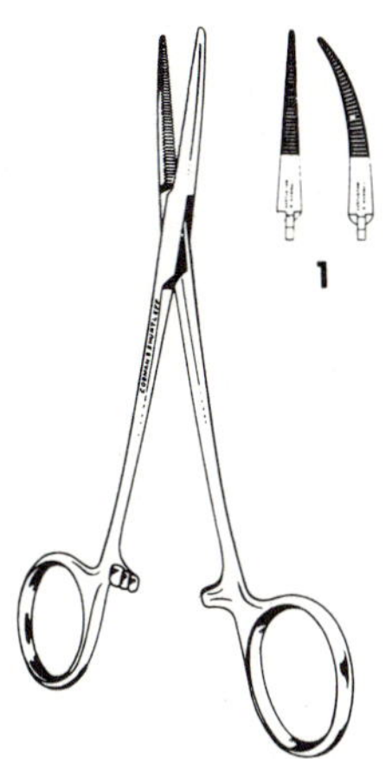

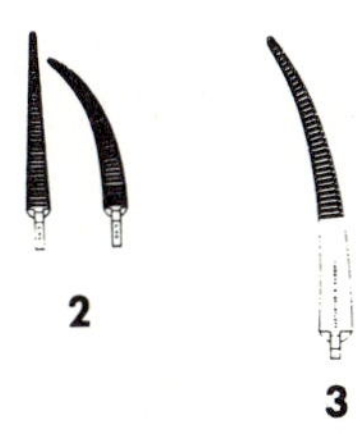

Fig. 22-38. Clamping instruments for operations on external nose and nasal cavity. *1,* Halsted hemostats, straight and curved; *2,* mosquito hemostats, straight and curved; *3,* Kelly hemostat, curved. (Courtesy Codman & Shurtleff, Inc., Randolph, Mass.)

Accessory items (Fig. 22-40)

1 Measuring instrument
2 Frazier nasal suction tubes and tubing
2 Antrum suction tubes
  Obturators for cleaning suction tube
1 Bulb syringe and saline solution
1 Mallet
4 Applicators, serrated end
1 Yankhauer tonsil suction tip

Postoperative care of instruments

Care of the instruments used in nasal surgery follow the general care regimen of any other surgical instruments. Chisels and gouges should be inspected carefully for any nicks and sent for repair as needed. Using damaged instruments may cause tissue damage in succeeding procedures. Rasps and files should be thoroughly cleaned and all bone debris removed. Special attention should also be given to suction tips. Lenses on head lights used during the procedure should be checked for cleanliness. Spatter on lenses should be removed according to the manufacturer's instructions.

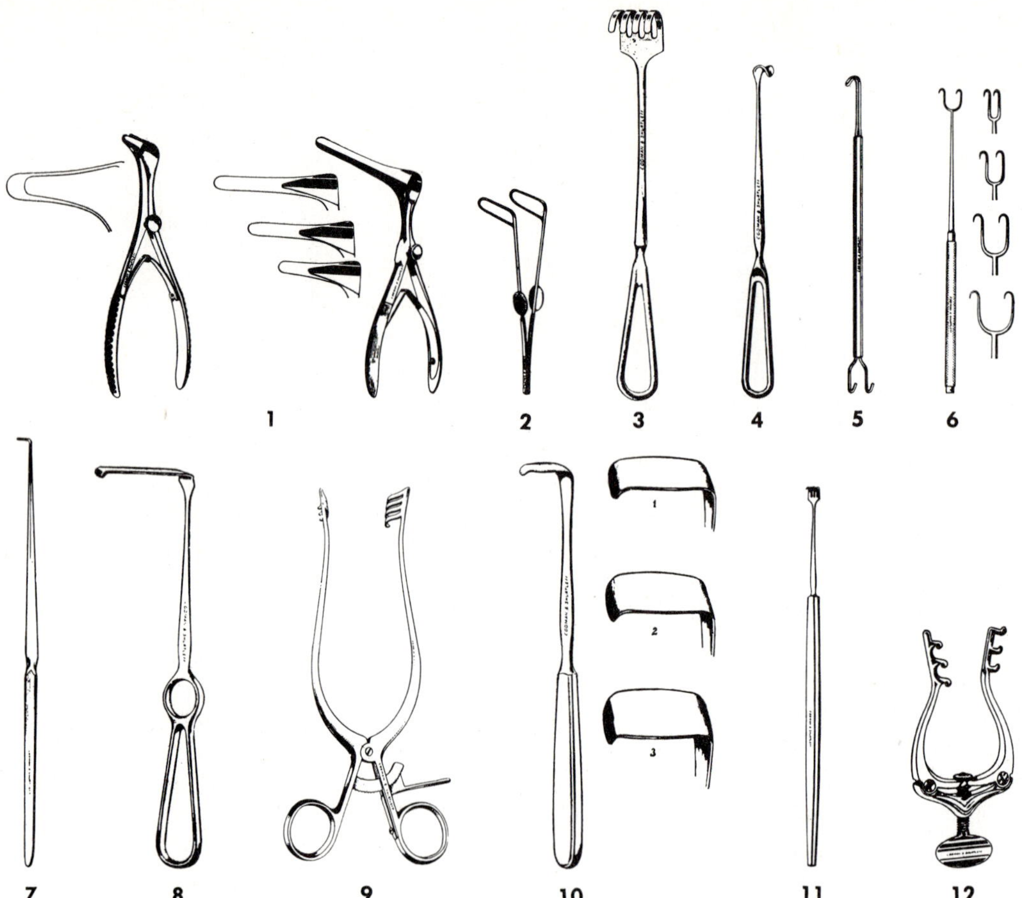

Fig. 22-39. Exposing instruments for operations on external nose, nasal cavity, and mastoid. *1,* Vienna and Killian nasal specula; *2,* Bosworth nasal wire speculum; *3,* Volkmann rake retractor; *4,* Cushing vein retractor; *5,* one- and two-pronged retractor, double-ended; *6,* two-pronged retractors, sharp, various sizes; *7,* Hoen nerve hook; *8,* Kocher retractor; *9,* Weitlaner self-retaining retractor; *10,* Langenbeck retractors, various sizes; *11,* delicate four-pronged retractor; *12,* Jansen mastoid retractor. (Courtesy Codman & Shurtleff, Randolph, Mass.)

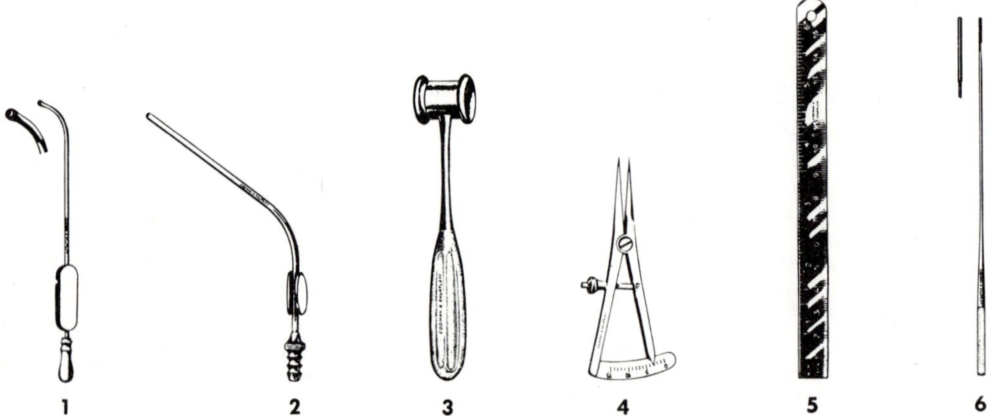

Fig. 22-40. Accessory instruments for operations on external nose and nasal cavity. *1,* Antrum suction tubes; *2,* Frazier suction tube; *3,* metal mallet; *4,* caliper; *5,* ruler; *6,* nasal applicators. (Courtesy Codman & Shurtleff, Inc., Randolph, Mass.)

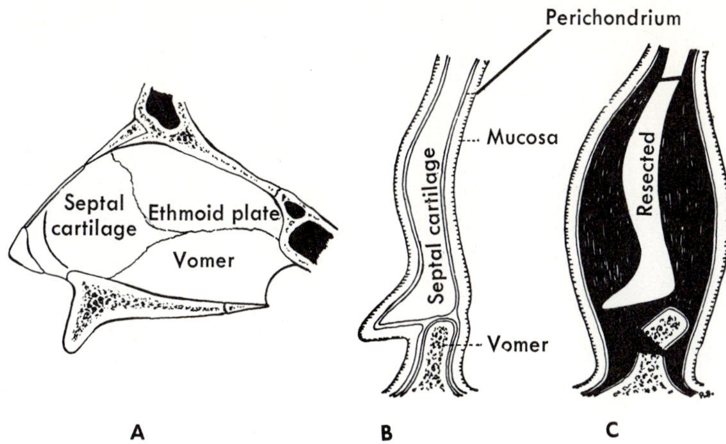

Fig. 22-41. A, Primary components of septum. Incision line is for Killian type of submucous resection. **B,** Septum with deviated cartilage and spur at junction of vomer and septal cartilage. **C,** Resection of obstructive parts after careful elevation of mucoperichondrium and mucoperiosteum. (From DeWeese, D.D., and Saunders, W.H.: Textbook of otolaryngology, ed. 3, St. Louis, The C.V. Mosby Co.)

OPERATIONS

Submucous resection of the septum

Definition. Removal of either the cartilaginous or osseous portions of the septum that lie between the flaps of the mucous membrane and the perichondrium.

Considerations. When the nasal septum is deformed, fractured, or injured, normal respiratory function and nasal drainage may be impaired. Deviations of the septum, involving cartilage, bony parts (spurs), or both, may block the meatus and compress the middle turbinate on that side, thereby resulting in an obstruction of the sinus opening. Septal deviations tend to produce sinus disease and nasal polyps.

The objective of a submucous resection is to establish an adequate partition between the left and right nasal cavities, thereby providing a clear airway of both the internal and external cavity and the parts of the nose.

Setup and preparation of the patient. As described in the general preparation for nasal surgery.

Operative procedure

1. The nostril is opened with a speculum. An incision is made through the mucoperichondrium and mucoperiosteum of the septum with a knife with no. 15 blade. The tissues are separated and elevated with a Freer knife (Fig. 22-41).

2. The cartilage is incised with a knife, and the mucous membrane is elevated with a Ballenger knife and a septal elevator; deviated cartilage and bony, thickened structures are removed with a septum punch and a nasal cutting forceps.

3. The mucous membrane is freed from the bony septal base by means of a chisel, gouge and mallet, or punch forceps. Bleeding is controlled by gauze sponges; suctioning is used to expose the field.

4. The perpendicular plate of the ethmoidal sinus may be removed, as well as the vomer, by means of the retractor, chisel and mallet, and suitable septum-cutting forceps (Fig. 22-36).

5. The incision may or may not be sutured with silk no. 3-0 swaged on a small needle.

6. Nostrils are packed with petrolatum gauze to keep the septal flaps in a midline position. The face is cleansed with both moist and dry compresses. A "moustache" dressing may be applied. External dressings or splints are dependent on the surgeon's preference, as is the application of a small ice bag to the nose. A surgeon's glove filled with ice makes an excellent ice bag because it is small and fairly lightweight.

Corrective rhinoplasty

Definition. Removal of the hump, narrowing and shortening of the nose, and reconstruction of the tip of the nose.

Considerations. Rhinoplasty may help in solving the patient's physiological, psychological, or economic problems.

Setup and preparation of the patient. The patient's face is prepped as described in the general preparation for nasal surgery. The patient is usually placed in a dorsal recumbent position. The head may be stabilized with sandbags. The nasal and plastic setups are shown in Figs. 22-42 and 22-43.

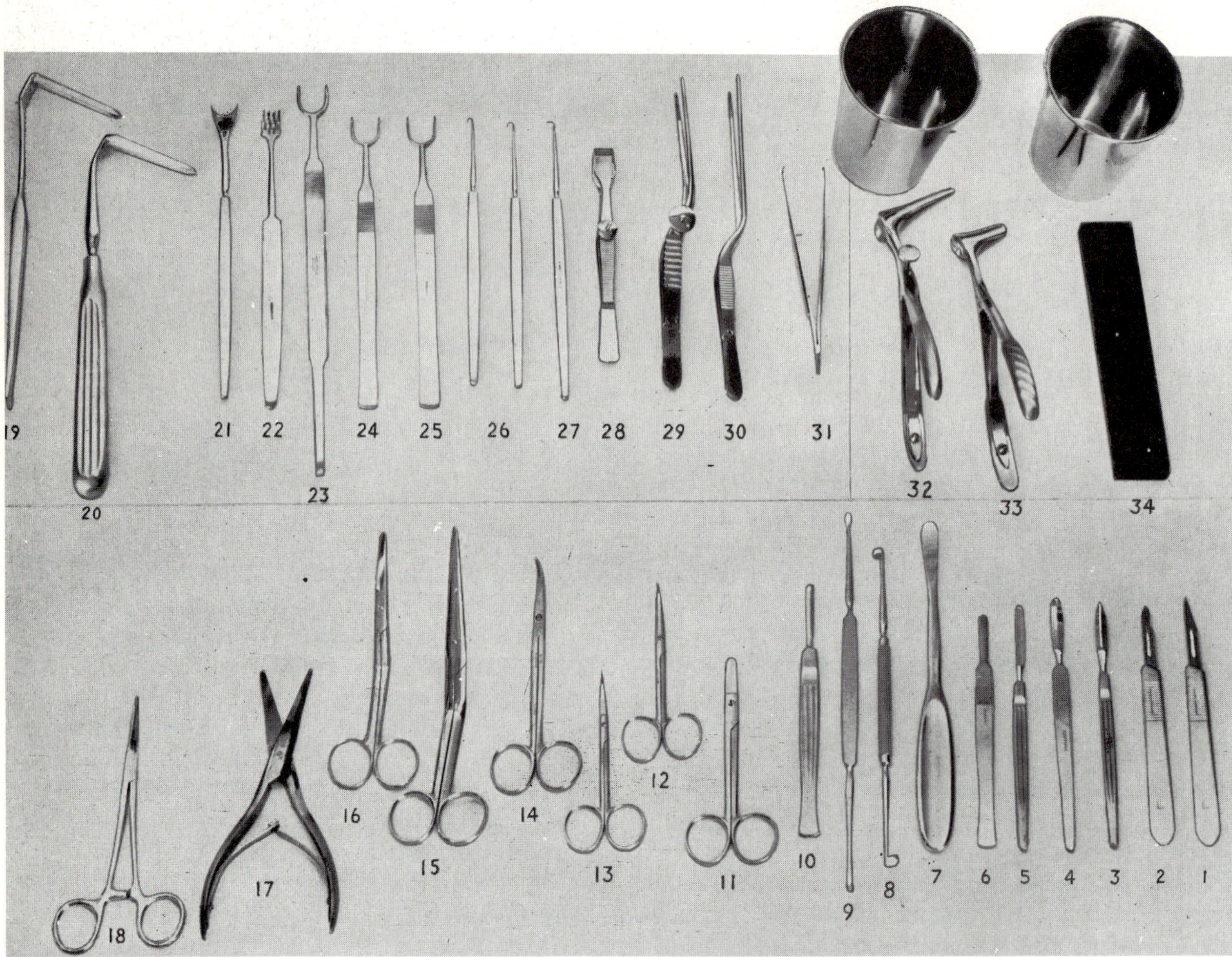

Fig. 22-42. Nasal and plastic setup used by Maurice H. Cottle, M.D. *1,* Bard-Parker knife handle no. 3 with blade no. 11; *2,* Bard-Parker knife handle no. 3 with blade no. 15; *3,* Cottle knife, double-edged, straight; *4,* Fomon knife, double-edged, curved; *5,* Joseph buttonhole knife, straight; *6,* Cottle knife, straight; *7,* Cottle skin elevator, curved; *8,* Pierce submucous dissector; *9,* Cottle elevator, graduated; *10,* MacKenty septum elevator; *11,* Cottle bulldog scissors, 4½ inches; *12,* Knapp strabismus scissors, curved; *13,* Knapp iris scissors, curved, sharp-pointed; *14,* Fomon upper lateral scissors, full curved; *15,* Cottle angular scissors, 6½ inches; *16,* Fomon angular scissors, light; *17,* scissors, straight, spring-action; *18,* Kelly artery forceps, straight; *19,* Aufricht nasal speculum, fenestrated; *20,* Aufricht nasal speculum solid; *21,* Cottle alar protector; *22,* Cottle four-pronged retractor, blunt; *23,* Cottle-Neivert retractor, double-ended; *24,* Cottle retractor, two-pronged, small; *25,* Cottle retractor, two-pronged, large, sharp; *26,* tenaculum, single, straight; *27,* Cottle tenaculum, single; *28,* Cottle columella clamp; *29,* Cottle lower lateral forceps, bayonet; *30,* Gruenwald nasal dressing forceps, 6¼ inches; *31,* Cottle-Graefe tissue forceps; *32,* Cottle-Killian nasal speculum; *33,* Vienna nasal speculum, medium; *34,* oil stone, for honing knives; stainless cups, for cartilage fragments. (From V. Mueller Armamentarium, no. 10, with permission of American V. Mueller, Chicago.)

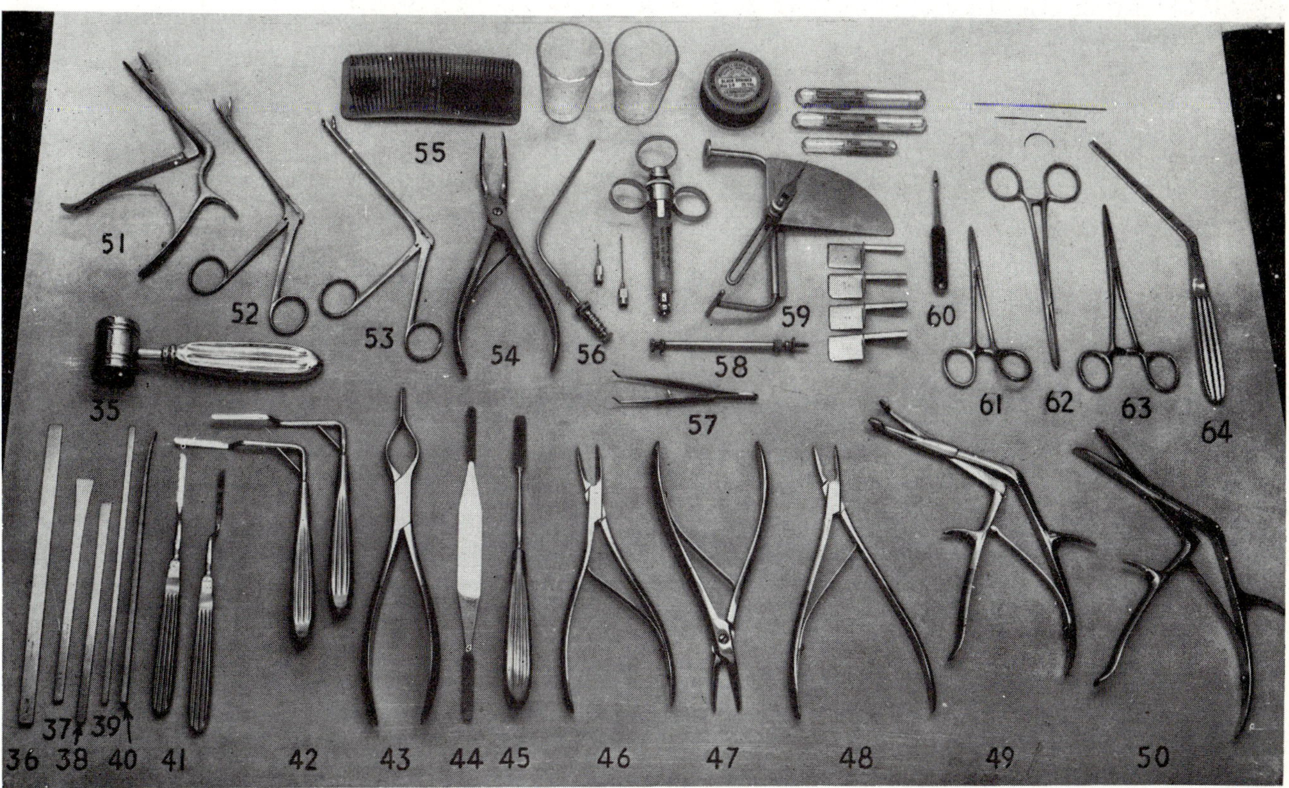

Fig. 22-43. Nasal and plastic setup used by Maurice H. Cottle, M.D., continued. *35,* Crane mallet, small, bronze head; *36,* Cottle bone lever, blunt end; *37,* to *39,* Cottle chisels, thin blade, rounded corners, 12, 8, and 4 mm; *40,* Cottle chisel, curved; *41* Joseph bayonet saws, right and left; *42,* Joseph-Maltz angular saws, right and left; *43,* Cottle-Walsham septum straightener; *44,* Fomon rasp, double-ended; *45,* Cottle nasal rasp (Sweeper); *46,* Cottle-Kazanjian cutting forceps: *47,* Kazanjian nasal hump-cutting forceps; *48,* Cottle-Lempert rongeur forceps; *49* and *50,* Cottle septal ridge–cutting forceps, right and left; *51,* Kofler-Lillie septum forceps; *52,* Ferris-Smith fragment forcps; *53,* Bruening septum forceps, alligator jaws, 6.5 mm wide; *54,* Cottle-Jansen rongeur forceps, angular jaws, with cupped portion of jaws straight; *55,* Turchiks instrument holder; *56,* Frazier nasal suction tube; *57,* Prince forceps, with teeth; *58,* Cottle cartilage holder; *59,* Cottle profilometer; *60,* Keyes cutaneous mucoperiochondrium punch, 2-mm diameter; *61,* Neivert needle holder; *62,* Allis tissue-holding forceps, 6 inches; *63,* Kelly artery forceps, straight; *64,* Joseph measuring instrument, angular; Keith needles, 4 inches and 2½ inches; cutting needle, curved, size 20; Sana-Lok control syringe, 5 ml; hypodermic needles, 22 gauge, 2 inches, and 25 gauge, ½ inch; medicine glasses for methylene blue. (From V. Mueller Armamentarium, no. 10, with permission of American V. Mueller, Chicago.)

Operative procedure

1. An incision is made through the skin of one nostril with a knife and no. 15 blade; a second incision is made in the other nostril and carried around the columella to join the first incision. A nasal speculum, sponges, and skin hooks are used.

2. The skin of the nose is undermined by elevators, knives, and scissors; the periosteum and perichondrium are freed with elevators, saws, and a periosteal dissector.

3. The nasal bone or upper lateral cartilage is fractured; the hump and possibly septal cartilage are removed by means of cutting forceps, such as the Jansen-Middleton; osteotomes, such as the Kazanjian action type; mallet; plastic scissors; and Adson forceps (Fig. 22-43). The field is cleaned by suctioning and by sponging with bayonet forceps.

4. The edges of the cartilages are trimmed by means of septum forceps and scissors (Fig. 22-43).

5. To prevent or control infection and the formation of a hematoma, the blood is suctioned from the nose, and the wound is cleaned.

6. The cartilage and bones are molded into proper position. The columella is sutured back onto the septum with fine silk sutures. The membranous septal edges are closed; dressings with a pressure splint are applied and are held in place with tape. A ''moustache'' dressing may be secured below the nares to absorb any bleeding. The head is elevated, and ice packs may be applied to the eyelids.

Intranasal antrostomy (antral window)

Definition. Opening made in the lateral wall of the nose under the middle turbinate and the removal of the anterior end of the inferior turbinate (Figs. 22-33 and 22-34).

Considerations. The patient suffers from headaches, edema, infection, or swelling of the lining membranes of the sinuses.

Setup and preparation of the patient. As described in the general preparation for nasal surgery. The instrument setup includes the following:

2 Towel clamps, 1 small and 1 large
1 Nasal speculum
2 Dean applicators
1 Side-biting mouth gag
1 Metal tongue depressor
1 Tonsil suction tip
2 Nasal suction tips
1 Universal handle with punches
2 Dean antrum trocar needles
1 Dean antrum rasp, concave
2 Dean rasps, blunt, 1 right and 1 left
2 Weiner rasps, 1 trocar point and 1 dull
2 Coakley curettes
1 Freer elevator
1 Knight nasal scissors
1 Bayonet forceps
1 Nasal dressing forceps
1 Bruening septal forceps
1 Knife handle no. 7 with no. 15 blade
2 Syringes, 10 ml, with 24-gauge needles

Accessory item

1 Postnasal plug or pack (Figs. 22-44 and 22-45)

Operative procedure

1. When the patient has been anesthetized, prepped, and draped, the postnasal plug is inserted (Fig. 22-45). The inferior turbinate is explored by means of bone-cutting forceps, elevators, and dissectors (Fig. 22-35).

2. An opening is made into the maxillary sinus (Fig. 22-33) beneath the inferior turbinate by means of a gouge, a perforator, or antrum cannulas (Fig. 22-36). The opening is enlarged with cutting forceps and antrum punches. Accessory polyps and degenerate mucosa are removed with a snare, septum forceps, and a suction (Figs. 22-35, 22-36, and 22-40).

3. The sinus is irrigated with saline solution and suctioned; the sinus is packed with petrolatum gauze, and the face is cleaned and dried.

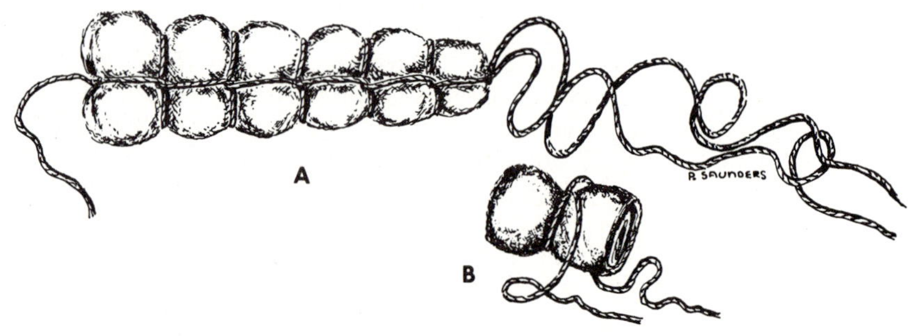

Fig. 22-44. Postnasal pack for hemorrhage. **A,** Three strings are needed. **B,** Pack also can be made from roller bandage or gauze; however, pack should not be too large, since it not only may obstruct both choanae but also may block eustachian tube. This pack should also have third string to dangle in nasopharynx to make removal easier. (From DeWeese, D.D., and Saunders, W.H.: Textbook of otolaryngology, ed. 5, St. Louis, 1977, The C.V. Mosby Co.)

Removal of nasal polyps

Definition. Removal of polyps from the nasal cavity (Fig. 22-46)

Considerations. The tissues become edematous, resulting in the formation of polyps that obstruct the free passage of air and make breathing difficult.

Setup and preparation of the patient. For polyps arising from the border of the middle turbinate, the instruments are as described for submucous resection. An intranasal setup is used if the polyps arise from above or from the semilunar hiatus. In some cases, polyps are removed in conjunction with a Caldwell-Luc operation, ethmoidectomy, enlargement of the frontal sinus, or opening of the sphenoidal sinus.

Operative procedure. As described for intranasal antrostomy or other types of operations on the sinuses with removal of the polyps and degenerated tissue.

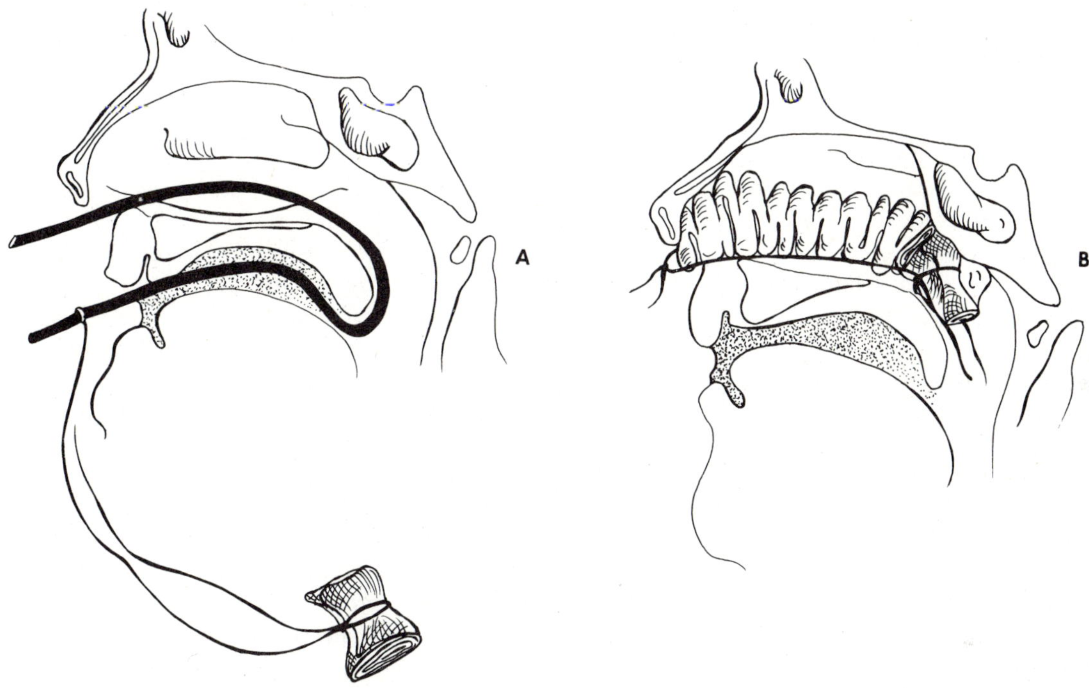

Fig. 22-45. Postnasal packing. **A,** First step. **B,** Second step. Anterior packing with ½-inch petrolatum gauze is then placed.

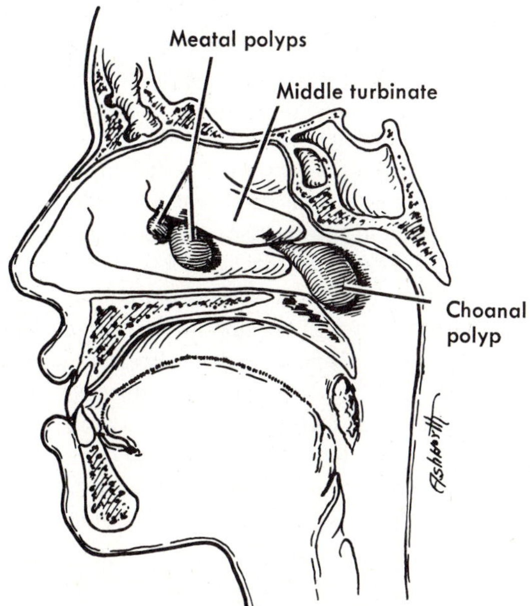

Fig. 22-46. Nasal polyps. Choanal polyp is usually single and originates in maxillary sinus; however, most polyps are found in middle meatus. (From DeWeese, D.D., and Saunders, W.H.: Textbook of otolaryngology, ed. 6, St. Louis, 1982, The C.V. Mosby Co.)

Radical antrostomy (Caldwell-Luc operation)

Definition. Use of an incision into the canine fossa of the upper jaw and exposure of the antrum for removal of bony diseased portions of the antral wall and contents of the sinus, or establishment of drainage by means of a counteropening into the nose through the inferior meatus (Fig. 22-47).

Considerations. In the presence of pus in an acute sinus disease, the mucous membrane may become thickened and polyps may form, resulting in an obstruction of the nasal cavity and external passageway. In such cases, the patient suffers from nasal catarrh, headaches, and cough. Chronic sinusitis may be associated with asthma.

The purpose of a radical antrostomy is to establish a large opening in the nasoantral wall of the inferior meatus, which ensures adequate gravity drainage and aeration and permits removal, under direct vision, of all diseased tissue in the sinus.

Setup and preparation of the patient. As described for intranasal antrostomy, plus the following:

2 Jansen-Middleton septum-cutting forceps
2 Kerrison rongeur (upbiting)
1 Citelli rongeur
1 Lempert rongeur
1 Olivecrona rongeur
1 Kofler septum forceps
1 Ferris-Smith forceps
1 Knoyes alligator forceps
1 Killian nasal dressing forceps
1 Weil nasal forceps
1 Nasal snare with wires
3 Mastoid curettes
1 Ethmoid curette
1 Chisel no. 6, curved
1 Chisel no. 8, straight
1 Orbital retractor
2 Caldwell-Luc retractors
1 Mallet
1 Self-retaining nasal speculum
2 Kelly forceps, medium
8 Mosquito forceps, curved
2 Allis forceps
8 Towel clamps
2 Tissue forceps, 1 with and 1 without teeth
1 Bayonet tissue forceps
1 Adson tissue forceps
1 Brown-Adson tissue forceps
1 Tracheal hook
1 Single skin hook
2 Freer elevators, 1 sharp and 1 dull
1 Pierce elevator
1 Pennington elevator
1 Periosteal elevator
1 Ball-tip elevator
1 Freer chisel
1 Ballenger V-shaped chisel
1 Knight nasal scissors
1 Metzenbaum scissors
2 Mayo scissors, curved and straight
2 Scissors, curved, small, 1 blunt and 1 sharp
2 Knife handles no. 3 with no. 15 blades

The patient may be given a general anesthetic.

Operative procedure (Fig. 22-47)

1. The upper lip is elevated with a Caldwell-Luc retractor, and a transverse incision is made in the gingivolabial sulcus just above the teeth; the incision is carried down to the underlying bone. Periosteum and soft tissue are elevated with dissectors and periosteal elevators.

2. The thin bony plate is perforated with a gouge, the antrum is entered, and its opening is enlarged with nasal rongeurs. The anterior angle of the sinus may be opened by enlarging the window with Jansen-Middleton septum-cutting forceps, double-action rongeurs, and Kerrison forceps (Fig. 22-36).

3. The mucous membrane of the antrum is removed with curettes (Fig. 22-36).

4. Nasoantral drainage may be established by removal of a portion of the nasoantral wall below the inferior turbinate by means of cutting forceps and rasps (Figs. 22-35 and 22-36).

5. Permanent communication between the oral cavity and the antrum may be established by removal of a portion of the hard palate and alveolar ridge with chisel and mallet. The edges of the palate are trimmed with a rongeur; the antrum is packed with petrolatum gauze or a ½-inch iodoform packing.

6. The labial incision may or may not be sutured with no. 3-0 chromic gut swaged on a small curved needle. The face of the patient is cleaned and dried. The patient should be advised that there may be a foul taste in the mouth postoperatively if iodoform packing is used.

Frontal sinus operation (external approach)

Definition. Making of an incision above the eyebrow of the affected side through the anterior wall and floor of the frontal sinus for removal of the diseased tissue, cleansing of the sinus cavity, and drainage.

Considerations. In an acute frontal sinusitis, in which the patient suffers from persistent headaches and edema of the upper lid, and in cases in which medical therapy has failed, surgical treatment may be indicated. Drainage of the frontal sinus may be performed by a simple trephine opening through the floor of the sinus. In the presence of chronic suppuration with repeated acute attacks of frontal sinusitis, surgery may be done to remove the diseased lining of the sinus and to reconstruct the nasofrontal duct, thereby ensuring adequate drainage.

Setup and preparation of the patient. As described for intranasal antrostomy, plus the following items:

1 Stryker saw with oscillating blade
2 Brawley or Spratt frontal rasps

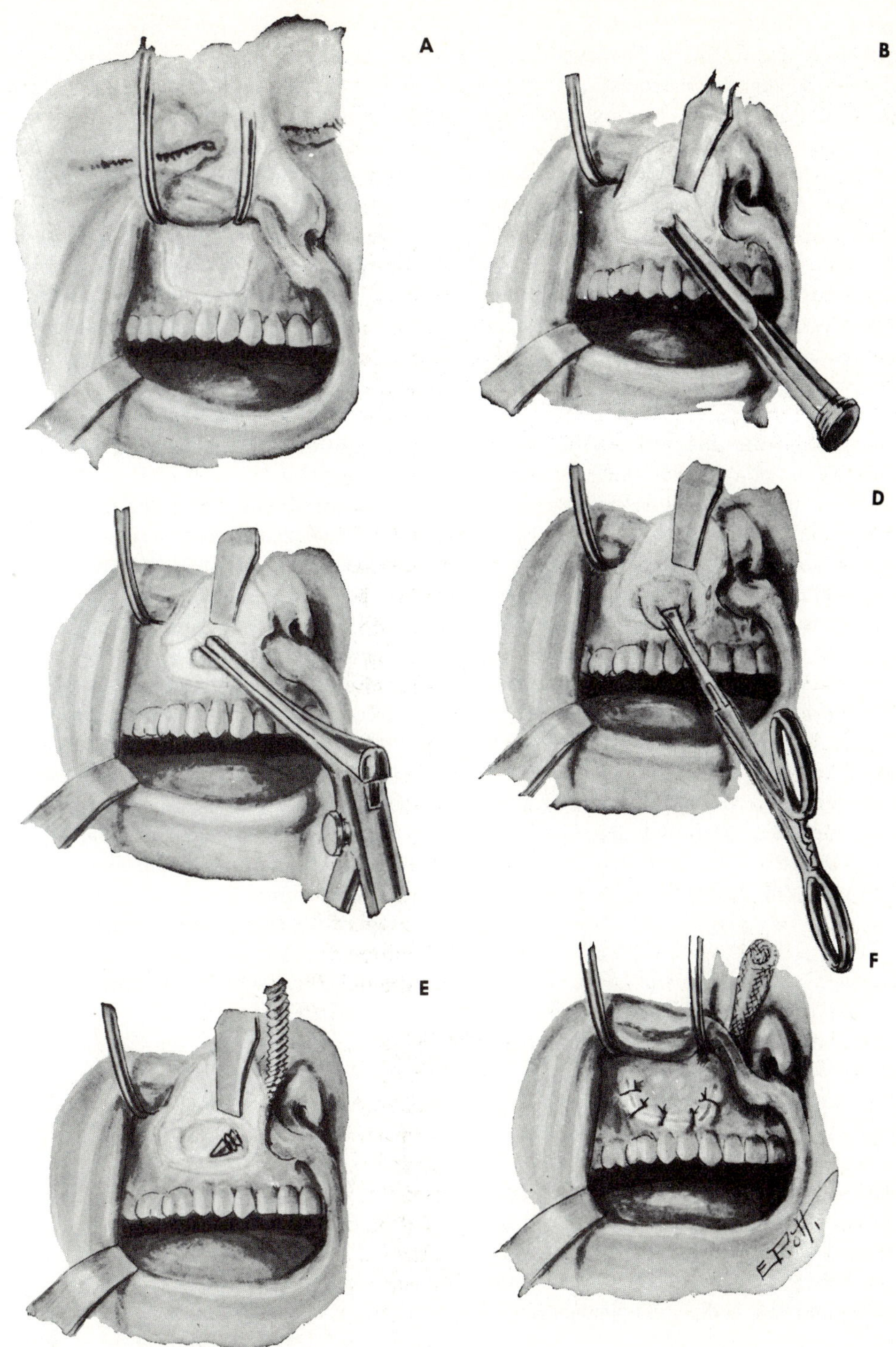

Fig. 22-47. Caldwell-Luc operation. **A,** Incision. **B,** Flap retracted and perforation made in canine fossa with gouge. **C,** Perforation enlarged with Kerrison forceps. **D,** Removal of diseased antral membrane. **E,** Trocar used to make nasoantral window. **F,** Incision closed. (From Thoma, K.H.: Oral surgery, ed. 5, St. Louis, The C.V. Mosby Co.)

1 Potts or Cushing nerve hook, blunt
2 Cushing forceps, straight, fine
2 Adson tissue forceps
1 Weitlaner self-retaining retractor (Fig. 22-39)

The patient usually is given a general anesthetic.

Operative procedure

1. An incision is made over the affected frontal sinus, extending from the base of the nose through the eyebrow as far as the supraorbital notch (Fig. 22-48). A self-retaining retractor, hook retractor, knife, sponges, fine hemostats, fine ligatures, and suction are needed.

2. Either the anterior wall of the frontal sinus or the floor of the sinus is opened by means of dental burs, chisel, mallet, gouges, septum-cutting forceps, curettes, and nasal forceps. Drainage is established by either the nasofrontal duct or the insertion of drains.

3. An ethmoidal incision is made behind the nasal process of the superior maxillary bone with a chisel and mallet. The lacrimal duct is identified and preserved. Ethmoidal cells are curetted.

4. A Penrose drain is introduced; the external wound is approximated with fine silk sutures, and a dressing is applied. The patient's face is cleaned and dried.

Ethmoidectomy

Definition. Removal of the diseased portion of the middle turbinate, removal of ethmoidal cells, and removal of diseased tissue in the nasal fossa through a nasal or an external approach.

Considerations. The purpose of an ethmoidectomy is to reduce the many-celled ethmoidal labyrinth into one large cavity to ensure adequate drainage and aeration (Fig. 22-31).

Setup and preparation of the patient. *For the nasal approach,* as described for intranasal antrostomy; *for the external approach,* as described for the frontal sinus operation.

Operative procedure. *For the nasal route,* the procedure is similar to intranasal antrostomy described previously. *For the external route,* the procedure is similar to the frontal sinus operation described previously (Fig. 22-48).

Sphenoidectomy

Definition. Making of an opening into one or both of the sphenoidal sinuses by the intranasal or external ethmoidectomy approach.

Considerations. In surgical treatment of sinusitis of the sphenoidal sinus, it is difficult to visualize the cavity because of its depth. Surgery of the sphenoidal sinus is usually done intranasally or through an external ethmoidectomy approach.

Setup and preparation of the patient. As described for intranasal antrostomy, with the addition of long sphenoid curettes, antrum rasps, and antrum punches (Figs. 22-35 and 22-36).

Operative procedure. As described for intranasal antrostomy.

Turbinectomy

Definitions

anterior inferior turbinectomy Removal of the anterior end of the inferior turbinate.

inferior turbinectomy Removal of the greater part of the lower border of the hypertrophied inferior turbinate.

anterior middle turbinectomy Removal of the anterior end of the middle turbinate body.

In all cases, turbinectomy may include removal of polyps (Fig. 22-46).

Considerations. A turbinectomy is performed to provide adequate ventilation and drainage and relieve pressure against the floor of the nose (Fig. 22-31).

Setup and preparation of the patient. As described for intranasal antrostomy.

Operative procedure. The nose is packed with petrolatum gauze on all sides of the turbinate. An incision is made. The affected turbinate is amputated and removed, the polyps are removed, and the cavity is packed, as described for intranasal antrostomy.

Repair of nasal fracture

Definition. Manipulation and mobilization of nasal bones.

Considerations. When the nose is struck by a direct frontal blow, usually both nasal bones are fractured, displaced outward, and depressed into the ethmoidal sinus (Fig. 22-33). The septal cartilage is usually broken or deviated, and lateral cartilages are displaced. Early reduction is done.

Setup and preparation of the patient. The patient is placed on the operating table in a dorsal recumbent position, and a topical anesthetic may be applied.

The setup includes a topical anesthesia set, plus a rubber-covered forceps (Salinger elevator) or Asch septum-straightening forceps, a straight hemostat, petrolatum gauze packing, a plastic mold or aluminum splint, and adhesive tape.

Operative procedure. A rubber-shod narrow forceps is inserted into the nostril; the nasal bones are elevated and molded into place by external manipulation.

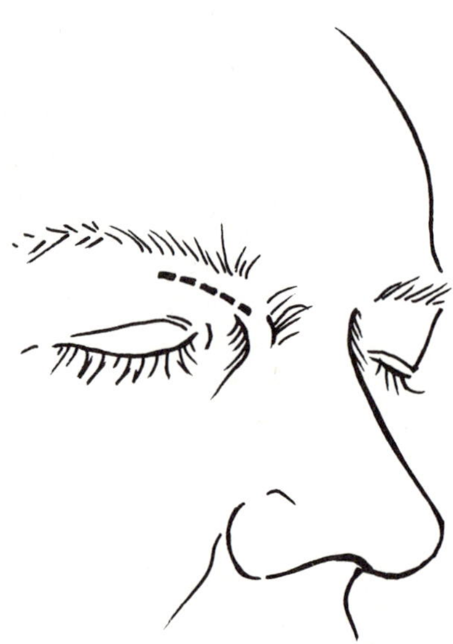

Fig. 22-48. Incision to expose ethmoidal and frontal sinuses. Resulting scar is almost invisible.

■ Throat, tongue, and neck

ANATOMY AND PHYSIOLOGY

The word *throat* refers to the structures of the neck in front of the vertebral column, including the mouth, tongue, pharynx, tonsils, larynx, and trachea (Fig. 22-31).

The *mouth* extends from the lips to the anterior pillars of the fauces. The portion of the mouth outside the teeth is known as the buccal cavity, and that on the inner side of the teeth as the lingual cavity. The tongue occupies a large portion of the floor of the mouth. The hard and soft palates form the upper and posterior boundaries of the oral cavity, separating it from the nasal cavity and the nasopharynx. The soft palate emerges from the posterior border of the hard palate to form the uvula, a finger-like movable projection. On either side, the uvula joins the base of the tongue anteriorly and the pharynx posteriorly.

The *pharynx* serves as a channel for both the digestive and respiratory systems. It is situated behind the nasal cavities, mouth, and larynx (Fig. 22-31). The food and air passages cross each other in the pharynx. The pharynx is a funnel-shaped structure, wider above and narrower below, about 12 cm in length. It is composed of muscular and fibrous layers and lined with mucous membrane. It is associated above with the sphenoidal sinus and the basilar part of the occipital bone, and it joins the esophagus below. Seven cavities communicate with the pharynx: the two nasal cavities, the two tympanic cavities, the mouth, the larynx, and the esophagus. The cavity of the pharynx may be subdivided from above downward into three parts: nasal, oral, and laryngeal. Infection may spread from the pharynx to the middle ear through the eustachian tube.

The nasopharynx communicates with the oropharynx through the pharyngeal isthmus, which is closed by muscular action during swallowing. The oropharynx and the laryngopharynx cannot be closed off from each other; both serve respiratory and digestive functions.

The pharynx comprises three groups of constrictor muscles (Fig. 22-49). Each muscle fits within the one below, and each inserts posteriorly in the median line with its mate from the opposite side. The constrictor muscles provide constriction of the pharynx for swallowing. Between the origins of the constrictor muscle groups are so-called intervals through which ligaments, nerves, and arteries pass (Fig. 22-49). The recurrent laryngeal nerve is closely associated with the lower portion of the pharynx.

The *tonsils* are situated one on each side of the oropharynx, lodged in a tonsillar fossa that is attached to folds of membrane containing muscle. One pair, the palatine tonsils, are the only lymphatic organs covered with stratified squamous epithelium. The lateral surface of each tonsil is usually covered with a fibrous capsule. The anterior and posterior tonsillar pillars join to form a triangular fossa, with the posterior lateral aspects of the tongue at its base. The so-called lingual tonsils are lodged in each fossa. The adenoids or pharyngeal tonsils are sus-

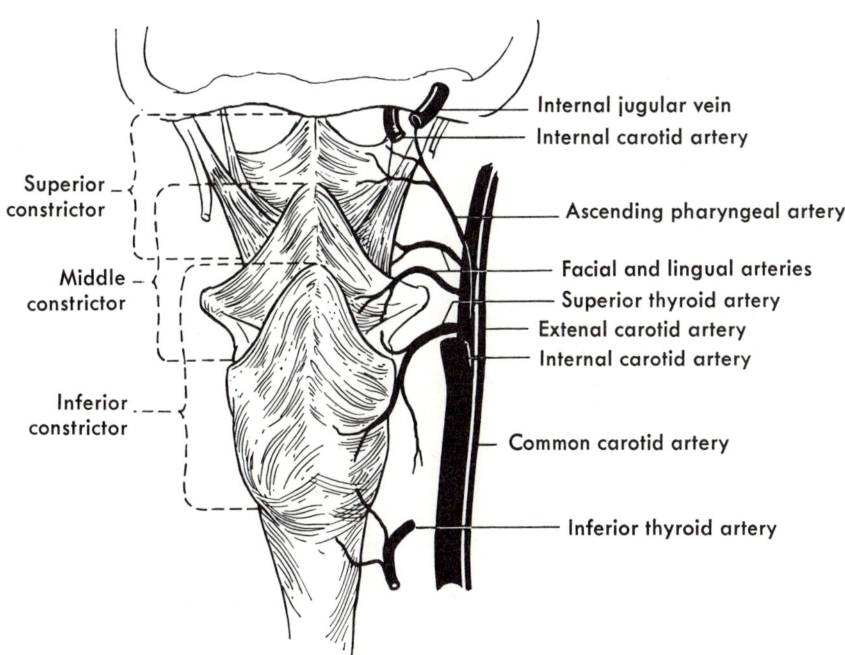

Fig. 22-49. Constrictor muscles and arteries of pharynx. (From Ryan, R.E., and others: Synopsis of ear, nose, and throat diseases, ed. 3, St. Louis, 1970, The C.V Mosby Co.)

pended from the roof of the nasopharynx and consist of an accumulation of lymphoid tissue.

The arteries of the tonsils enter the upper and lower poles. The tonsils are supplied with blood by tonsillar branches of the ascending palatine branch of the facial artery (branches of the external carotid artery). The external carotid artery on each side lies behind and lateral to each tonsil. The nerves supplying the tonsils are derived from the middle and posterior palatine branches of the maxillary and glossopharyngeal nerves.

Larynx and associated cartilages and muscles

Larynx. The larynx is located at the upper end of the respiratory tract. It is situated between the trachea and the root of the tongue, at the upper front part of the neck (Fig. 22-31). The larynx has three main functions: as a passageway for air, as a valve for closing off air passages from the digestive system and the pharynx, and as a voice box on which sound and speech depend to a degree.

The larynx is a cartilaginous box situated in front of the fourth, fifth, and sixth cervical vertebrae. The upper portion of the larynx is continuous with the pharynx above, and its lower portion joins the trachea. The skeletal structure provides for patency of the enclosed airway. The complex muscle action and arrangement of tissues within the structure provides for closure of the lumen for protection against trauma and entrance of foreign bodies and for speech.

Cartilages. The skeletal framework of the larynx consists of cartilages and membranes. There are nine separate cartilages—three of them single and six arranged in pairs. The main cartilages of the larynx include the thyroid, cricoid, epiglottis, two arytenoid, two corniculate, and two cuneiform. The thyroid cartilage, or Adam's apple, forms the anterior portion of the voice box. The cricoid cartilage, which resembles a signet ring, rests beneath the thyroid cartilage and within the laryngotracheal space (Fig. 22-50). The epiglottis is a slightly curled, leaf-shaped, elastic fibrous membrane. It is prolonged below into a slender process, attached in the midline to the upper border of the thyroid cartilage. When the cricothyroid muscle contracts, it pulls the thyroid cartilage and the cricoid cartilage, thereby tightening the vocal cords and, if unopposed, closing the glottis. The arytenoid cartilages, which rest above the signet ring portion of the cricoid cartilage, support the posterior portion of the true vocal cords.

Laryngeal ligaments. The extrinsic ligaments of the larynx are those connecting the thyroid cartilage and epiglottis with the hyoid bone and the cricoid cartilage with the trachea. The intrinsic ligaments of the larynx are those connecting several cartilages of the organ to each other. They are considered the elastic membrane of the larynx (Fig. 22-50).

The mucous lining of the larynx blends with the fibrous tissue to form two folds on each side of the larynx. The upper set is known as the false cords. The lower set is called the *true vocal cords* because they are primarily concerned with the speaking voice and protection of the lower respiratory channels against the invasion of food and foreign bodies.

Laryngeal muscles. The laryngeal muscles perform two distinct functions: the extrinsic muscles open and close the glottis, and the intrinsic muscles regulate the degree of tension on the vocal cords (Fig. 22-51).

It should be noted that the spoken voice also depends on the sphincter action of the soft palate, tongue, and lips. The muscle action of the larynx permits the glottis to close either voluntarily or involuntarily by reflex action. The closure of the inlet by this mechanism protects the respiratory passages. The closure of the glottis and the action of the vocal cords are precisely coordinated to produce the spoken voice.

Two branches of the vagus nerve supply the intrinsic muscles. The recurrent laryngeal nerve branch of the vagus nerve is the important motor nerve of the intrinsic muscles of the larynx. The sensory nerve, which is derived from the branches of the superior laryngeal nerve, supplies the mucous membrane of the larynx.

When both the recurrent laryngeal nerves become divided or paralyzed, the glottis remains closed so tightly that air cannot be drawn into the lungs. As a life-saving measure, an endotracheal or tracheostomy tube is inserted immediately.

The larynx derives its blood supply from the branches of the external carotid and subclavian arteries.

Trachea

The trachea, a cylindrical tube about 15 cm in length and from 2 to 2.5 cm in diameter, begins in the neck and extends from the lower part of the larynx, on a level with the sixth cervical vertebra, to the upper border of the fifth thoracic vertebra. The tube descends in front of the esophagus, enters the superior mediastinum, and divides into right and left main bronchi. The trachea is composed of a series of incomplete rings of hyaline cartilage. The carina is a ridge on the inside at the bifurcation of the trachea. It is a landmark during bronchoscopy and separates the upper end of the right main branches from the upper end of the left main branches of the bronchi. Branches given off from the arch of the aorta—the brachiocephalic (innominate) and left common carotid arteries—are in close relation to the trachea. The cervical portion of the trachea is related anteriorly to the sternohyoid and sternothyroid muscles and to the isthmus of the thyroid gland.

Salivary glands

The salivary glands consist of three paired glands: the sublingual, submaxillary, and parotid. They communi-

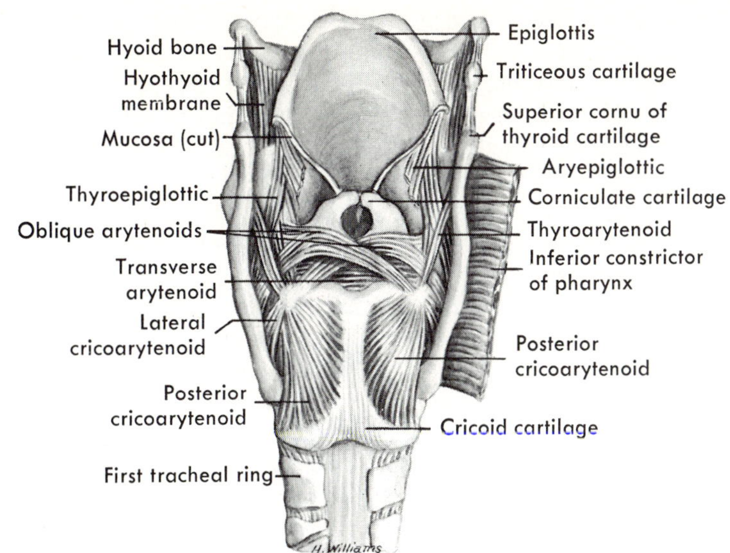

Fig. 22-50. Intrinsic muscles and general structure of larynx, viewed from behind. (From Francis, C.C., and Martin, A.H.: Introduction to human anatomy, ed. 7, St. Louis, 1975, The C.V. Mosby Co.)

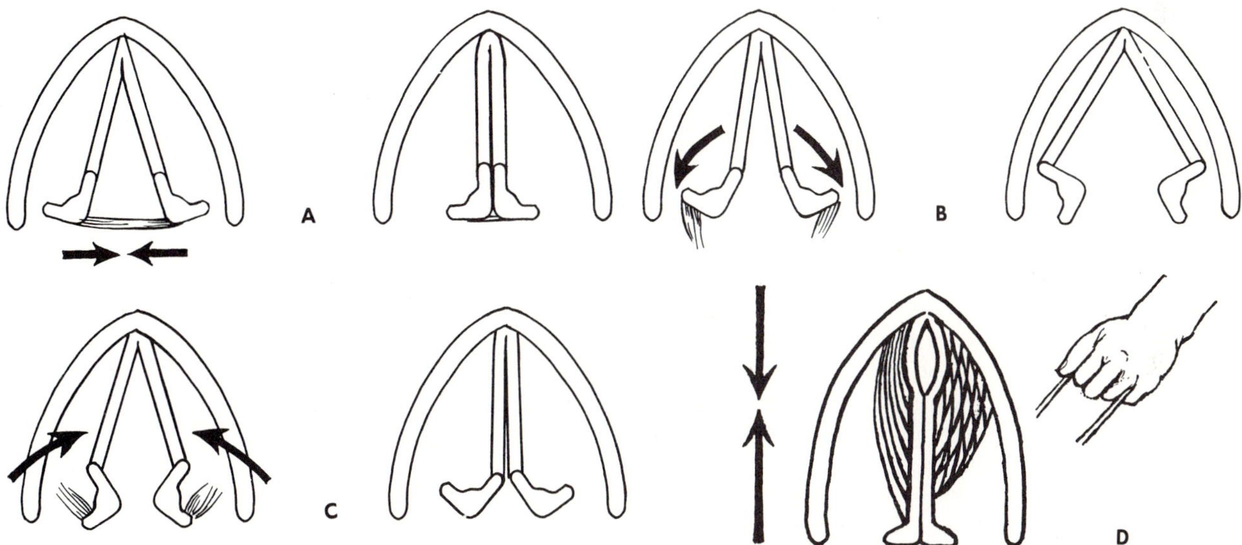

Fig. 22-51. Action of laryngeal muscles. **A,** Transverse arytenoid muscle. **B,** Posterior cricoarytenoid muscles. **C,** Lateral cricoarytenoid muscles. **D,** Thyroarytenoid, or vocalis, muscles. (From Ryan, R.E., and others: Synopsis of ear, nose, and throat diseases, ed. 3, St. Louis, 1970, The C.V. Mosby Co.)

cate with the mouth and pour their secretions into its cavities. The combined secretion of all these glands is termed *saliva*. The salivary glands consist of tissues found in the mucosa of the cheeks, tongue, palates, floor of the mouth, pharynx, lips, and paranasal sinuses. A tumor of a salivary gland may occur in any of these structures.

The external carotid artery supplies the salivary glands and divides into its terminal branches: the internal maxillary and superficial temporal. The superficial temporal and internal maxillary veins unite to form the posterior facial vein.

The *sublingual* gland lies on the undersurface of the tongue beneath the mucous membrane of the floor of the mouth at the side of the tongue, in communication with the sublingual depression on the inner surface of the mandible.

The sublingual gland is supplied with blood from the submental arteries. Its nerves are derived from the sympathetic nerves. The many tiny ducts of each gland separately enter the oral cavity on the sublingual fold.

The *submandibular* gland lies partly above and partly below the posterior half of the base of the mandible and on the mylohyoid and hyoglossus muscles. This gland is closely associated with the lingual veins and the lingual and hypoglossal nerves. The external maxillary artery lies on the posterior border of the gland. Its duct (Wharton's duct) enters the mouth at the frenulum of the tongue.

The *parotid* gland, the largest of the salivary glands, lies below the zygomatic arch in front of the mastoid process and behind the ramus of the mandible. This gland is enclosed in fascia, attached to surrounding muscles, and divided into two parts—a superficial and a deep portion—by means of the facial nerve. The parotid duct (Stensen's duct) pierces the buccal pad of fat and the buccinator muscle, finally opening into the oral cavity opposite the crown of the upper second molar tooth. The superficial temporal artery and small branches of the external carotid artery arise in the parotid gland behind the neck of the mandible.

General structures of the neck

The general topography of the organs lying in front of the prevertebral fascia has been described. A layer of deep cervical fascia surrounds the neck like a collar and is attached to the trapezius and sternocleidomastoid muscles. In front of the neck, the deep fascial layer is attached to the lower border of the mandible.

The *pretracheal fascia* of the neck lies deep in the strap muscles (sternothyroid, sternohyoid, and omohyoid) and partially encloses the thyroid gland, trachea, and larynx. The pretracheal fascia is pierced by the thyroid vessels. It fuses with the front of the carotid sheath on the deep surface of the sternocleidomastoid muscle. The carotid sheath consists of a network of areolar tissue surrounding the carotid arteries and vagus nerve.

Laterally, the carotid sheath is fused with the fascia on the deep surface of the sternocleidomastoid muscle; anteriorly, it is fused with the middle cervical fascia along the lateral border of the sternothyroid muscle. Lying between the floor and roof of this triangular formation of muscles are the lymph glands and the accessory nerve. Arteries and nerves traverse and pierce this triangle.

Lymphatic system of the neck

The lymph glands of the neck are closely associated with the salivary glands and the lymph plexus. The submaxillary nodes, located in the submaxillary triangle, drain the cheek, side of the nose, upper lip, side of the lower lip, gums, side of the tongue, and medial palpebral commissure. Lymph from the facial and submental nodes also drains to these glands. The superficial cervical nodes, following the external jugular vein, drain the ear and parotid area to the superior deep cervical nodes. The cervical nodes are in close contact with the larynx, thyroid gland, nasal cavities, ear, nasopharynx, palate, esophagus, and skin and muscles of the neck.

OPERATIONS

Laryngoscopy

Definition. Direct visual examination of the interior of the larynx by means of a lighted speculum known as a laryngoscope (Fig. 22-52) to obtain a specimen of tissue or secretions for pathological examination or to instill a drug.

Considerations. To facilitate the examination, the patient should be sufficiently relaxed by psychological reassurance and drug preparation. Sedatives are usually ordered before surgery.

Immediate preoperative assessment should include the presence of any dental appliances and condition of dental work and loose teeth. Any stiffness or immobility of the neck or shoulders should be evaluated. Respiratory problems such as asthma must receive careful attention.

The patient should be cautioned about not eating or drinking after surgery until the gag reflex has returned and swallowing occurs without difficulty.

Setup and preparation of the patient. Infants usually do not require an anesthetic; children and adults who cannot relax are given a general anesthetic; adults who are well prepared do very well with the application of a local anesthetic of lidocaine (Xylocaine), tetracaine (Pontocaine), or cocaine.

The setup includes the following:

Local anesthesia setup

Gauze sponges, 4 × 4
Laryngeal mirror
Cotton applicator stick, curved (Sawtell)
Cotton balls
Small cup for hot water (to warm the laryngeal mirror so that it does not fog when inserted into the mouth to view the vocal cords)
Emesis basin
Syringe, 5 ml, and Abraham cannula
Medication cup
Cetacaine spray, with angulated tip, or other topical anesthetic for the oral mucosa

Instrument setup

1 Head light
1 Bite block
1 Laryngoscope (surgeon's choice), size suitable to the patient (adult, child, or infant)
2 Aspirating tubes
1 Light carrier and extra bulb
2 Laryngeal biopsy forceps, 1 straight and 1 upbiting
2 Sponge-carrier forceps with extra sponges

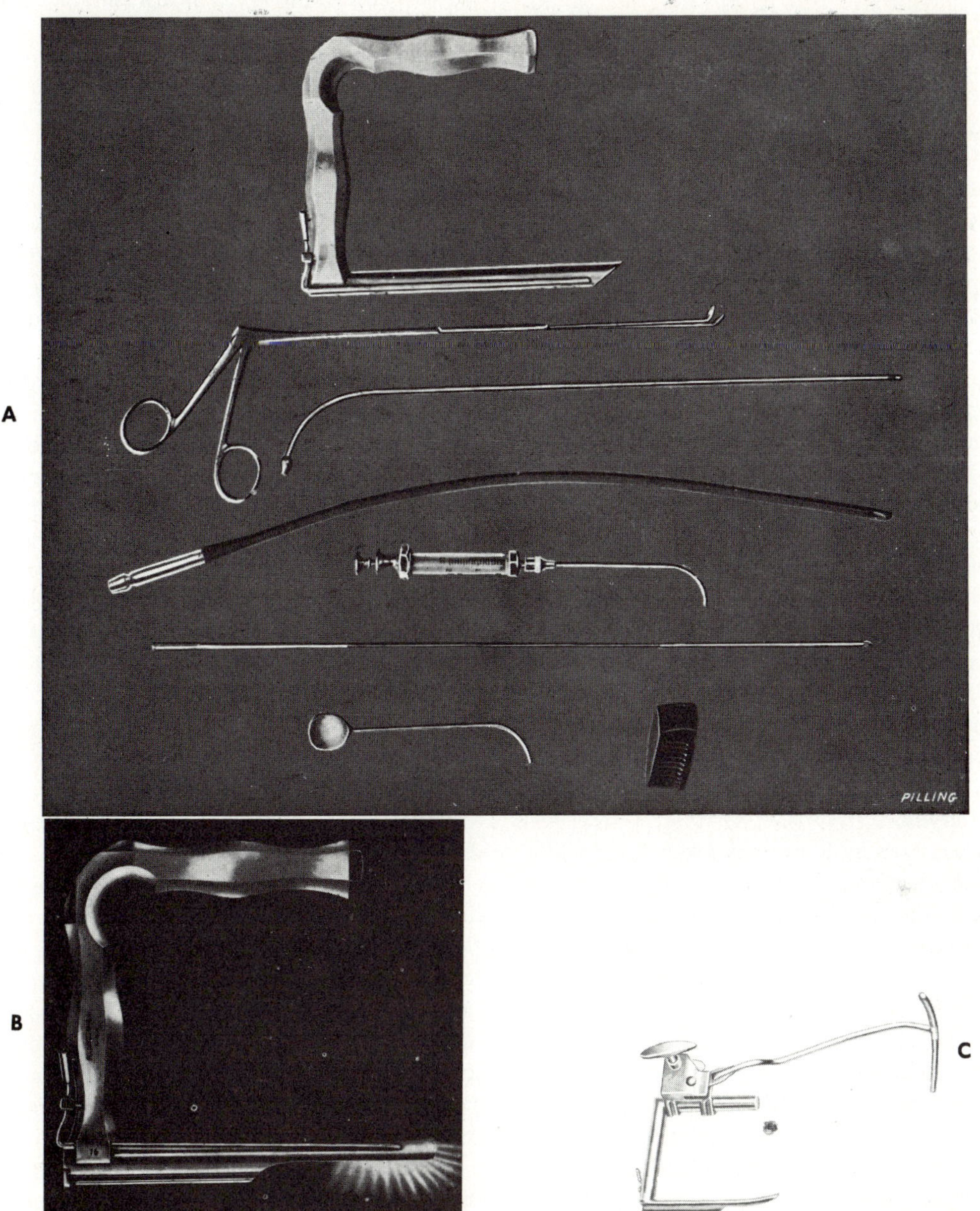

Fig. 22-52. A, Instruments for diagnostic laryngoscopy. *Top to bottom,* Anterior commissure laryngoscope (C.L. Jackson model); tissue forceps (laryngeal grasping forceps should be included, similar to tissue forceps but with straight alligator jaws); aspirating tube, metallic; aspirating tube, silk-woven; laryngeal syringe (Lukens model); sponge carrier for secure holding of gauze sponges for swabbing, hemostasis, and obtaining smear specimens; mouth opener (C.L. Jackson model); bite block of suitable size. **B,** Laryngoscope for introduction of bronchoscope. Slide permits removal of this necessarily rather heavy displacing instrument in trachea for safe exploration of tracheobronchial tree and for passage of bronchoscope. **C,** Lewy self-retaining laryngoscope holder, which allows surgeon to have both hands free. (**A** and **B** from Jackson, C., and Jackson, C.L.: Bronchoesophagology, Philadelphia, 1950, W.B. Saunders Co.; **C** courtesy American V. Mueller, Chicago.)

Accessory items

Specimen jars
Basin of sterile water (to flush suction)
Paper tissues
Pack of sterile towels

If the surgeon wishes to do a suspension laryngoscopy, the Lewy laryngoscope holder is added to the instrument table (Fig. 22-52, *C*). A sterile half-sheet or folded towels may be placed on the patient's chest to act as a support for the holder. The surgeon may request the operating microscope for use during the laryngoscopy.

The patient is placed in a supine position, and an assistant holds the patient's head in the proper position for good visualization of the vocal cords.

Operative procedure

1. Moist gauze pads should be put over the patient's eyes to protect them from the light of the instrument and to prevent possible injury and any irritation from secretions during the procedure. The head may also be wrapped in a sterile towel. Some surgeons may request a sterile drape to cover the patient.

2. The spatula end of the laryngoscope is introduced into the right side of the patient's mouth and directed toward the midline; then the dorsum of the tongue is elevated, exposing the epiglottis.

3. The patient's head is first tipped backward and then elevated and lifted upward as the laryngoscope is advanced into the larynx.

4. The larynx is examined, a biopsy taken, secretions aspirated, and bleeding controlled.

5. The patient's face is cleansed. The patient is reassured and then taken to own room or recovery room.

Microlaryngoscopy

Definition. Microlaryngoscopy facilitates improved diagnoses and allows the laryngologist to view with relative ease areas that were previously inaccessible or difficult to visualize. It may also be used for minor surgery of the larynx, especially for the removal of polyps or nodes on the vocal cords.

Considerations. If the procedure is done to remove polyps or nodes from the vocal cords, the patient must be cautioned about not speaking for a period of time postoperatively. Any necessary speaking should be done only in a whisper. The patient should be provided with a pencil and paper or a Magic Slate to aid in communication. Notations must be made at the nursing station about the patient's restriction on speaking.

Setup and preparation of the patient. The basic setup for laryngoscopy is used; however, the patient may receive a general anesthetic instead of a local. Microlaryngeal instruments are to be added to the setup and include the following (Fig. 22-53):

Lewy laryngoscope holder (Fig. 22-52, *C*)
Jako microlaryngeal grasping forceps
Jako microlaryngeal cup forceps, straight and upbiting cups (Fig. 22-53)
Jako microlaryngeal scissors, straight and angled
Jako microlaryngeal knives, straight and curved
Laryngeal probes, straight and curved
Jako laryngeal mirror
Jako open-ended microlaryngeal suction tip
Laryngoscope (twin light channel is instrument of choice)

The aforementioned instruments have a length of 22 cm to allow use with the microscope, but they are long enough to keep the surgeon's hands out of the visual field.

The microscope is used. The head will be adjusted to allow visualization of the larynx. The surgeon will usually do the adjustments on the microscope.

The microscope lens should be changed to one with a 400-mm focal length. Focal length is the distance from the lens to the operative area and is the point at which the field can be clearly viewed through the microscope. Beyond this point the field becomes fuzzy. The 400-mm lens gives the surgeon a 40-cm focal length, or working distance. A general rule for determining focal length of a particular lens is to divide the millimeter power, for example, 400 mm, by 10. In this instance it is 40 cm.

Care of endoscopic equipment

Endoscopic equipment is fragile and should be handled carefully. Rigid endoscopes should be thoroughly cleaned and lumens checked for cleanliness. Long, narrow brushes and long pipe cleaners are available for cleaning the lumen, suction, and light channels. The scopes should be dried carefully before storing. The light carriers are stored in the endoscope. The endoscope should be checked for any dents, roughened edges, or deep scratches on the surface. Any of these can cause tissue damage and/or lead to corrosion of the instrument. Endoscopes should be handled individually.

Fiberoptic equipment is also very fragile. The light cables should be handled with care and not allowed to drop or swing free while being carried. This can break the filaments inside the cords, rendering them unusable. Most cables can be autoclaved, but according to manufacturer's instructions only. They should be coiled loosely when not in use, and care should be taken not to put anything heavy on top of the cables. Kinking and sharp bending of the cables must be avoided.

The main advantage of fiberoptic light is that the light, although very bright, remains cool when used over a relatively long period of time. A simple test that can be performed by the operating room nurse to check the integrity of the cable is to hold one end of the cable to a bright light and visually inspect the opposite end of the

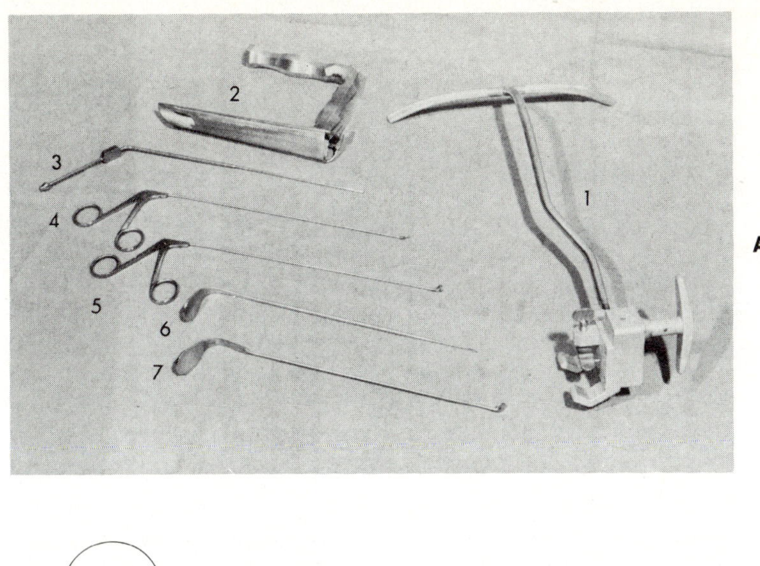

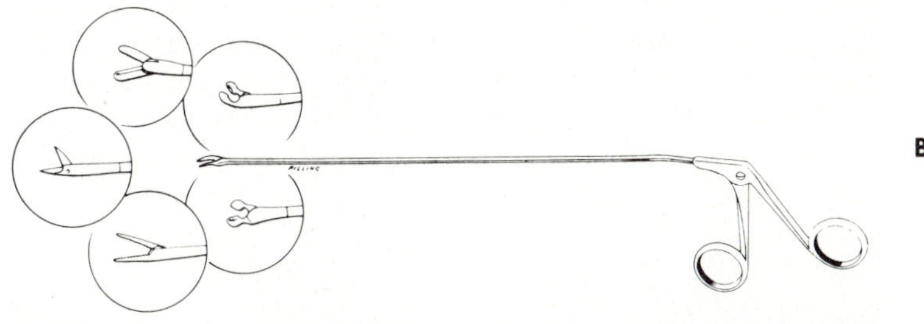

Fig. 22-53. Jako microlaryngeal instrumentation. **A,** Basic setup *1,* Lewy self-retaining laryngoscope holder; *2,* Jako laryngoscope; *3,* suction tip; *4,* grasping forceps; *5,* cup forceps; *6,* probe; *7,* mirror. **B,** Closeup of working ends of instruments. (**A** from DeWeese, D.D., and Saunders, W.H.: Textbook of otolaryngology, ed. 6., St. Louis, 1982, The C.V. Mosby Co.; **B** courtesy Pilling Co., Philadelphia.)

cable. Dark spots are an indication that some of the fibers are broken. If more than 25% of the fibers are broken, the cable should be sent for repair or replacement should be considered.

Telescopes for rigid equipment should also be handled very carefully to prevent damage. The telescope should be cleaned carefully, thoroughly dried, and returned to its case for protection during storage. Telescopes may be sterilized, but strict adherence to manufacturer's instructions must be followed. Gas sterilization is the method of choice. If a telescope is either dropped or hit against another object, it should be sent to the manufacturer for examination and repair if required.

Suction tips should be flushed thoroughly with running water. An instrument cleaning solution may also be used for this purpose. The lumen should be cleaned with a long pipe cleaner to remove remaining debris. The tip is then rinsed again, and the lumen dried with a clean dry pipe cleaner. The suction tip should be inspected for dents or nicks, especially on the end, to prevent damage to delicate tissues.

Biopsy forceps should be thoroughly cleaned, and the edges of the cups inspected for chips or nicks. They should also be checked periodically for sharpness. If the forceps become dulled, nicked, or chipped, tissue will be torn or ripped instead of cut cleanly when a biopsy is taken, resulting in more bleeding than usual. It is a good practice to rotate the use of biopsy forceps on a regular basis depending on the frequency of use. All forceps should be thoroughly cleaned, dried, and inspected for damage after use and should be sent for repair if necessary.

Proper care of endoscopic equipment can extend the service life of these instruments indefinitely.

Carbon dioxide laser surgery of the larynx

Definition. The advent of the carbon dioxide laser has added a new dimension to the laryngologist's methods of treatment for lesions of the larynx and vocal cords. The carbon dioxide laser is efficient and has a high power output. It uses a combination of carbon dioxide, nitrogen, and helium gases that become energized to a high degree by an electric current. As the energy level subsides, light beams are produced and are reflected off the mirror-lined walls of the laser tube. These beams eventually form a single beam of light that has a high intensity in the ultraviolet range and that is therefore invisible

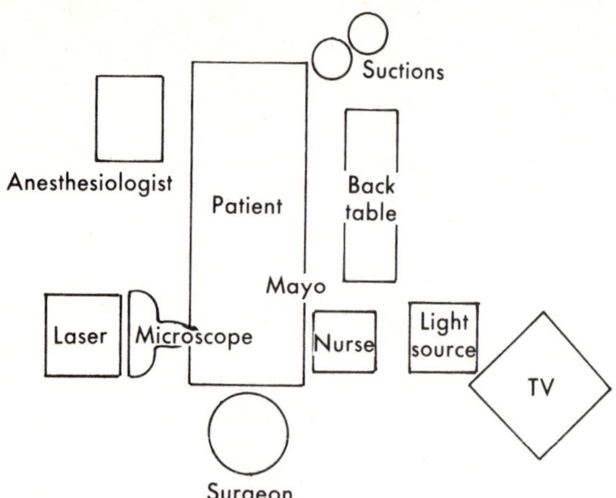

Fig. 22-54. Operating room arrangement of equipment for laser surgery. (From Pilcher, L.: AORN J. **33:**1402, 1981.)

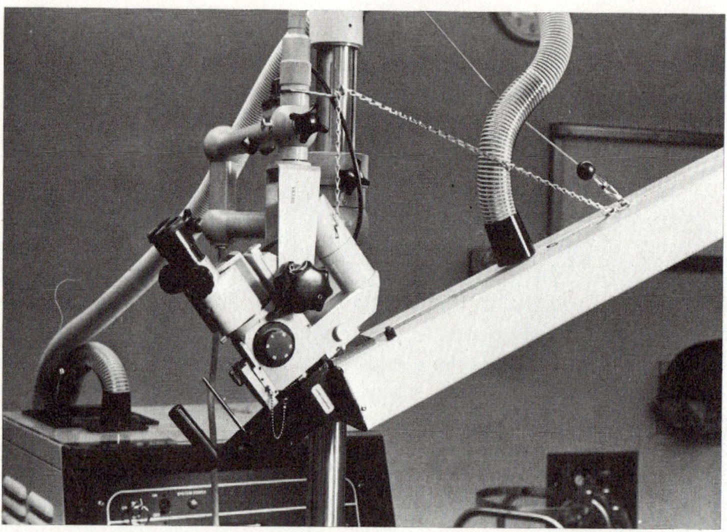

Fig. 22-55. Operating microscope with laser head attached. (From Pilcher, L.: AORN J. **33:**1402, 1981.)

to the eye. For this reason, a red beam from a helium-neon laser is added to the carbon dioxide beam so that it can be properly aimed at the affected tissue. The beam destroys tissue at a precise point with minimal tissue destruction in the surrounding area. It is especially useful in surgeries such as removal of webs in the larynx, vocal cord papillomas, and carcinoma in situ of the larynx.

Setup and preparation of the patient. The basic setup for laryngoscopy and microlaryngoscopy is used. General anesthesia is usually given. Suggested equipment placement is shown in Fig. 22-54.

The operating microscope with the 400-mm lens is used. The laser head is attached to the microscope head (Fig. 22-55). The manufacturer's instructions for attaching the head must be followed. The beam should also be tested for proper working order. Signal lights on the console illuminate if there is any malfunction in the equipment or if the gas supply is low. Extreme care should be used when handling this equipment because it is very delicate.

Precautions. Because of the pinpoint tissue destruction, specific precautions are necessary:

1. Laser light is reflected by shiny surfaces or absorbed by moisture. Because silicone, polyvinylchloride (PVC), latex, and red rubber endotracheal tubes are combustible, they must be protected, if used, by being carefully wrapped with adhesive aluminum foil. In addition, saline-soaked gauze is placed just above the tube cuff. These precautions eliminate the possibility of the tube and/or cuff being punctured or set afire by a stray laser beam. A safer alternative is the use of copper (Carden) or stainless steel (Porch) endotracheal tubes and a jet ventilation system.

2. Because of the ability of the laser beam to destroy tissue, healthy tissue must be protected. This is best done by covering the areas such as the eyes, the oral cavity,

and the peritracheal area by the application of *wet* gauze pads or cottonoid sponges. Cottonoid sponges covering the balloon on the endotracheal tube are effective in preventing rupture of the cuff. *It is imperative that all gauze pads be kept wet during the surgery to prevent damage to healthy tissue from stray or reflected beams of light.* Water is the most effective barrier to stop the laser energy from penetrating healthy tissue and/or igniting materials in the area. Should the endotracheal tube ignite for some reason (not a common occurence but the most dangerous of complications) during the procedure, a ventilating bronchoscope, grasping forceps of some type, and a tracheostomy tray should be available.

3. Operating room personnel in the room must wear eyeglasses or special plastic protective goggles. Contact lenses do not protect the eyes. The corneas of the eyes are especially vulnerable to stray laser radiation and must be protected. If the corneas are left unprotected and energy is absorbed, corneal opacification can result.

4. Signs should be placed on the operating room door during the procedure to keep extra people out of the room while the laser is in use. Any windows or other such openings should also be covered for the duration of the procedure.

5. If, for any reason, the equipment does not test properly before the procedure, it should be checked immediately by the manufacturer before being used.

The use of this equipment requires thorough education of operating room nursing personnel, anesthesia staff, and surgeons. The teaching should include the assembly and disassembly of the equipment, proper techniques for the immediate preoperative testing of the equipment, precautions that must be taken while in use, and a basic explanation of the principles of the laser beam itself. These points should be thoroughly understood by all involved to prevent any undue tissue damage to the patient or injury to personnel.

Tonsillectomy and adenoidectomy

Definition. Removal of the tonsils and adenoids by sharp or blunt dissection.

Considerations. Enlarged tonsils and adenoids are usually associated with difficulty in breathing and hearing, chronic colds, enlarged glands of the neck, otitis media, and pressure on the eustachian tubes because of adenoiditis. Rheumatism, bronchitis, and deafness may be associated with diseased tonsils.

Special preoperative teaching and orientation sessions for pediatric patients have decreased the stress of hospitalization for children undergoing this surgery. During these sessions, parents are instructed in the essentials of postoperative care.

Setup and preparation of the patient. If a general anesthetic is to be administered, the patient is anesthetized first, then placed in slight Trendelenburg's position. The neck is hyperextended by placing a roll under the shoulders. If a local anesthetic is to be administered, the patient is placed in a sitting position.

The patient's face may be cleaned with an antimicrobial solution. The patient is draped as follows:

1. An opened sheet with two opened towels on top is placed under the head of the patient.

2. The uppermost towel is wrapped around the head and secured by a forceps, and the free ends of the towel are tucked under the head.

3. A second sheet is placed over the patient.

The instruments and supplies required include the following (Fig. 22-56):

1 Knife handle no. 7 with no. 15 blade
1 Tonsil knife, single-edged
1 Tonsil knife, double-edged, if desired
2 Eves snares with wires or Tydings snares and wires
2 LaForce or Sluder tonsil guillotines, if desired
1 Metzenbaum scissors, curved or flat, 7½ inches
1 Mayo scissors, straight
2 Adenoid curettes, suitable size
1 Adenoid punch, suitable size
1 LaForce adenotome, suitable size
1 Hurd dissector and pillar elevator
2 Robb sponge-holding forceps
1 Towel clamp
1 Adson tissue forceps
2 Allis forceps
2 Pillar-grasping forceps
2 Tenacula for seizing tonsils
2 Boettcher tonsil hemostats
2 Mayo-Pean hemostats, curved, 6¼ inches
2 Dean hemostatic forceps
1 Jennings mouth gag, suitable size
1 Uvula retractor
1 Tongue depressor
1 Needle holder, 7 inches
Plain gut ligatures, no. 0
Plain gut sutures, no. 2-0, swaged to ½-circle tonsil needle
2 Yankauer suction tubes with tubing
1 Pharyngeal tube
Minor throat pack, including tonsil sponges, gauze compresses, and tonsil tampons
Minor drape pack

Operative procedure

1. When a general anesthetic is used, an endotracheal tube is inserted, the mouth is retracted open with a self-retaining retractor, and the tongue is depressed with a blade retractor. An efficient suction is most important. The metal suction tube is introduced gently and passed along the floor of the mouth, over the base of the tongue, and into the pharynx. During the procedure the suctioning ensures adequate exposure of the operative site and prevents blood from reaching the lungs.

2. The tonsil is grasped with a pair of tonsil-grasping

forceps, and the mucous membrane of the anterior pillar is incised with a knife; the tonsil lobe is freed from its attachments to the pillars with a tonsil dissector, curved scissors, and gauze sponges on a holder. The tonsil is withdrawn with forceps (Fig. 22-57).

3. The posterior pillar is cut with scissors, and the tonsil is removed with a snare (Fig. 22-57). In some cases the LaForce or Sluder tonsil guillotine clamp may be used.

4. A tonsil sponge or tampon (cottonoid or gauze tied securely to silk) is placed in the fossa by means of a hemostat.

5. Bleeding vessels are clamped with tonsil forceps and tied with slipknot ligatures of plain no. 0, and the free ligature ends are cut.

6. The adenoids are removed with an adenotome or curette. Bleeding is controlled by pressure with sponges.

7. The fossa is carefully inspected, and any bleeding vessels are clamped and tied. Retractors and endotracheal tube are removed, the patient's face is cleaned, and the head turned to one side. The patient is kept in the semi-recumbent (Fowler's) position or on one side, horizontally, to prevent aspiration of blood and venous engorgement.

Surgery of the oral cavity

Definition. Excision of benign or malignant lesions of the tongue, floor of the mouth, alveolar ridge, buccal mucosa, or tonsillar area.

Considerations. Benign or small malignant tumors of the oral cavity may be excised without neck dissection. In the presence of tongue cancer without evidence of metastasis, a ''prophylactic'' neck dissection may be performed in an effort to control a cancerous growth in the upper jugular chain of the neck.

In the treatment of typical carcinoma of the floor of the mouth with involvement of the mandible, a portion of the tongue is removed in the combined operation—a

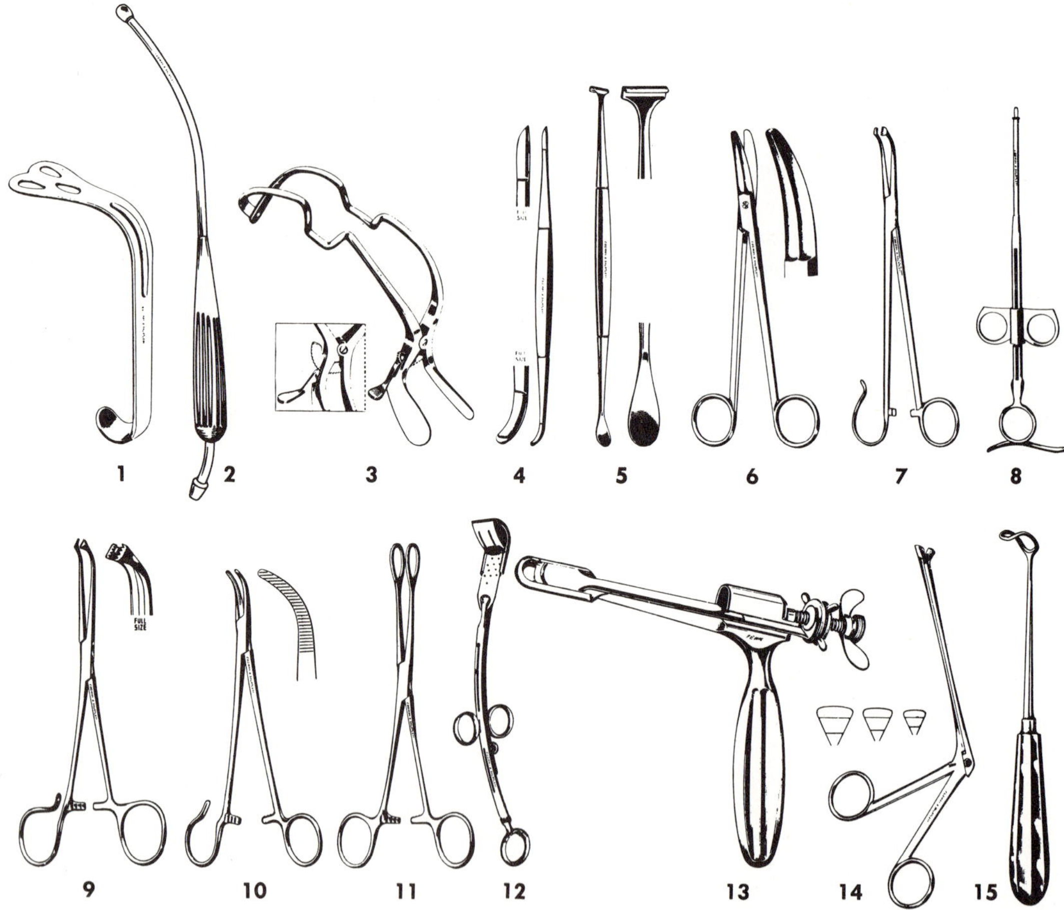

Fig. 22-56. Instruments for tonsillectomy and adenoidectomy. *1,* Tongue depressor; *2,* Yankauer suction tube; *3,* Jennings mouth gag; *4,* tonsil knife; *5,* Hurd dissector and pillar retractor; *6,* Boettcher tonsil scissors; *7,* White tonsil-seizing forceps; *8,* Eves tonsil snare and wire; *9,* Allis-Coakley forceps, straight and curved; *10,* Dean hemostatic forceps; *11,* Ballenger sponge-holding forceps, serrated jaw; *12,* LaForce adenotome; *13,* Daniel tonsillectome; *14,* adenoid punch; *15,* Barnhill adenoid curette. (Courtesy Codman & Shurtleff, Inc., Randolph Mass.)

radical neck dissection and resection of both the mandible and the tongue. When the primary intraoral lesion is confined to the tongue, a neck dissection and a hemiglossectomy are performed without resection of the mandible.

In the presence of a lesion of the tonsil or an extensive lesion at the base of the tongue with pharyngeal wall involvement, a resection of the ascending ramus of the mandible is necessary, and portions of the base of the tongue, pharyngeal wall, and soft palate are removed to secure an adequate margin of normal tissue around the lesion.

Psychological preparation of the patient is extremely important, since these procedures may be done for a minor lesion in the oral cavity or they may be the first part of much more extensive surgery in the head and neck area. A supportive and accepting family is most important to the patient at this time because of the possibility of disfigurement after surgery.

Setup and preparation of the patient. The patient is placed in a dorsal recumbent position with shoulders elevated. Generally, endotracheal anesthesia is used, and a pharyngeal pack of moist gauze is inserted in the mouth.

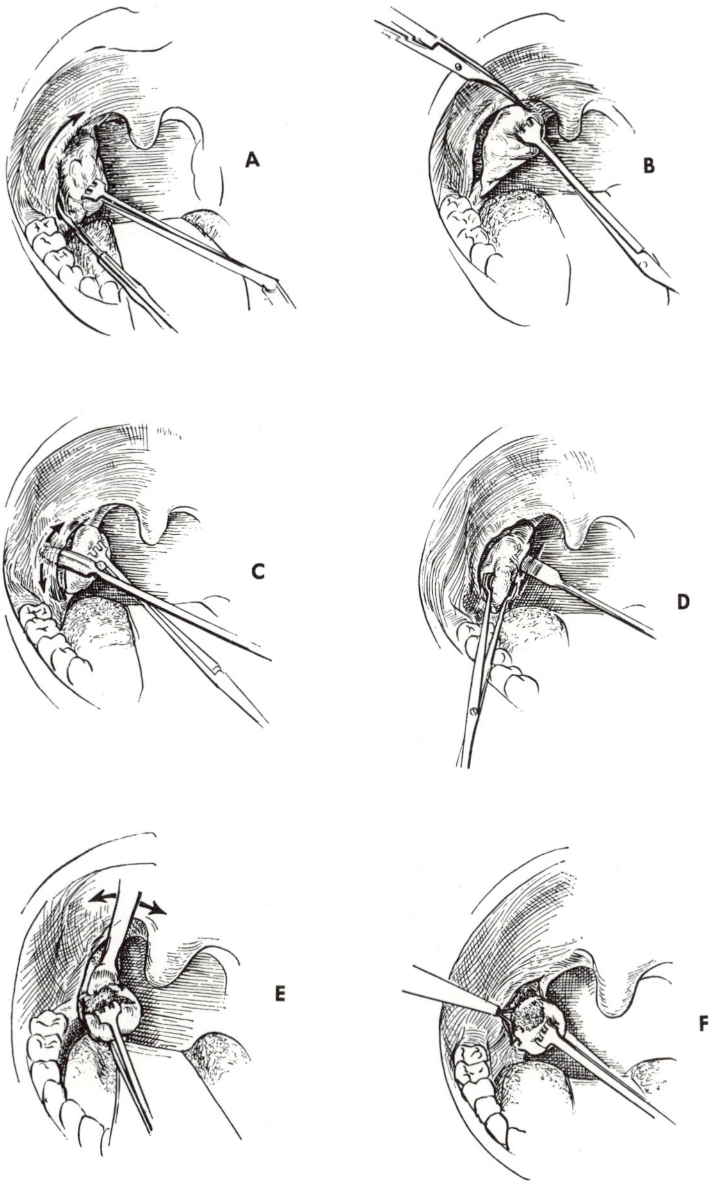

Fig. 22-57. Dissection method of tonsillectomy. **A,** Incision of mucous membrane along edge of anterior pillar. **B,** Extension of mucosal incision along its superior and posterior attachments. **C,** Separation of tonsil from anterior pillar. **D,** Separation of tonsil from posterior pillar. **E,** Completion of dissection along superior and lateral walls. **F,** Application of snare for removal of tonsil (From Ryan, R.E., and others: Synopsis of ear, nose, and throat diseases, ed. 3, St. Louis, 1970, The C.V. Mosby Co.)

Instruments and supplies include the following items:

2 Knives, nos. 3 and 7, with nos. 10 and 15 blades
1 Metzenbaum scissors, curved, 7¼ inches
1 Mayo scissors, straight
1 Mayo scissors, curved
1 Suture scissors
4 Foerster or Ballenger sponge-holding forceps
6 Towel clamps
2 Tissue forceps without teeth, 5½ inches
2 Tissue forceps with teeth, 5½ inches
2 Adson forceps
2 Brown-Adson forceps
2 Nasal dressing forceps
4 Allis forceps, 3 and 4 teeth
6 Mayo-Pean hemostats, curved, 6½ inches
3 Mayo-Pean hemostats, curved, 9¼ inches
6 Crile hemostats, straight
2 Rochester-Carmalt hemostats, 8 inches
3 Tonsil artery forceps
1 Metal anesthesia tube
1 Mouth gag
2 McBurney retractors
3 Bosworth tongue depressors
1 Cheek retractor
2 Parker retractors
1 Cushing loop retractor
1 Nerve hook
1 Crile-Wood needle holder, 8 inches
1 Crile-Wood needle holder, 5½ inches
Chromic gut, nos. 2-0 and 3-0, for ligatures
Silk, no. 3-0, taper point needles
Silk, no. 4-0 swaged to cutting-edge needles
Silk, no. 3-0, taper point needles (Murphy type)
1 Catheter, whistle-tipped, with open end, 14 Fr
1 Roll folded gauze packing with petrolatum
1 Postnasal plug set (Figs. 22-44 and 22-45)
2 Yankauer suction tubes and tubing
1 Tracheostomy set
1 Local anesthesia set for nerve block, if desired
1 Minor throat pack, including gauze compresses, pads, and tonsil sponges
1 Minor neck drape pack
Electrosurgical unit

Operative procedure. Although the procedure may be scheduled as a local excision, frequently lesions of the oral cavity require more extensive excisions than planned preoperatively. The setup should be designed to include the instruments for a neck dissection, or they should be readily available.

In most tumors of the oral cavity a tracheostomy is performed to ensure an airway after surgery.

Excision of the submaxillary gland

Definition. Removal of the gland and tumor through an incision made in the neck, just beneath the chin (Fig. 22-58, *A*).

Considerations. This operation is performed to remove mixed tumors and multiple calculi associated with extensive chronic inflammation.

Setup and preparation of the patient. The patient is placed on the table in a dorsal recumbent position, with the affected side uppermost, and prepared as for neck surgery.

The instruments include a minor neck dissection setup. A tracheostomy tube should be available. A set of lacrimal probes should also be added to the instrument setup if exploration of the submaxillary (Wharton's) duct is necessary during surgery.

Operative procedure

1. A small skin incision is made below and parallel to the mandible, extending forward to beneath the chin. The platysma is incised with scissors; the skin flaps and undersurface of the platysma and cervical fascia covering the gland are undermined with fine hooks, tissue forceps, and Metzenbaum scissors (Fig. 22-58, *B*).

2. The mandibular branch of the facial nerve is retracted away with a small loop retractor.

3. The submaxillary gland is elevated from the mylohyoid muscle (Fig. 22-58, *C*). The edge of the muscle is retracted to expose the lingual veins and nerve and the hypoglossal nerve.

4. The gland is freed by blunt dissection, and the submaxillary duct is clamped, ligated, and divided.

5. The external maxillary artery is clamped, ligated, and divided. The submaxillary gland is removed (Fig. 22-58, *D* and *E*).

6. The wound is closed with interrupted fine silk or chromic gut sutures. The skin edges are approximated with nylon sutures. A Penrose drain is inserted in the submaxillary bed and secured to the skin. Dressings are applied.

Parotidectomy

Definition. Removal of the tumor and a portion of or the entire parotid gland through a curved incision in the upper neck and behind the lobe of the ear or through a Y type of incision in both sides of the ear and below the angle of the mandible (Fig. 22-59).

Considerations. The majority of benign tumors of the salivary glands occur in the parotid gland. These benign tumors are of the same types as are those found in soft tissues in other parts of the body. In the parotid gland, the closeness of the facial nerve makes it difficult to remove the entire tumor. Parotidectomy is indicated for removal of all benign and some malignant tumors, for inflammatory lesions, for vascular anomalies, and for metastatic cancer involving lymph nodes overlying the gland.

In the removal of malignant tumors involving adjacent structures, such as the mandible or cheek, the operation may become a radical removal of the involved structures.

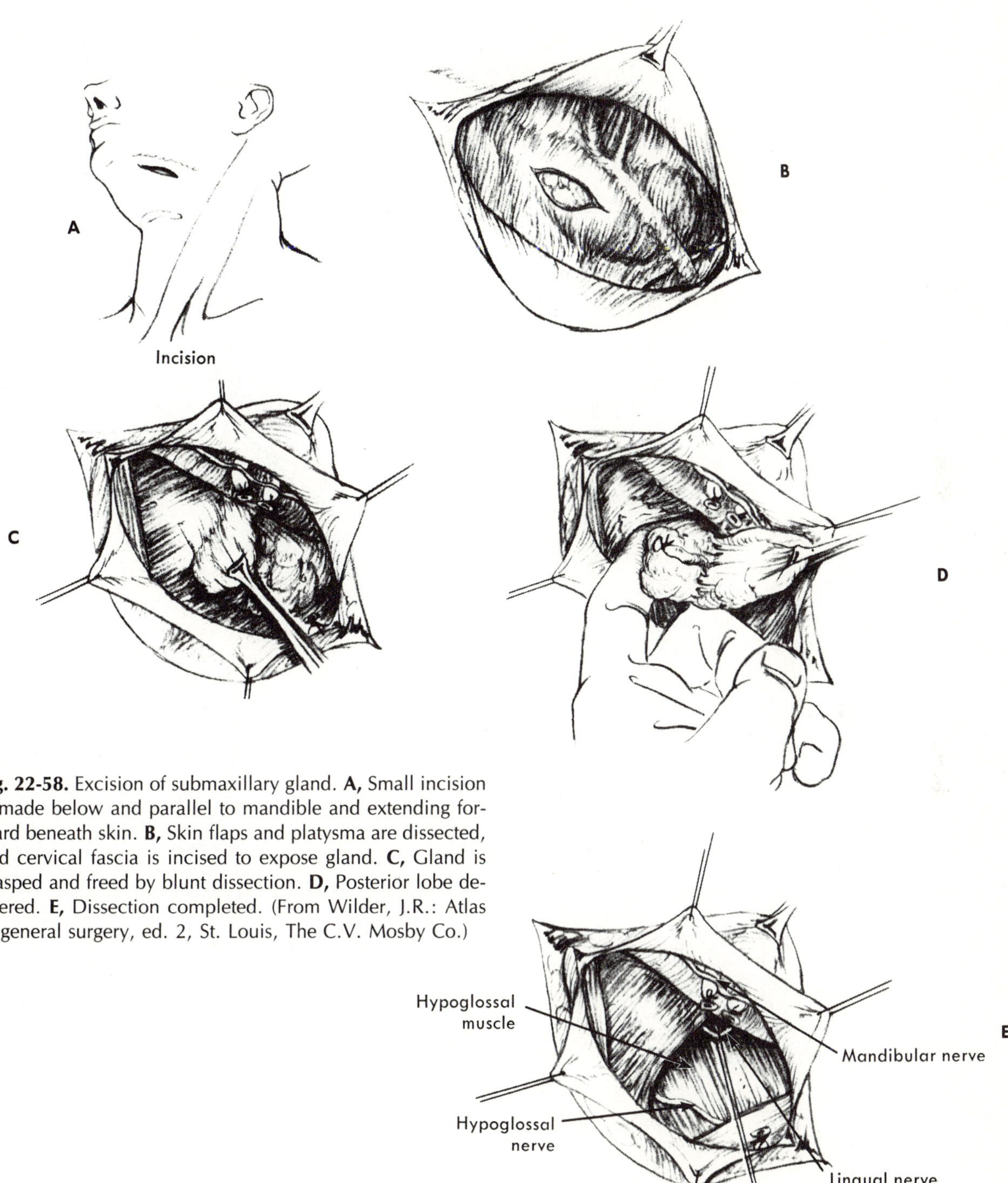

Fig. 22-58. Excision of submaxillary gland. **A,** Small incision is made below and parallel to mandible and extending forward beneath skin. **B,** Skin flaps and platysma are dissected, and cervical fascia is incised to expose gland. **C,** Gland is grasped and freed by blunt dissection. **D,** Posterior lobe delivered. **E,** Dissection completed. (From Wilder, J.R.: Atlas of general surgery, ed. 2, St. Louis, The C.V. Mosby Co.)

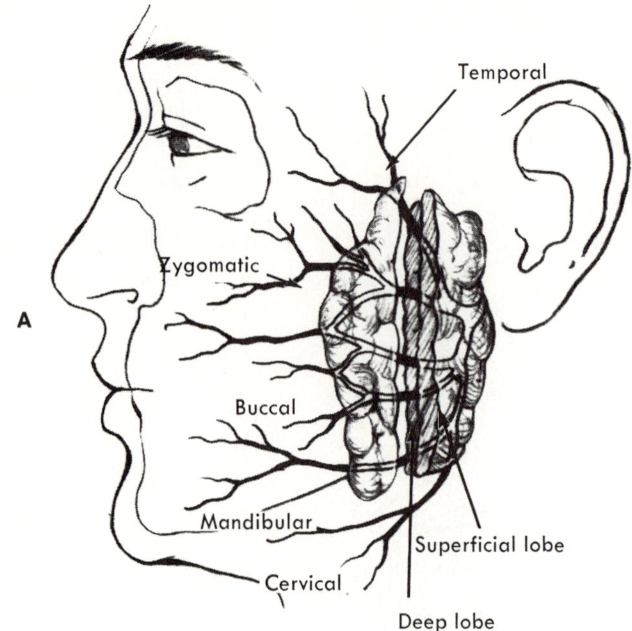

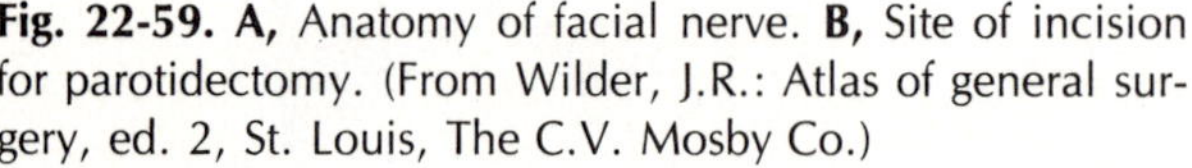

Fig. 22-59. A, Anatomy of facial nerve. **B,** Site of incision for parotidectomy. (From Wilder, J.R.: Atlas of general surgery, ed. 2, St. Louis, The C.V. Mosby Co.)

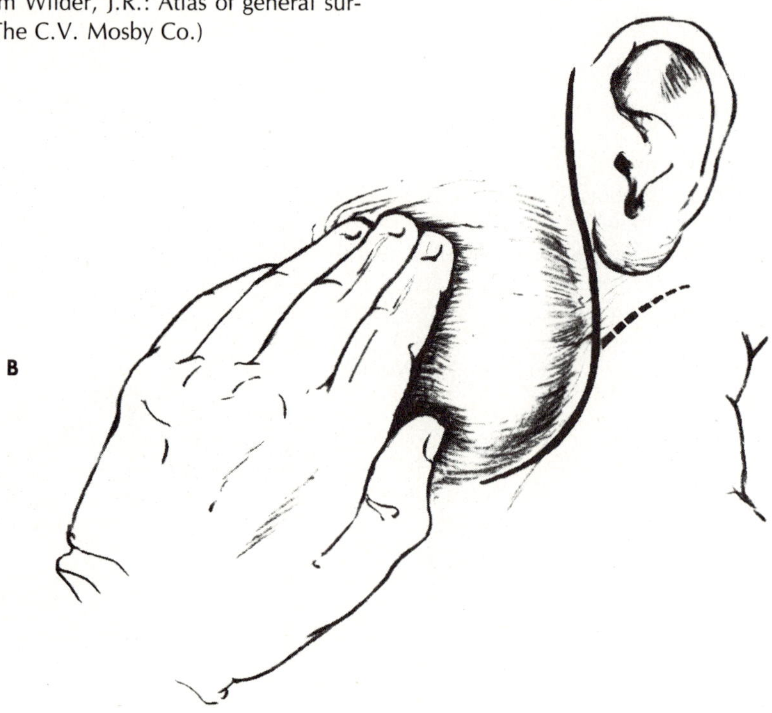

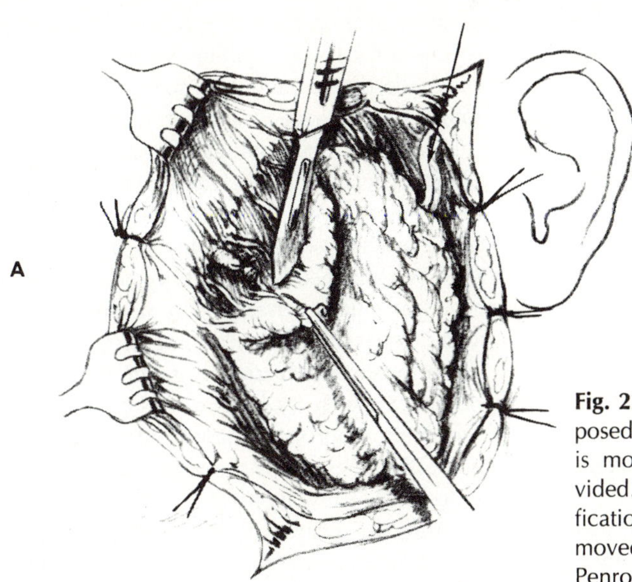

Fig. 22-60. Excision of parotid gland. **A,** Parotid duct is exposed and identified. By sharp and blunt dissections, duct is mobilized and ligated with fine gut suture and is divided. **B,** Following anterior lobe mobilization and identification of facial nerve and vessels, posterior lobe is removed. **C,** Wound is cleansed, and bleeding is controlled. Penrose drain is inserted, and wound is closed. (From Wilder, J.R.: Atlas of general surgery, ed. 2, St. Louis, The C.V. Mosby Co.)

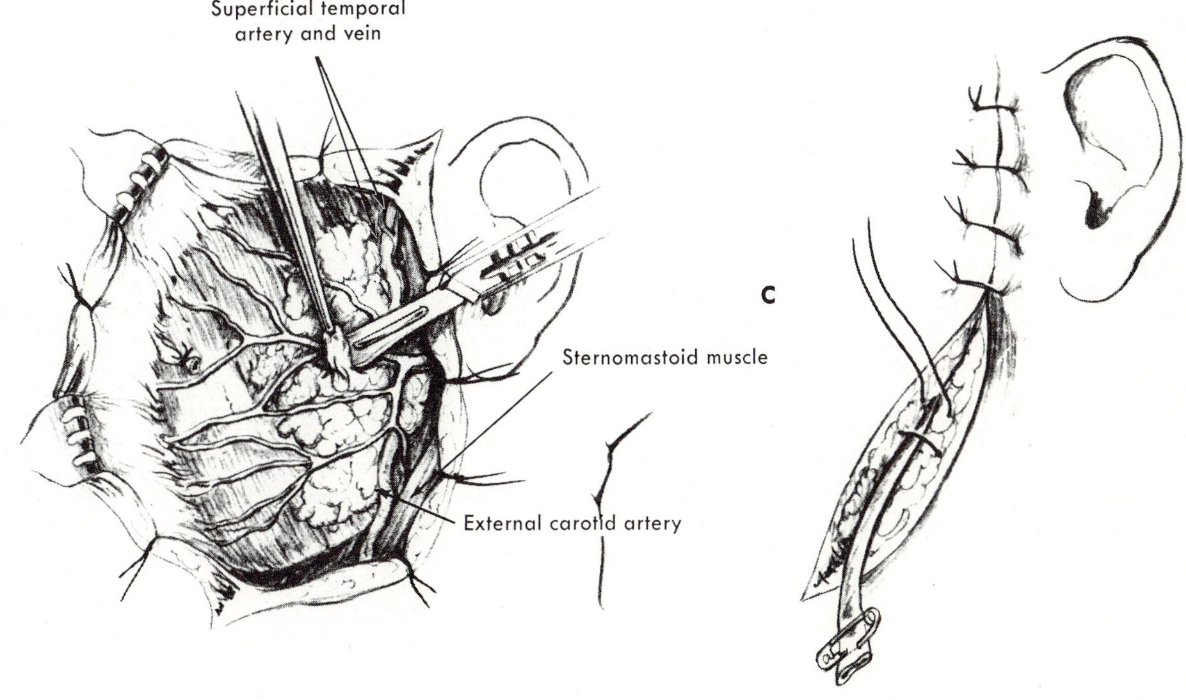

Setup and preparation of the patient. The patient is placed on the operating table in a dorsal recumbent position with the entire affected side of the face uppermost. The entire side of the face, the mouth, the outer canthus of the eye, and the forehead are prepared and left exposed.

The instrument setup is a neck dissection set. A nerve stimulator should be set up and ready for use. A set of lacrimal probes should be included in the setup if exploration of the ductal system of the parotid is necessary during the course of surgery.

Operative procedure (Fig. 22-60)

1. The incision may extend from the posterior angle of the zygoma downward in front of the tragus of the ear and behind the lobule of the ear backward over the mastoid process, then downward and forward on the neck parallel to and below the body of the mandible (Fig. 22-59). (A chin incision may be used.) Bleeding vessels are controlled by hemostats and fine ligatures.

2. With fine-toothed tissue forceps and scissors, the skin flaps are elevated as described for thyroidectomy. The skin wound edges are retracted by means of silk sutures fastened to the clamps.

3. The upper portion of the sternocleidomastoid muscle is exposed and retracted, the auricular nerve is identified, and the lower part of the parotid gland is elevated with curved hemostats.

4. The superficial temporal artery and vein and external jugular vein are identified by means of blunt dissection.

5. The parotid tissue is dissected from the cartilage of the ear and the tympanic plate of the temporal bone. The temporal, zygomatic, and mandibular and cervical branches of the facial nerve are identified and preserved.

6A. The superficial portion of the parotid gland containing the tumor is removed. In some cases, the entire superficial portion is removed, followed by ligation and division of the parotid duct.

6B. When the deep portion of the parotid gland must be removed, the facial nerve is retracted upward and outward by nerve hooks; then the parotid tissue is removed from beneath the nerve. Kocher retractors are used to retract the mandible. The external carotid artery is identified. In many cases the internal maxillary and superficial temporal arteries are clamped, ligated, and divided.

7. The wound is closed in layers with fine silk sutures. A small Penrose drain is inserted, and a pressure dressing is applied.

Tracheostomy

Definition. Opening of the trachea and insertion of a cannula through a midline incision in the neck, below the cricoid cartilage.

Considerations. Tracheostomy is used as an emergency procedure to treat upper respiratory tract obstruction and as a prophylactic measure in the presence of chronic lung disease in which an obstruction could occur. A prophylactic tracheostomy is performed at the time of surgery, thus providing for easy and frequent aspiration of the tracheobronchial tree and diminishing the dead space that exists from the opening of the mouth down to the supraclavicular region. The creation of a new clearance (tracheostomy) nearer to the functional areas in the lung provides for a greater volume of air for the patient with a partly destroyed lung. Anesthesia may be maintained through a prophylactic tracheostomy.

The patient's psychological status should be carefully evaluated because of the altered body image and physical status, which may be either temporary or permanent depending on the disease entity involved. Tracheostomy care should be explained very carefully and thoroughly so that the patient will understand why it must be done so frequently, especially the suctioning of the tube.

Reinforcement should be given about the ability to communicate with others by means of a pencil and paper. As recovery progresses, the patient can be shown how to occlude the opening of the tube for brief periods to be able to speak a few words.

Setup and preparation of the patient. The patient is placed in a dorsal recumbent position, with the shoulders raised by a folded sheet to hyperextend the neck and head. The neck is prepped, and sterile drapes applied. Along with a basic minor pack, the following instruments should be included:

2 Knife handles no. 3 with nos. 10 and 15 blades
1 Metzenbaum scissors, curved
1 Mayo scissors, straight
1 Suture scissors
2 Allis forceps, straight
1 Needle holder
2 Tissue forceps, fine teeth
2 Tissue forceps without teeth
2 Adson forceps
4 Towel clamps
2 Sponge-holding forceps
4 Mosquito hemostats, straight
4 Kelly hemostats, curved
1 Mayo-Pean hemostat, curved
2 Crile hemostats, curved
2 Volkmann rake retractors
2 Cushing loop retractors
2 Frazier skin hooks
1 Jackson tracheal retractor
1 Cushing nerve hook
2 Brophy tenaculum hooks
Plain no. 3-0 sutures
Chromic no. 4-0 sutures swaged to fine, ½-circle, taper point needles
Silk no. 2-0 sutures swaged to ⅜-circle, cutting-edge needles
2 Catheters, whistle-tipped, open-ended, 14 Fr

1 Yankauer suction tube
1 Frazier suction tube
2 Suction tubings
Tracheostomy tubes (Figs. 22-61 and 22-62), appropriate for age and size of patient, and Martin extension on inner cannula, if desired, for use with bulky dressing
Cardiac arrest setup, oxygen, and thiopental (Pentothal) sodium setup
Local anesthesia set
Minor drape pack

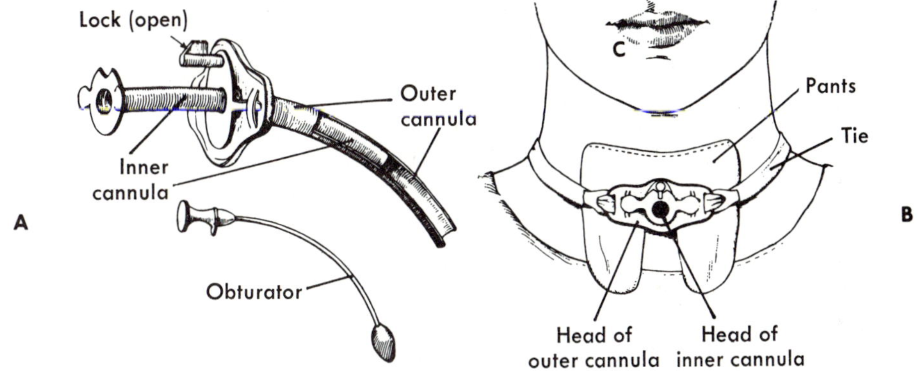

Fig. 22-61. A, Parts of metal tracheostomy tube. **B,** Tracheostomy ties and gauze pants in place. (From Work, W., and Smith, M.F.W.: Postgrad. Med. **34:**479.

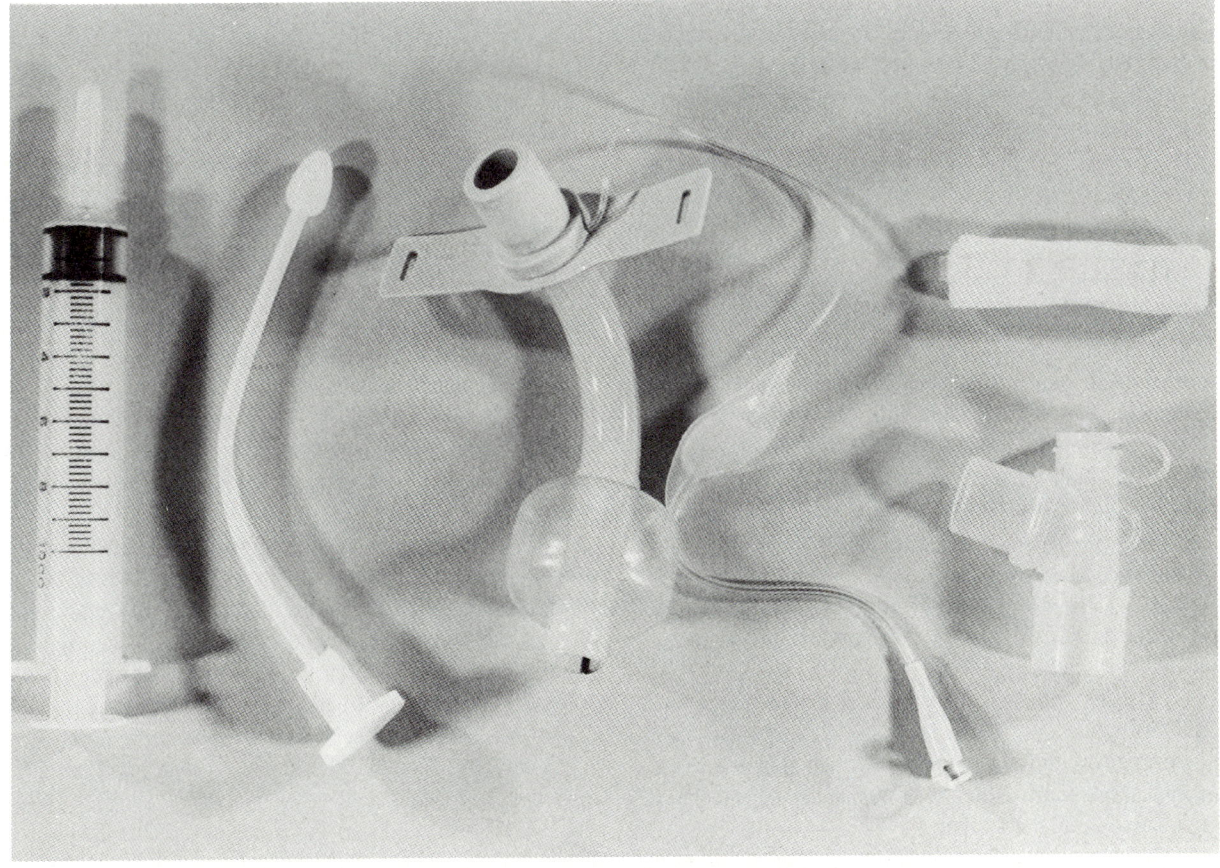

Fig. 22-62. Portex tracheostomy tube with cuff inflated: obturator, syringe, adaptor, and neck ties.

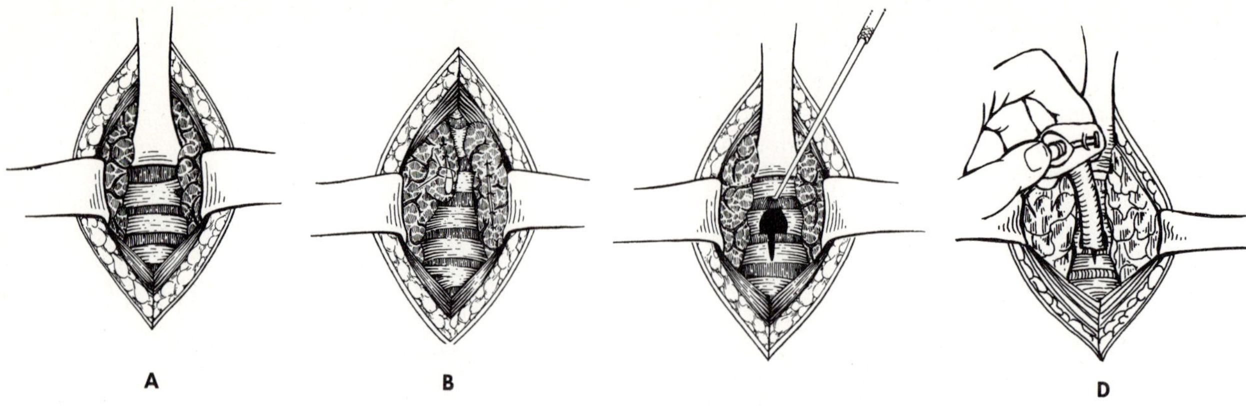

Fig. 22-63. Operative technique for elective tracheostomy. **A,** Retractor exposing trachea by drawing isthmus of thyroid upward. **B,** Alternate method to that shown in **A:** isthmus of thyroid is divided to expose trachea. **C,** Two tracheal rings are cut, and upper ring is partially resected. Tracheal hook pulls trachea from depth of wound nearer surface. **D,** Insertion of tube. (Adapted from DeWeese, D.D., and Saunders, W.H.: Textbook of otolaryngolgy, ed. 6, St. Louis, 1982, The C.V. Mosby Co.)

Operative procedure

1. A vertical or transverse incision may be used. A vertical incision is made in the midline from approximately the cricoid cartilage to the suprasternal notch. When a transverse incision is made, it extends approximately one fingerbreadth above the suprasternal notch parallel to it and from the anterior border of one sternocleidomastoid muscle to the opposite side. Soft tissues and muscle are divided, and the isthmus of the thyroid gland that joins both lobes of the gland in the midline over the trachea is retracted in an upward direction with Cushing retractors, thus resulting in exposure of the underlying tracheal rings, usually the third and fourth (Fig. 22-63). In some cases two curved clamps may be inserted through this incision across the isthmus and the isthmus transected (Fig. 22-63). The transected ends of the isthmus are secured with chromic gut sutures.
2. Lidocaine, 1% (1 or 2 ml), may be instilled into the trachea to reduce the coughing reflex when the tube is inserted. Air is first drawn into the syringe to ensure that the needle point is located in the lumen. With a knife and no. 15 blade, a vertical incision is made in the trachea directly across the two tracheal rings. The cut ends of the cricoid cartilage are retracted with a hook (Fig. 22-63).
3. A tracheostomy tube is inserted into the trachea, the obturator is quickly removed, and the trachea is suctioned with a catheter.
4. The wound edges are lightly approximated with silk sutures no. 2-0, or the wound edges are allowed to fall together around the tube. One or two skin sutures are inserted above the tube. The lower angle of the wound may be left open for drainage.
5. The tracheostomy tube is held in place with tapes tied with a square knot behind the neck. The inner tube is then inserted. A gauze dressing split around the tube is applied to the wound (Fig. 22-61, *B*).
6. The obturator of the tracheostomy tube should be taped to the patient's shoulder during transport of the patient to the recovery room or the unit so that it will not become misplaced. The obturator is needed to reinsert the tube if it becomes dislodged.

Laryngofissure

Definition. Opening of the larynx for exploratory, excisional, or reconstructive procedures.

Considerations. A laryngofissure is performed whenever access to the intrinsic larynx is necessary. The thyroid cartilages are split in the midline, and the true vocal cords and false vocal cords are incised at the midline anteriorly.

Setup and preparation of the patient. A neck dissection set is required, plus a Stryker power saw.

Operative procedure

1. A tracheostomy is performed, and an endotracheal tube inserted. A general anesthetic is administered. (This procedure can be done with the patient under local anesthesia.)
2. A transverse incision is made through the skin and first layer of the cervical fascia and platysma muscles, approximately 2 cm above the sternoclavicular junction or in the normal skin crease. The upper skin flap is undermined to the level of the cricoid cartilage; then the lower flap is undermined to the sternoclavicular joint.
3. Bleeding vessels are clamped with mosquito hemostats and ligated. The strap muscles are elevated and incised in the midline.
4. The thyroid cartilages are cut with a Stryker saw, and the true vocal cords are visualized through an incision into the cricothyroid membrane. The true vocal cords

are divided in the midline (anterior commissure), and the interior of the larynx is exposed.

5. The tracheostomy tube must be left in place after surgery to ensure an airway.

Partial laryngectomy

Definition. Removal of a portion of the larynx.

Considerations. A partial laryngectomy is done to remove superficial neoplasms that are confined to one vocal cord or to remove a tumor extending up into the ventricle on the anterior commissure or a short distance below the cord. Cancers confined to the intrinsic larynx (Figs. 22-50 and 22-64) are generally of a low grade of malignancy and tend to remain localized for long periods.

Setup and preparation of the patient. The patient is placed in the dorsal recumbent position. The operative site is prepped and draped as described for thyroidectomy.

The setup for partial laryngectomy includes a neck dissection setup, Stryker saw, and tracheostomy tubes. Electrocautery should be available.

Operative procedure

1. A tracheostomy is performed as previously described, and an endotracheal tube is inserted.

2. A vertical incision or a thyroid incision with elevation of a flap may be employed (Fig. 22-64).

3. The sternothyroid muscles are separated in the midline and retracted by means of Green retractors.

4. The fascial covering over the thyroid cartilage is incised with a knife, and with a Freer periosteal elevator the perichondrium is elevated from the cartilage on the side of the tumor.

5. The thyroid cartilage is divided longitudinally in the midline by means of a Stryker power saw.

6. The cartilages are retracted, and the cricothyroid membrane is incised with a knife. A blunt-nosed laryngeal scissors is introduced between the vocal cords to divide the mucosa of the anterior wall of the glottis.

7. The divided cartilages are retracted with Kocher retractors to expose the interior of the larynx. A small moist gauze pack may be placed in the trachea to prevent aspiration of blood or mucus. A small amount of a topical anesthetic may be applied to the larynx to prevent laryngeal muscular spasm. The extent of the intrinsic laryngeal tumor is determined.

8. With a small periosteal elevator, the mucosa on the involved side of the larynx is freed; the false cord and mucosal layer of the region are lifted by means of a periosteal elevator and hooks. The involved cord is excised with straight scissors (Fig. 22-64).

9. In some cases, the thyroid cartilage may be removed with a knife and straight scissors. Bleeding is controlled with hemostats and fine chromic gut ligatures and sutures.

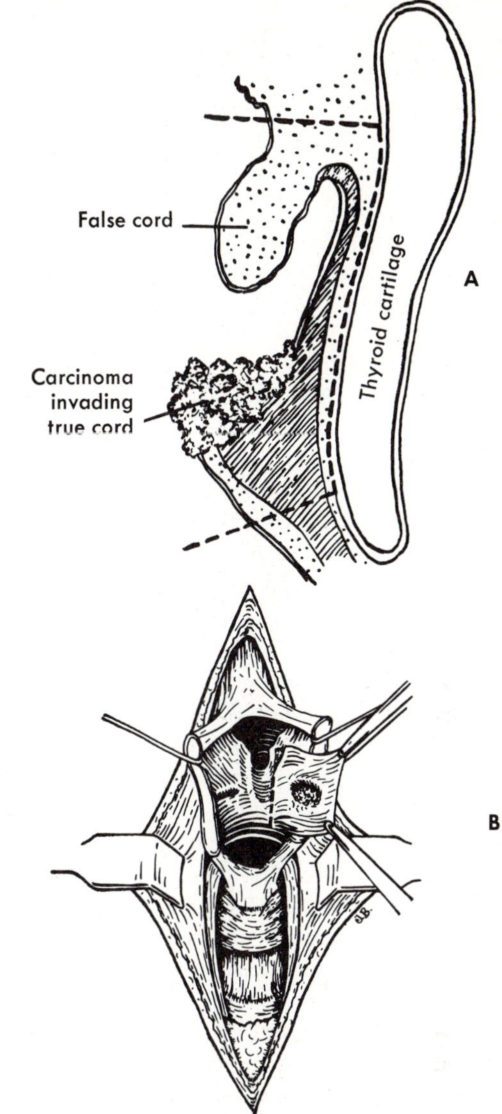

Fig. 22-64. Partial laryngectomy. **A,** Lesion suitable for removal. Dotted line indicates wide margin of normal tissue removed along with tumor. When limits of tumor are known, false cord may not be excised. **B,** Incision into larynx is from thyroid notch above to cricoid below. Drawing shows excision of lesion on true cord along with wide margin of normal tissue. (Adapted from DeWeese, D.D., and Saunders, W.H.: Textbook of otolaryngology, ed. 6, St. Louis, 1982, The C.V. Mosby Co.)

10. The gauze pack is removed from the trachea. The perichondrium is approximated with chromic gut no. 2-0 sutures. The strap muscles are approximated in the midline with chromic gut no. 2-0 sutures; then the platysma and the skin edges are approximated separately with fine silk sutures.

11. A tracheolaryngeal tube is left in place and removed at a later date when the airway is adequate. Dressings are applied to the wound and around the tube.

Supraglottic laryngectomy

Definition. Excision of the laryngeal structures above the true vocal cords.

Considerations. Supraglottic laryngectomy is indicated in cancer of the epiglottis and false vocal cords. It is designed to remove the cancer, yet preserve the phonatory, respiratory, and sphincteric functions of the larynx. A neck dissection is always performed.

Setup and preparation of the patient. As described for neck dissection.

Total laryngectomy

Definition. Complete removal of the cartilaginous larynx, the hyoid bone, and the strap muscles connected to the larynx and possible removal of the preepiglottic space with the lesion.

Considerations. A wide-field laryngectomy is done when there is a loss of mobility of the cords and to treat cancer of the extrinsic larynx and hypopharynx. Malignant tumors of the extrinsic larynx are more anaplastic and tend to metastasize. When laryngeal carcinoma involves more than the true cords, a prophylactic (preventive) radical neck dissection if done to remove the lymphatics. In the presence of malignant tumors, the patient usually has no previous hoarseness, and the first symptom is usually the appearance of a lump in the neck.

Laryngectomy presents many psychological problems. The loss of voice that follows total laryngectomy is psychologically traumatic for the patient and family. The patient may be taught to talk either by using esophageal voice or with an artificial larynx. Esophageal voice is produced by the air contained in the esophagus rather than by that in the trachea. Speech requires a sounding air column. With instruction and practice, the patient is able to control the swallowing of air into the esophagus and reintroduction of this air into the mouth with phonation. The sounding air column is then transformed into speech by means of the lips, tongue, and teeth.

Because the stump of the trachea is brought out to the skin of the neck, all the patient's breathing is done directly into the trachea. This air is no longer moistened by the nose. Drying and crusting of the tracheal secretions occur. Humidification may be provided by covering the opening with a moist gauze compress.

The patient will be anxious to know about postoperative voice quality. This depends on the specific procedure performed. Table 4 lists surgical procedures and associated predictions of postoperative voice qualities.

Setup and preparation of the patient. The patient is placed on the table in a dorsal recumbent position with neck extended and shoulders raised by a rubber block or folded sheet.

An endotracheal anesthetic is administered. An effective suction apparatus is most essential.

The proposed operative site, including the anterior neck region, lateral surfaces of the neck down to the outer aspects of the shoulders, and the upper anterior chest region, is prepped and draped in the usual manner.

The instrument setup is a neck dissection set.

Operative procedure

1. A tracheostomy may be performed to control the airway.

2. A midline incision is made from the suprasternal notch to just above the hyoid bone. Skin flaps are undermined on each side. The sternothyroid, sternohyoid, and omohyoid muscles (strap muscles) on each side are divided by means of curved hemostats and a knife.

3. The suprahyoid muscles are severed from the portion of the hyoid to be divided. The hyoid bone is divided at the junction of its middle and lateral thirds with bone-cutting forceps. Bleeding vessels are clamped and ligated.

4. The superior laryngeal nerve and vessels are exposed and ligated on each side with long curved fine hemostats and fine chromic gut or silk ligatures.

5. The isthmus of the thyroid gland is divided between hemostats. Each portion of the thyroid gland is dissected from the trachea with fine dissection Stevens and Metzenbaum scissors and fine tissue forceps. The superior pole of the thyroid is retracted. The superior thyroid vessels are freed from the larynx by sharp dissection.

6. The larynx is rotated. The inferior pharyngeal constrictor muscle is severed from its attachment to the thyroid cartilage on each side (Fig. 22-49).

7. The endotracheal tube is removed. The trachea is transected just below the cricoid cartilage over a Kelly or Crile hemostat previously inserted between the trachea and esophagus. The upper resected portion of the trachea and the cricoid cartilage are held upward with Lahey forceps (Fig. 22-65). A balloon-cuffed tube (endotracheal) or a Foley catheter is inserted in the distal trachea.

8. The larynx is freed from the cervical esophagus and attachments by sharp and blunt dissection. A moist pack is placed around the endotracheal tube to help prevent leakage of blood into the trachea.

9. The pharynx is entered. In most cancers of the intrinsic larynx, the pharynx is entered above the epiglottis. The mucosal membranous incision is extended along either side of the epiglottis; the remaining portion of the pharynx and cervical esophagus is dissected well away from the tumor by means of fine-toothed tissue forceps, Metzenbaum scissors, knife, and fine hemostats. The specimen is removed en masse.

10. A nasal feeding tube is inserted through one nare into the esophagus; closure of the hypopharyngeal and esophageal defect is begun with continuous, inverting fine sutures of chromic gut no. 3-0. The nasal tube is guided down past the pharyngeal suture line.

11. The pharyngeal suture line is reinforced with interrupted sutures; the suprahyoid muscles are approximated to the cut edges of the inferior constrictor muscles.

12. The diameter of the tracheal stoma is increased by means of a knife and heavy straight scissors. The two portions of the thyroid behind the tracheal opening are approximated with interrupted silk sutures, thereby obliterating dead space posterior to the upper portion of the trachea (Fig. 22-65).

13. A small Penrose drain or catheter may be inserted through two separate stab wounds, one on each side of the neck just below the pharyngeal suture line (Fig. 22-65). If a closed wound drainage system is used, the suction drains are appropriately placed (Fig. 22-66).

14. The edges of the deep cervical fascia and the platysma are closed separately with interrupted, fine silk sutures. When a great amount of the fascia and platysma has been removed, the wound edges are approximated with silk sutures.

15. A laryngectomy tube of desired size is inserted into the tracheal stoma; a pressure dressing is applied to the wound and neck.

Radical neck dissection

Definition. Removal of the tumor, surrounding structures, and lymph nodes en masse, through a Y-shaped or trifurcate incision in the affected side of the neck.

Considerations. Radical neck dissection is done to remove the tumor and metastatic cervical nodes present in malignant lesions, as well as all nonvital structures of the neck. Metastasis occurs through the lymphatic channels by way of the bloodstream. Disease of the oral cavity, lips, and thyroid gland may spread slowly to the neck. Radical neck surgery is done in the presence of cervical node metastasis from a cancer of the head and neck, which has a reasonable chance of being controlled.

A prophylactic neck dissection implies elective radical neck surgery when there is no clinical evidence of metastatic cervical cancer. This may be done in the presence of cancer of the tongue.

Setup and preparation of the patient. The patient is placed on the table in a dorsal recumbent position. General endotracheal anesthesia is used. The anesthetic is administered before the patient is positioned for surgery. During the operation, the anesthesiologist works behind a sterile barrier, away from the surgical team. The

Table 4. Surgical procedures for laryngeal carcinomas and predictions of vocal quality after surgery

Structures removed	Structures left	Postoperative condition
Total laryngectomy		
Hyoid bone Entire larynx (epiglottis, false cords, true cords) Cricoid cartilage Two or three rings of trachea	Tongue Pharyngeal walls Lower trachea	Loses voice Breathes through tracheostomy stoma No problem swallowing
Supraglottic or horizontal laryngectomy		
Hyoid bone Epiglottis False vocal cords	True vocal cords Cricoid cartilage Trachea	Normal voice May aspirate occasionally, especially liquids Normal airway
Vertical (or hemi) laryngectomy		
One true vocal cord False cord Arytenoid One-half thyroid cartilage	Epiglottis One false cord One true vocal cord Cricoid	Hoarse but serviceable voice Normal airway No problem swallowing
Laryngofissure and partial laryngectomy		
One vocal cord	All other structures	Hoarse but serviceable voice; occasionally almost normal voice No airway problem No swallowing problem
Endoscopic removal of early carcinoma		
Part of one vocal cord	All other structures	May have a normal voice No other problems

From Saunders, W.H., and others: Nursing care in eye, ear, nose, and throat disorders, ed. 4, St. Louis, 1979, The C.V. Mosby Co.

head is moderately extended with the entire affected side of the face and neck facing uppermost. During surgery, the face of the patient is turned away from the surgeon.

The preoperative skin preparation is extensive. The patient's neck is draped, leaving a wide operative field. The thigh area is also prepared and draped with sterile towels in readiness for obtaining a skin graft before closure of the neck wound; it is usually more convenient to use the thigh on the same side as the neck dissection.

The instrument setup includes the following:

50 Mosquito hemostats, curved
8 Allis forceps
8 Kelly forceps, medium
8 Pean forceps
4 Thyroid tenacula
4 Babcock forceps
2 Right-angle clamps
Needle holders, assorted
12 Towel clamps
2 Tonsil suction tubes
1 Trousseau tracheal dilator
2 Rake retractors
2 Army-Navy retractors
2 Richardson retractors
2 Vein retractors
4 Skin hooks, 2 single and 2 double
1 Gelpi retractor
4 Knife handles no. 3 and nos. 10 and 15 blades
1 Tracheal hook
1 Upper-lateral scissors
1 Cartilage scissors
2 Mayo scissors, straight and curved
2 Metzenbaum scissors
2 Scissors, small, curved, sharp and dull
4 Tissue forceps, 2 with and 2 without teeth
2 Adson tissue forceps
2 Brown-Adson tissue forceps
1 Periosteal elevator
2 Freer elevators
1 Bayonet forceps
Brown or Stryker dermatome

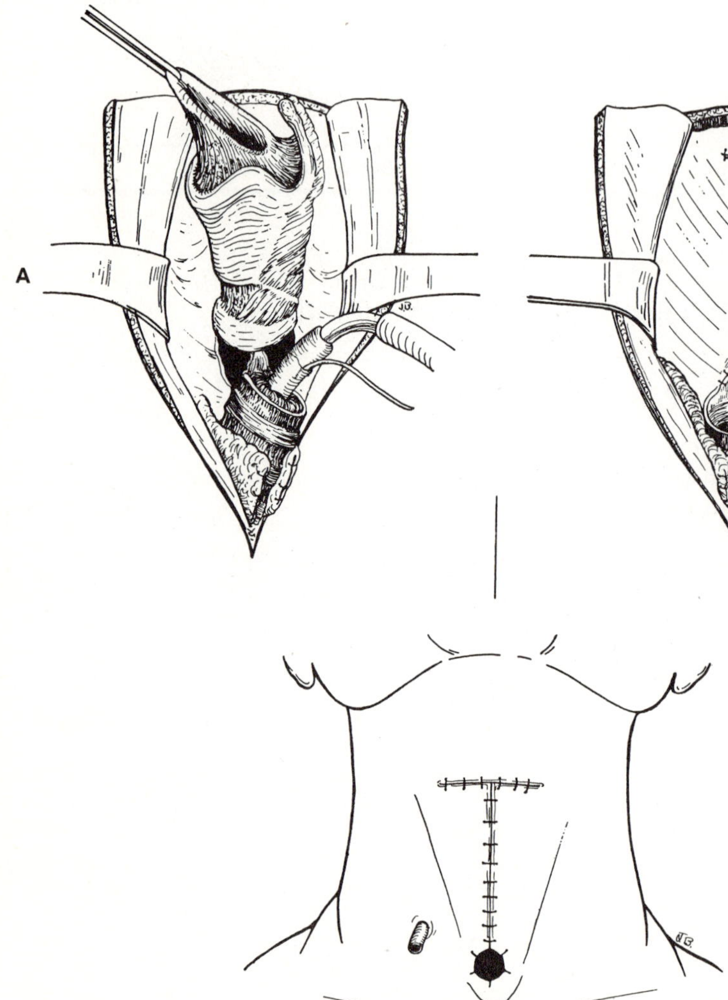

Fig. 22-65. Total laryngectomy. **A,** Usually one or two tracheal rings and hyoid bone are included with specimen. **B,** Mucous membrane and muscles of pharynx are closed in layers. **C,** Tracheostomy. Trachea is sutured to skin. (From DeWeese, D.D., and Saunders, W.H.: Textbook of otolaryngology, ed. 6, St. Louis, 1982, The C.V. Mosby Co.)

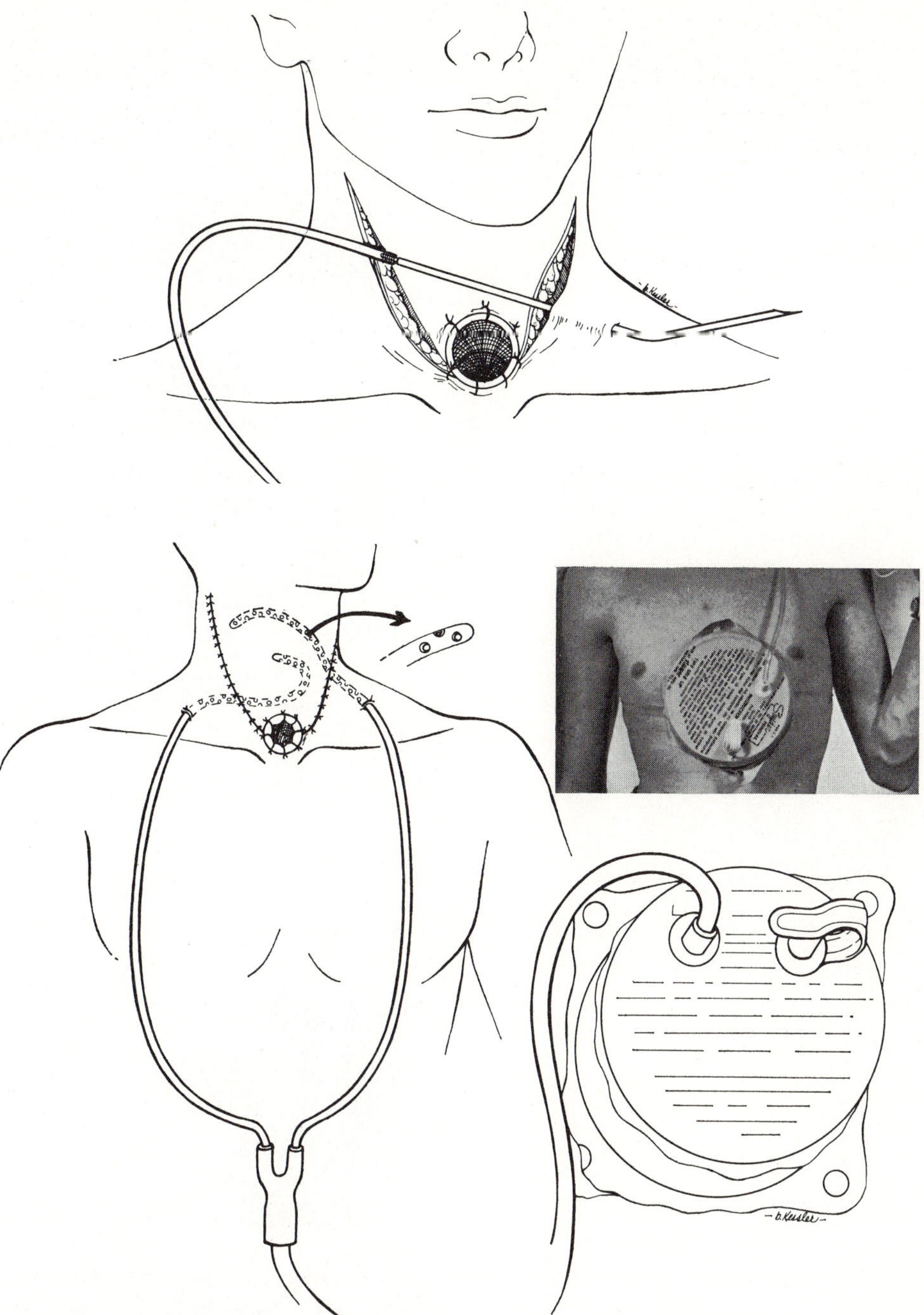

Fig. 22-66. Hemovac apparatus for constant closed suction. In this system of wound drainage, suction is maintained by plastic container with spring inside that forces apart lids and thereby produces suction, which is transmitted through plastic tubing. Neck skin is pulled down tight, and no external dressing is required. Container serves as both suction source and receptacle for blood. It is emptied as required, and drainage tubes are left in neck for 3 days. (From DeWeese, D.D., and Saunders, W.H.: Textbook of otolaryngology, ed. 6, St. Louis, 1982, The C.V. Mosby Co.)

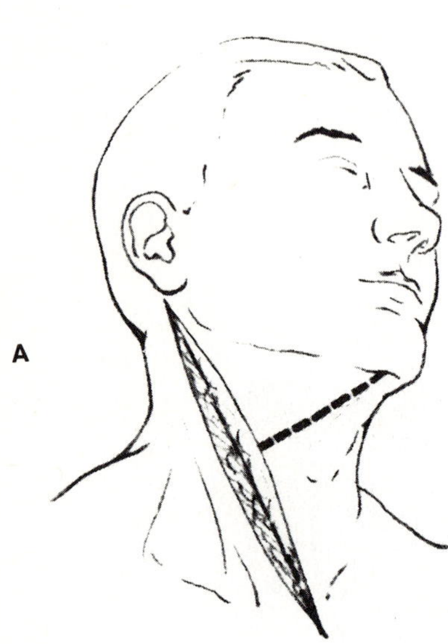

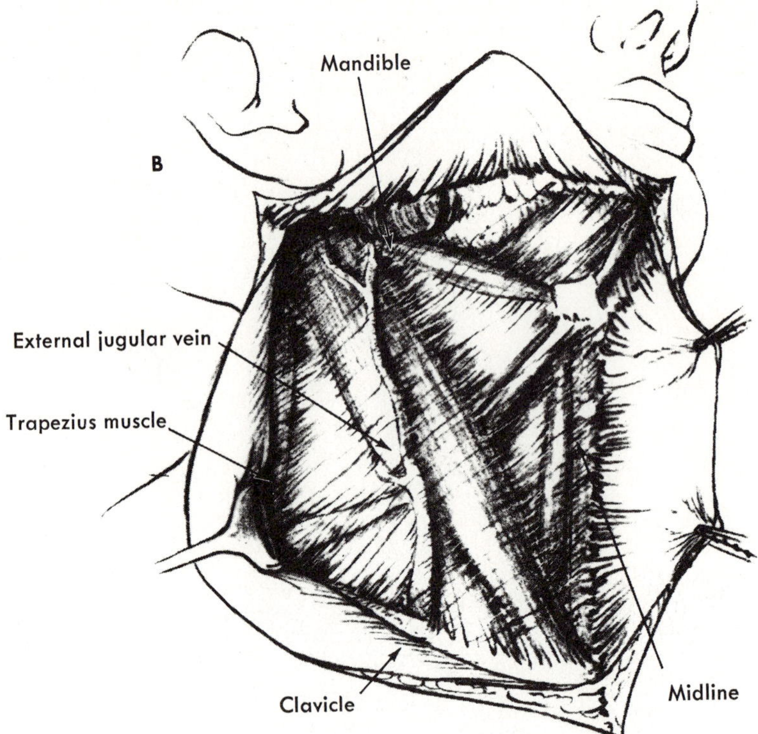

Fig. 22-67. For legend see opposite page.

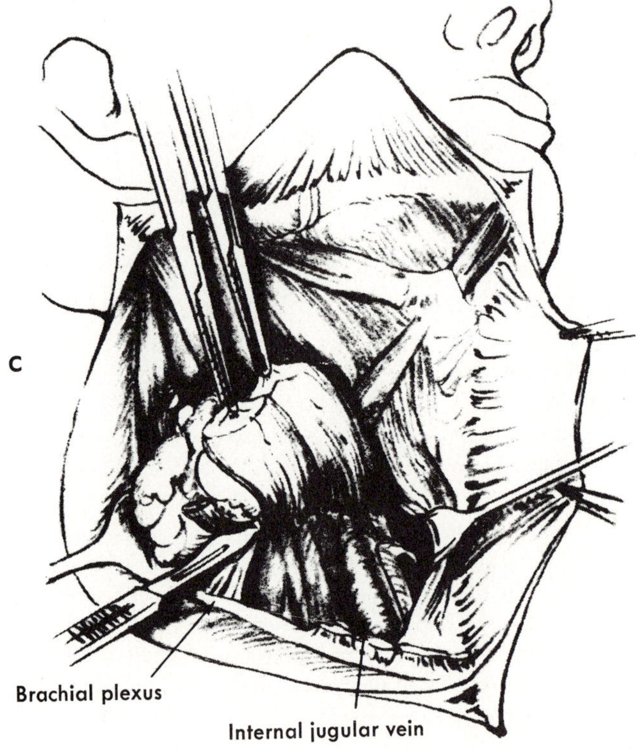

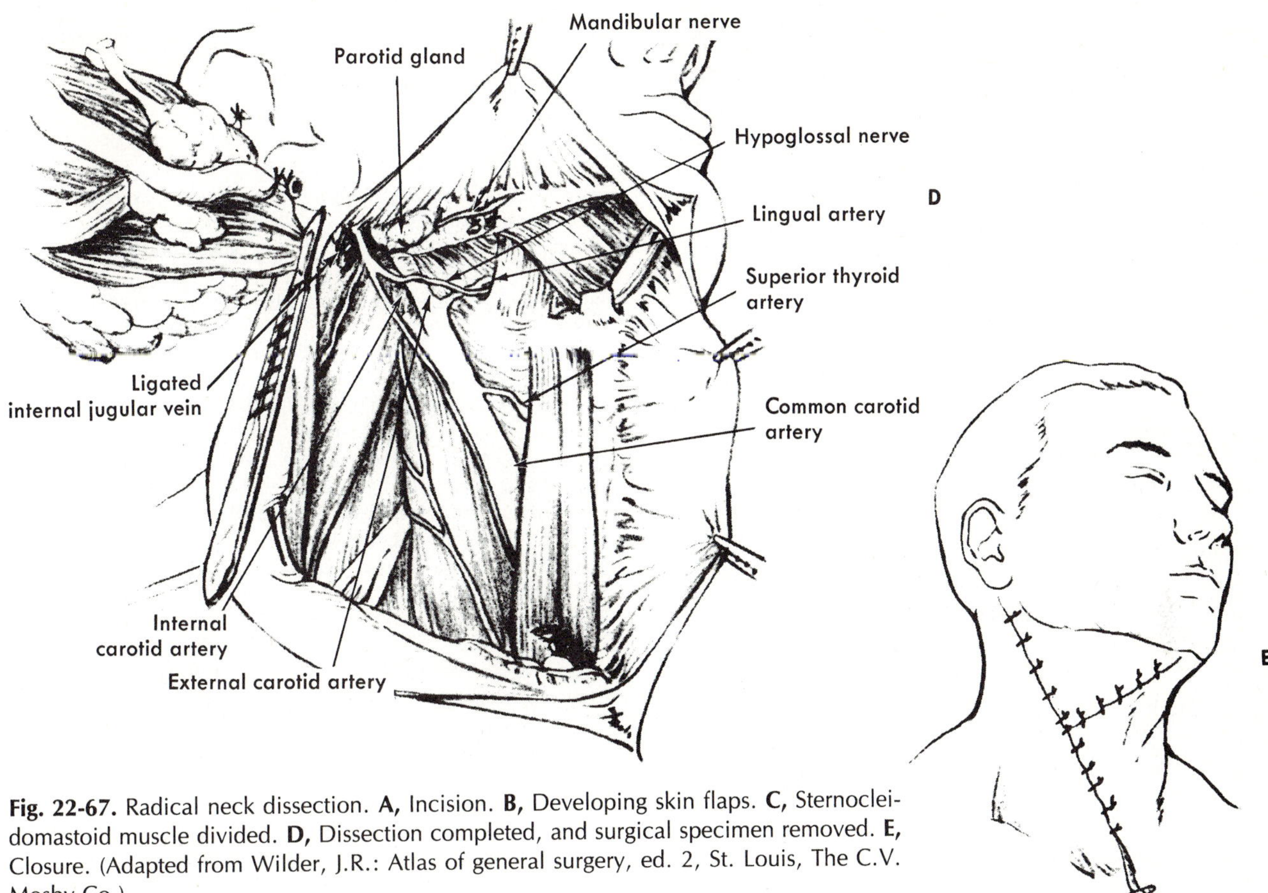

Fig. 22-67. Radical neck dissection. **A,** Incision. **B,** Developing skin flaps. **C,** Sternocleidomastoid muscle divided. **D,** Dissection completed, and surgical specimen removed. **E,** Closure. (Adapted from Wilder, J.R.: Atlas of general surgery, ed. 2, St. Louis, The C.V. Mosby Co.)

Operative procedure

1. One of several types of incisions may be used, including the Y-shaped, H-shaped, or trifurcate incision (Fig. 22-67, *A*).

2. The upper curved incision is made through the skin and platysma with a knife, tissue forceps, and fine hemostats and ligatures for bleeding vessels. The upper flap is retracted; then the vertical portion of the incision is made, and the skin flaps retracted anteriorly and posteriorly with retractors. The anterior margin of the trapezius muscle is exposed by means of curved scissors. The flaps are retracted to expose the entire lateral aspect of the neck (Fig. 22-67, *B*). Branches of the jugular veins are clamped, ligated, and divided.

3. The sternal and calvicular attachments of the sternocleidomastoid muscle are clamped with curved Pean forceps and then divided with a knife. The superficial layer of deep fascia is then incised. The omohyoid muscle is severed between clamps just above its scapular attachment (Fig. 22-67, *C*).

4. The internal jugular vein is isolated by blunt dissection and then doubly clamped, ligated with medium silk, and divided with Metzenbaum scissors. A transfixion suture is placed on the lower end of the vein.

5. The common carotid artery and vagus nerve are identified. The fatty areolar tissue and fascia are dissected away, using Metzenbaum scissors and fine tissue forceps. Branches of the thyrocervical artery are clamped, divided, and ligated.

6. The tissues and fascia of the posterior triangle are dissected, beginning at the anterior margin of the trapezius muscle, continuing near the brachial plexus and the levator scapulae and the scalene muscles. During the dissection, branches of the cervical and suprascapular arteries are clamped, ligated, and divided.

7. The anterior portion of the block dissection is completed. The omohyoid muscle is severed at its attachment to the hyoid bone. Bleeding is controlled. All hemostats are removed, and the operative site is covered with warm, moist laparotomy packs.

8. The sternocleidomastoid muscle is severed and retracted. The submental space is dissected free of fatty areolar tissue and lymph nodes from above downward.

9. The deep fascia on the lower free edge of the mandible is incised; the facial vessels are divided and ligated.

10. The submaxillary triangle is entered. The submaxillary duct is divided and ligated. The submaxillary glands with surrounding fatty areolar tissue and lymph nodes are dissected toward the digastric muscle. The facial branch of the external carotid artery is divided. Portions of the digastric and stylohyoid muscles are severed from their attachments to the hyoid bone and on the mastoid. The upper end of the internal jugular vein is elevated and divided. The surgical specimen is removed (Fig. 22-67, *D*).

11. The entire field is examined for bleeding and then irrigated with warm saline solution. A skin graft is placed, covering the bifurcation of the carotid artery extending down approximately 4 inches, and sutured with no. 4-0 chromic gut on a very small cutting needle. Closed-wound suction drains are placed in the wound (Fig. 22-66).

12. The flaps are approximated with interrupted, fine silk sutures (Fig. 22-67, *E*). A bulky pressure dressing is applied to the neck. Gauze dressings are applied to the wound edges and covered with sterile fluffed gauze to provide even pressure. A wide gauze roller bandage is wrapped snugly around the neck, and in some cases encircles the head. The dressing may then be covered with elastic bandage that is wrapped around the neck and anchored to the chest wall.

SUGGESTED READINGS

Baida, M.R.: Nursing care in use of local anesthesia, AORN J. **28:**855, 1978.

Bush, E., Hunt, L., and Tarwater, W.: Care and use of microscope in OR, AORN J. **20:**392, 1974.

Davis, H., and Silverman, S.R., editors: Hearing and deafness, ed. 3, New York, 1970, Holt, Rinehart & Winston, Inc.

DeWeese, D.D., and Saunders, W.H.: Textbook of otolaryngology, ed. 6, St. Louis, 1982, The C.V Mosby Co.

Grubb, R.D., and Ondov, G.: Operating room guidelines: an illustrated manual, St. Louis, 1979, The C.V. Mosby Co.

Gruendemann, B.J.: The impact of surgery on body image, Nurs. Clin. North Am. **10:**635, 1975.

Guyton, A.C.: Textbook of medical physiology, ed. 5, Philadelphia, 1976, W.B. Saunders Co.

Hood, G.H., and Dincher, J.R.: Total patient care: foundations and practice, ed. 5, St. Louis, 1980, The C.V. Mosby Co.

Huber, H.L.: Draining the "fluid ear" with myringotomy and tube insertion, Nursing '78 **8**(7):28, 1978.

Last, R.J.: Anatomy: regional and applied, ed. 5, Baltimore, 1972, The Williams & Wilkins Co.

Montgomery, W.: Surgery of the upper respiratory system, vols. 1 and 2, Philadelphia, 1973, Lea & Febiger.

Paparella, M., and Shumrick, D.: Otolaryngology, vol. 3, Head and neck, ed. 2, Philadelphia, 1980, W.B. Saunders Co.

Pilcher, L.: Carbon dioxide lasers in laryngeal surgery, AORN J. **33:**1402, 1981.

Protocol for laser surgery described, Anesth. News **8**(7):1, 1982.

Sabiston, D.C., Jr., editor: Davis-Christopher textbook of surgery: the biological basis of modern surgical practice, ed. 12, Philadelphia, 1981, W.B. Saunders Co.

Safety precautions of CO_2 laser surgery, Cavitron Lasersonics News **1**(1), 1981.

Saunders, W.H., and others: Nursing care in eye, ear, nose, and throat disorders, ed. 4, St. Louis, 1979, The C.V. Mosby Co.

Shambaugh, G.E.: Surgery of the ear, ed. 2, Philadelphia, 1967, W.B. Saunders Co.

Thoma, K.H.: Oral surgery, ed. 5, St. Louis, 1969, The C.V. Mosby Co.

White, N.: OR nursing in otomicrosurgery, AORN J. **22:**889, 1975.

23 Ophthalmic surgery

Sight is the most precious sensory possession of humans. Aristotle said, "The eye is the chief organ through which objective reality is appreciated," and, "Sight is the most comprehensive of all the senses."

Ophthalmology is closely associated with general medicine because many diseases affect the eyes. Many ocular disorders are manifestations of systemic diseases, such as endocrine disturbances, diabetes, brain tumor, nephritis, and syphilis.

In the time of Hippocrates, surgery of the eye was confined to the eyelids. Because of the advent of asepsis and advances in ophthalmology and anesthesia, many eye disorders are now treated by surgery. The success of the surgeon's plan of treatment depends to a degree on the knowledge and skill of the members of the nursing team as they perform their functions before, during, and after surgery.

ANATOMY AND PHYSIOLOGY

General knowledge of the anatomical structures involved in an operation provides for understanding of the surgeon's plan of treatment and the need for specific instruments.

Bony orbit

The two orbital cavities are situated on either side of the midvertical line of the skull between the cranium and the skeleton of the face. Above each orbit is found the anterior cranial fossa and the frontal sinus; medially, the nasal cavity; below, the maxillary sinus; and laterally, from behind forward, the middle cranial and temporal fossae (Figs. 23-1 and 23-2).

The seven bones that form the orbit are the maxilla, palatine, frontal, sphenoidal, zygomatic, ethmoidal, and lacrimal bones. The margins of the bony orbit may be subdivided into four continuous parts: supraorbital, lateral, infraorbital, and medial.

The orbit may be considered as a four-sided pyramid, its base directed forward, laterally, and slightly downward, with its apex facing posteriorly. The periosteum of the orbital walls is continuous with the dura mater.

The orbit is essentially a socket for the eyeball and the muscles, nerves, and vessels that are necessary to proper functioning of the eye. The orbit also serves as a distribution center for the transmission of certain vessels and nerves that supply the areas of the face around the orbital aperture.

Globe

The eyeball (globe) is delicately poised in the orbital cavity on a cushion of fat supported by fascia (Fig. 23-3). The eye occupies a third or less of the cavity of the orbit. The eyeball has three concentric layers: (1) the external, protective fibrous tunic, comprising the cornea and sclera; (2) the middle, vascular, pigmented tunic, comprising the iris, ciliary body, and choroid; and (3) the internal tunic, called the retina (Fig. 23-3).

External tunic. The *cornea* is the anterior, transparent, avascular part of the external tunic and is, for the most part, continuous with the sclera. The cornea serves as a window through which light rays may pass to the retina. The branches of the ophthalmic division of the fifth cranial nerve supply the cornea.

The junction of the clear cornea and the opaque sclera is called the *limbus*.

The *sclera* is the posterior opaque part of the external tunic. A portion of the sclera can be seen through the conjunctiva as the white of the eye. The sclera consists of collagenous fibers loosely connected with fascia, which receives the tendons of the muscles of the globe. The sclera is pierced by the ciliary arteries and nerves and posteriorly by the optic nerve (Fig. 23-3).

Middle tunic. The middle covering of the eye comprises the choroid, ciliary body, and iris from behind forward. The *choroid* is a brownish coat, comprising three layers itself, that lines the greater part of the sclera. The choroid contains many blood vessels and is the main source of nourishment of the receptor cell and pigment epithelial layers of the retina.

The *ciliary body* consists of an extension of the choroidal blood vessels, a mass of muscle tissue, and an extension of the neuroepithelium of the retina. The ciliary muscle acts in effecting accommodation. The neuroepithelium becomes secretory in nature and is responsible for the formation of the aqueous humor.

The *iris,* a thin membrane, is the anterior portion of the middle tunic and is situated in front of the lens. The peripheral border of the iris is attached to the ciliary body, whereas its central border is free. The iris aperture is located slightly nasal to its center, known as the *pupil* (Fig.

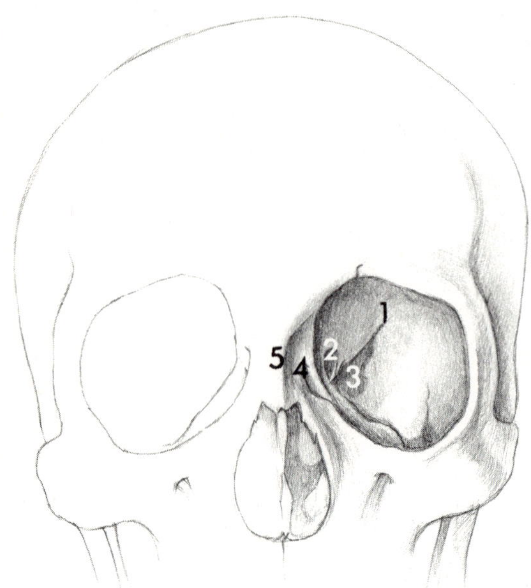

Fig. 23-1. Bony orbital cavity, *1,* communicates with brain through optic foramen; *2,* transmits optic nerve and superior orbital fissure; *3,* transmits most of other nerves and vessels entering orbit (lacrimal fossa); *4,* contains lacrimal sac; and *5,* is bounded medially by nasal bone.

23-3). The iris divides the space between the cornea and the lens into an anterior and a posterior chamber. Both chambers are filled with aqueous humor.

The iris with its many striations regulates the amount of light entering the eye and assists in obtaining clear images. The movement of the iris takes place by means of smooth muscle fibers situated within the connective tissue. The sphincter pupillae contract the pupil, and the dilatator pupillae dilate the pupil. As more light strikes the eye, the sphincter constricts the pupil.

Internal tunic. The innermost tunic, sometimes called the nervous covering, is the *retina*. This thin network of nerve cells and fibers receives images of external objects and transfers the impression via the optic nerve, optic tracts, lateral geniculate body, and optic radiations to the occipital lobe of the cerebrum. The retina lies at the back of the eyeball (Fig. 23-3). The nerve fibers from the retina converge to form the optic nerve, which pierces the eyeball almost at its posterior point, slightly to the inner side. This point is called the *optic disc* (Fig. 23-4). In field testing, this is the anatomical blind spot.

The retina is composed of many layers. The receptor cell layer, which consists of the rods and cones, contains the photosensitive pigments that respond to light energy and initiate the neural response, which is eventually interpreted in the occipital cortex. The point of highest resolution is the foveal pit, which exists in the center of the area that takes on a yellow hue after death (the macula lutea).

An inverted image of the object is focused on the

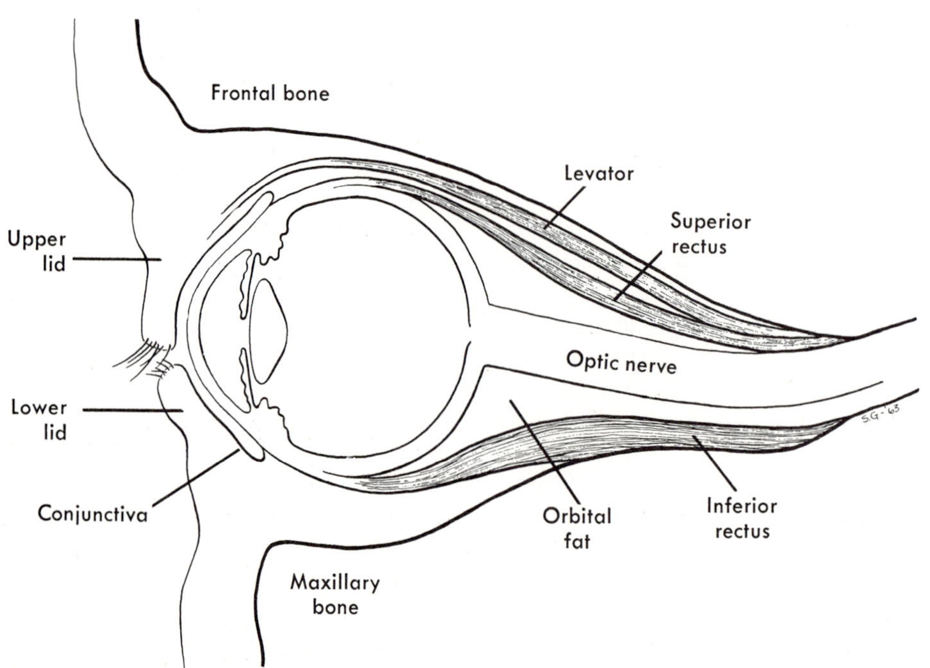

Fig. 23-2. Diagrammatic section of orbit. (From Saunders, W.H., and others: Nursing care in eye, ear, nose, and throat disorders, ed. 4, St. Louis, 1979, The C.V. Mosby Co.)

retina. The nerve fibers leaving the retina by the way of the optic nerve travel to the lateral geniculate body of the thalamus. The fibers nasal to the foveal pit cross in the optic chiasma to go to the contralateral geniculate body. Thus all fibers composing the same half of the visual field project to the same geniculate body, from which fibers project to the ipsilateral occipital cortex for interpretation.

Refractive apparatus of the eye. The refractive apparatus comprises the cornea, the aqueous humor, the lens, and the vitreous body (Fig. 23-3).

The *lens* of the eye is biconvex and has a diameter of 1 cm (Fig. 23-3). It is suspended behind the iris and connected to the ciliary body by means of zonular fibers. Its anterior and posterior surfaces are separated by a rounded

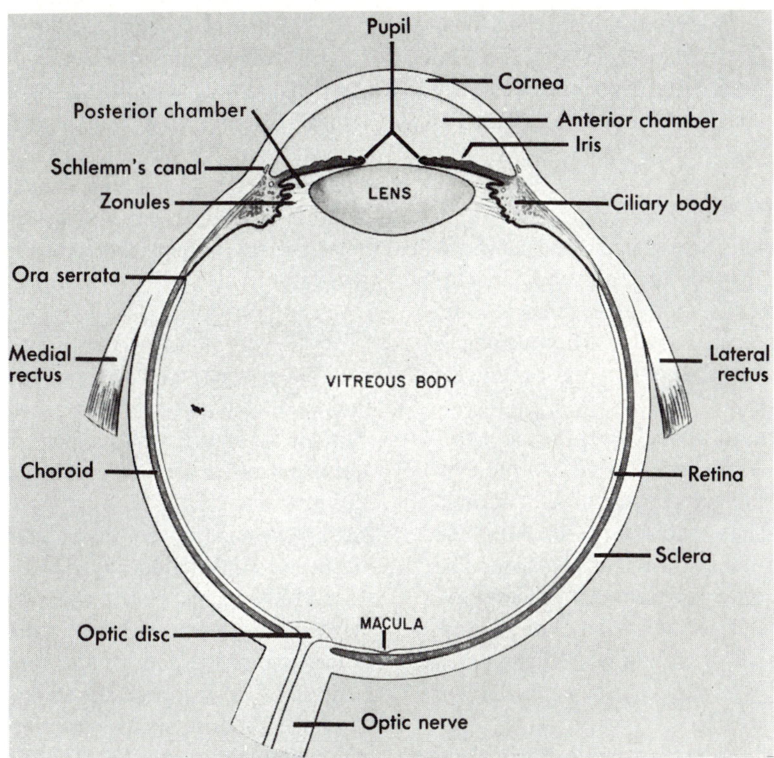

Fig. 23-3. Diagrammatic cross section of eye. (From Saunders, W.H., and others: Nursing care in eye, ear, nose, and throat disorders, ed. 4, St. Louis, 1979, The C.V. Mosby Co.)

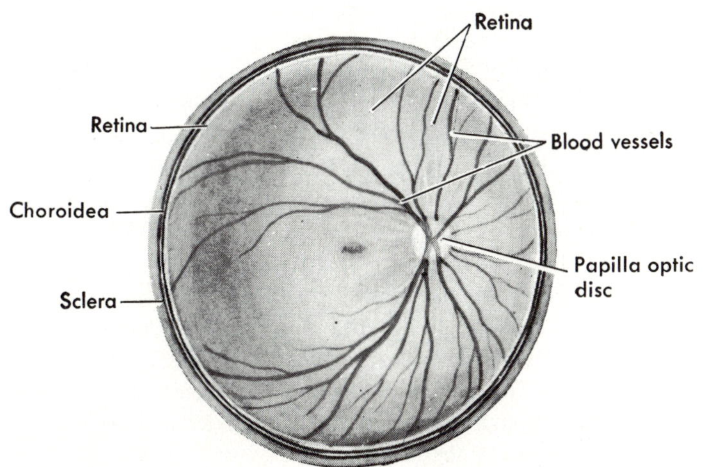

Fig. 23-4. Normal fundus of eye: view of eye seen through ophthalmoscope. (From Anthony, C.P., and Kolthoff, N.J.: Textbook of anatomy and phsiology, ed. 9, St. Louis, 1975, The C.V. Mosby Co.)

border known as the *equator*. The lens hardens with age and therefore cannot respond to accommodative effort with an increase in power. This is why many older persons need bifocals. An opacity of the lens is termed *cataract*.

The *vitreous body* is a glass-like, transparent, gelatinous mass, of which 98.8% is water. It fills the posterior four fifths of the eyeball and is adherent to the margin of the retina.

The central components of a light wave enter the eyes perpendicularly and at the sides obliquely. For clear vision the oblique rays must converge and come to a focus with the central rays on the retina. Light rays from an object pass through the system of refractory devices—the cornea, aqueous humor, lens, and vitreous—and are refracted so that rays strike the macular area.

Conjunctiva and lacrimal apparatus

The *conjunctiva* is a thin, transparent mucous membrane that lines the back surface of the eyelids and the front surface of the globe. The conjunctiva forms a sac (conjunctival sac) that is open in front. The opening is called the *palpebral fissure*. When the eye is closed, the fissure becomes a mere slit.

The conjunctiva is divided into a palpebral and a bulbar part. The palpebral portion lines the back of the eyelids and contains the openings (puncta) of the lacrimal canaliculi, which establish a passageway between the conjunctival sac and the inferior meatus of the nose. The bulbar part of the conjunctiva is transparent, thereby allowing the sclera, termed the white of the eye, to show through. The central portion of the bulbar conjunctiva is continuous at the limbus with the anterior epithelium of the cornea.

The *lacrimal apparatus* comprises the lacrimal gland and its ducts, the lacrimal passages, the lacrimal canaliculi and sac, and the nasal lacrimal duct. The lacrimal gland produces tears and secretes them through a series of ducts into the conjunctival sac. The tears then make their way inward to the puncta, from which they are conducted by the canaliculi to the lacrimal sac, to finally pass into the nasal duct. When the lacrimal glands secrete too profusely, this normal process becomes insufficient and overflow tearing results.

Eyelids

The eyelids are two movable musculofibrous folds in front of each orbit that protect the globe and rest the eye from light.

The upper eyelid is more mobile and larger than the lower. The upper and lower lids meet at the medial and lateral angles (canthi) of the eye. The palpebral fissure, as previously mentioned, is located between the margins of the two eyelids. When the eye is closed, the cornea is completely covered by the upper eyelid. The eyelids are closed by the orbicular muscle of the eye, which is arranged in a circular fashion and acts as a sphincter. When the fibers contract, the eyes close. The upper lid is opened by the levator muscle, which is innervated by the third cranial nerve, as well as by relaxation of the orbicular muscle.

The eyelid consists of several layers, moving from anterior backward. The lid consists of skin, subcutaneous tissue that contains lymphatics, and muscles. Dense fibrous tissue, called *tarsal cartilage,* forms the framework of the lids. The tarsus is anchored to the walls of the orbit by the medial and lateral palpebral ligaments.

The free margins of each eyelid possess two or three rows of hairs called *cilia,* or eyelashes. Posterior to the lashes is a row of glandular orifices of the meibomian glands. Near the medial ends, the free margin of each eyelid presents an opening known as the *punctum lacrimale*. The eyelids serve to distribute all adnexal secretions, thereby keeping the cornea moist and washing away any dust.

Muscles

The extrinsic ocular muscles of the eyeball are the four recti and two oblique muscles. These six striated muscles are inserted into the sclera by means of tendons. These muscles arise, except for the inferior oblique muscle, from the back of the orbit. All the muscles are supplied by cranial nerves: third (oculomotor), fourth (trochlear), and sixth (adducens). All of the muscles work in pairs. Movements of the eyes are brought about by an increase in the tone of one set of muscles and a decrease in the tone of the antagonistic muscles. According to the position of the recti muscles in the eyes, they are referred to as the superior rectus, inferior rectus, medial rectus, and lateral rectus muscles. The oblique muscles insert on the back of the eye and are designated the superior oblique and inferior oblique muscles.

Nerve and blood supply

The optic nerve (second cranial nerve) extends between the posterior eyeball and the optic chiasma (Fig. 23-5). This nerve carries visual impulses, as well as the sensations of pain, touch, and temperature from the eye and its surounding structures to the brain. The third cranial nerve (oculomotor) is the primary motor nerve to all rectus muscles except the lateral rectus, which is innervated by the sixth cranial nerve (abducens). The fourth cranial nerve (trochlear) innervates the superior oblique muscle.

The ophthalmic artery, the main arterial supply to the orbit and globe, is a branch of the internal carotid artery. It divides into branches supplying the globe, muscles, and eyelids. The central retinal artery and central retinal vein travel through the optic nerve and provide an independent circulation for the inner retina.

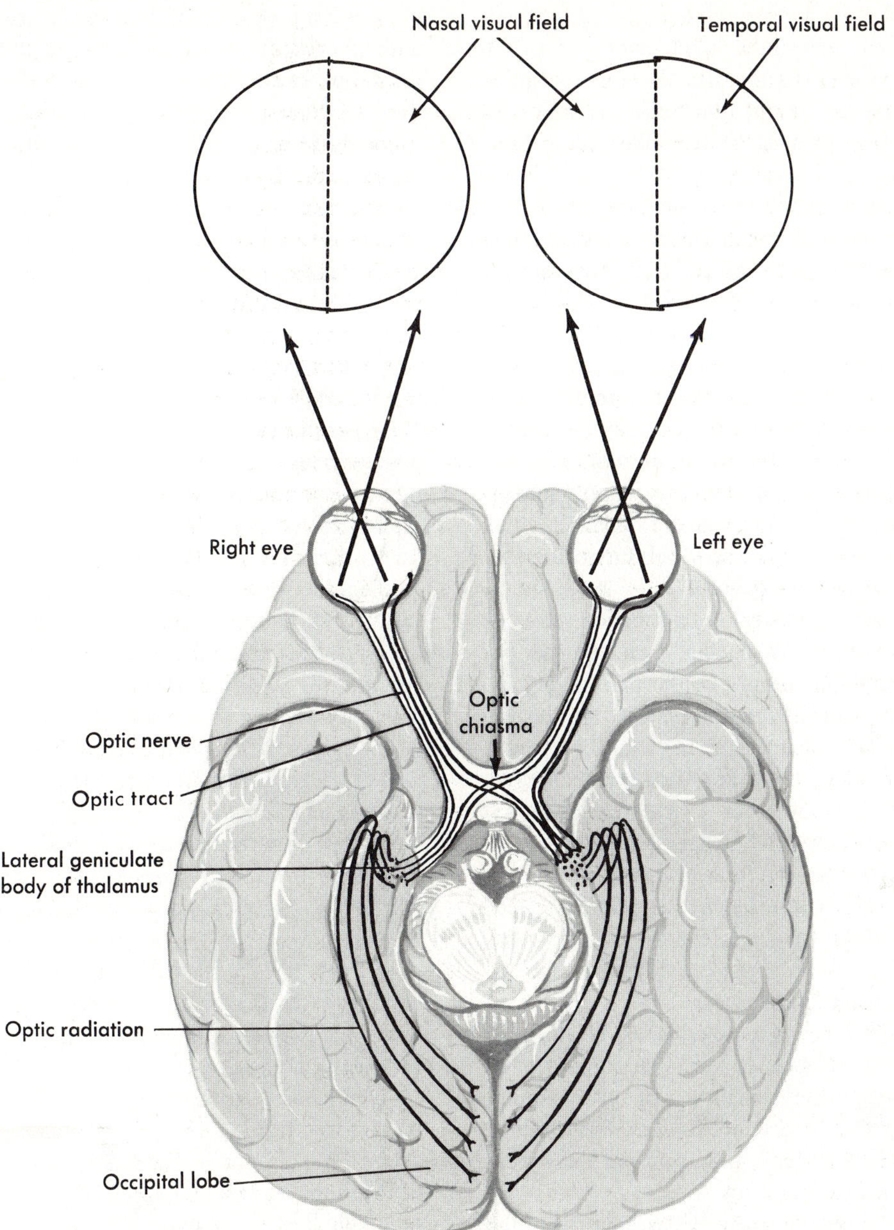

Fig. 23-5. Visual pathways. Note structures that compose each pathway: optic nerve, optic chiasma, lateral geniculate body of thalamus, optic radiations, and visual cortex of occipital lobe. Fibers from nasal portion of each retina cross over to opposite side at optic chiasma, hence terminating in lateral geniculate body of opposite side. Location of lesion in visual pathway determines resulting visual defect. For example, destruction of an optic nerve produces permanent blindness in same eye, and pressure on optic chiasma (by pituitary tumor, for instance) produces bitemporal hemianopsia, or more simply, blindness in both temporal visual fields because it destroys fibers from nasal sides of both retinas. (From Anthony, C.P., and Kolthoff, N.J.: Textbook of anatomy and physiology, ed. 9, St. Louis, 1975, The C.V. Mosby Co.).

NURSING CONSIDERATIONS

Preoperative care

Patients entering the hospital for eye surgery exhibit many different emotions and reactions to the experience: hostility, anger, fear, grief, and helplessness are just a few. Their prime concern is the success of the surgical procedure. Although the initial preparation is begun in the physician's office, it must be continued on the patient's admission to the hospital.

It is preferable to locate all ophthalmic patients in one area to decrease the risk of cross-contamination and also to provide specialized care. The staff must be prepared to meet the specific needs of each patient.

Admission assessment

On admission to the unit, the patient should be fully oriented to the physical surroundings. It may be helpful to walk with the patient to familiarize him with areas of the room and nursing unit. Constant description and reinforcement are important to the visually impaired. Consistency in nursing personnel is very helpful so that the patient can recognize a familiar voice.

In addition to routine admission information, an ocular history must be obtained. It should include the patient's primary complaint, history of the present illness, nature of symptoms, and limitations imposed on the patient by the disease or problem. A medical history should also be obtained because ocular problems are sometimes directly related to other diseases. An external examination of the eye, including lids, lashes, conjunctiva, and lacrimal apparatus, should be done to detect any deviations from normal. The corneal reflex should be tested, and the cornea inspected for superficial irregularities. Pupil size and contour should be noted as well as pupillary reaction, both direct and consensual.

Function of the extraocular muscles should be checked. Movement should be synchronous, and visual lines should meet on a fixed object. Documentation of this examination must be descriptive, accurate, and concise. It may be of value later in assessing the outcome of the procedure.

Close attention to other areas of the assessment of the patient, such as a systems assessment and medications the patient is currently taking, will be of value throughout the hospitalization.

After the assessment information has been compiled and patient problems identified, the plan of care will be developed.

Patient education

Planning to meet the patient's educational needs should play an equal role with meeting other needs. The ophthalmic patient should be informed of the purpose and desired results of preoperative eyedrops and sedation. An explanation of what to expect from the local anesthetic will help decrease the level of anxiety and enable the patient to cooperate better. The operating room nurse should discuss the activities and routines of the intraoperative period. A brief description of the operating room and its equipment will help allay the patient's fears on arrival in the operating suite.

The patient should be informed of what to expect immediately after surgery so that the initial adjustment will be less stressful. Reassurance is especially important for patients whose eyes will be patched postoperatively.

A thorough preoperative preparation will play a vital role in the successful outcome of the surgical procedure.

Ophthalmic pharmacology

Preoperative sedatives and dilating drops

To allay anxiety and reduce general muscle tone, the patient is usually given a barbiturate-narcotic combination as a preoperative medication. On arriving in the operating room suite, the patient receives repeated instillation of topical anesthetic drops.

Dilating drops (mydriatics and cycloplegics) are used to dilate the pupil in order to examine the retina objectively, to test refraction, or to facilitate the removal of the lens. Mydriatic drugs dilate the pupil but permit the patient to focus. The most commonly used mydriatic is phenylephrine 10% (Neo-Synephrine).

A cycloplegic drug dilates the pupil and also prevents focusing of the eye. This type of drug is used to aid in refraction. Commonly used cycloplegics are tropicamide (Mydriacyl) 1%, atropine 1%, and cyclopentolate 1% (Cyclogyl). Atropine has a long-lasting effect.

Drugs for diagnosis and treatment

Drugs for diagnosing and treating eye disorders are extremely potent. One error could result in total, irreversible blindness.

The patient's medical and ocular histories play an important role in the selection of an appropriate ophthalmic agent. This information should be included in the patient's initial nursing assessment.

Following an established protocol for medication administration will greatly reduce the incidence of medication errors:

1. Of prime importance is the nurse's knowledge of the specific medication ordered, including purpose, strength, action and duration, adverse reactions, route of administration, and contraindications.
2. The medication label must be checked during preparation and again immediately before administration. This is especially important, since many ophthalmic drugs are distributed in single-dose units that closely resemble one another.
3. The patient must be positively identified, and the site of administration clearly defined from the physician's

orders. The abbreviations OD, OS, and OU indicate right eye, left eye, and both eyes, respectively.

4. Ensuring that the precise dosage of medication be given at its scheduled time will greatly enhance its effectiveness.

The patient should be made aware of the expected effect of each medication to be able to evaluate the effectiveness, detect signs and symptoms of adverse reactions, and know when to notify the physician concerning problems. The patient should also be well informed of special considerations associated with specific medications so that appropriate safety precautions can be taken. One example of this is protection of the cornea after application of a topical anesthetic.

Selection of specific medications is influenced by the physician's previous training and experience and the patient's disease condition. Following is a classification of ophthalmic medications and specific examples of use.

Constricting drops. Miotic drugs cause the pupil of the eye to contract. Commonly used miotics are pilocarpine 1% to 4% and phospholine iodide 0.012% to 0.25%. Miotics improve the ease with which the aqueous fluid escapes from the eye, independent of their action on the pupil, thereby resulting in decrease of intraocular pressure. Miotics are used in the treatment of glaucoma. These drugs increase contraction of the sphincter of the iris, thus causing the pupil to become smaller. Phospholine iodide is usually discontinued before intraocular surgery is performed.

Pilocarpine is often used after the extraction of a cataractous lens to cause sustained pupillary contraction and to prevent vitreous rupture.

The natural cholinergic transmitter released by the parasympathetic nerves to the iris sphincter is acetylcholine. It is relatively unstable in solution. Acetylcholine (Miochol) is often used intraocularly to produce rapid pupillary contraction, especially after the insertion of an artificial lens (pseudophake). Acetylcholine is prepared immediately before use.

Corticosteroids. A great number of corticosteroid preparations exist. Corticosteroids are used to prevent the normal inflammatory response to noxious stimuli. Corticosteroids reduce the resistance of the eye to invasion by bacterial viruses and fungi. Presence of active infection is therefore an important contraindication to therapy with cortisone and its derivatives in the treatment of allergic eye conditions and chronic inflammations.

Hyperosmotic agents. Hyperosmotic drugs increase the osmolarity of the serum and, by the effect of the induced osmotic pressure gradient, shrink the vitreous body and reduce the intraocular pressure. These drugs are used routinely in the preoperative medication of patients undergoing ophthalmic surgery, as well as therapeutically in cases of uncontrolled glaucoma (usually angle-closure glaucoma).

The commonly used agents may be divided into those given orally (glycerol and isosorbide) and those given parenterally (mannitol and urea). These drugs by their nature induce a diuresis; the nursing personnel must be aware of this and have urinals available, as well as sterile urethral catheters.

Antibiotics, lubricants, and stains. The method or route of administration of the antibiotic depends on the location of the problem. Selection of the drug involves the nature and sensitivity of the isolated organism, the physician's clinical experience, the sensitivity and response of the patient, and the disease. Topical antibiotics are used in the treatment of lid and surface infections and often used prophylactically to prevent infection. Bacitracin and neomycin sulfate are frequently used antibiotic ointments.

Systemic administration of an antibiotic is prescribed for an infection in the posterior portion of the eye or orbit. An infection of this nature can threaten sight. Selection of the specific antibiotic follows the aforementioned criteria.

Ophthalmic lubricants are used to provide corneal protection as a result of problems such as faulty lid closure, complications of lacrimal gland disease, and prominence of the corneal surface in thyroid disease. Methylcellulose 0.5% is considered an excellent ophthalmic lubricant.

Fluorescein sodium is a topical stain commonly used for diagnostic purposes. The use of fluorescein strips is preferred over the use of solution, since the solution can become contaminated easily. In its dilute form, fluorescein is yellow-green and temporarily stains the areas of denuded corneal epithelium. The staining is used to determine the extent of corneal abrasion or infection and is also helpful in locating superficial foreign bodies.

Preparation of the patient

Members of the nursing team have several important responsibilities in the admission of the patient to the operating room and in the preparation of the room and the equipment.

The factors relating to cross infection, safety, comfort, and the well-being of the patient before, during, and after surgery are evident in practice. The duties of the nursing team include the following:

1. Identifying the patient by name if the patient is awake; seeking to gain patient cooperation and confidence by speaking softly, kindly, yet in a confident manner; and endeavoring to keep the patient quiet and relaxed by staying close by, perhaps holding a hand
2. Checking the patient's name on the wristband with the name on the chart and on the surgical schedule
3. Reviewing the surgeon's preoperative orders and nurses' notes to determine if the operative eye has

been prepared properly and other procedures have been carried out according to hospital policies

4. Reaffirming preoperative orders with the surgeon, if necessary
5. Preparing the operating table, making sure all the necessary attachments for the table are in proper readiness
6. Starting an intravenous drip, placing the blood pressure cuff, recording the baseline blood pressure, and attaching the cardiac monitor

Preparation of the face

The preparation of the patient is done under aseptic conditions. Topical anesthetic drops are administered first, if the patient is to be given a local anesthetic. A sterile prep tray containing sterile normal saline solution, irrigation bulbs, basins, cotton, sponges, towels, and antimicrobial skin disinfectant should be near the operating table.

The clipping of eyelashes or shaving of eyebrows is not routinely done. When eyelashes are clipped, it is done before the skin preparation. A thin film of petrolatum is smoothed over the cutting surfaces of the curved eyelash scissors so that the free lashes will adhere to the blades rather than fall into the eyes or onto the face.

The preparation includes cleansing the eyelids of both eyes, lid margins, lashes, eyebrows, and surrounding skin with an appropriate antimicrobial solution (Fig. 23-6, *A*). To prevent the solution from entering the patient's ears, they may be temporarily plugged with cotton pledgets or a plastic cap may be taped over the head and ears. Care is taken to keep the agent out of the eyes. The operative area is washed with warm sterile water, using soft-textured gauze or cotton sponges (Fig. 23-6, *B*), and painted with an aqueous nonirritating skin antiseptic.

When toxic chemicals or small particles of foreign matter must be removed, the eyes may be irrigated with tepid sterile normal saline solution. The conjunctival sac is thoroughly flushed, using an irrigating bulb or an Asepto syringe.

Draping

In some cases the local anesthetic may be injected before completion of the draping procedure. The aseptic principles in draping a patient for an operation are discussed in Chapter 5.

For general eye surgery the basic draping procedure is shown in Fig. 23-7.

1. The head is draped with a double-thickness half sheet and two towels.

2. A large folded sheet is needed to cover the patient and operating table.

3. A fenestrated disposable plastic eye sheet is placed over the operative site.

Anesthesia

Local or standby anesthesia is frequently preferred and indicated for eye surgery in elderly individuals and in those with circulatory and other systemic diseases. A sedative is given the night before and again an hour before surgery. An analgesic is administered 1 to 1½ hours before surgery, followed by topical tetracaine immediately prior to surgery.

The circulating nurse assembles the sterile local anesthesia setup as ordered by the surgeon before the patient enters the operating room and checks the bottles of drugs to make sure they are the correct medications and of the proper strengths.

Suitable needles and syringes of proper sizes and gauges are necessary. For example, the following may be used:

Subcutaneous injection and infiltration—two Luer-Lok 2-ml syringes and two 25-gauge needles, ½ inch long
Subconjunctival injection—two Luer-Lok 2-ml syringes and two 26- or 27-gauge needles, 1 or 1½ inches long
Retrobulbar injection—two Luer-Lok 2- or 5-ml syringes or one 10-ml syringe and two 24-gauge needles, 1 or 1½ inches long

Drugs frequently used. Tetracaine (Pontocaine) in a 0.5% solution may be instilled into the eye before surgery. For local anesthesia in adults, lidocaine 2% (Xy-

A 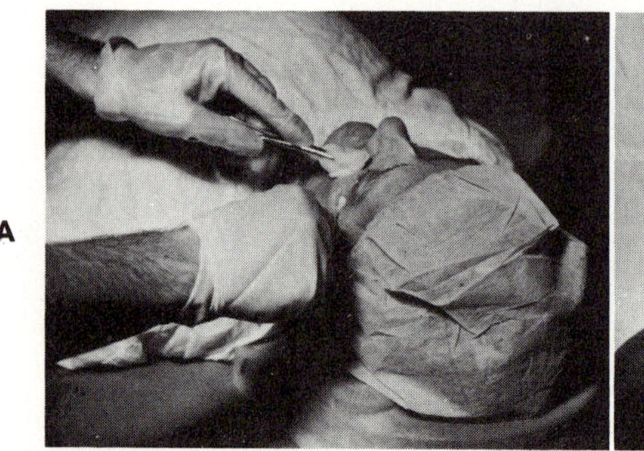

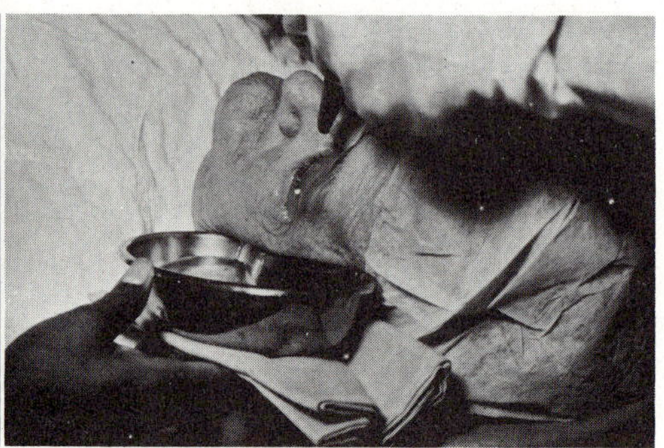 B

Fig. 23-6. Preparation of operative site. **A,** Cleaning of skin area around eye. **B,** Irrigation of cul-de-sac.

locaine) with epinephrine in a 1:150,000 or 1:200,000 dilution is frequently used.

Hyaluronidase is commonly mixed with the anesthetic solution (75 units/10 ml). The enzyme increases the diffusion of the anesthetic through the tissue, thereby improving the effectiveness of the anesthetic nerve block. Hyaluronidase is nontoxic and effective over a wide range of concentrations.

For cataract surgery, an effective retrobulbar injection reduces intraocular pressure by preventing muscle contraction, thus becoming a surgical safeguard against vitreous loss.

In cataract surgery, alpha chymotrypsin (Zolyse) in a 1:5000 or 1:10,000 solution may be used to dissolve the zonular fibers that suspend the cataract within the eye.

Epinephrine in a 1:1000 solution may be applied topically to mucous membranes to decrease bleeding. Cocaine 4% or 10% solution may similarly be used. Epinephrine in a 1:50,000 to 1:200,000 solution may be combined with injectable anesthetics to prolong the duration of anesthesia. Epinephrine in a 1:1000 solution is not used with local anesthetics because it can cause cardiac arrhythmia.

Methods used for administration of local anesthetics. The three methods of administration are instillation of eyedrops, infiltration, and block or regional anesthesia.

Instillation of eyedrops (Fig. 23-8). With the patient's face tilted upward, the first drop is placed in the lower cul-de-sac, and the following drops (number depends on the type of operation to be performed) may be placed from above, with the patient looking downward and the upper lid raised. However, the natural blinking of the lids distributes the drug evenly on the eye surface, regardless of where the drop is placed. When a toxic drug is instilled, the inner corner of the eyelids should be dried of excessive fluid with a tissue or clean cotton ball after each instillation drop, thereby minimizing systemic absorption of the drug. The tip of the applicator must not touch the patient's skin or any part of the eye.

Infiltration method. The surgeon injects the anesthetic solution beneath the skin, beneath the conjunctiva, or into Tenon's capsule, depending on the type of surgery.

Retrobulbar injection is usually performed 10 to 15 minutes before surgery to produce a temporary paralysis of the extraocular muscles.

Block or regional anesthesia. The solution is injected into the base of the eyelids at the level of the orbital margins or behind the eyeball to block the ciliary ganglion and nerves. For eyelid repairs, the solution is introduced through the lower lid. For operations on the lacrimal apparatus, the anesthetic is injected at the level of the anterior ethmoidal foramen to anesthetize the internal and external nasal nerves. In the Van Lint block method, procaine or another local anesthetic is injected

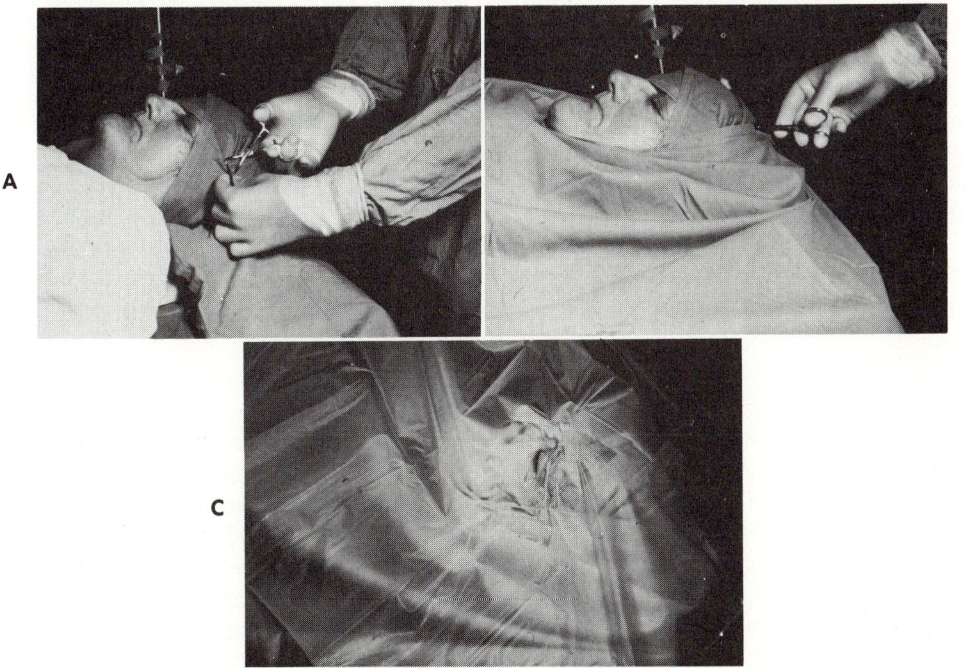

Fig. 23-7. Draping for ophthalmic surgery. **A,** Two sheets are placed under head; uppermost sheet is brought around head to cover eyebrows and nonoperative eye. **B,** Large body sheet is placed and secured over head drape. **C,** Disposable plastic drape sheet is placed over head and operative eye. Patient is completely draped.

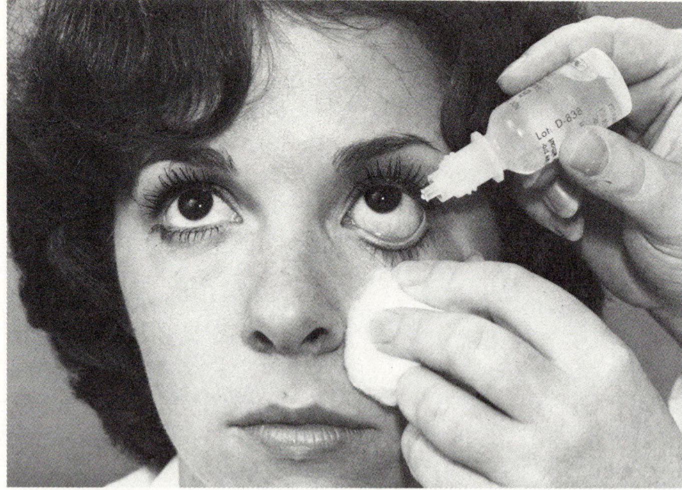

Fig. 23-8. Proper position of head for instillation of eyedrops. Gentle retraction of lower lid is necessary for drop to be placed in lower cul-de-sac.

into the orbicular muscle and reaches the ends of the facial nerve.

General anesthesia. A general anesthetic, with or without intravenous injection of thiopental (Pentothal) sodium, is used when a patient is unable to cooperate because of youth, dementia, nervousness, or extensive operation of the orbit. To produce eye-muscle paralysis in intraocular surgery, tubocurarine chloride may be administered intravenously by the anesthesiologist. Mannitol 20% may be used to lower intraocular pressure, and/or any one of a number of solutions, such as 5% glucose in water or isotonic saline, may be infused intravenously during surgery. A sedative is given the night before surgery, and a drying agent—atropine, scopolamine, or glycopyrrolate (Robinul)—and an analgesic are given 1 to 1½ hours before surgery. The patient must not eat or drink anything for 6 hours prior to induction.

Intraoperative care

General duties of the nursing team are discussed in previous chapters. However, some considerations are particular to the ophthalmic patient. Since many ophthalmic procedures are performed under local anesthesia, the circulating nurse or an additional monitor nurse, if available, must be prepared to provide support to the patient. These patients are self-oriented and have increased sensitivity to both noise and activities within the room. The atmosphere of the room should remain quiet and relaxed to help decrease the patient's anxiety. Patient cooperation is definitely greater in the patient with a decreased level of anxiety.

The scrub nurse has the additional responsibility of monitoring instruments and supplies used during the procedure. It is imperative that foreign substances are not introduced intraocularly. Lint-free barriers should be used to create the sterile field on the instrument table; gloved hands must be rinsed with sterile water to remove any powder particles before the procedure begins. The portion of an instrument used in an intraocular wound should not be touched by gloved hands, and debris should be cleansed from instruments with cellulose sponges. All solutions on the sterile field must be clearly labeled, and intraocular solutions must be separated from others.

The entire surgical team must be knowledgeable of their roles and be prepared to function quickly in the event of a complication.

At completion of the operation

At completion of the operation, the operative area is cleansed with saline sponges.

Antibiotic ointment may be thinly spread over the skin and eyelashes to prevent adhesion of the bandage. This is frequently done after plastic procedures on the lids or lacrimal duct.

Dressings are applied to prevent palpebral movements, protect the operative wound from dust and external contaminants, and absorb any blood and tears that are produced.

The initial dressing usually consists of a piece of fine cotton. It is generally moistened in saline solution before it is applied to the operative site. An eye pad that is commercially prepared and sterilized is applied over the cotton splint. The eye dressing is held in place by means of plastic, paper, or cellophane strips (Fig. 23-9).

After intraocular operations, when external pressure on the eyes might be harmful, the initial dressing is covered with a protector such as a wire gauze cap, perforated aluminum plate, convex perforated metal cup, convex flexible celluloid plate, or another variety of shield (Fig. 23-10).

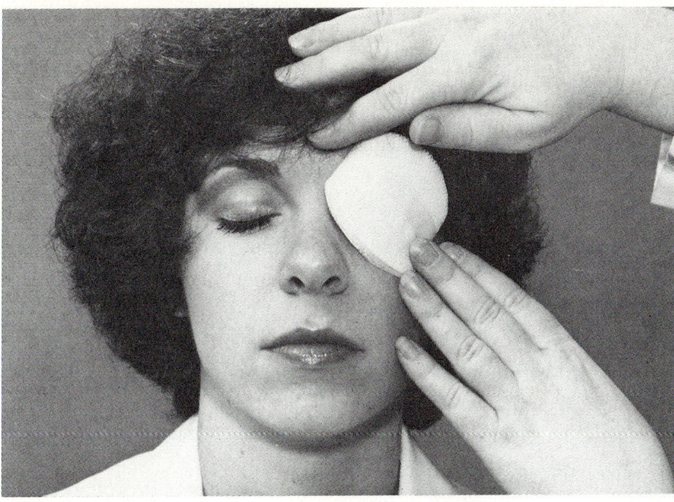

Fig. 23-9. Eye dressing should be held in place by plastic, paper, or cellophane strips. Lids should be gently closed before patch is applied.

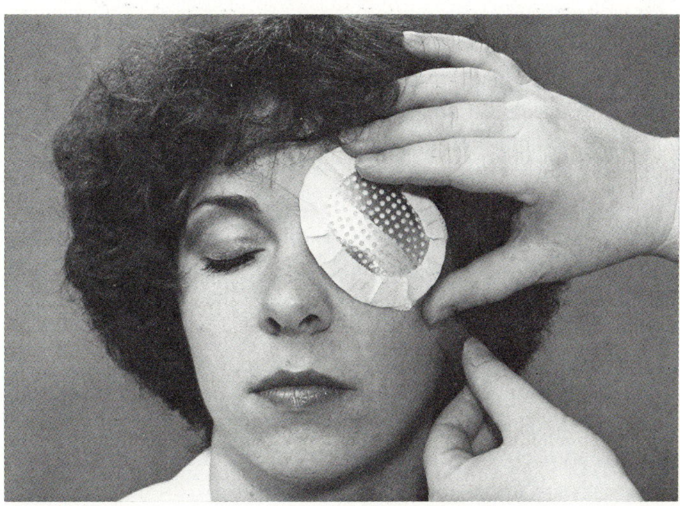

Fig. 23-10. Protection of wound is provided by application of metal shield over dressing.

A pressure bandage may be used in some cases when a compression effect is desired. The gauze roller bandage is applied over the initial dressing, encircling the head.

Postoperative care

The postoperative routine varies depending on (1) the type of procedure, (2) the anesthetic agent, and (3) the physician's specific orders. However, the main goal is to prevent infection and ensure the best healing of the eye. The nursing staff must be knowledgeable of the specific procedure performed, possible complications, and signs and symptoms of these complications.

Patients should be evaluated for the quality of vision in the unaffected eye, and appropriate measures taken to provide safety and assistance to the patient. Elderly patients should be assisted with ambulation as soon as permitted to enhance the circulatory status.

Patients should be informed of the purpose and importance of following the postoperative orders. The nurse should be certain that the patient and/or family can perform procedures to be continued after discharge, such as wound care, dressing changes, and medication administration.

Written discharge instructions should be reviewed and given to the patient and family. These should include specific instructions for dressing changes, wound care, medication administration, activity limitations, and a follow-up office visit. The patient should be instructed to contact the physician immediately if a problem arises.

BASIC INSTRUMENTS

The frequent changes in surgical techniques and instrument patterns make selection of basic instruments individualized. Exacting performance of these instruments is crucial to the success of the procedure. Increased use of the microscope has brought about changes in the design of ophthalmic instruments.

Care and handling. To maintain quality, precision microsurgical instruments, strict criteria must be followed for their care and handling. Racks are available for storage and sterilization to provide protection to instrument tips and cutting surfaces. The instruments should be inspected under magnification when purchased and before and after each use, observing for burs on tips, nicks on cutting surfaces, and alignment of jaws. They should be cleaned during use with nonfibrous sponges to prevent damage to delicate instrument tips. Personnel handling the instruments should know the identity and purpose of each instrument. Tissue can be damaged by use of an inappropriate instrument; instruments can also be damaged by inappropriate use. After use, the instruments should be cleaned by hand and thoroughly dried before storage. It is recommended that microsurgical instruments undergo ultrasonic cleaning with distilled water and an appropriate cleansing agent. They can be hand-held individually or immersed together as long as they are not touching each other. Instruments should be rinsed with distilled water and thoroughly dried. A hot air blower can be used for drying instruments, since a towel should never be used. Gas sterilization is preferred; a washer/sterilizer should be avoided.

In addition to basic care and handling, a routine preventive maintenance program should be established for sharpening, realigning, and adjusting these precision instruments. Keeping an instrument in good repair is much less costly than purchasing a new one.

Basic setup. Each ophthalmic operating room should have sufficient number of basic standard eye surgery setups that can be supplemented to meet specific needs. Instruments routinely needed for a particular type of operation and each surgeon's personal preferences should be listed on cards and kept on file (Chapter 2).

Ophthalmic sutures. Sutures used in ophthalmic surgery are very fine, ranging in size from nos. 4-0 to 10-0. They produce minimum reaction and discomfort for the patient. Suture should be handled as little as possible to avoid weakening or fraying. Surgical gut and collagen suture, plain and chromic, should be rinsed before use to prevent introducing a possible irritant into the eye. Ophthalmic needles are also very delicate and must be handled with extreme care. Needles must be inspected before use for evidence of burs.

SURGICAL PROCEDURES ON THE EYELIDS

The most common procedures performed on the eyelids are for treatment of chalazion, entropion, and ectropion and excisional biopsy and repair of traumatic injuries.

Removal of chalazion

Definition. Incision and curettage of a chalazion, a chronic granulomatous inflammation of one or more of the meibomian glands in the tarsal plate of the eyelid.

Setup and preparation of the patient. The following instruments should be available:

- 2 Chalazion clamps, 1 large and 1 small
- 1 Lester fixation forceps
- 2 Chalazion curettes, 1 medium and 1 large
- 1 Iris scissors
- 1 Bard-Parker no. 9 knife handle with no. 15 blade

The patient is prepared as described for general ophthalmic surgery. A local anesthesia setup is also needed.

Operative procedure

1. The affected lid is everted with a lid retractor to expose the chalazion.
2. A cruciate incision is made on the inner lid surface, using a sharp knife; corners of the tarsal plate are resected (Fig. 23-11).

The contents of the chalazion are removed with a curette. The affected eye is dressed and patched.

Canthotomy

Definition. Lengthening of the opening (slit) between the eyelids prior to cataract surgery when exposure of the globe is inadequate or when necessary to correct ankyloblepharon or blepharochalasis.

Setup and preparation of the patient. The following instruments should be available:

- 1 Straight hemostat
- 1 Blunt scissors, small

The patient is prepared as described previously for general ophthalmic surgery.

Operative procedure

1. The hemostat is clamped over the full thickness of the outer canthus and left in place for 60 seconds.
2. The skin and conjunctiva are incised. For canthoplasty the adjacent bulbar conjunctiva is dissected, and its borders and those of the skin are sutured together with fine silk sutures.
3. The affected eye is dressed and patched.

Surgery for positional defects of the eyelids

Several techniques are followed to treat faulty position of the eyelids. Plastic surgery is effective in the treatment of entropion, ectropion (Fig. 23-12), and blepharochalasis of the eyelids.

Plastic repair of entropion

Definition. Surgical correction of muscular fibers of the lid to evert the lid margins and eyelashes.

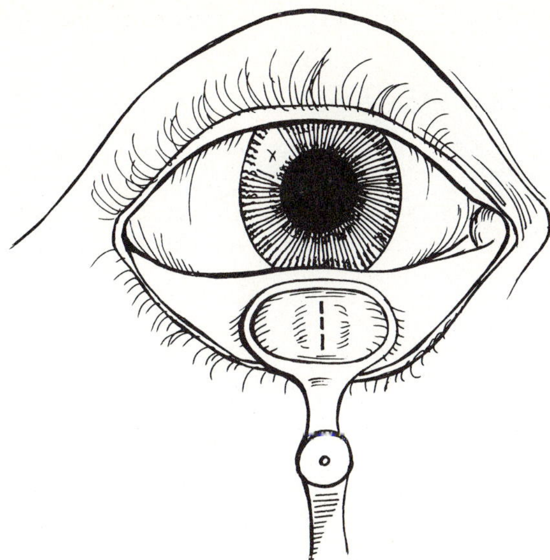

Fig. 23-11. Clamp everts eyelid during surgery for chalazion. Incision has been made on inner lid surface to avoid scarring. Viscous contents of chalazion will be removed with curette.

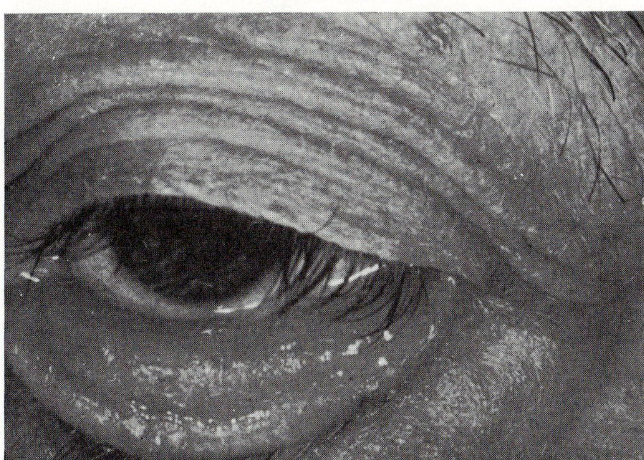

Fig. 23-12. Ectropion, or turning out of lid, is most commonly caused by senile relaxation of eyelid framework. (From Saunders, W.H., and others: Nursing care in eye, ear, nose, and throat disorders, ed. 4, St. Louis, 1979, The C.V. Mosby Co.)

Considerations. Entropion (turning inward of the lid) usually affects the lower lid but may affect the upper lid. It seldom occurs in persons under 40 years of age. There are two types: spastic and cicatricial. Spastic entropion results from degeneration of fascial attachments between the pretarsal muscle and the tarsus, which permits the former to override the lid margin during contraction. Cicatricial entropion is a complication of spastic entropion resulting from scarring of either the upper or lower tarsus and its conjunctiva, turning in the lashes (trichiasis) so that they rub on the cornea.

Setup and preparation of the patient. The following plastic tray and local anesthetic set are needed:

6 Mosquito hemostats
1 Kelly forceps, large
1 Razor blade breaker
2 Desmarres lid retractors
1 von Graefe muscle hook
1 Skin hook, double-pronged
2 Skin hooks, single-pronged
1 Ruler
1 Conjunctival forceps with teeth
1 Serrated conjunctival forceps
1 Quevedo utility forceps
1 Lester fixation forceps
2 McCullough suture forceps
1 Adson forceps with teeth
1 Jeweler's forceps
1 Storz suturing forceps
1 Straight iris forceps
2 Bishop-Harmon iris forceps
2 Bard-Parker no. 9 knife handles with no. 15 blades
1 Stevens scissors
1 Iris scissors, small
1 Iris scissors, large
1 Metzenbaum scissors
1 Kalt needle holder
1 Plastic needle holder
2 Castroviejo needle holders
1 Nasal suction tube
1 Disposable cautery
2 Senn retractors
1 Beaver no. 3H knife handle with no. 64 blade
1 Rubber band
2 Richardson retractors
1 Freer elevator, sharp
1 Metal bone plate
2 Sempken tissue forceps
1 Double fixation hook, small
1 Ribbon retractor
1 Special bone plate with suture holder
1 Rake retractor, small

Operative procedure. The treatment of entropion involves either removing a base-down triangle of skin, muscle, and tarsus and suturing the edges together to evert the lid margin or exposing the orbicular muscle, dividing it, and suturing it to the lower border of the tarsus.

Plastic repair of ectropion

Definition. Plastic operation to shorten the lower lid in a horizontal direction (Figs. 23-12 and 23-13).

Considerations. Ectropion (sagging and eversion of the lower lid), which is usually bilateral, is common in older persons. Ectropion may be caused by the relaxation of the orbicular muscle. Symptoms are tearing, conjunctival infection, and irritation. Minor ectropion may be treated by electrocautery penetrations through the conjunctiva. Surgery is indicated when facial paralysis is permanent or when scarring follows lacerations, lesions, or penetrating injuries and the cornea becomes exposed, resulting in ulceration and photophobia.

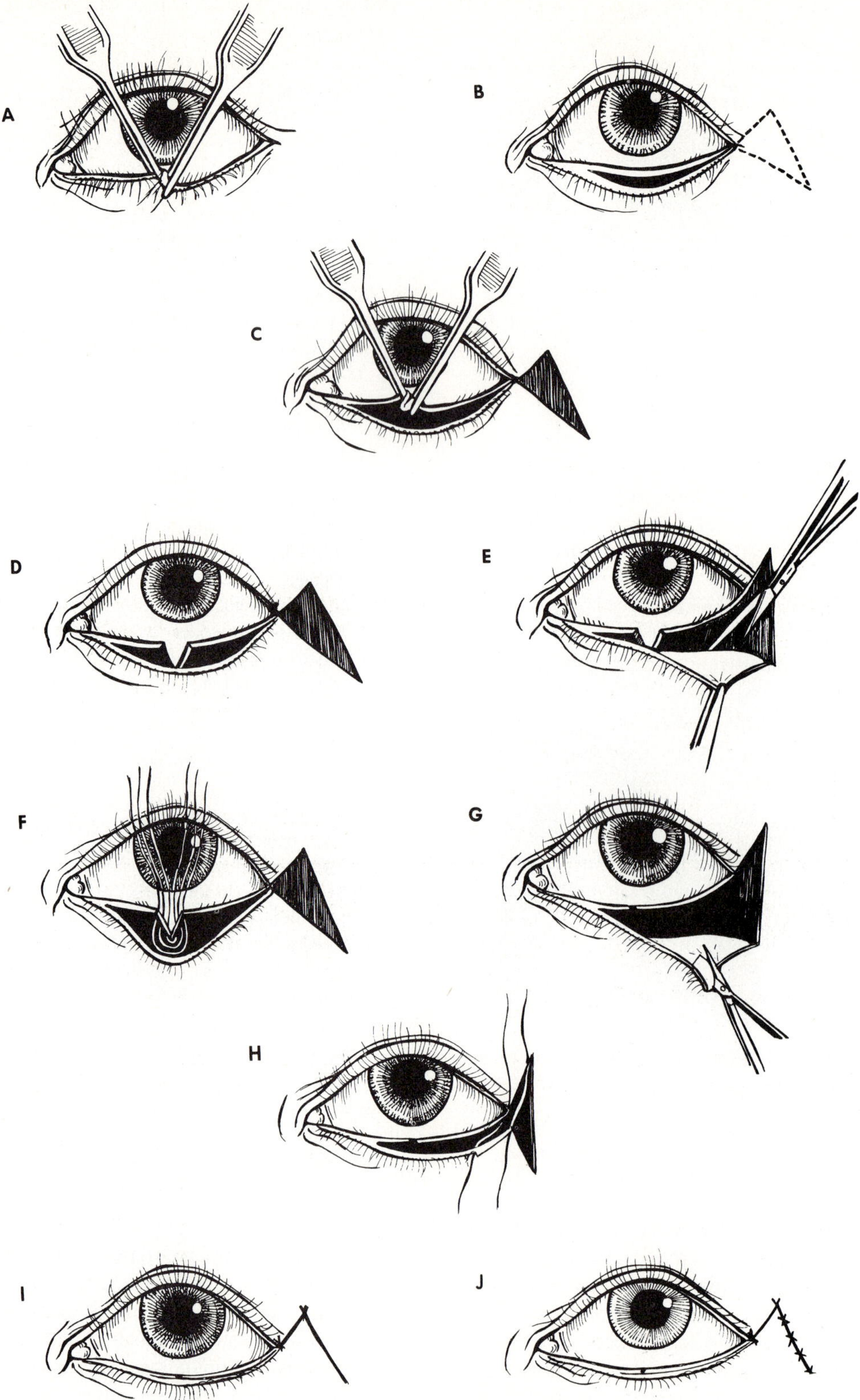

Fig. 23-13. Kuhnt-Szymanowski operation for atonic ectropion. **A,** Lower lid picked up with two smooth forceps, and amount of lengthening needed gauged. **B,** Lateral skin triangle marked, and lid split. **C,** Lateral triangle resected, and amount of tarsoconjunctiva to be excised gauged. **D,** Tarsoconjunctival triangle receded. **E,** Skin-muscle lamina dissected free. **F,** Tarsal wound closed. **G,** Excess cilia resected. **H,** Sutures placed to form a new canthus. **I,** Sutures tied. **J,** Final closure done. (Adapted from Fox, S.A.: Ophthalmic plastic surgery, ed. 3, New York, Grune & Stratton, Inc.)

Setup and preparation of the patient. As described for entropion. A pressure dressing and a local or general anesthesia setup should be prepared.

Operative procedure. Correction of cicatricial ectropion is accomplished either by mobilization of the surrounding skin or by free grafting. Many procedures have been devised, such as the *Wharton Jones* V-Y *procedure,* free whole skin graft, or epidermis graft. The operation includes removal of scar tissue and approximation of layers, small sliding grafts from the immediate area by means of Z-plasty or V-Y incision if loss is minimal, and free graft from the upper lid for the lower lid by means of tarsorrhaphy.

The *Kuhnt-Szymanowski procedure* is performed to treat senile or full-blown atonic ectropion. The external two-thirds or the entire lid is split, the tarsoconjunctival triangle is resected, and the wound is closed by means of sutures in such a manner that a new canthus is performed (Fig. 23-13).

Plastic repair for blepharochalasis

Definition. Removal of redundancy of skin of the upper eyelids.

Considerations. Blepharochalasis causes the upper lids to hang down over the eyes, sometimes obscuring vision. It may occur in older persons who have lost normal elasticity of the skin of the upper lids or in persons who have suffered from persistent angioneurotic edema with stretching of the skin of the eyelids.

Setup and preparation of the patient. As described for entropion.

Operative procedure. An elliptical segment of skin of the upper lid is removed by plastic surgical technique.

Surgery for unilateral or bilateral ptosis

Considerations. Drooping of the upper lid is considered to be congenital, acquired, or senile. In congenital ptosis, there is frequently weakness of the superior rectus muscle. Acquired ptosis is generally caused by laceration of the third cranial nerve or the levator muscle or both. Tumors may cause ptosis. Senile ptosis is the result of poor muscle tone of the levator.

The objective of ptosis surgery is to achieve a perfect cosmetic result by creating a good upper lid fold with elevation of the lid. The many surgical procedures that have been devised are based on the advancement of the levator muscle, the frontalis muscles, or the superior rectus muscle. These muscles are the elevating forces of the upper lids. Some of the techniques involve resection of the levator (Iliff method), use of the superior rectus muscle (Berke method), or modification of other methods such as the Motais or the Crawford frontalis collagen sling procedure.

Iliff method (resection of the levator)

Definition. Creation of an effective upper lid by shortening the levator muscle and reapproximating the conjunctiva and muscles to reestablish the correct relationship of the involved structures.

Setup and preparation of the patient. The plastic tray setup previously described is used. The patient is prepared as described previously for eye surgery. General anesthesia is preferred.

Operative procedure

1. The upper lid is everted over the lid clamp. With a sharp-pointed scissors, two buttonhole incisions are made through the conjunctiva medial and lateral to the superior edge of the tarsus.
2. Blunt scissors are directed through the buttonhole incisions and spread open to enlarge the incisional opening. As scissors are withdrawn, the angular, rubber-shod, jawed ptosis clamps are positioned to contain the conjunctiva, superior edge of the tarsus, superior arcuate artery, aponeurosis of the levator, and orbital septum.
3. Another incision is made with scissors distal to the clamp and through all structures held by the clamp.
4. The orbital septum is freed from the clamp. Structures between the orbital septum and levator are dissected by means of blunt instruments.
5. Traction is applied to the clamp. Double-armed chromic gut sutures no. 4-0 are inserted from the cut tarsal edge through all structures held by the clamp. The tissues distal to the suture line are excised.
6. The free end of each of the double-armed sutures is passed through the orbital septum, between the skin and tarsus, and brought out through the skin at the cilia margin.
7. Sutures are tied over a silicone strip or small beads. Redundant skin is invaginated with a peg to form a good lid fold.
8. The eye is closed by fastening a single suture that is passed through the skin of the lower lid to the forehead by means of an adhesive strip. Bland eye ointment is applied, and then eye pads are secured to the eyes by means of nonallergenic adhesive tape.

Silver-Hildreth Supramid suspension

Definition. Attachment of the lid by Supramid sutures anchored in the periosteum to the frontalis muscle.

Considerations. This procedure may be done in the total absence of levator and superior rectus action.

Setup and preparation of the patient. Plastic tray, Wright fascia needle, and no. 4-0 Supramid suture are required.

Operative procedure

1. An incision is made in the lid fold exposing the tarsus. An incision is made over the eyebrow centrally to the frontalis muscle.

2. A double-armed Supramid suture is woven through the tarsus.

3. The needles are removed from the suture, and the suture is threaded on the fascia needle.

4. The fascia needle is passed under the skin of the lid through the periosteum of the orbital rim and out through the brow incision. This is repeated so that both ends of the suture are now in the brow incision.

5. The suture is tied as it lies on the frontalis muscle.

6. The skin is closed with a nylon, subcuticular, continuous suture no. 6-0.

7. The conjunctival sac is filled with antibiotic ointment. A double-armed, silk suture no. 4-0 is passed through the center of the lower lid margin and fastened to the brow with adhesive tape, thus covering the exposed cornea. A pressure dressing is applied.

Excisional biopsy

Definition. Removal of lesions either neoplastic (benign or malignant) or viral in nature.

Considerations. Basal cell carcinomas account for 95% of neoplastic lesions of the lid; the treatment of choice is excisional biopsy. Viral lesions such as papilloma and molluscum contagiosum are also treated in this way.

Setup and preparation of the patient. A plastic tray is needed.

Operative procedure. Through-and-through excision of skin, muscle, tarsus, and conjunctiva is followed by careful structural closure of anatomical spaces.

Surgery for traumatic injuries

Definition. Repair of lacerations of the lids, including damage to the inferior canaliculus.

Considerations. Tantamount to success is the careful approximation of the borders of the lid margin and the ends of a torn canaliculus.

Setup and preparation of the patient. A plastic tray, a pigtail probe, Verhuff rods, and a Supramid suture are needed.

Operative procedure

1. Lacerations of the lid margin are closed with a silk suture no. 5-0 to align the gray line of the lid that lies between the lash follicles and the orifices of the meibomian glands. Once this anatomical line has been approximated, all other sutures are placed, maintaining this relationship.

2. If the canaliculus has been lacerated, a pigtail probe is passed through the uninvolved punctum, through the sac, and carefully through the proximal and distal ends of the lacerated structure to emerge from the involved punctum. A Supramid suture no. 4-0 is hooked onto the probe and, by reversing the previous procedure, is pulled out of the uninvolved punctum, thus establishing continuity of the system. Careful plastic closure of the lid defect is then carried out.

SURGERY OF THE LACRIMAL GLAND AND APPARATUS

Considerations. Surgery of the lacrimal gland and apparatus is concerned generally with cure or diagnosis of tumors of the lacrimal fossa or with deficient drainage with overflow of tears. Chronic dacryocystitis in adults (Fig. 23-14) requires dacryocystorhinostomy because of resistant obstruction of the nasolacrimal duct. The dacryocystorhinostomy operation is done when the lower canaliculus is patent but the tear duct is blocked, thus causing epiphora, which cannot be tolerated. This deformity frequently follows malunited fracture of the medial wall of the orbit. Dacryocystorhinostomy creates a new, large opening between the lacrimal sac and the nose.

Surgery of the lacrimal fossa

Definition. Biopsy of any structure in the lacrimal fossa and possibly removal of the lacrimal gland (extirpation) for excess tearing.

Setup and preparation of the patient. A plastic tray is required.

Operative procedure

1. The lacrimal fossa, which is in the upper temporal quadrant of the orbit, may be approached directly through the lid or through the conjunctiva by everting the upper lid. The lacrimal gland is divided into a palpebral and orbital part by the orbital septum. All drainage ducts go through the palpebral portion; therefore surgery performed on this part alone affects tearing because, although the orbital part is intact, no access to the eye is available.

2. Routine surgical closure procedures are followed.

Probing

Considerations. The opening of the lacrimal drainage system posterior and below the inferior nasal conchae is closed in approximately 35% of newborns. In most cases this closure opens spontaneously within the first 2 or 3 months of life. In cases in which the lacrimal drainage system does not open spontaneously, an acute infectious process involving the lacrimal drainage system becomes obvious. The infectious process is treated with antibiotics, and then probing is carried out.

Setup and preparation of the patient. A plastic tray, plus the following, is required:

Punctum dilators, assorted sizes
Safety pins
Probe set, assorted sizes
Lacrimal needles
Syringe

In a child under 6 months of age, this procedure may be done with mummification, using topical anesthesia. After this age, the procedure is done with the patient under general anesthesia.

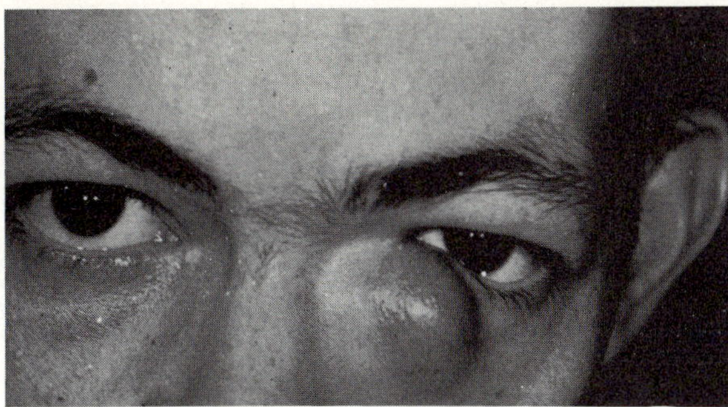

Fig. 23-14. Chronic infection of lacrimal sac (dacryocystitis) causes swelling of inner lower corner of eye socket. (From Saunders, W.H., and others: Nursing care in eye, ear, nose, and throat disorders, ed. 4, St. Louis, 1979, The C.V. Mosby Co.)

Operative procedure

1. Manipulation is done through the upper punctum and canaliculus to prevent trauma to the inferior part of the system, which carries 90% to 95% of the total amount of secretions.

2. The upper punctum is dilated first with a safety pin and then with a punctum dilator. A lacrimal probe is then passed through the upper punctum and canaliculus into the sac, at which time the resistance is met from the lacrimal bone. The probe is rotated 90 degrees, passed through the bony canal, and forced through the imperforate opening into the nose. A small amount of blood may regurgitate at this time. The procedure may be repeated with a larger probe.

3. With the blunt lacrimal needle, a fluorescein solution is used as irrigation to ensure the patency of the system.

Dacryocystorhinostomy

Definition. The establishment of a new tear passageway for drainage directly into the nasal cavity.

Setup and preparation of the patient. A basic eye surgery setup is needed, including the following:

4 Towel clamps
16 Mosquito hemostats
1 Kelly forceps
1 Allis forceps
1 Stevens scissors
1 Iris scissors, straight
1 Graefe fixation forceps
2 McCullough suture forceps
2 Lester fixation forceps
2 Bayonet forceps
1 Adson forceps with teeth
1 Adson forceps without teeth
1 Quevedo utility forceps
2 Skin hooks, fine, double-pronged
2 Skin hooks, fine, single-pronged
1 Skin hook, medium, double-pronged
2 Senn retractors
2 Desmarres lid retractors
1 Paul lacrimal retractor
1 Ballen-Alexander orbital retractor
3 Freer elevators, 2 sharp and 1 blunt
1 Jameson muscle hook
1 Chisel, small
1 Periosteal elevator
2 Malleable retractors, narrow
2 Curettes, small
2 Gouges
1 Mallet
2 Angled suction tubes
1 Goldstein lacrimal retractor
2 Nasal specula
Assorted rongeurs
2 Kerrison punches, small
1 Cittelli punch, small
1 Alligator forceps
1 Kalt needle holder
1 Castroviejo needle holder
2 Bard-Parker no. 9 knife handles with no. 15 blades
1 Gold lacrimal needle
1 Silver lacrimal needle
Set of assorted Bowman lacrimal probes
Assorted Wilder dilators
Stryker saw trephines or high-speed dental drill and bits
Chromic gut no. 4-0 on ½-circle needle
Catheters, 10 to 16 Fr

The nasal cavity is anesthetized topically with cocaine just before surgery, and a general anesthetic is administered in the operating room. The patient is prepared as described for eye surgery.

Operative procedure (Fig. 23-15)

1. An incision is made on the nasal side of the orbital rim. With blunt-pointed, curved, or flat scissors, knife, retractors, and forceps, dissection is carried down to the periosteum, which is separated from the bone with elevators.

2. Through the lower canaliculus, the sac is probed, identified, and displaced laterally.

3. The anterior lacrimal crest is perforated by a Stryker saw, dental drill, or mallet and chisel. The hole is enlarged with rongeurs. During this time, the cornea is protected by a metal retractor or plastic contact lens.

4. Irregular fragments of bone and fibrous tissue are removed, and hemostasis is obtained with bone wax if necessary.

5. The lacrimal sac and nasal mucosa are incised with H incisions with the long line vertical.

6. The mucous membrane of the nose is sutured to that of the lacrimal sac with no. 4-0 chromic sutures. A probe is passed through the nostril into the base of the wound to test the opening from the sac into the nose. A French catheter may be passed from the nose and sutured into the roof of the sac with no. 4-0, chromic sutures. It remains in place until the sutures dissolve, thereby acting

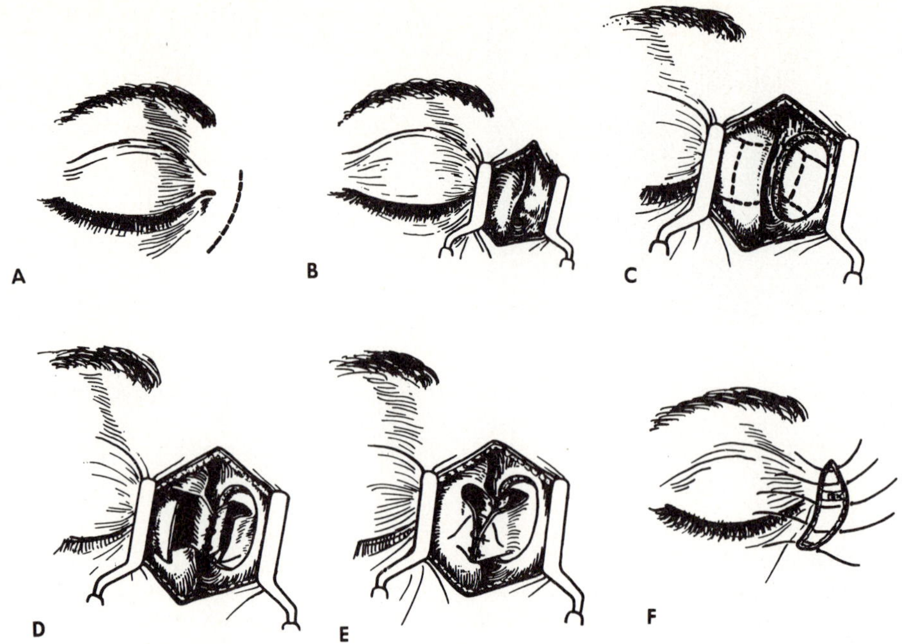

Fig. 23-15. Dacryocystorhinostomy. **A,** Skin incision for dacryocystorhinostomy or dacryocystectomy. **B,** Lacrimal sac and lacrimal bone exposed. **C,** Opening made in lacrimal bone and lacrimal crest, with dotted lines indicating incision to be made in wall of sac and in nasal periosteum and mucosa. **D,** Posterior flap of wall of sac sutured to posterior flap of nasal mucosa. **E,** Anterior flap of wall of sac sutured to anterior flap of nasal mucosa. (Drawing somewhat distorted for visualization of relative positions.) **F,** Reattachment of medial canthal ligament, and wire sutures in position for closure of skin incision. (From Allen, J.H., editor: May's manual of the diseases of the eye, ed. 23, Baltimore, The Williams & Wilkins Co.)

as a stent about which epithelial union can occur between the lacrimal and nasal mucosa.

7. The interior flap of mucous membrane from the nose and sac is sutured with interrupted, chromic no. 4-0 sutures; skin margins are approximated and closed with silk sutures no. 6-0; interpalpebral sutures are placed to maintain position of the eyelids under the dressing. The wound is dressed.

SURGERY FOR STRABISMUS

Strabismus (squint) is the inability to direct the two eyes at the same object because of lack of coordination of the extraocular muscles. Corrective surgery is performed to change the relative strength of individual muscles, therefore improving coordination (Fig. 23-2).

The deviation of the eye may be inward, outward, upward, or downward. The amount of deviation is a measurement of the angle formed by the visual axis of the two eyes. The lateral rectus muscle abducts the eye, the medial rectus muscle adducts the eye, and the other ocular muscles have both primary and secondary functions regarding elevation, depression, intorsion, and extorsion, according to the position of the eye.

Basically, there are two surgical approaches to the correction of strabismus: strengthening is usually accomplished by a resection procedure, and weakening is usually by a recession procedure. It may be necessary to operate on three or more muscles, in two stages. To some extent, the type of strabismus influences the type of surgery (Fig. 23-16).

Resection

Definition. Removal of a portion of muscle and attachment of cut ends (Fig. 23-16).

Setup and preparation of the patient. The following muscle set is used (Fig. 23-17):

1 Williams lid speculum
1 Castroviejo caliper
1 Hartmann hemostat, curved
1 Quevedo utility forceps
1 Serrated conjunctival forceps, delicate
1 Conjunctival forceps, delicate, with teeth
1 Thorpe forceps
2 Lester fixation forceps
2 McCullough suture forceps
1 Guist fixation forceps
1 Graefe iris forceps
1 Graefe fixation forceps
2 Bulldog clamps, serrefine
2 Jameson muscle forceps

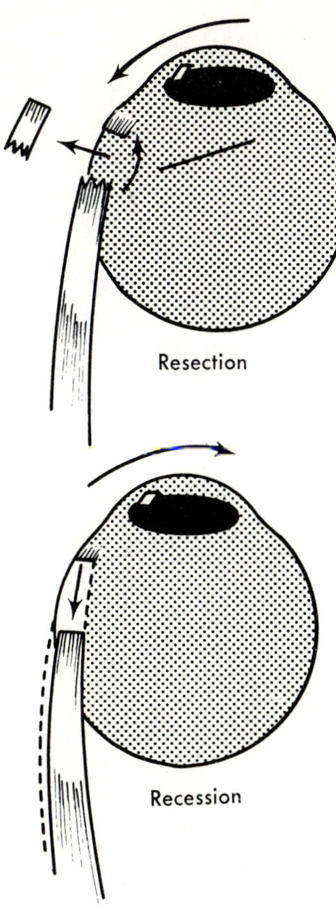

Fig. 23-16. In surgery for strabismus, resection of part of ocular muscle tendon rotates eye toward operated muscle, whereas recession moves muscle tendon backward on eye, permitting eye to rotate away from operated muscle. (Adapted from Havener, W.H.: Synopsis of ophthalmology, ed. 5, St. Louis, 1979, The C.V. Mosby Co.)

2 Jameson muscle hooks
1 von Graefe muscle hook
1 Castroviejo needle holder
1 Kalt needle holder
1 Stevens scissors
1 Hildreth cautery with tip

Suture material varies according to the surgeon's preference, but usually the suture is on a spatula needle. The patient is prepared as described for general ophthalmic surgery; local or general anesthesia is used.

Operative procedure

1. A speculum is inserted, and the conjunctiva is incised at one border of the muscle to be resected.

2. The muscle insertion is hooked with a muscle hook, and the conjunctiva over the insertion is opened.

3. Double-armed sutures are passed through the muscle belly at the desired position of shortening, and the muscle is incised anterior to this suture.

4. The stump of the muscle is excised from the insertion, and the muscle is now sutured to the insertion using the double-armed suture.

5. The conjunctiva is closed with an absorbable suture.

Recession

Definition. Severence of the muscle from its original insertion and its reattachment more posteriorly on the sclera (Fig. 23-16).

Setup and preparation of the patient. As described for strabismus resection.

Operative procedure

1. The insertion of the muscle is exposed as described previously.

2. Sutures are passed through the muscle tendon at its insertion into the globe, and the tendon is severed distal to the suture.

3. With calipers, marks are made on the globe at the desired distance behind the insertion, and the muscle is anchored to the globe at that point.

4. The conjunctiva is closed with absorbable suture.

Myectomy

Definition. Method of weakening the action of the muscle. This may be done as a lengthening procedure such as a Z marginal tenotomy or myectomy, an intersheath tenotomy of the superior oblique tendon, or as a complete severance of a muscle, such as an inferior oblique myectomy procedure.

Setup and preparation of the patient. A muscle tray is needed.

Operative procedure

1. The involved muscle is isolated as in the case of a Z marginal tenotomy.

2. Cuts from opposite sides of the muscle are made through approximately three fourths of the width of the muscle, effectively lengthening the muscle.

3. In the case of the superior oblique muscle, the tendon sheath is opened, and graded sections of tendon are excised according to the needs of the individual patient.

4. Myectomy of the inferior oblique muscle is done in a graded manner by placing two Kelly clamps across the muscle belly lateral to the inferior rectus muscle and excising the isolated strip of muscle. The ends of the muscle are cauterized with a Hildreth cautery and released. Because of the peculiar anatomy of this muscle, lateral discontinuity weakens the muscle but does not paralyze it.

Tuck

Definition. Method of shortening a muscle and thus strengthening it.

Considerations. Tucking is performed primarily on the superior oblique muscle.

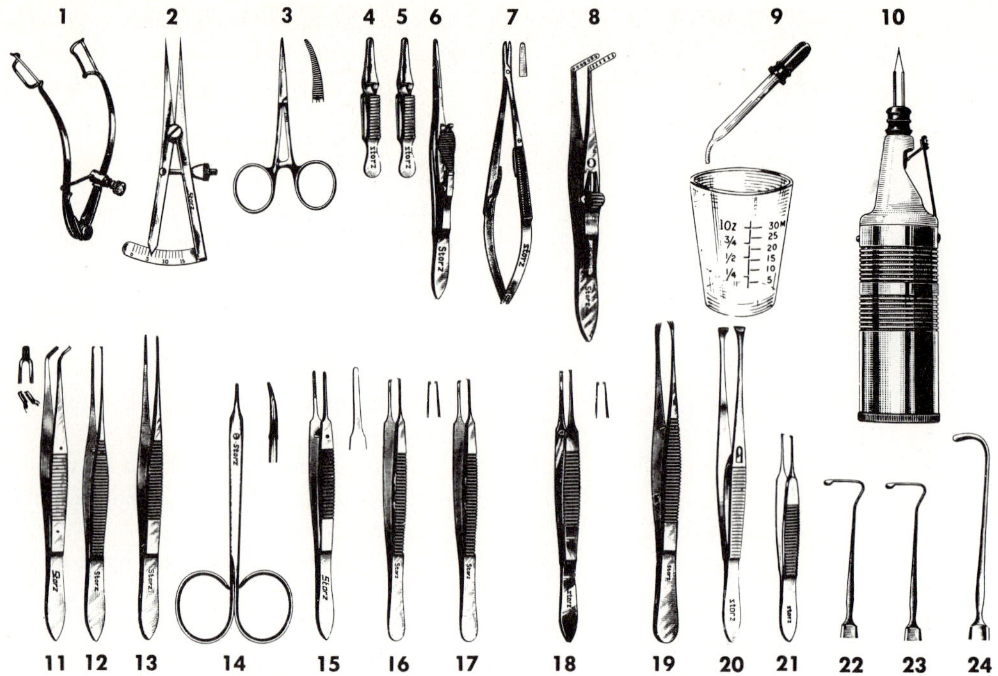

Fig. 23-17. Instruments for eye-muscle operations. *1,* Williams lid speculum; *2,* Castroviejo caliper; *3,* Hartmann curved, short, delicate hemostat; *4* and *5,* small bulldog clamps (serrefine); *6,* Kalt needle holder; *7,* Castroviejo needle holder; *8,* Jameson muscle forceps; *9,* medicine glass with dropper; *10,* Hildreth cautery with white tip; *11,* Quevedo suturing and utility forceps; *12,* heavy serrated straight dressing forceps; *13,* heavy straight tissue forceps with mouse teeth; *14,* Stevens tenotomy scissors; *15,* Thorpe conjunctiva-fixation forceps; *16* and *17,* Lester fixation forceps; *18,* McCullough suture-tying forceps; *19,* Guist fixation forceps; *20,* Graefe fixation forceps; *21,* Graefe iris forceps; *22* and *23,* Jameson muscle hook; *24,* von Graefe muscle hook. (Courtesy Storz Instruments Co., St. Louis.)

Setup and preparation of the patient. A muscle setup, a Fink-Scobie hook, and a Fink tucker are required.

Operative procedure

1. An incision is made in the conjunctiva medial to the superior rectus muscle. The Fink-Scobie hook is passed posteriorly into the orbit, and the superior oblique muscle is hooked and brought into the incision. The Fink tucker is placed over the tendon, and a graded doubling of the tendon, like looping a rope, is completed. A double-armed Supramid suture is passed through the base of the loop, effectively shortening the muscle. The tip of the loop is sutured to the sclera. (The surgeon often may attempt to tuck the muscle lateral to the superior rectus muscle.)
2. The conjunctiva is closed with absorbable sutures.

SURGERY OF THE GLOBE AND ORBIT

Considerations. Rupture of the eyeball may be direct at the site of injury or, more frequently, indirect from an increase in intraocular pressure, causing the wall of the eyeball to tear at weaker points such as the limbus. When the intraocular contents have become deranged so that useful function is prohibited, removal of the eye contents (evisceration procedure) or of the entire eyeball (enucleation) is indicated. If either procedure is required, implantation of an inert globe may be used as a space filler and to aid in the movement of a prosthesis (artificial eye) Fig. 23-18).

Fractures of the walls of the orbit (Fig. 23-19) may be caused by direct blows or by extension of a fracture line from adjacent bones (Figs. 23-19 and 23-20). Isolated orbital-floor, or blowout, fractures usually follow injury to the region of the eye by an object the size of an apple or an adult's fist. Orbital contents herniate into the maxillary sinus, and the inferior rectus or inferior oblique muscle may become incarcerated at the fracture site. A Caldwell-Luc antrostomy (Chapter 22) may be done with reduction of the fracture from below, or the fracture site may be approached directly through the lower lid along the orbital floor and the prolapsed tissue reduced, the orbital floor reduced, and the orbital-floor defect bridged with a graft of bone, cartilage, or plastic material.

Repair of laceration. The preferred method of closing corneal lacerations is the use of direct appositional suturing with the aid of an operating microscope. The suture material used is generally no. 8-0 or finer.

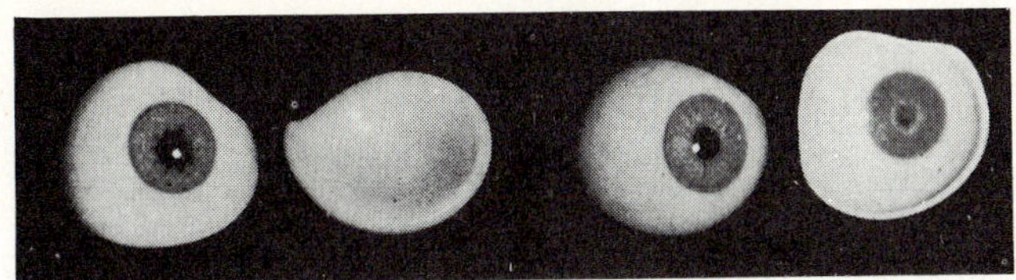

Fig. 23-18. Artificial eyes. Shell prosthesis is seen at right. (From Allen, J.H., editor: May's manual of the diseases of the eye, ed. 23, Baltimore, The Williams & Wilkins Co.)

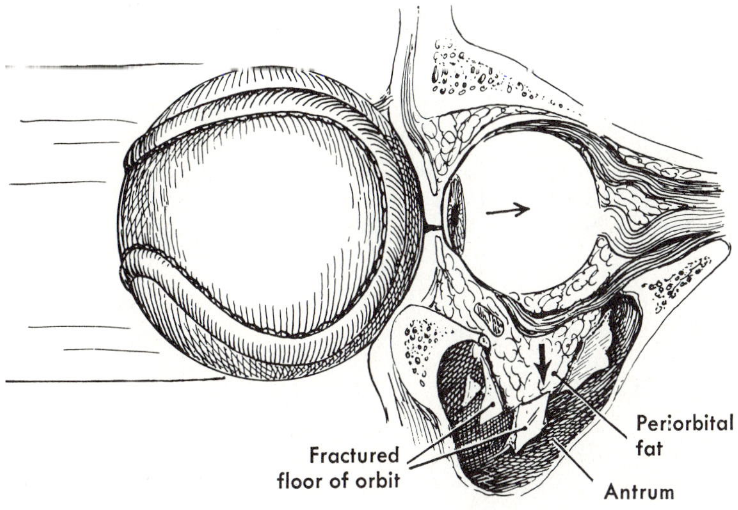

Fig. 23-19. Ball has struck rim of orbit and has pressed orbital contents backward, displacing fragments of bone into maxillary sinus. Inferior rectus muscle is incarcerated in fracture. At times, inferior oblique muscle may also be involved. (From Paton, R.T., and Katzin, H.M.: Atlas of eye surgery, ed. 2, New York, McGraw-Hill Book Co.)

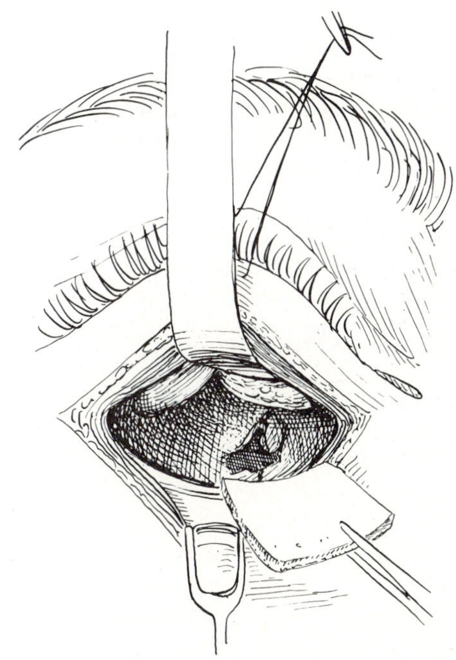

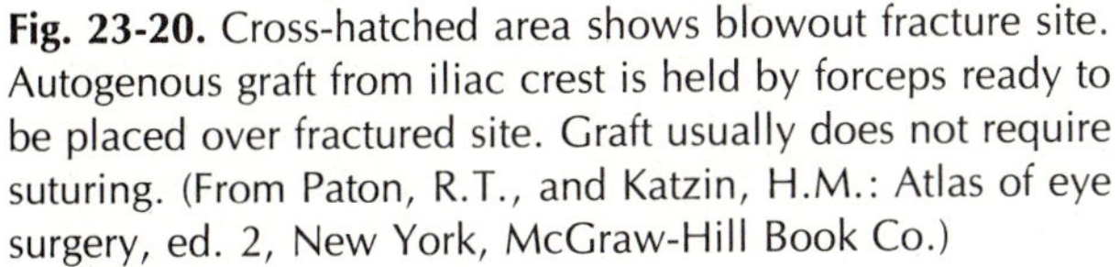

Fig. 23-20. Cross-hatched area shows blowout fracture site. Autogenous graft from iliac crest is held by forceps ready to be placed over fractured site. Graft usually does not require suturing. (From Paton, R.T., and Katzin, H.M.: Atlas of eye surgery, ed. 2, New York, McGraw-Hill Book Co.)

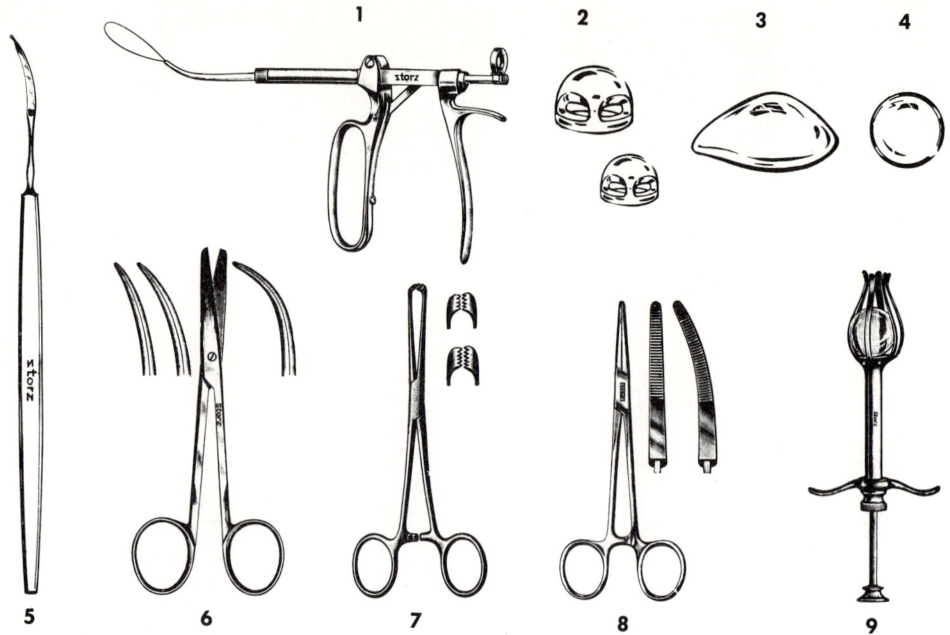

Fig. 23-21. Instruments for enucleation. *1,* Castroviejo enucleation snare; *2,* Allen implants, large and small; *3,* conformer; *4,* mule eye sphere; *5,* canaliculus knife; *6,* enucleation scissors; *7,* Allis forceps; *8,* Kelly forceps; *9,* Carter sphere introducer. (Courtesy Storz Instrument Co., St. Louis.)

Experimentally, tissue adhesives, that is, cyanoacrylate monomers, are being used. The tissue adhesive is applied to the well-dried tissue that has been properly oriented anatomically, and it polymerizes and seals the wound on contact with the tissue. The tissue adhesive is supplied in packaged sterile vials (Co-Apt).

Cultures are usually obtained at the time of surgery, and subconjunctival antibiotics are injected postoperatively before the dressings are applied.

Enucleation

Definition. Removal of the entire eyeball.

Setup and preparation of the patient. A muscle setup is needed, plus the following (Fig. 23-21):

- 1 Enucleation snare
- 1 Implant, as desired
  - Conformer
  - Mule eye sphere
- 1 Weber canaliculus knife
- 1 Enucleation scissors
- 1 Allis forceps
- 1 Kelly clamp, large
- 1 Eye sphere with introducer and holder

Operative procedure

1. A speculum retractor is introduced into the palpebral fissure.
2. The conjunctiva is divided around the cornea with a curved Weber canaliculus knife and forceps.
3. The medial, lateral, inferior, and superior rectus muscles are divided, leaving a stump of medial rectus muscle. The globe is separated from Tenon's capsule with blunt-pointed, curved scissors, retractors, hemostats, and forceps.
4. The eye is rotated laterally, using the stump of the medial rectus muscle.
5. A large curved hemostat is passed behind the globe, and the optic nerve is clamped for 60 seconds. The hemostat is removed, enucleation scissors are passed posteriorly, and the optic nerve is transected. The oblique muscles are severed as the eye is lifted out of the socket by the stump of the medial rectus muscle.
6. The muscle cone is packed with saline sponges to obtain hemostasis.
7. The muscle cone is filled with an implant, and careful closure of Tenon's capsule and conjunctiva is completed.
8. A socket conformer with ointment is placed in the cul-de-sac.
9. A pressure dressing, usually of the head roll type, is applied.

Evisceration

Definition. Removal of the contents of the eye, leaving the sclera intact and the muscles attached to the sclera.

Setup and preparation of the patient. As described for enucleation (Fig. 23-21).

Operative procedure

1. The conjunctiva is not separated from the sclera as it is for enucleation. A sharp-pointed knife is inserted through the limbus anterior to the iris.

2. The contents of the eye (iris, vitreous, lens) are removed.

3. The choroid adhering to the sclera is removed with curettes.

4. Bleeding is controlled with delicate hemostatic forceps, electrocoagulation, and sutures.

5. A plastic implant is now placed within the empty shell.

6. The conjunctival scleral edges are brought together with silk sutures no. 4-0 or 5-0, and a pressure bandage is applied.

Repair of fracture of the orbit (blowout)

Definition. Repair of the fractured orbit by means of graft or realignment of contents of the orbit (Fig. 23-20).

Setup and preparation of the patient. The setup is as for dacryocystorhinostomy, plus a graft set (for implantation of an autogenous graft or synthetic graft materials of various sizes and thicknesses) and a flexible, narrow-width retractor. The patient is prepared as described for eye surgery. A general anesthetic is usually administered.

Operative procedure

1. The maximum ocular rotation is tested by exerting traction with a forceps on the tendon of the inferior rectus muscle to determine if the inferior muscle sling is trapped in the fracture.

2. To distribute tension over the lower lid and put the orbicular muscle on stretch, a traction suture is inserted through the lower lid margin.

3. With a Bard-Parker no. 3 knife handle and no. 15 blade, the lower lid is incised in the lid fold above the orbital rim.

4. The skin is separated from the orbicular muscle, and the orbital septum is identified by blunt dissection. Dissection is continued down to the periosteum of the orbital rim by means of scissors, loop retractors, elevators, and forceps.

5. The periosteum of the orbital rim is incised with a no. 15 blade. With periosteal elevators, the floor of the orbit is exposed and explored. When the fracture site is identified, bone spicules are removed, and the herniated contents are freed from the maxillary antrum. The contents of the orbit are elevated by means of narrow-width, flexible retractors, and a traction suture of black silk no. 4-0 is placed around the tendon of the inferior rectus muscle.

6. An autogenous graft is taken from the iliac crest, or an alloplastic material of proper size is used to repair the bony defect. The material may or may not be anchored to the orbital rim by wire sutures.

7. The periosteum is carefully closed with chromic sutures no. 4-0.

8. The skin is closed with black silk no. 6-0, and a pressure dressing is applied.

Exenteration

Definition. Removal of the entire orbital contents, including periosteum, for certain malignancies of the globe or orbit.

Setup and preparation of the patient. As described for fracture of the orbit. General anesthesia is usually employed.

Operative procedure

1. Depending on circumstances, exenteration of the eye may or may not include the removal of the lids. An incision is made down to the orbital rim, through the periosteum, and around the entire orbit.

2. With periosteal elevators, the periosteum is freed from the orbital walls and the apex of the orbit.

3. The optic nerve is clamped, and the entire contents of the orbit are removed en bloc.

4. Hemostasis is obtained by the use of cautery and bone wax.

5. A skin graft or temporal muscle implant may be used to fill the orbital cavity, but this is not usually done.

6. Iodoform gauze is used to fill the cavity, a pressure dressing is put in place, and the cavity is allowed to granulate.

Corneal transplant (keratoplasty)

Definition. Grafting of corneal tissue from one human eye to another (Figs. 23-22 and 23-23).

Keratoplasty may be classified as follows: (1) lamellar (partial-thickness) graft, (2) penetrating (whole thickness) graft, (3) keratectomy (peeling of the cornea), and (4) tattooing (simulation of a pupil—rarely done).

Considerations. A corneal transplant is performed in the presence of corneal thickening and opacification. Impairment of the transparency of the cornea may be the result of infection, thermal or chemical burns, or certain diseases of unknown cause.

A corneal transplant is done to improve vision in cases in which the basic visual structures of the eye, that is, the retina and the optic nerve, are properly functioning.

Corneas are obtained from recently deceased persons. Eye banks help coordinate services for such operations.

Setup and preparation of the patient. The basic cataract set plus special transplant instruments is used (Fig. 23-24).

1 Needle, blunt, 30 gauge
2 Katzin corneal transplant scissors, 1 right and 1 left
1 Paton double-ended spatula
1 Castroviejo double-ended spatula
1 Allis forceps
1 Castroviejo corneal trephine (surgeon will state size needed)

1 Corneal carrying case
1 Barraquer wire speculum
1 Double Flieringa-LeGrand fixation ring
1 Barraquer needle holder
1 Bonn forceps, 0.12-mm teeth
2 Jeweler's forceps
Operating microscope (Fig. 23-25)

Lamellar transplant

Castroviejo electrokeratome with shims
1 Gill corneal splitter
1 Paufique knife
1 Bard-Parker no. 3 knife handle with no. 15 blade
1 Beaver no. 3H knife handle with no. 64 blade

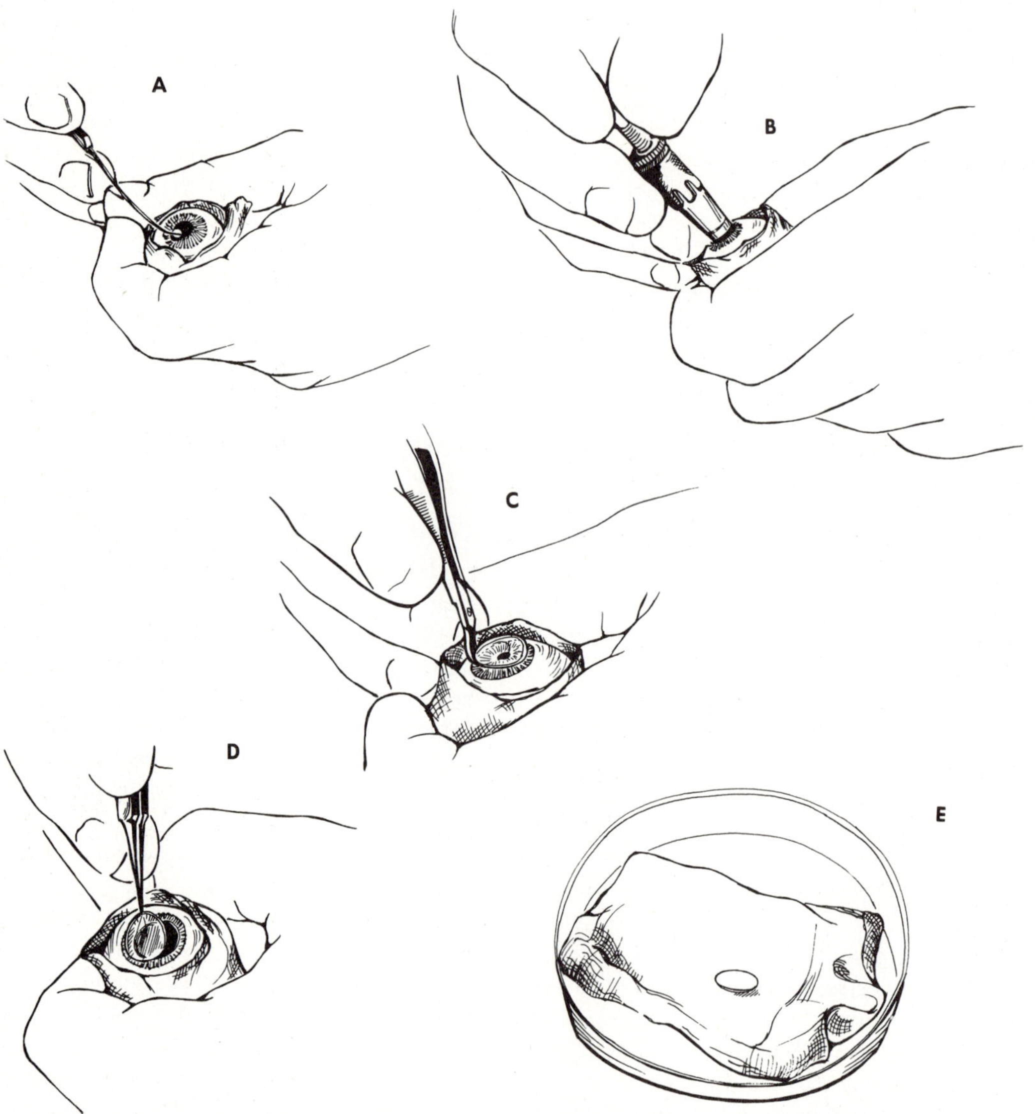

Fig. 23-22. A, Epithelium from donor cornea is being removed by abrading with iris spatula. Donor eye is wrapped in smooth cloth dressing. **B,** Donor eye is firmly grasped in surgeon's left hand, and corneal trephine is centered on donor eye. With twisting motion, cornea is cut through its entire thickness. **C,** Corneal scissors are used to cut any areas of corneal tissue that have not been penetrated by trephine. **D,** Corneal button is removed with fine forceps, with care taken not to touch endothelial surface. **E,** Donor corneal button is stored on moistened gauze pad, endothelial side up in covered Petri dish to preserve moisture.

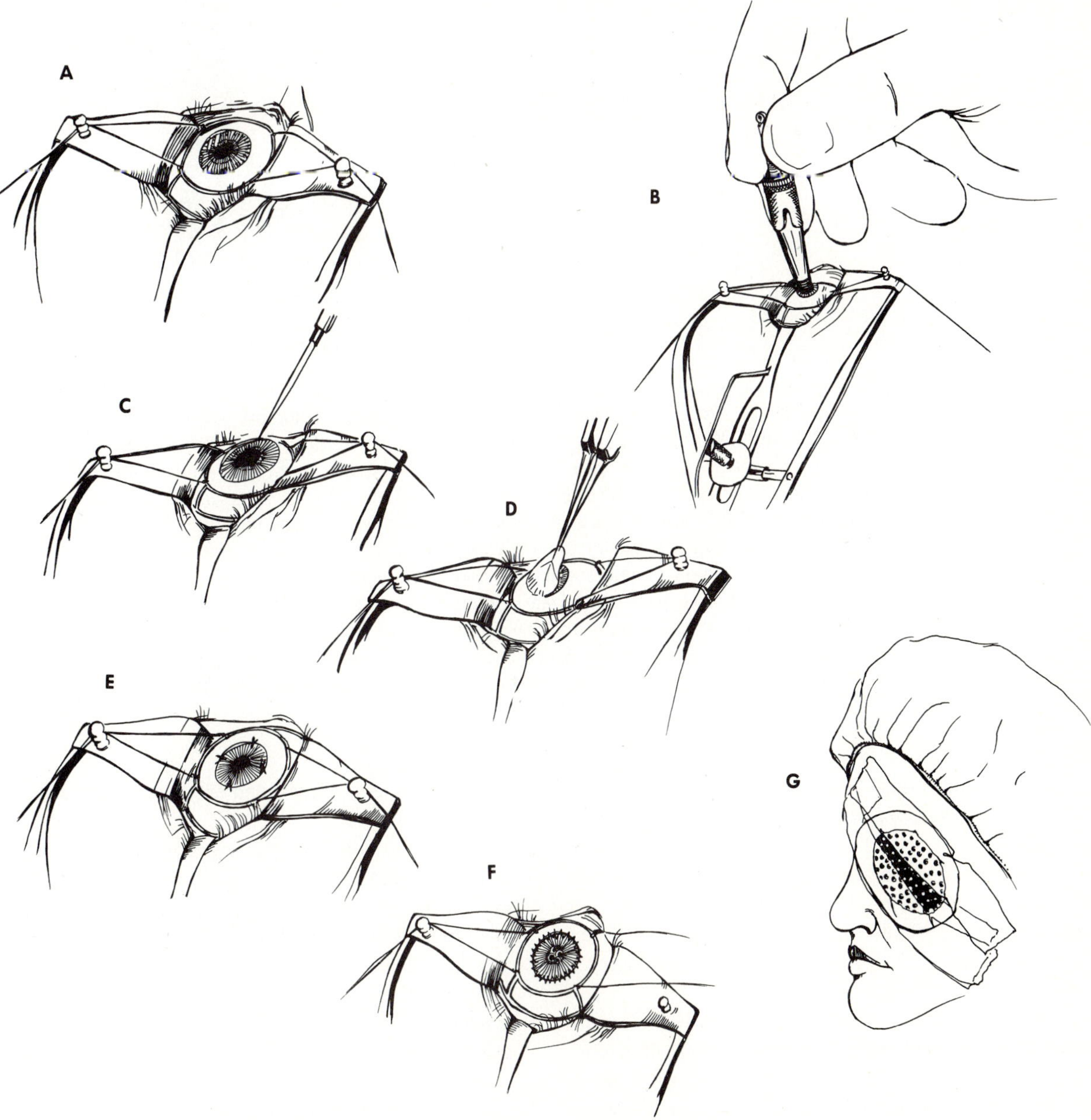

Fig. 23-23. A, Eye of patient who will undergo combined procedure including corneal transplantation and cataract extraction. Double Bonaccolto-Flieringa fixation ring is sutured in place with no. 5-0 Dacron sutures posted over solid bladed eye speculum. **B,** Corneal trephine is placed on recipient cornea, and partial penetration is made approximately three fourths through stroma. **C,** Anterior chamber is entered through groove with Wheeler knife. Remainder of button is excised with right and left micro–Katzin corneal scissors. **D,** Corneal button is removed. **E,** Donor button sutured in place with four no. 8-0 black silk sutures. **F,** Cornea sutured in place with continuous no. 10-0 suture with air in anterior chamber. **G,** Patient postoperatively with Fox shield properly applied on bony margins.

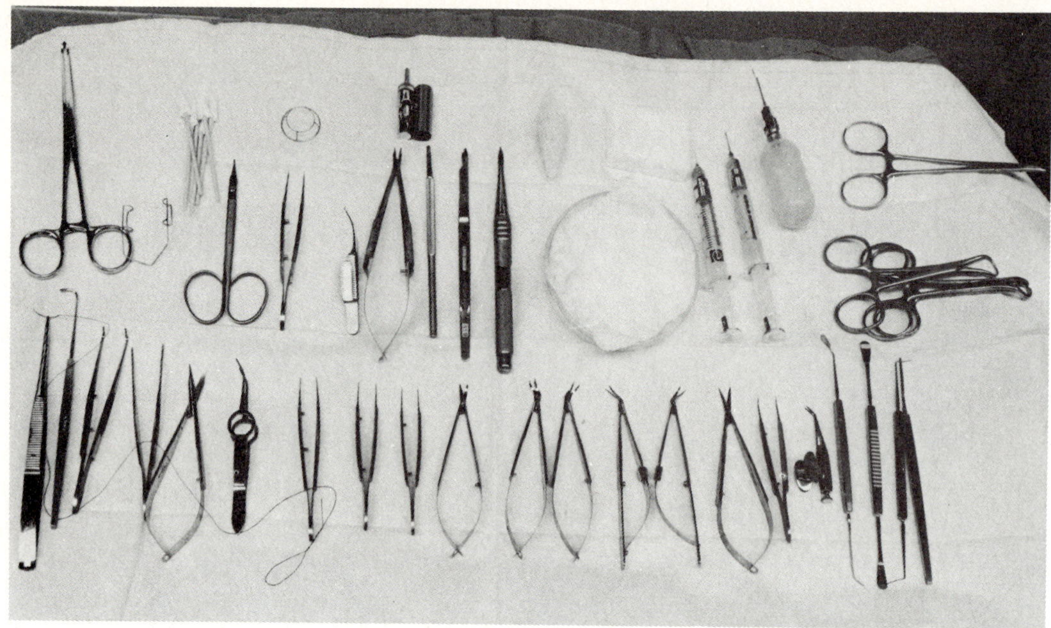

Fig. 23-24. Instruments used in corneal transplant. *Top row, left to right,* Allis forceps; Barraquer lid speculum; Weck-cel spears; Stevens scissors; Flieringa-LeGrand fixation ring; Bonn forceps, 0.12 mm; Colibri forceps, 0.12 mm; Barraquer needle holder; Castroviejo corneal trephine with metal guard; Beaver knife with no. 64 blade; Bard-Parker knife with no. 15 blade; razor blade breaker and holder; Petri dish; Silastic block; 2-ml syringe with air injection cannula; 2-ml syringe with 19-gauge blunt needle; Bishop-Harmon AC irrigator with cannula; mosquito hemostat; small towel clamps. *Bottom row, left to right,* Castroviejo needle holder; von Graefe strabismus hook; Quevedo utility forceps; serrated conjunctival forceps; Wescott scissors; Schaaf forceps; two straight McPherson forceps; small, curved Castroviejo scissors; right and left Castroviejo scissors; right and left Troutman scissors; fine-stitch scissors; angled McPherson scissors; angled McPherson forceps; Barraquer iris scissors; Paton spatula; Green spatula; Castroviejo double-ended spatula; iris repositor.

Operative procedure

Penetrating keratoplasty (performed with operating microscope)

1. The eye speculum is put in place, and superior rectus and inferior rectus bridle sutures are placed, if a double Flieringa-LeGrand ring is not to be used. If a ring is used, it is sutured in place with four Dacron sutures no. 5-0.

2. The eye from the eye bank is removed from its container and washed in Neosporin solution, or a corneoscleral button that has been stored in tissue culture medium or that has been frozen (and is thawed) is removed from its container.

3. The donor eye is then wrapped in surgical dressing for stabilization. The cornea is excised from the donor eye by means of a corneal trephine cataract knife, corneal scissors, and forceps after the epithelium is removed with a sponge. The graft is placed, epithelial side down, in a Petri dish containing a saline-moistened gauze (Fig. 23-22, *E*). Some surgeons preplace sutures in the graft. Others place the corneoscleral button epithelial (outside) surface down in a sterile Teflon block. The corneal trephine is then used as a punch, and the donor button is pressed out centrally.

4. The section of cornea removed from the recipient's eye is the same size as the graft taken from the donor's eye. A groove is made with the identical trephine used to obtain the donor button set at 0.3 to 0.4 mm. The anterior chamber is entered with one of the variety of cataract knives, and the button is excised with corneal scissors. (Care must be taken to close the guard on the trephine after use to prevent damage to the cutting surface.)

5. Peripheral iridectomies or iridotomies may be performed at this time according to the surgeon's discretion, or a cataract extraction may be completed if the lens is opaque.

6. The graft is placed into the opening of the recipient's eye and anchored in place by means of four to eight single-armed black silk sutures no. 8-0 placed at the four cardinal meridians, using an operating microscope. The graft is now sutured to the host with either continuous or interrupted nylon sutures no. 10-0 (Fig. 23-23, *F*).

7. Air may be injected into the anterior chamber of

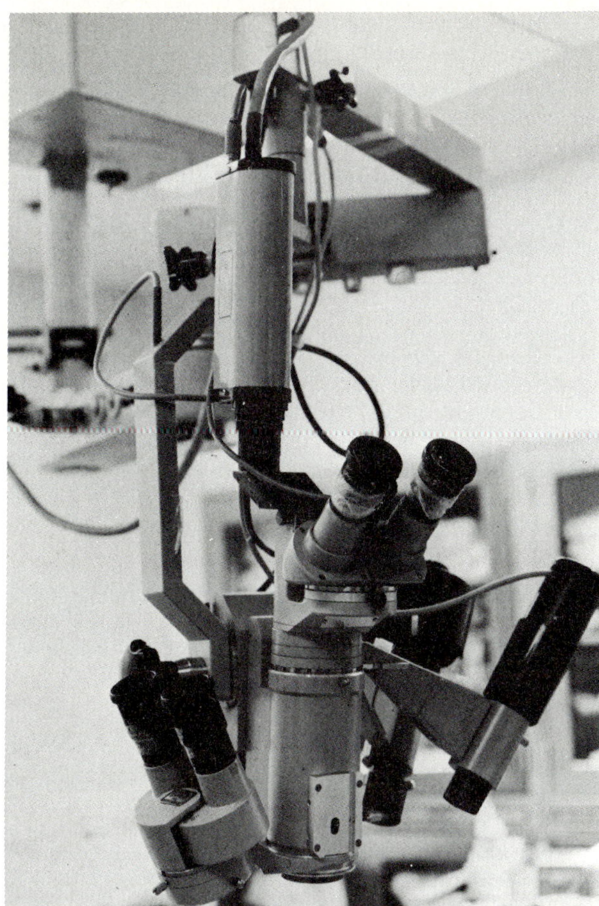

Fig. 23-25. General operating microscope with television attachments.

the recipient's eye to keep the iris from sticking to the suture line. Mydriatic or miotic solutions are used at the surgeon's discretion.

8. A subconjunctival injection of antibiotic solution or a topical application of antibiotic drops may be used at the completion of the procedure. A splint, eye patch, and metal guard are applied.

Lamellar keratoplasty

1. The eye speculum and superior rectus and inferior rectus bridal sutures are placed.

2. The eye from the eye bank is removed from its container and washed in Neosporin solution.

3. The eye is wrapped in surgical dressing. A groove is made at the desired depth in the cornea with the trephine. The Castroviejo keratome is now set at the desired depth and the lamellar sheet of cornea is removed and placed in a Petri dish.

4. The recipient cornea is grooved with the same trephine to the appropriate depth. Using the operating microscope, the surgeon performs a lamellar resection, that is, removes the anterior part of the cornea at a predetermined depth with a Gill knife, Beaver knife blade no. 64, or other corneal splitter.

5. The donor tissue is sutured in place with a continuous 10-0 nylon suture.

6. A mydriatic agent and subconjunctival or topical antibiotics may then be used.

7. The eye is patched.

Eye bank procedure

Definition. Removal of eyes immediately after death in accordance with legal regulations.

Considerations. The bank may be a central community agency or may be maintained by the hospital. The containers for eyes and regulations for the procedure are generally obtained from the bank. The enucleations are usually done in the hospital morgue under aseptic conditions.

A special consent form is required and should be signed by the authorized next of kin and by the hospital administrative office.

Setup and preparation of the donor. The instrument setup consists of a modified enucleation set, including the following:

1 Stevens scissors
1 Suture scissors
1 Enucleation scissors
1 Knife handle no. 3 with no. 15 blade
2 Lester forceps
2 Conjunctival forceps
2 Muscle hooks
1 Allis clamp, short
3 Towel clamps
2 Mosquito hemostats
1 Modified Guyton-Park speculum
1 Medicine glass
2 Eye specimen bottles

The eyes are washed and irrigated in the routine manner of preparation for eye surgery. The sterile field, drapes, and instruments are essentially the same as for an enucleation on a living patient.

Operative procedure

1. Eye specimen bottles are labeled for right and left eyes. The speculum is inserted, and after routine enucleation the donated eye is placed in the sterile specimen bottle with the cornea up. The eye is supported on a sponge that has been soaked in saline solution. An antibiotic solution may be placed on the cornea. The eye sockets are packed with cotton and the lids closed.

2. Specimen bottles are sealed with tape and labeled with the donor's name, time and cause of death, time of enucleation, and date.

Appropriate specimens may be placed in tissue culture medium for short-term storage (9 to 10 days) or frozen for long-term storage after appropriate manipulation.

Radial keratotomy

Definition. Series of spoke-like superficial incisions from the edge of the cornea toward the center, leaving the visual axis intact. The result is a flattening of the cornea that will reduce the refractive error and improve vision. Correction can be seen in as little as 24 hours but can fluctuate up to 4 months.

Considerations. Radial keratotomy has been performed in Japan since 1953 but has only recently been introduced in the United States. The procedure is designed to improve vision for myopia and is being performed on a limited basis.

Although limited knowledge is available on long-term effects, some complications that can occur from surgery are corneal epithelial healing defects, corneal perforation, lack of permanent corneal curvature change, and variable visual acuity.

As more data is gathered in the next several years, radial keratotomy may gain wide acceptance in the treatment of myopia.

Setup and preparation of the patient. Since this is a superficial procedure, it can be performed under local anesthesia. Skin preparation and draping are as previously described.

The operating microscope is employed, and the following instruments are required:

1 Lid speculum
2 Corneal trephines, 3 mm and 2.5 mm
1 Castroviejo forceps, 0.12 mm
Keratotomy blades
Micrometer, capable of measuring 0.02 mm increments

Operative procedure

1. By use of the operating microscope, the central visual axis of the cornea is marked and stained.
2. A 3-mm blunt trephine is used to inscribe the area around the axis.
3. The outer perimeter of the cornea is inscribed in the same manner.
4. Radial incisions are made, joining the two rings. The number and depth of the incisions are predetermined according to the amount of correction desired.
5. Subconjunctival injections of steroid and antibiotic are given, and a patch is applied.

Surgery of the lens (cataract operation, generally with operating microscope)

Definition. Extraction of the opaque lens from the interior of the eye.

Considerations. The lens consists of 64% to 65% water, 34% to 35% protein, and a trace of other body minerals. The disorders of the lens are opacification and dislocation, resulting in blurred vision without pain or inflammation.

Cataracts (opacification) vary in degree of density, size, and location and are usually caused by aging or trauma.

Various methods, basically intracapsular or extracapsular extraction, are used to remove the lens.

The intracapsular method of cataract removal consists of removing the lens within its capsule.

In the extracapsular method, the anterior portion of the capsule is first ruptured and removed, and the lens cortex and nucleus are expressed from the eye, leaving the posterior capsule behind. The intracapsular method is the procedure of choice in most cases.

Setup and preparation of the patient. A basic setup for eye surgery is needed, plus the following (Fig. 23-26):

Weck-cel sponges
1 Guyton-Park lid speculum
1 Castroviejo corneal forceps
1 Quevedo utility forceps
1 Conjunctival forceps with teeth
1 Conjunctival forceps, serrated
1 Allis fixation forceps
1 Graefe iris forceps, curved, with teeth
2 McCullough suture forceps
1 Arruga capsule forceps
1 Straight iris forceps
2 Kalt needle holders
1 Iris repositor
1 Spoon
1 Lens expressor
1 von Graefe muscle hook
1 Lens loop
1 Cyclodialysis spatula
1 Hildreth cautery with tips
1 Plastic anterior chamber irrigator with tip
1 Stevens scissors
1 Westcott scissors
1 Iris scissors
1 Corneal scissors
1 von Graefe knife
1 Keratome knife
1 Bard-Parker no. 9 knife handle with no. 15 blade
1 Beaver no. 3H knife handle with no. 64 blade
1 Bonn forceps
1 Operating microscope (Fig. 23-25)

The patient is prepared as described for general ophthalmic surgery.

Operative procedure

Intracapsular method (Fig. 23-27)

1. A speculum is placed in the eye to hold the lids apart.
2. The globe is held by transfixion with a silk suture no. 4-0, which is inserted under the tendon of the superior rectus muscle and clamped to the drape. A conjunctival flap, either limbal or fornix based, may be prepared with the use of scissors. Some surgeons do not dissect a flap.
3. Bleeding points are controlled by means of bipolar cautery, which provides maximum cauterization with minimum tissue necrosis. Partially penetrating incisions (grooves) are made at the limbus or in the cornea.
4. Corneoscleral or corneocorneal sutures are passed

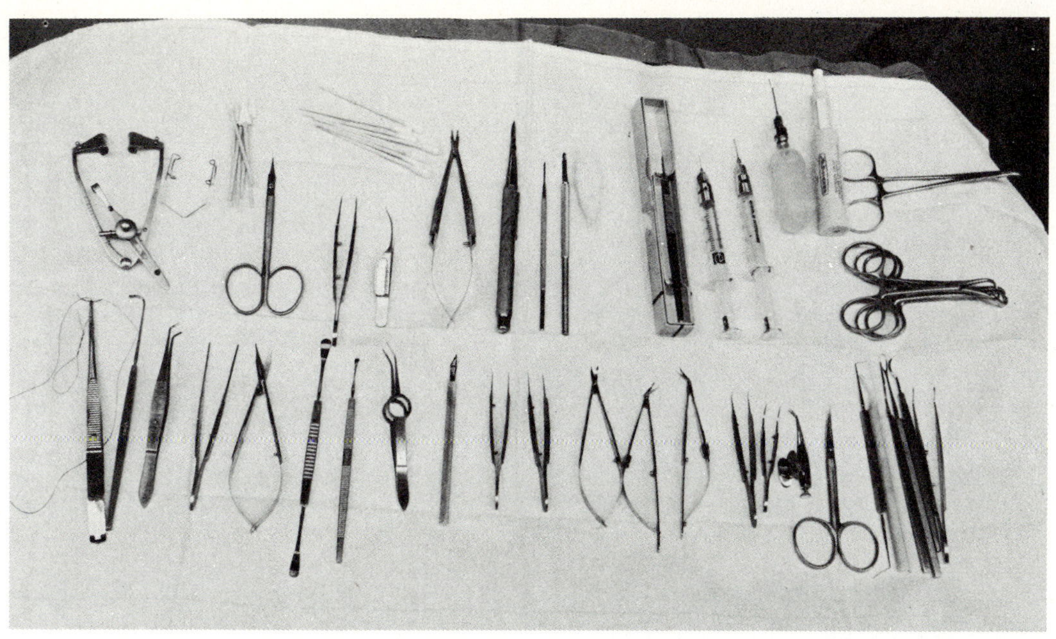

Fig. 23-26. Cataract-extraction instruments. *Top row, left to right,* Guyton-Park eye speculum; Barraquer lid speculum; Weck-cel spears; Stevens scissors; Bonn forceps, 0.12 mm; Colibri forceps, 0.12 mm; Barraquer needle holder; razor blade breaker and holder; twist-grip scleral fixator; Beaver knife with no. 64 blade; von Graefe knife; 2-ml syringe with air-injection cannula; 2-ml syringe with 19-gauge blunt needle; Bishop-Harmon AC irrigator with cannula; disposable cautery; mosquito hemostat; small towel clamps. *Bottom row, left to right,* Castroviejo needle holder; von Graefe strabismus hook; Quevedo utility forceps; serrated conjunctival forceps; Wescott scissors; Green spatula; Gill corneal dissector; Schaaf forceps; Drews suture pickup; two straight McPherson forceps; small, curved Castroviejo scissors; right and left Troutman scissors; angled McPherson forceps; Jervey iris forceps; Barraquer-De Wecker iris scissors; Knapp scissors; Castroviejo double-ended spatula; Rosebaum-Drews iris retractor; straight iris repositor; Wilder lens loop; Berens lens expressor; Arruga forceps.

through the lips of the wounds. These sutures are looped out of the groove and set in an orderly manner around the margins of the incision.

5. With the keratome, von Graefe, or razor knife, the anterior chamber is entered, and the limbal wound is enlarged with corneal scissors.

6. A peripheral iridectomy or sector iridectomy is performed. Alpha chymotrypsin (Zolyse) is injected through the iridectomy. The lens is grasped, in most cases with a cryoextractor, and extracted slowly from the eye (Fig. 23-28).

7. For the past 10 to 15 years, many surgeons in the United States have been following the lead of their European counterparts and have been implanting artificial lenses of methyl methacrylate (pseudophake) that ride in the iris plane. Basically, two types of lenses are currently in use: (1) lenses that are sutured to the iris with various fine, nonabsorbable materials, such as 9-0 or 10-0 Ethilon, Supramid, or Perlon, and (2) lenses that depend on their design and the integrity of the pupillary sphincter to hold the lens in place. The lenses are available in various powers at 0.5-diopter steps. Depending on the manufacturer of the lens to be used, different procedural steps must be followed before insertion. Nursing personnel must become familiar with directions associated with each lens type in use at their institution (Fig. 23-29). After insertion of an intraocular lens, it is common to use acetylcholine (Miochol) to cause rapid pupillary constriction.

8. The corneoscleral sutures are tied, and the conjunctival flap is reapproximated with either absorbable or nonabsorbable sutures of the desired size.

9. Pilocarpine 2% or atropine 1% is topically administered. Antibiotics may be used topically or subconjunctivally. The eye is dressed and patched.

10. If, at any time during the operation, vitreous gel is extruded from the eye, a partial vitrectomy is performed to prevent vitreous from becoming incorporated into the wound, which can lead to various postoperative complications. The first step usually involves an attempt to aspirate liquefied vitreous from the eye with a 19-gauge blunt needle on a 2-ml syringe. Once this is accomplished, solid vitreous may be removed by the use of Weck-cel sponges and scissors (Wescott) or by using any of the various vitrectomy instruments available (Fig. 23-30).

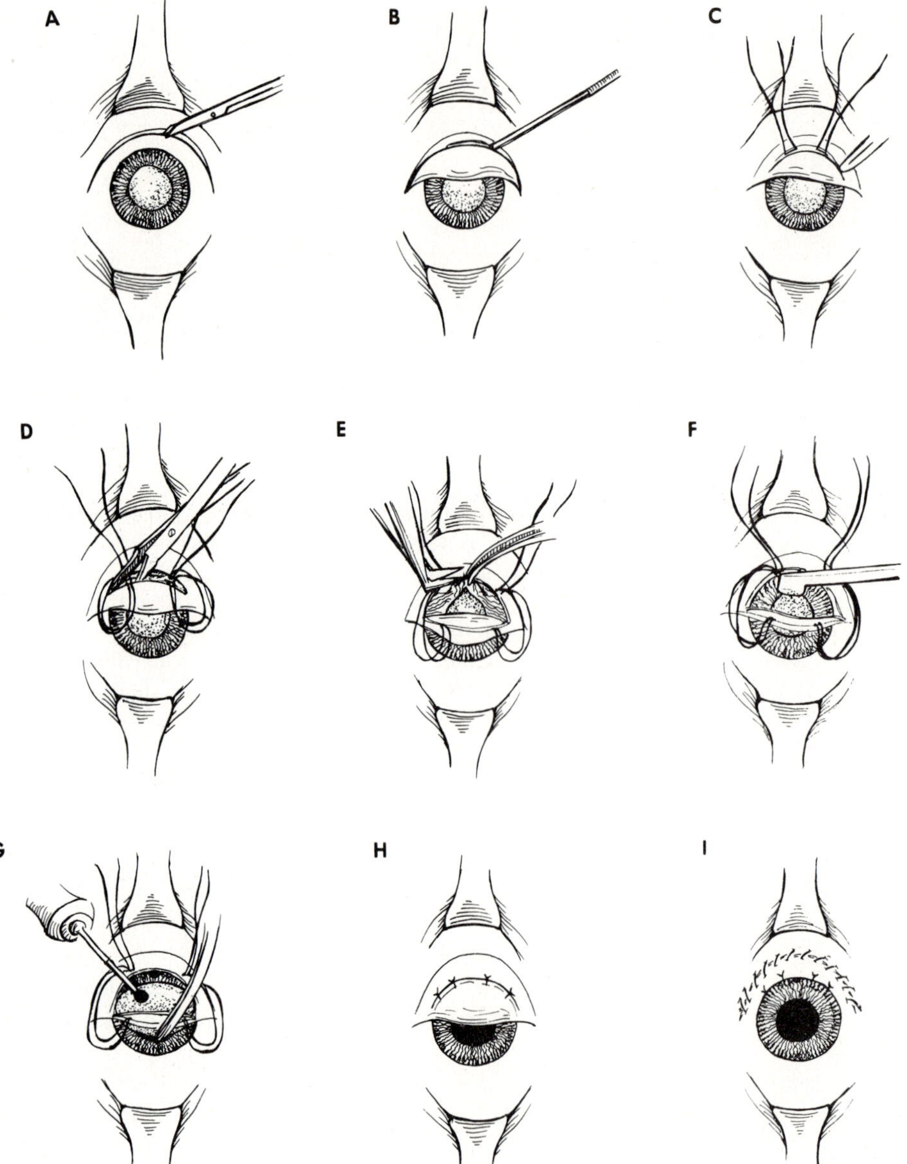

Fig. 23-27. Intracapsular lens extraction. **A,** Preparation of conjunctival flap with scissors. **B,** Nonpenetrating (partial-thickness) incision made at limbus or in cornea. **C,** Corneoscleral sutures are placed. **D,** Limbal incision completed with scissors. **E,** Peripheral iridectomy is performed. **F,** Iris retractor in place for delivery of lens. **G,** Lens grasped and pulled slowly from eye with cryostat unit. **H,** Corneoscleral sutures tied. **I,** Conjunctival flap reapproximated and sutured. (Adapted from King, J.H., and Wadsworth, J.A.C.: An atlas of ophthalmic surgery, ed. 2, Philadelphia, 1970, J.B. Lippincott Co.)

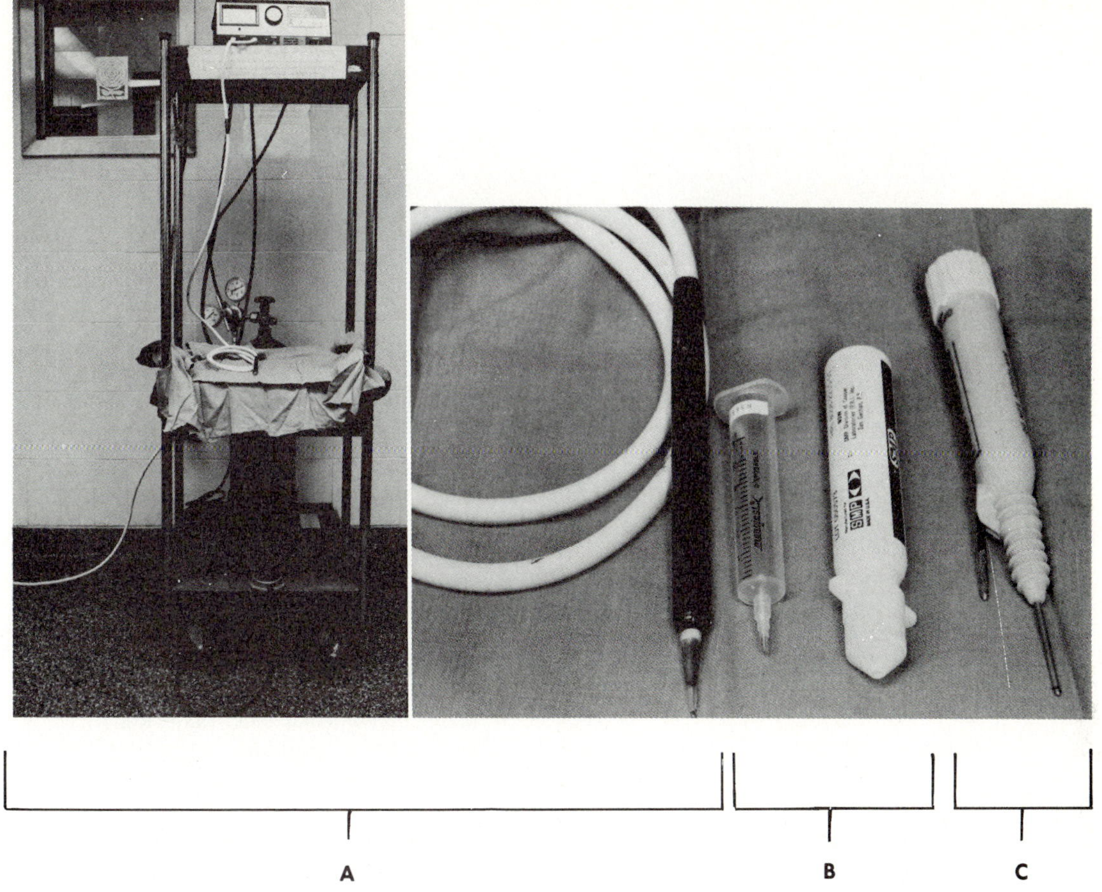

Fig. 23-28. Cryoextractors. **A,** Amoils electrical cataract cryoextractor. **B,** SMP disposable cryoextractor. **C,** Frigitronics disposable cryoextractor.

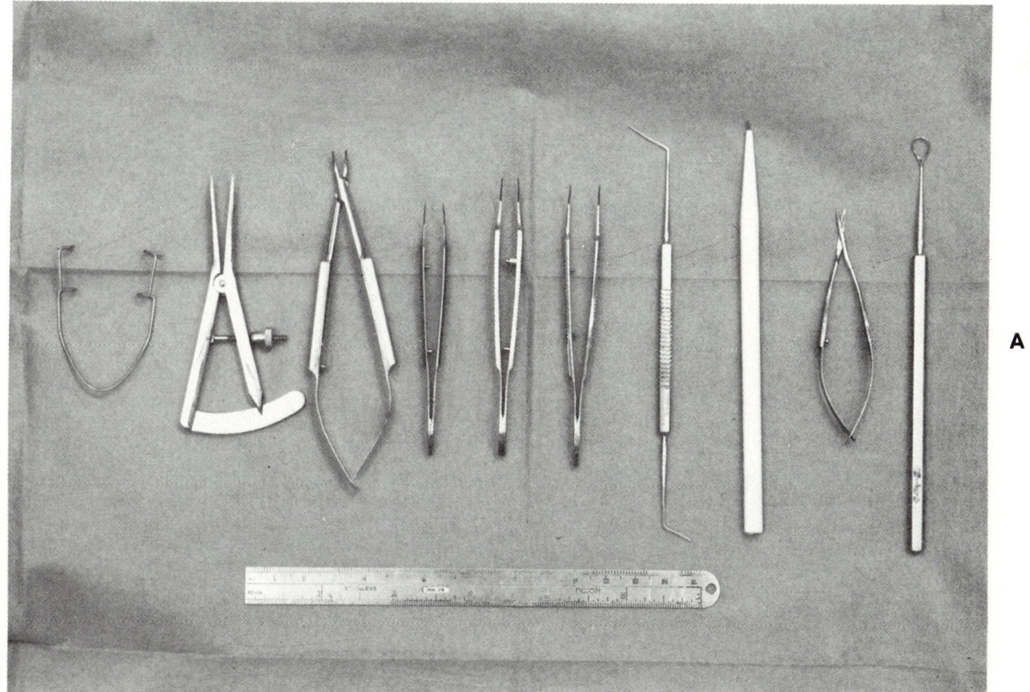

Fig. 23-29. A, Extra instruments for lens implants. *Left to right,* Wire speculum, caliper, needle holder, straight McPherson forceps, angled McPherson forceps with teeth, smooth angled McPherson forceps, Castroviejo spatula, Super blade, corneal scissors, lens loop, ruler.

Continued.

B

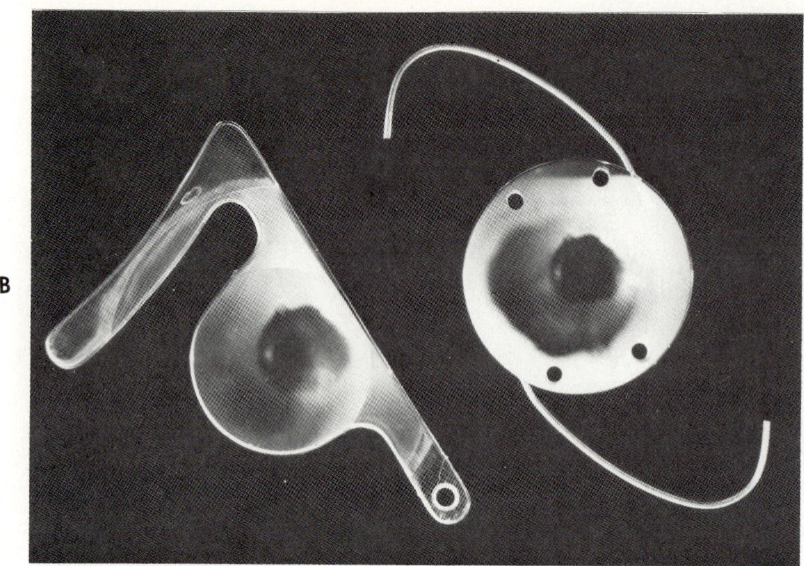

Fig. 23-29, cont'd. B, *Left,* Kelman type II anterior chamber intraocular lens; *right,* Kratz variation posterior chamber intraocular lens, elliptical open loop.

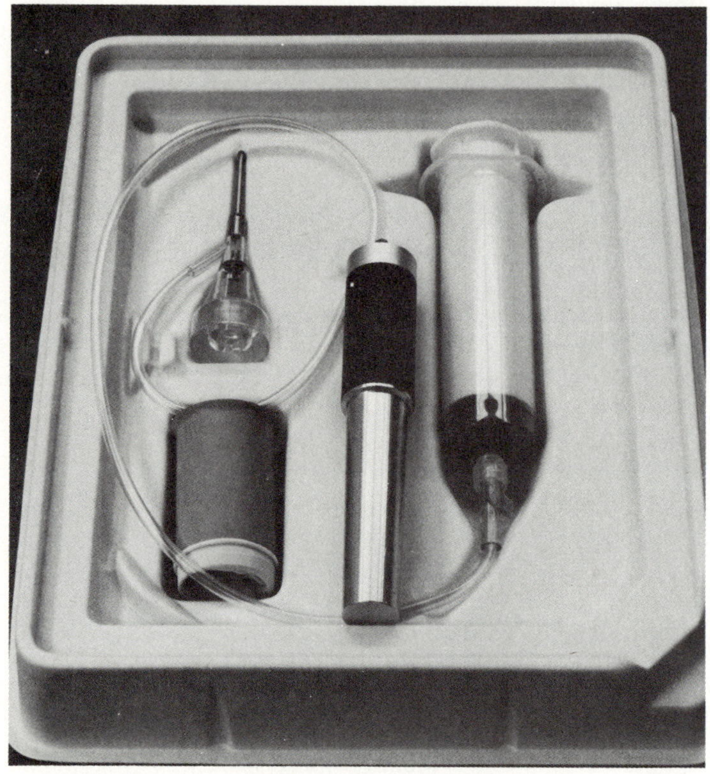

Fig. 23-30. Disposable Kaufman vitrector.

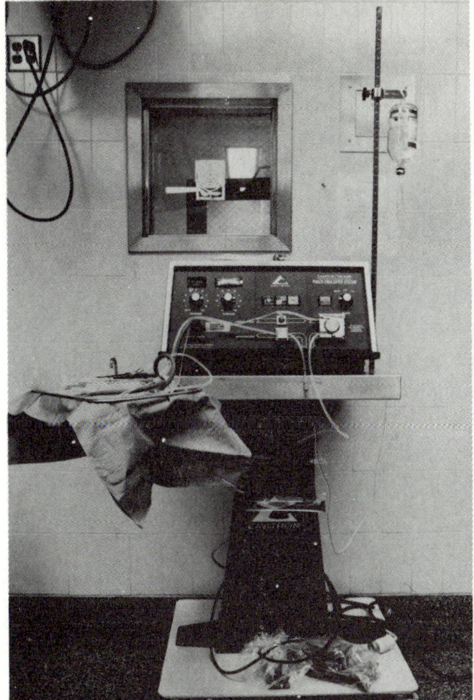

Fig. 23-31. Phacoemulsifier system with water-resistant covers on foot pedals.

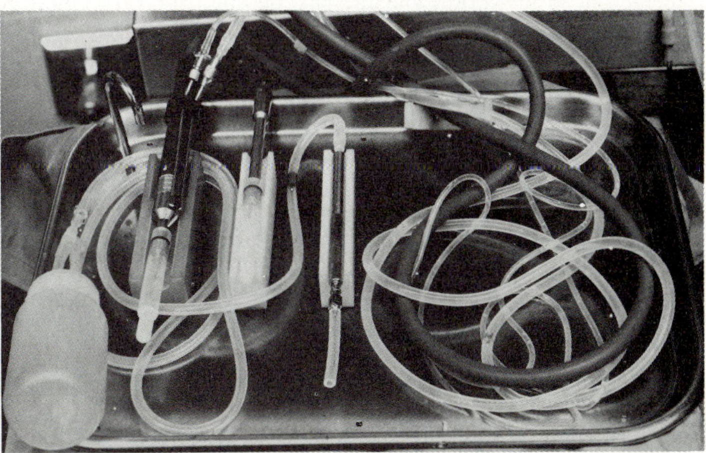

An ophthalmosurgical aid, *Healon,* may be used in intraocular lens implantation to protect the corneal endothelium from possible damage resulting from the removal of the cataractous lens. Healon is a viscoelastic preparation of sodium hyaluronate that is injected into the anterior chamber before or after delivery of the lens. It may also be used as a vitreous replacement after vitrectomy and retinal detachment surgery.

Extracapsular method. The routine procedure for the extracapsular method is essentially similar to an intracapsular extraction up to the step of removal of the lens. At this point the capsule of the lens is opened by means of a cystotome or capsule forceps; the lens cortex is removed from the eye by irrigation; and the nucleus of the lens, if present, is removed by expression with a lens expressor and a lens loop. Cycloplegic agents are generally used. The remainder of the procedure is as outlined previously for intracapsular extraction.

Phacoemulsification. Over the past years, a number of microsurgical techniques have been developed for lens removal through a small incision. Basically, each technique involves the opening of the lens capsule and the use of ultrasonic energy to produce a fragmentation of hard lens material, which can then be aspirated from the eye.

The subsequent description and illustrations relate to the use of the Cavitron unit (Fig. 23-31). All personnel who are to be involved with the use of the instrument must have special training in its use.

The operative procedure is as follows:

1. After a superior rectus bridle suture is placed, a small limbal-based flap is dissected superiorly.
2. The surgical lumbus is cleaned by sharp dissection with a Beaver knife blade. Hemostasis is obtained with a disposable cautery.
3. A 3-mm incision is made into the eye with either a keratome or razor knife and calipers.
4. At this point, air or 1 drop of 1:1000 epinephrine without preservative may be injected into the anterior chamber.
5. The lens capsule is opened, using either a cystotome or capsule forceps. The anterior chamber may be kept formed with either air or irrigating solution.
6. The nuclear-cortical fragment is then shelled out of its capsule with either the cystotome or a blunt cyclodialysis spatula.
7. The large ultrasonic handpiece is checked by the physician for appropriate vacuum control. *This check should be repeated before either handpiece is introduced into the eye.*
8. The ultrasonic handpiece is then introduced into the eye. Three positions are related to the operation of the foot pedal under the surgeon's control: (a) on—irrigation alone, (b) on—irrigation and aspiration, and (c) on—irrigation, aspiration, and ultrasound power. As the machine enters the various positions, and they vary during the case, the surgeon should be informed in an appropriate manner; for example, "one, two, three, two, three." In addition, it is the responsibility of the operating room team to inform the surgeon as to whether there is ade-

quate flow of aspirate through the transparent tubes toward the pump.

9. When the majority of the lens material has been removed, the surgeon asks for the 0.3-mm irrigation-aspiration handpiece. The scrub nurse makes the appropriate unit changes and hands the instrument to the surgeon for a preentry vacuum check. The small handpiece is then introduced into the eye, and the remaining cortex in the anterior chamber and in the fornices of the lens capsule are removed by irrigation and aspiration.

10. A peripheral iridectomy may then be performed. Acetylcholine may then be introduced into the eye to produce pupillary constriction.

11. The corneoscleral wound is now closed with one or two nonabsorbable sutures.

12. At this point, if the posterior lens capsule is not clear, a capsulectomy is performed with one of a number of sharp instruments, such as a burred 27-gauge needle. Air may or may not be injected.

13. The conjunctival flap is sutured closed.

14. The eye is appropriately dressed.

Surgical procedures for glaucoma

Iridectomy

Definition. Removal of a section of iris tissue.

Considerations. Peripheral iridectomy is done in the treatment of acute, subacute, or chronic angle-closure glaucoma when extensive peripheral anterior synechiae have not formed. This operation is done to reestablish communication between the posterior and anterior chambers, thus relieving pupillary block and permitting the iris root to drop away from the trabecular meshwork to reestablish the outflow of aqueous through Schlemm's canal.

Setup and preparation of the patient. A basic cataract setup is needed.

Operative procedure

1. The speculum is introduced. The globe is fixed with a black silk suture no. 4-0 passed under the superior rectus tendon with a fixation forceps and needle holder. The suture is fastened to the drape with a hemostat.

2. A small peritomy is performed at the superior limbus. The corneoscleral junction is scraped clean of epithelium. With a Beaver knife handle and no. 64 blade, a limbal groove is made down to Descemet's membrane. A preplaced suture, usually of black silk no. 7-0, is set in place.

3. The wound is spread apart with the preplaced sutures, and the anterior chamber is entered with a Bard-Parker no. 15 blade. There is an attempt to make the incision into the anterior chamber as large as possible. Pressure is placed on the posterior lip of the wound, and the iris usually prolapses spontaneously. The iris is grasped, and either peripheral or complete iridectomy is performed. The iris spontaneously retracts into the anterior chamber without assistance, but gentle stroking of the corneal surface may be necessary.

4. The preplaced suture is passed through the conjunctiva and tied. Subconjunctival antibiotics may be administered, and an eye dressing applied.

Iridencleisis

Definition. Creation of a tract lined with iris tissue to serve as a wick to accomplish filtration, thus reducing abnormal pressure in glaucoma.

Considerations. Iridencleisis is rarely used, but when it is, it is used in open-angle glaucoma and in chronic angle-closure glaucoma when extensive anterior synechiae have formed. The objective is to establish an artificial method of draining aqueous. By using the iris as a wick in a scleral opening, the surgeon permits the aqueous to drain into the subconjunctival space for reabsorption by the bloodstream.

Setup and preparation of the patient. The iridectomy setup is needed, plus scleral trephines, including interchangeable cutting blades. Routine instillation of drops to prevent excessive mydriasis and retrobulbar injection or general anesthesia may be used.

Operative procedure

1. A conjunctival flap is dissected from above the superior limbus.

2. A keratome is introduced into the anterior chamber through the superior limbus. An iris forceps is introduced into the chamber, and the iris is grasped and pulled outward.

3. After an iridectomy is performed, the iris is incarcerated in the wound. The operative site is covered by suturing the conjunctival flap.

4. Cycloplegic agents and an eye dressing are applied.

Elliot trephination

Definition. Formation of a drainage channel to the subconjunctival space in the treatment of chronic glaucoma.

Considerations. The object of Elliot trephination is to establish a route of aqueous drainage to subconjunctival space for absorption. The operation is similar to iridencleisis and is done primarily for open-angle glaucoma. Postoperatively, the aqueous escapes through the scleral hole into the subconjunctival space, where it is absorbed into the bloodstream.

Setup and preparation of the patient. As described for iridencleisis. The patient is prepared as described for general ophthalmic surgery; a subconjunctival injection is carried out.

Operative procedure

1. A superior rectus bridal suture of black silk no. 4-0 is set in place and clamped to the drape.

2. A sub–Tenon capsule injection of a solution consisting of 2 ml of saline and 1 drop of 1:1000 epinephrine (Adrenalin) is injected superiorly to dissect a flap from the underlying sclera.

3. The conjunctiva is incised to the sclera. The flap is dissected anteriorly into clear cornea.

4. With the conjunctival flap raised by means of forceps, the trephine is applied at the corneal limbus.

5. After completion of the trephining, the scleral disc is cut at its hinge, if it is not free.

6. An iridectomy is performed with iris forceps and De Wecker scissors.

7. The operative area is cleansed of blood, and the conjunctival flap is resutured with a silk suture no. 6-0 or 7-0. Cycloplegic agents are administered. The eye is dressed with a splint, patch, and metal guard.

Anterior and posterior lip sclerectomies

Definition. Formation of a drainage channel to the subconjunctival space in the treatment of chronic glaucoma.

Considerations. As described for iridencleisis and Elliot trephination.

Setup and preparation of the patient. As described for iridencleisis, plus one Holt or Gass punch to the set.

Operative procedure

1. Proceed as described for Elliot trephination through the dissection of the conjunctival flap (steps 1 to 3).

2A. *For thermal sclerectomy,* a scleral flap is made approximately 3 mm from the limbus with a Beaver no. 64 blade. The disposable cautery with a transilluminating head is used to outline the anterior chamber. The disposable cautery is used to apply heat energy to the posterior wound edge under the scleral flap. The anterior chamber is entered with a clean sweep of the cautery. The iris usually spontaneously prolapses, or an iris forceps is used to grasp the iris, and a peripheral or radial iridectomy is performed.

2B. *For punch sclerectomy,* an incision is made into the anterior chamber either at the anterior or posterior margin of the limbus after the anterior chamber has been outlined with a transilluminator. A punch is introduced, and sections of either the anterior or posterior lip are removed, depending on which incision has been made. An iridectomy is performed.

3. A careful closure of conjunctiva and Tenon's capsule is accomplished with black silk suture no. 6-0, leaving both ends free.

4. Air is introduced under the flap with a blunt 30-gauge needle on a 2-ml syringe.

5. The conjunctival flap is closed with a continuous suture. The free ends may be used to delimit the bleb. Atropine sulfate 1% is dropped on the eye, and an eye dressing is put in place.

Cyclodialysis

Definition. Formation of a communication between the anterior chamber and the space located between the sclera and the choroid to reduce aqueous secretion and thus induce lower pressure.

Considerations. By means of this surgical procedure, aqueous secretion is reduced, and absorption is increased into the suprachoroidal space. This operation is usually reserved to treat glaucoma associated with peripheral anterior synechiae.

Setup and preparation of the patient. A basic cataract setup is needed. A local anesthetic is used.

Operative procedure

1. A superior rectus bridal suture of black silk no. 4-0 is put in place and clamped to the drape.

2. In one of the superior quadrants between the rectus muscles, the conjunctiva is incised and dissected from the sclera. An incision is made through the sclera to the suprachoroidal space with the use of a Beaver no. 64 blade.

3. A cyclodialysis spatula is introduced through the scleral opening, and the anterior chamber is entered in the neighborhood of the iris root; thus the ciliary body is detached from the sclera by means of the spatula. The scleral incision is closed.

4. The conjunctiva is closed with fine sutures. A dressing is applied.

Trabeculectomy

The term *trabeculectomy* is really a misnomer because it implies that part of the trabecular meshwork is necessarily removed during surgery. Any of the previously described operations for glaucoma may be performed and may be called a trabeculectomy, with the addition of the dissection of a partial thickness, limbal-based scleral flap before the anterior chamber is entered. This scleral limbal flap may or may not be loosely sutured before the conjunctival flap is closed.

Setup. A basic cataract setup, plus instruments as shown in Fig. 23-32, and the operating microscope are required.

Goniotomy

Definition. Opening of a congenital membrane from the iris surface to Schwalbe's line, thus allowing aqueous humor to reach the trabecular meshwork in cases of congenital glaucoma.

Setup and preparation of the patient. A general anesthesia is used. The setup (Figs. 23-33 and 23-34) is as follows:

Tonometer	Utility forceps
Calipers	Castroviejo needle holder
Indirect ophthalmoscope	Gonioprism
Eye speculum, pediatric	Maumenee irrigating knife

Barkan knife	Syringe, 2 ml
Bond forceps, 0.12 mm	Needle, blunt, 30 gauge
Barraquer needle holder	Operating microscope

Operative procedure

1. The patient is anesthetized without intubation.

2. An examination under anesthesia is performed, and corneal clarity and size, intraocular pressure, microscopic examination of the anterior segment (including gonioscopy), and examination of the posterior pole of the eye (especially the optic disc) are recorded.

3. The patient is then intubated, if indicated, and prepared and draped in the usual manner.

4. A pediatric eye speculum and superior (and inferior rectus) bridle suture are put in place.

5. Under microscopic control with an appropriate gonioprism in place, the Maumenee irrigating knife is introduced ab externo through the temporal limbus. The anterior chamber is kept formed by constant irrigation through the knife. The anterior chamber is crossed, and the membrane covering the iris and angle structures is cut without damaging the trabecular meshwork. The knife is removed.

6. Air may be introduced into the eye, and a suture may or may not be used.

7. A cycloplegic agent may be used topically.

8. The eye is splinted and dressed in the usual manner.

SURGERY FOR RETINAL DETACHMENT (SEPARATION)

Retinal detachment is actually a separation of the neural retinal layer from the pigment epithelium layer of the retina. Retinal detachment may occur because of the presence of intraocular neoplasms originating in the retina or choroid (exudative type) or, more commonly, secondary to retinal tears or holes associated with injury, degeneration, or rhegmatogenous detachment.

This condition usually causes the sudden onset of the appearance of floating spots before the eye, caused by freeing of pigment or blood cells into the vitreous. The vitreous humor of the eye is a gelatinous liquid possessing an ultrastructure of fine protein fibers in a network arrangement, with some attachments to the retina. Fluid from the vitreous cavity may seep through the retinal tears and separate the retinal components. This condition progresses as the liquid seeps behind the retina. The part of the retina that has become separated from its nutritional source becomes damaged and relatively nonseeing. Prompt treatment of retinal detachment is aimed at preventing permanent loss of central vision. Reattachment of the retina can be accomplished only by surgery. Repair is done from outside the globe. The principle involved in surgery is that of sealing off the area at which the tear or hole has been located with or without drainage of the subretinal fluid (Fig. 23-35).

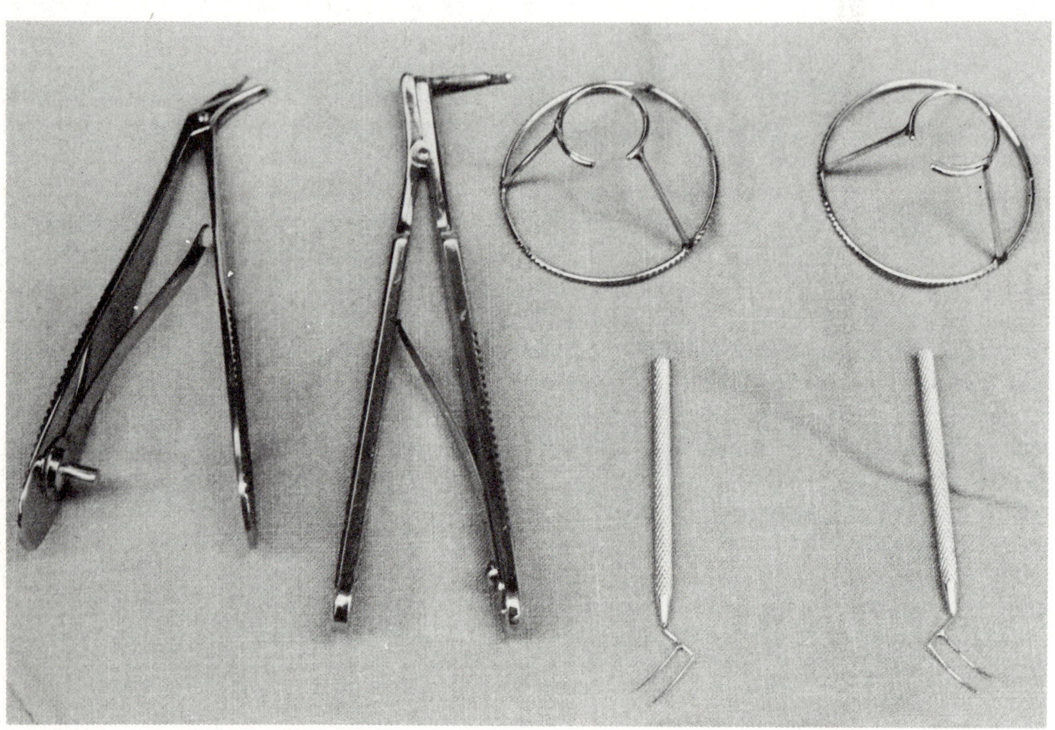

Fig. 23-32. Instruments for sclerectomy and trabeculotomy. *Left to right,* Holt corneoscleral punch; Gass sclerotomy punch; right and left trabeculotomes; ring trabeculotomes.

Surgical procedures performed in the treatment of retinal detachment include scleral buckling using episcleral and intrascleral techniques with diathermy or cryotherapy. Cryosurgery or light coagulation may be used alone or in combination with buckling procedures.

Considerations. The purpose of surgery for retinal detachment is to cause an intrusion or push into the eye at the site of the pathological cause. Treatment by diathermy or cryotherapy causes an inflammatory reaction that leads to a permanent adhesion between the detached retina and underlying structures. In the treatment of retinal detachment, the aim is to return the retina to its normal anatomical position.

Setup and preparation of the patient

1 Williams lid speculum
1 Cibis double muscle hook
4 Mosquito hemostats
1 Quevedo utility forceps
2 Serrated conjunctival forceps, heavy
1 Thorpe forceps
3 Lester forceps
1 McCullough suture forceps
1 Cyclodialysis spatula
2 Jameson muscle hooks
1 von Graefe muscle hook
1 Graefe iris forceps, straight, with teeth
1 Stevens scissors
2 Beaver knife handles no. 3 with no. 64 blades
2 Bulldog clamps (serrefine)
1 Diathermy pencil with cord and electrodes
1 Watzke forceps
1 Caliper
1 Tonometer
1 Loop no. 20
3 Silastic sponges, 3, 5, and 7 mm
1 Silastic band no. 40 and sleeve
Preserved sclera
Indirect ophthalmoscope
Diathermy unit
Cryosurgical unit
Dacron suture no. 5-0
Supramid sutures no. 4-0

The patient is prepared as described for general ophthalmic surgery.

Operative procedure. A detailed drawing of the retina is made before surgery and is displayed in the operating suite. On the basis of this drawing, the conjunctiva is opened to whatever extent has been previously determined, that is, 90 degrees for a simple horseshoe tear or 360 degrees for an aphakic detachment. With the indirect ophthalmoscope, the abnormality is localized under di-

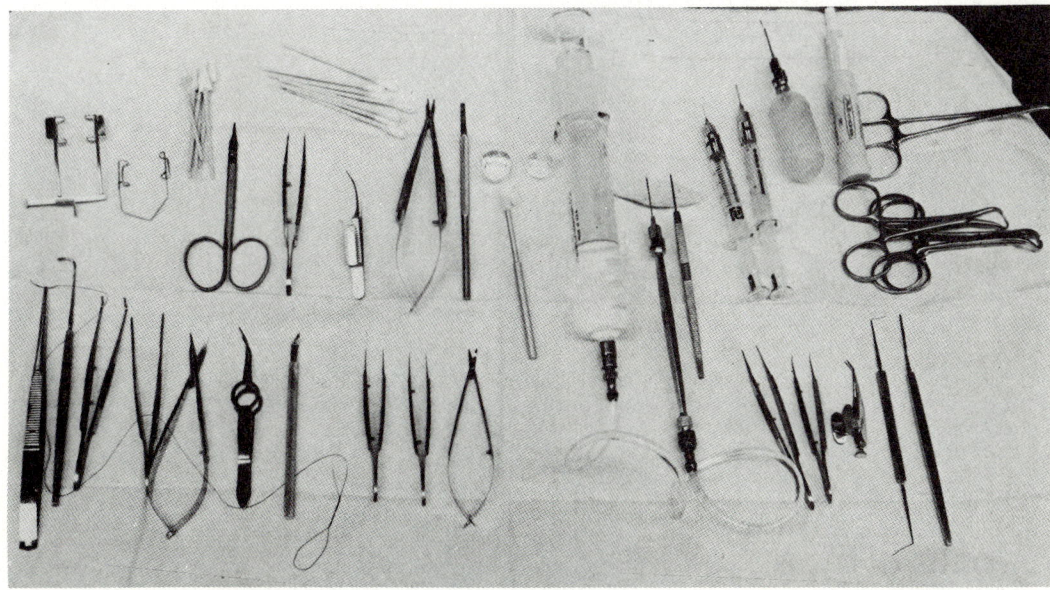

Fig. 23-33. Goniotomy instruments. *Top row, left to right,* Wiener eye speculum; Barraquer eye speculum; Weck-cel spears; Stevens scissors; Bonn forceps, 0.12 mm; Colibri forceps, 0.12 mm; Barraquer needle holder; Beaver knife with no. 64 blade; Barkan gonioscopic lens; modified Troncoso lens; Swan gonioprism; Maumenee goniotomy knife cannula; Barkan goniotomy knife; 2-ml syringe with air-injection cannula; 2-ml syringe with 19-gauge blunt needle; Bishop-Harmon AC irrigator with cannula; disposable cautery; mosquito hemostat; small towel clamps. *Bottom row, left to right,* Castroviejo needle holder; von Graefe muscle hook; Quevedo utility forceps; conjunctival forceps; Wescott scissors; Schaaf forceps; Drews suture pickup; 2 pairs of straight McPherson iris forceps; small, curved Castroviejo scissors; Thorpe forceps; angle McPherson iris forceps; Barraquer-De Wecker iris scissors; cyclodialysis spatula; iris repositor.

rect visualization, and nonpenetrating diathermy marks are made over the site by indentation.

Episcleral technique

1. Cryotherapy is applied to the pathological areas under direct visualization (an iceball is seen to form in the proper areas until all of the lesion has been treated).

2. If a localized plombage (push) is to be used, Dacron sutures are set in the sclera surrounding the lesion and tied over Silastic sponges, causing the outer shell of the eye to be pushed toward the elevated retina. If an encircling band is to be used, belt loops are made in the sclera in four quadrants with nos. 64 and 66 Beaver blades. A no. 40 Silastic band is passed 360 degrees around the eye through the belt loops, and a self-holding Watzke sleeve or sutures are applied to the band to maintain a predetermined circumference. This causes a 360-degree constriction of the outer coats into the eye.

3. If drainage of subretinal fluid is desired, an area is chosen under direct visualization, where a significant fluid level exists under the retina, and a diathermy mark is made on the sclera. The sclera is split to the choroid, and a preplaced suture is put in place. A small amount of diathermy is applied to the choroid bed. A needle is then used to puncture the choroid into the subretinal space with subsequent drainage of fluid. The preplaced suture is tied.

Scleral resection. An incision is made into the sclera, and a scleral flap is dissected both anteriorly and posteriorly from the original incision. Diathermy can be used in this bed, or cryotherapy can be used under direct visualization. Preserved eye bank sclera or a groove piece no. 20 may be sutured into the bed, using a Supramid suture no. 4-0 or Dacron sutures no. 5-0 with or without an encircling band as previously described. Drainage of subretinal fluid may be accomplished as previously described. Air or other replacement or ballast fluids may be introduced into the eye after the drainage of subretinal fluid. This is usually done through the pars plana under direct visualization.

A culture is taken at the end of surgery, and a subconjunctival injection of penicillin and gentamicin is given routinely unless contraindicated. The conjunctiva is closed with a selected suture material, and the eye is patched.

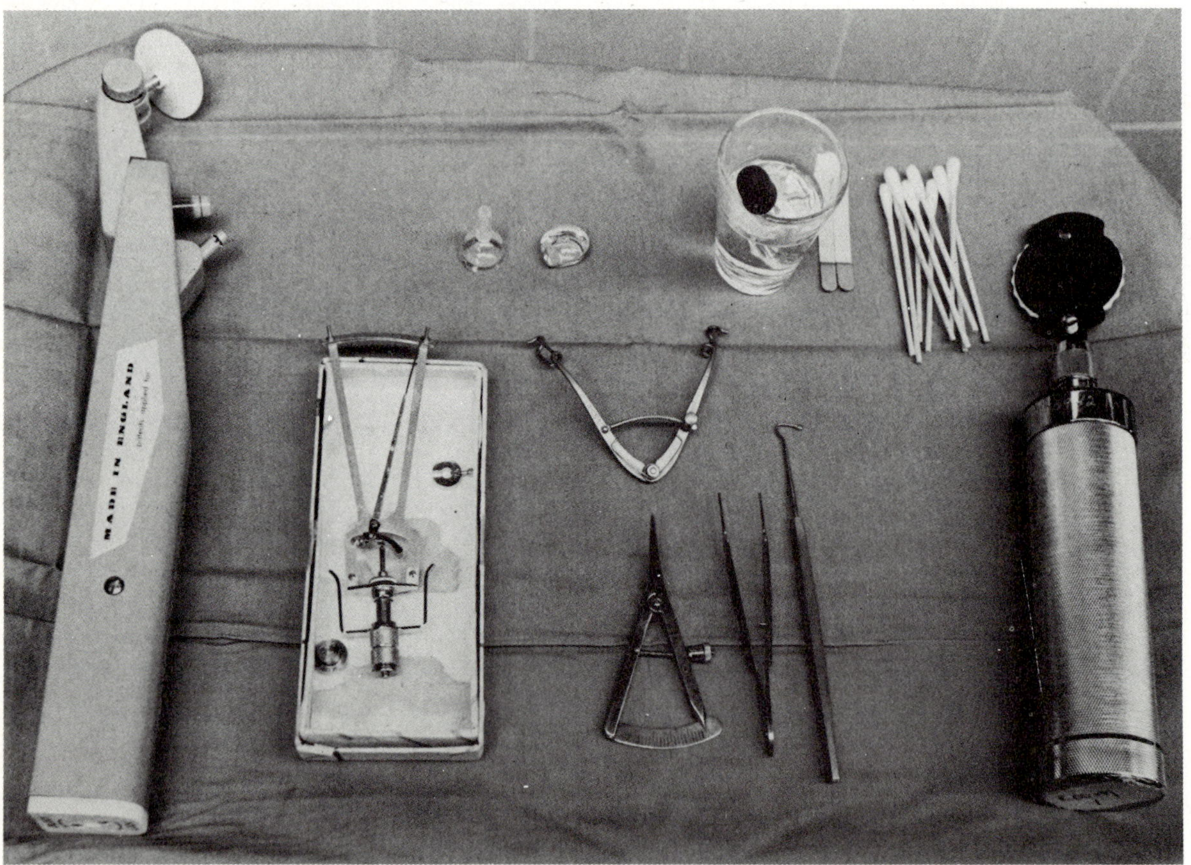

Fig. 23-34. Instruments used for eye examination. *Top row, left to right,* Modified Troncoso gonioscopic lens, Barkan gonioscopic lens, fluorescein solution in medicine glass, fluorescein strips, cotton applicators. *Bottom row, left to right,* Perkins tonometer, Storz-Schiotz tonometer, Castroviejo caliper, Williams eye speculum, Lester fixation forceps, Jameson muscle hook, ophthalmoscope.

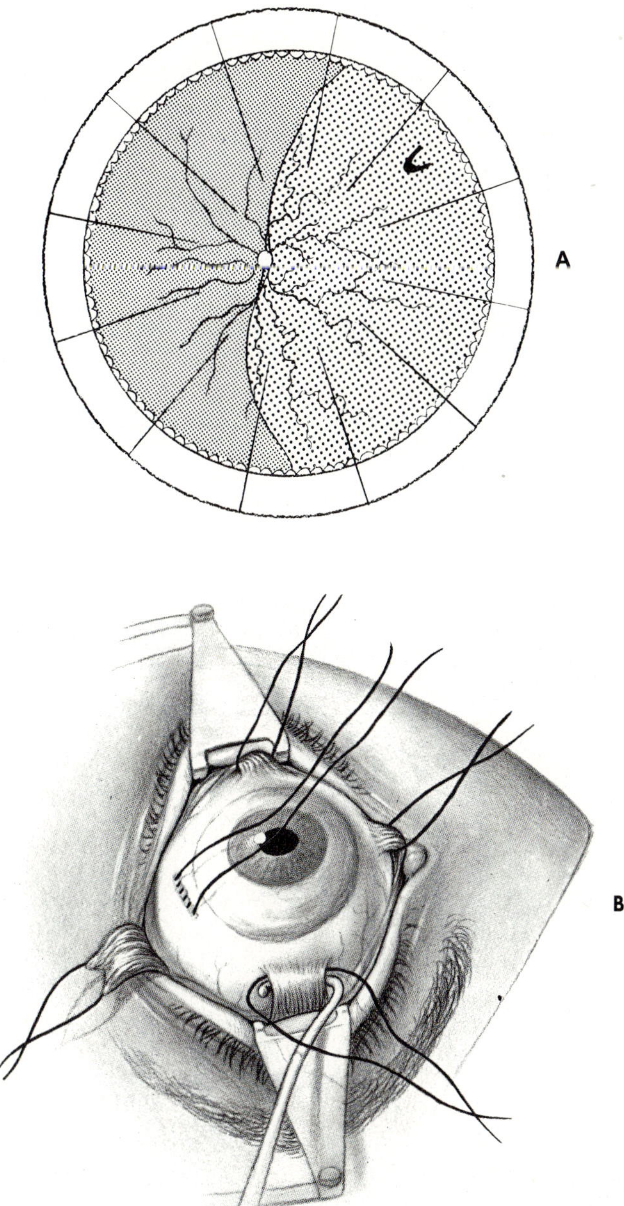

Fig. 23-35. Scleral buckling operation for treatment of retinal detachment. **A,** Diagram of retina showing detachment of retina of temporal half of left eye, with retinal tear at equator of globe at 1:30 o'clock. **B,** Bulbar conjunctiva and Tenon's capsule are opened to explore sclera. Stay sutures are placed under involved rectus muscles so that eye may be rotated to expose area to be treated. In some cases more than one rectus muscle is temporarily detached from globe to permit adequate exposure. *Continued.*

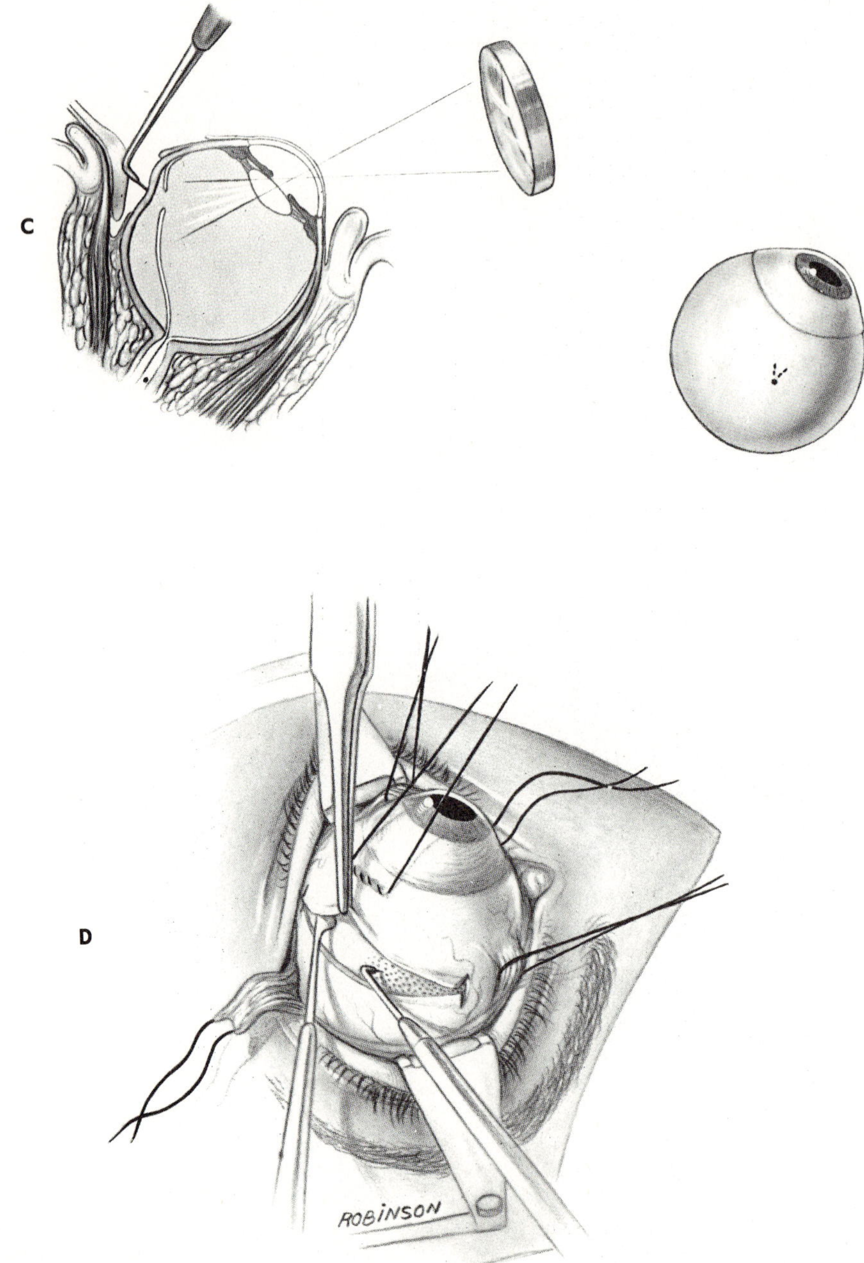

Fig. 23-35, cont'd. C, Examination of fundus by means of ophthalmoscope and depression of sclera with diathermy electrode. Surgeon visualizes field and directs assistant in placement of electrode beneath retinal tear; burn mark is made on sclera at site of retinal tear with diathermy electrode. **D,** Cut or groove is made in sclera along equator of eye. Each edge of groove is undermined.

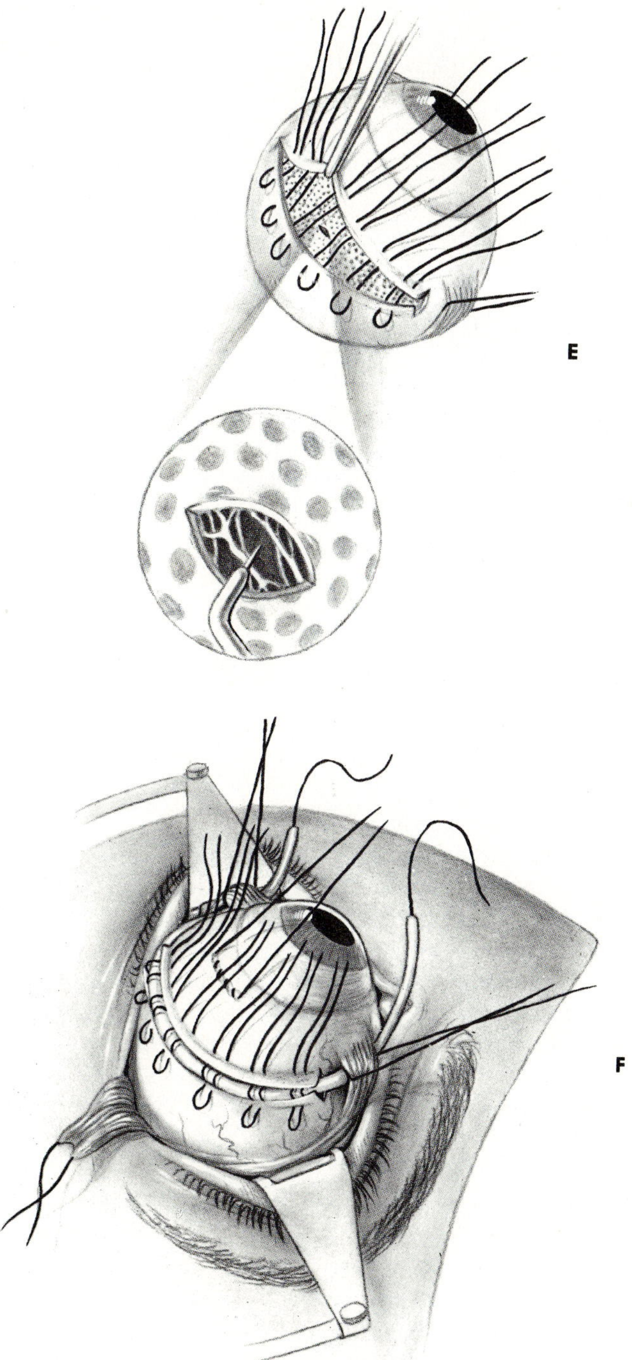

Fig. 23-35, cont'd. E, Mattress sutures of surgeon's preference are placed across scleral groove. Small incision is made through remaining layer of sclera down to choroid. Choroid is punctured with fine electrode to allow subretinal fluid to drain. **F,** A no. 40 Silastic band is laid in bed of scleral groove under mattress sutures. When retinal tears are large, a silicone patch may be placed under band.

Continued.

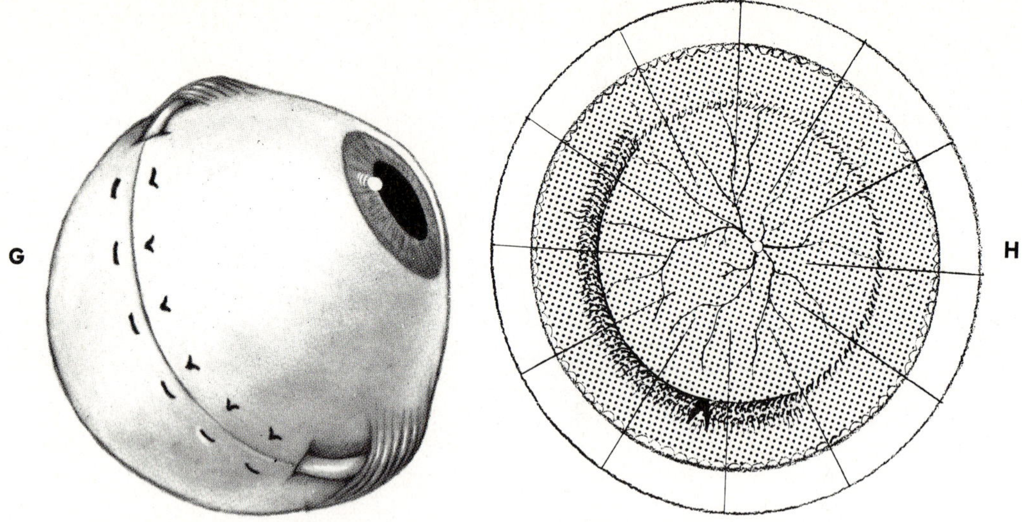

Fig. 23-35, cont'd. G, Edges of scleral groove are closed over Silastic band. **H,** Diagram of fundus with retina in place and 1:30 o'clock retinal tear on buckle. Diathermy reaction is seen on buckle from 12 to 5:30 o'clock. (From Advancing with surgery, Somerville, N.J., Ethicon, Inc.)

VITRECTOMY

Definitions. In the circumscribed sense, removal of all or part of the vitreous gel (body). In the broader clinical sense of the term, it also includes the cutting and removal of fibrotic membranes, the removal of epiretinal membranes, and cauterization of bleeding vessels.

Considerations. In its normal state, the vitreous gel of the eye is transparent. In certain disease states, bleeding from damaged or newly formed vessels may cause the vitreous to become opaque and may severely decrease vision. In addition to the inability of the patient to see is an associated inability of the ophthalmologist to visualize the retina and therefore to treat the underlying pathological condition before permanent damage can occur. In these cases, vitrectomy is indicated to allow the patient to see and to allow the surgeon to institute treatment, if indicated.

Certain ophthalmic diseases are associated with the formation of membranes, which in themselves may block the visual axis and cause decreased vision. Contraction of these membranes may produce either traction-type or rhegmatogenous retinal detachment. In these cases vitrectomy is indicated to relieve the underlying pathological processes leading to decreased vision.

Setup and preparation of the patient. General anesthesia is used because absolute control of patient position at all times is needed. The patient is prepped and draped with barrier drapes, and adequate drainage precautions for the irrigating fluid are taken.

Instrumentation is as follows:

Eye speculum
Utility forceps
Castroviejo needle holder
Wescott scissors
Thorpe forceps
Conjunctival forceps
Bonn forceps, 0.12 mm
Castroviejo forceps, 0.5 mm
Beaver knife with no. 64 blade
von Graefe knife
Barraquer needle holder
Weck-cel sponges
Fundus lens, three mirror
Fundus lens, posterior pole
Operating table with X, Y, Z axis control
Operating microscope with X, Y, Z axis control and coaxial illumination
Vitrectomy instrumentation
Retinal detachment instruments

Operative procedure

1. Appropriate fixation sutures are set in place.
2. A limbal flap is dissected temporally.
3. A pars plana incision is made, and Dacron sutures are preplaced.
4. The operating microscope (Fig. 23-36) is aligned, and a fundus lens is set on the anterior surface of the cornea.
5. With the surgeon controlling the infusion and cutting action of the vitrectomy instrument and the first assistant controlling the relative vacuum in the line, the vitreous and membranes are removed under direct visualization.

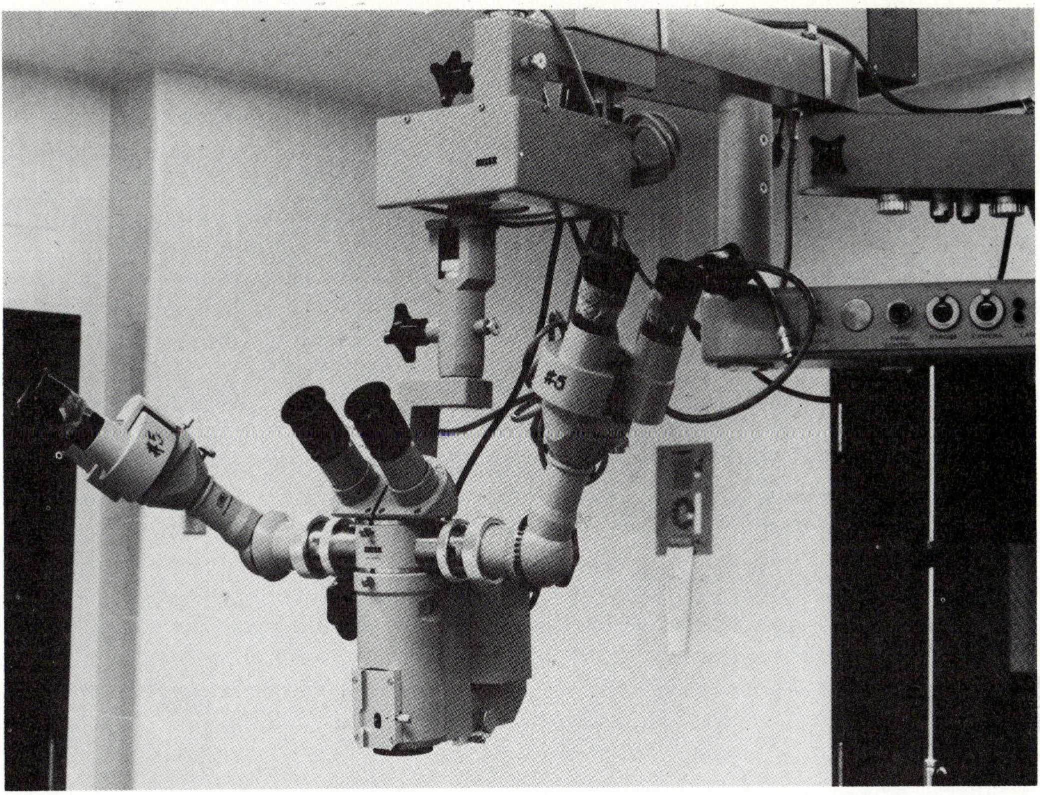

Fig. 23-36. Vitrectomy microscope with X, Y, Z axis control.

If the lens is opaque, it may be removed by the vitrectomy instrument through the pars plana incision, but this maneuver is to be avoided if possible because it is not an efficient way of removing a cataractous lens. The procedure is tedious and may add additional hours of operating time.

6. An additional pars plana opening may be required in order to have two intraocular instruments available for manipulation of membranes.

7. Once the media have been removed and the retinal condition can be visualized, direct repair using vitrectomy instrumentation or a routine scleral buckling procedure may be performed.

8. The pars plana incisions are closed, and the conjunctival flap is sutured appositionally. Cultures are usually obtained at this point.

9. Subconjunctival or topical antibiotics may be used. The eye is then splinted and dressed, and a protective eye guard is taped in place.

Photocoagulation, laser, and cryotherapy treatments

Considerations. Certain localized detachments, sites of potential pathological conditions, tumors, and some vascular proliferative diseases, for example, diabetic retinopathy, can be treated without opening the conjunctiva. The mode of therapy is selected by the surgeon according to the location and type of lesion that is being treated. The patient's pupil is dilated preoperatively, and a retrobulbar anesthetic is used. The purpose is to form an adhesion between the retina and pigment epithelium or to destroy proliferating blood vessels or tumors.

SURGERY OF THE CONJUNCTIVA

Considerations. The conjunctiva of the eye is transparent and elastic, and there is an abundance of it. Traumatic lacerations caused by injury and deficits resulting from excision of tumors, cysts, nevi, or pterygium can usually be repaired by simple undermining and suturing.

Pterygium excision

Definition. A pterygium is a fleshy, triangular encroachment onto the cornea, which occurs nasally and tends to be bilateral. When the pterygium encroaches on the visual axis, it is removed surgically (Fig. 23-37).

Setup and preparation of the patient

Williams lid speculum
Mosquito hemostat
Quevedo utility forceps
Conjunctival forceps, fine, with teeth
Lester forceps

Bard-Parker no. 3 knife handle with no. 15 blade
Beaver knife handle with no. 64 blade
Stevens scissors
Castroviejo needle holder
Disposable cautery with white (hot) tip

Operative procedure. The major steps in the McReynolds technique are described in Fig. 23-37.

Pterygium can also be excised totally, and the limbus treated with a cautery. The conjunctiva can then be closed, or the sclera can be left bare.

Excisional biopsies

Any suspicious lesion of the conjunctiva can be removed by simple elliptical excision for pathological examination. The conjunctiva may or may not be closed, depending on the surgeon's particular technique.

Reformation of cul-de-sacs (mucous membrane graft)

Considerations. Infections, trachoma, or chemical burns, for example, may cause severe scarring and contractures of the conjunctiva and underlying tissues leading to motility problems, exposure problems, and the like. Simple dissection is usually not satisfactory, and extra mucous membrane is required. This may be obtained from excess conjunctiva from the opposite eye, if available, or a mucous membrane graft from the oral cavity.

Setup and preparation of the patient. A basic pterygium set is needed, plus a plastic tray for obtaining the mucous membrane graft.

A local or general anesthetic is used.

Operative procedure

1. An anesthetic solution is injected into the mucous membrane of the lower lip or the lateral wall of the mouth with a separate set of instruments. An elliptical incision is made with a no. 15 knife blade (if the incision is made into the lateral wall, the opening of the parotid duct must be avoided), and a thin, full-thickness layer of mucous membrane is removed by sharp dissection. The wound is approximated with black silk suture no. 4-0.

A second method is the use of an electric Castroviejo dermatome. The mucous membrane is then always obtained from the lower lip.

2. The mucous membrane graft is placed in a Neosporin solution, the surgeon is regowned in a sterile gown, and another set of sterile instruments is used for reconstruction of the cul-de-sac.

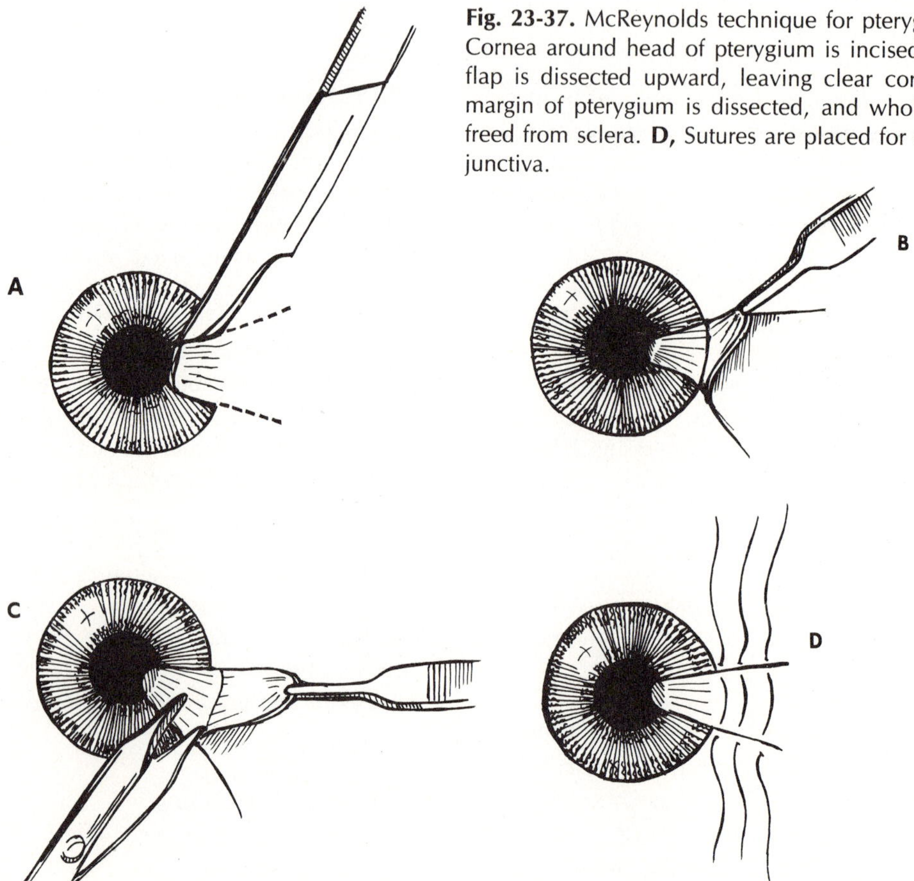

Fig. 23-37. McReynolds technique for pterygium repair. **A,** Cornea around head of pterygium is incised. **B,** Pterygium flap is dissected upward, leaving clear cornea. **C,** Lower margin of pterygium is dissected, and whole pterygium is freed from sclera. **D,** Sutures are placed for closure of conjunctiva.

SUGGESTED READINGS

Atkinson, L.J., and Kohn, M.L.: Berry and Kohn's introduction to operating room techniques, ed. 5, New York, 1978, McGraw-Hill Book Co.

Baida, R.: Nursing care in use of local anesthesia, AORN J. **28:**855, 1978.

Boyd-Monk, H.: Cataract surgery, Nursing '77 **7**(6):56, 1977.

Boyd-Monk, H.: Helping the corneal transplant patient to see again, Nursing '78 **8**(2):47, 1978.

Care and handling of surgical instruments, Randolph, Mass., 1981, Codman & Shurtleff, Inc.

Dahle, J.S.: Caring for the patient with local anesthesia, AORN J. **27:**985, 1978.

Foster, C.G., and others: Effects of surgical positioning, AORN J. **30:**219, 1979.

Fyodorov, S.: Dissection of corneal circular ligament in cases of myopia of mild degrees, Ann. Ophthalmol. **11:**1885, 1979.

Gaston, N.C.: Kerato refractive surgery: new horizons, AORN J. **33:**1068, 1981.

Gruendemann, B.J., and others: The surgical patient: behavioral concepts for the operating room nurse, ed. 2, St. Louis, 1977, The C.V. Mosby Co.

Hahn, A.B., Barkin, R.L., and Oestreich, S.J.K.: Pharmacology in nursing, ed. 15, St. Louis, 1982, The C.V. Mosby Co.

Havener, W.H.: Ocular pharmacology, ed. 4, St. Louis, 1978, The C.V Mosby Co.

Jennings, B.: Intraocular lens for cataracts, AORN J. **23:**664, 1976.

Jennings, B.: Outpatient posterior capsulotomy, AORN J. **23:**270, 1976.

Jennings, B.: Combined ophthalmic implant and transplant, AORN J. **28:**41, 1978.

Kwitko, M.L.: Artificial lens implantation, AORN J. **28:**47, 1978.

Lach, J.: O.R. nursing: preoperative care and draping technique, Chicago, 1974, The Kendall Co.

LeMaitre, G., and Finnegan, J.: The patient in surgery: a guide for nurses, ed. 4, Philadelphia, 1980, W.B. Saunders Co.

Low, C.R.: Outpatient cataract surgery, AORN J. **28:**35, 1978.

Luckmann, J., and Sorensen, K.C.: Medical-surgical nursing: a psychological approach, ed. 2, Philadelphia, 1980, W.B. Saunders Co.

MacFadyen, J.S.: Caring for the patient with a primary retinal detachment, Am. J. Nurs. **80:**920, 1980.

Mazzocco, T.R.: Microsurgery of cataracts, AORN J. **24:**1091, 1976.

Perrin, E.D.: Laser therapy for diabetic retinopathy, Am. J. Nurs. **80:**664, 1980.

Saunders, W.H., and others: Nursing care in eye, ear, nose, and throat disorders, ed. 4, St. Louis, 1979, The C.V Mosby Co.

Scheie, H.G., and Albert, D.M.: Textbook of ophthalmology, ed. 9, Philadelphia, 1977, W.B. Saunders Co.

Schneeman, Y.T., and Taylor, J.A.: A technical look at vitrectomy, AORN J. **33:**867, 1981.

Schrader, E.S.: Perioperative nurses reassure ophthalmologic patients, AORN J. **30:**1066, 1979.

Schrader, E.S.: Surgeons summarize progress, AORN J. **33:**73, 1981.

Shurtz, A.: The pediatric strabismus patient in surgery, AORN J. **30:**639, 1979.

Smith, J.F., and Nachazel, D.P., Jr.: Ophthalmologic nursing, Boston, 1980, Little, Brown & Co.

Suggested instrument setups for ophthalmic procedures, Storz Eye Instruments, ed. 14, St. Louis, 1973, Storz Instrument Co.

Suture use manual: use and handling of sutures and needles, Somerville, N.J., 1981, Ethicon, Inc.

Waddleton, C.A.: Eye openers: uses and precautions, Nurses' Drug Alert **2:**132, Nov. 1978.

Wong, E.K., Wang, S., and Leopold, I.H.: How ophthalmic drugs can fool you, RN **43:**36, March 1980.

24 Neurosurgery

Nurses in the operating room must understand the structure and function of the nervous system to provide intelligent, safe, humanistic care for neurosurgical patients. They should know the range of variables of normal development and identify those which are critical for each patient. They must recognize and respond to a variety of dependency needs such as the normal response to preoperative sedation, age, and pathological conditions, for example, paralysis, aphasia, or coma. They must understand many pathological conditions that result in surgical intervention. They should be able to plan and manage patient care for many complex surgical procedures. They must be familiar with the use, care, working order, and safety factors of sophisticated instrumentation. They need to appreciate the limitations and stresses facing neurosurgeons. They should anticipate and respond to potential complications inherent in specific patients and procedures. They must respond in neurosurgical emergencies with greater speed but with the same care and precision as in elective situations. Basic general information to assist nurses to function effectively in their own clinical settings is presented here.

ANATOMY AND PHYSIOLOGY

The nervous system, the single most complex and least understood of all body systems, has been subdivided in various ways to simplify study. Structural divisions are the central nervous system (brain and spinal cord) and the peripheral nervous system (cranial and spinal nerves).

Nervous system tissue is composed of neurons and neuroglial cells that support the neurons. The brain and spinal cord are protected by bony structures. The cranial nerves originate within the brain and emerge through openings in the skull to run peripherally. The spinal nerves that emerge from the spinal cord through the vertebral foramina also run peripherally. Peripheral nerves, in this chapter, therefore, are those outside the cranial cavity and vertebral canal.

Functionally, the nervous system is divided into voluntary and autonomic (involuntary) systems. The nervous system functions as the communication system for the rest of the body. The functions of all body systems are dependent, in part, on nervous system function. In turn the nervous system is directly dependent on circulatory system function for life-sustaining glucose and oxygen. Nervous system functions include orientation, coordination, conceptual thought, emotion, memory, and reflex response.

Within the framework of neurosurgical techniques, logical divisions of the nervous system are the head, or cranium; the back, or spine; and the peripheral nerves. These subdivisions lend themselves to meaningful discussion of supporting structures, body positions, instrumentation, and other considerations useful to the nurse providing care for neurosurgical patients during the intraoperative phase of care.

Head

Scalp layers of the head (Fig. 24-1) include skin, subcutaneous tissue, galea, and occipitofrontal musculature. The skin is thick. The subcutaneous tissue, which is exceptionally dense, tough, and vascular, is firmly attached to the galea. Most of the blood vessels lie superficial to the galea. The subgaleal space contains loose areolar tissue that permits mobility of the scalp. The pericranium, or outer periosteum of the skull, separates the galea from the cranium.

The arterial supply of the scalp comes from the external carotid artery through the superficial temporal, posterior auricular, occipital, frontal, and supraorbital branches. Most veins roughly follow the course of the arteries, except emissary veins that drain directly through the skull into the intracranial venous sinuses. Unlike the arteries, the surface veins of the brain have many large anastomoses. The scalp, the extracranial arteries, and portions of the dura mater are the only pain-sensitive structures that cover the brain, which itself is insensitive.

The skull is formed by twenty-four bones, joined by serrated bony seams called *sutures*. Eight bones form the walls of the cranial cavity, which houses the brain. There are four single bones—frontal, occipital, ethmoid, and sphenoid—and four paired bones—temporal and parietal (Fig. 24-2). The coronal suture joins the frontal and parietal bones. The squamous sutures border the squamous part of the temporal bones. The lambdoidal suture joins the occipital and parietal bones. The sagittal suture lies in the medial plane and joins the two parietal bones (Fig. 24-3).

At the top of the skull in front of and behind the parietal bones are the anterior and posterior fontanelles,

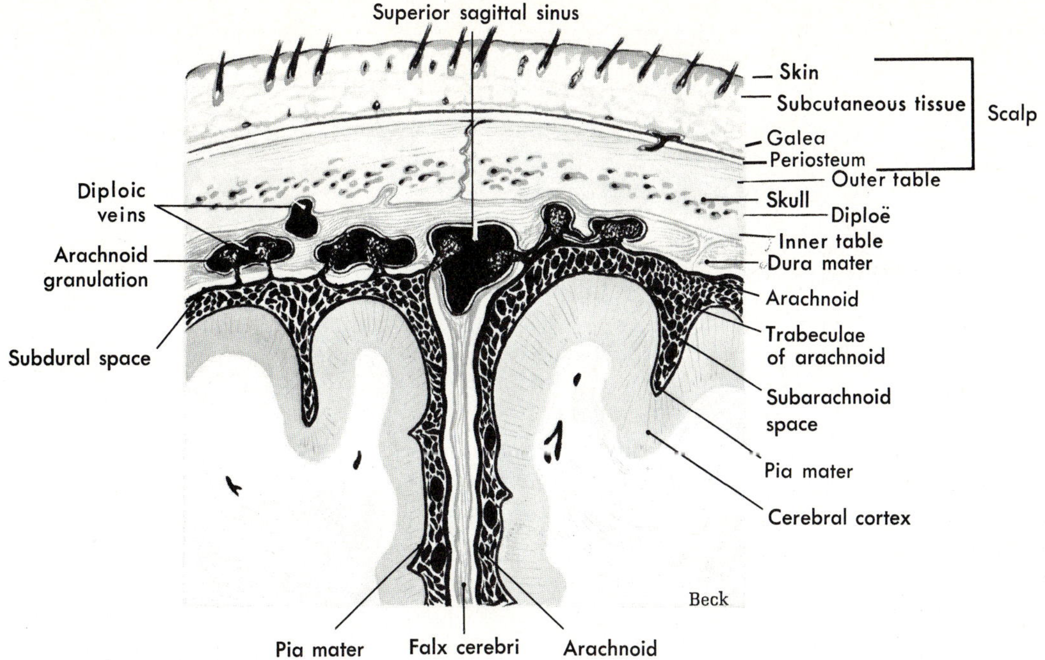

Fig. 24-1. Scalp is composed of following layers: skin, subcutaneous tissue, galea, and periosteum of the skull. Skull bone has three tables: outer, diploë or spongy layer, and inner. Dura mater lies beneath skull and completely encapsulates brain. Other structures are identified for reference and are described in text. (Adapted from Anthony, C.P., and Kolthoff, N.J.: Textbook of anatomy and physiology, ed. 9, St. Louis, 1975, The C.V. Mosby Co.)

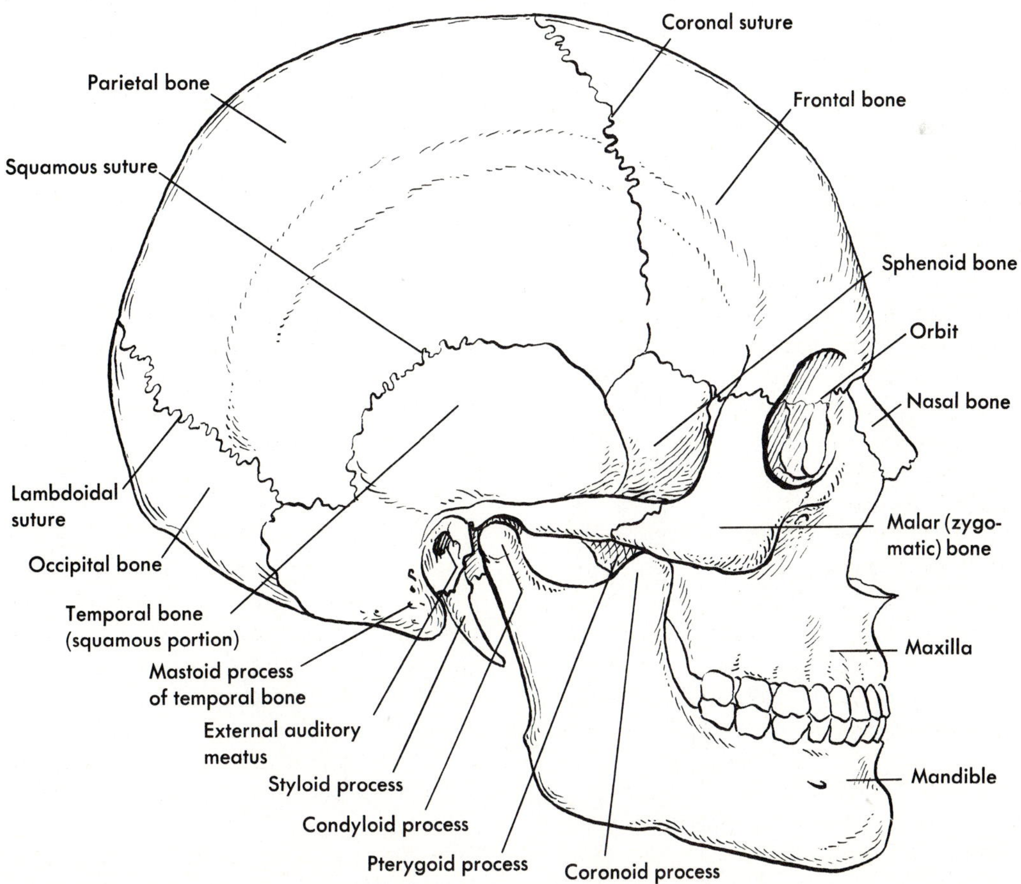

Fig. 24-2. Skull viewed from right side. (From Anthony, C.P., and Kolthoff, N.J.: Textbook of anatomy and physiology, ed. 9, St. Louis, 1975, The C.V. Mosby Co.)

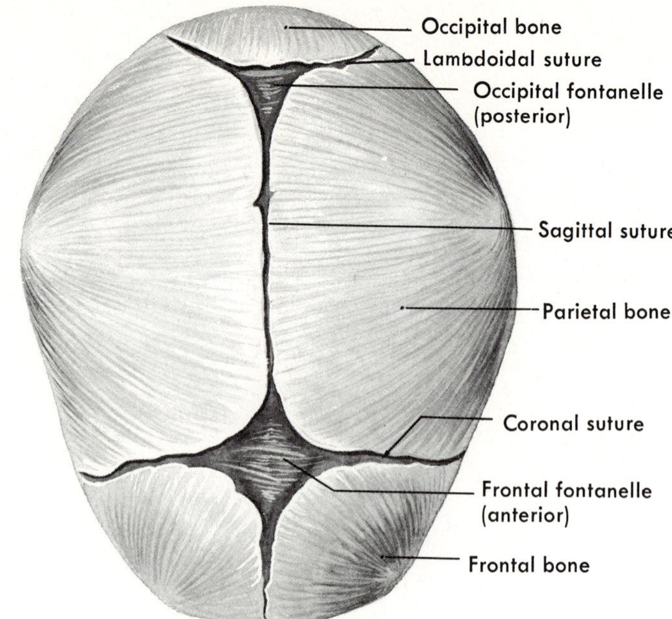

Fig. 24-3. Skull at birth viewed from above. (Adapted from Anthony, C.P., and Kolthoff, N.J.: Textbook of anatomy and physiology, ed. 9, St. Louis, 1975, The C.V. Mosby Co.)

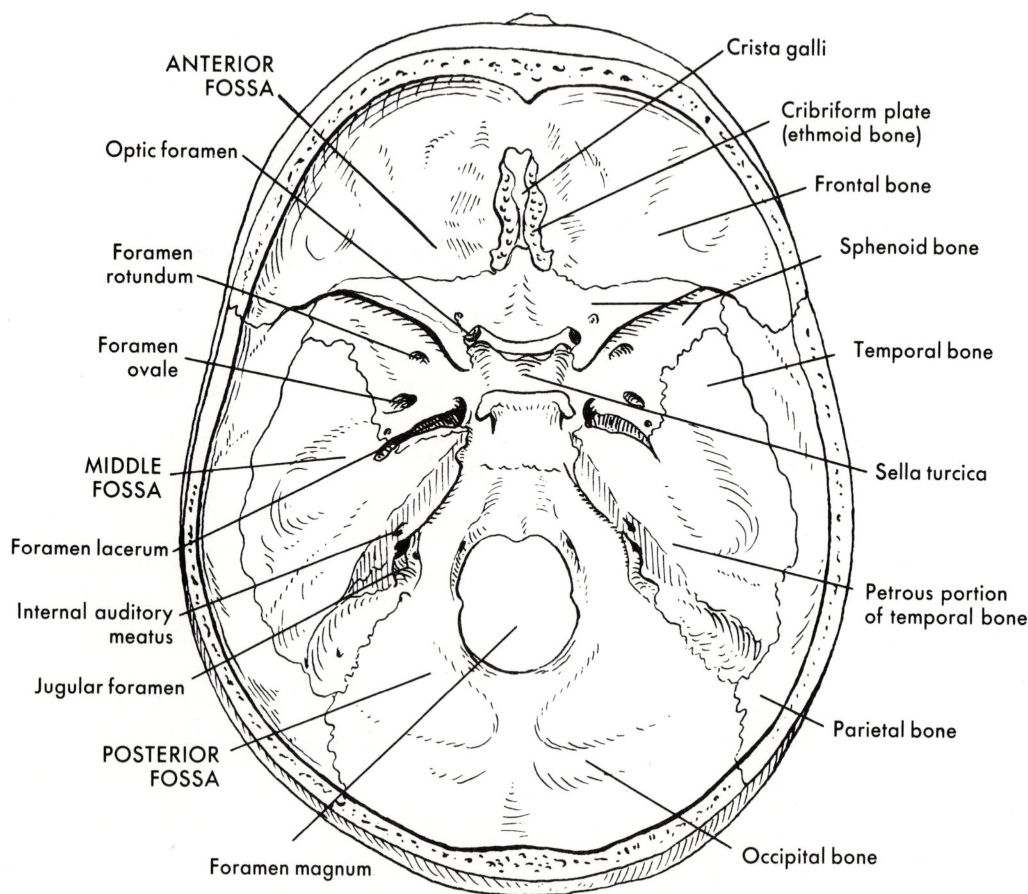

Fig. 24-4. Floor of cranial cavity. (Adapted from Anthony, C.P., and Kolthoff, N.J.: Textbook of anatomy and physiology, ed. 9, St. Louis, 1975, The C.V. Mosby Co.)

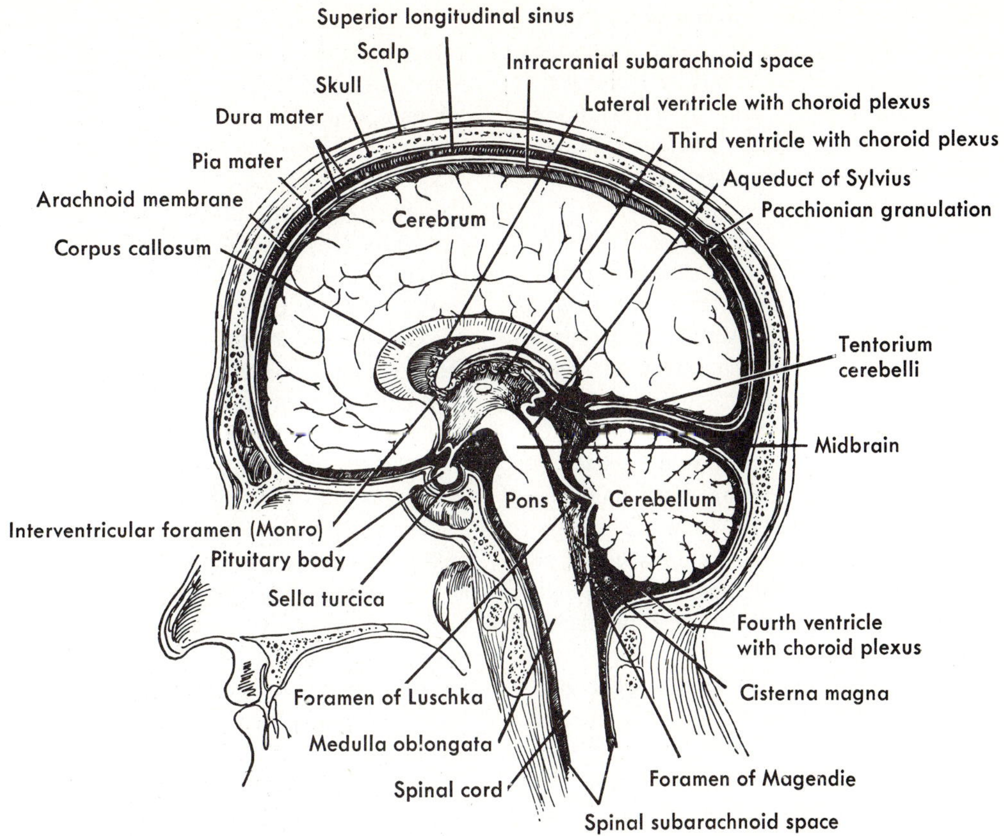

Fig. 24-5. Diagram of sagittal section of head showing cerebrospinal fluid spaces and their relationship to venous circulation and principal subdivision of the brain and its coverings. (From Conway-Rutkowski, B.L.: Carini and Owens' neurological and neurosurgical nursing, ed. 8, St. Louis, 1982, The C.V. Mosby Co.)

which are open at birth. The posterior fontanelle is closed by 2 months and the anterior by about 18 months after birth (Fig. 24-3). If the suture lines close prematurely, the skull cannot expand as the brain grows. This condition, *craniosynostosis,* demands early surgical intervention.

The skull is oval shaped and is wider in back than in front. The flattened, irregular bones consist of two tables of compact bone that enclose a layer of spongy bone, or *diploë* (Fig. 24-1).

The interior of the skull is anatomically divided into three cranial fossae: anterior, middle, and posterior (Fig. 24-4). The anterior fossa is limited posteriorly by the sphenoid ridge, along which pituitary tumors and aneurysms of the circle of Willis are generally approached. The frontal lobes and olfactory bulbs and tracts lie in the anterior fossa. The temporal lobes lie in the middle fossa, which is shaped like a butterfly. The sella turcica, formed by the sphenoid bone, is the most central part of the middle fossa and houses the pituitary gland. The floor and lateral walls of the middle fossa are shaped from the greater wings of the sphenoid bone and parts of the temporal bone, which house the internal and middle ear structures (Fig. 24-4). The posterior fossa, the largest and deepest fossa, is formed by the occipital, sphenoid, and petrous portions of the temporal bones; the cerebellum, pons, and medulla lie here, as do many cranial nerves. The foramen magnum, the largest opening in the skull, permits the spinal cord to join the brainstem in the posterior fossa. There are numerous other openings in the base of the skull for passage of arteries, veins, and cranial nerves (Fig. 24-4).

Between the skull and brain are the meninges, three covering membranes: the dura mater, arachnoidea, and pia mater (Fig. 24-1).

The *dura mater* is a tough, shiny, fibrous membrane close to the inner surface of the skull that folds to separate the cranial cavity into compartments. The largest fold is the falx cerebri (Fig. 24-1), an arch-shaped, vertically placed, midline structure separating the right and left cerebral hemispheres. A smaller fold of dura mater, the falx cerebelli, separates the cerebellar hemispheres vertically. A transverse fold, the tentorium cerebelli, forms the roof of the posterior fossa. The tentorium supports the occipital lobes of the cerebral hemispheres. Below the tentorium lie the cerebellum and brainstem. Structures above the tentorium are referred to as supratentorial, those below as infratentorial (Fig. 24-5).

At the margins of these dural folds lie large venous

sinuses that drain blood from the intracranial structures into the jugular veins. Several arteries also lie within the layers of the dura. The largest is the middle meningeal, a source of serious hemorrhage if torn by an overlying fracture of the skull. The rigid skull makes hemorrhage and swelling in the brain critical. Pressure on brain tissue may cause irreparable damage.

Beneath the dura mater is a fine membrane, the *arachnoidea*. The outer layer of arachnoidea closely approximates the dura mater. The inner layer forms innumerable web-like filaments that bridge to the surface of the brain (Fig. 24-1). The outer surface of the arachnoid membrane is closely adhered to the dura mater with no space normally between two membranes. The inner surface is separated from the pia mater beneath it by the subarachnoid space, which is filled with cerebrospinal fluid that bathes the brain. Around the base of the brain particularly, this space becomes enlarged to form cisterns. The major intracranial nerves and blood vessels pass through these compartments. Intracranial approaches can be charted in terms of the basal cisterns.

The *pia mater,* the innermost membrane, is like gossamer and attaches to the gray matter, dipping into the sulci and gyri. The pia mater has a rich vascular network that helps form the choroid plexus of the ventricles.

The brain is divided into the cerebral cortex, basal ganglia, hypothalamus, midbrain, brainstem, and cerebellum (Figs. 24-5 and 24-6).

The right and left cerebral hemispheres are the largest parts of the brain. Each hemisphere is composed of cerebral cortex and is divided into frontal, parietal, occipital, and temporal lobes; insula; rhinencephalon; basal ganglia; and hypothalamus. The two hemispheres are divided by a longitudinal fissure and joined underneath the falx by a large transverse bundle of nerve fibers, the corpus callosum (Fig. 24-6). Each of the cerebral hemispheres controls sensation and motor activity to and receives sensory stimuli from the opposite half of the body.

The surfaces of the hemispheres form convolutions called *gyri* and intervening furrows called *sulci*. Two sulci of anatomical importance to the surgeon are the central sulcus, or fissure of Rolando, which separates the motor from the sensory cortex, and the lateral sulcus, or fissure of Sylvius, which marks off the temporal lobe (Fig. 24-7). The insula (island of Reil) lies deep within the fissure of Sylvius and can be exposed by separating the upper and lower lips of the fissure. The frontal lobe is anterior to the fissure of Rolando and controls the higher functions of intellect and abstract reasoning. The motor cortex lies anterior to the fissure of Rolando. Destruction leads to loss of voluntary motor function on the opposite side of the body (Fig. 24-8).

Posterior to the fissure of Rolando is the parietal lobe, extending back to the parietooccipital fissure. This area contains the final receiving and integrating station for

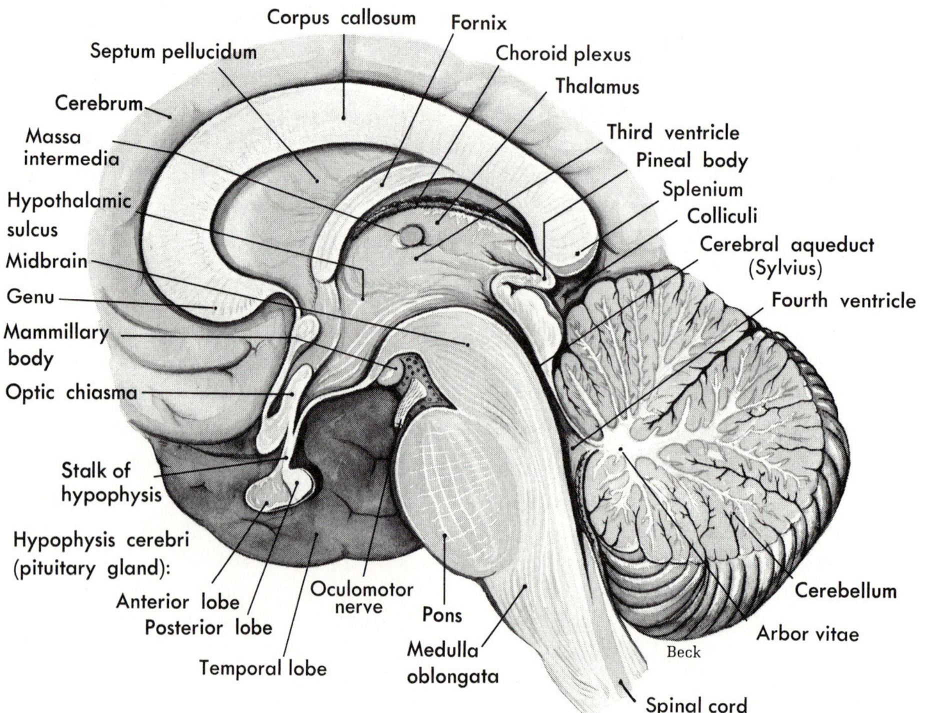

Fig. 24-6. Sagittal section through midline of brain showing structures around third ventricle including corpus callosum, thalamus, and hypothalamus. (From Anthony, C.P., and Kolthoff, N.J.: Textbook of anatomy and physiology, ed. 9, St. Louis, 1975, The C.V. Mosby Co.)

sensory impulses from the contralateral side of the body. The occipital lobe lies posterior to the parietooccipital fissure. It receives and integrates visual impulses and registers them as meaningful images (Figs. 24-7 and 24-8).

Inferior to the fissure of Sylvius, in the middle fossa, is the temporal lobe. Lesions of the left temporal lobe in right-handed individuals and in many left-handed persons often affect the comprehension and the verbalization of words, resulting in aphasia. Rhinencephalic structures such as the anterior limbic area may exert an inhibitory effect on brain mechanisms in the expression of emotions such as anger. Restlessness and hyperactivity may result from lesions of this area. The rhinencephalon has many connections with the hypothalamus. Malfunctions may affect sexual behavior, emotions, and motivation. Loss of recent memory may indicate a lesion of this area.

The convoluted surface of the cerebrum consists of gray matter, the *cerebral cortex,* which contains the cell bodies of the many nerve pathways of the brain. The underlying white matter contains millions of myelinated nerve axons and is relatively avascular compared with the cortex. The nerve pathways, or fiber tracts, are of three types: (1) commissural fibers, which pass from one cerebral hemisphere to the other; (2) association fibers, which connect gyri regions and lobes longitudinally within a cerebral hemisphere; and (3) projection fibers, including the great motor and sensory systems, which run vertically to connect the cortical regions with other portions of the central nervous system.

In prefrontal lobotomy, association fibers in the frontal lobe are divided, to effect changes in personality that may be beneficial in certain psychiatric disorders. *Cingulumotomy,* in which the cingulum is interrupted, also may be performed for treatment of these disorders.

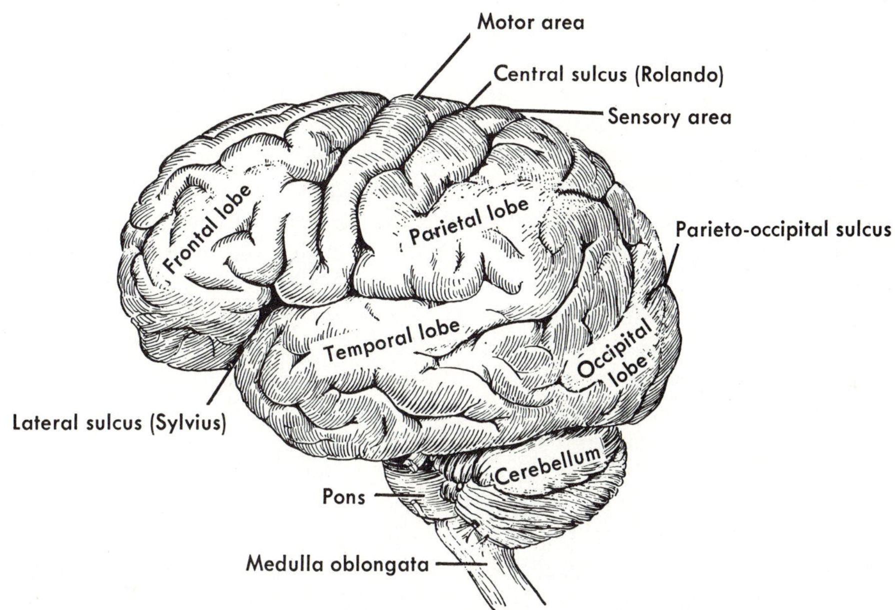

Fig. 24-7. Lateral view of cerebral hemisphere (showing lobes and principal fissures), cerebellum, pons, and medulla oblongata. (From Conway-Rutkowski, B.L.: Carini and Owens' neurological and neurosurgical nursing, ed. 8, St. Louis, 1982, The C.V. Mosby Co.)

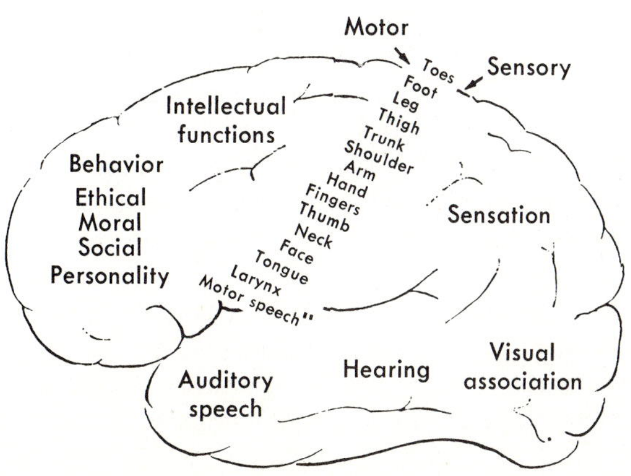

Fig. 24-8. Principal functional subdivisions of cerebral hemispheres. (Adapted from Conway, B.L.: Carini and Owens' neurological and neurosurgical nursing, ed. 7, St. Louis, 1978, The C.V. Mosby Co.)

Deep in the brain are five *basal ganglia,* or collections of nuclei, of the extrapyramidal system. Three of them, the caudate nucleus, putamen, and globus pallidus, associate with the thalamus for motor control (Fig. 24-6). Lesions here cause rigidity of the skeletal muscles and various types of spontaneous tremors. The basal ganglia and thalamus can be selectively destroyed surgically in an effort to relieve the tremors and rigidity associated with multiple sclerosis, Parkinson's disease, various forms of cerebellar degeneration, and late effects of severe brain trauma. The thalamus is the great receiving station of incoming sensory stimuli. Many of these stimuli are subsequently relayed to a final destination in the parietal cortex. Because of its central role in perception of body sensations, surgical lesions can be made in the thalamus in an attempt to alleviate pain.

Along the floor of the third ventricle is the *hypothalamus* (Fig. 24-6), which is principally concerned with the autonomic regulation of the body's internal environment and is intimately connected with the pituitary gland.

The short, stocky portion of the brain, between the cerebral hemispheres and pons, is called the *midbrain* (Fig. 24-5). It is made up of the cerebral peduncles, numerous nerve tracts and nuclei, and association centers that control the majority of eye movements. The hindbrain, or *brainstem,* immediately below the midbrain, consists of the pons and medulla oblongata (Fig. 24-7). The midbrain and brainstem form the floor of the fourth ventricle in the posterior fossa of the skull and contain many large efferent and afferent tracts and nuclei of most cranial nerves. The brainstem contains the cardiovascular and respiratory regulatory centers. Direct surgery on the brainstem is extremely dangerous.

The *cerebellum,* which occupies most of the posterior fossa, forms the roof of the fourth ventricle (Figs. 24-6 and 24-7). It has two lateral lobes and a medial portion, the *vermis.* The fissures of the cerebellum are small and run transversely. The cerebellum is principally concerned with balance and coordination of movement. It has many complex connections with higher and lower centers and exerts its influence homolaterally, in contrast to the cerebral hemispheres, which act contralaterally. At least half the brain tumors in children originate in the cerebellum. In adults and children the most common surgical lesions in this area are tumors and abscesses. By splitting the vermis in the exact midline, a satisfactory exposure of tumors that lie in the fourth ventricle is obtained without sacrificing the important cerebellar functions.

Within the brain are four communicating cavities, or *ventricles,* filled with cerebrospinal fluid. In the lower medial portion of each cerebral hemisphere lies a large lateral ventricle, which resembles a wishbone and is separated anteriorly from its counterpart by a thin pellucid septum (Fig. 24-9). Each lateral ventricle has a body and three horns: frontal, occipital, and temporal. Below the bodies of the lateral ventricles is a central cleft, or third ventricle. It communicates anteriorly with the lateral ventricles through the foramen of Monro and posteriorly with the fourth ventricle through the aqueduct of Sylvius, a long narrow channel passing through the midbrain. The fourth ventricle is a rhomboid-shaped cavity in the posterior fossa, between the cerebellum and the brainstem. In the roof of the fourth ventricle is an opening into the cisterna magna, the foramen of Magendie; at the lateral margins are the two foramina of Luschka, which open into the cisterna pontis.

Much of the cerebrospinal fluid originates in the *choroid plexuses* of the ventricles. These are tufted, vascular structures that allow certain fluid elements of the blood to pass through their ependymal linings. A choroid plexus is found along the floor in each lateral ventricle, on the roof of the third ventricle, and in the posterior portion of the fourth ventricle. Most of the fluid is formed in the lateral ventricles, flowing through the interventricular foramen of Monro to the third ventricle, and through the aqueduct of Sylvius to the fourth ventricle, where it escapes into the subarachnoid space of the basal cisterns through the foramina of Magendie and Luschka. From the basal cisterns, the fluid flows around the spinal cord, over the cerebellar lobes, around the medulla and the base of the brain, and over the cerebral hemispheres in the subarachnoid space. The fluid is absorbed into the bloodstream through little projections of the arachnoidea (pacchionian granulations) into the great dural venous sinuses, particularly the superior sagittal sinus, and by diffusion through perivascular, perineural, and periradicular channels (Fig. 24-1).

The total content of circulating cerebrospinal fluid averages 125 to 150 ml in the adult. Each lateral ventricle contains 10 to 15 ml, the rest of the ventricular system contains 5 ml, the cranial subarachnoid space averages about 25 ml, and the spinal subarachnoid space contains about 75 ml. The ventricular fluid normally has 5 to 15 mg/100 ml protein content, whereas the spinal fluid has 25 to 45 mg/100 ml. These values may be considerably elevated in pathological conditions of the central nervous system.

The function of the cerebrospinal fluid is mainly mechanical. It bathes the brain and spinal cord, helps support the weight of the brain, and acts as a cushion for the brain and spinal cord by absorbing some of the force of external trauma. By variation in its volume, it aids in keeping intracranial pressure relatively constant. If the brain atrophies, the cerebrospinal fluid increases in amount to fill the dead space; if the brain swells, the cerebrospinal fluid decreases in amount to compensate for the increase in brain mass. The fluid can carry certain drugs to diseased parts of the brain. It does not, however, play a significant role in supplying nutrition to the structures that it bathes.

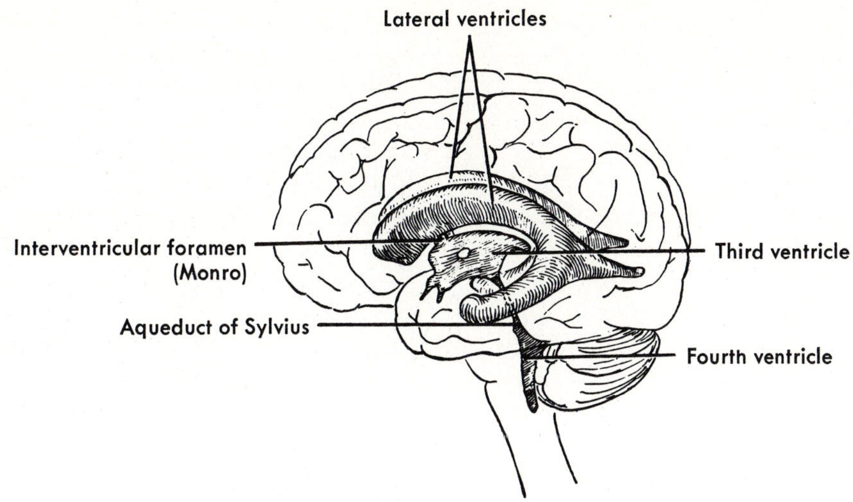

Fig. 24-9. Diagram of ventricular system showing its relationship to various parts of the brain. (From Conway-Rutkowski, B.L.: Carini and Owens' neurological and neurosurgical nursing, ed. 8, St. Louis, 1982, The C.V. Mosby Co.)

The rate of formation and absorption of cerebrospinal fluid is related to the osmotic and hydrostatic pressure of the blood. When intracranial pressure rises, an intravenous injection of hypertonic mannitol or urea or a nonosmotic diuretic is employed to dehydrate the blood and decrease the volume of cerebrospinal fluid.

Elevations in cerebrospinal fluid pressure can be caused by an expanding mass within the skull, such as a tumor, hemorrhage, or cerebral edema; an increase in formation of fluid, as in meningitis, encephalitis, and other febrile conditions; and increase in venous pressure within the skull from an obstruction to normal venous drainage; a blockage of absorption by inflammatory conditions of the arachnoidea and perivascular spaces; and any mechanical obstruction of the ventricular or subarachnoidal fluid pathways. Some of these conditions are amenable to surgical intervention.

The arterial supply of the brain comes from the internal carotid arteries anteriorly and the vertebral arteries that join to form the basilar artery posteriorly. The arterial circle of Willis, at the base of the brain, links the anterior and posterior arterial supply. The circle of Willis is a ring of blood vessels around the stalk of the pituitary gland and the optic chiasma. The branches of the circle are of two types: (1) small central terminal arteries, which dip perpendicularly into the brain and do not anastomose with one another, and (2) three large cortical branches on either side, named the anterior, middle, and posterior cerebral arteries, respectively (Fig. 24-10). The latter have a fairly free communication with each other peripherally, so that occlusion of one may be partly compensated for by its neighbor. The cortical branches do not, however, anastomose with their counterparts, except through the often inefficient communicating branches of the circle of Willis (Fig. 24-11).

The circle of Willis is of particular interest surgically because of the development of aneurysms there. An aneurysm is a weakness in the wall of a large artery. Aneurysms usually develop in or near the crotch of a bifurcation of the circle of Willis. It is thought that the weakness develops because of the superimposition of two lesions: a congenital absence of the media and a degeneration of the internal elastic lamina that normally strengthens the arterial wall. Erosion of the lamina results from the wear and tear of pulsatile pressure.

The most common sites of intracranial aneurysms are as follows: (1) adjacent to the anterior communicating artery, (2) at the junction of the posterior communicating artery and the internal carotid artery, (3) at the origin of the anterior cerebral arteries, and (4) at the first bifurcation of the middle cerebral artery.

The cerebral veins do not parallel the arteries as do the veins in most other parts of the body. The external cortical veins anastomose freely in the pia mater, forming larger cerebral veins, and as such they pierce the arachnoid membrane, cross the subdural space, and empty into the great dural venous sinuses. A subdural hemorrhage following head trauma may arise from disruption of these bridging vessels; an epidural hemorrhage often results from lacerations of the middle meningeal artery, a branch of the external carotid artery that supplies the dura mater. The deep cerebral veins, which drain the interior of the hemispheres, empty principally into the great vein of Galen and the inferior sagittal sinus (Figs. 24-12 and 24-13).

The blood transports oxygen, nutrients, and other substances necessary for the proper functioning of living tissue. The needs of the brain for oxygen and glucose are critical. The brain can store only very limited amounts of oxygen and energy-producing nutrients. Constant flow of blood to the brain must be maintained.

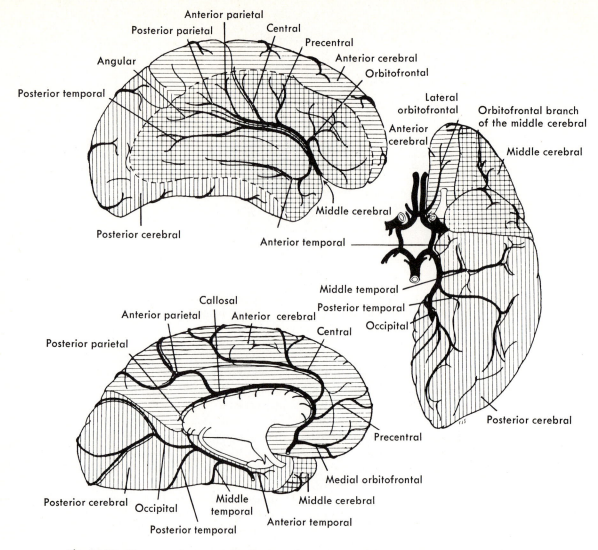

Fig. 24-10. Diagram of areas of distribution of anterior, middle, and posterior cerebral arteries. (From Mettler, F.A.: Neuroanatomy, ed. 2, St. Louis, The C.V. Mosby Co.)

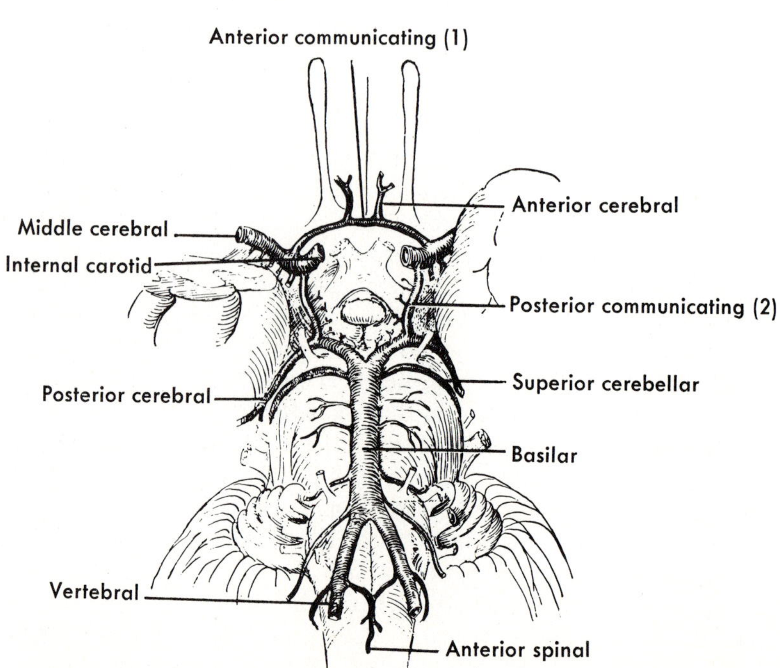

Fig. 24-11. Diagram of principal cerebral arteries and circle of Willis. (From Conway-Rutkowski, B.L.: Carini and Owens' neurological and neurosurgical nursing, ed. 8, St. Louis, 1982, The C.V. Mosby Co.)

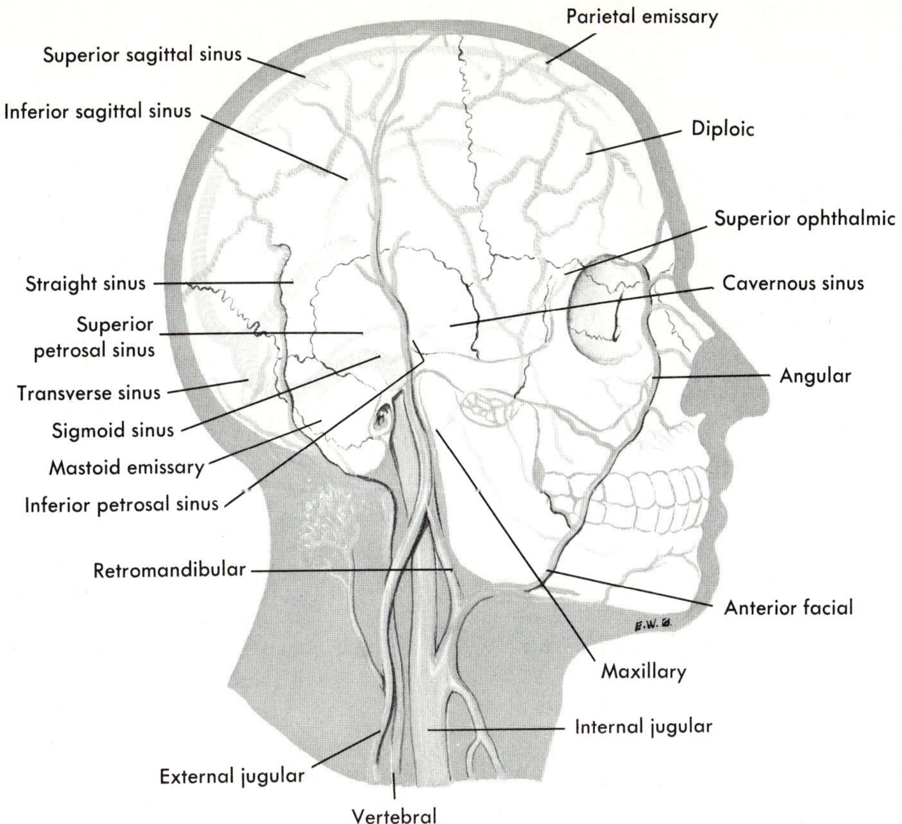

Fig. 24-12. Semischematic projection of large veins of head. Deep veins and dural sinuses are projected on skull. Note connection (emissary veins) between superficial and deep veins. (From Anthony, C.P., and Kolthoff, N.J.: Textbook of anatomy and physiology, ed. 9, St. Louis, 1975, The C.V. Mosby Co.)

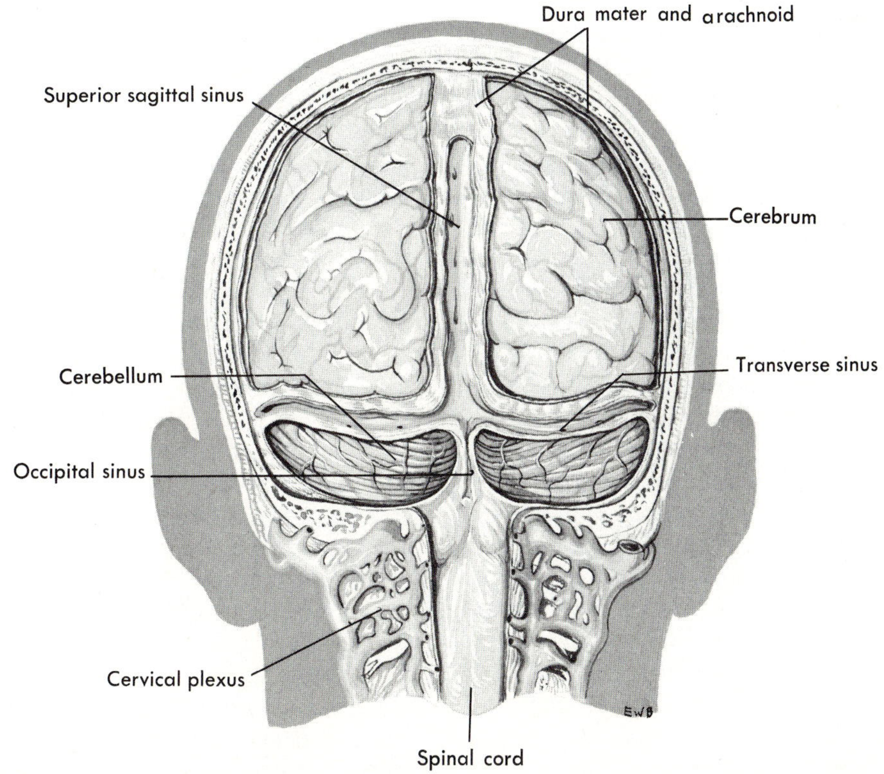

Fig. 24-13. Venous sinuses shown in relation to brain and skull. (From Anthony, C.P., and Kolthoff, N.J.: Textbook of anatomy and physiology, ed. 9, St. Louis, 1975, The C.V. Mosby Co.)

The brain uses oxygen in the metabolism of glucose, the chief source of energy. Protein and fat metabolism play little part in energy production. In the face of an oxygen deficit, the survival time of central nervous system tissue is very short. In the face of low blood sugar, central nervous system function is compromised, and unconsciousness results.

Generally, all factors affecting the systemic blood pressure indirectly affect the cerebral circulation. Twenty percent of the cardiac output normally goes to the brain. The cerebral blood flow is kept constant by an autoregulation phenomenon. When the mean arterial pressure falls below 60 mm Hg, the autoregulation mechanism usually fails. Thus controlled hypotension may be safely used in intracranial surgery.

The blood-brain barrier prevents many substances in the blood from reaching the brain. It may influence brain function by determining composition of brain fluids. Some types of abnormal brain functions could result from an abnormal blood-brain barrier.

Cranial nerves

Twelve pairs of cranial nerves arise within the cranial cavity (Fig. 24-14). From a surgical standpoint, they are considered with the head.

First cranial nerve. The olfactory nerve, a fiber tract of the brain, is located under the frontal lobe on the cribriform plate of the ethmoid bone. It governs the sense of smell. Frontal lobe tumors, fractures of the anterior fossa of the skull, and lesions of the nasal cavity may affect the olfactory nerve.

Second cranial nerve. The optic nerve is a fiber tract of the brain. Originating in the ganglion cells of the retina, it passes through the optic foramen in the apex of the orbit to reach the optic chiasma, where a partial crossing of the fibers occurs, so that the fibers from the nasal half of each retina pass to the opposite side. Posterior to the chiasma, the visual pathway is called the *optic tract;* still further back, it becomes the optic radiation. Lesions in various parts of this pathway produce characteristic defects in the visual fields. For example, a lesion of the chiasma usually destroys the temporal vision of each eye (bitemporal hemianopia), whereas a lesion of the occipital lobe produces impairment of vision (homonymous hemianopia) affecting the right or left halves of the visual fields of both eyes.

Lesions that affect the optic nerve and are treated by neurosurgery include primary gliomas of the nerve, pituitary tumors that press on the optic chiasma, and, occasionally, meningiomas in the region of the sella turcica and olfactory groove. The optic nerves and chiasma are best exposed through a frontal craniotomy, along the floor of the anterior fossa, or through a frontotemporal approach along the sphenoid ridge.

Third, fourth, and sixth cranial nerves. These three pairs of nerves—the oculomotor, the trochlear, and the abducens, respectively—are conveniently considered together because they are the motor nerves to the muscles of the eyes. They are affected by many toxic, inflammatory, vascular, and neoplastic lesions. The third nerve may be affected by aneurysms of the internal carotid artery, and pressure against this nerve accounts for pupillary dilatation when temporal lobe herniation resulting from increased intracranial pressure is present.

Fifth cranial nerve. The trigeminal nerve has two functions: (1) sensory supply to the forehead, eyes, meninges, face, jaw, teeth, hard palate, buccal mucosa, and tongue and (2) motor innervation of the muscles of mastication. The sensory fibers that arise from cells in the gasserian ganglion travel along the medial wall of the middle cranial fossa and then extend peripherally in three divisions: ophthalmic, maxillary, and mandibular. Behind the ganglion, the fibers enter the brainstem by way of the sensory root. The motor root, which originates from cells in the brainstem, follows the course of the larger sensory component.

Trigeminal neuralgia (tic douloureux) is characterized by excruciating, piercing paroxysms of pain, affecting one or more of the major peripheral divisions. The recurrent attacks are usually brought on by stimulation of trigger zones present about the face, nares, lips, or teeth. This affliction, of unknown cause, tends to occur unilaterally and in older persons. Medical treatment is frequently unsuccessful. A great variety of neurosurgical procedures have been proposed for its control. Peripheral neurectomies of the supraorbital or infraorbital nerves may easily be performed with the patient under local anesthesia, but the effect is temporary because the nerves regenerate. A more certain method of relief is retrogasserian neurectomy. When the nerve root is divided behind the ganglion, no regeneration can occur, and the pain is permanently obliterated (Fig. 24-15). However, some patients complain about the postoperative numbness of the face, and a few are disturbed by annoying paresthesia. Anesthesia of the cornea may lead to keratitis; differential section of the root has been sufficiently perfected to preserve a few sensory fibers to the cornea and prevent this complication. In most cases, the motor root can be saved.

Retrogasserian neurectomy may be performed through a temporal approach along the floor of the middle fossa or by a posterior fossa craniectomy, in which case the nerve root is sectioned in the cerebellopontine angle where it emerges from the pons. By the posterior fossa approach, the surgeon can more easily spare the motor root, but this advantage is countered by slightly greater morbidity than with the temporal operation.

Trigeminal neuralgia can also be treated by retrogasserian rhizotomy with radiofrequency current. With the patient under local anesthesia, an electrode is placed by

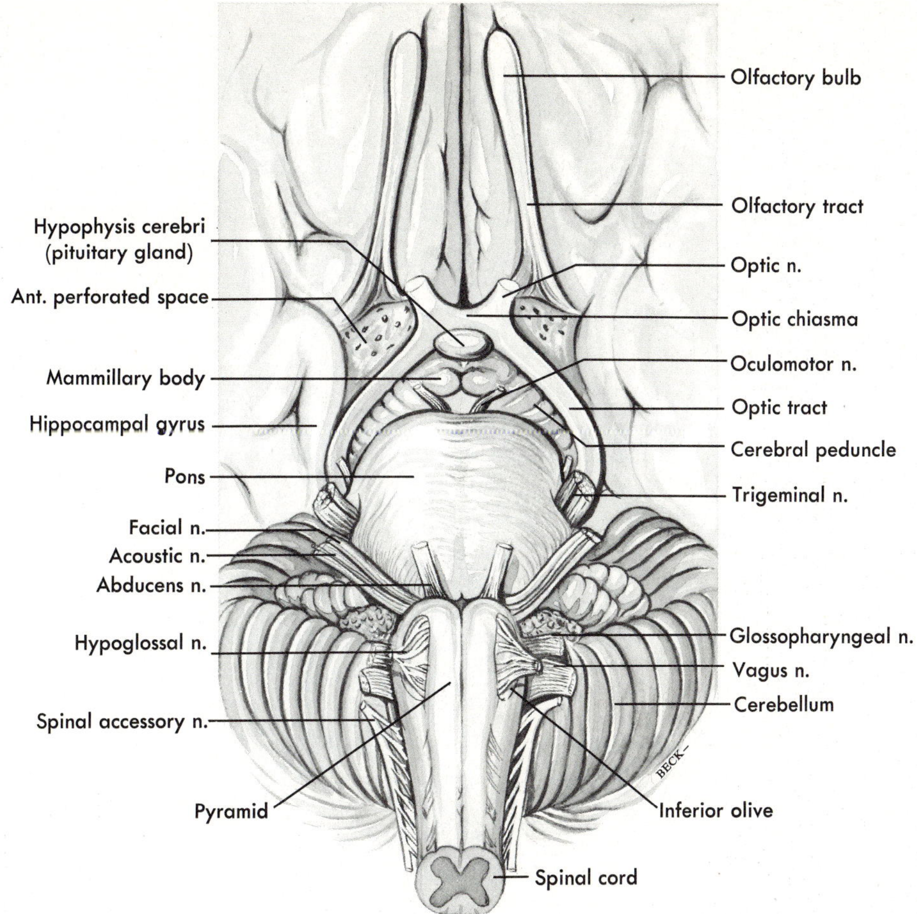

Fig. 24-14. Ventral surface of brain showing attachment of cranial nerves. (From Anthony, C.P., and Kolthoff, N.J.: Textbook of anatomy and physiology, ed. 9, St. Louis, 1975, The C.V. Mosby Co.)

x-ray vision. Lesions are made in the ganglion to achieve the desired results (Fig. 24-15).

Seventh cranial nerve. The facial nerve supplies the musculature of the face and the anterior two thirds of the tongue (for taste). It originates in the brainstem, passes through the skull with the eighth nerve by way of the internal acoustic meatus, continues along the facial canal, and exits just posterior to the parotid gland. The nerve may be damaged by acoustic neurinomas, fractures at the base of the skull, mastoid infections, or surgical procedures in the vicinity of the parotid gland. When permanent interruption occurs, useful operations for restoration of function include spinofacial or hypoglossofacial anastomosis. These operations are performed high in the neck behind the parotid gland, using the operating microscope.

Eighth cranial nerve. The acoustic nerve has two parts, both sensory—the cochlear for hearing and the vestibular for balance. The former receives stimuli from the organ of Corti, the latter from the semicircular canals. The major surgical lesion of the eighth nerve is acoustic neurinoma, a histologically benign tumor growing from the nerve sheath at its entrance into the internal auditory meatus. This tumor arises deep in the angle between the cerebellum and pons. Symptoms may include unilateral deafness, tinnitus, unilateral impairment of cerebellar function, occasionally numbness of the face from involvement of the fifth cranial nerve, and, late in the course, papilledema caused by pressure on the pons. The operative approach is usually through a unilateral suboccipital craniectomy. Great care must be taken to prevent injury to the pons, and an attempt is made to preserve the facial nerve.

Ménière's disease is an affliction of the eighth nerve characterized by deafness and tinnitus, with episodic attacks of severe vertigo and vomiting. These episodes may pitch the patient violently to the floor without warning and force the patient to bed for days. When simple medical measures fail to alleviate the problem, section of the eighth nerve may be performed; there have been consistently excellent results with this procedure.

Ninth cranial nerve. The glossopharyngeal nerve supplies the sense of taste to the posterior third of the

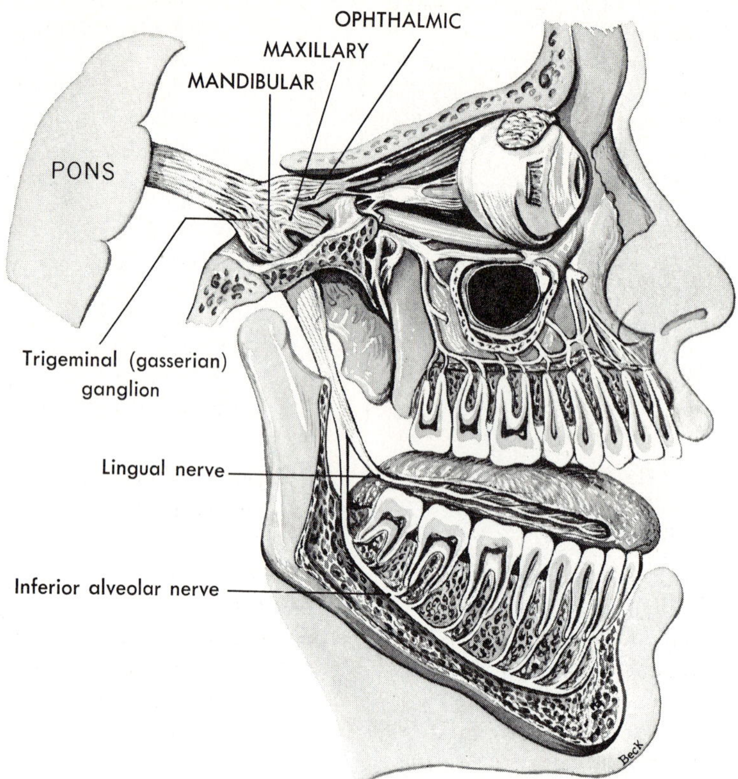

Fig. 24-15. Trigeminal (fifth cranial) nerve and its three main divisions. (From Anthony, C.P., and Kolthoff, N.J.: Textbook of anatomy and physiology, ed. 9, St. Louis, 1975, The C.V. Mosby Co.)

tongue and sensation to the tonsils and pharyngeal region and partially innervates the pharyngeal muscles. Rarely, it is involved in a painful tic similar to trigeminal tic. Its sensory component can be sectioned for this reason, to treat a hypersensitive carotid sinus, or, along with the fifth nerve, to treat painful malignancies of the face, mouth, and pharynx. The ninth nerve lies near the eighth nerve in the posterior fossa and is exposed in a similar way.

Tenth cranial nerve. The vagus nerve has many functions, chief among which are innervation of pharyngeal and laryngeal musculature, control of heart rate, and regulation of acid secretion of the stomach. In neck surgery, the surgeon carefully avoids the recurrent laryngeal branch; in gastric surgery, the surgeon severs the nerve at the lower end of the esophagus to treat a peptic ulcer. The neurosurgeon is mainly concerned with preventing damage to the vagus nerve during posterior fossa surgery.

Eleventh cranial nerve. The spinal accessory nerve is a motor nerve to the sternocleidomastoid and trapezius muscles. To restore mobility to the face, it may be anastomosed to the peripheral end of a damaged facial nerve.

Twelfth cranial nerve. The hypoglossal nerve innervates the musculature of the tongue. Its neurosurgical interest is similar to that of the spinal accessory nerve.

Pathological lesions of the brain

Brain tumors are neither as rare nor their prognosis as poor as is often believed. Early diagnosis simplifies surgical treatment because increased intracranial pressure and severe neurological changes are not usually present.

Brain tumors are either malignant or benign, depending on the cell type. Primary tumors generally do not resemble the carcinomas and sarcomas found elsewhere in the body and rarely metastasize outside the central nervous system. However, carcinomas or sarcomas growing elsewhere in the body metastasize to the central nervous system.

If both primary and metastatic tumors of the brain and its covering membranes are included in the term *intracranial tumors,* such tumors may be classified pathologically as congenital, mesodermal, ectodermal, metastatic, and miscellaneous as follows:

A. Congenital tumors
   1. Epidermoid
   2. Dermoid
   3. Teratoma
   4. Chordoma
   5. Craniopharyngioma occurs in children and adults and arises from the region of the pituitary stalk. It is

usually cystic, and calcification above the sella turcica is often seen on x-ray films. Diabetes insipidus and visual field changes are common.

B. Mesodermal tumors
   1. Meningioma usually is encapsulated and easily separated from nervous tissue. It is very vascular and may adhere to the dural venous sinuses or major arteries.
   2. Neurinoma usually arises from neurilemma sheath cells of the vestibular portion of the eighth cranial nerve within the auditory meatus. It grows to fill the cerebellopontine angle and may indent the brainstem.
   3. Vascular tumors
      a. Angioma is regarded as a malformation. Most of these are arteriovenous malformations.
      b. Hemangioblastoma is usually cystic and likely to occur in the cerebellar hemispheres. It is sometimes present in association with angiomas of the retina and other organs.
      c. Aneurysm is a saccular dilatation or out-pouching of the cerebral arteries. It may rupture, producing subarachnoid hemorrhage.

C. Ectodermal tumors
   1. Gliomas
      a. Glioblastoma multiforme is an infiltrative, fast growing, rapidly recurring cerebral tumor that occurs most frequently in middle age. It may invade both cerebral hemispheres by crossing in the corpus callosum. Areas of necrosis are characteristic. Astrocytomas, astroblastomas, and oligodendrogliomas may transform into this malignant tumor with time.
      b. Medulloblastoma is a fast growing, rapidly recurring tumor of the vermis of the cerebellum and fourth ventricle that usually occurs in young children. It characteristically metastasizes in the subarachnoid spaces, usually spreading to the base of the brain by this route.
      c. Ependymoma occurs most frequently in children and is likely to arise in or near the ventricular walls. It commonly occurs in the fourth ventricle, where it abuts or involves vital medullary centers. It also frequently metastasizes in the subarachnoid spaces.
      d. Astrocytoma usually occurs in the cerebellum of children and the cerebrum of adults. It is often cystic and discrete in children, infiltrating and ill defined in adults.
      e. Oligodendroglioma is usually found in the cerebral hemispheres and is infiltrating but occasionally moderately well defined.
      f. Astroblastoma is a rare glioma occurring in the cerebral hemisphere of middle-aged adults. It may share the growth characteristics of astrocytoma and glioblastoma multiforme.
      g. Spongioblastoma occurs predominantly in the optic chiasma and nerves of children and in the pons. This lesion grows in vital structures and is rarely amenable to even partial removal.
   2. Pituitary tumors
      a. Chromophobe tumor is relatively common in the anterior pituitary glands of adults. It causes compression of the pituitary, adjacent optic chiasma, and hypothalamus. The latter may lead to diabetes insipidus.
      b. Chromophile tumor is often secreting (as are some chromophobe tumors). Acromegaly or, less commonly, Cushing's syndrome may occur and cause the patient to seek help long before the tumor has expanded sufficiently to compromise the optic chiasma.

D. Metastatic tumors usually arise from carcinoma, more rarely from sarcoma, and occasionally from melanomas and retinal tumors. The most common sources are bronchogenic carcinoma and carcinoma of the breast.

Tumors not discussed here are eosinophilic granuloma, tuberculomas, and other granulomas; brain abscesses; pinealomas; colloid cysts; choroid plexus papillomas; microgliomas; fibrous dysplasia; and lymphomas.

A brain lesion is diagnosed by history, neurological examination, and diagnostic studies. The manifestations of an intracranial tumor fall into two classes: those resulting from irritation or impairment of function in specific areas of the brain directly affected by the tumor and those resulting from diffuse increased intracranial pressure.

Lesions that are situated in the left frontotemporal region, where motor speech originates, lead to aphasia; occipital tumors produce hemianoptic visual defects; large frontal lobe tumors may cause striking personality changes. Cortical tumors frequently produce focal seizures of diagnostic value. The onset of epileptiform seizures in the adult is often associated with an intracranial neoplasm. Pituitary tumors characteristically press on the optic chiasma and impair the temporal vision of each eye. They disturb pituitary glandular function, resulting in hypopituitary states, pituitary dwarfism, or acromegaly. Posterior fossa tumors often manifest their presence by blocking the cerebrospinal fluid circulation, but they may also destroy cerebellar function, resulting in incoordination, ataxia, and scanning speech.

Back

The spinal column consists of thirty-three vertebrae: seven cervical, twelve thoracic, five lumbar, five sacral (fused as one), and one coccygeal (fused from four small vertebrae) (Fig. 24-16).

The first cervical vertebra, or atlas, supports the skull. The second cervical vertebra, or axis, can be identified by its odontoid process, a vertical projection extending into the foramen of the atlas like a stick in a hoop, and rests against the anterior tubercle. Ligaments hold the two together but allow considerable rotational movement. When these ligaments are torn, as in a hanging, or when the odontoid is fractured by trauma, the atlas may slip on the axis and crush the cord, resulting in immediate death.

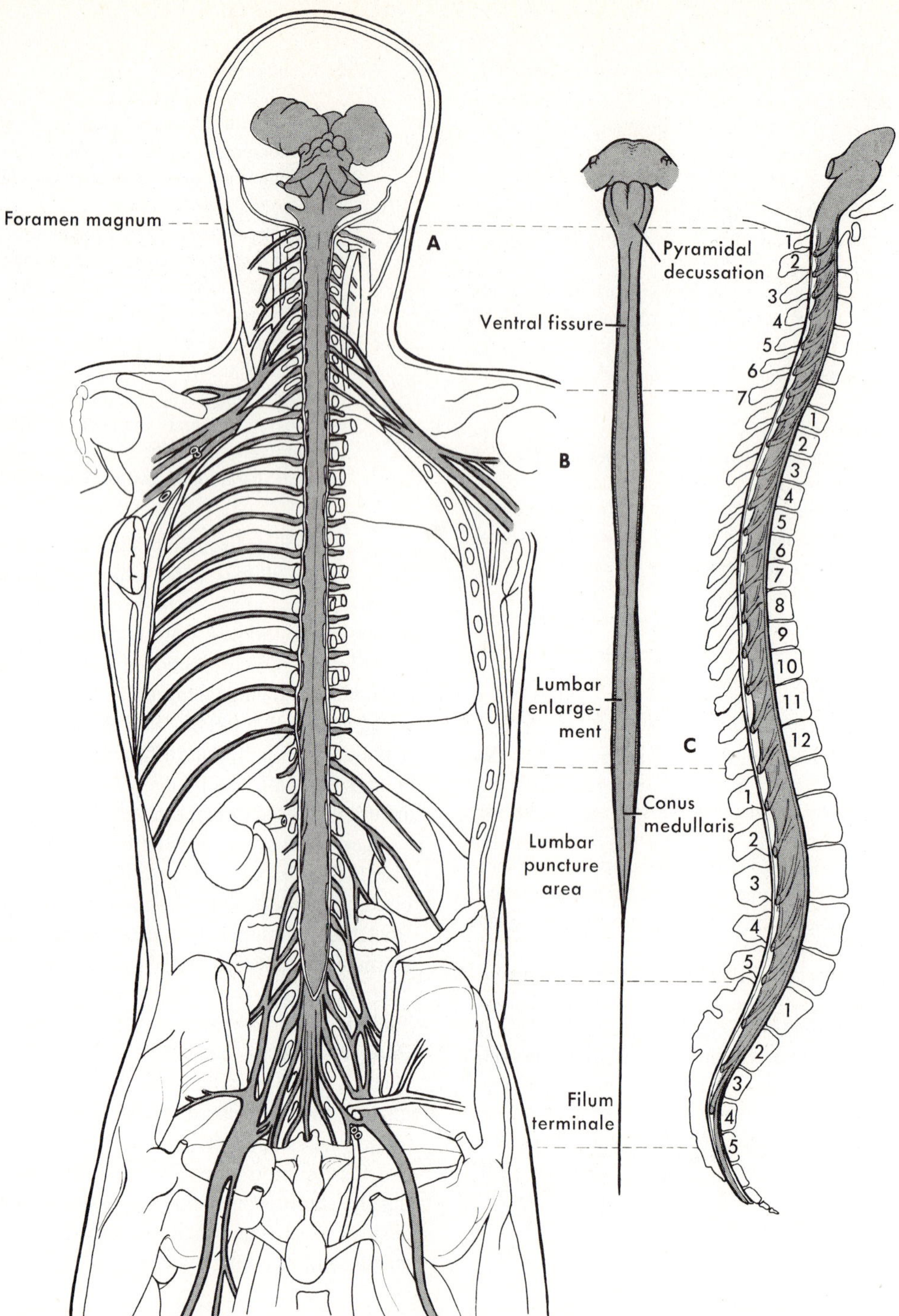

Fig. 24-16. Posterior view of brainstem and spinal cord. **A,** Torso dissected from back is shown. Dura mater has been opened and cord exposed. Levels concerned can be easily determined by referring to ribs on left side of thorax. Cord proper terminates opposite body of second lumbar vertebra (**B**) as conus medullaris. **B,** Ventral surface of cord stripped of dura mater and arachnoidea. It is symmetrical in structure, two halves of which are separated by ventral fissure. This fissure stops at foramen magnum. Caudally, pia mater leaves conus medullaris as glistening thread or filum terminale. **C,** Cord is exposed from lateral side. Dura mater has been opened. Since cord is shorter than canal and spinal nerves leave through intervertebral foramina, one at a time, lowest portion of canal is occupied only by a bundle-like accumulation of nerve roots, the cauda equina. Caudal end of dural sac, enclosing spinal cord and cauda equina, lies somewhere between bodies of first and third sacral vertebrae. Size and position of the three views correspond, and delimitation of major vertebral levels is indicated by transverse lines for all three figures. (Adapted from Mettler, F.A.: Neuroanatomy, ed. 2, St. Louis, The C.V. Mosby Co.; from Conway-Rutkowski, B.L.: Carini and Owens' neurological and neurosurgical nursing, ed. 8, St. Louis, 1982, The C.V. Mosby Co.)

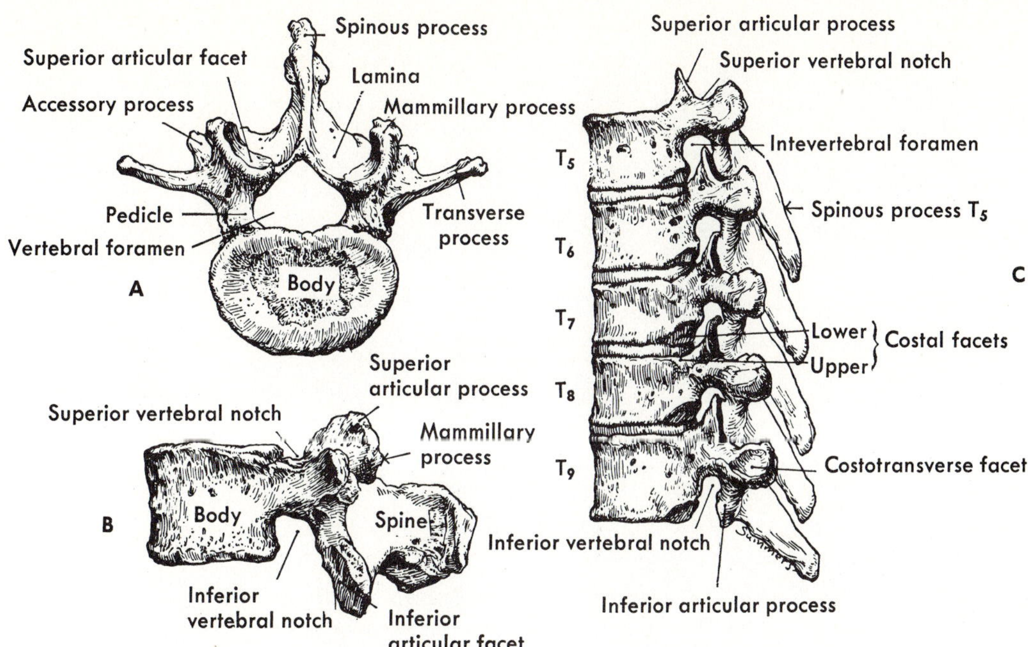

Fig. 24-17. A, Fourth lumbar vertebra from above. **B,** Fourth lumbar vertebra from side. **C,** Fifth to ninth thoracic vertebrae, showing relationships of various parts. (From Mettler, F.A.: Neuroanatomy, ed. 2, St. Louis, The C.V. Mosby Co.)

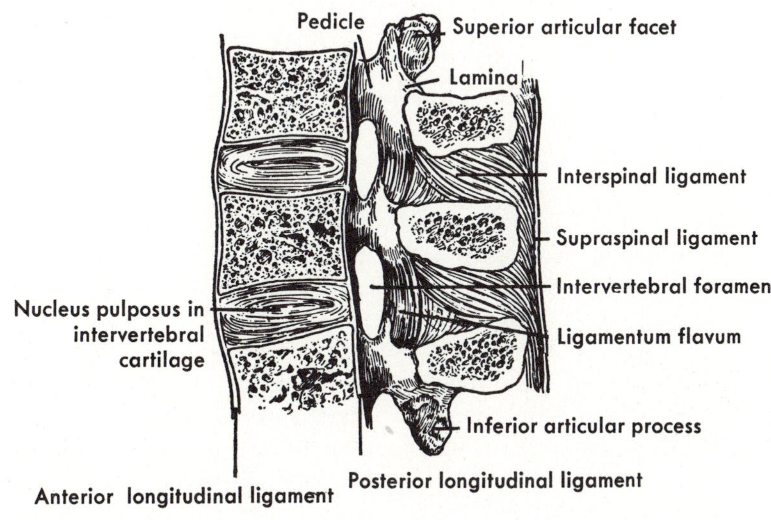

Fig. 24-18. Median section through three lumbar vertebrae, showing intervertebral discs (nuclei pulposi). (From Mettler, F.A.: Neuroanatomy, ed. 2, St. Louis, The C.V. Mosby Co.)

The other cervical, thoracic, and lumbar vertebrae are more alike in structure. Each has a body, an oval block of spongy bone situated anteriorly. An intervertebral disc, a fibrocartilaginous elastic cushion, separates one body from another (Figs. 24-17 and 24-18). The spinal cord lies in a canal formed by the vertebral bodies, pedicles, and laminae. Articular surfaces or facets project from the pedicles and form joints with the facets of the vertebrae above and below. Transverse processes extend laterally and serve as hitching posts for muscles and ligaments. Spinous processes extend posteriorly and can be palpated in all except obese persons (Fig. 24-17). The vertebrae are held together by multiple ligaments and muscles. Motion of the spine occurs at the articular facets and through the elastic intervertebral discs (Fig. 24-18).

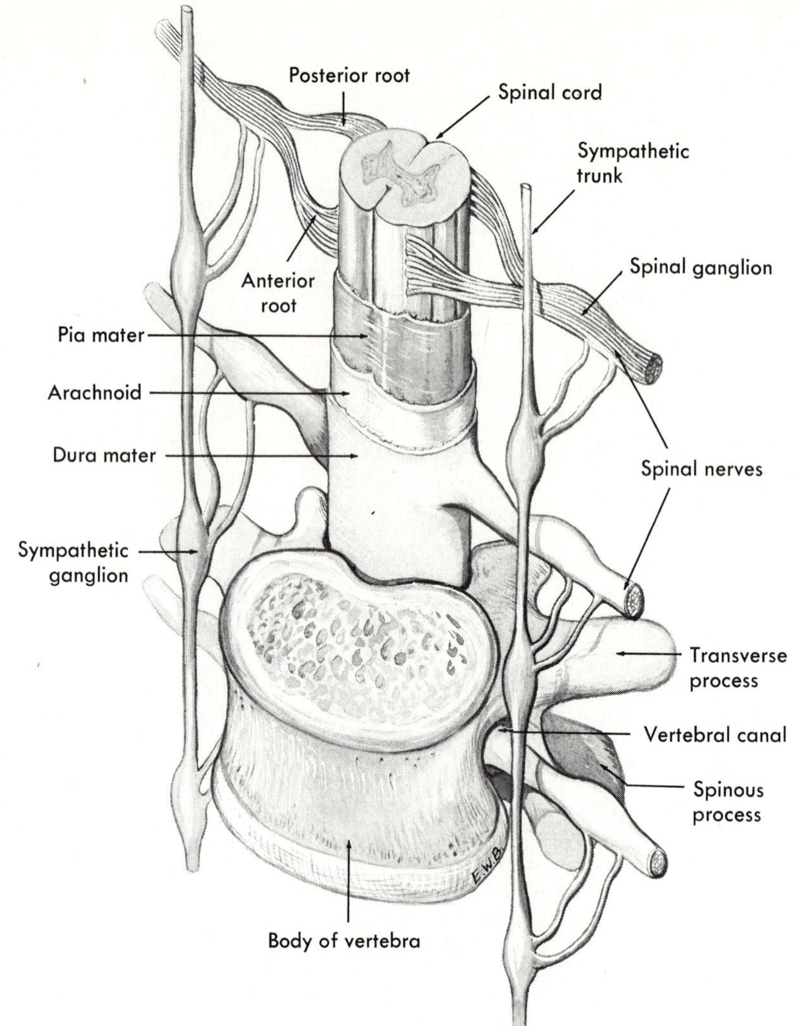

Fig. 24-19. Spinal cord, showing meninges, formation of spinal nerves, and relations to vertebra and to sympathetic trunk and ganglia. (From Anthony, C.P., and Kolthoff, N.J.: Textbook of anatomy and physiology, ed. 9, St. Louis, 1975, The C.V. Mosby Co.)

The spinal cord is protected by this bony framework. The dura mater is separated from its bony surroundings by a layer of epidural fat. Beneath the dura mater is the arachnoidea, a continuation of the same structure in the head. The subarachnoid space contains spinal fluid. A thin layer of pia mater adheres to the cord, and cerebrospinal fluid also circulates from the fourth ventricle into the central canal of the cord.

The spinal cord is a downward prolongation of the brainstem, starting at the upper border of the atlas and ending at the upper border of the second lumbar vertebra. The cord is oval in cross section. It is slightly flattened in the anteroposterior diameter. A cross section looks like a gray H surrounded by a white mantle split in the midline, anteriorly and posteriorly, by sulci.

The peripheral white matter carries long myelinated motor and sensory tracts; the central gray matter consists of nerve cell bodies and short unmyelinated fibers (Figs. 24-16 and 24-19). The principal long pathways are the laterally placed pyramidal tracts, carrying impulses down from the cerebral cortex to the motor neurons of the cord; the dorsal ascending columns, mediating sensations of touch and proprioception; and the anterolaterally placed spinothalamic tracts, carrying pain and temperature sensations to the thalamus, the sensory receiving station of the brain (Fig. 24-20).

At each vertebral level are two pairs of spinal nerves (Fig. 24-19): an anterior or motor root, the cell bodies of which lie in the anterior horn of the spinal gray matter, and a posterior root, the cell bodies of which lie in the spinal ganglia in the intervertebral foramina, through which the nerves exit from the spinal canal and emerge from the cord. Each pair of roots forms one spinal nerve. The cervical nerves pass out horizontally, but at each lower level they take on an increasingly oblique and downward direction. In the lumbar region, the course of the nerves

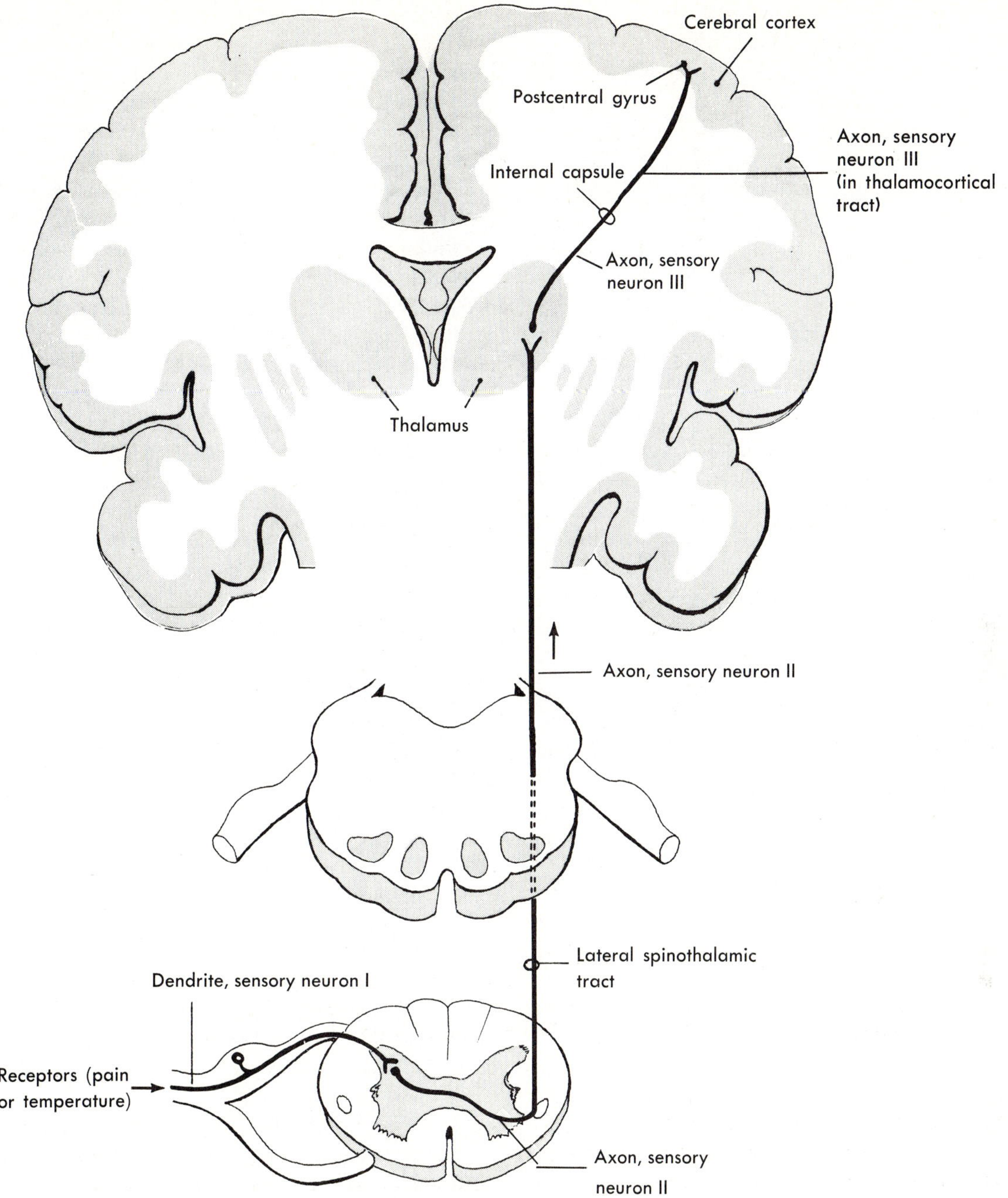

Fig. 24-20. Lateral spinothalamic tract relays sensory impulses from pain and temperature receptors up cord to thalamus. Thalamocortical tract fibers relay them to somatic sensory area of cortex (postcentral gyrus). (From Anthony, C.P., and Kolthoff, N.J.: Textbook of anatomy and physiology, ed. 9, St. Louis, 1975, The C.V. Mosby Co.)

is nearly vertical, forming the cauda equina (Fig. 24-16). This phenomenon is explained by the fact that the spinal cord, which fills the entire spinal canal in the fetus, grows at a slower rate than the bony spine, thus leaving the lower nerves a progressively longer course to their exit.

The vasculature of the spinal cord and vertebral column is a rich, delicate network. The arterial blood supply to the spinal cord arises from the vertebral arteries as the anterior spinal artery and the posterior spinal arteries. These vessels branch and anastomose on both sides of the cord and within the substance of the cord. They also branch into anterior and posterior radicular arteries that form spinal rami as they accompany the spinal nerve roots through the intervertebral foramina.

A series of venous plexuses surround and innervate the spinal cord at each level in the vertebral canal. They anastomose with each other and form the intervertebral veins as they exit through the intervertebral foramina with the spinal nerves to join the intercostal, lumbar, and sacral veins. The lateral longitudinal veins near the foramen magnum empty into the inferior petrosal sinus and cerebellar veins. The venous network innervates the bony structures and musculature as well as the spinal cord and nerve roots. Venous bleeding during spinal surgery is always a potential problem for which the nurse must be prepared.

Pathological lesions of the spinal cord and adjacent structures

Operations are performed to correct the following conditions: congenital malformations, injuries, tumors, herniated and degenerative intervertebral discs, abscesses, and intractable pain.

The most common congenital lesion encountered is a lumbar *meningocele,* or *meningomyelocele,* a failure of union of the vertebral arches during fetal development. The fluid-filled, thin-walled sac often contains neural elements. Surgical correction is necessary when the sac lining is so thin that there is a potential or actual cerebrospinal fluid leak. The operation consists of excising the sac wall to preserve adhering nerves, closing the dura mater, and reinforcing the closure with fascial flaps swung from the paraspinal muscles. Skin closure without tension is essential for primary healing. Large skin and subcutaneous flaps must occasionally be fashioned to ensure healing.

Injuries to the spinal cord are serious. No regeneration of destroyed or divided nerve tracts occurs. Recovery may take place with lesser degrees of injury, such as contusion or compression. Surgery can be of value in preventing further damage by debridement of penetrating wounds, removal of foreign bodies, relief of pressure on the cord or roots, open reduction of certain dislocations and fractures, and measures aimed at stabilizing the spine. In cervical injuries, skeletal traction by means of tongs applied to the skull is often the preferred treatment.

Spinal cord tumors are classified according to location as extradural (outside the dura mater) or intradural (inside the dura mater). Intradural tumors may be either extramedullary (outside the cord) or intramedullary (within the cord). Extradural tumors include sarcomas and carcinomas, which may be metastatic (from adjacent structures in or about the vertebrae). Other extradural lesions include Hodgkin's disease, lipomas, neurofibromas, chondromas, angiomas, abscesses, and granulomas.

Intradural tumors can be extramedullary, which are usually benign and originate from the dura mater and arachnoidea surrounding the cord and from the root sheaths of spinal nerves. Neurinomas are especially common in the thoracocervical area and may be part of generalized neurofibromatosis. Meningiomas also commonly occur in intradural extramedullary locations. Less frequently, lipomas or other types of tumors are found. Gliomas are the most common intramedullary tumors and have a less favorable prognosis. These tumors infiltrate the cord tissue and are much more difficult to remove than extramedullary tumors.

The majority of intradural tumors are extramedullary and benign and, if diagnosed early, before severe neurological deficits occur, offer an excellent prognosis. They manifest their presence by pain of a radicular nature and various motor and sensory disabilities below their segmental locations. Cord tumors frequently produce spinal fluid block and can be pinpointed accurately by intraspinal injection of a radiopaque oil (myelography). A standard laminectomy is used for exposure and removal.

The rare surgical infections of the spinal cord take the form of extradural abscesses and granulomas. Treatment consists of a combination of excision, drainage, chemotherapy, and occasionally spinal fusion.

The most frequently encountered neurosurgical problem is the herniated intervertebral disc. Because of weakness or rupture of the circular ligament (annulus fibrosus), which confines the soft center of the disc (nucleus pulposus), herniation of the latter may occur and give rise to pain from nerve root compression. When pain is severe or nerve damage excessive, surgical excision of the disc offers the most satisfactory relief. The procedure entails interlaminar exposure and piecemeal removal of the displaced nucleus. If the spine is unstable or there are other incontrovertible reasons for operative stabilization of the bony spine, a fusion of one type or another may be combined with the disc surgery (Chapter 20).

Certain painful lesions, usually of a malignant nature, can be controlled by dividing the pain fibers supplying the affected area. This may be accomplished by sectioning the sensory roots intraspinally (posterior rhizotomy) or by incising the spinothalamic tracts (anterolateral cordotomy) that carry pain and temperature impulses. A laminectomy is necessary for exposure.

Peripheral nerves

Within the context of this discussion, the peripheral nervous system includes the cranial nerves outside the cranial cavity, the spinal nerves, the autonomic nerves, and the ganglia. This division is artificial and only for the purpose of delineating surgical approaches. The cranial nerves have been described under the section on the head because all arise within the cranial cavity, and most are usually approached neurosurgically through the head.

There are thirty-one pairs of spinal nerves, each pair numbered for the level of the spinal column at which it emerges: cervical one (C-1) through eight (C-8), thoracic one (T-1) through twelve (T-12), lumbar one (L-1) through five (L-5), sacral one (S-1) through five (S-5), and coccygeal one. The thoracic region is sometimes referred to as the dorsal region with D-1 synonymous with T-1. The first pair of cervical spinal nerves emerges between C-1 and the occipital bone. The eighth cervical nerves emerge from the intervertebral foramina between C-7 and T-1. The first thoracic nerves emerge between T-1 and T-2.

In the cervical and lumbosacral regions, the spinal nerves regroup in a plexiform manner before they form the peripheral nerves of the upper and lower extremities; those in the thoracic region form cutaneous and intercostal nerves. The principal nerves of the upper plexus include the musculocutaneous, median, ulnar, and radial; those of the lumbosacral plexus include the obturator, femoral, and sciatic.

Each spinal nerve divides into anterior, posterior, and white rami. Anterior and posterior rami contain voluntary fibers; white rami contain autonomic fibers. Posterior rami further branch into nerves going to the muscles, skin, and posterior surfaces of the head, neck, and trunk. Most anterior rami branch to the skeletal muscles and the skin of extremities and anterior and lateral surfaces. In the process, they form plexuses, such as the brachial and sacral plexuses. Spinal nerves contain sensory dendrites and motor axons; some have somatic axons, and some have axons of preganglionic autonomic motor neurons.

The autonomic (involuntary) nervous system consists of all the efferent nerves, through which the cardiovascular apparatus, viscera, glands of internal secretion, and peripheral involuntary muscles are innervated (Plate 1). A major anatomical difference between the somatic and autonomic nervous systems is that in the former an impulse from the brainstem or spinal cord reaches the end organ through a single neuron, whereas in the latter an impulse passes through two neurons—the first ending in an autonomic ganglion and the second running from the ganglion to the end organ. Some of the ganglia lie adjacent to the vertebral column to form the sympathetic trunks or chains; others are closely associated with the end organs.

The preganglionic neurons from the brainstem, which go out along the cranial nerves, and those from the second, third, and fourth sacral segments to the pelvic viscera end in ganglia in proximity to their end organs; thus their postganglionic fibers are very short. This is known as the *parasympathetic* or craniosacral division of the autonomic nervous system. The preganglionic fibers from the thoracic and lumbar spinal cord end in the paravertebral ganglia, making up the sympathetic chain, and their postganglionic fibers are relatively long. This is termed the *sympathetic* or thoracolumbar division of the autonomic nervous system.

The two divisions are distinct anatomically and physiologically. The chemical substance mediating transmission of impulses at most postganglionic sympathetic nerve endings is norepinephrine, and at all parasympathetic and preganglionic sympathetic neurons, acetylcholine.

The majority of organs have dual innervation, part from the craniosacral and part from the thoracolumbar divisions. The functions of these two systems are antagonistic. Together they work to maintain homeostasis. In general, the thoracolumbar division functions as an emergency protective mechanism, always ready to combat physical or psychological stress. The craniosacral division functions to conserve energy when the body is in a state of relaxation.

Stimuli arising from internal organs or from outside the body traverse visceral and somatic afferent nerve fibers to make reflex connections with preganglionic autonomic neurons in the brainstem and spinal cord. Such stimuli trigger activity of these involuntary systems automatically. When these automatic mechanisms break down or overact, surgery may be indicated. Thoracolumbar sympathectomy was once performed in hypertension to try to decrease blood vessel tone and lower the blood pressure. Vagotomy is done to decrease acid secretion to the stomach in peptic ulcer patients. Lumbar sympathectomy is used to relieve vasospastic disorders of the legs.

Diagnostic procedures

Most diagnostic procedures are performed before arrival of the patient in the operating room. Studies of most significance to the operating room nurse are radiological studies that produce either positive or negative images that the surgeon can use during the operation to assist in locating the pathological condition. It is the responsibility of the nurse to have these images in the operating room before the procedure begins. These studies include the following:

myelography Injection of contrast medium into the spinal subarachnoid space to demonstrate a defect, by radiography

pneumoencephalography (PEG) Injection of air into the subarachnoid space, usually through a lumbar or cisternal puncture, to outline the ventricular system and the cranial subarachnoid space to identify deviations from normal

ventriculography Injection of air directly into the lateral ventricles when a block exists between the spinal canal and the lateral ventricles; ventricular needles or cannulas can be inserted through open fontanelles in infants and by way of a twist drill (7/64-inch bit) hole in adults; or the patient may be brought to the operating room where the minor surgical procedure of bur holes is performed, the ventricles tapped, air injected, needles removed, incisions closed, and the patient taken to the radiology department for the x-ray films; or after the ventricles are tapped, flexible cannulas such as Scott or Seletz are sutured in place, incisions are closed, and air is injected as the patient is exposed to x rays

angiography (arteriography) Injection of contrast medium into the brachial, carotid, or vertebral arteries to study the intracranial blood vessels for size, location, and configuration to diagnose space-occupying lesions and vascular abnormalities

computed tomography (CT scan) Use of x rays with or without contrast medium and computer technology to produce a sequential series of positive images of transverse sections of the brain in which differences in tissue density can be detected and deviations from normal identified

brain scan Injection of radioactive substance intravenously to demonstrate brain lesions

echoencephalography Use of sound to identify a shift of midline structures (not a radiological technique)

NURSING CONSIDERATIONS

Nurse-surgeon communication, either direct or through a knowledgeable person, such as a clinical nurse specialist, operating room supervisor, or resident who has direct communication with the surgeon, is essential for intelligent planning of care for the neurosurgical patient in the operating room. Information the nurse needs before the arrival of the patient in the operating room includes the diagnosis; the diagnostic studies done and reports needed at the time of operation; the age, size, level of consciousness, physical disabilities resulting from neuropathological conditions (as well as those from other causes), and communication problems of the patient; the specific surgical approach and body position to be used; the need for any special equipment, instruments, or supplies not usually used; the amount of blood ordered and available; the method or methods planned to reduce intracranial pressure in the case of cranial surgery; the need for radiological support during the procedure; and the planned preliminary procedures, such as carotid ligation, ventriculogram, lumbar puncture, cutdown for placement of right atrial line, and Foley catheter insertion. This information permits the nurse to plan for needed equipment, instruments, and supplies ahead of time. Such preparation can significantly reduce both anesthesia and intraoperative time for the patient and physical and psychological stress for the neurosurgeon and the nurse.

Patients and families

Neuropathological conditions requiring surgical intervention can be found in any age group.

The most common problems requiring neurosurgical procedures in infants and children include meningocele, myelomeningocele, encephalocele, craniosynostosis, hydrocephalus, brain tumors, and trauma. The nurse plays a vital role in maintaining blood volume, body temperature, and fluid balance in pediatric patients. The nurse's role functions in maintaining blood volume include planning for minimizing and monitoring blood loss, as well as for blood replacement. The surgeon may minimize blood loss by infiltrating the tissues at the site of incision with normal saline solution; minimizing or eliminating periosteal stripping and carefully attending to intracranial emissary veins and sinuses; and using electrocautery, bone wax, Gelfoam, thrombin, or Surgicel. The surgeon's preferences must be prepared and ready for use before needed. Sponges from the operative field must be continuously placed within view of the anesthesiologist or weighed as they are discarded from the field. Blood for transfusion must be in the surgery department and divided into units of 100 or 250 ml, rather than in the usual 500-ml units used for adults. A blood warmer must be set up and ready to use as careful, accurate replacement is carried out. When the anesthesiologist is unable to see the operative field (which is usually the situation during *any* cranial surgery), the nurse must inform the anesthesiologist immediately of active bleeding at the operative site.

The nurse must place a warming blanket on the operating table before the pediatric patient arrives. The nurse who is able to control the room temperature can regulate the thermostat to a temperature above 22.2° C (72° F) after consultation with the anesthesiologist. The child's temperature should be monitored with a rectal, intraaural, or esophageal thermister probe. The thermister unit must be previously calibrated and placed within the view of the anesthesiologist.

Some means to control and monitor fluid intake and output must be planned with the anesthesiologist and neurosurgeon: microdrip intravenous tubing or an electronic drip regulator such as an I-vac unit may be used for regulating intravenous intake; a Foley catheter may be inserted into the bladder and attached to a urinometer and closed drainage system if the child is to undergo a prolonged procedure; output should be recorded at time intervals decided on by the nurse and anesthesiologist and based on the general condition of the child. Irrigation fluid and suction bottle contents are measured and recorded.

Parents of infants and children are usually extremely anxious, as are the families of most surgical patients. Arrangements by which families can have contact with the patient through a nurse who has direct access to the operating room during the operation and the postanesthesia recovery relieves anxiety and diminishes perceived waiting time for them.

Older children and adolescents, as well as adults, come to the operating room with a great deal of fear and apprehension about the outcome of the surgical procedure and what it will mean to them and their life-style. Both male and female patients are devastated by having their hair removed. This procedure is best done by a nurse who can provide psychological support and give realistic reassurance and information to both conscious, responsive patients and patients who may be incoherent or unconscious but who may still hear what is going on around them and feel what is being done to them. Head hair removal, like all other forms of preoperative preparation, should be done as close to the time of skin incision as possible to decrease the possibility of postoperative wound infection. Complete hair removal is preferred by some surgeons because dressings are easier to apply, hair regrowth is more even, a better wig fit can be obtained, and it is far easier to prepare a sterile field around such an operative site. However, because of the severe alterations in body image caused by total hair removal, an effort should be made to facilitate a compromise between patient and surgeon. Whenever possible, minimal hair removal is recommended. There may be a relationship between hair removal and postoperative recovery, especially in the areas of orientation, social interaction, and compliance. Also, giving consideration to the patient's wishes permits some degree of control by the patient over what is happening. Hair should be removed in a holding area or induction room after the patient has left the family unless contraindicated by the neurological status of the trauma patient. If hair is removed in the operating room, care must be taken to ensure that it will not be carried by air currents and contaminate the sterile field. Hair is always placed in a plastic bag, marked with the patient's name, and kept with the patient until discharge.

The aged person undergoing neurosurgical intervention brings a potential range of problems such as hearing, sight, or mobility deficiencies unrelated to the neuropathological condition. Responses to stimuli generally are slower in the elderly. The skin is more prone to pressure sores. The ability to heal may be impaired. More time and greater care must be taken with older patients. Communication can be established and reassurance given by touching and by being nearby while the patient is conscious. Vigilant monitoring of blood loss, temperature, and urine output is also required in caring for the older patient in the operating room. Surgery may be performed under local anesthesia, and the nurse may be responsible for monitoring vital signs, as well as for providing a human communication link for the patient. Sitting with the patient and explaining the procedure and the sensations that will be experienced will make the patient more comfortable and cooperative and will diminish fears.

Among neurosurgical patients are those who have little or no apparent loss of function, those who are coping with chronic pain and are looking forward to the operation for the relief it will bring, and those who are totally or partially dependent for everything because they are unconscious, quadriplegic, or aphasic, for example. If pain is present, the nurse should know the type and site of the pain and aim to make the patient as comfortable as possible while conscious. If the patient is acutely and severely traumatized, the nurse must be aware of injuries other than those for which the patient is being treated neurosurgically so that these injuries can be taken into consideration also. A nurse with prior knowledge of a given situation can be better prepared to cope with that situation and can plan individualized care based on that knowledge.

Basic neurosurgical maneuvers

Scientific advances that enable surgeons to control pain, hemorrhage, infection, and other physiological responses have contributed largely to the neurosurgeon's ability to operate successfully on the nervous system. The extent of a modern neurosurgical operation may be determined not so much by the physiological hazards involved as by the degree of neurological disability that may be expected after surgery. Knowing the hazards and having everything ready in advance will enhance the ability of the surgeon to achieve a favorable outcome.

Preliminary procedures

A number of procedures or therapeutic measures may be performed by the neurosurgeon or other member of the team in a holding or induction room before positioning, preparing, and draping take place. It is important that the nurse know why these procedures are done in order to anticipate them and be prepared to facilitate them.

A Foley catheter is often inserted into the bladder to monitor urinary output during the procedure. It is essential for prolonged procedures and when urea or mannitol is to be given intravenously, so that the bladder does not become distended. A Foley catheter is also required when hypothermia or hypotension will be induced, when excessive bleeding is anticipated, and in trauma patients to continuously assess kidney function.

A right atrial or central venous pressure line is required for management of air embolism. An air embolus can occur in operations on the head and neck when the patient is in an upright position. A venous cutdown and placement of this line may be done in the operating room immediately before the surgical procedure is begun.

When excessive intracranial bleeding is a possibility, the neurosurgeon may choose carotid cutdown and temporary ligation or tourniquet placement for occlusion of the carotid arteries during bleeding. Carotid cutdown is a separate surgical procedure and requires a special sterile setup, including drapes and instruments. Procedures that may require such management include intracranial vascular surgery and removal of meningiomas.

In some situations, cerebrospinal fluid drainage may be required. This can be done by placement of a ventricular cannula, such as the Scott or Seletz, or by placement of a spinal needle in the lower lumbar spinal canal. The stylet of either needle is left in place until drainage is required. The surgeon can remove the ventricular stylet, but the nurse must be able to remove the spinal needle stylet. When the lumbar puncture method is used, the patient is placed in a semilateral position and stabilized so as not to roll onto the needle so the nurse can remove the stylet without contaminating it during the procedure. An extension tubing and stopcock can be attached to the needle at the time of lumbar puncture. When this is done, the tubing and stopcock are supported so that traction is not put on the needle and are placed where they are accessible to the nurse or anesthesiologist. The stopcock can be opened when drainage is required.

Induced hypotension may be required to manage bleeding. Intracranial vascular surgery and removal of some tumors also may require induced hypotension. Sodium nitroprusside (Nipride) is an effective agent. Very little of the drug is required to produce an immediate and dramatic hypotensive state. Recovery from the effects of the drug is immediate. When mixed in solution for intravenous administration, sodium nitroprusside is unstable in light. The nurse must have a roll of aluminum foil available to cover the intravenous bottle and tubing completely when the drug is hanging and in use or ready for immediate use; an electronic device to measure and control the amount administered must also be set up.

Skin preparation

Head hair is best removed after the patient has arrived in the surgery department but before arrival in an operating room. The hair is first clipped with an electric clippers, which is cleaned and disinfected after each use. The hair is placed in a bag, labeled with the patient's name, and kept with the patient after surgery. The scalp is then shaved, using warm, soapy water and either a straight razor or several disposable safety razors. As soon as the patient experiences any pulling, the razor blade should be changed. The nurse should explain to the patient exactly what is being done and what sensations to expect during the procedure.

For surgery on the cervical spine, it is possible to secure long hair on top of the head and remove neck hair with a clippers to a level even with the top of the ears or just below the occipital protuberance. Postoperatively, patients with long hair can comb it down over the shaved area until the hair regrows.

Patients undergoing thoracic or lumbar spine surgery may not need to be shaved. If hair is present, it can be removed by depilatory or a shave can be done in the surgery department immediately before surgery.

After the shave, the skin should be inspected carefully for any signs of inflammation or infection. If any such signs are noted, they should be reported to the surgeon immediately.

An antiseptic skin preparation is done after the patient is positioned and before draping. The agent or agents used are dictated by the hospital procedure. Skin preparation may be done by the circulating nurse, surgeon, or resident. General principles and precautions cited in Chapter 5 apply to neurosurgical preparations, regardless of who performs them.

Many neurosurgeons mark the incision line with a marking pencil, a marking solution and wooden stick, or a scalpel. If a marking solution is used, indigo carmine, gentian violet, or brilliant green is recommended. Methylene blue should *never* be found in a neurosurgical operating room because it produces an inflammatory reaction in central nervous system tissue and could be disastrous if accidently injected into the subarachnoid space, for example.

After marking, the surgeon may inject the incision site and the sites for application of towel clamps with a local anesthetic agent or with normal saline solution. Any solution will apply pressure within the tissues and decrease bleeding at the time of incision. The local anesthetic agent has the additional effect of decreasing the effect of the stimulus of the skin incision.

Positioning

The basic body positions and their modifications are used in neurosurgery. The nurse must know the position for each procedure, the hazards and precautions of each position, and the equipment, support, and time necessary to place a patient in a given position (Chapter 6). General considerations of special importance in positioning for neurosurgery include protecting the eyes from pressure, chemical burns, and corneal scratches; maintaining joints in functional alignment with no pressure or tension on superficial nerves and vessels; and checking the Foley catheter for tension and kinks to ensure drainage.

The dorsal recumbent, or supine, position or some modification of it is used for supratentorial craniotomy, subtemporal decompression, and anterior cervical fusion. The lateral recumbent position is used for thoracic and lumbar laminectomy by some surgeons and for lumbar sympathectomy. Modifications of the prone position can be used for lumbar, thoracic, and cervical laminectomy and for posterior fossa craniectomy. The sitting, or upright, position can be used for cervical laminectomy, posterior fossa craniectomy, temporal craniectomy, and ventriculogram. Only specific aspects of the sitting position for neurosurgical procedures and the knee-chest position, a modification of the prone position, are covered in this chapter.

The extreme sitting, or upright, position may be the neurosurgeon's choice for infratentorial cranial surgery and posterior cervical laminectomy when acute trauma is not the cause of cervical cord disease. Advantages of this position include optimum visibility of the operative field and decreased blood loss because of the lowered arterial and venous pressures. The latter advantage also poses potential problems: some patients cannot tolerate the upright position under general anesthesia; thus the patient is slowly placed in this position as the anesthesiologist monitors the blood pressure. Most patients have a drop in pressure but rapidly adapt to the position; those who do not are placed in the prone position. In the sitting position, the venous pressure in the head and neck may be negative, predisposing to air embolism. Other poten-

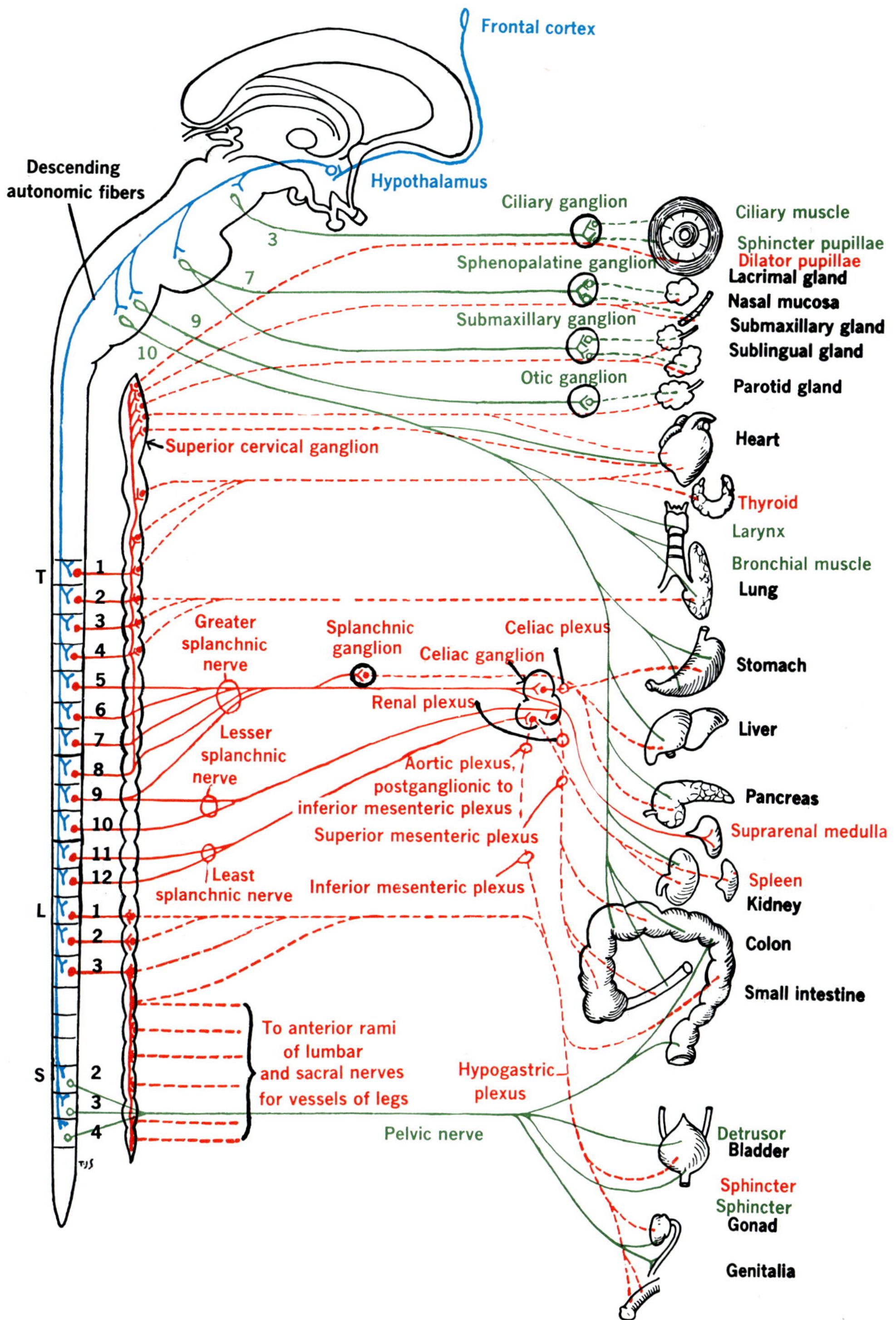

Plate 1. Diagram of autonomic nervous system. (From Mettler, F.A.: Neuroanatomy, ed. 2, St. Louis, The C.V. Mosby Co.)

tial problems with this position include neck flexion with airway compromise and difficulty in achieving and maintaining functional alignment.

Before anesthesia induction the patient's legs are wrapped from toes to groin with elastic bandages, or special tensor stockings, such as TED hose, are worn by the patient to the operating room to prevent venous stasis in the lower extremities and help maintain the blood pressure. In addition, the legs and feet are elevated slightly.

Other precautions during positioning and throughout the procedure include checking heels, soles of feet, and popliteal areas to prevent pressure; checking male genitals to ensure that pressure will not compromise circulation and cause necrosis; preventing thighs from contacting the metal crossbar table attachment; and stabilizing the head in the head rest and shoulders and torso to prevent neck flexion.

Preparations should be made in collaboration with the anesthesiologist to manage air embolism if this complication should occur. Sometimes this is done by placing the patient in a G-suit before positioning is begun. The G-suit also assists in maintaining the blood pressure. Usually, however, a right atrial line is placed under direct vision fluoroscopy either in the cardiac catheterization laboratory or radiology department, before arrival of the patient in the operating room, or in the operating room, using the image intensifier. After anesthesia induction, the anesthesiologist may place an esophageal stethoscope or attach the patient to a Doppler unit to hear air entering the right atrium. The air can be withdrawn through the atrial line with a 50-ml syringe and three-way stopcock connection. If the plan for management of air embolism includes repositioning the patient with the surgical wound open, the plan should be shared with the surgeon, the surgeon's assistant, the nurses, and any other team members present by the anesthesiologist so that this can be accomplished quickly and without endangering the patient in other ways, such as contaminating the surgical wound, displacing a joint, or dislodging the endotracheal tube.

The most common position for lumbar and thoracic laminectomy is prone. Both legs are wrapped with elastic bandages, or tensor hose are used to prevent venous stasis in the extremities. Anesthesia induction and intubation take place on the transport gurney. The patient is then placed on the operating room table in the prone position. Special table attachment supports or a chest roll must be placed under the chest on each side from the shoulder to the iliac crest to permit lung expansion during the procedure. The bottom of the table is dropped to about a 25-degree angle. The patient's knees are flexed, and the lower legs elevated and supported on two large pillows and the table mattress, under which the footboard is placed at right angles to the table. The knees are padded with foam. The arms are flexed at the elbows and supported by pillows on wide armboards. Care is taken to prevent pressure or tension on the brachial plexus. For surgery on the neck and posterior skull, the foot of the table is not dropped; the ankles and feet are supported on a large pillow, and the arms are secured at the patient's sides protecting the ulnar, median, and radial nerves. A horseshoe headrest may be used.

The major problems encountered in this position include increase in venous pressure and bleeding at the operative site, peripheral venous stasis, and decrease in vital capacity. Precautions include checking female breasts, male genitals, and knees to prevent pressure on these areas; avoiding hyperextension of shoulders and pressure on the brachial plexus when turning the patient to begin positioning and during the procedure; preventing abduction of the arms and occlusion of the subclavian and axillary arteries; and protecting the eyes from pressure, corneal scratches and chemical burns.

The knee-chest, or ''tuck,'' position is also used for lumbar laminectomy. This is a modification of the prone position, in which the patient's hips and knees are flexed so that the body is supported on the thighs and lower legs, with the abdomen and chest hanging free or supported on chest rolls. Advantages of this position include decreased bleeding because of the collapse of epidural veins, better exposure resulting from hyperflexion of the spine, absence of pressure on the vena cava, and increased ease of ventilation. Operating time is usually reduced when this position is used.

Disadvantages include the difficulty of maintaining physical stability on the operating table, hypotension, and pooling of blood in the lower extremities.

Draping

Most neurosurgeons do their own draping. Draping for some procedures is complex and requires the cooperation of surgeon, assistant, and nurse. Four or more towels are placed around the operative site. They may be secured by small towel clamps or by silk sutures on a heavy cutting needle. When sutures are used, the surgeon also needs a heavy, 6-inch toothed forceps and a suture scissors. Forceps, scissors, needle holders, and needles are discarded after towels have been secured in place.

A plastic adhesive drape may be placed either before or after the towels. The skin must be completely dry for the drape to adhere tightly to the skin.

Disposable barrier drape sheets and towels are essential. If an overhead instrument table is used, it should be covered with a sheet that is large enough so that the front edge can be fanfolded at the front edge of the table until the table is brought forward over the patient toward the operative site. The fanfolded sheet can then be secured at the lower border of the operative site to bridge the gap between the unsterile undersurface of the table and the sterile field. Mayo stands should also be covered with barrier towels or parchment paper. The particulars of draping for neurosurgical procedures vary and are influenced by the patient's position, the surgeon's preferences, and what is available in each hospital. Therefore a detailed description of the draping for each procedure is not provided here. The particulars of draping for each procedure should be clearly described on the neurosurgeon's preference card. Doubts can be clarified by communication with the neurosurgeon, preferably before the time of operation.

As a general rule, neurosurgeons prefer to have all equipment ready before making the incision. Therefore they can be very helpful to the nurse in attaching and hooking up suction tubings, cautery cords, and other equipment that will be needed for the operation.

Hemostasis

Meticulous hemostasis is of particular importance in neurosurgical technique. The first consideration is control of hemorrhage from the highly vascular scalp. Compression of the edges of the wound with gauze sponges and fingers during the initial incision is followed by application of hemostatic clips and clamps. When clips are used, they are applied so that they include the galea and skin edge, whereas clamps are attached directly to the galea and then everted. Normal saline solution or a local anesthetic agent may be injected before making the incision to minimize scalp bleeding.

Bone wax, a hemostatic material, is prepared for all cranial and spinal cord operations as described in Chapter 7. The surgeon firmly rubs the wax into the bleeding surface of the bone after all periosteum has been scraped off. When the skull flap has been elevated, bone wax is also rubbed into the diploë to control bleeding from the bone edge. During spinal surgery, bone wax is used on the cut edges of the laminae.

Electrocoagulation is routine for neurosurgical procedures. Nursing personnel must understand the uses and hazards of the electrosurgical unit and be familiar with the safety measures. Electrocoagulation may be used to stop bleeding in the galea, in the periosteum, on the surface of the dura, on the spinal cord, and in the brain. The coagulation current seals the blood vessels. The electrical current is applied to the forceps, a metal suction tip, or other instrument, which acts as a conducting tool. To be effective, the cauterizing current must contact the vessel in a dry field. For this reason, suctioning is necessary to remove the blood as the contact is made between the instrument carrying the current and the bleeding point.

Bipolar coagulation units are frequently used. Bipolar units provide a completely isolated output with negligible leakage of current between the tips of the forceps, permitting use of coagulating current in proximity to structures where ordinary unipolar coagulation would be hazardous. Ringer's lactate or normal saline irrigation is used

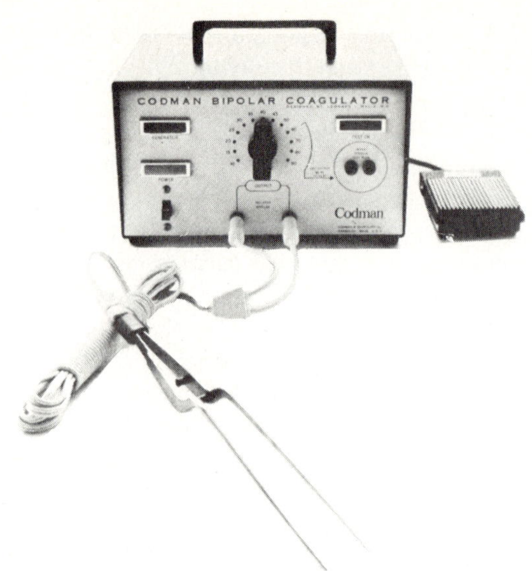

Fig. 24-21. Malis bipolar coagulation unit with forceps. (Courtesy Codman & Shurtleff, Inc., Randolph, Mass.)

during bipolar coagulation, minimizing tissue heating, shrinkage, drying, and sticking to the forceps (Fig. 24-21). Need for a ground plate is eliminated. The use of the bipolar coagulation technique allows hemostasis of almost any size vessel encountered. Vessels as large as the superficial temporal artery, as well as those too small for suture or clip ligation, may be coagulated.

Electrocautery is also used for cutting with a lower power setting. When the surgeon is using a cutting electrode to remove a tumor, the circulating nurse should stand by the machine to adjust the current as needed. As the surgeon uses the cutting electrode, an assistant holds a suction tip to one side of the area of dissection to remove smoke.

Gauze sponges are used to control bleeding before entering the skull or spinal canal, as in any general surgical procedure. Coarse gauze sponges will injure fragile tissues such as the brain or spinal cord, so wet compressed rayon cotton (cottonoid) pledgets or strips are used in place of gauze sponges to control bleeding beneath the skull and around the spinal cord. Cottonoid strips and pledgets, or "patties," must be available in a variety of sizes (Fig. 24-22).

At one time making these strips and patties from large sheets of cottonoid material was a part of the routine of every nurse working in neurosurgery. Today the strips and pledgets can be purchased sterile and ready to use. Strips are usually 6 inches long, although some surgeons prefer them 3 inches in length. The standard widths are ¼, ½, ¾, and 1 inch. Strips may or may not have x-ray–detectable markers or strings attached. Pledgets should have both x-ray–detectable markers and strings attached. Standard sizes for pledgets are ½ × ½ inch, ¾ × ¾

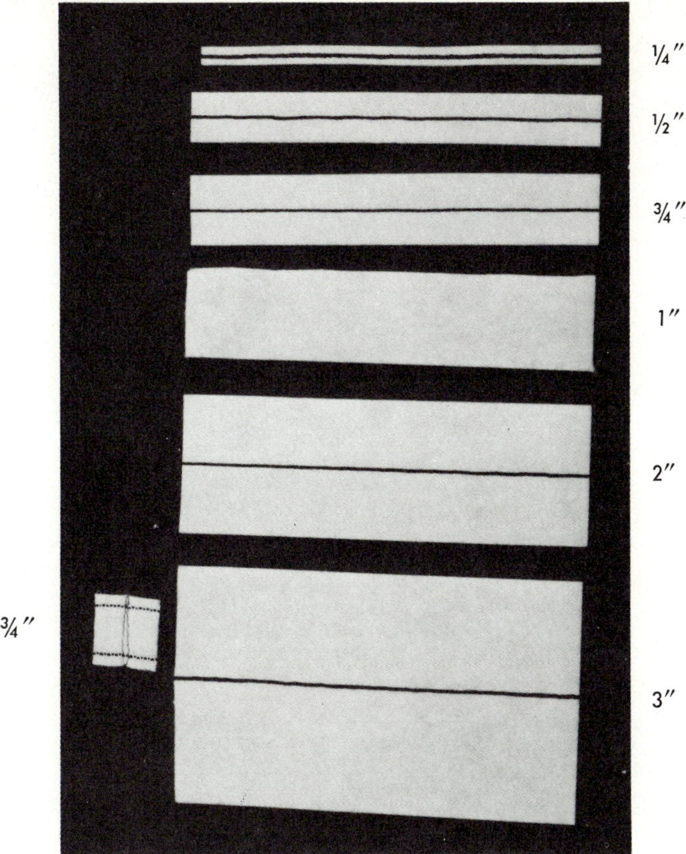

Fig. 24-22. Cottonoid strips and pledgets.

inch, and 1 × 1 inch. All strips and pledgets must be counted. Some surgeons prefer to use Telfa strips, which the nurse cuts to size before use. During the procedure, the nurse maintains a supply of these special neurosurgical sponges, thoroughly soaked with normal saline solution or Ringer's lactate solution, within reach of the surgeon's forceps. They may be displayed on a waterproof surface, such as towel drape, a sterile metal basin (emesis basin, small bowl), a plastic towel drape such as 3M or Vi-drape, or a piece of rubber clipped to a folded towel. The surgeon may prefer that the nurse keep a supply of these moist sponges on the palm or back of one hand and extend them toward the surgeon as needed. The sponges are aligned on the display surface in order of size. As soon as one is used, the nurse replaces it.

Loose wet cotton balls may be used as a temporary pack or tamponade in a bleeding tumor bed after a tumor has been removed. The gentle pressure of the cotton balls along with time and patience on the part of the surgeon may stop bleeding not controllable by other means. The scrub nurse is responsible for counting the number of cotton balls placed in the tumor bed and to make sure that none is left behind at closure.

A variety of hemostatic clips are available and used by neurosurgeons to occlude both superficial and deep vessels. The original clip used by Cushing and later modified by McKenzie is made of silver. Newer clips such as the Samuels Hemoclip and the Ligaclip are of tantalum or stainless steel. The nurse removes the clips from a special cartridge with the appropriate applicator and passes them to the surgeon for application to a vessel. Such clips enable the surgeon to occlude vessels in areas difficult to reach by other means and to ligate superficial vessels of the brain before cutting them and without destroying any surrounding tissues. Clips can be obtained in a variety of sizes.

Hemostatic scalp clips include Autoclips, Michel, Raney, Adson, and LeRoy clips (Fig. 24-23). Raney and Adson clips are reusable. There are also plastic disposable scalp clips similar to the Raney. Each type of clip has a specific clip applicator by which the clips are placed on the scalp edges. At time of closure, clips are removed by either a hemostat or a special clip remover. A minimum of two clip applicators is essential; the nurse loads one clip applicator while the surgeon is using the other to place the clip on the scalp. The Adson clips are loaded on the applicators from a special rack. After use, they must be reshaped before replacement on the clip rack.

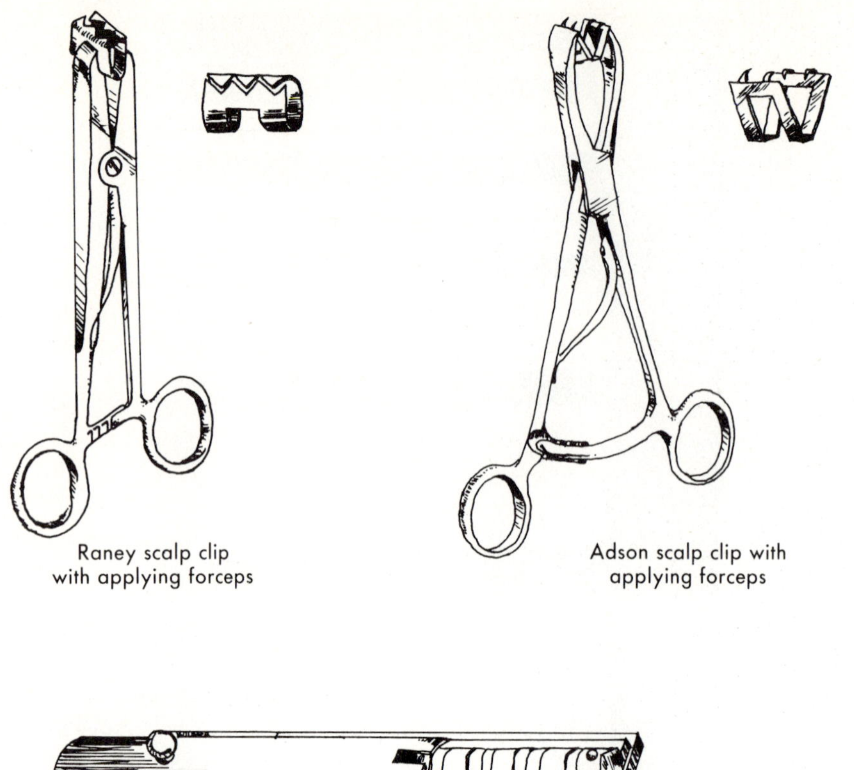

Fig. 24-23. Scalp clip applicators and clips.

There is a special instrument for this purpose. The Raney and Michel clips are loaded by hand. Raney clips are very difficult to clean by hand and should be placed in a sonic cleaner or soaked in hydrogen peroxide.

Numerous special clips are used to permanently or temporarily occlude vessels or an aneurysm neck in the surgical treatment of intracranial aneurysm. These are discussed under microneurosurgery.

Neurosurgeons almost routinely use certain hemostatic agents in addition to mechanical hemostasis. Gelfoam is one of these agents. It comes in two forms: a powder and a compressed sponge. The sponge is produced in three sizes: nos. 12, 50, and 100. The sponge form can be applied to an oozing surface dry or saturated with saline solution or topical thrombin. The larger pieces of Gelfoam are cut into a variety of sizes of strips and pledgets. The surgeon's perference dictates the exact method of preparation and use. Gelfoam is absorbable and can be left in the body.

Surgicel, a rayon-like cellulose gauze, and Oxycel, an absorbable hemostatic agent that comes in both cotton and gauze forms, are used to control bleeding from oozing surfaces, vessels, and sinuses in the brain and spinal canal. These hemostatic substances are also cut into suitable sizes and shapes and are handed to the surgeon dry, followed by a moist cottonoid strip or patty. The hemostatic material adheres to the bleeding area as gentle pressure is applied to the cottonoid material for several minutes.

Pieces of fresh muscle tissue can be used to tamponade and control bleeding where the usual forms of hemostasis are not possible.

Most neurosurgeons use silk suture material for traction sutures and wound closure. Occasionally silk is used to ligate blood vessels by suture ligature or on a ligature carrier.

Irrigating the wound with Ringer's lactate or normal saline solution may facilitate hemostasis. This procedure definitely helps the surgeon identify active bleeding points. Two completely filled bulb or Asepto syringes should always be within reach of the surgeon. Suction is the best means of keeping the wound dry and permitting control of bleeding. Therefore, suction and irrigation are used together.

Metal suction tips, such as the Cone, Sachs, Frazier, Bucy, or Adson (Fig. 24-24), are used because they not only keep the wound dry, but also can be used to conduct coagulation current from a monopolar unit to the bleeding point. The Bucy-Frazier tip is insulated and attached to both suction and electrocautery to become the active

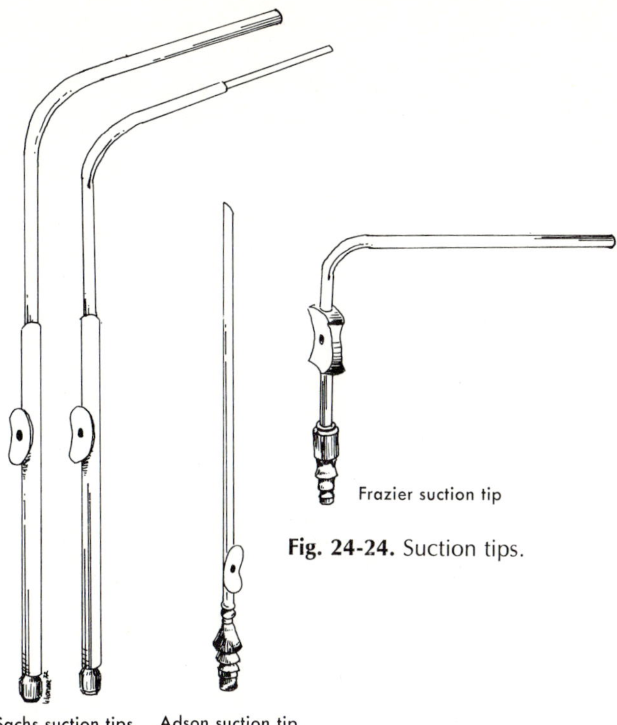

Fig. 24-24. Suction tips.

coagulating electrode. Use of the suction-coagulation unit is limited to areas in which gross coagulation can be done safely, for example, during the opening phase of a surgical procedure.

Suction can be used to remove necrotic or traumatized brain tissue or soft brain tumors rapidly after a sample has been obtained for pathological examination. It is also useful in evaluation of abscess cavities, removal of fluid from a ventricle or the subarachnoid space, holding a solid tumor during its removal, and applying compression to a bleeding vessel.

Many neurosurgeons irrigate surgical wounds with an antibiotic solution before wound closure. The antibiotic must be mixed with irrigation solution according to the surgeon's preference so that it is ready for use when needed. Gelfoam may be soaked in antibiotic solution before use.

EQUIPMENT

An operating room used for neurosurgical procedures should be large enough to accommodate equipment necessary to perform procedures done by the neurosurgeons on the hospital staff. A wider variety of procedures is usually done in research and teaching centers than in the average community hospital; therefore space and equipment needs will be greater in research and teaching centers. The emphasis of this discussion is equipment that is *necessary* for neurosurgery in any setting.

Essential built-in equipment includes a minimum of two electrical outlets per wall, four overhead spotlights with autoclavable handles to permit persons at the operative field to adjust the lights as needed, and a minimum of six single or three double x-ray view boxes and four wall or ceiling vacuum suction outlets capable of high negative pressure. Other equipment that can be built in if the situation demands includes a two-way telephone communication line, a ceiling-mounted operating microscope with camera, a closed-circuit television unit with monitor, an electrocardiogram-electroencephalogram monitor with readouts, and a wall or ceiling source of nitrogen or compressed air to operate air-powered equipment.

Some basic mobile equipment is needed for any setting in which neurosurgery is done. An operating room table and complete set of table attachments and neurosurgical headrests is essential. The best headrest is one that can be adapted for use in any body position, such as the AMSCO multipoise, the Gardner, and the Mayfield (Fig. 24-25, *B*). Each of these headrests has a three-pin suspension and skull clamp that attaches to a headrest table attachment to securely fixate the skull during the operation. This is especially useful when the patient is placed in a sitting position. Two or three sterile pins are placed in the head after preparing the insertion sites with an antiseptic, such as an iodophor. The headrest skull clamp is first attached to the pins and then to the table attachment. Precautions during insertion of the pins include avoiding the frontal sinuses and superficial temporal arteries. Other headrests, such as the Light-Veley (Fig. 24-25, *A*), that are of more limited use may be preferred by the individual neurosurgeon. In many instances, especially for supratentorial craniotomy, the head can be stabilized by a rubber donut wrapped in Kling or Webril. It is recommended that a mobile cart be used for storage of the neurosurgical headrests and table parts, as well as any other positioning devices and aids used by the neurosurgeon.

At least one portable spotlight should be available. One special neurosurgical overhead instrument table, such as the Mayfield table (Fig. 24-26), is preferable, but two large Mayo trays can be used for any neurosurgical procedure. One large instrument back table is a must. It is recommended that it be at least 6 to 8 inches higher than the standard table because the scrub nurse must frequently work on a high lift to be able to see the operative field and work effectively. The extra height of the back table enables the nurse to maintain a sterile field and to work more comfortably.

Eight to ten footstools are needed. They can be arranged side by side or on top of each other for the safety, efficiency, and comfort of the personnel. Four kickbuckets are needed for trash and sponges. Three are positioned around the sterile field. For head surgery, the fourth can be placed under the head of the table so that the drapes can be gathered together and funneled into it as a trough for irrigation fluid and blood. Also useful are two

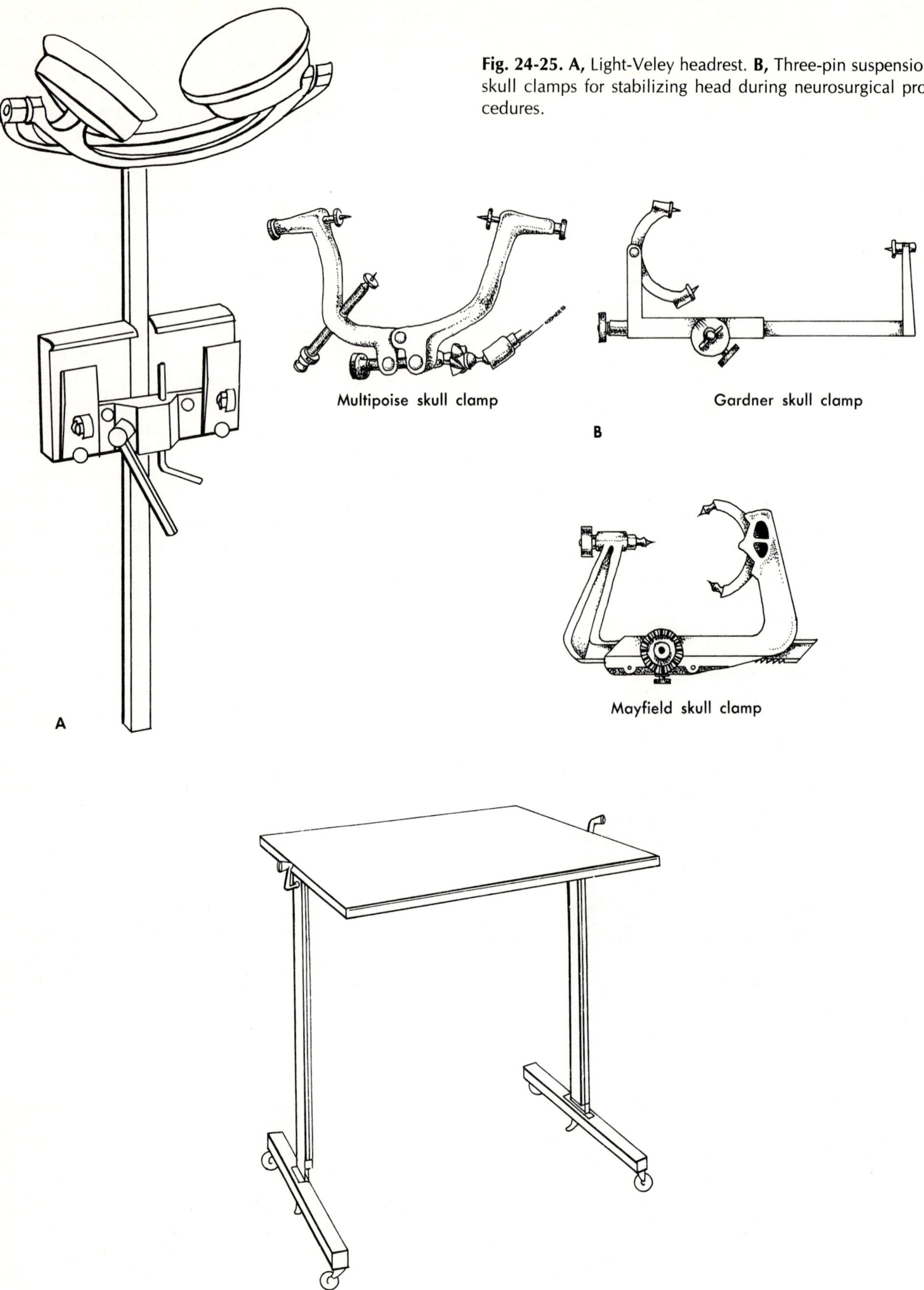

Fig. 24-25. A, Light-Veley headrest. **B,** Three-pin suspension skull clamps for stabilizing head during neurosurgical procedures.

Fig. 24-26. Mayfield overhead instrument table.

small utility tables for preparation and special equipment and supplies.

A cooling-heating unit with two blankets, such as the K-thermia unit, should be available for use. An electronic temperature monitoring device with esophageal, intraaural, and rectal probes is essential.

Other essential equipment includes a monopolar electrocautery unit, a bipolar electrocautery unit, at least one fiberoptic headlight, and one fiberoptic light source for lighted retractors and telescopes, if they are used. Also needed is an operating microscope such as the Zeiss, a portable tank of nitrogen with a special pressure gauge for operating air-powered instruments, four inflatable cuffs and bulb pumps for infusion of blood, two blood-warming units, one or two electronic intravenous rate control units such as I-vac units, a solution warmer, and a nerve stimulator. A cryosurgical unit, an image intensifier, and a stereotaxic apparatus may be needed if surgical procedures requiring them are performed.

Specialized instruments

Scientific developments in other fields have been applied to the health care delivery system in general. Some of the developments with application to neurosurgery in the forms of specialized instrumentation and equipment have been discussed previously. A few items require further discussion.

Air-powered instrumentation has become popular with neurosurgeons over the years since the first Hall air drill was developed. Modifications of the original instrument continue today. These instruments decrease open wound time and anesthesia time for the patient and conserve energy for the surgeon.

The basic air driver has been adapted by means of special attachments for neurosurgery. Because of the history of improvements and new developments in air-powered instruments, it is recommended that specific instructions for use and care of such equipment be obtained from the manufacturer at the time of purchase. Basic general information is included here.

The Air Drill 100 (Fig. 24-27) has replaced the Surgairtome or Hall II air drill for precision cutting, shaping, and repair of bone. Its use increases the ease of bone work and reduces operating time. Compressed nitrogen is the power source as with other air-powered equipment. The Air Drill 100 can be used to widen the graft area in anterior fusions and to unroof the auditory canal in eighth cranial nerve surgery. For use in less accessible areas, such as the sphenoidal sinus, pituitary fossa, and vertebral bodies, 20-degree and 90-degree angle attachments are available. A range of burs and guards is available.

The Craniotome C-100 (Fig. 24-28) is the newest adaptation of the original Hall Neurairtome. A perforator driver attachment reduces the speed to 1000 rpm for drilling bur holes. Both 12-mm and 7-mm perforators are available. The perforator driver attachment can be removed, and a saw blade and dura guard attached to adapt the instrument for cutting a craniotomy bone flap. The

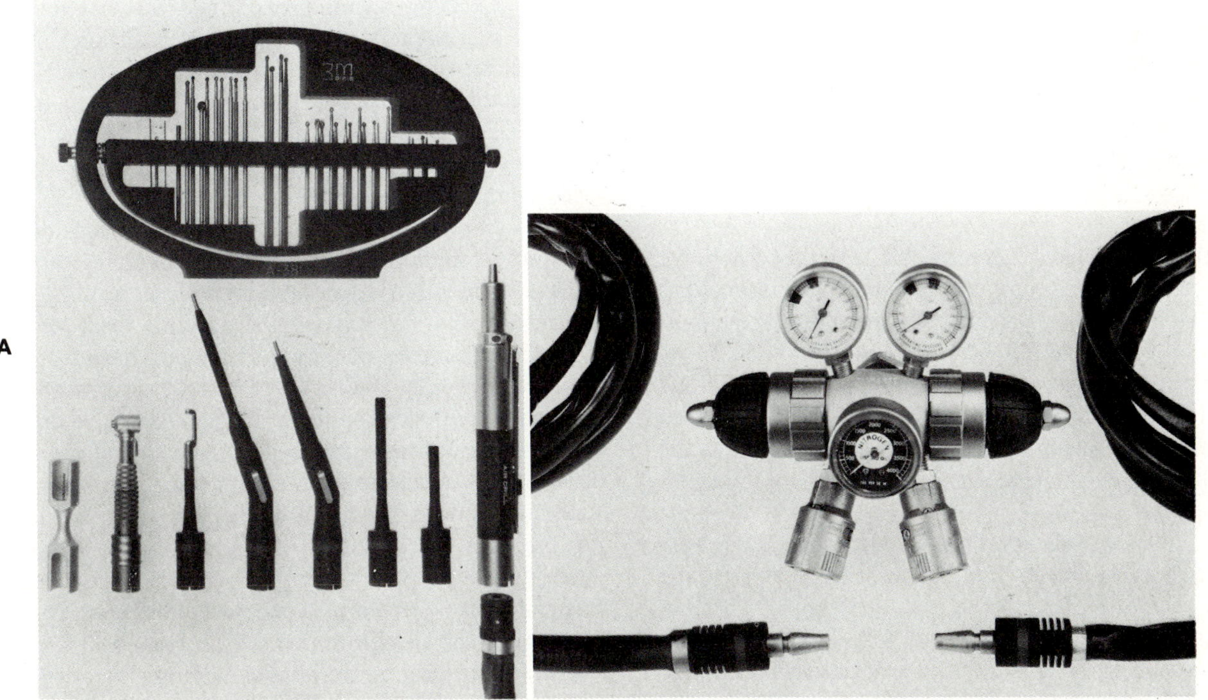

Fig. 24-27. A, Air Drill 100 with attachments. **B,** Dual nitrogen regulator. (Courtesy 3M Co., St. Paul.)

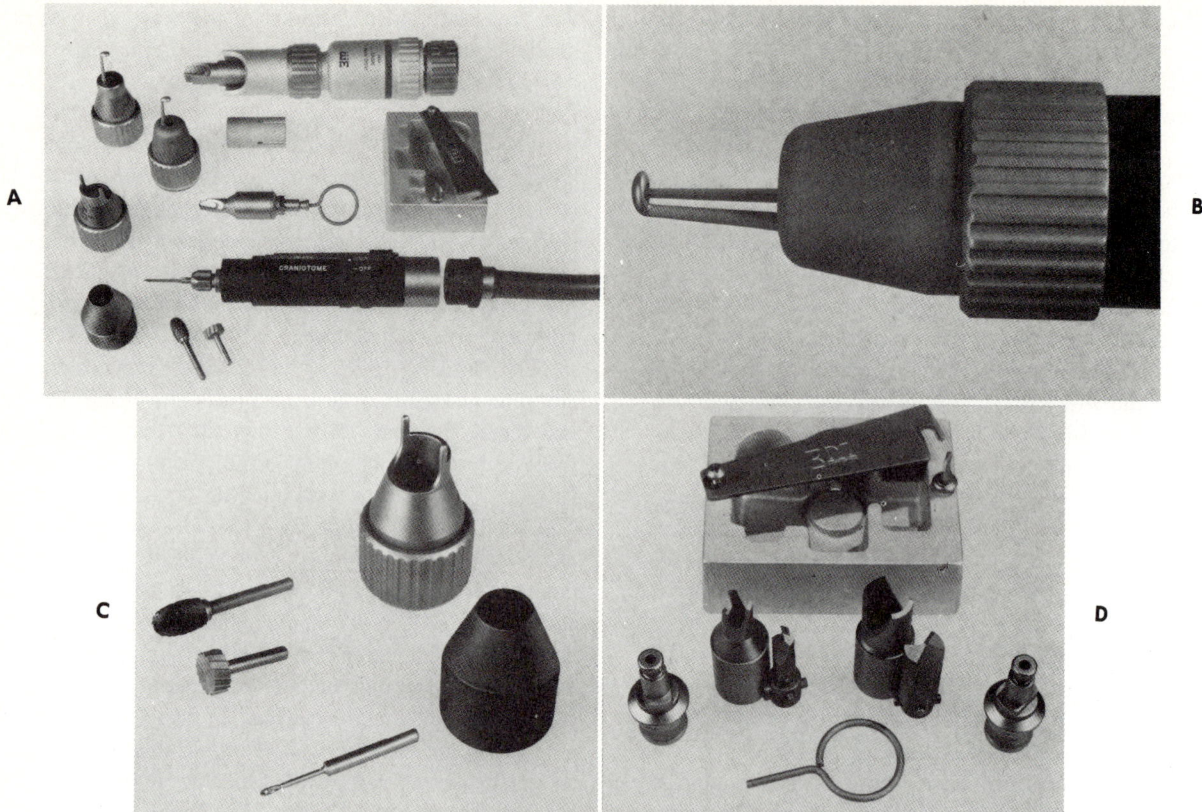

Fig. 24-28. **A,** Craniotome C-100 with attachments. **B,** Craniotome with neuroblade. **C,** Cranioplasty and wire-pass attachments. **D,** Skull perforators. (Courtesy 3M Co., St. Paul.)

saw blade is interchangeable with a wire-pass drill bit for drilling holes and placing wires, when a bone flap is to be wired in place. A cranioplasty bur and skull contour bur as well as guards for each type of bur are available.

The Ronjair (Fig. 24-29), an air-powered rongeur used in surgery of the spine, has interchangeable attachments for Leksell, Luer, and Kerrison rongeurs. This instrument is operated by a squeeze trigger with a built-in locking device.

The manufacturer makes specific recommendations for use, care, cleaning, and sterilization. These instructions must be followed to maintain the instruments in the most efficient working order.

Electrically powered instruments were popular and widely used before the introduction of the air-powered models. Some surgeons prefer power drills such as the Light-Veley or the Codman-Shurtleff drills with Smith perforator.

Another versatile pneumatic tool is the Midas Rex Whirlwind instrument. The variety of disposable cutting tools of this foot-controlled instrument and its attachments provides the neurosurgeon with a wide capability in bone cutting, including small rectangular holes in place of bur holes, bone flaps of any size and shaping, and unroofing areas such as the sphenoid wing. Manufacturer's,precautions and instructions must be followed.

The operating microscope (Chapter 23) has revolutionized neurosurgery, making possible procedures never done before, such as endarterectomy of small vessels and vessel grafting to improve intracranial circulation. It has also made other neurosurgical procedures on vessels, such as aneurysm surgery and surgery on nerves, more precise and, therefore, more successful.

The lens system for neurosurgery and the angle of the microscope are different from that used in otological surgery. If a microscope is shared by neurological and otological services, the nurse must be able to adapt the microscope for use in neurosurgery by attachment of the appropriate pieces, and the surgeon must check it for focal length and focus before scrubbing. Disposable drapes are available for the microscope. Assistant and observer lenses are available for the Zeiss microscope. Cameras and closed-circuit television monitors are also available for use with the operating microscope, if the situation warrants such sophisticated equipment. The House-Urban vacuum rotary dissector is a combination of rotating cutting blades and suction device that provides both suction and tissue resection in conjunction with the operating microscope (Fig. 24-30).

The routine use of video cameras, recorders, and tele-

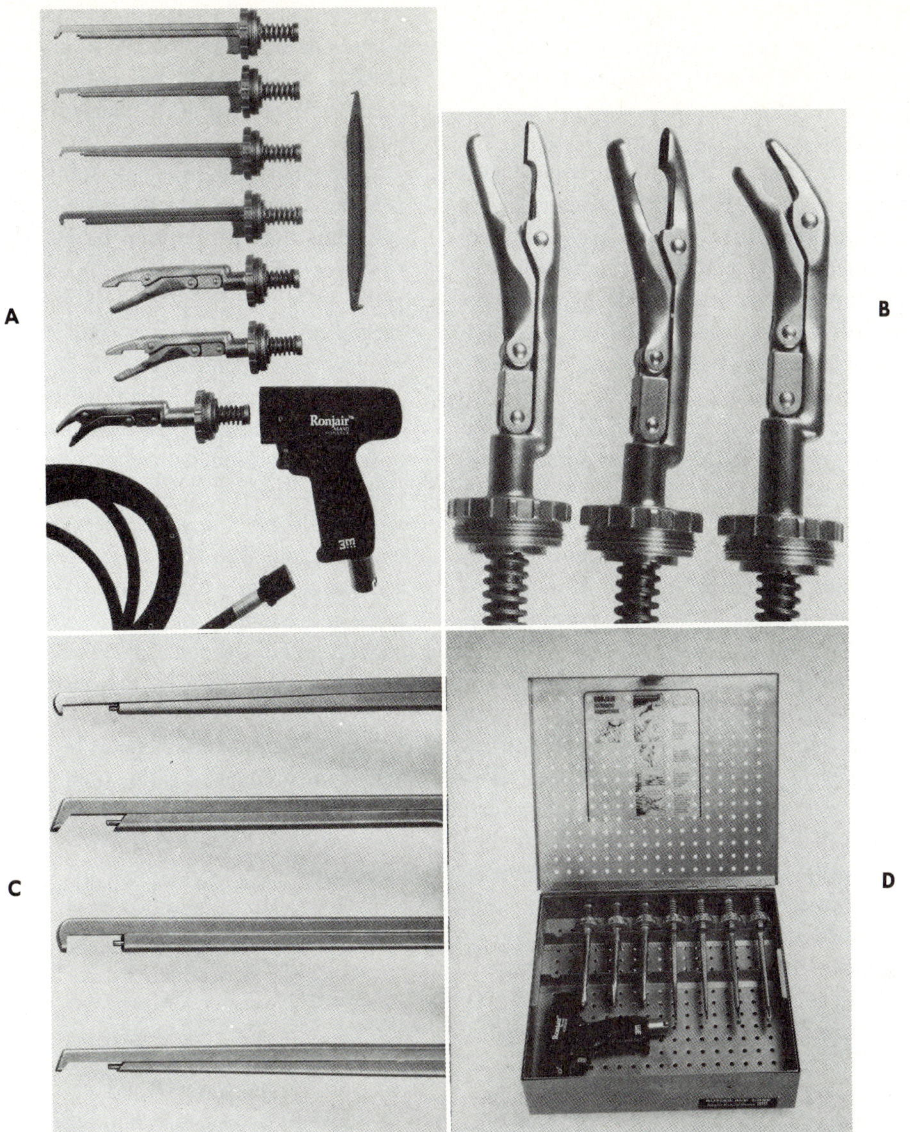

Fig. 24-29. A, Ronjair with attachments. **B,** Leksell and Luer rongeur attachments. **C,** Kerrison blades. **D,** Sterilizing and storage case.

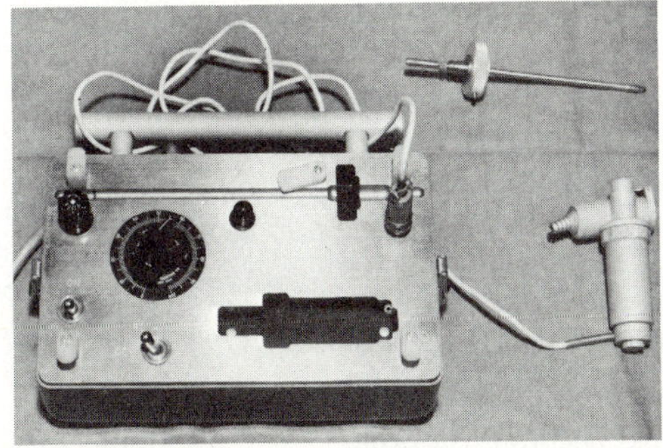

Fig. 24-30. House-Urban vacuum rotary dissector. (Courtesy Urban Engineering Co., Inc., Burbank, Calif.)

vision monitors, if available, is invaluable to teach staff and enhance interest and understanding of the surgical procedure by nurses who are otherwise unable to directly visualize the surgeon's actions.

The surgical carbon dioxide laser is used routinely by many surgeons for precision dissection and hemostasis. The laser produces a concentrated infrared energy beam generated by carbon dioxide that can be precisely focused on any point at which it is aimed. The beam, which is made visible by a superimposed red aiming light, causes flash vaporization of cellular water at 100° C. Advantages of the laser include improved hemostasis and healing with decreased tissue trauma, swelling, and risk of metastatis. Postoperative morbidity is minimal. The laser is especially advantageous in microvascular surgery and is used to occlude vessels less than 0.5 mm in diameter in operations for aneurysms and arteriovenous malformations as well as to remove tumors with minimal or no damage to surrounding structures. Tissue damage depends on amounts of energy generated and exposure duration.

Precautions include the need to wear protective glasses or plastic goggles to prevent accidental damage to eyes of personnel in the room and the need to keep all cottonoid, sponge, and towel materials thoroughly damp to prevent fire that could result from contact between a dry combustible material and the beam. The carbon dioxide source must be checked before use to ensure adequate supply for the procedure. Of course, nonflammable anesthetic gas mixtures must be used.

Direct image intensification is essential for an increasing number of neurosurgical procedures such as placement of nerve stimulator electrodes in brain or spinal areas and stereotaxic procedures. If possible, a C-arm and monitor should be available in the operating room. Otherwise these procedures can be done in the radiology department, although it does not usually provide an adequate aseptic environment. The sterile field can be prepared in the operating room and transported to radiology, or the supplies can be taken to radiology and the sterile field prepared there. Both situations are less than ideal. The sterile field must be covered for transportation. In both situations the conditions in radiology, including control of environment and personnel, require compromise of surgical aseptic technique. Each situation must be analyzed, and the most acceptable compromise from the perspective of patient safety determined and implemented. Procedures requiring use of the CT scan have to be done in radiology.

Basic instrumentation for craniotomy

Choice of instrumentation for a given neurosurgical procedure is largely controlled by the operating surgeon or, in some settings, by the chief of the department. Exactly what the neurosurgeon needs for a specific procedure is highly individual. Factors that influence the choices include training, experience, type of setting in which the surgery is performed, pathological condition of the patient, surgical approach planned, and equipment available.

Some hospitals provide a full range of highly specialized neurosurgical instrumentation; some supply only instruments that can be used in orthopedic, otological, or nasal surgery as well as in neurosurgery. Many neurosurgeons in private practice carry some or all of their own special instruments from hospital to hospital.

Two instrumentation cards are necessary for a neurosurgical procedure: one listing all basic instruments needed (a basic dissecting set) and one listing general and special instruments preferred by the specific surgeon for a specific procedure.

Usually several instruments can be used to perform one function. The choice depends on what is available and the surgeon's preference. Therefore only instrument types and examples of each type are listed here. The exact instrument list for any neurosurgeon for each procedure must be written by the nurse in collaboration with that surgeon.

Basic instruments include the following list (specific names in parentheses are examples):

1 Hudson brace (or craniotome) with burs and perforators
1 Drill guide
1 Hand drill with drill points and key
2 Cranial saw handles
2 Cranial saw guides (Cushing, Bailey, Poppen)
6 Cranial saws (Gigli, Tyler)
2 Double-action rongeurs, 9¾ inches (Stille gooseneck, Leksell)
2 Double-action rongeurs, 6¾ inches (Zaufel-Jansen, Beyer, Fulton)
2 Single-action rongeurs (Adson, Stookey, Lempert)
2 Cloward punches, 40-degree, 5 mm and 3 mm
1 Raney punch
1 Kerrison rongeur, 5 mm
5 Penfield dissectors, nos. 1, 2, 3, 4, and 5
2 Bone curettes, nos. 0 and 00
2 Four-prong rake retractors, dull
2 Cushing subtemporal decompression retractors
4 Self-retaining retractors, dull, 8 inches (Cone, Weitlaner, Anderson-Adson)
1 Jansen mastoid retractor
36 Scalp clips (Adson, Raney, Michel)
2 Scalp clip applicators for the specific clip used
1 Scalp clip remover (Adson, Michel)
4 Bayonet forceps, smooth, 7¼ inches
2 Tissue forceps with teeth, 6 inches
2 Cushing forceps, smooth, 7 inches
2 Cushing forceps with teeth, 7 inches
2 Adson tissue forceps, 5 inches
18 Towel clamps, Backhaus type, 3½ inches
18 Halstead mosquito forceps, 12 curved and 6 straight
36 Hemostatic scalp forceps (Dandy, Crile, Kolodney, Kelly)

10 Rochester-Pean hemostat forceps
4 Kochers forceps, straight, 6 inches
12 Towel clamps, Peers type
6 Fish-hook retractors
4 Periosteal elevators (Cushing, Adson, Langenbeck)
1 Dura separator (Sachs, Frazier, Hoen)
1 No. 3 Adson elevator
2 Freer dissectors (Olivecrona, Woodson)
4 Ventricular needles with obturators, 3½ inches (Cone, Seletz, Scott)
1 Brain-aspirating needle with cannula
1 Aneurysm needle
2 Brain spoons, 1 small and 1 large (Cushing)
6 Suction tips, 2 each large, medium, and small (Frazier, Bucy, Sachs, Cone, Adson)
2 Suction tubings
1 Active cautery electrode pencil with spatula tip
6 Gerald bayonet forceps: 2 fine with teeth; 2 fine, smooth; and 2 heavy with teeth
6 Davis brain retractors, 2 each narrow, medium, and wide
4 Clip applicators, 2 medium and 2 small (Hemoclips, Ligaclips, McKenzie)
4 Clip cartridges, 2 each medium and small
1 Clip rack
2 Alligator clip applicators (Penfield, Samuels-Weck)
1 Stainless steel metric ruler
2 Dura hooks, 6 inches
6 Needle holders: 2 each fine, 7½ inches; fine, 6 inches; and heavy, 7¼ inches
3 Adson (tonsil) hemostatic forceps, straight, 7¼ inches
3 Nerve hooks, 7¾ inches, 1 each small, medium, and large
3 Copper pituitary spoons, 1 each small, medium and large (Cushing)
1 Self-retaining brain retractor with assorted blades (Leyla-Yasargil, Edinborough, DeMartel, Hamby)
6 Knife handles, 2 each nos. 3, 4, and 7
1 Mayo scissors, curved, 7 inches
2 Metzenbaum scissors, 5 and 7 inches
5 Alligator pituitary/disc rongeurs with assorted cup sizes
1 Bipolar cautery forceps and cord
3 Irrigating syringes (Asepto, ear bulb)
6 Glass syringes, 10 ml, 2 each plain tip, Luer-Lok, and control grip
1 Devilbiss bone-cutting instrument with 2 blades

The foregoing instrument list is very basic and is compiled to help the nurse in the general hospital rather than the nurse in the large neurosurgical center. A hospital with an active neurosurgical service has its own basic craniotomy instrument list. The nurse should use that list and add the special preferences of a given neurosurgeon.

In addition to the basic types of instruments essential for supratentorial craniotomy (Figs. 24-31 to 24-34), su-

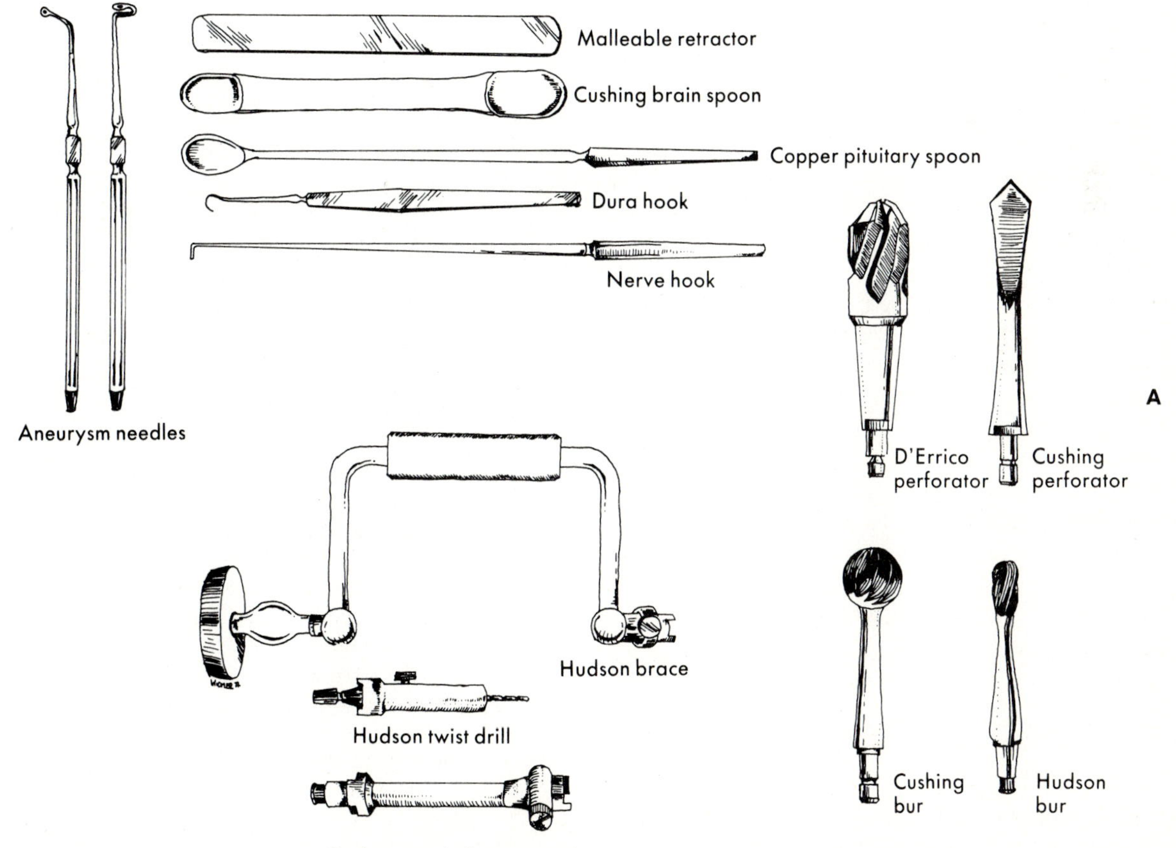

Fig. 24-31. A, Some basic instruments for craniotomy.

Continued.

B

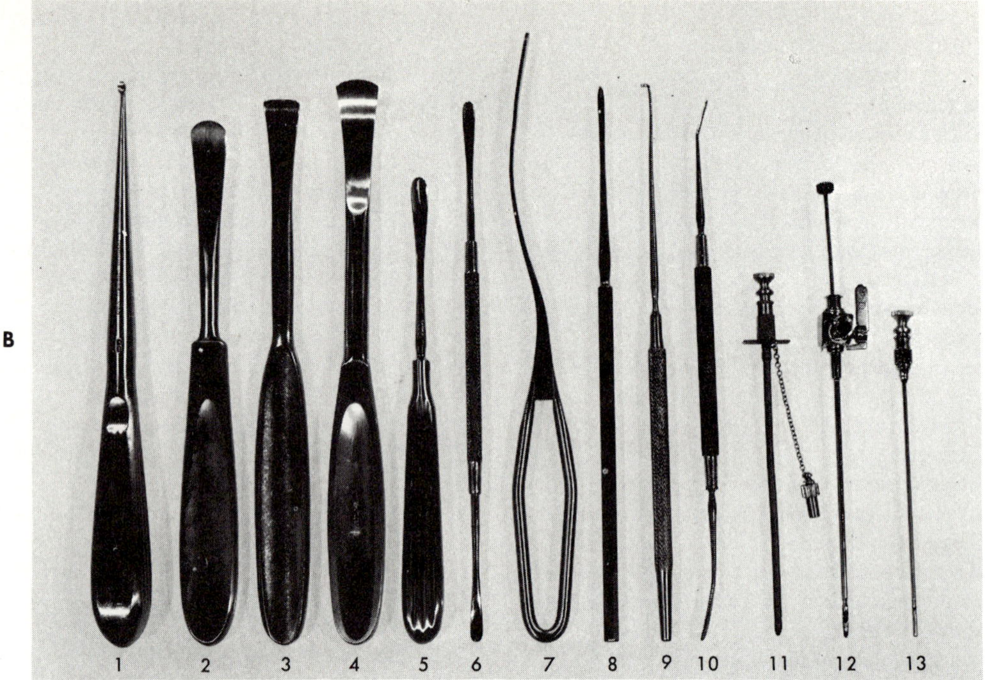

Fig. 24-31, cont'd. B, *1,* Spinal curette, straight; *2,* Cushing periosteal elevator, blunt; *3,* Cushing periosteal elevator, sharp; *4,* Adson periosteal elevator, wide; *5,* Adson elevator no. 3 (Joker); *6,* Freer elevator; *7,* Sachs dura separator; *8,* Sunday staphylorrhaphy elevator; *9,* nerve hook; *10,* Olivecrona double-ended dissector; *11,* Scott ventricular cannula; *12,* Seletz ventricular cannula; *13,* Cone ventricular needle.

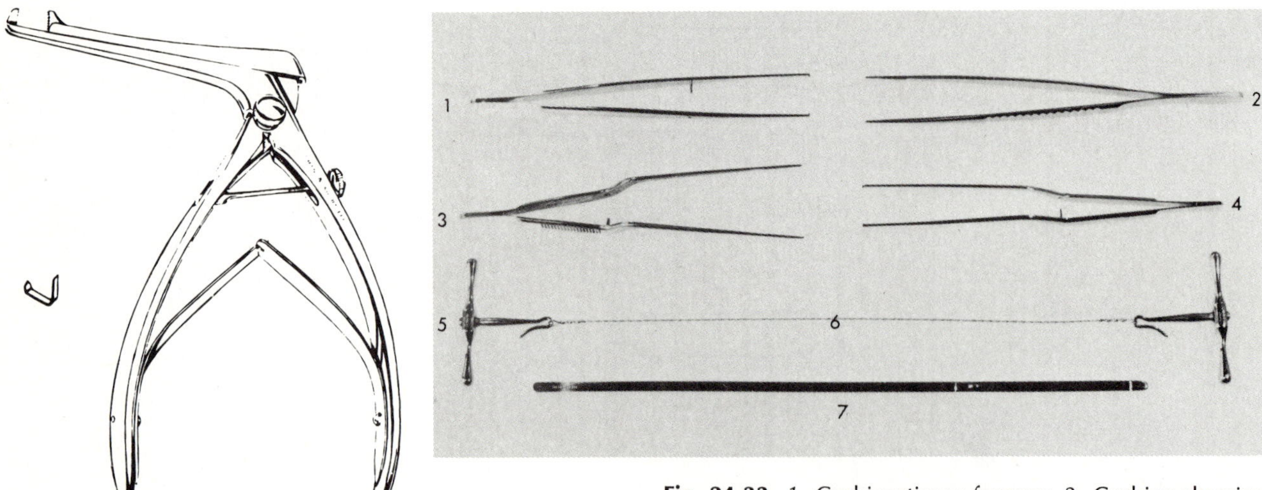

Fig. 24-33. *1,* Cushing tissue forceps; *2,* Cushing dressing forceps; *3,* Cushing bayonet dressing forceps; *4,* Cushing bayonet tissue forceps; *5,* Gigli saw handle; *6,* Gigli saw wire; *7,* Bailey saw guide.

Fig. 24-32. Setup for craniosynostosis may include Ingraham-Fowler tantalum clips, Ingraham-Fowler guillotine applicators, and preformed silicone strip. (Courtesy Codman & Shurtleff, Inc., Randolph, Mass.)

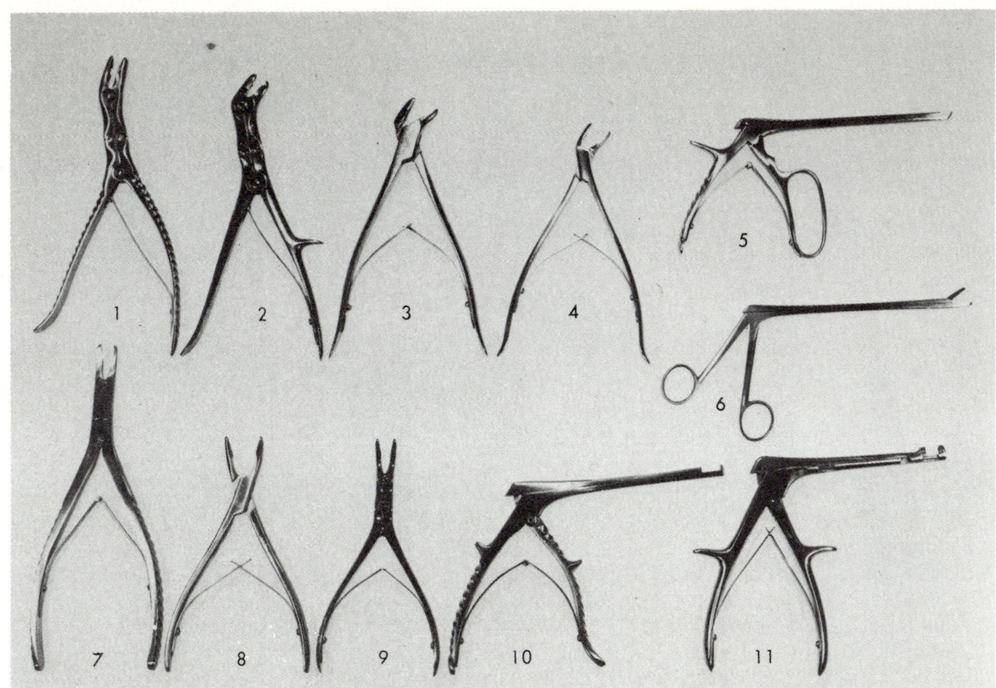

Fig. 24-34. *1,* Leksell rongeur; *2,* Stille gooseneck rongeur; *3,* Bacon rongeur; *4,* Stookey cranial rongeur; *5,* Cloward 40-degree angle punch rongeur; *6,* pituitary disc rongeur; *7,* Fulton rongeur; *8,* Lempert rongeur; *9,* Zaufal-Jansen rongeur; *10,* Kerrison rongeur; *11,* Raney punch.

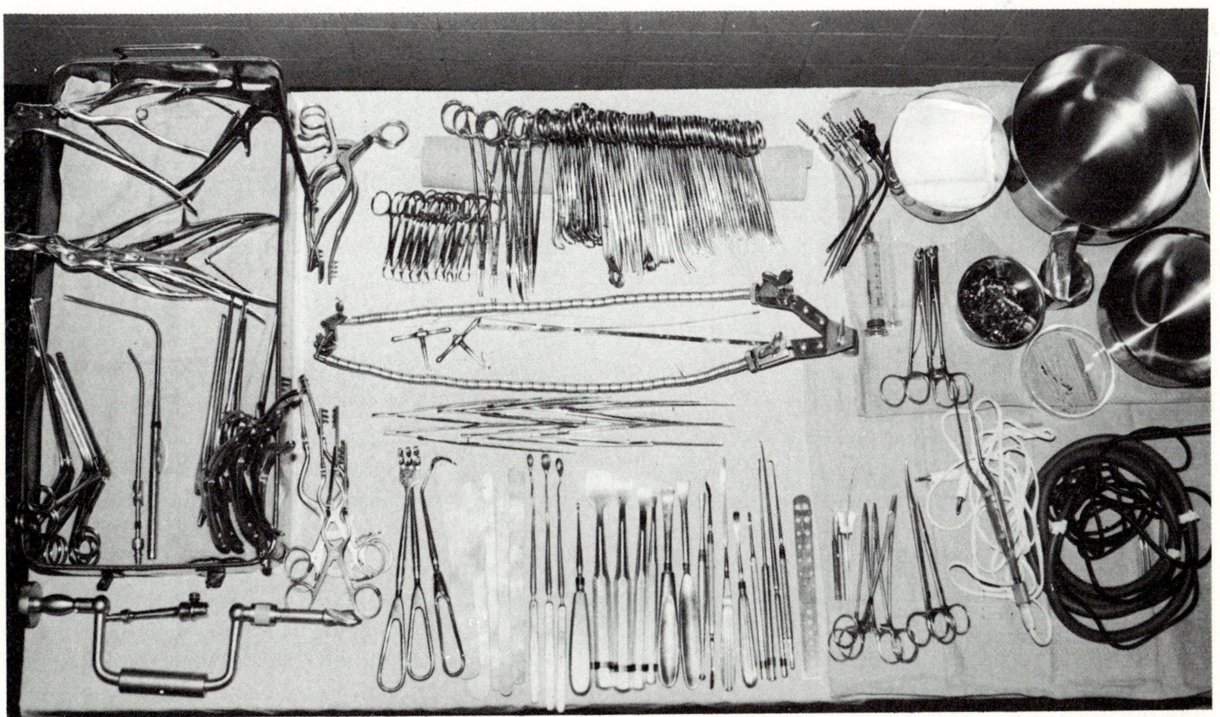

Fig. 24-35. Back table instrument setup for craniotomy.

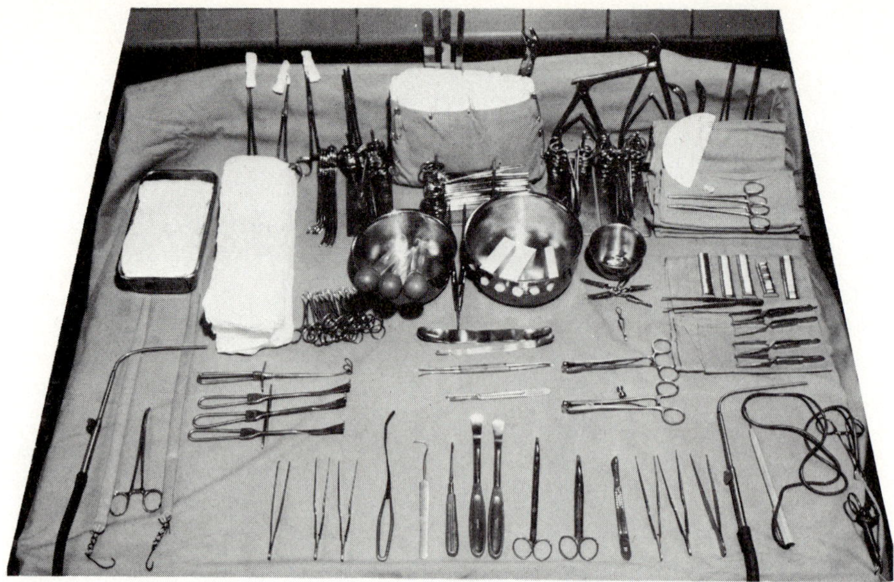

Fig. 24-36. Craniotomy instruments arranged on overhead table.

ture scissors, a wire scissors, and a 6-inch Russian forceps should be included. A bone punch (Cone or Ingram), a drill guide and dura protector (Adson or Hamlin), a twist drill that fits the Hudson brace or a Raney brace and perforator, McKenzie silver clips and applicators, trephines, bur hole covers (Silastic, such as the Todd-Crue buttons, or tantalum), Ray pituitary curettes, a Rayport dura knife, pituitary forceps (Adson or D'Errico), Bonney forceps, Penfield watchmaker's forceps, Hartmann forceps, monopolar cautery bayonet forceps (Davis, Raney, Hoen, Jansen), bulldog clamps, angled dura scissors (Taylor, Frazier, DeBakey, Potts-Smith), or a myriad of other instruments that a given neurosurgeon may desire can be included.

Many neurosurgeons prefer Allis forceps, rather than towel clamps, or Peers clamps to attach suction, cautery, and other devices to the drapes. Allis forceps used for this purpose should not be used for any other surgical procedures. They can be marked for neurosurgery and kept with the special neurosurgical instruments. They will not hold tissue such as the edge of the small bowel effectively after continued use on drape materials.

Glass syringes are usually preferred by neurosurgeons. Two 10-ml Luer-Lok and two 10-ml plain tip syringes should be included in every craniotomy setup. Also included should be six to twelve rubber bands, one or two Penrose drains, two medicine cups, suture material and needles of the surgeon's choice, and dressing headrolls (Kling or Kerlix).

Most neurosurgeons own magnifying loupes. They should be available.

Posterior fossa or infratentorial craniectomy requires the same instrumentation as supratentorial craniotomy, minus saws, saw handles, and saw guides. A cerebellar extension for the Hudson brace must be included as well as a larger assortment of double-action and Kerrison rongeurs. The Ronjair rongeur is especially useful, if available.

Additional instruments required for laminectomy, anterior fusion, surgery of peripheral nerves, microsurgery, and aneurysm surgery are included in the descriptions of the surgical procedures.

An example of a back-table setup for craniotomy is shown in Fig. 24-35. Arrangement of instruments on the overhead table can be seen in Fig. 24-36.

OPERATIONS

It is not possible in this chapter to provide a detailed approach to each neurosurgical procedure. Specific neurosurgical procedures are numerous, and each has a number of modifications or variations. The operating surgeon decides exactly which procedure and what variation will be performed. Basic general approaches, however, are limited and can be described in detail. Therefore only a few step-by-step descriptions of basic approaches are presented. The nurse who is familiar with neurosurgical anatomy and pathological conditions can learn these basic approaches and adapt them to the specific procedure.

Bur holes

Bur holes are placed to remove a localized fluid collection beneath the dura mater. Fluid not composed of clot can be easily evacuated through a bur hole. Bur holes are also made to tap a lateral ventricle to relieve pressure. Bur holes are used by many surgeons when treating a

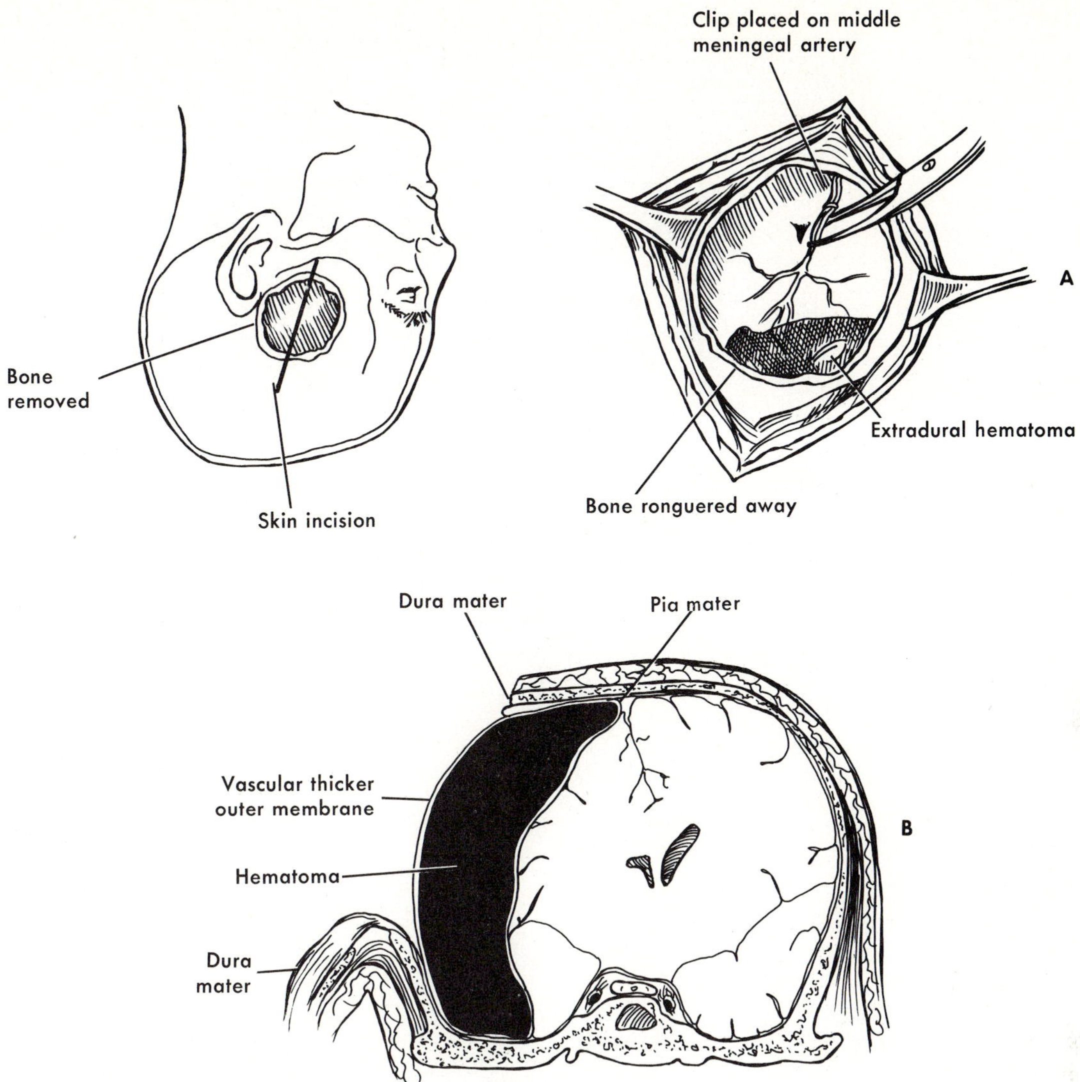

Fig. 24-37. A, Extradural hemorrhage. **B,** Subdural hematoma. (From Richards, V.: Surgery for general practice, St. Louis, The C.V. Mosby Co.)

brain abscess. The abscess may be aspirated, and antibiotics instilled. Other surgeons prefer to treat abscess by craniotomy. Occasionally, bur holes are used to locate or drain subdural hematomas. However, a craniectomy is usually necessary to gain adequate exposure in these cases (Fig. 24-37). A bur hole is one of the steps in procedures to shunt ventricular fluid to another body system for absorption or elimination.

Bur holes are placed to introduce air into the lateral ventricles for ventriculography (Fig. 24-38). The air makes the ventricles visible in x-ray studies.

Trephination

Trephination is the formation of an opening into the skull. This term usually applies when the opening is larger than the average bur hole. A plug of bone is cut with a circular saw that attaches to the Hudson brace. Procedures performed by trephination include prefrontal lobotomy, topectomy, cingulumotomy, and leukotomy. In these procedures, nerve pathways in the frontal lobe of the cerebral cortex are selectively interrupted to correct psychosis or relieve intractable pain. Surgical approach can be either transorbital or frontal by way of a trephine or bur hole (Fig. 24-39). A leukotome is used to selectively divide areas of frontal white matter, interrupting transmission pathways. In prefrontal lobotomy or leukotomy, the medial third of the frontal white matter is interrupted bilaterally. In the transorbital approach, the thalamofrontal radiation is interrupted. In topectomy, specific cortical areas for social behavior and personality are resected. The cingulate gyrus is the target in cingulumotomy.

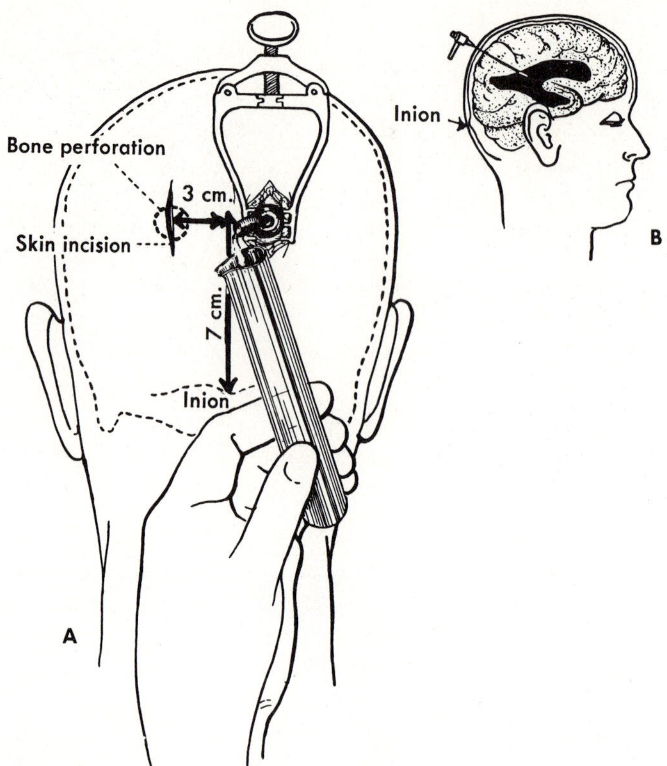

Fig. 24-38. Occipital bur holes for ventriculography. (From Richards, V.: Surgery for general practice, St. Louis, The C.V. Mosby Co.)

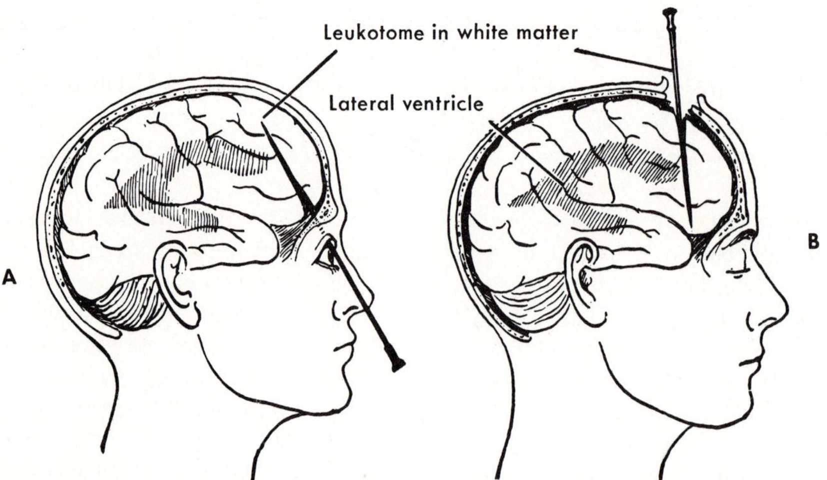

Fig. 24-39. A, Transorbital leukotomy (Fiamberti). **B,** Classic frontal leukotomy (Moniz). (From Carini, E., and Owens, G: Neurological and neurosurgical nursing, ed. 6, St. Louis, 1974, The C.V. Mosby Co.)

Craniotomy

Definition. Incision into the skull to expose and surgically treat intracranial disease.

Considerations. Depending on the location of the pathological condition, the craniotomy may be frontal, parietal, occipital, temporal, or a combination of two or more of these. Craniotomy is the term usually used when the bone flap is cut out with a saw. When turning a scalp flap for a craniotomy, the surgeon may peel the scalp back off the periosteum (osteoplastic) or the periosteum may be stripped off the skull as the scalp is being lifted off the bone (osteoclastic).

The bone plate may be separated from the soft tissues, removed from the skull, and set aside for replacement at the end of the procedure. It may be placed in an antibiotic solution or wrapped in a sponge that has been saturated with an antibiotic solution. The bone plate is not removed from the sterile field. If it is not replaced, it may be frozen in a sterile container or saved and stored in a marked, unsterile container to use as a template for forming a cranioplastic plate at a later date. The defect can be repaired without use of this template, however. If the bone is not separated from the soft tissues, it is turned back with the temporal muscle and soft tissues.

Operative procedure. After draping and attachment of suctions and cauteries the procedure is begun:

1. The surgeon and the assistant apply digital pressure over folded 4 × 4–inch Raytex sponges on both sides of the incision line. The skin and galea are incised in segments, the length of each segment being equal to that over which the finger pressure is applied. The tissue edges are held with a 6-inch toothed forceps as scalp clips are placed on the flap edges. Hemostats are placed on the outside edge of the incision in adults and are grouped in segments and secured together by rubber bands placed around the handles or by a Penrose drain or open 4 × 4–inch sponge threaded through the handles and tied or clamped together with a heavy clamp, such as a Pean (Fig. 24-40). Any remaining active arterial bleeding is controlled by electrocoagulation. If the incision extends into the temporal area, bleeding in the temporal muscle is managed by cautery, hemostats, tamponade, or suture ligature. A Mayo scissors may be used to incise temporal muscle and fascia.

2. The soft tissue is peeled off the periosteum by sharp or blunt dissection or by electrodissection (Fig. 24-40). The scalp flap is turned back over folded sponges and retracted by use of small towel clamps and rubber bands or muscle hooks on rubber bands. In either case the traction is maintained by securing the rubber band to the drapes with heavy forceps. The flap may be covered with a moist sponge or Telfa strips and a sterile towel. Bleeding is controlled by electrocautery.

3. When a free bone flap is planned, the muscle and periosteum are incised. Muscle and periosteum are elevated with the skin-galea flap, turned back, and retracted as a unit, as described previously.

4. The periosteum and muscle are incised with a scalpel or cautery knife except at the inferior margins, which are left intact to preserve blood supply to the bone flap. The periosteum is stripped from the bone at the incision line with a periosteal elevator. Bone wax is used to control bleeding.

5. The scalp edges and muscle are retracted from the bone incision line by a Sachs or Cushing retractor. Two or more bur holes are made with either a hand or power cranial drill (Fig. 24-41). As each hole is drilled, the patient's head must be held by the assistant to diminish the agitation and prevent displacement from the headrest. A great deal of heat is generated by the friction of the perforator or bur against the bone. The nurse or assistant must irrigate the drilling site to counteract the heat and remove bone dust, which collects as the holes are made. Some surgeons prefer that the nurse collect the bone dust for replacement in the bur holes at closure. The dust is placed in a medicine glass and kept moist with a small amount of normal saline solution. A large-gauge suction tip is used to remove both irrigating solution and debris from the field. As the inner table is perforated and the dura exposed, the bur hole may be temporarily tamponaded with bone wax and/or a cottonoid strip or patty. Each hole is eventually debrided by a no. 0 or 00 bone curette or small joker. The dura mater is freed at the margins with a no. 3 Adson elevator, no. 3 Penfield dissector, or right-angle Frazier elevator or similar instrument. The hole is irrigated, and suction applied simultaneously. Active bleeding points in the bone are identified, and bone wax is applied.

6. When all bur holes have been made, the bone flap is cut by sawing between holes after the dura mater has been separated from the bone by a dural separator, such as the Sachs or Horsley, or by a no. 3 Penfield dissector. Dural separation is done to prevent tearing of the dura mater, especially over venous sinuses. Using a rongeur, the surgeon may cut channels in the two bur holes at the inferior edge of the planned bone flap under the muscle. When the rest of the bone flap has been sawed, this segment can be easily cracked as the bone is elevated and turned back. If the sawing is done by hand, a dural separator is passed from one hole to the next under the bone. A saw guide-passer with a saw attached is passed from one hole to the next in the same manner (Fig. 24-42). The saw is detached from the guide, saw handles are attached to both ends of the saw, and the bone is incised by sawing in a back and forth motion. Friction generates heat, so irrigation and suction must be used during the process. The procedure is repeated until all segments but the one under the muscle have been cut. Usually a new saw is used each time.

When a power saw or craniotome is used, only two

bur holes may be necessary. Irrigation and suction are required as the bone flap is cut. Soft tissue edges are retracted with Sachs or Cushing retractors.

7. The bone flap with muscle attached is lifted off the dura mater by two periosteal elevators. As it is forced up and back, the bridge of bone under the muscle cracks. Bleeding from the bone is controlled with bone wax. A double-action rongeur is used to remove sharp, irregular edges where the bone cracked (Fig. 24-43). The bone flap is covered with a moist sponge, cottonoid material, or Telfa pads, and a clean sterile towel and is retracted in the same manner as the scalp flap.

8. The dura mater is irrigated. Moist cottonoid strips or patties or Telfa pads may be inserted between the dura mater and bone and folded back to cover the exposed bone edges. Clean sterile towels may be placed around the operative site.

9. The dura mater is opened (Fig. 24-44). A dura hook may be used to elevate the dura mater from the brain, and a small nick is made in the dura mater with a no. 15 blade on a no. 3 scapel handle, or a small opening may be made in the dura mater without elevating it, after which the dural edges are grasped with straight mosquito forceps or two Adson or Cushing forceps with teeth and are elevated. A narrow, moist cottonoid strip is inserted with a smooth forceps (bayonet, Cushing) into the opening to protect the brain as the dura mater is incised and elevated. The dural incision can be made with a Metzenbaum scissors, special dura scissors, or a Rayport dura knife. Usually traction sutures are placed at the outer edge of the dura mater and are tagged with small bulldog clamps or mosquito forceps. Sometimes the tag instruments are attached to the drapes to increase traction and keep tension on them. As the dural veins are approached during dural opening, they are ligated or coagulated before cutting. Ligation is done with hemostatic clips such as Weck Hemoclips, Ligaclips, or McKenzie clips. The brain surface is protected by moist cottonoid strips.

10. Cottonoid strips and brain retractors, self-retaining (Fig. 24-45) and manual, are placed appropriately by the surgeon while working toward visualizing the particular pathological entity.

11. Brain spoons, Cushing pituitary spoons, and Ray curettes, as well as pituitary rongeurs or other tumor forceps, must be available for tumor removal. Also, a selection of dissectors, Cushing and Gerald forceps, and a bipolar coagulation unit are used. Completely filled irrigating syringes and a full range of moist cottonoid patties and strips must be within easy reach of the surgeon and the assistant. Following correction of the pathological condition and control of bleeding, the brain may be irrigated with an antibiotic solution of the surgeon's choice.

12. The dura mater may be left open, or it may be closed. If closure is done, it is usually by interrupted sutures of no. 4-0 silk. A drain may or may not be used; drains range from those such as the Jackson-Pratt closed system to a Robinson catheter to a Penrose.

13. The bone flap may or may not be replaced. If swelling is anticipated, it is usually not replaced. If free and replaced, holes may be drilled in the flap and the skull and wires inserted to secure the flap in place. Usually no. 28 or 26 wire is used. The craniotome can be used for this purpose. During drilling, a dura protector is used on the skull side. A brain spoon can serve as a dura protector. Holes for wires can also be made with a skull punch, such as the Cone punch.

14. Periosteum and muscle are approximated with no. 2-0 or 3-0 silk. The galea is closed with no. 3-0 silk. Skin closure can be interrupted or continuous and of silk or some synthetic suture material, such as nylon.

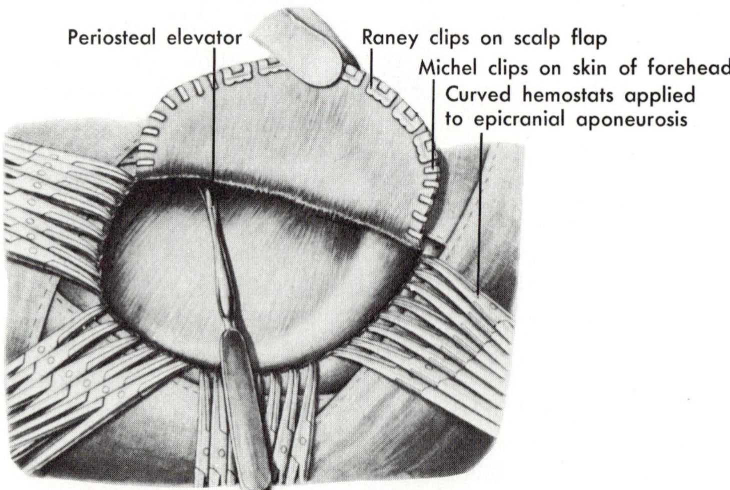

Fig. 24-40. Elevation of scalp flap. Hemostats on outer rim of incision and Raney clips and Michel clips on scalp flap. (From Kempe, L.G.: Operative neurosurgery, vols. 1 and 2, New York, Springer-Verlag New York, Inc.)

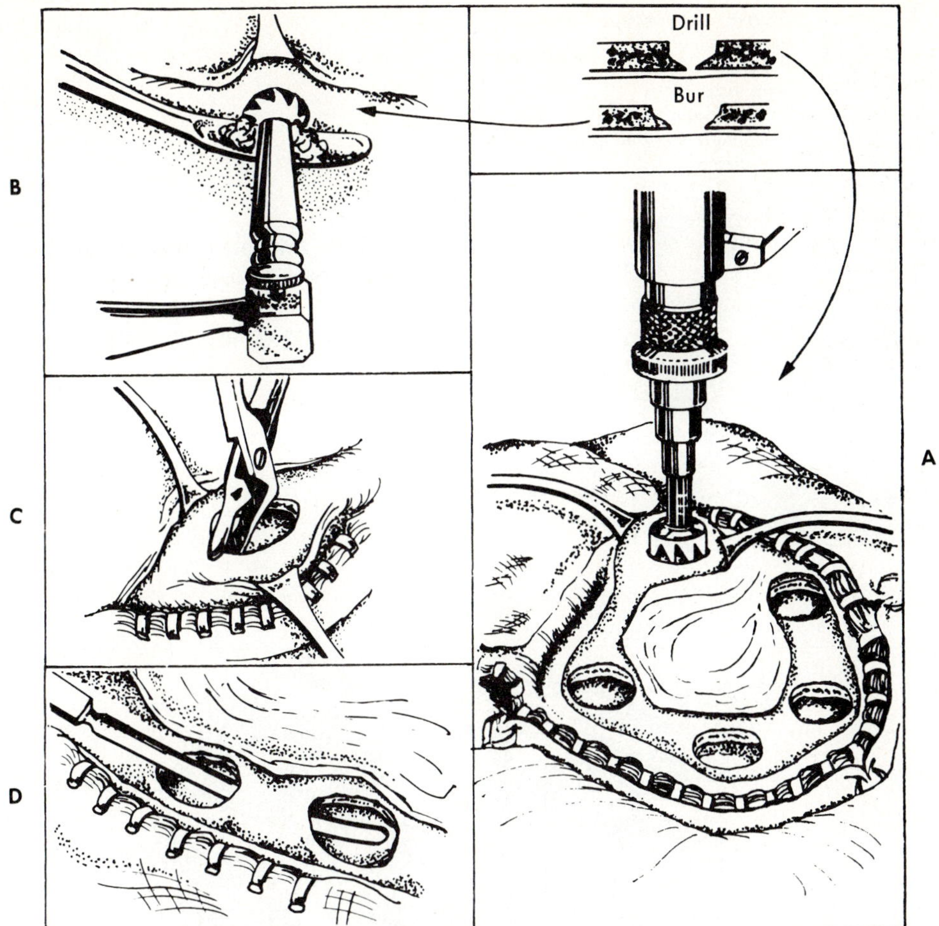

Fig. 24-41. Methods of making osteoplastic flap (craniotomy). **A,** Using electric drill to make bur hole. **B,** Using hand perforator to make bur hole. **C,** Using rongeur to enlarge bur hole. **D,** Separating dura mater from skull. (From Carini, E., and Owens, G.: Neurological and neurosurgical nursing, ed. 6, St. Louis, 1974, The C.V. Mosby Co.)

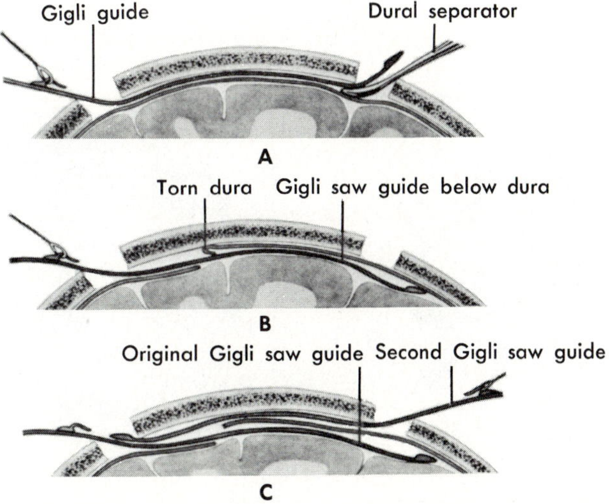

Fig. 24-42. Gigli saw insertion. **A** to **C,** Steps to be taken if Gigli saw tears dura mater. (From Kempe, L.G.: Operative neurosurgery, vols. 1 and 2, New York, Springer-Verlag New York, Inc.)

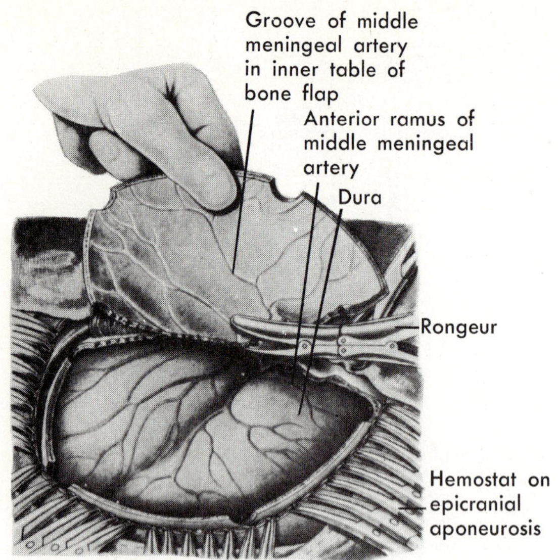

Fig. 24-43. Frontotemporal craniotomy, opening and closure. Removal of rough bone edge from fracture site. (From Kempe, L.G.: Operative neurosurgery, vols. 1 and 2, New York, Springer-Verlag New York, Inc.)

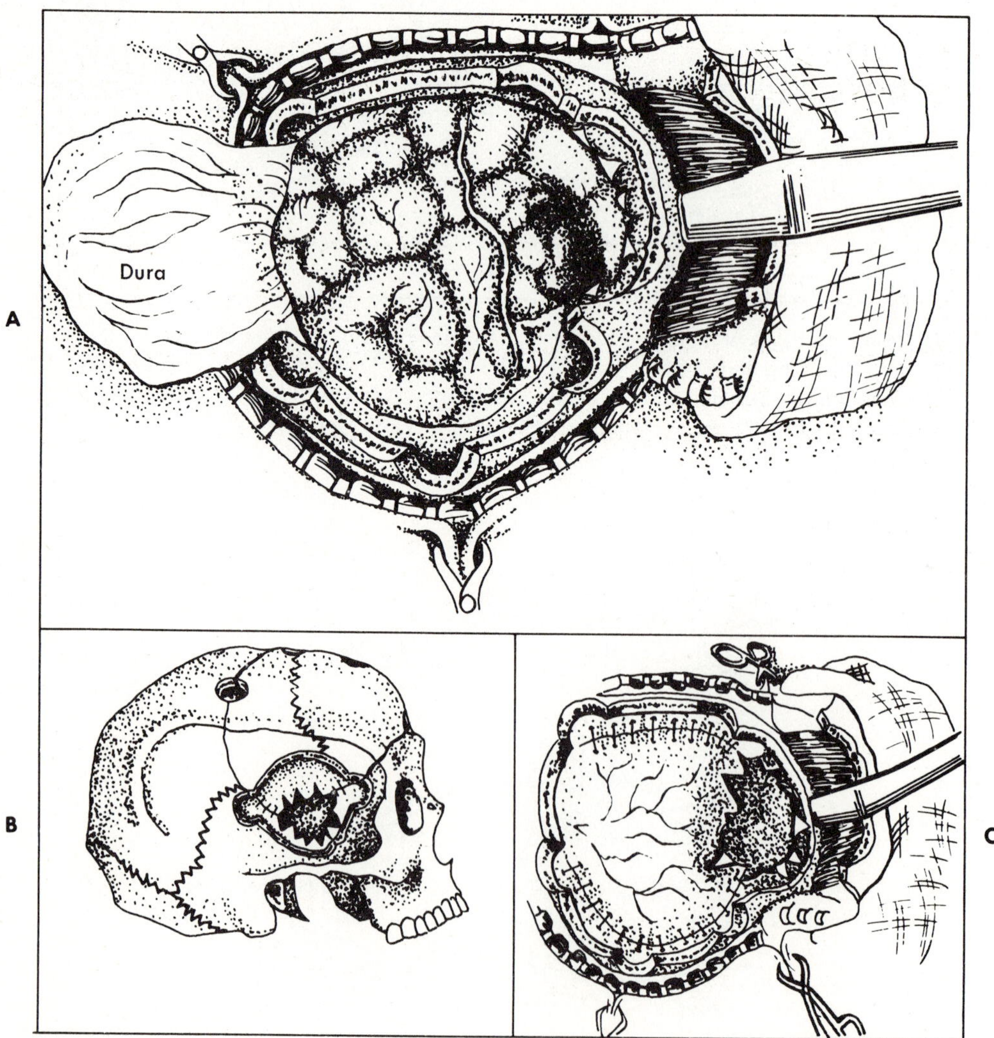

Fig. 24-44. Craniotomy with subtemporal decompression. **A,** Malignant cerebral tumor exposed. **B,** Bony defect. **C,** Dural defect. (From Carini, E., and Owens, G.: Neurological and neurosurgical nursing, ed. 6, St. Louis, 1974, The C.V. Mosby Co.)

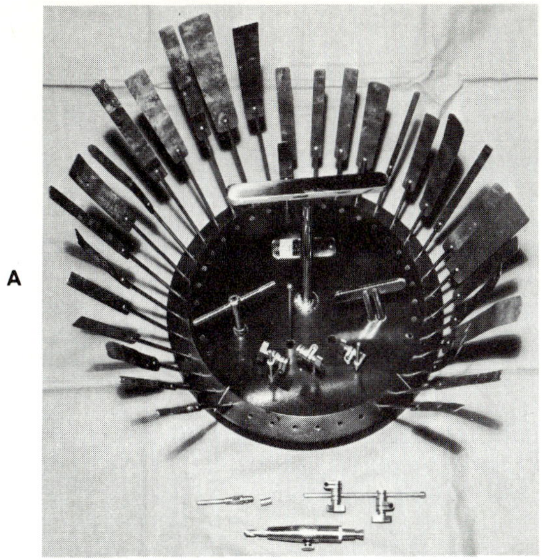

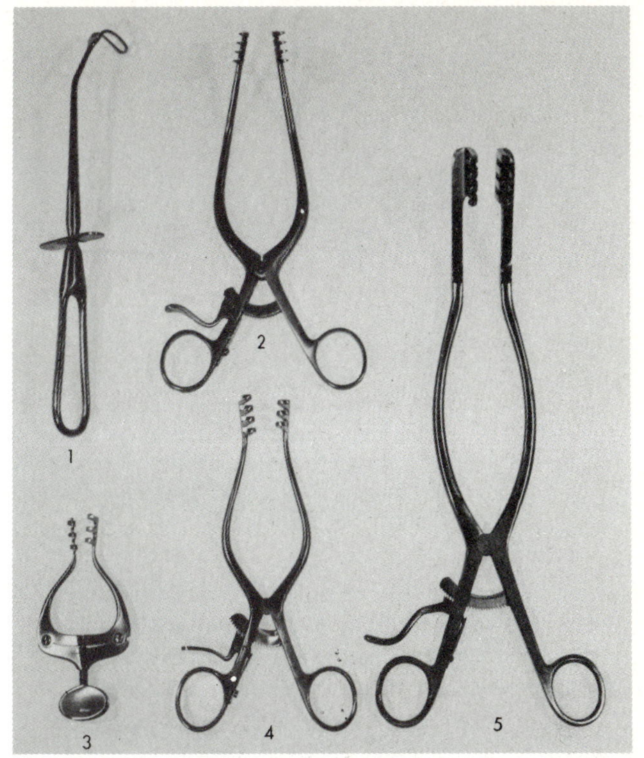

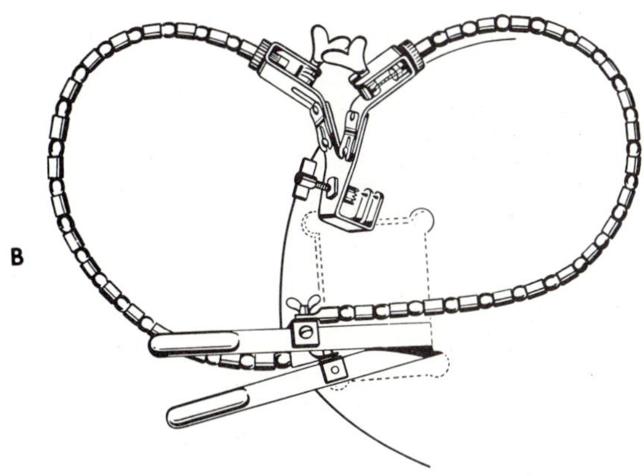

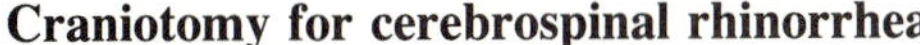

Fig. 24-45. A, Edinborough retractor with blades, poles, screws, and adapters. **B,** Leyla-Yasargil self-retaining retractor. **C,** Retractors: *1,* Cushing subtemporal decompression retractor; *2,* Adson cerebellar retractor; *3,* Jansen mastoid retractor; *4,* Weitlaner retractor; *5,* Beckman laminectomy retractor. (**A** courtesy American V. Mueller Chicago; **B** courtesy Holco Instrument Corp., New York.)

Craniotomy for cerebrospinal rhinorrhea

Considerations. Cerebrospinal rhinorrhea is a rupture of the dura mater, with evagination of the torn arachnoidea through the dura mater into a hole or fracture in the skull communicating with one of the nasal sinuses or the nasal cavity. This results in leakage of spinal fluid from the nose. It is necessary to repair the defect to prevent air from being trapped under pressure in the brain and to prevent intracranial infection.

Operative procedure

1. Usually, a frontal craniotomy is carried out, and the dura mater is opened. The frontal lobe is elevated until the defect can be visualized. The surgeon may elect to use the microscope.
2. The dura mater is dissected from the orbital and cribriform plates.
3. The defect in the bone is defined, and the bony defect may be filled with methyl methacrylate or covered with tantalum mesh.
4. The dural defect may be closed with sutures, but usually some type of patch is placed over it. A piece of muscle, pericranium, fascia, gelatin foam, or silicone sheeting may be used. These may be sutured or glued. Some surgeons do not fasten the patch into place.
5. The dural incision is sutured, and the wound closed.

A similar procedure is carried out in the temporal or suboccipital region to repair a defect in cerebrospinal otorrhea.

Craniotomy for intracranial aneurysm

Considerations. An aneurysm is a vascular dilatation usually caused by a local defect in the vascular wall. Within the cranial cavity, an aneurysm may impinge on the third nerve or the optic chiasm. Hemorrhage is generally the first evidence of an intracranial aneurysm.

Modern neurosurgical techniques have made operations on intracranial aneurysms more feasible. Fatal hemorrhage is the greatest hazard of the condition and of the

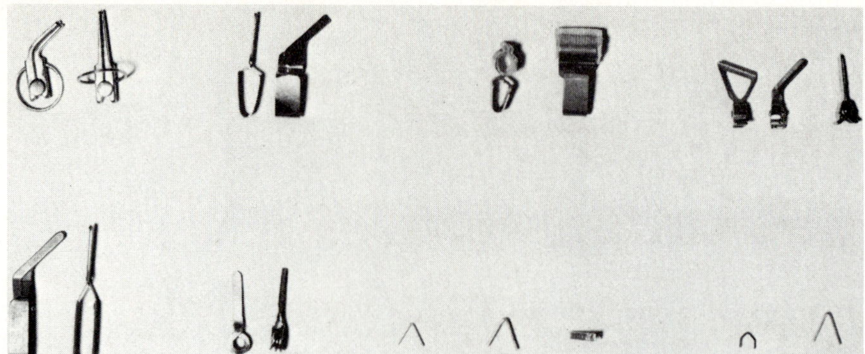

Fig. 24-46. Some types of vascular clips and clamps available. *Left to right: top,* Kerr clip, Mayfield clip, Sundt-Kees clip, Heifetz clip; *bottom,* Schwartz temporary clamp, Scoville clip, McKenzie silver clip, Olivecrona clip (wide), Weck Hemoclip, Olivecrona clip (narrow). (Courtesy K. Cramer Lewis, Department of Illustrations, Washington University School of Medicine, St. Louis.)

operation. To prevent this, control of the blood pressure, as well as the vascular supply to the region well beyond the limits of the lesion, may be required. Occasionally, control of the cerebral circulation at the level of the cervical carotid artery is desired. The artery may be exposed and controlled by means of preplaced ligatures or clamps that can be tightened to occlude the vessel if bleeding occurs at the site of the aneurysm during the operation. This is a separate preliminary surgical procedure.

Setup and preparation of the patient. Aneurysm clips and applicators of the surgeon's choice must be included with the instrumentation. Figs. 24-46 and 24-47 illustrate a few of the clips and applicators available. A minimum of two applicators for each type of clip must be included; both temporary and permanent clips must be available. Temporary clips include Mayfield, McFadden, Drake, and Schwartz. Heifetz, Sundt-Kees, Olivecrona, Housepian, and Scoville are types of permanent aneurysm clips. The Yasargil clips can be used as either temporary or permanent clips (Fig. 24-48). Permanent clips can be removed from the vessel if necessary. The clip applicators serve as clip removers.

Aneurysm clips should never be compressed between the fingers. Clips should be compressed only when seated in their applicators. Once a clip has been compressed, it should be discarded. Clips that have been compressed may be sprung and may slip, causing complications, such as bleeding or compression of another vessel or of a nerve.

The full armamentarium of aneurysm occlusion tools should be available for the surgeon. Besides clips, fast-setting aneuroplastic resinous material, a piece of temporal muscle, ligature carriers, latex spray, or any other material, such as linen or gold foil, requested by the surgeon should be in the room and ready to use. Iron-impregnated silicone is also being used to obliterate aneurysms. Fine silk ligatures and hemostatic clips, with or without bipolar coagulation of the neck of the aneurysm, have also been used successfully.

A basic craniotomy setup is required in addition to the special items mentioned. Supplementary suction must be immediately available on the field to prevent hemorrhage from obscuring the surgeon's vision if the aneurysm dome ruptures during operation and for removing smoke resulting from laser dissection.

Operative procedure

1. A frontal, frontotemporal, or bifrontal craniotomy may be done to approach an aneurysm in the area of the circle of Willis. The bifrontal approach requires extra scalp clips and hemostatic forceps. All aneurysm instruments preferred by the surgeon must be included.

2. After the dura mater has been opened, a self-retaining brain retractor is placed, and the optic nerve and subarachnoid cisterns are exposed. The olfactory nerve may be coagulated and divided with a long scissors for better exposure.

3. The operating microscope is positioned. Microinstruments, including a microbipolar cautery bayonet, are used (Figs. 24-49 to 24-59).

4. Bridging veins are coagulated with bipolar cautery.

5. The covering arachnoidal webs are dissected away with microdissectors, hooks, elevators, scissors, knives, and forceps. A Scarff bipolar suction cautery may be used.

6. Careful dissection of the arachnoidea and clear visualization of the neck of the aneurysm without rupture of the dome are the aims of the surgeon.

7. The parent arteries are identified and freed so that they can be occluded with a temporary clip if necessary. Other structures, such as the optic chiasma and optic nerves, are identified.

8. As the surgeon works slowly toward the dome and neck of the aneurysm, the patient's blood pressure is lowered for easier control of hemorrhage should the aneurysm rupture.

9A. If the neck of the aneurysm can be isolated, a clip is placed across it. Clips such as the Sundt-Kees and Heifetz have Teflon linings and can be used to approach

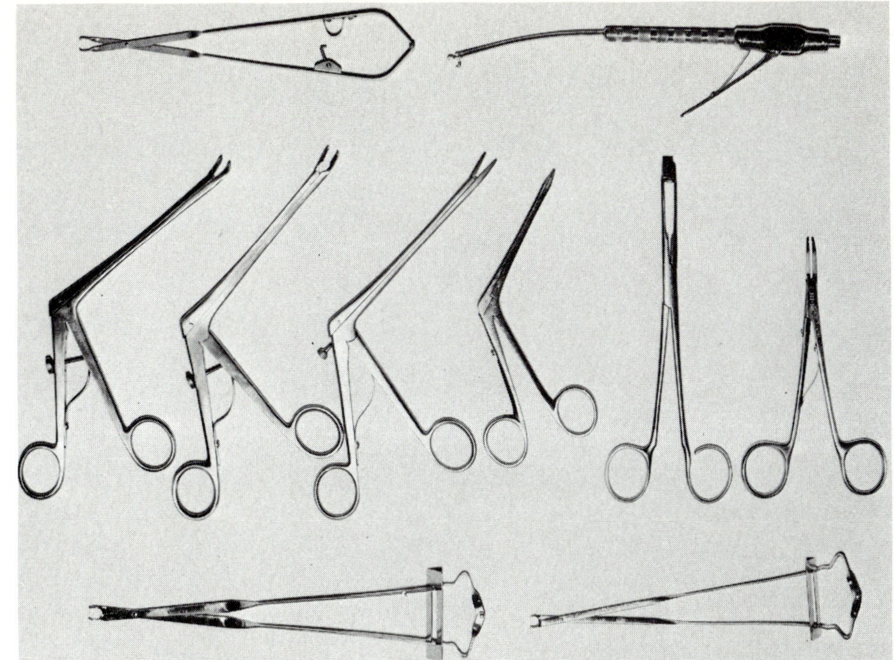

Fig. 24-47. Some types of vascular clip applicators. *Left to right: top,* Heifetz and Kerr clip applicators; *center,* right-angled Hamby, right-angled Mount-Olivecrona, Scoville-Drew, Scoville, Schwartz, and Weck Hemoclip applicators; *bottom,* Mayfield and small Mayfield clip applicators. (Courtesy K. Cramer Lewis, Department of Illustrations, Washington University School of Medicine, St. Louis.)

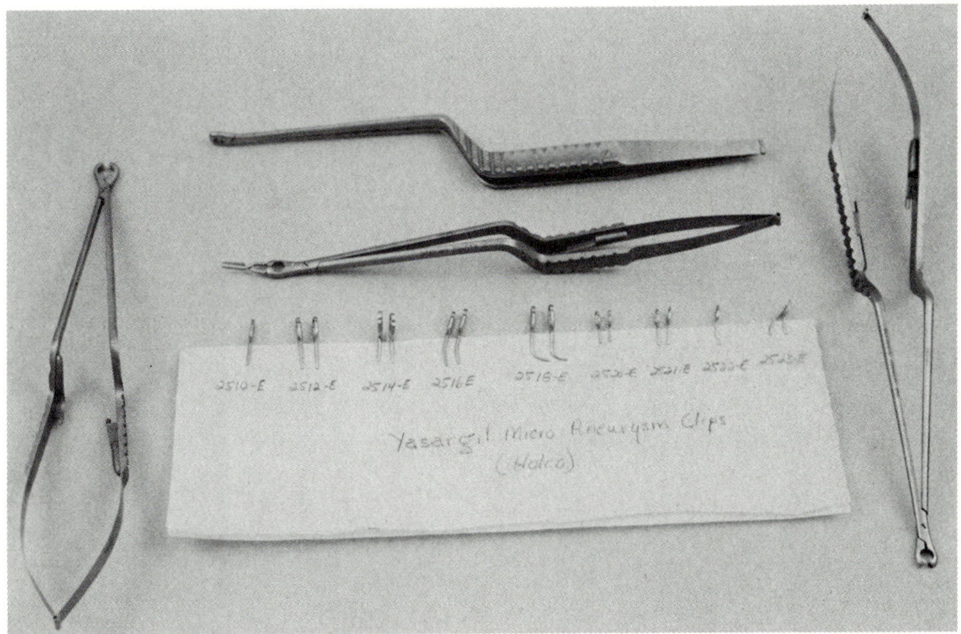

Fig. 24-48. Yasargil microaneurysm clips and applicators.

the aneurysm from a 180-degree angle to avoid excessive manipulation and traction of the parent vessel, if the neck is on the underside of the vessel. These clips support the vessel and serve as a clip graft.

9B. When clipping is not feasible, coating the aneurysm with fast-drying methyl methacrylate has good results. The chemicals are mixed, and, before the chemical hardens, it is applied to the surface of the aneurysm with a disposable plastic syringe and the plastic cannula from a large (16- or 14-gauge) angiocath. All surrounding tissues must be walled off with cottonoid material before the acrylic substance is mixed and applied.

10. As soon as the aneurysm has been occluded, the blood pressure is returned to normal, and the aneurysm site is checked for bleeding. When the surgeon is satisfied that the operative field is dry, wound closure is begun.

Text continued on p. 751.

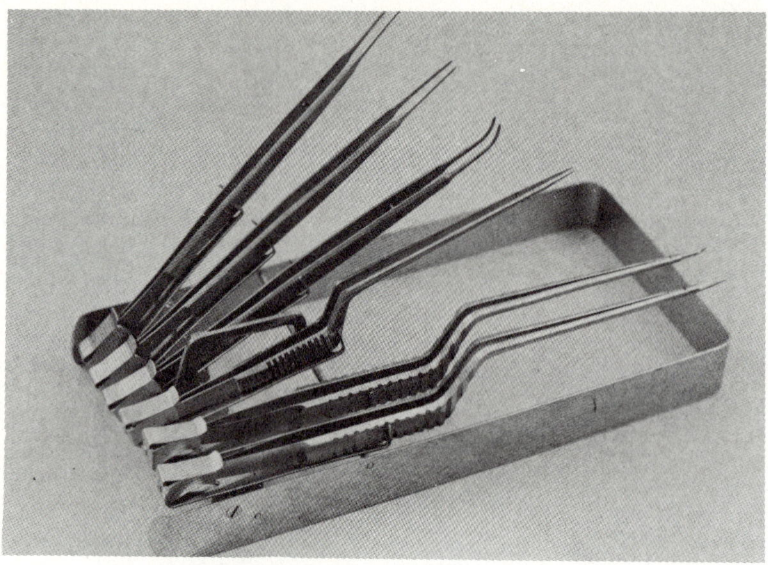

Fig. 24-49. Microscissors and forceps in rack.

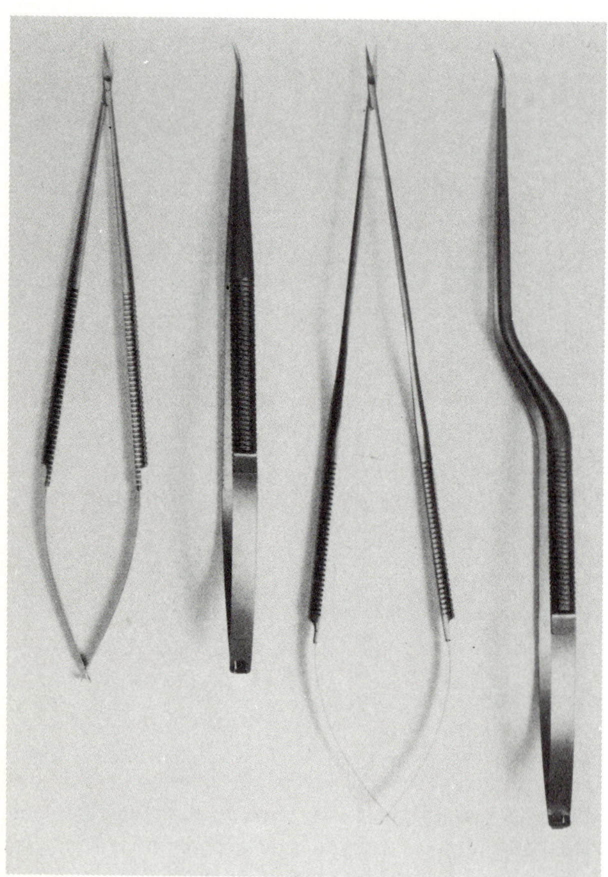

Fig. 24-50. Rhoton titanium microscissors. (Courtesy Codman & Shurtleff, Inc., Randolph, Mass.)

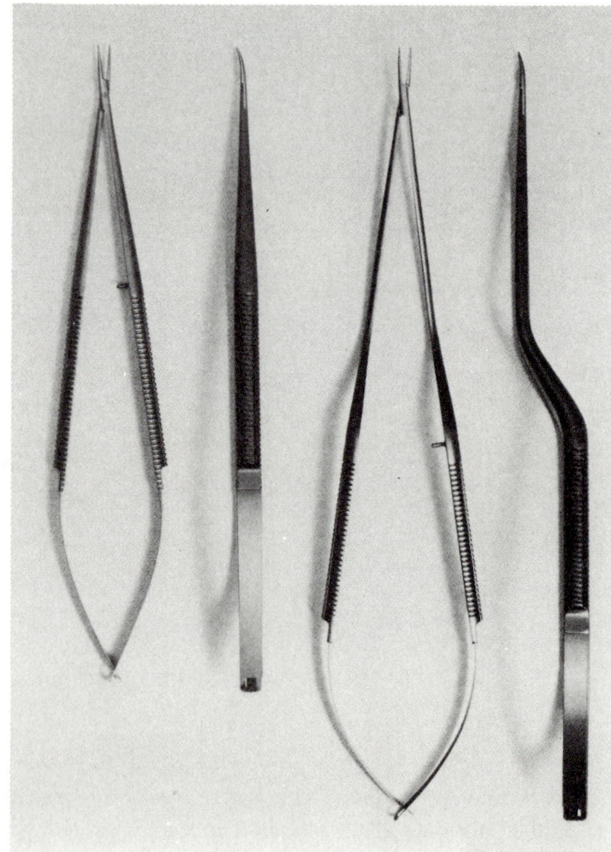

Fig. 24-51. Rhoton microsurgical needle holders. (Courtesy Codman & Shurtleff, Inc., Randolph, Mass.)

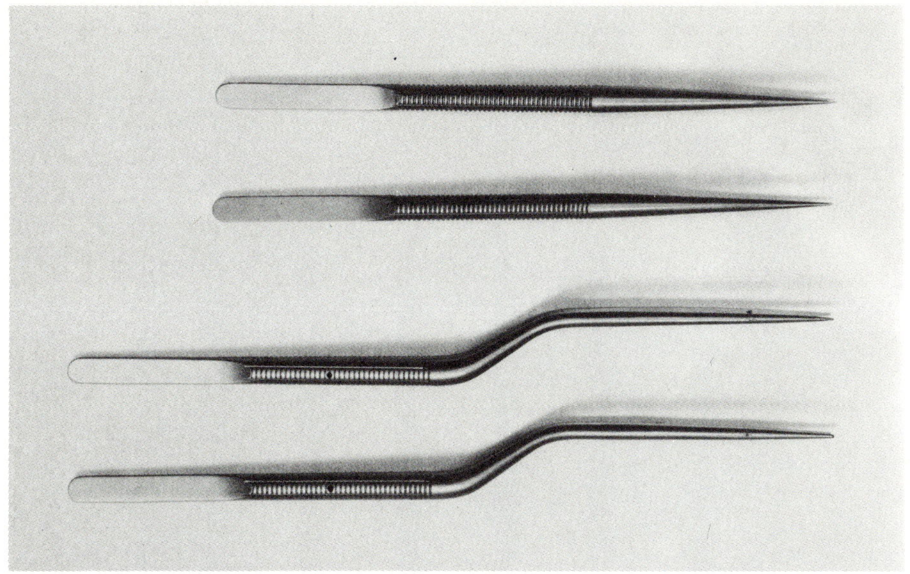

Fig. 24-52. Rhoton microsurgical forceps, straight and bayonet. (Courtesy Codman & Shurtleff, Inc., Randolph, Mass.)

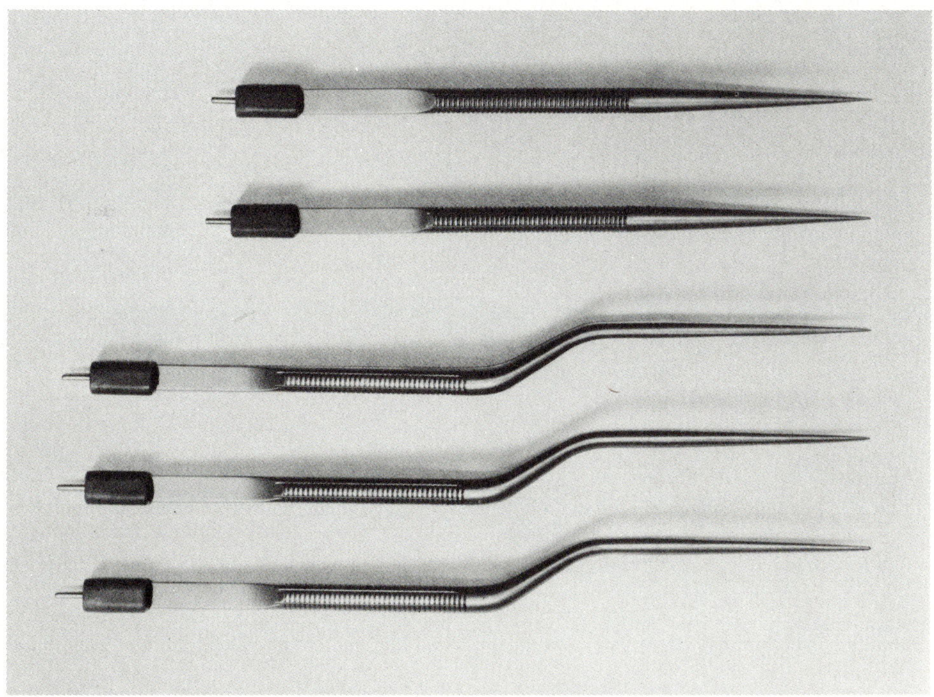

Fig. 24-53. Rhoton microsurgical bipolar forceps, straight and bayonet. (Courtesy Codman & Shurtleff, Inc., Randolph, Mass.)

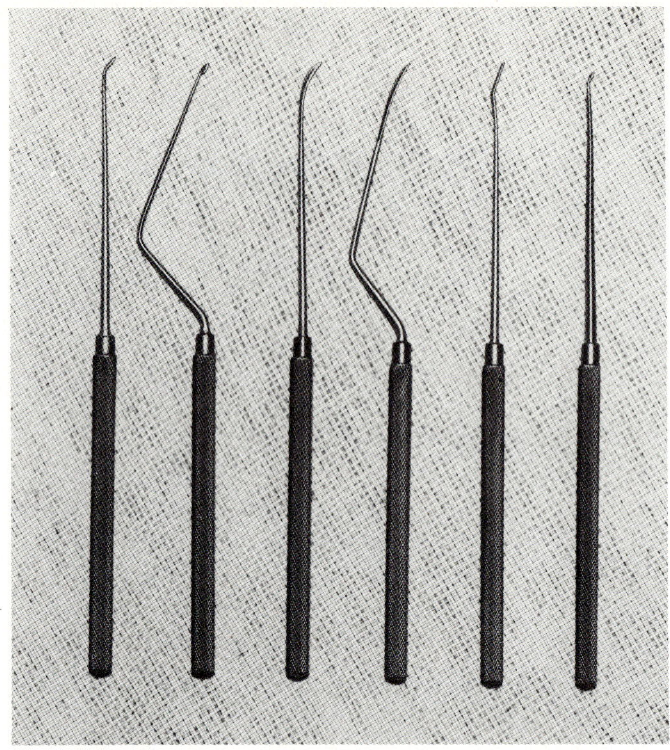

Fig. 24-54. Malis microsurgical instruments. *Left to right,* Semisharp dissector, curette, two elevators, sharp dissector, round dissector. (Courtesy Codman & Shurtleff, Inc., Randolph, Mass.)

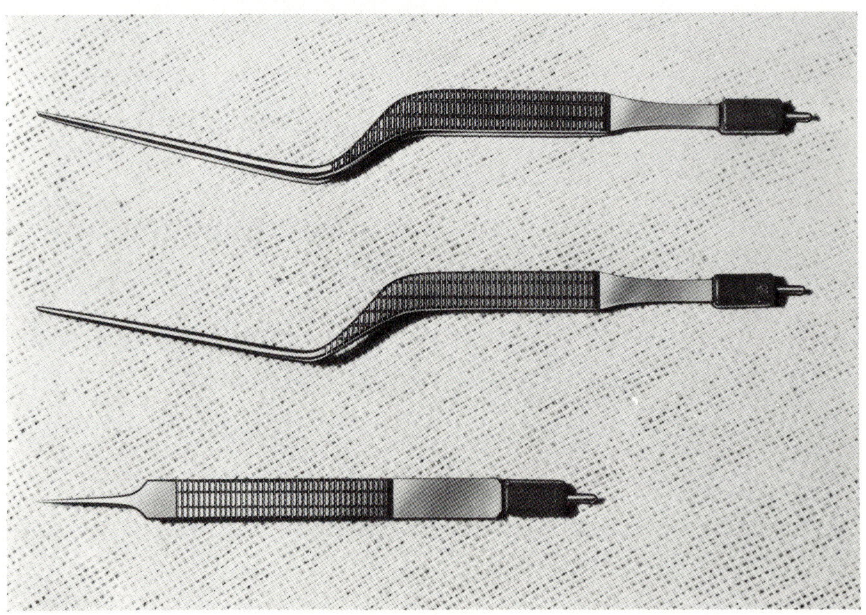

Fig. 24-55. Malis titanium bipolar forceps. (Courtesy Codman & Shurtleff, Inc., Randolph, Mass.)

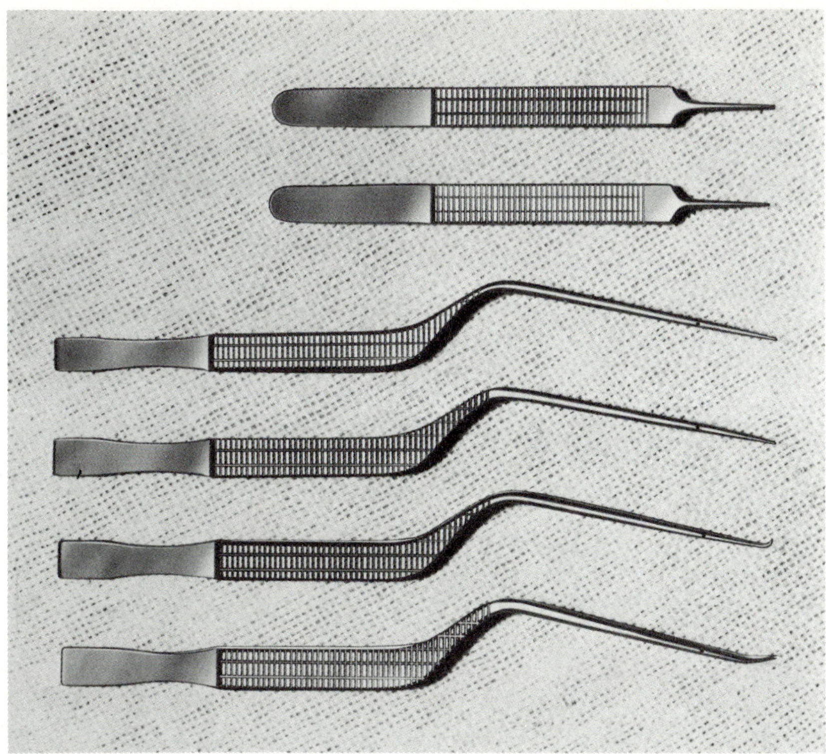

Fig. 24-56. Malis microforceps (titanium), straight and bayonet. (Courtesy Codman & Shurtleff, Inc., Randolph, Mass.)

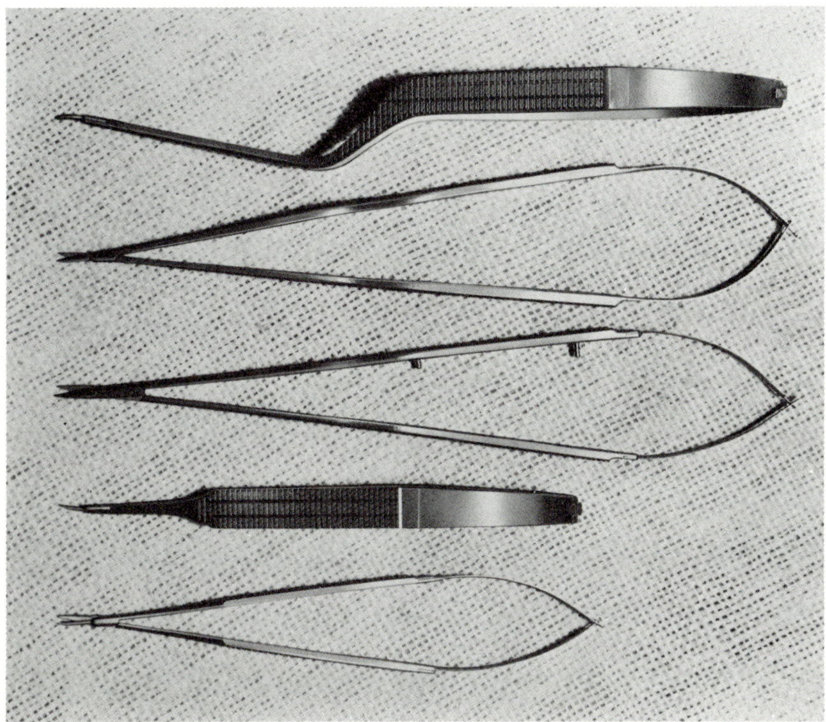

Fig. 24-57. Malis microsurgical scissors. (Courtesy Codman & Shurtleff, Inc., Randolph, Mass.)

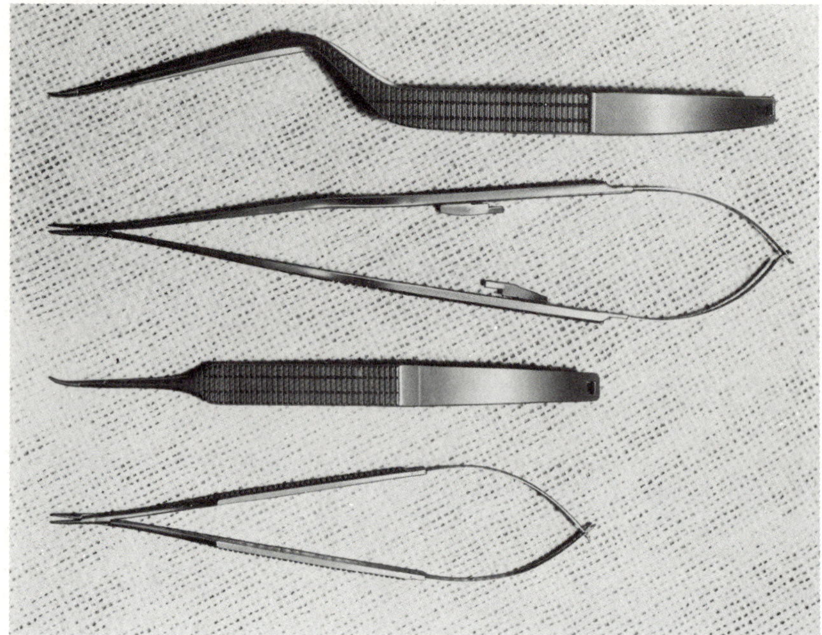

Fig. 24-58. Malis microsurgical needle holders. (Courtesy Codman & Shurtleff, Inc., Randolph, Mass.)

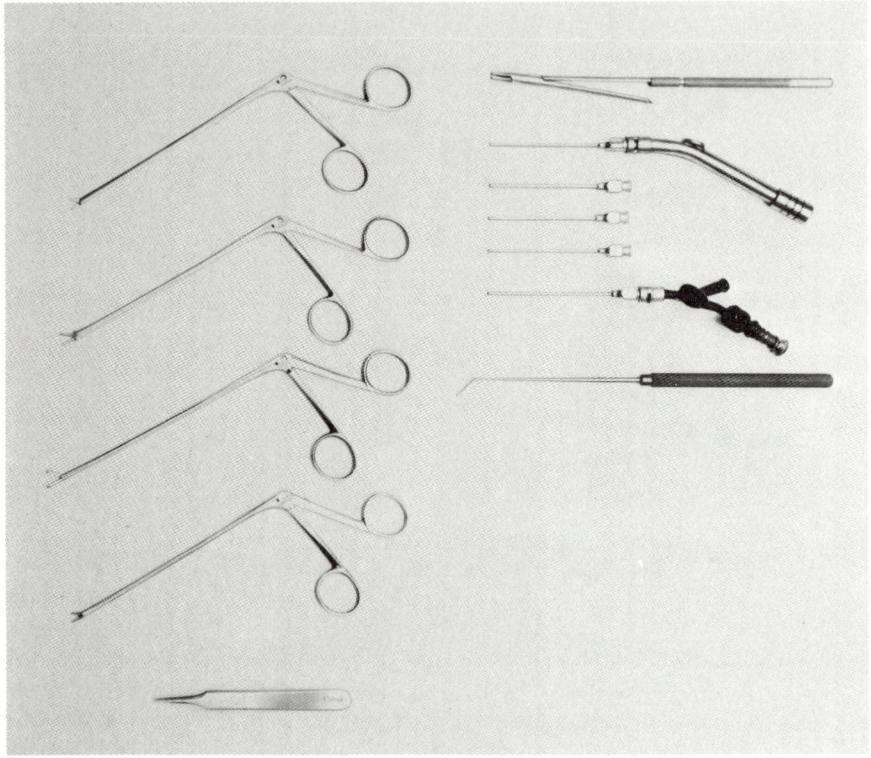

Fig. 24-59. Microinstruments for neurosurgical procedures. *Bottom to top: left,* Forceps, rongeurs, and scissors; *right,* arachnoid knife, Malis suction-coagulation handle and four tips, Cadac microsuction handle and tip, blade breaker and holder. (Courtesy Codman & Shurtleff, Inc., Randolph, Mass.)

Craniotomy for arteriovenous malformation

Considerations. An arteriovenous malformation consists of thin-walled vascular channels that connect arteries and veins without the usual intervening capillaries. These vascular lesions may be microscopic or massive.

Malformations vary widely in size, area of involvement, and structure. Arteriovenous fistulas may be congenital or may result from trauma or disease. Vascular anomalies may also give rise to subarachnoid or intracerebral hemorrhage or may have extensive irritative effects and cause focal or generalized seizures.

These lesions are difficult to treat successfully. Feeding vessels can be clipped with or without partial removal of the lesion. Total removal, when possible, gives best results. Microsurgical techniques and the laser have made total removal without devastating injury to surrounding brain tissue and vessels possible in many cases.

Other methods of treating these malformations have been tried. Among them are the injection of shot pellets into the malformation through a vessel in the neck. More recently, barium-impregnated spheres, ranging from 0.5 mm to 4 mm in diameter, have been used for artificial embolization (Fig. 24-60).

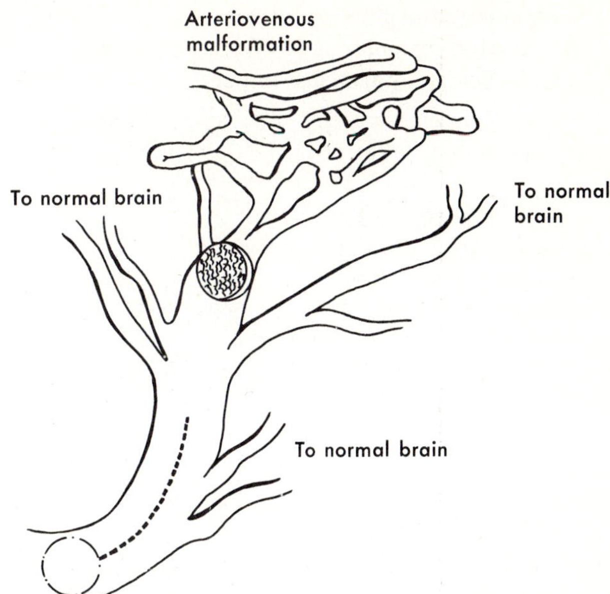

Fig. 24-60. Barium-impregnated spheres in arteriovenous malformation.

Operative procedure

1. A supratentorial or infratentorial craniotomy is done, depending on the location of the lesion.

2. The feeding arteries are exposed a distance from the malformation, then traced toward it, and occluded a short distance before they penetrate its substance. This spares as many of the arteries to the brain as possible. The feeding arteries may be occluded by clipping, coagulation, ligation, or laser beam coagulation.

3. The malformation is dissected out with suction and bayonet forceps. Additional vessels are clipped or coagulated along the way. Usually one or more draining veins are left to be ligated as the last step in the removal.

4. Closure and dressing are as described for craniotomy.

Craniotomy for intracranial revascularization

Definition. Microbypass technique developed in 1967 used to shunt blood flow around an occluded portion of the internal carotid artery or the middle cerebral artery by anastomosing the superficial temporal artery to the middle cerebral artery distal to the occlusion.

Operative procedure. Craniotomy for intracranial revascularization, though brief in description, is long and tedious; 7 hours is not unusual. Positioning is crucial to prevent pressure on superficial nerves, vessels, and vulnerable skin areas. Blood gas monitoring and arterial pressure readings are done routinely during the procedure. An arterial line may be placed before the patient's arrival in the surgery department or as a preliminary procedure in the operating room.

The procedure occurs in two steps:

1. The *first stage* is reflection of the scalp flap on the operative side to expose the superficial temporal artery for dissection. Care must be taken in placing the hemostatic scalp clips to make sure they are further apart than usual to prevent compromise of the scalp circulation following diversion of the flow of the temporal artery. Care also must be taken to prevent injury to the temporal artery as the scalp incision is made and the flap reflected.

2. After the superficial temporal artery is identified, the microscope is positioned, and the microinstrumentation is put into use.

3. The portion of the temporal artery to be used is freed but not occluded until the time of anastomosis. It may be supported and covered with Gelfoam or cottonoid material soaked in a papaverine solution. Papaverine aids in preventing vessel spasm.

4. The temporal muscle is incised and retracted with fish hooks to begin the *second stage* of the procedure.

5. A bur hole is made in the frontotemporal area and enlarged with a rongeur.

6. The dura mater is opened and anchored over the bone edges with silk sutures. The self-retaining brain retractor is used.

7. The middle cerebral artery is located, and a branch suitable for anastomosis is isolated. Flow is occluded by temporary microvascular clips, such as Heifetz or Yasargil.

8. Flow also is occluded in the superficial temporal artery; the artery is cut, and an end-to-side anastomosis is completed with very fine suture material, such as no. 10-0 monofilament nylon.

9. The temporary microvascular clips are removed. The vessels are observed for patency and flow.

10. The wound is closed, and dressings are applied.

Craniotomy for pituitary tumor (craniopharyngioma, optic glioma, and other suprasellar and parasellar tumors)

Setup. The setup is as for craniotomy with these additional pituitary instruments:

Ray curettes (ring, sharp)
Spinal needles, no. 22 or 24
Luer-Lok syringe, 10 ml
Angulated suction tips, right, left; large, small
Curettes, small, nos. 0 through 4-0

Operative procedure

1. Either a bifrontal or unilateral incision is made in the frontal or frontotemporal region. Most unilateral approaches are carried out from the right side.

2. Wet brain retractors over moist cottonoids are inserted for exposure of the optic chiasma and the pituitary gland. The frontal and often the temporal lobes are retracted. The olfactory nerve may be coagulated and divided with scissors.

3. A DeMartel, Edinborough, or Yasargil self-retaining retractor is placed to maintain exposure. Aneurysm clips and applicators should be available to control unexpected bleeding from major vessels. The microscope may be moved into place.

4. Using a syringe with moistened plunger and a no. 22 or 24 spinal needle, the surgeon attempts to aspirate the contents of the tumor to guard against inadvertently entering an aneurysm or vessel.

5. The tumor capsule is coagulated for hemostasis and incised with a no. 11 blade on a long knife handle. With a pituitary rongeur or cup forceps, the tumor is removed.

6. Small stainless steel, copper, or Ray curettes, as well as suction, may be used during the tumor removal.

7. A wide Olivecrona clip may be applied to the stalk of the pituitary, which may then be cut distally. A long angulated scissors is especially helpful for this.

8. If the tumor capsule is to be removed, bayonet forceps, cup forceps, nerve hooks, and suction aid in the dissection. If the tumor capsule is not removed, Zenker's solution may be placed in the capsule of a pituitary adenoma after the adjacent structures are walled off with cottonoid.

9. Closure and dressing are as described for craniotomy.

In case of a pituitary adenoma with a prefixed chiasma, the surgeon may elect to remove the anterior wall of the sphenoidal sinus and sella turcica with an air drill to gain access to the tumor.

In the case of craniopharyngioma, extreme caution must be used in removing fluid from the capsule because the fluid is extremely irritating and may cause chemical leptomeningitis. Calcified pieces of tumor are dissected and removed in the same manner as the capsule of a pituitary adenoma. This is an extremely difficult procedure because of deposits on the carotid arteries, the optic nerves, and optic chiasma. The tumor capsule is often left behind on the hypothalamus to avoid stripping off blood vessels supplying this structure. Many moist cottonoid strips are used to protect the surrounding areas from the cystic contents.

Suprasellar meningiomas usually arise from the tuberculum sella just anterior to the optic nerves and chiasma. Tumor removal is similar to that of a pituitary adenoma except that the cutting loop of the electrocautery may be used to excavate the interior of the tumor. After the tumor has been removed, the site of its attachment to the dura is thoroughly coagulated to prevent recurrence. Other meningiomas arising at the base of the skull are treated by similar techniques.

Transsphenoidal hypophysectomy

Considerations. Endocrine pituitary disorders, such as Cushing's syndrome, acromegaly, malignant exophthalmos, and hypopituitarism resulting from intrasellar tumors, as well as nonpituitary disorders, such as advanced metastatic carcinoma of the breast and prostate, diabetic retinopathy, and uncontrollable severe diabetes, have been successfully treated by transsphenoidal hypophysectomy.

Rapid access to the sella turcica is achieved. Complete extracapsular enucleation of the pituitary in cases of hypophysectomy and possible complete removal of small pituitary tumors, with the remaining normal portion of the gland left intact can be obtained. Patients are relatively free of pain after surgery. No visible scar remains.

Setup and preparation of the patient. Transsphenoidal hypophysectomy is performed with the patient under light general endotracheal anesthesia, combined with a local anesthetic. The patient is placed in a semisitting position, with head against the headrest and positioned in a portable image intensifier. The horizontal beam is centered on the sella turcica. A subnasal midline rhinoseptal approach is used.

The face, mouth, and nasal cavity are prepared with an antiseptic solution. Infiltration of the nasal mucosa and the gingiva with a local anesthetic agent containing 1:2000 epinephrine is helpful in initiating sumucosal elevation, as well as diminishing oozing from the mucosa. A sterile adhesive plastic drape is applied to the entire face with additional sterile drapes to ensure a relatively sterile operative field. Sterile sponges or cotton are placed in the patient's mouth, so that only the upper gum margin is exposed.

A biopsy setup is required, as well as special instruments (Fig. 24-61). The operating microscope is used for the cranial portion of the procedure.

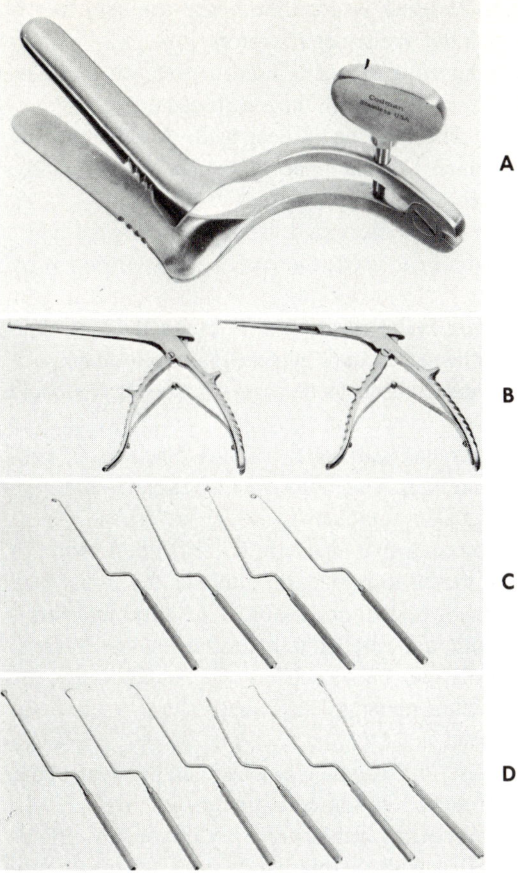

Fig. 24-61. Special instruments for transsphenoidal hypophysectomy. A, Hardy's modified Cushing bivalve speculum. B, Angell James punch forceps, extra small, upbiting, and Angell James punch forceps, extra small, downbiting. C, Hardy modifications of Bronson-Ray curette. D, *Left to right,* Hardy's fork with bayonet handle, Hardy's enucleator (right), Hardy's dissector, angled knife handle, Hardy's enucleator (left), Hardy's modification of Cushing's malleable pituitary spoon. (Courtesy Down Bros. and Mayer & Phelps, Ltd., Toronto, and Codman & Shurtleff, Inc., Randolph, Mass.)

Operative procedure

1. Using the biopsy setup on a separate small Mayo table, the surgeon takes a small piece of muscle from the previously prepared thigh to be used later in the procedure. This is kept in a moist sponge.
2. An incision is made in the middle of the upper gum margin. The soft tissues of the upper lip and nose are elevated from the bone with an elevator, and the nasal septum is exposed. The nasal mucosa is elevated from either side of the nasal septum, which is flanked by the blades of a Cushing bivalved speculum. The inferior third of the anterior cartilaginous septum and osseous vomer are resected, as is the floor of the sphenoidal sinus, exposing the sinus cavity. The floor of the sella turcica can be identified.
3. The floor is opened with a sphenoidal punch, and the dura mater is incised. The hypophyseal cavity should be opened only in patients undergoing surgery for pituitary adenoma. In these patients, the gland is explored, and the tumor is identified and removed.
4. The extracapsular cleavage plane is identified, and the superior surface of the pituitary is dissected until the stalk and the diaphragmatic orifice are found. Cotton pledgets are applied for exposure, hemostasis, and protection of structures.
5. The stalk is sectioned low with a "sickle" knife, and the lateral posterior and inferior surface of the pituitary is dissected with an enucleator.
6. The gland is removed in toto, and the sellar cavity is packed with muscle obtained previously from the thigh. The floor is reconstructed with cartilage from the nasal septum.
7. Antibiotic powder may be used and a nasal packing introduced for 2 days. The gingiva incision is closed with catgut.

Some surgeons prefer to do this operation by means of a lateral rhinotomy with a transantral-transsphenoidal approach.

Craniectomy

Definition. Incision into the skull and removal of bone by enlarging one or more bur holes, using rongeurs to gain access to the underlying structures.

Considerations. A craniectomy procedure may be required to remove tumors, hematomas, scars, or infections of the bone. Craniectomy is also indicated as treatment for craniosynostosis in infants and to relieve pressure on the brain from depressed bone or internal hemorrhage resulting from trauma.

Craniectomy with evacuation of epidural or subdural hematoma

Definition. Following trauma, decompression of the brain, as well as removal and drainage of blood clots and collections of liquefied blood from outside or beneath the dura mater.

Operative procedure

1. A linear or small horseshoe incision is made over the site of the lesion. The initial procedure is similar to craniotomy. One or more bur holes are made. A bone flap is not turned.
2. If a blood clot or collection of bloody fluid is found outside or beneath the dura mater, the bur hole is further enlarged, with a Kerrison or double-action rongeur, until adequate exposure is obtained. Bone edges are waxed, and cotton strips placed along the edges.
3. Clot and fluid are evacuated, and hemostasis is accomplished with coagulation or the use of hemostatic clips.
4. In cases of chronic subdural hematoma, the inner and outer membranes are stripped and coagulated.

5. The brain is irrigated with catheters or directly with an Asepto or bulb syringe. Large amounts of solution are used until the return is clear.

6. A silver or a hemostatic clip may be placed on the cortex at the site of a small incision. Another clip is placed on the dura mater. These are tag clips that are visible on postoperative x-ray films to check the bleeding site.

7. A small Penrose drain or a polyethylene or red rubber catheter may be inserted subdurally for additional drainage, or a closed drainage system, such as the Jackson-Pratt, may be used through a separate stab wound in the skin posterior to the incision.

Additional bur holes are made during the course of the procedure to be sure that clots in other areas do not remain undetected and untreated.

Craniectomy for craniosynostosis

Considerations. Craniectomy for craniosynostosis is performed on infants whose suture lines have closed prematurely. Synthetic material such as silicone is used to keep the edges of the cranial sutures from reuniting and preventing brain growth. Careful attention to blood volume is mandatory.

Operative procedure. After the scalp incision is made over the appropriate skull suture, the dura mater is stripped off the underside of the skull. A generous strip of the bone edges joining to form the fused suture is then removed with heavy scissors, a craniotome, a rongeur, or a Kerrison punch. The bone edges are waxed. Preformed Silastic sheeting (Fig. 24-45) is inserted over the bone edges bordering the craniectomy and sutured or stapled in place. When sutures are used, holes must be placed in the bone edges bordering the craniectomy before the sheeting is placed.

Suboccipital craniectomy or posterior fossa exploration

Definition. Perforation and removal of the posterior occipital bone and exposure of the foramen magnum and arch of the atlas for removal of the lesion in the posterior fossa (Fig. 24-62).

Considerations. Depending on the type and size of the lesion, the exposure may be unilateral or bilateral. The operation may include the removal of the arch of the atlas. This approach gives the surgeon access to the fourth ventricle, the cerebellum, the brainstem, and the cranial nerves.

Setup and preparation of the patient. The sitting position is preferred for surgery of the posterior fossa. An extra-high instrument table and standing stool are necessary for the nurse.

Operative procedure

1. The incision may be made from mastoid tip to mastoid tip, in an arch curving upward 2 cm above the external occipital protuberance.

2. Scalp bleeding is controlled, and the skin flap is retracted with the Weitlaner retractors.

3. A periosteal elevator is used to free the muscles, which are then divided with the electrocautery, using cutting current. The incision is deepened. A self-retaining retractor is used. The laminae of the first two or three cervical vertebrae may be exposed.

4. One or more holes are drilled in the occipital bone. If a Hudson brace is used, the cerebellar extension is attached.

5. The dura mater is stripped from the bone. A double-action rongeur, Raney punch, Kerrison punch, or Leksell rongeur is used to enlarge the hole and smooth the edges.

6. Osseous and cerebellar venous bleeding is controlled at each step with bone wax, Gelfoam, and cautery, to prevent air embolism.

7. The dura mater is opened. A small brain spoon or cotton strip is used to protect the brain as the initial nick is extended with scalpel or scissors. The dural incision is continued until the cerebellar hemispheres, the vermis, and the tonsils can be visualized. Hemostatic clips are used on the dura mater as necessary. Dural traction sutures are placed.

8. The cisterna magna is opened, emptied of spinal fluid, and protected with a cotton strip.

9. The cerebellar hemispheres are inspected. Bleeding is controlled with the bipolar cautery. A needle may be introduced through a small coagulated incision in the cerebellar hemisphere in an attempt to palpate or tap a deep lesion.

10. Brain retractors over cotton strips are placed for exposure. The handle of the retractor must be kept dry to avoid slippage in the surgeon's hand. However, the inserted edge should be wet to prevent damage or tears in the brain surface. These retractors may be positioned in areas that control respiration or other vital functions, so every effort must be made to avoid jarring these instruments in the operative field. When the pathological entity is identified, a self-retaining retractor may be placed.

11. Long bayonet forces, bayonet cup forceps, pituitary forceps, suction, and the electrocautery loops may be used to remove the lesion. Clips may be used to aid in hemostasis. A nerve stimulator may be used to identify cranial nerves.

12. After the lesion has been removed and bleeding controlled, further checking for adequate hemostasis is required. Venous pressure in the head is increased by the anesthesiologist.

13. The dura mater may be partially or completely closed. The muscle, fascia, and skin are closed. A dressing is applied.

14. The patient must remain anesthetized until the supine position is achieved and the prongs of the headrest are removed. Particular attention must be given to the

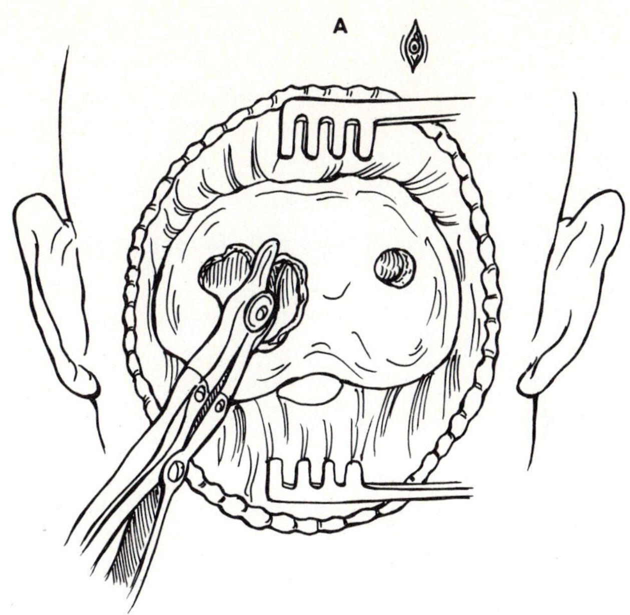

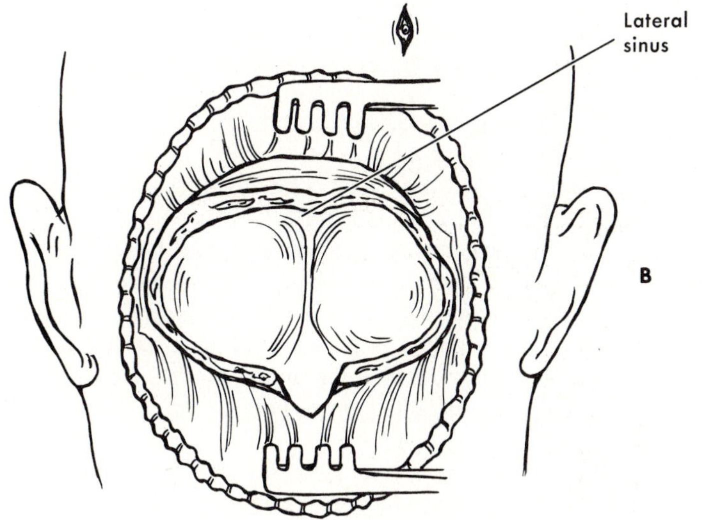

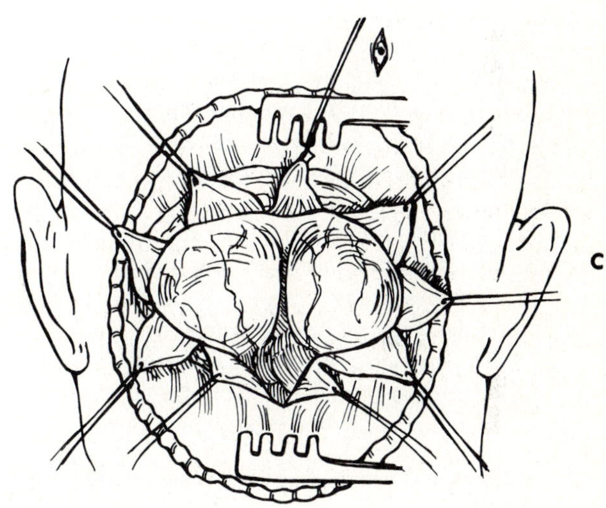

Fig. 24-62. Suboccipital craniectomy. **A,** Craniectomy being performed. **B,** Dura mater exposed. **C,** Dura mater incised and cerebellum exposed. (From Sachs, E.: Diagnosis and treatment of brain tumors and the care of the neurosurgical patient, ed. 2, St. Louis, The C.V. Mosby Co.)

patient's head when removing these prongs to prevent tearing the scalp or endangering the eyes.

Subtemporal craniectomy for trigeminal rhizotomy

Considerations. Trigeminal neuralgia (tic douloureux, fifth cranial nerve pain) is a condition characterized by brief, repeated attacks of excruciating pain in the face. Temporary relief of trigeminal neuralgia may be obtained by interruption of branches of the nerve divisions (ophthalmic, maxillary, and mandibular) by means of alcohol injection or surgical sectioning.

The patient may be placed in the supine or sitting position, depending on the preference of the surgeon.

Operative procedure

1. A vertical temporal incision extending from the zygomatic process and through the temporal muscles and periosteum is made.
2. The soft tissue is freed from the bone with a periosteal elevator. The bone exposure is maintained with a self-retaining retractor.
3. A bur hole is made. The dura mater is freed from the underside of the temporal bone.
4. The bur hole is enlarged to a diameter of about 2½ inches, with a double-action rongeur.
5. With a moist brain retractor, the dura mater overlying the temporal lobe is retracted upward. By means of blunt dissection with cottonoids held in bayonet forceps, the dura mater is elevated from the bony floor of the middle fossa.

6. The brain retractor is replaced by a self-retaining brain retractor placed deeper into the wound to hold up the temporal lobe and dura mater. The microscope provides light as well as magnification.

7. As the dura mater is elevated, the middle meningeal artery is seen as it leaves the foramen spinosum to join the dura mater. It is coagulated with bipolar bayonet forceps and may be clipped before being divided. A cottonoid, wood, or wax plug is packed into the foramen spinosum.

8. Additional blunt dissection uncovers the mandibular division of the trigeminal nerve and finally the trigeminal (gasserian) ganglion within its own dural sheath (dura propria). Bleeding is controlled with cottonoid and a hemostatic material such as Gelfoam and thrombin.

9. Some surgeons terminate the procedure after stripping the ganglion and its dura mater from that of the overlying temporal lobe. (The ganglion may be injected with saline solution, and the dura mater may be split.)

10. If a root section is to be performed, a no. 11 blade on a long scalpel handle is used to make an incision into the lateral rim of the dura propria. The sensory and motor roots of the nerve are defined with a fine nerve hook. The mandibular and maxillary sections of the root are usually then divided. These are elevated with a nerve hook and divided with a fine scissors or a fine blade. The ophthalmic portion of the root is spared, as is the motor root.

11. Absolute alcohol may be injected into the affected divisions of the nerve just distal to the ganglion.

12. Saline solution is injected into the dura mater overlying the temporal lobe to distend it.

13. The incision is closed, and dressings are applied.

Some surgeons prefer to section the posterior root of the trigeminal nerve by the suboccipital route.

Suboccipital craniectomy for trigeminal rhizotomy

Considerations. The position of the patient for suboccipital craniectomy may be sitting, prone, or semilateral. To be prepared, the nurse must know during the planning phase (usually the day before the procedure is scheduled) which position the surgeon plans to use.

Operative procedure

1. The incision is made vertically behind the mastoid process. A trephine or bur hole is made and enlarged with a rongeur.

2. The dura mater is opened. The cisterna magna is pierced to empty the cerebrospinal fluid and permit backward retraction of the cerebellum. A brain spoon, brain spatula, or lighted retractor over moist strips of cotton are used to gently lift the cerebellar hemisphere. The eighth nerve is readily seen. The fifth nerve is approached by opening the arachnoidea of the cisterna pontis and sucking out the fluid. Veins are protected and bleeding controlled by pressure over cotton strips.

3. The nerve is elevated on a hook and carefully dissected. Some sensation in the face may be preserved by partial sectioning or crushing rather than by complete section of the nerve. The motor root medial and anterior to the sensory root is preserved.

4. The wound is closed.

Suboccipital craniectomy and glossopharyngeal nerve section

Posterior fossa exploration for glossopharyngeal neuralgia is occasionally necessary. The same posterior fossa approach is used as for trigeminal neuralgia. The cerebellar hemisphere of the affected side is gently elevated upward and toward the midline. The ninth, tenth, and eleventh nerves are identified and defined with bayonet forceps, nerve hooks, and fine dissectors. The ninth nerve and a portion of the tenth are consecutively elevated with a nerve hook and divided with a fine-tipped scissors.

Suboccipital craniectomy for acoustic neuroma

Considerations. Usually the acoustic neuroma arises from the vestibular portion of the eighth cranial nerve within the auditory meatus. Although it is not always possible, it is desirable to remove the complete tumor without damage to the facial nerve.

Operative procedure

1. The posterior fossa approach is used. A unilateral straight paramedian incision is made.

2. The cerebellum is retracted gently upward with brain retractors and is cushioned with moist cottonoids. The lower cranial nerves are defined with a nerve or aneurysm hook. A cottonoid is placed over these nerves to protect them. Veins draining the tumor into the superior petrosal sinus are identified and either clipped or coagulated and cut.

3. The tumor is excavated and resected by methods similar to those employed to remove a pituitary adenoma.

4. A nerve stimulator may be used to identify the facial nerve. Use of the operating microscope is advantageous because of the many nerves and vessels in the area.

5. A high-speed air drill may be used to unroof the auditory canal and expose the remaining tumor. Constant irrigation is mandatory during drilling.

More recently, very small tumors confined to the auditory canal have been approached by drilling directly through the temporal bone to open the auditory canal within the bone and avoid the posterior fossa.

Suboccipital craniectomy for Ménière's disease

Considerations. Ménière's disease is characterized by recurrent explosive attacks of vertigo associated with nausea, vomiting, tinnitus, and progressive deafness. It is usually unilateral. The cause is obscure, and in intractable cases surgical section or partial section of the eighth cranial nerve (acoustic) may be performed for relief.

However, surgery is not often performed for Ménière's disease.

Operative procedure

1. The cerebellum is approached through a lateral vertical incision behind the ear. The cerebellum on the affected side is retracted.

2. The eighth nerve is exposed with bayonet forceps and gentle manipulation. The nerve is freed from the arachnoidea of the lateral cistern. It is separated from the underlying structures with a blunt nerve hook. Care is taken to prevent traction on the nearby seventh nerve (facial).

3. With fine scissors the vestibular fibers in the anterior half of the nerve are divided over a nerve hook. If the patient has useful hearing, the posterior auditory branches are preserved. Tinnitus may be relieved by section of the anterior fibers of the auditory portion of the nerve.

4. The dura mater and wound are closed.

Cranioplasty

Definition. Repair of a skull defect (Fig. 24-44) resulting from trauma, malformation, or a surgical procedure. Cranial defects covered by muscular areas need not be repaired.

Considerations. The purpose of cranioplasty is to relieve headache, vertigo, fear of injury, or local tenderness or throbbing; to prevent secondary injury to the underlying brain; and for cosmetic effect.

Setup and preparation of the patient. Many materials have been used to repair skull defects, including bone and cartilage; celluloid; metals, such as Vitallium and tantalum; and the synthetic resins, such as methyl methacrylate and silicone rubber. All involve technical problems. The use of commercially prepared cranioplastic synthetics that supply the needed chemicals and mixing containers has, to a large extent, simplified the procedures of shaping and molding the prosthesis. Sometimes heavy wire mesh is cut to the shape of the defect, and the methyl methacrylate molded over the mesh.

Operative procedure

1. A scalp flap is turned, and the bony defect exposed.

2. The edges of the defect are trimmed, and a ledge is formed to seat the prosthesis.

3. After the bone defect has been prepared so that it is slightly saucerized, the methyl methacrylate is mixed by adding one volume of liquid monomer to one volume of the powdered polymer. When this has formed a doughy mass, it is dropped into a sterile polyethylene bag. The soft plastic is then rolled on a flat surface into the desired shape, leaving the thickness to the approximate depth of the skull edges. A sterile test tube, syringe barrel, or other round object can be used, although a stainless steel roller is preferred because of its weight and ease of use.

4. The soft cranioplastic material in the bag is then placed over the skull defect and, through light pressing with the ends of the fingers, is fitted into the missing skull area. The plastic bag is stretched by assistants as the surgeon molds the plate into the defect and forms an overlapping bevel edge. This overlapping fringe keeps the plate from falling inside the skull, as does the skull saucerization.

5. When the heat of the chemical reaction begins, the plate is lifted out of the bony wound and removed from the polyethylene bag.

6. When cool enough to handle, the excess material is trimmed away with bone rongeurs or cut with a saw and placed in the cranial defect.

7. A sterile carborundum wheel attached to the electrical bone saw or craniotome is used to smooth the rough spots and bevel the edges so that the plate will blend gradually with the skull.

Mixing and fitting the plate takes about 7 minutes, as does hardening. Screws, wire, or no. 2-0 silk sutures may be used to hold the plate in place, generally at three or more points.

Microneurosurgery

Adaptation of the operating microscope for neurosurgery has resulted in improvement of many neurosurgical procedures and made new procedures possible. For years neurosurgeons have worn magnifying loupes to see small structures. Loupes usually have a magnification of 2 or 2.8. The microscope has a variety of magnifications ranging from 6 to 40, providing flexibility and precision. The coaxial illumination overcomes the difficulties of lighting neurosurgical wounds.

Use of the microscope restricts the surgeon's field of vision and mobility; therefore, the scrub nurse must be proficient. The operative field, unless video monitoring is available, cannot be seen. The scrub nurse must understand the surgical procedure, know the anatomy, know the names and uses of all the microinstruments, and be able to place each instrument in the surgeon's hand without delay, so that the surgeon will be able to use the instrument without readjusting it. The nurse must make it possible for the surgeon to perform the operation without averting his eyes from the operative field. Instruments must be kept free of blood and tissue during use, since the microscope also magnifies debris on the instruments, occluding the structure the surgeon is about to approach. The nurse must understand the degree of stress these difficult procedures place on the neurosurgeon.

Microneurosurgical instruments are expensive and delicate. Instructions for handling, cleaning, sterilizing, and storing these instruments should be followed. An instrument that is sprung, bent, dulled, hooked, or in any way damaged must never be handed to a surgeon for use but must be repaired or replaced.

Existing microsurgical instruments have been modified and adapted to the requirements of neurosurgery. These instruments often possess the following characteristics: bayonet shape, so that the hand of the surgeon remains outside the line of vision and the beam of the microscope light; finely sprung and fluted grip; long length for access to deep structures; and slender and delicate tips that take up as little space as possible.

Very fine microsutures are available. The neurosurgeon may want to open the suture pack and ready the suture for use. However, the scrub nurse should be able to open and handle a delicate suture without damaging it. Each time the surgeon must look away and then back to the surgical field, open wound time and anesthesia time are increased for the patient while the surgeon becomes reoriented to the field. Therefore any assistance the nurse gives the surgeon saves time and directly benefits the patient.

Microsurgical techniques have been applied to cranial, spinal, and peripheral nerve operations. Perhaps microneurovascular surgery is the area in which the most progress has been made. However, patient outcomes following microsurgical procedures on cranial nerves, spinal nerves, and cord tumors and especially for repair of peripheral nerve injuries have all been enhanced.

Some procedures in which microsurgery is of value are posterior fossa explorations, especially for tumors of the fourth ventricle or cerebellopontine angle; translabyrinthine and transpetrosal removal of small acoustic neuromas, with resulting preservation of the facial nerve; and transsphenoidal hypophysectomy and transsphenoidal operations for small intracranial tumors, such as pituitary adenomas or even craniopharyngiomas. Transclival operations are also performed. Small vessel endarterectomy, cerebral arterial bypass, cerebral aneurysm surgery, and excision of arteriovenous malformations are done under the microscope. There are also advantages to microsurgery in the treatment of tumors and arteriovenous malformations of the spinal cord.

Stereotaxic procedures

Definition. Use of complex mechanisms to locate and destroy target structures in the brain. Predetermined anatomical landmarks are used as guides. Special head-fixation devices have been developed by surgeons and engineers for use with radiography, fluoroscopy, and CT scans to permit accurate placement of a probe directed at the target area. Stereotaxic procedures can also be done on the spinal cord.

Considerations. Common target areas for the stereotaxic approach include tumors, the basal ganglia, the thalamus, the hypophysis, aneurysms, and anterolateral spinal tracts. Target areas are biopsied or destroyed by chemical or mechanical means or electrically stimulated to control intractable pain. Stereotaxic procedures are also done to place electrodes in various regions of the brain to determine the site of origin of seizures. Lesions in target areas are made to biopsy and remove tumors; alleviate pain; abolish movement disorders; change endocrine balance to reverse such conditions as retinopathy, acromegaly, and endocrine-sensitive cancers; and obliterate aneurysms.

Operative procedure. The patient's head is placed in a special head holder, and the probe is introduced into the brain through a bur hole along one axis of the head holder. The probe is placed in position for insertion, and radiography, fluoroscopy, and/or CT scans are used to check the axis along which the probe is to be introduced. The position of the probe is checked by the same method after it is believed to rest on target (Fig. 24-63).

Hollow cannulas, coagulating electrodes, cryosurgical probes, wire loops, and other lesion-producing or biopsy instruments have been introduced for the destruction of areas in the brain. Temporary and permanent nerve-stimulator electrodes are also introduced to augment the pain control function of the central nervous system. These instruments are introduced through a bur hole or twist-drill hole in the skull.

Surgery of the globus pallidus, basal ganglia, and thalamus

Definitions

pallidotomy Incision into the globus pallidus, usually by electrocautery.

chemopallidectomy Introduction of a sclerosing solution through a rigid catheter or cannula to produce a lesion.

thalamotomy Incision into the thalamus.

chemothalamectomy Creation of a lesion in the region of the ventrolateral nucleus of the thalamus by means of a chemical solution such as alcohol with iophendylate.

Considerations. The surgical intervention is intended to interrupt the nerve pathways and alleviate the crippling locomotor symptoms of persistent, intractable tremor or rigidity associated with multiple sclerosis, severe brain trauma, Parkinson's disease, and various types of cerebellar degeneration. Operations of this type are also performed on the thalamus in an attempt to relieve pain.

Setup and preparation of the patient. The patient must be conscious and cooperative to permit careful examination and observation of response to the procedure and the effects on the symptoms. Local anesthesia is used. The patient may be in a supine or semisitting position.

Operative procedure

1. The patient's head is positioned and secured in the stereotactic frame.

2. A skin incision and bur hole are completed as for ventriculography.

3. It may be necessary to take ventriculograms, in addition to viewing the position of the cannulas or needles.

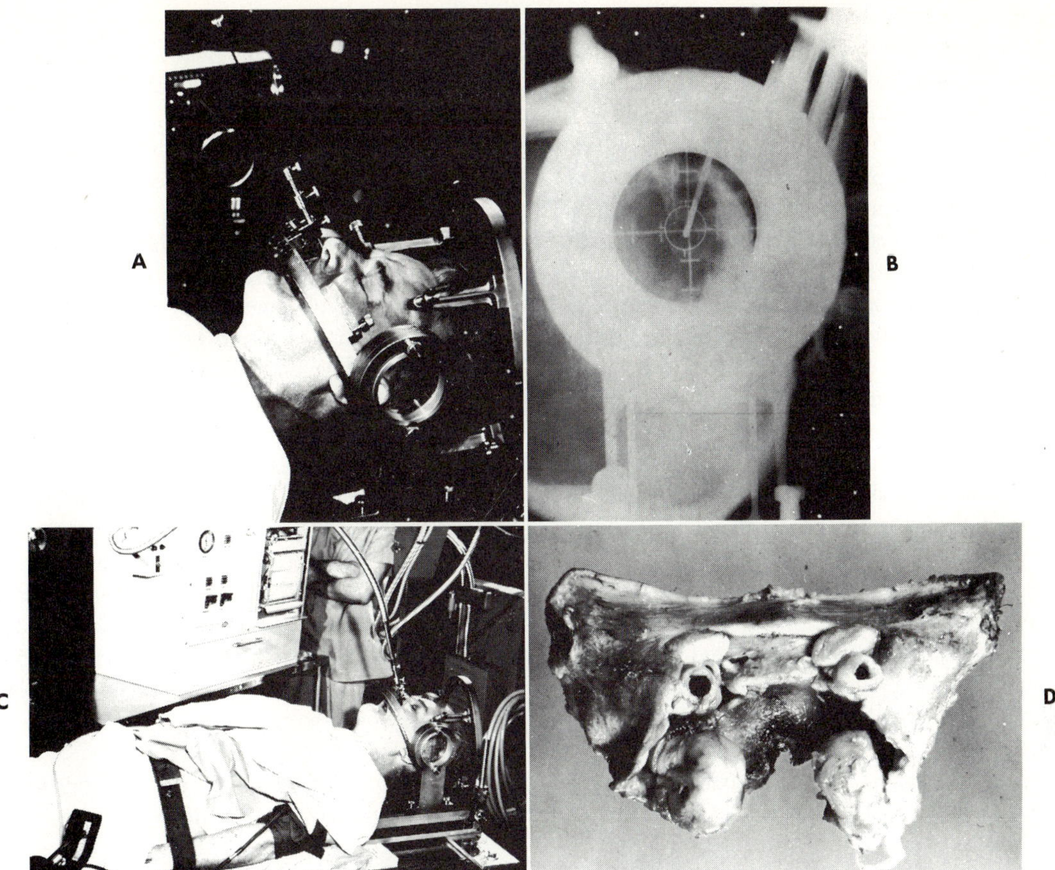

Fig. 24-63. Stereotaxic procedure. **A,** Patient's head is fixed to stereotaxic unit. Twist drill is inserted into anterior wall of sphenoidal sinus by way of left nostril into nasopharynx. **B,** Lateral x-ray film demonstrating freezing unit properly placed in target area (pituitary gland). Circle and cross hairs are positioned at target point before insertion of cannula. **C,** Cannula in patient's left nostril is attached to freezing unit on table. X-ray equipment is seen in upper left background. Since procedure is performed with patient under local anesthesia, body straps are used to immobilize patient. **D,** Sella turcica viewed from above, demonstrating bone perforation at base through which cannula was inserted. To either side of sella turcica, internal carotid arteries are seen (below, siphon; above with open lumen, cranial extension). Above sectioned arteries, optic nerves are seen passing into orbits. (From Conway-Rutkowski, B.L.: Carini and Owens' neurological and neurosurgical nursing, ed. 8, St. Louis, 1982, The C.V. Mosby Co.)

4. When the correct position has been achieved, tests or reversible lesions may be attempted. The patient's response is observed. Finally, the definitive lesion is created at the selected site by means of electrocautery, chemical solutions, or a cryogenic unit.

5. The dura mater and incision are closed.

Cryosurgery

Cryosurgery is the use of subfreezing temperatures to create a lesion in the treatment of disease. It is used in neurosurgery for transsphenoidal destruction of the pituitary gland in patients with acromegaly, diabetic retinopathy, and metastatic breast carcinoma. It can also be used for the destruction of the posterior portion of the thalamus for the treatment of Parkinson's disease or other involuntary movement disorders.

Transsphenoidal cryosurgery of the pituitary gland

Considerations. Transsphenoidal cryosurgery is of special benefit to the patient suffering from metastatic carcinoma of the breast. These patients are more likely to respond if they have benefited from previous hormonal therapy or oophorectomy. In the patient with diabetic retinopathy, transsphenoidal cryosurgery is indicated when further laser beam coagulation of retinal lesions is considered useless. With acromegaly, if optic nerve or chiasma compression is present, a craniotomy is usually necessary.

All patients should undergo retrograde jugular venography before surgery to outline the cavernous sinuses and carotid arteries. The patients with tumors must also have pneumoencephalography with polytomography.

Advantages

1. Candidates in poor physical condition tolerate this procedure better than a craniotomy because it is less traumatic. Local rather than general anesthesia may be used.
2. Mortality and morbidity rates are low.
3. Complete destruction can be achieved with fair certainty in neoplastic glands and good certainty in normal glands.

Setup and preparation of the patient. The surgery is performed with fluoroscopic control. The patient is under local anesthesia supplemented with neuroleptanalgesia. Transtracheal anesthesia is used before insertion of an endotracheal tube for maintenance of a patent airway during the procedure. The patient is instructed to answer questions with hand signals.

Operative procedure

1. A topical local anesthetic administered with cotton applicators and 1% lidocaine injections through long needles are used to anesthetize the nasal and nasopharyngeal mucosa.
2. The head is placed in the stereotaxic head holder and fixed after injection of local anesthetic in the skin at the points of fixation.
3. Preliminary x-ray films of the skull are taken to be sure that proper positioning has been achieved.
4. A guide is introduced, and a hole is drilled into the sphenoidal sinus and the floor of the sella turcica through the nasal vault. The guide is positioned fluoroscopically.
5. A cryoprobe is introduced through the guide into the pituitary gland, and its position is confirmed with x-ray films. The temperature of the probe is lowered to −18° to −19° C for 12 to 15 minutes. The probe can be used to feel the exact location of the dura mater surrounding the pituitary gland laterally and the diaphragm of the sella turcica superiorly.
6. The probe may be introduced to several depths of penetration into the sella turcica and additional lesions made. Additional holes may be drilled for further lesions.
7. The probe is withdrawn, and the nasal vault is inspected for bleeding. It can be packed with nasal packing. Antibiotics can be instilled before packing.

Patients are kept supine for 2 to 3 days and placed on a regimen of prophylactic antibiotics and cortisone replacement. Complications are meningitis secondary to a cerebrospinal fluid leakage, extraocular palsy, damage to the optic nerve, and injury to cranial vessels such as the carotid and cavernous sinus. These can be prevented by an accurate preoperative evaluation and precise probe placement during surgery.

Cryothalamectomy

Definition. Cryogenic destruction of the posterior aspect of the thalamus for treatment of pain or movement disorder.

Considerations. The following steps are necessary to obtain a good result: (1) placement of a probe with x-ray control, (2) localization of the lesion by clinical findings, and (3) gradual production of the lesion in a conscious, cooperative patient (so that the neurosurgeon can detect the point at which involuntary movements or pain perceptions are abolished and prevent the undesirable neurological and psychological results of too large a lesion).

Operative procedure

1. The patient is placed on the operating table, and the special head holder is applied as in the cryohypophysectomy procedure. The head holder is attached to the operating table.
2. After injection of a local anesthetic, an incision is made with a no. 15 blade on a no. 3 knife handle at the level of the coronal suture.
3. Scalp clips are placed on the skin edges, and a Weitlaner or mastoid retractor placed for exposure.
4. Trephination of the skull is performed with a special large bur.
5. The dura mater is opened, and stay sutures of no. 4-0 silk are placed for retraction. Hemostasis is obtained.
6. The cortex is coagulated with a bayonet forceps or dural elevator. It is incised with a no. 11 blade.
7. A Scott cannula is inserted into the frontal horn of the ipsilateral ventricle, and air is exchanged for cerebrospinal fluid. Radiopaque oil may be injected.
8. X-ray films are taken and compared with previous ones for positioning.
9. The basal ganglia guide is attached to the head holder. This guide permits adjustments of cannula position as to direct it to the target area, as well as to hold it firmly during the production of the lesion.
10. The cryosurgical cannula is fixed in the guide, and the tip is brought to the surface of the cerebral cortex. It is directed at the thalamus but is not inserted until its correct aim has been verified by x-ray film, with anteroposterior and lateral projections.
11. The cannula is advanced gently until its tip rests in the thalamus. Verification of placement by x-ray study is obtained. The flow of refrigerant is started, and the patient is checked regularly as the lesion is being produced.
12. Motor and sensory functions of the patient's limbs, as well as tremor, rigidity, or ability to perceive painful stimuli, are evaluated by the neurosurgeon. Speech and consciousness are also checked.
13. After a satisfactory lesion is created, the flow of the refrigerant to the cannula is stopped. Cannula position is verified by final x-ray films.
14. The cannula is removed, and the incision closed.

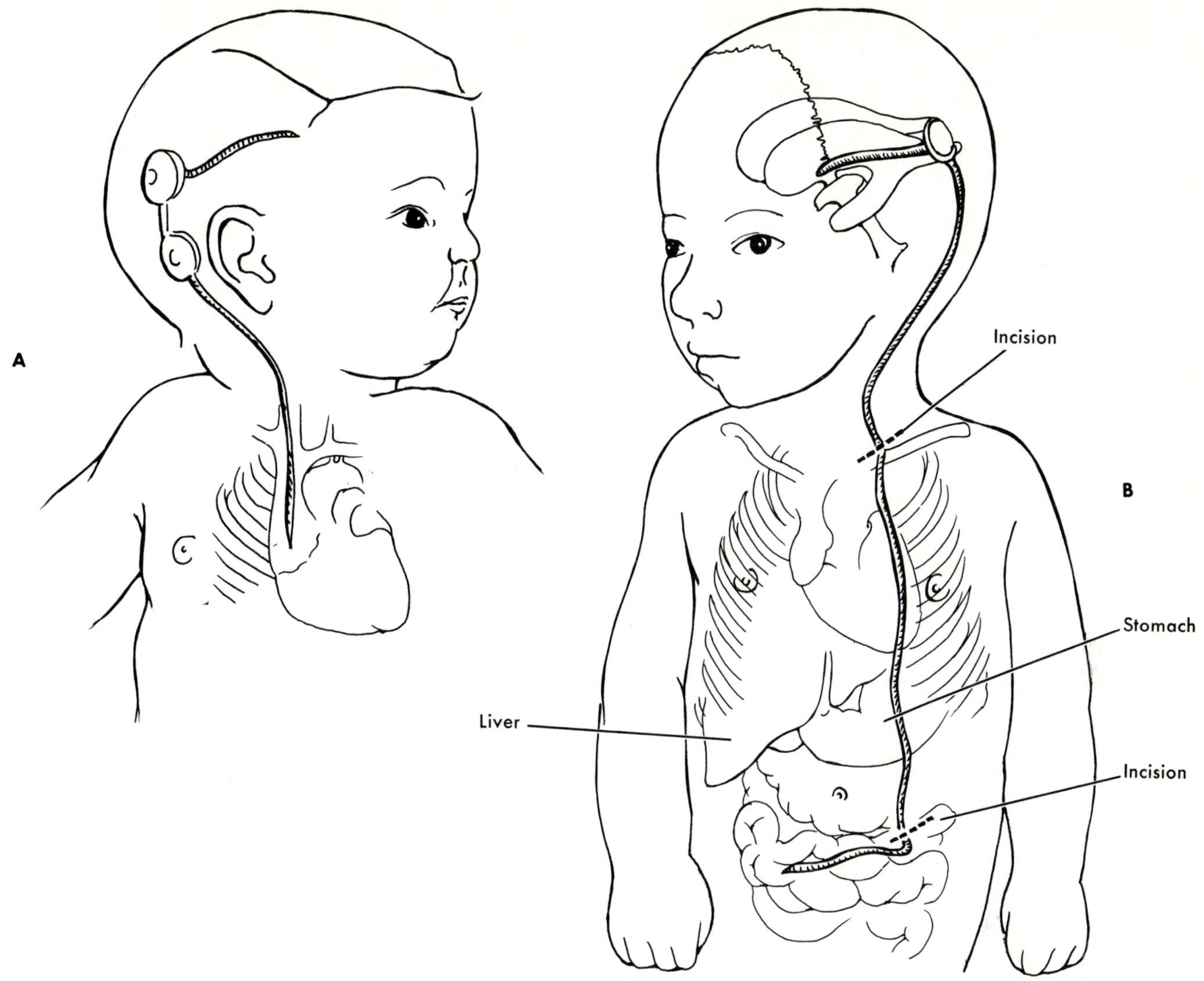

Fig. 24-64. A, Placement of ventriculoatrial shunt. **B,** Placement of ventriculoperitoneal shunt catheter.

Shunt operations

Hydrocephalus is a pathological condition in which there is an increase in the amount of cerebrospinal fluid in the cranial cavity because of excessive production of cerebrospinal fluid, inadequate absorption of cerebrospinal fluid, or an obstruction that interferes with the flow of fluid through the ventricular system.

Noncommunicating or internal hydrocephalus results from obstruction within the ventricular system. Ventricular fluid does not communicate with subarachnoid fluid.

Communicating or external hydrocephalus results from an obstruction outside the ventricular system. All the ventricles are enlarged, and ventricular and subarachnoid fluids freely communicate.

Currently, the two most widely used methods to divert excessive cerebrospinal fluid from ventricles to other body cavities from which it can be absorbed are ventriculoatrial (ventriculocardiac) and ventriculoperitoneal shunts. A catheter is inserted into the ventricular system (usually a lateral ventricle) and connected to a distal catheter that is placed in the right atrium of the heart or the peritoneal cavity (Fig. 24-64).

A valve system is used to direct the flow of cerebrospinal fluid and regulate the ventricular fluid pressure by opening within a preset range and draining the excess fluid into the atrium or peritoneum. The valve system may be a separate unit, such as the Holter valve, which is placed between the ventricular and distal catheters under the scalp just behind the ear (Fig. 24-65), or the valve may be incorporated into the distal catheter (Fig. 24-66).

Usually a reservoir is inserted into the system between the ventricular catheter and the valve. The reservoir is also placed under the scalp just behind the ear or in a bur hole that was made to tap the lateral ventricle. The reservoir can be punctured through the scalp with a 25- or 26-gauge Huber needle to irrigate and clear an ob-

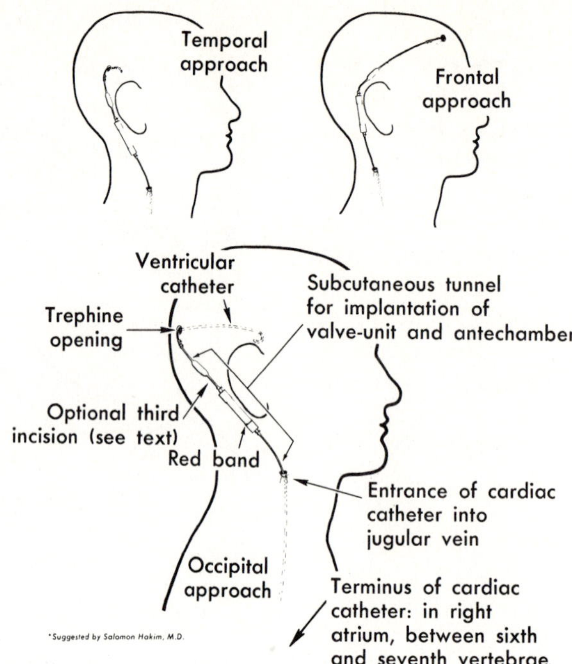

Fig. 24-65. Diagram of placement of Hakim ventriculoatrial shunt. (Courtesy Cordis Corp., Miami.)

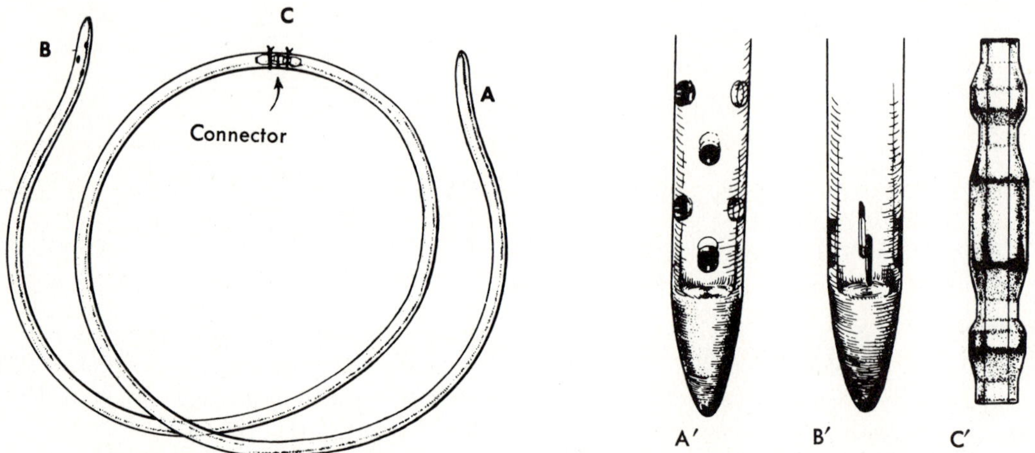

Fig. 24-66. Shunt is made from silicone tubing of special formula and consists of three component parts: **A,** cardiac tube with slit valve in side wall near tip; **B,** ventricular tube with side perforations; and **C,** nylon connector. Materials used in shunt can be sterilized in autoclave. Slit valve is designed to allow cerebrospinal fluid to flow freely when pressure in tube exceeds predetermined pressure specified by manufacturer for particular model used. When intraventricular pressure falls below specified level, valve slits remain closed and prevent escape of fluid. Before implantation in patient, valve should be checked by filling it with sterile, physiological saline solution and holding it in vertical position to determine if fluid column level reaches specified pressure level within time limitation required as stated in manufacturer's instructions. Although valve slits are coated with compound to prevent sticking, heat sterilization may increase adhesion. If this occurs, film may be broken by rolling valve end gently between thumb and index finger. (Courtesy Codman & Shurtleff, Inc., Randolph, Mass.)

struction in the ventricular catheter, to introduce a contrast medium for an x-ray check of patency, to inject medication into the ventricle, or to serve as a flushing device when digital compression is applied (Fig. 24-67).

The valve assembly must be checked for patency and pressure before implantation. Each manufacturer provides specific instructions, which must be followed. As with all implantable devices, the shunt assembly must be kept free of lint, glove powder, or other potential foreign bodies that could cause a reaction by the patient's tissues.

Neurosurgeons and engineers frequently modify and improve shunt assemblies used today, as in the examples in Figs. 24-66 and 24-67. Valves are manufactured with pressure ranges of high, medium, low, and extra low. Slit-valve catheters have three pressure ranges: high, medium, and low. All shunt systems and parts can be purchased sterile.

Other procedures that are sometimes done to correct hydrocephalus include cauterization of the choroid plexus of the lateral ventricles by placing a lensed endoscopy instrument and resectoscope into the ventricle through a bur hole to visualize and destroy the production site of cerebrospinal fluid by electrocautery; ventriculoureteral shunts (requiring nephrectomy); lumbar subarachnoid shunt, in which a laminectomy is done and the cerebrospinal fluid is diverted into the peritoneal cavity or a ureter (the latter requiring nephrectomy); and ventriculocisternostomy, or Torkildsen procedure, in which a catheter is placed to shunt fluid from a lateral ventricle to the cisterna magna (Fig. 24-68).

Ventriculoatrial shunt

Setup and preparation of the patient. Insertion of a ventriculoatrial shunt is carried out with the patient in a modified supine position. The head is usually slightly elevated and turned to the left and may be supported on a donut. An x-ray film of the chest is taken to validate correct placement of the distal catheter, or the catheter can be placed under direct vision fluoroscopy with the image intensifier.

Operative procedure. When the distal slit-valve catheter is used, an incision is made in the neck to isolate the facial or the internal or external jugular vein. The atrial (distal) catheter is filled with normal saline solution, clamped with a bulldog clamp to prevent air from entering the circulatory system, and threaded into the right atrium through the isolated vein. Most catheters have a radiopaque tip for easy identification of placement during radiography. The catheter should lie at the T-6 or T-7 level.

Access is gained to the right lateral ventricle through a bur hole or twist-drill hole. The ventricular catheter is placed and connected to a reservoir. A tunnel is made under the skin from the bur hole to the neck incision with a uterine packing forceps or special tunneling device ap-

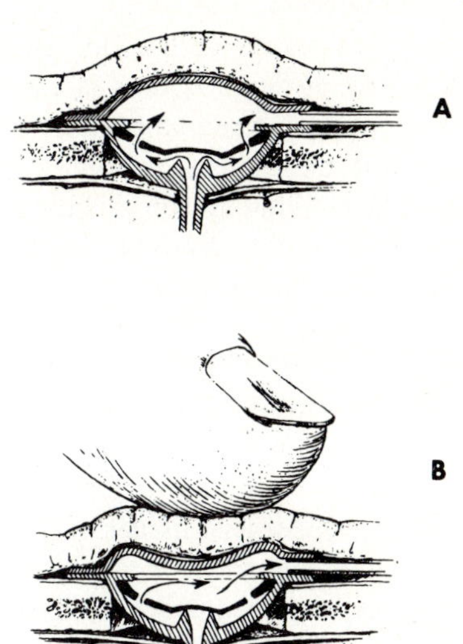

Fig. 24-67. Pudenz valve flushing device for ventricular shunts. **A,** Flanged silicone capsule and diaphragm valve shaped to fit into bur hole in skull. **B,** Pressure on capsule closes ventricular inlet and flushes shunt tube. (Courtesy Codman & Shurtleff, Inc., Randolph, Mass.)

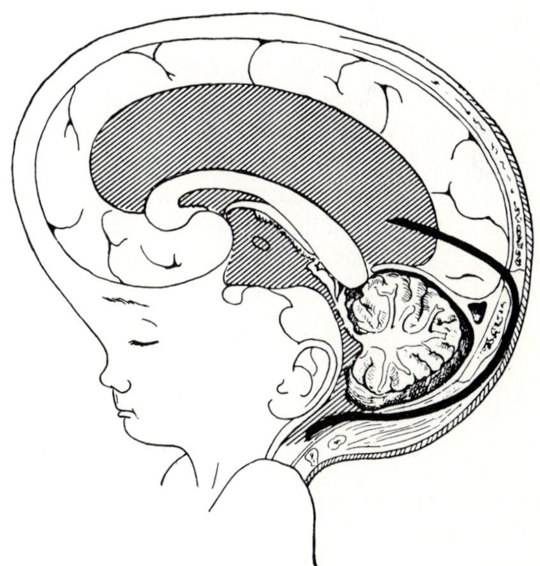

Fig. 24-68. Torkildsen operation (ventriculocisternostomy) showing catheter in place: one end in occipital horn of lateral ventricle, the other in cisterna magna. (From Conway-Rutkowski, B.L.: Carini and Owens' neurological and neurosurgical nursing, ed. 8, St. Louis, 1982, The C.V. Mosby Co.)

propriate for the specific assembly being used. The atrial catheter is pulled through the tunnel to the bur hole and connected to the reservoir.

When a separate valve, such as the Holter, is used, the ventricular part of the procedure is carried out first. A special valve introducer and tube passer have been designed for use with the Holter assembly.

A single-catheter shunt system without a reservoir is also available. The distal end is a slit valve, and the proximal end is a ventricular catheter.

Ventriculoperitoneal shunts

The ventricular portion of this procedure is the same as for ventriculoatrial shunts. The distal catheter is much longer and is threaded from the ventricular puncture site under the scalp and superficial tissues of the neck, chest, and abdomen to an abdominal incision. The tip of the distal catheter may be placed under the liver.

Some precautions that must be taken during the valve implant procedures include the following:

1. Trapping of air in the valve assembly unit should be prevented.

2. Storage fluid surrounding the valve should be removed, pumped out of the valve, and replaced with Ringer's solution.

3. Extreme care should be used in handling the unit. It should never be placed on gauze or linen, to avoid lint or other foreign body. *The unit is always placed in a basin.*

4. Lubricants should never be used on the unit. The patient's body fluid adequately lubricates the device.

5. The valve must be properly oriented. It permits only one-way passage of fluid.

6. The valve system must not be pumped excessively immediately after surgery. This can cause too rapid a fluid loss, leading to a rapid decrease in ventricular size. This is poorly tolerated and may lead to subdural hemorrhage.

Frequently, shunts must be revised. Some shunts become obstructed. Others become disconnected or malfunction mechanically in some way. The growth of infants and children may require revision of distal tubings.

Operations on the back

Definitions

laminectomy Removal of one or more of the vertebral laminae to expose the spinal cord. Laminectomy, hemilaminectomy, and interlaminar approach are performed to reach the spinal cord and its adjacent structures to treat compression fracture, dislocation, herniated nucleus pulposus, and cord tumor. Section of the spinal nerves, including cordotomy, and rhizotomy require similar surgical exposure. Laminectomy is also done to insert subarachnoid shunts for hydrocephalus or pseudotumor cerebri.

cordotomy Surgical division of the anterolateral tracts of the spinal cord for intractable pain.

rhizotomy Interruption of the roots of the spinal nerves within the spinal canal.

anterior rhizotomy Division of the anterior or motor spinal nerve roots for the relief of spasm.

posterior rhizotomy Division of the posterior or sensory spinal nerve roots for the relief of intractable pain.

Laminectomy

Considerations. Laminectomy can be done with the patient in the prone, lateral, knee-chest, or sitting position. It is performed on the cervical, thoracic, or lumbar spine.

Setup and preparation of the patient. Laminectomy instruments (Fig. 24-69) include the basic neurosurgical set and the following:

- 3 Scoville hemilaminectomy retractors
- 4 Beckman-Adson self-retaining laminectomy retractors, sharp, 12 inches, 2 regular and 2 large
- 4 Key periosteal elevators, ¼, ½, ¾, and 1 inch
- 2 Adson self-retaining cerebellum retractors, angled
- 1 Horsley bone cutter, large, 10½ inches
- 2 Spurling-Kerrison laminectomy rongeurs, downbiting, 3 and 5 mm
- 2 Schlesinger cervical punches, thin-lipped rongeur, 3 and 5 mm
- 2 Love nerve root retractors
- 1 Angled curette, no. 1
- 2 Diamond-jawed needle holders, 9 inches
- 6 Cone ring curettes

Laminectomy for herniated disc (nucleus pulposus)

1. A midline vertical or transverse incision is made at the operative site.

2. Hemostatic forceps are placed on the under side of the skin edge and everted for hemostasis. Deeper vessels are usually coagulated.

3. Two self-retaining retractors (Cone, Weitlaner, or Adson) are inserted for exposure.

4. The fascia is incised in the midline with Mayo scissors or electrocautery current.

5. One side of the spinous processes is exposed by sharp dissection.

6. The paraspinous muscles and periosteum are stripped off the laminae with a knife and sharp periosteal elevators. Cutting current dissection with the electrocautery may be used.

7. As each area is stripped, a gauze sponge is packed around the bony structures with a periosteal elevator to aid in blunt dissection and to tamponade bleeding. The paraspinous muscles are dissected from all the laminae. In disc surgery this may be done only on one side, the side of the lesion (Fig. 24-70).

8. A laminectomy retractor is then placed in position. Either a Scoville (1 blade on tissue side and a slightly

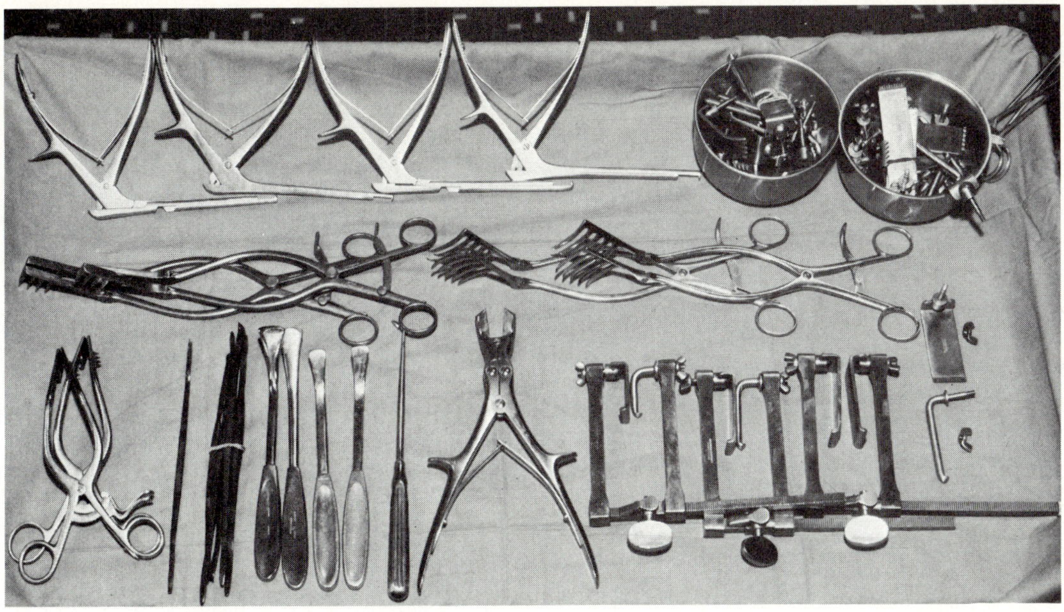

Fig. 24-69. Back table setup displaying some special laminectomy instruments. *Left to right: top,* Spurling-Kerrison laminectomy rongeurs, Schlesinger cervical punches, basins with assorted retractor blades and hooks; *center,* Beckman-Adson retractors, two regular and two large; *bottom,* Adson self-retaining cerebellum retractors, copper nerve root retractors, Campbell angled periosteal elevators, angled curette, Horsley bone cutter, Scoville hemilaminectomy retractors with blades. (Courtesy K. Cramer Lewis, Department of Illustrations, Washington University School of Medicine, St. Louis.)

shorter hook on bone side) or Beckman-Adson retractor can be used.

9. Cotton strips are placed in the extremes of the field for hemostasis.

10. The edges of the laminae overlying the interspace with the herniated disc are defined with a curette. A partial hemilaminectomy of these laminal edges extending out into the lateral gutter of the spinal canal is performed with a Schwartz-Kerrison rongeur. The bone edges are waxed.

11. The flaval ligament is grasped with a vascular or a bayonet forceps with teeth, and a no. 15 blade on a no. 7 scalpel handle is used to incise it as close to the midline as possible. Cotton strips are passed through this incision to protect the underlying dura, and a window is cut in the flaval ligament with a no. 15 blade on a no. 7 scalpel handle (Fig. 24-71).

12. Additional ligaments out in the lateral gutter of the spinal canal may be removed with a large curette or a Cloward punch after first protecting the dural sac and nerve root with a cottonoid.

13. A dural elevator and a Love or copper nerve root retractor are used to retract the nerve root and dural sac to expose the disc space (Fig. 24-71).

14. Epidural veins are controlled by packing with narrow cotton strips and if necessary by careful coagulation with bipolar cautery bayonet.

15. Any herniated fragment of disc is removed with a pituitary rongeur.

16. After coagulation of its surface, an opening is cut into the posterior aspect of the interspace with a no. 11 blade on a no. 7 scalpel handle.

17. Pituitary rongeurs, straight and angled, narrow and wide, are used to remove the disc material from the interspace.

18. Straight and angled ring curettes help to further clean out the interspace. Disc material so loosened is removed with the pituitary rongeurs.

19. The area is irrigated with Ringer's or normal saline solution, and the interspace is explored with a suction tip.

20. The nerve roots and extradural space are explored with a nerve hook.

21. If no further specimen is obtained, hemostasis is secured with cotton strips. If possible, neither gelatin sponge nor gauze or other hemostatic material is used.

22. The cotton strips are removed from the epidural space, the table is unflexed, and the area is further irrigated. A change of position sometimes causes more disc material to protrude, and the interspace is reexposed with a root retractor to rule out this possibility.

23. All cotton strips and retractors are removed, and the wound is closed.

For cervical or thoracic discs, only the protruding

fragment is removed and limited if any exploration of the interspace is performed. This is because attempts at adequate interspace exploration require retraction of the dural sac, which contains the spinal cord at these levels. Such retraction would result in cord injury and paralysis.

Laminectomy for spinal cord tumors

1. The fascial incision is made in the midline, both sides of the spinous processes are dissected out, and the paraspinous muscles are taken down bilaterally, one side at a time.

2. One or more double-bladed Scoville or Beckman-Adson self-retaining retractors are placed to maintain the bony exposure.

3. A midline laminectomy is performed, with the spinous processes excised with a Horsley bone cutter. Various rongeurs (such as Leksell, double-action, Cloward) are used to remove the laminae after defining the edges with a curette. The bone edges are waxed.

4. The remaining flaval ligament is removed with scissors, scalpel, and Kerrison or Cloward rongeurs. Epidural fat is coagulated and, if necessary, removed with dissecting scissors, so that the dura mater is exposed fully.

5. A wide moist cottonoid is placed over the superficial soft tissues and muscle down to the bone bordering the exposed dura mater. This provides additional hemostasis.

6. The dura mater is elevated with a small hook and nicked with a no. 15 scalpel blade. A grooved director is inserted beneath the dura mater, and the dural incision is extended over it, using long forceps and fine scissors. Alternatively, the incision may be lengthened by pulling apart the two edges of the dural incision with bayonet forceps or by pushing at the ends of this incision with the edge of a dural elevator. Traction sutures of no. 4-0 silk on dura needles are placed in the dural edges, and the cord is exposed (Fig. 24-72).

7. The cord is explored for the pathological area. Aspiration through a no. 22 needle on a plain-tipped syringe may be carried out. The tumor may be encountered extradurally or intradurally. Whenever possible, the tumor mass is dissected free and removed by suction, dissecting scissors, the cutting electrocautery, forceps, cottonoid, small (pituitary) scoops, curettes, and pituitary rongeurs. Bleeding is controlled with a moist cottonoid, hemostatic clips, gelatin gauze, and gelatin sponge. Bipolar cautery is used around the nerves and spinal cord. The spinal subarachnoid space may be explored with a small rubber catheter to detect blockage.

8. The wound is irrigated with normal saline or Ringer's solution, Asepto syringes, and suction.

9. Hemostasis is obtained; the dura mater is closed with no. 4-0 or 5-0 silk.

10. The incision is checked for further bleeding, and the paraspinous muscles are approximated with no. 2-0 silk. The remainder of the wound is closed.

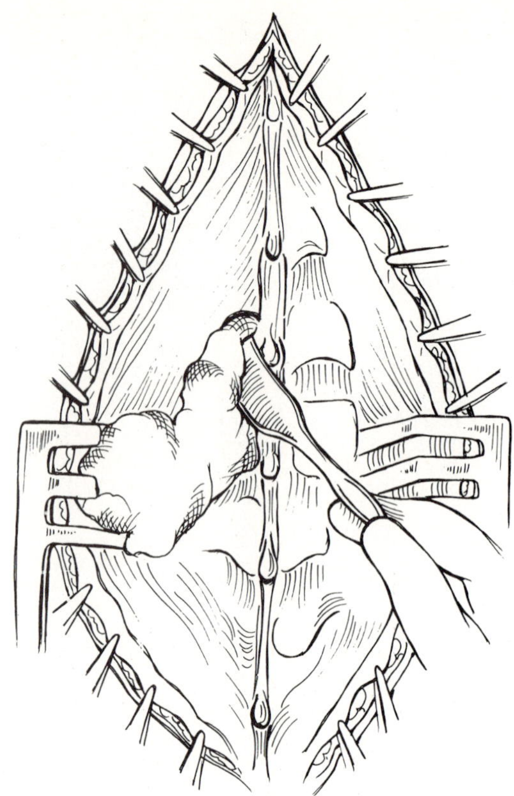

Fig. 24-70. Laminectomy: exposing vertebrae by dissecting muscle away from spine. (From Sachs, E.: Diagnosis and treatment of brain tumors and the care of the neurosurgical patient, ed. 2, St. Louis, The C.V. Mosby Co.)

In the case of extradural tumors, intradural exploration is omitted.

The operating microscope may be used, especially on intradural tumors and vascular anomalies.

Laminectomy for meningocele

Considerations. Malformations such as meningoceles are usually congenital. They are a threat to the life of the newborn infant, since the defect may predispose to infection or spinal cord damage. Defects of the cord and spinal nerves are often associated with the condition. There also may be spina bifida, a congenital defect resulting from incomplete closure of the vertebral canal.

Operation for repair of meningocele is directed at preserving intact the neural elements involved and at closing the cutaneous, muscular, and dural defects.

Setup. For surgery on infants, small hemostats, retractors, and other instruments are provided. Large bone-cutting instruments may be omitted. The nerve stimulator may be needed.

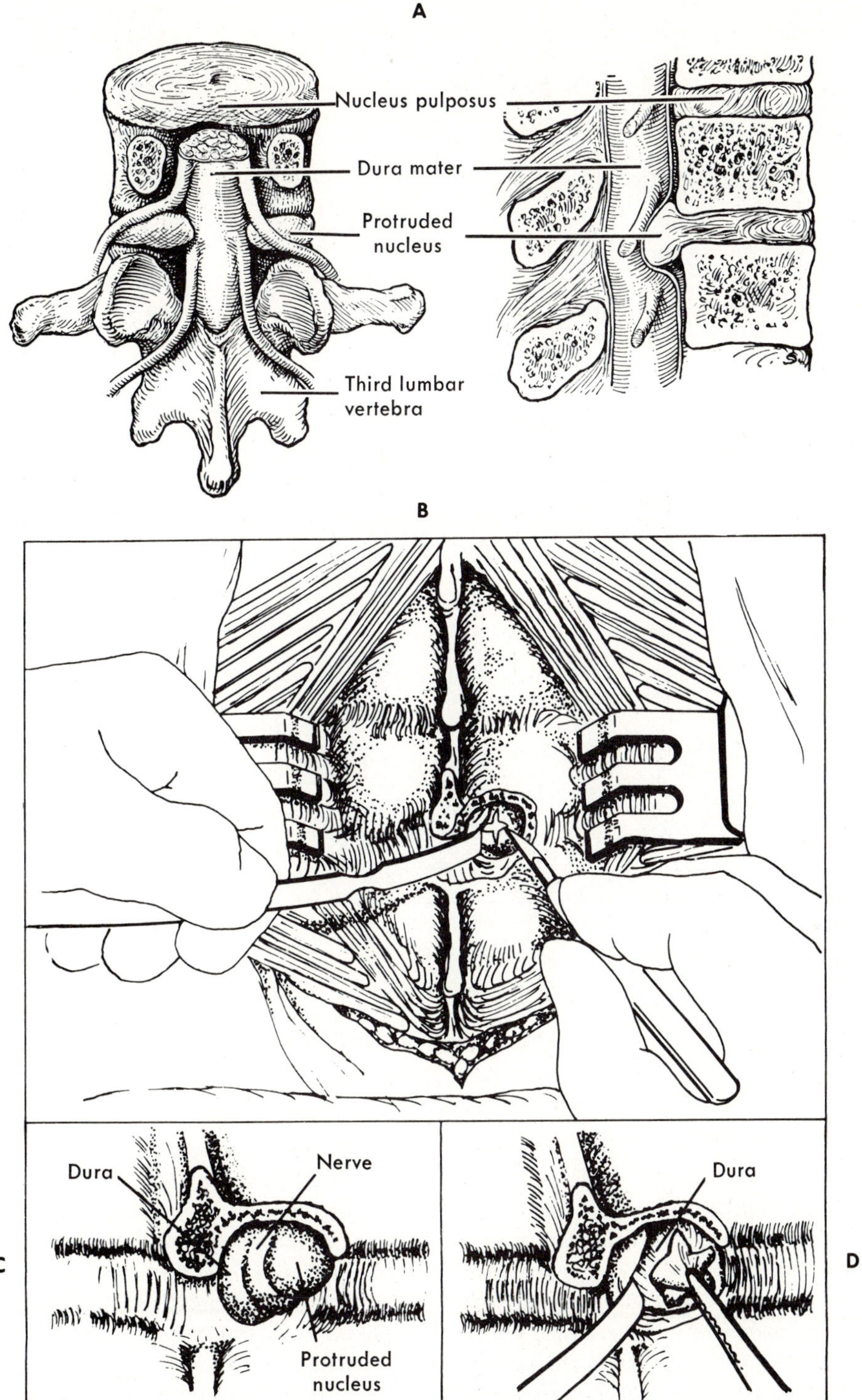

Fig. 24-71. A, Normal and herniated nucleus pulposus (disc). **B,** Window has been made in lamina, and ligament has been incised to expose underlying dura mater and nerve root. **C,** Relationship of dura mater, nerve root, and protruded nucleus pulposus (disc). **D,** Retraction of nerve root over dura mater and removal of disc. (From Carini, E., and Owens, G.: Neurological and neurosurgical nursing, ed. 6, St. Louis, 1974, The C.V. Mosby Co.)

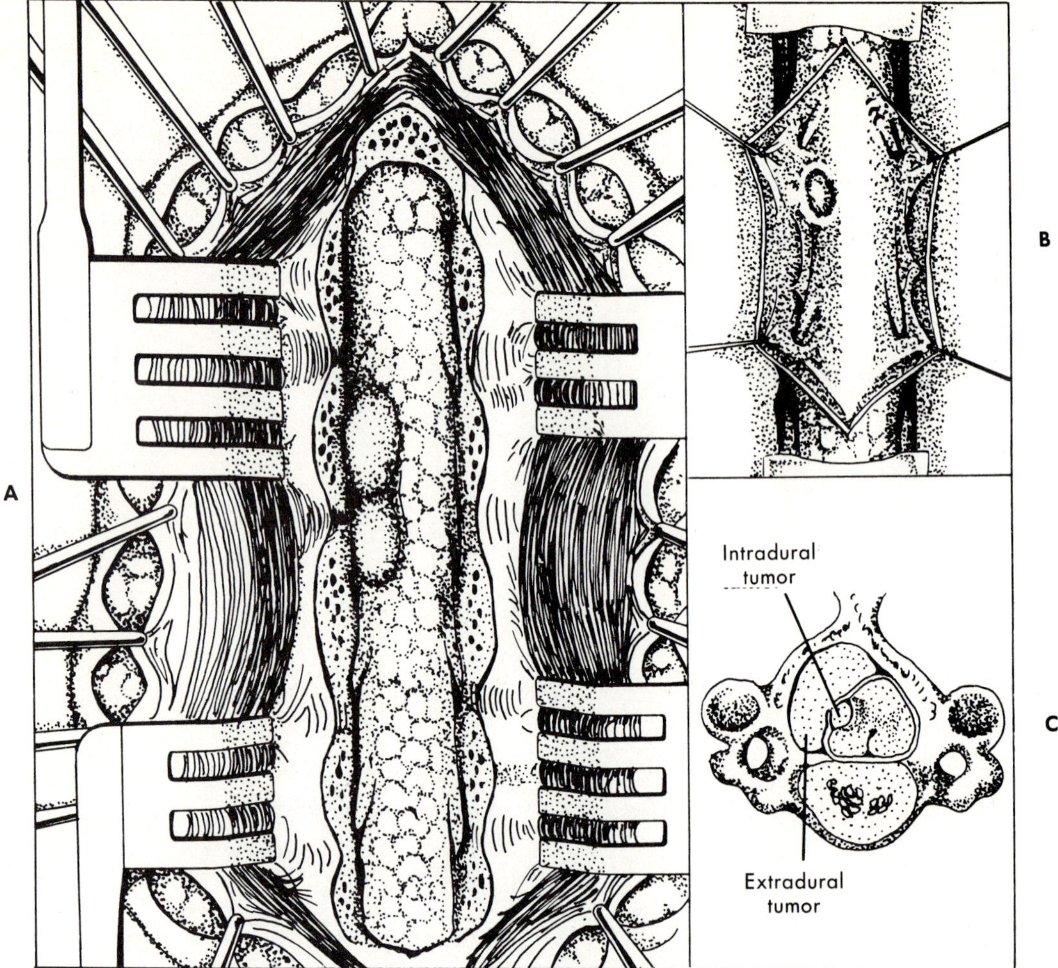

Fig. 24-72. A, Laminectomy completed: dura mater and tumor exposed. **B,** Dura mater incised and retracted, revealing pia arachnoidea over spinal cord and part of tumor. **C,** Diagram of cross section of tumor site and location of extradural and intradural pathological areas. (From Carini, E., and Owens, G.: Neurological and neurosurgical nursing, ed. 6, St. Louis, 1974, The C.V. Mosby Co.)

Cervical cordotomy (Schwartz technique, thoracic cordotomy, rhizotomy)

Definition. Division of the spinothalamic tract for the treatment of intractable pain. High cervical cordotomy is a most effective and frequently used procedure.

Considerations. Cervical cordotomy may be performed with the patient under general anesthesia, but, to permit intraoperative testing of the level of analgesia achieved, local anesthesia is preferred. The nurse should keep an accurate account of the amount of local anesthetic agent used. In a very ill or apprehensive patient, a drop in blood pressure or cardiac symptoms may develop if too much local anesthetic is injected.

Setup and preparation of the patient. The patient is placed in a prone position, with head slightly flexed to a level below the horizontal level of the cervical spine. It is essential to keep the patient as comfortable as possible and to offer reassurance frequently.

Operative procedure

1. The skin is infiltrated with the local anesthetic agent, the incision line is marked, and longer needles are used to block the second and third cervical nerves at their points of emergence from the spinal canal.

2. A midline incision is used. Hemostatic forceps are placed to control bleeding, and the Weitlaner retractor is inserted for exposure.

3. Using the electrocautery (cutting current) with the spatula blade, the surgeon separates the muscles from one side of the arches and laminae of the first and second cervical vertebrae. An angled periosteal elevator may be used for further dissection. A gauze sponge may be packed into the wound to enhance the dissection as well as to aid hemostasis (Fig. 24-70).

4. A Scoville hemilaminectomy retractor with short hook and longer blade is inserted between the midline structures and the reflected paraspinous muscles. The

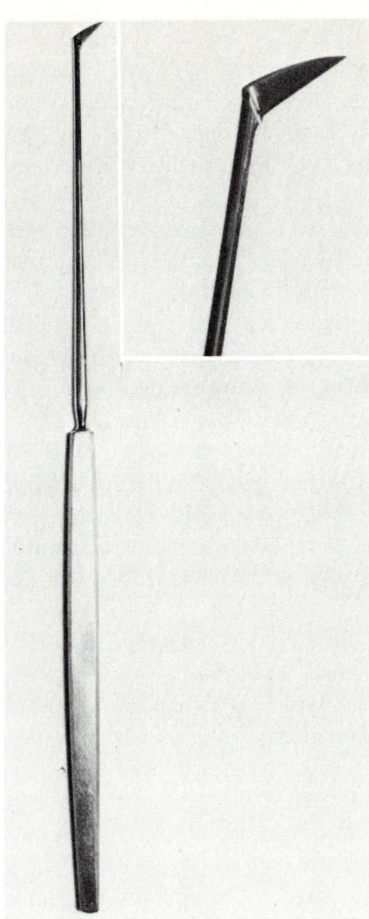

Fig. 24-73. Schwartz cordotomy knife. (Courtesy K. Cramer Lewis, Department of Illustrations, Washington University School of Medicine, St. Louis.)

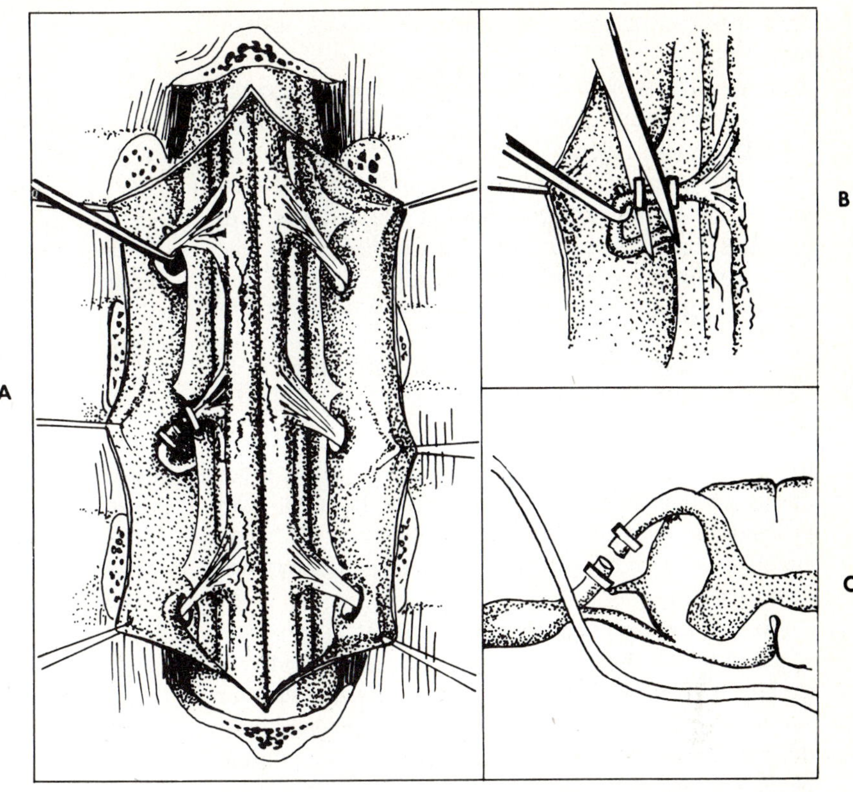

Fig. 24-74. Posterior rhizotomy after laminectomy. **A,** Spinal cord and roots exposed. **B,** Posterior root identified. **C,** Diagram showing cross section of spinal cord and divided posterior root. (From Carini, E., and Owens, G.: Neurological and neurosurgical nursing, ed. 6, St. Louis, 1974, The C.V. Mosby Co.)

flexion of the head is increased when the retractor is inserted.

5. The Schwartz self-retaining retractor (modified Gelpi) is placed, with the multitoothed end in the occipital bone and the sharp point penetrating the spinous process of C-2 to widen the interlaminar space between C-1 and C-2 vertebrae. (For additional exposure, it may be necessary to remove some of the laminae with a Kerrison rongeur.)

6. Large moist cotton strips are placed over the superficial tissues and muscle down to the bone bordering the exposed dura mater.

7. With the use of a dural hook, the dural incision is made with a no. 7 scalpel and a no. 15 blade. A vascular or Metzenbaum scissors is used to lengthen the incision.

8. With no. 4-0 silk stay sutures on an ophthalmic needle, the dural edges are retracted and secured with curved mosquito or straight hemostatic forceps.

9. While suctioning is being performed on cotton strips to remove spinal fluid, the dentate ligament is identified at its dural attachment with bayonet forceps and followed to the cord and left attached to prevent distortion of the cord.

10. A fine bayonet forceps (Gerald) is used to elevate the dentate attachment to provide visualization of the anterolateral quadrant of the cord and the anterior nerve rootlets.

11. The cord is incised with a slightly curved cordotomy knife (Fig. 24-73).

12. After the incision is made, the patient is checked for adequacy of the level of analgesia. If the level is not satisfactory, the cord incision is deepened.

13. Hemostasis is obtained, the dural incision is closed, retractors are removed, and the wound is checked for bleeding and is closed.

For *bilateral cordotomy,* the muscles are separated from both sides of the arches and laminae of the vertebrae. A double-bladed Scoville retractor is used, and the Schwartz retractor (modified Gelpi) is placed according to the side of the cord being approached. The cordotomy is performed on one side and then on the other. With bilateral high cervical cordotomy, falls in blood pressure and respiratory difficulty may occur.

High thoracic cordotomy is performed unilaterally or bilaterally in a similar manner, but a hemilaminectomy or total laminectomy at two levels must usually be performed to gain adequate exposure. The lateral position may be used.

Rhizotomy is performed through a similar exposure with the appropriate nerve roots dissected free of any large radicular vessels, held up with a nerve hook, crushed with a hemostatic forceps, and divided with fine-tipped scissors. A silver clip may be placed on the distal ends of the roots before division. This aids in hemostasis and permits subsequent radiological visualization of the extent and precise level of the root section (Fig. 24-74).

Removal of anterior cervical disc with fusion (Cloward technique)

Considerations. This procedure is done to relieve pain in the neck, shoulder, and arm caused by cervical spondylosis or herniated disc by removal of the disc, with fusion of the vertebral bodies. Bone dowels for the fusion are obtained from the patient's iliac crest or from a bone dowel bank.

Setup and preparation of the patient. The patient is placed in the supine position, with the head turned very slightly to the left and with the right hip elevated for exposure of the iliac crest (if the bone dowel comes from the iliac crest). The basic minor dissecting set is used, plus the following instruments (Fig. 24-75):

- 4 Cloward self-retaining retractors, 2 large and 2 small, with assorted blades (with and without teeth)
- 4 Sizes of drill guards, cervical drills, and dowel cutters
- 1 Cloward bone graft holder and impactor
- 1 Cloward bone graft impactor, double-ended
- 6 Cloward hand retractors
- 4 Cloward vertebral spreaders, 2 regular and 2 self-retaining
- 2 Deaver retractors, narrow
- 1 Rasp
- 1 Mallet
- 2 Adson cerebellum retractors, angled
- Assorted spinal fusion curettes, straight and angulated, nos. 0 to 4-0
- Meyerding finger retractors

Operative procedure

1. A transverse skin incision is made on one side of the neck (usually the right) directly over the involved disc space; curved mosquito forceps or Michel clips are placed on the skin edges for hemostasis.
2. A Weitlaner retractor is placed, and the platysma muscle is divided with Metzenbaum scissors and tissue forceps with teeth or with the cutting electrocautery.
3. The medial edge of the sternocleidomastoid muscle is defined with the scissors by blunt and sharp dissection.
4. A vertical plane of dissection between the carotid sheath laterally and the trachea and esophagus medially is created by blunt finger dissection. This plane is held open with Cloward hand retractors, Meyerding finger retractors, or U.S. Army retractors.
5. The anterior surface of the spine is identified, and the long muscles of the neck are peeled off the anterior surface of the spine with periosteal elevators. Bleeders are coagulated with a dural elevator or bayonet forceps.
6. A short needle is inserted a short distance into the disc space, and a lateral x-ray film is taken to determine the level of the exposure.
7. While x-ray films are being developed, the neck incision is covered, an incision is made over the iliac crest, and straight hemostats are applied and retracted.
8. Soft tissue is dissected until the crest is reached, using Mayo scissors, tissue forceps, cutting electrocautery, and Richardson retractors for exposure.
9. A Hudson brace with the Cloward dowel cutter is used to remove the bone graft. (Care must be exercised to use dowel cutter, Cloward guide, and cervical drill guards matched for size.) The dowel obtained should have cortex at both ends. The dowel hole is inspected and waxed if needed. The incision is packed with gauze sponges and covered.
10. The Cloward self-retaining retractors (two long and two short) are inserted into the neck incision. The right blade should be slightly longer than the left. Care is used to protect the carotid artery and the esophagus. A combination of sharp and dull blades is used to acquire the best retraction. If a toothed blade is used, the teeth are carefully hooked beneath the long muscle of the neck.
11. A no. 15 or 11 blade on a no. 7 scalpel handle is used to cut into the disc space; a fine pituitary rongeur is used to remove the disc material, which is saved and weighed as a specimen. A vertebral spreader is inserted into the vertebral space to widen the area, and further disc material is removed with the rongeur or small curettes (angled or straight, nos. 0 to 4-0) until the entire surfaces of both vertebrae are clean. A Surgairtome with a small bur may also be used.
12. The Cloward bone guide is inserted into the disc space to measure its depth.
13. After the drill guard is adjusted so that the drill can protrude no farther than the measured depth of the interspace, the cervical drill guard is inserted around the disc space, with the aid of a mallet, until the points catch the vertebral bodies above and below the interspace.
14. After the guard is in place, the vertebral spreader is removed or spread to a more limited degree.
15. The Cloward drill on a Hudson brace is inserted into the guard, and the hole is drilled. (The bone dust on the drill point is inspected and saved in a medicine glass.) Cotton strips or gelatin sponge is used for active bleeders. Bone wax should not be used on the walls of the disc hole. Thrombin-soaked cottonoid pledgets may help control bleeding.
16. The bottom of the hole is checked for further disc or cartilaginous material, which is removed. The guide may be removed and replaced, and drilling may be done several times until the desired depth is reached. The drill and guide are then removed.

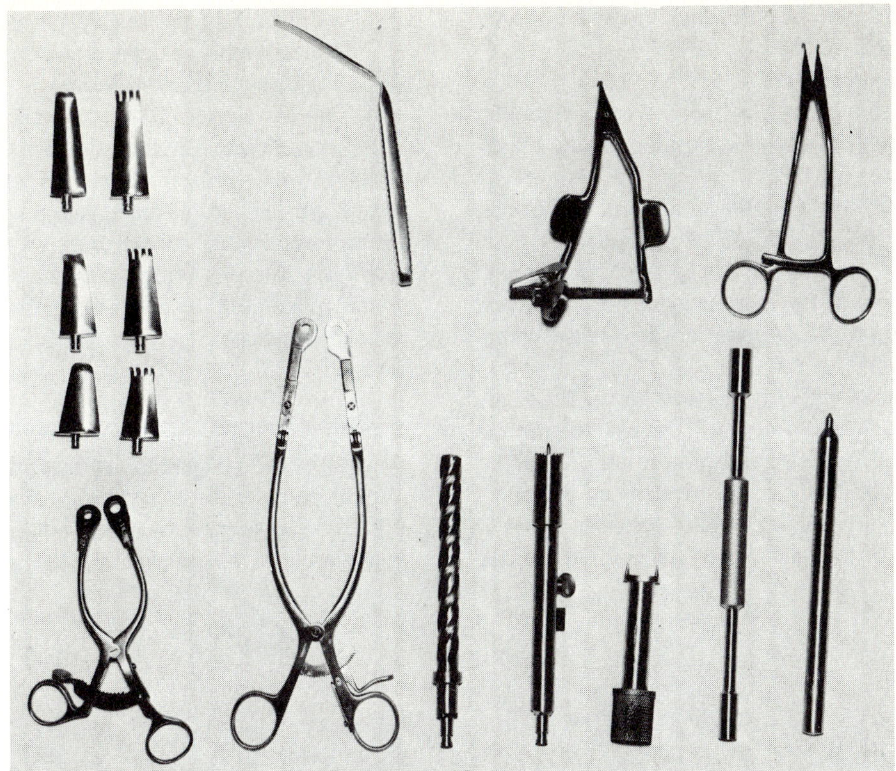

Fig. 24-75. Instruments for anterior cervical disc removal with fusion. *Left to right: top,* Cloward retractor blades, small Cloward hand retractor, Cloward cervical vertebral self-retaining spreader, Cloward cervical vertebral spreader; *bottom,* Cloward small cervical self-retaining retractor, Cloward large cervical self-retaining retractor, Cloward cervical drill, Cloward dowel cutter, Cloward guard guide, Cloward impactor, Cloward drill guard. (Courtesy Codman & Shurtleff, Inc., Randolph, Mass.)

17. Further bone is removed by use of the Cloward cervical punch or curettes until complete anterior decompression of the nerve root or dural sac is obtained. Nerve hooks may be used here for demonstration of adequate dissection. The Air Drill 100 may also be used.

18. The depth of the hole is measured and compared with the dowel. The dowel may be trimmed with a drill, rongeur, or rasp. The shaped dowel attached to the impactor is inserted into the hole and tapped into place. The double-edged impactor is used to drive the dowel in deeper if necessary. The spreader is removed, and bone dust may be applied.

19. Hemostasis is obtained and the wound irrigated; the vertebral spreader and retractors are removed, and both incisions closed.

Carotid surgery of the neck

Carotid artery ligation

Considerations. Carotid artery ligation is performed to occlude the internal carotid artery.

It may be done to control anticipated hemorrhage during intracranial surgery for vascular anomalies. A permanent occlusion may be necessary for the control of intracranial hemorrhage or small, repeated strokes from an intracranial lesion that is not amenable to direct attack. Special clamps, such as the Selverstone (Fig. 24-76), Selibi, and Crutchfield carotid artery clamps (Fig. 24-77) are available for gradual occlusion of the artery. Occlusion may protect the patient from debilitating or fatal intracranial hemorrhage from aneurysm and may be used to treat carotid-cavernous fistula.

Setup. Only a basic minor instrument set is used.

Operative procedure

1. The skin is incised, and a Weitlaner retractor is inserted for exposure.

2. The carotid artery is freed. A small Penrose tubing or umbilical tape is passed around the vessel for retraction.

3. *For temporary control* of the carotid artery (during procedures for very large aneurysms or arteriovenous anomalies): an umbilical tape is passed around the vessel and fixed, using the Roper-Rumel tourniquet in such a manner that occlusion can be accomplished immediately if necessary.

4. *For permanent occlusion:* two heavy silk ligatures are used, and the artery may be divided between liga-

tures. Transfixing suture ligatures may be used as well if the artery is divided.

5. *For gradual occlusion:*
   a. A carotid clamp, such as the Selverstone, Selibi, or Crutchfield, is placed in position around the artery.
   b. A small stab wound is made adjacent to the incision.
   c. The control assembly with cap is passed through the stab wound. By loosening the locking screw and pressing down on the screwdriver, the operator can remove the cap.
   d. The control assembly is snapped on the lid of the clamp, and with a hemostatic forceps holding the clamp, each flange is gently forced into position.
   e. Using the dot on the screwdriver as an indicator, the number of turns for complete occlusion is noted. The clamp is then unscrewed a measured number of turns, and the screwdriver is locked. The control assembly is capped and left in place, protruding through the stab wound.
6. The incision is closed, and a dressing is applied.

After the procedure the carotid artery clamp tools are packaged and sterilized. They are kept at the patient's bedside for daily adjustments and returned to the operating room or central service for resterilization after each use. They must be returned to the patient's bedside as soon as possible to be available if the patient cannot tolerate the occlusion and the clamp must be opened immediately.

Carotid surgery for carotid-cavernous fistula

Ligation of the common carotid artery is one mode of surgical treatment for a carotid-cavernous fistula. Another form of surgical treatment is to embolize the fistula with muscle or other material. The segment of external

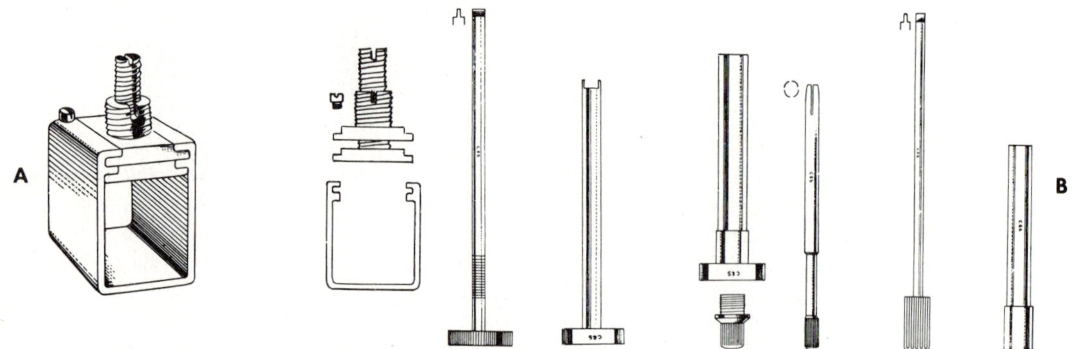

Fig. 24-76. A, Selverstone carotid artery clamp. **B,** Selverstone carotid artery clamp tools. (Courtesy Codman & Shurtleff, Inc., Randolph, Mass.)

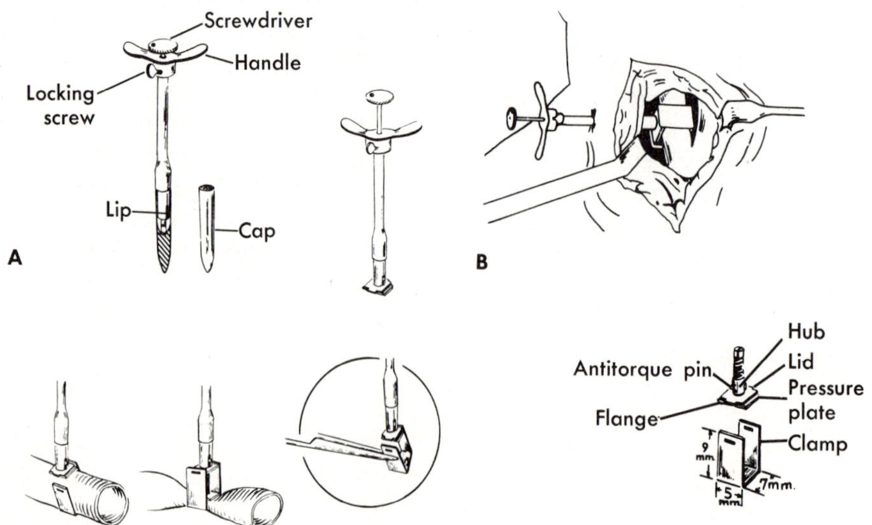

Fig. 24-77. Crutchfield clamp. **A,** Control assembly. **B,** Clamp assembly. (Courtesy Codman & Shurtleff, Inc., Randolph, Mass.)

carotid artery just distal to the carotid bifurcation is occluded with vascular clamps and incised as a point of entry. A piece of muscle is labeled with a metal clip and attached to a length of silk so that it can be visualized by radiography and withdrawn if necessary. It is introduced into the internal carotid artery through the arteriotomy in the external carotid artery after the internal and common carotid artery after the internal and common carotid arteries are occluded and after the proximal external carotid artery clamp is removed. The internal and then common carotid artery clamps are released as the clamp is removed. The proximal external carotid artery clamp is reapplied, leaving a small proximal opening in the arteriotomy unclamped for the protrusion of the tag suture on the embolus. The blood flow in the common internal carotid artery system then pushes the embolus up to the fistula.

Alternatively, an appropriately controlled internal carotid artery may be embolized by forcing the muscle plug up into the area of the fistula with saline solution injected through polyethylene tubing.

In either case, internal carotid ligation is usually done after satisfactory placement of the embolus. In some cases, a frontotemporal craniotomy is also performed, and the internal carotid artery clipped intracranially as well.

Peripheral nerve surgery

Sympathectomy

Definition. Excision of a portion of the sympathetic division of the autonomic nervous system.

Considerations. Most sympathectomies are performed on the paravertebral chain and are named for the region resected, for example, cervical, thoracolumbar, and lumbar. The periarterial sympathectomy, vagotomy, and presacral neurectomy are other procedures that are occasionally performed on the autonomic system.

The principal diseases treated by sympathectomy are vascular disorders of the extremities and intractable pain from certain nerve injuries and/or chronic abdominal conditions.

Setup and preparation of the patient. The position of the patient depends on the region to be resected.

Basic dissecting instruments are used, plus the following:

For *retropleural and transthoracic approaches,* Doyen rib raspatories, rib cutters, and rongeurs are added (Fig. 24-78).

For *thoracic and lumbar approaches,* the following are added:

2 Volkmann rake retractors, large, eight-pronged, blunt
3 Malleable copper retractors
2 Richardson retractors, large
2 Weinberg retractors
2 Deaver retractors
2 Harrington retractors
2 Beckman retractors

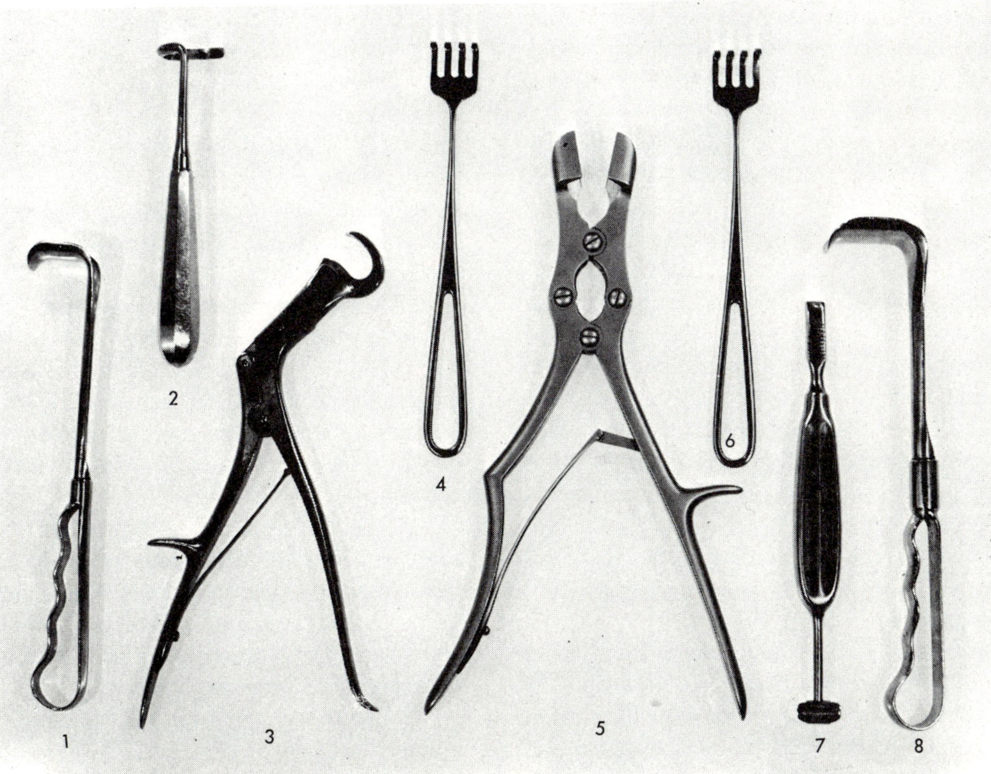

Fig. 24-78. Instruments for rib resection. *1,* Richardson retractor; *2,* Doyen rib raspatory; *3,* Stille rib shears; *4,* blunt rake retractor; *5,* Sauerbruch rib rongeur; *6,* blunt rake retractor; *7,* Alexander costal periosteotome; *8,* Richardson retractor.

For the *thoracic approach,* Beckman or Scoville laminectomy retractors are added.

For the *abdominal approach,* Balfour retractors are added.

Cervicothoracic sympathectomy (dorsal)

Definition. Removal of the cervicothoracic chain, often from the fourth cervical to the third thoracic ganglion.

Considerations. Sympathetic denervation of the upper extremities and heart may be accomplished by cervicothoracic sympathectomy. The vasospastic phenomenon of Raynaud's disease is relieved by this procedure. It also may be beneficial in relieving intractable angina pectoris.

Setup and preparation of the patient. For the anterior approach, both the laminectomy set and rib instruments are used, plus deep retractors and a nerve stimulator. The setup for the posterior approach is as for the anterior approach, plus rib-cutting instruments, periosteal elevators, small rib retractors, a firm rubber pad, and operating table attachments for the posterolateral position.

Operative procedure

Anterior approach

1. The patient is placed in a supine position with head rotated to the opposite side as in mastoidectomy (Chapter 22). General endotracheal anesthesia is necessary, since there is a possibility of puncturing the pleura.

2. A transverse incision is made one fingerbreadth above the clavicle, the clavicular head of the sternocleidomastoid muscle is severed, and the deep cervical fascia is divided.

3. The phrenic nerve and the jugular vein are protected, and the anterior scalene muscle is divided to expose and isolate the underlying subclavian artery. The thyroid axis, one of its branches, is ligated and divided.

4. The stellate ganglion, deep against the vertebral body, is then brought into view and lifted on a nerve hook. The sympathetic chain is traced upward to the middle cervical ganglion and divided. Deep dissection behind the pleura exposes the upper thoracic ganglia, which are removed to below the third thoracic ganglion. Clips may be placed on the sympathetic nerves before their division.

5. The wound is closed according to the surgeon's preference.

Posterior approach

1. The patient is placed in the lateral position, and a paravertebral incision is centered over the third rib. The trapezius muscle is divided, and the rhomboid is split in line with its fibers. The third and fourth ribs are isolated extrapleurally, and the posterior 4 to 5 cm is resected. The transverse processes may be removed, to provide better exposure.

2. The sympathetic trunk, which lies on the anterolateral aspect of the vertebral body, is reached by carefully reflecting the pleura. The trunk is picked up on a nerve hook, traced up and down, and removed, usually from the stellate ganglion to the fourth thoracic ganglion. Clips may be applied to the nerve before severing the fibers.

3. A firm rubber tube may be left in the wound during closure. Suctioning apparatus is applied to this tube as the last deep fascial suture is drawn tight; all air is aspirated, and the tube is quickly withdrawn.

4. The subcutaneous tissue and skin edges are closed.

Thoracolumbar sympathectomy and splanchnicotomy

Definition. Through a paravertebral incision, dissection of the greater splanchnic nerve and removal of the lower sympathetic nerves from the diaphragm down to the third lumbar ganglion.

Considerations. This extensive procedure, which denervates the majority of the viscera, reduces vascular tone over such a large area that the blood pressure is markedly reduced. It has been used in the treatment of essential hypertensions. A more limited resection is used occasionally to interrupt the visceral pain pathways from the upper abdomen and to relieve the intractable pain involving the biliary tract.

Setup and preparation of the patient. The patient may be placed in a prone position, with face resting in the cerebellum headrest and shoulders slightly elevated, or in a lateral decubitus position.

Operative procedure. The operation is carried out bilaterally, usually in two stages, 10 days apart. A retropleural or retroperitoneal approach is commonly used, although some surgeons prefer a transpleural or transdiaphragmatic exposure. The classic Smithwick procedure is described.

1. A paravertebral incision is made downward from the ninth rib and curved anteriorly toward the iliac crest.

2. The latissimus dorsi muscle is divided in line with the skin incision, and the sacrospinal muscle is retracted medially to expose the eleventh and twelfth ribs. These two ribs are resected subperiosteally, leaving the intercostal neurovascular bundle intact.

3. The pleura is gently stripped off both the inner chest wall and the diaphragm by blunt dissection. The renal fascia is incised, and the retroperitoneal space is opened and enlarged to expose the undersurface of the diaphragm. The latter structure is divided down to its attachment to the vertebral bodies.

4. The greater splanchnic nerve is dissected out with a staphylorrhaphy elevator at the level at which it pierces the diaphragm. The nerve is divided as it enters the celiac plexus. It is then traced upward to the ninth rib and avulsed.

5. The sympathetic chain is similarly dissected out and traced upward, with each ramus clipped in turn with silver clips. The communicating rami are divided. Attention is directed to removing the lower sympathetic nerves from the diaphragm down to the third lumbar ganglion.

6. When all bleeding has been controlled, a large, firm rubber tube is placed in the retropleural space, and the wound is closed. A purse-string suture, which is placed around the exit of the tube, is tightened. The suction apparatus is applied to the tube to remove any remaining air in the retropleural space, and the tube is rapidly removed as the purse-string suture is tied down.

7. If the pleura has been opened during the operation, an indwelling chest tube may be inserted into the chest cavity and connected to an underwater-seal drainage set.

Lumbar sympathectomy

Considerations. Through a midflank or lower abdominal incision a lumbar sympathectomy is performed to treat such vasospastic disorders as Buerger's disease and some selected cases of vascular insufficiency secondary to peripheral arteriosclerosis. It may also be of benefit in combating excessive sweating of the feet.

Setup and preparation of the patient. The patient may be placed in a supine position if an anterior approach is to be used or in a lateral position for a posterolateral incision.

Operative procedure

1. Lumbar sympathectomy may be done transperitoneally or retroperitoneally, but the latter is more commonly used. A long McBurney type of incision or a straight or curved paramedian incision is employed.

2. The muscles are split in line with their fibers, or portions are divided to expose the retroperitoneal space.

3. The sympathetic chain is picked up on a long nerve hook and resected from above the second to below the third lumbar ganglion, clipping the rami as in a thoracolumbar sympathectomy. Deep retractors usually are necessary for adequate exposure; care is taken not to tear the lumbar veins that lie over the nerves.

4. The wound is closed in layers and dressed as for hernia repair.

Nerve repairs

Considerations. Peripheral nerve injuries are the most common indication for this surgery. Nerve tumors are rare in comparison. During wartime, injuries of nerves assume particular importance because of their frequency and disabling results.

When the continuity of a nerve is destroyed, function distal to the site of injury is lost. Recovery will occur only if regeneration of nerve axons takes place from the healthy proximal segments. These axons must grow down the axis cylinders of the nerve beyond the injury if they are to reinnervate their end organs and allow function to return.

When a nerve is divided, the cut ends retract, become scarred, and form neuromas. Regenerating axons from the proximal segment cannot bridge such a gap or penetrate the scar tissue. An unobstructed path down the axis cylinder must be made available if nerves are ever again to move muscles or transmit sensation. All procedures are directed toward obtaining the best possible conditions for regeneration.

Setup and preparation of the patient. A basic dissecting instrument set is used. Special items include the following:

Nerve stimulator
Jeweler's nerve forceps
Microsutures
Loupes
Operating microscope
Microforceps
Microscissors
Microneedle holders
Microdissectors
Tongue blades
Sterile double-edged razor blades (can be sterilized in their paper wrappers with ETO)

For lesser procedures such as spinofacial anastomosis in the neck, division of the volar carpal ligament for median nerve compression at the wrist, or repair of a small digital nerve, suitable modification may be made.

The positioning, skin preparation, and draping of the patient depend on the site of the injury. A large area is prepped.

General anesthesia is usually preferred, with the patient positioned for maximum accessibility to the injured nerve. Exposure must be adequate, since considerable mobilization of the nerve is often necessary. A dry field may be achieved by using a tourniquet on the extremities.

Operative procedure. The site of injury is explored with careful attention to hemostasis. Nerve ends are dissected from surrounding scar tissue, and neuromas are excised. Moist umbilical tapes or Penrose tubing may be passed about the nerve to handle it more easily and with less trauma.

The nerve repair (anastomosis) is made with multiple fine sutures placed only through the nerve sheath or epineurium (Fig. 24-79). Tension at the suture line is eliminated by such maneuvers as freeing up a long length of nerve on either side of the point of injury, transposition of the nerve in order to shorten its course, appropriate positioning of the extremity with plaster splinting during the postoperative period and, rarely, use of a nerve graft. Some surgeons apply a cuff of inert material such as silicone about the anastomosis.

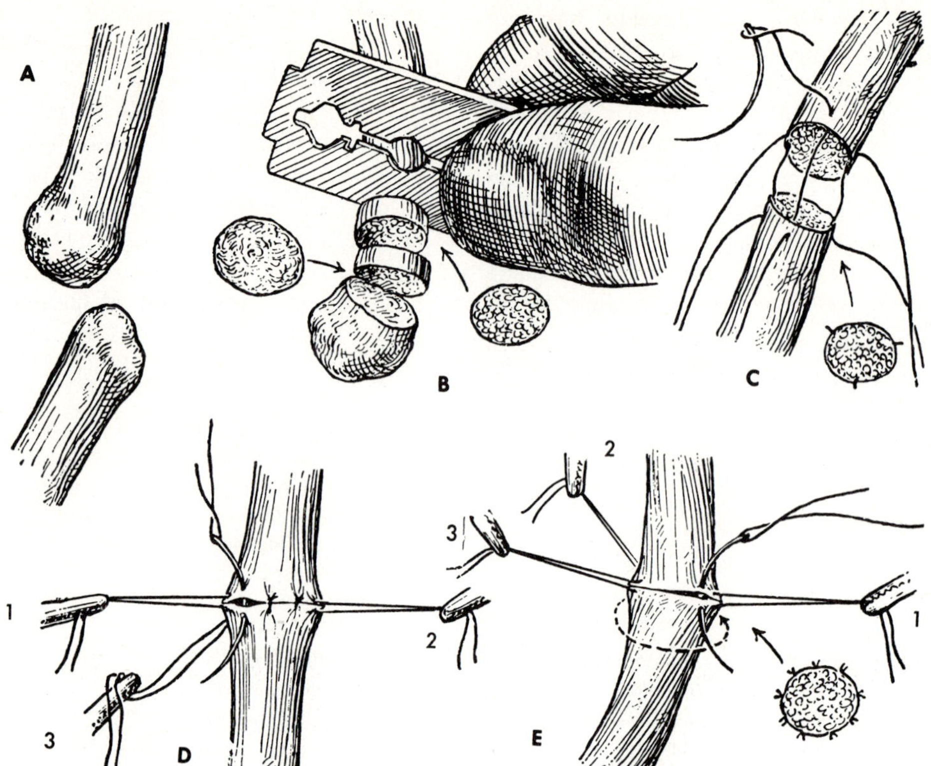

Fig. 24-79. Nerve repair. **A,** Divided nerve with neuroma. **B,** Serial resection of neuroma to healthy nerve fibers. **C,** Placement of sutures in epineurium. **D** and **E,** Approximation and tying of sutures. (From Sachs, E.: Diagnosis and treatment of brain tumors and care of the neurosurgical patient, ed. 2, St. Louis, The C.V. Mosby Co.)

Hypoglossal facial nerve anastomosis

Definition. Anastomosis performed to restore function to an injured facial nerve.

Considerations. With certain lesions in the posterior fossa and during some procedures on the posterior fossa, the facial nerve may be damaged.

Operative procedure. An incision is made over the anterior edge of the sternocleidomastoid muscle, extending from the mastoid process downward for a distance of approximately 11 to 12 cm. The fascia and muscles are divided, and further dissection is carried out until the hypoglossal nerve is exposed and divided distally. The facial nerve is exposed and divided close to its exit from the stylomastoid foramen deep to the front of the mastoid process. The proximal end of the hypoglossal nerve is anastomosed to the distal end of the facial nerve with fine arterial or nerve sutures, and the wound is closed.

Occasionally the surgeon may elect to use the accessory nerve or even the phrenic nerve instead of the hypoglossal nerve. Microsurgical techniques and instruments are used.

Carpal tunnel syndrome

Considerations. Carpal tunnel syndrome is a condition in which the median nerve is compressed by the transverse carpal ligament or by displacement of the lunate bone or a volar carpal ganglion. Decompression of the nerve is done by removing part of the roof of the fibrous sheath of the ligament or the offending bone or ganglion.

Setup and preparation of the patient. The patient is placed in the supine position with the operative arm extended on a hand table. Local, regional, or general anesthesia may be used.

Operative procedure

1. A longitudinal skin incision is made in the thenar palm crease. This runs perpendicular to and stops at the most distal transverse skin crease in the wrist. This incision generally suffices but may be extended into an L or a T.
2. A Weitlaner or mastoid retractor is placed.
3. The fibers of the carpal ligament are divided transversely in blunt fashion at the most proximal point of

exposure. A hemostat is introduced through this opening in the ligament, pointed distally, and spread. This protects the underlying median nerve. The ligament is divided between the jaws of the hemostat with a Mayo scissors.

4. After this incision has been carried well into the palm, the remaining proximal fibers of the ligament are divided in the same fashion. A small vein retractor is placed on the proximal skin edges to facilitate this step.

5. A biopsy of the ligament may be obtained.

6. The incision is closed with silk or nylon, and a bulky dressing is applied, with the fingers visible.

Ulnar nerve transposition at the elbow

Considerations. Because of traumatic or anatomical problems, the ulnar nerve may be predisposed to irritation resulting in chronic discomfort. In such instances, the position of the nerve can be changed to provide protection and comfort.

Setup and preparation of the patient. The patient is placed in the supine position. The arm may be supported in a functional position, with Webril and elastic bandages to attach it to the anesthesia screen, or it may be left free for the surgeon to manipulate during the procedure. The inner, posterior aspect of upper and lower arm must be exposed for the operation.

Operative procedure. A long incision is made, and the nerve is dissected free from the surrounding soft tissues with Metzenbaum scissors and hemostatic forceps. Moist umbilical tapes or Penrose tubing is passed around the freed segments of the nerve to aid in handling them for further dissection until a satisfactory length of nerve has been freed from above to below the elbow. The muscle and fascia entered by the nerve at each end of the field may be slit with a scissors to prevent tethering and kinking at these points after the nerve has been transposed. A flap of facia overlying the medial epicondyle of the humerus is cut and elevated, and the nerve is transposed beneath it. The fascia is then loosely reapproximated to the fascial edge remaining on the epicondyle with no. 3-0 silk. The wound is closed in layers.

An alternative procedure, medial epicondylectomy, is sometimes performed. In this case, the nerve is not dissected out, but the medial epicondyle of the humerus is removed with a rongeur, and the residual bone is waxed. The fascia and muscle tending to tether or kink the nerve, particularly distally, may be slit with a scissors, as in the transposition procedure.

SUGGESTED READINGS

Anthony C.P., and Thibodeau, G.A.: Textbook of anatomy and physiology, ed. 10, St. Louis, 1979, The C.V. Mosby Co.

Barraquer, J.: The history of the microscope in ocular surgery, J. Microsurg. **1:**288, 1980.

Batzdorf, U.: Neurosurgical approaches to the treatment of pain in cancer patients, UCLA Cancer Center Publication, p. 4, Aug./Sept. 1976.

Behrends, E.: Revascularization for intracranial stroke, AORN J. **20:**405, 1974.

Blount, M., and Kinney, A.B., editors: Symposium on neurologic and neurosurgical nursing, Nurs. Clin. North Am. **9:**591, 1974.

Buncke, H.J., Jr., and others: Techniques of microsurgery, Somerville, N.J., Ethicon, Inc.

Camunas, C.: Transsphenoidal hypophysectomy, Am. J. Nurs. **80:**1820, 1980.

Chalk, V.A.: Anterior approach to cervical fractures, dislocations and herniated nucleus pulposis, J. Neurosurg. Nurs. **5:**56, Dec. 1973.

Cloward, R.B.: Surgical techniques for lumbar disc lesions, Signature Series 3, Randolph, Mass., 1973, Codman & Shurtleff, Inc.

Cloward, R.B.: Ruptured cervical intervertebral discs, Signature Series 4, Randolph, Mass., 1974, Codman & Shurtleff, Inc.

Conway-Rutkowski, B.L.: Carini and Owens' neurological and neurosurgical nursing, ed. 8, St. Louis, 1982, The C.V. Mosby Co.

D'Agostino, J., and Pelczynski, L.: An overview of cyclotron treatment, Bragg peak proton hypophysectomy and Bragg peak radiosurgery for arteriovenous malformation of the brain, J. Neurosurg. Nurs. **11:**208, Dec. 1979.

Doolittle, N.: Arteriovenous malformations: physiology, symptomatology, and nursing care, J. Neurosurg. Nurs. **11:**221, Dec. 1979.

Ehni, G.: The surgical nurse and neurological surgery, J. Neurosurg. Nurs. **6:**7, July 1974.

Eliasson, S.G., and others: Neurological pathophysiology, New York, 1974, Oxford University Press.

Evans, J.P., and Keegan, H.R.: Danger in the use of intrathecal methylene blue, J.A.M.A. **174:**116, 1966.

Guyton, A.C.: Structure and function of the nervous system, ed. 2, Philadelphia, 1976, W.B. Saunders Co.

Handa, H., editor: Microneurosurgery, Baltimore, 1975, University Park Press.

Hardy, J.: Transsphenoidal operation of the pituitary, Signature Series 7, Randolph, Mass., 1975, Codman & Shurtleff, Inc.

Harris, L.O.: The specialized role of the neurosurgical operating room nurse, J. Neurosurg. Nurs. **12:**128, Sept. 1978.

Heidt, C.S.: The OR nurse's role in transseptal transsphenoidal hypophysectomy, RN **36:**1, July 1973.

Hoerenz, P.: The operating microscope. I. Optical principles, illumination systems, and support systems, J. Microsurg. **1:**364, 1980.

Hoerenz, P.: The operating microscope. II. Individual parts, handling, assembling, focusing, and balancing, J. Microsurg. **1:**419, 1980.

Hoerenz, P.: The operating microscope. III. Accessories, J. Microsurg. **2:**22, 1980.

Jackson, F.E., and others: A new neurosurgical drain: the Jackson-Pratt subdural "brain drain," Surg. Team, p. 23, May/June 1975.

Jackson, P.L.: Ventriculo-peritoneal shunt, Am. J. Nurs. **80:**1104, 1980.

Kaminski, D.: The microsurgical approach to acoustic neuroma, Point of View **12**(5):13, 1975.

Kildea, J., Jr.: Conquering an obstacle: pituitary, Point of View **12**(5):3, 1975.

Lamb, S.: Neuroaugmentation for the chronic pain patient, J. Neurosurg. Nurs. **11:**215, Dec. 1979.

Lamb, S.: Interstitial radiation for the treatment of brain tumors using the stereotactic method, J. Neurosurg. Nurs. **12:**138, Sept. 1980.

LeMaitre, G., and Finnegan, J.: The patient in surgery: a guide for nurses, ed. 3, Philadelphia, 1975, W.B. Saunders Co.

Mullaney, C.N.: Laser surgery in otolaryngology, Point of View **17:**6, Oct. 1980.

Netter, F.H.: Nervous system, New York, 1962, Ciba Parmaceutical Co.

Nursing care of the patient in the O.R., Somerville, N.J., 1972, Ethicon, Inc.

Ostrow, L.F.: New hope for patients with trigeminal neuralgia, Am. J. Nurs. **76**(8):130, 1976.

Pian, R.A., and others: Microsurgical treatment of 10 arteriovenous malformations in critical areas of the cerebrum, J. Microsurg. **1:**305, 1980.

Pincus, J.H., and Tucker, G.J.: Behavioral neurology, New York, 1974, Oxford University Press.

Raimondy, A.J.: Ventriculo-peritoneal shunting, Signature Series 6, Randolph, Mass., 1975, Codman & Shurtleff, Inc.

Senna, N.: Thalamotomy-stereotaxic neurosurgery, Point of View **10**(1):2, 1973.

Slaughter, J.D.: Preoperative neurosurgical diagnostic studies, Point of View **12**(5):6, 1975.

Sperry, R.W.: The great cerebral commissure, Sci. Am. **210**(1):42, 1964.

Tedesco, M.B., and others: Total nursing care of the vestibular nerve section patient, J. Neurosurg. Nurs. **12:**2, March 1980.

Weck/Heifetz intracranial aneurysm clips, Long Island City, N.Y., 1975, Edward Weck & Co., Inc.

Weisenberg, M., editor: Pain: clinical and experimental perspectives, St. Louis, 1975, The C.V. Mosby Co.

Williams, R.W.: Surgical techniques: microlumbar discectomy, Randolph, Mass., 1975, Codman & Shurtleff, Inc.

Yasargil, N.G., and others: Anatomical observations of the subarachnoid cisterns of the brain during surgery, J. Neurosurg. **44:**290, 1976.

25 Pediatric surgery

At the turn of the century the practice of medicine was conducted so that little distinction was made between the treatment of surgical conditions of the child and those of the adult.

The care of ill children has developed into a specialized area of practice known as pediatrics. Within this area, the field of pediatric surgery has evolved more recently as a concomitant discipline in health care for children. Pediatric surgery revolves around congenital malformations or defects in the newborn and diseases, primarily seen in infants and young children, that are amenable to surgical intervention. Pediatric surgery is no longer restricted to general surgery but encompasses all surgical disciplines.

The successful and rapid advancements in pediatric surgery can be attributed to the following:

1. Improved diagnostic procedures and techniques
2. A better understanding of physiological, psychological, and sociological problems affecting infants, small children, teenagers, and adolescents
3. Improved knowledge about fluid and electrolyte balance, pharmacology, and nutrition and their effects on the various pediatric age groups
4. Increased knowledge about the cause and physiology of the congenital malformations
5. Improved anesthetic agents and techniques, along with better understanding of the effects on pediatric patients
6. Improved surgical techniques with more appropriate instrumentation and support equipment
7. Implementation of more effective medical and nursing care before, during, and after surgery

The development of high-risk pregnancy centers for mothers with problem pregnancies has resulted in earlier detection of malformations in fetuses, as well as other problems. This has resulted in development of lifesaving operative procedures that can be performed in utero or immediately after delivery.

Pediatric patients are generally classified according to the following age groupings in most hospitals:

1. Neonate, or newborn: birth to 1 month of age; however, a premature infant may remain in this category until about 3 months of age
2. Infant: up to 1 year of age
3. Toddler: 1 to 3 years of age
4. Preschooler: 3 to 6 years of age
5. School-aged child: 6 to 11 years of age
6. Teenager (adolescent): 11 to 18 years of age; many hospitals consider 16 years as the upper age limit, with patients over this age considered as adults

NURSING CONSIDERATIONS

A preoperative assessment is necessary for collecting and analyzing data to be used to prepare the nursing care plan. The preoperative visit with the child and parent yields information relative to size, age, weight, physical condition, and allergies; reduces fears of the child and parent; secures their trust and cooperation; and provides an opportunity for the operating room nurse to become involved in the total care of the child.

The preoperative assessment provides the basic data by which the operating room nurse selects instruments, supplies, and equipment to be used during the surgical procedure. Although all aspects of the assessment are essential to good planning for pediatric patient care, three areas that deserve primary attention are age, weight, and height. This information is essential to modify basic routines to meet the patient's individual needs.

Many hospitals employ a multidisciplinary approach in caring for children and use parent-patient educators, play therapists, and clinical specialists to help lessen the trauma of hospitalization and surgery for the child and parents. The operating room nurse should be aware of the services available in the hospital and coordinate the multidisciplinary teaching. It is most disturbing for parents and older children to have the same questions asked over and over. The notes and other chart observations of the primary care nurse should be reviewed carefully before visiting with the child and parents.

The operating room nurse must realize that hospitalization and illness can have a profound effect on the child and other siblings. The child is primarily dependent on the parents for emotional support, and the preoperative visit must satisfy the parents as well as the child. Also, a child's thinking tends to be characterized by fantasy, which can contribute to disparity between what will actually happen and what the child thinks will happen. Parents and siblings play a significant role in helping prepare the child for the surgical experience. They should be involved in teaching that helps the patient care for himself at home, at school, or in the community.

Teaching aides such as dolls, puppets, and coloring books are most helpful in imparting information to the child. It is important to talk in a language the child understands and on the same eye level. A trip to the surgical suite is recommended for the child and parent so that they can see where the child will be during the period of separation. If such a visit is not possible, some form of audiovisual presentation is an acceptable substitute.

In addition to providing an opportunity to gather data for the operating room nursing care plan for the child, the visit should focus on alleviating fears of the unknown of the child and parents. The child's questions should be answered truthfully with no embellishments. The child will ask what he wants to know, so good judgment must be exercised when volunteering additional information.

The nurse must determine, through questioning, how much the child and parents know about the anticipated procedure. The actual operative techniques are not discussed, since each procedure is different; however, the nurse may wish to consult with the surgeon if it appears there are too many descrepancies between the parent's understandings and the projected procedure. The nurse will want to ensure that the parents and child, if old enough, understand the importance of no food and drink orders and other routines.

The trend is toward psychological preparation instead of pharmalogical preparation so parents and child must understand that the child may not be sleepy or drowsy when taken to surgery. However, the child must be assured that he will be asleep before the surgeon begins the operation and that he will not feel anything. The child should be aware of the levels of discomfort that he will feel after surgery and assured that he will feel better a few days later, if that is realistic. Parents need to be assured that the child's pain will be kept within tolerable limits. Positive, accurate reinforcement must be given. The child who knows what to expect will be less fearful of the surgical experience. The child must be able to trust the physicians and nurses and retain trust in his parents; therefore the answers to his questions must be truthful. This is especially important if the child faces several surgical experiences before the condition is corrected.

The child will normally want to know where his parents will be waiting during the surgery and why they will not be with him. An honest explanation must be given. Parents will want to know how soon and where they can see their child after surgery and where and when the surgeon will visit and discuss the results.

The operating room nurse caring for pediatric patients must be knowledgeable about the needs of patients ranging from the newborn to the adolescent. The child's physiological responses are geared toward rapid growth and development. This means that illness and the response to an operation affect and are affected by this young physiological state. Metabolic rates of children are high and necessitate corresponding increases in calories and fluids. The stress of surgery adds to these demands.

Moreover, the child is undergoing continued developmental psychological and emotional changes. These changes may be heightened by illness and surgery. All events in the life of a child become integral parts in the cycle of growth and development. Therefore, to minimize the disruptive effect of surgical intervention on the child's life, participation in pediatric surgery requires knowledge of advanced operating room nursing practices, the effects of anesthetic agents on children of various ages, and an understanding of the child's normal growth and developmental pattern.

The operating room must be in total readiness before the arrival of the child. Since a child is never left unattended in the operating suite, it is best to leave the child with the parents until all team members have completed preliminary preparations.

The child should be met on arrival in the suite by the operating room nurse, who will need to do an immediate assessment of the child's condition, establish positive identification, verify the proposed operative site, and check for a legal informed operative consent signed by the parents or guardian before taking the child into the operating room. The nurse must be free to administer nursing care and give gentle and sensitive emotional support to the child during the preparatory and induction stages of anesthesia.

The goals, considerations, and nursing actions that should be a basic part of the nurses' planning for each child are outlined in Table 5.

Ambulatory surgery

Many pediatric patients can be safely managed as ambulatory or day surgery patients. This type of management is normally used with essentially well children who have a physical defect that needs correcting. Since the child is not required to spend the night in the hospital, the emotional aspects associated with hospitalization and surgery, as well as separation anxiety, are lessened. Among the procedures acceptable for this type of care are repair of hernias; circumcisions; cystoscopy; eye muscle procedures; adenoidectomy; myringotomy with placement of grommets; extraction of molars; dental procedures; repair of hydroceles; examinations under anesthesia; closed reduction of fractures; excision of moles, skin tumors, and lesions; and minor scar revisions.

On the day before surgery, the child receives a preoperative workup that includes laboratory tests, a medical history, a physical examination, and the reason for an operation. A nursing assessment is performed, and teaching for home care by parents is started. The parent receives detailed written preoperative instructions, especially related to the last time for food and drink.

After the operation, the child is taken to the recovery room for monitoring until vital signs are stable and the effects of anesthesia have diminished. Normally the child is ready to go home after discharge from the recovery room.

While the child is recovering from anesthesia, the parents receive oral and written instructions for home care.

Table 5. Nursing goals, considerations, and actions in pediatric surgery

Goals	Considerations	Nursing actions
A. To maintain body temperature at a normal level during the surgical experience	1. An infant's shivering reflex is underdeveloped and therefore he may be unable to control body temperature. 2. Body temperature of 37° C (98.6° F) should be maintained to prevent hyperthermia or hypothermia. 3. Young children adjust rapidly to external temperatures; therefore constant monitoring of body temperature is essential. Wide temperature variations may occur. Anesthesia can cause vasodilatation and heat loss. 4. Infants to 1 month of age should be monitored by way of the axilla to lessen danger of rectal perforation. 5. Prepping and draping procedures can require total body exposure, in some instances, to the room temperature.	1. Adjust room air conditioning to acceptable temperature approximately an hour before arrival of patient: 26° to 27° C for infants and newborns; 23° to 24° C for older child. 2. Place circulating water mattress on operating table, and adjust water temperature to circulate at 38° to 40° C. 3. Provide radiant heat lamp for use during placement of monitoring lines, induction of anesthesia, positioning, prepping, and draping. 4. Transport critically ill infants in incubator to lessen danger of temperature fluctuation. 5. Warm blankets, prepping towels, and irrigation and other solutions to body temperature before using. 6. Provide stockinette covers for arms and legs during preparatory procedures to help reduce heat loss. 7. Use blood warmer for administration of blood and blood products; temperature setting should not exceed 38° C. 8. Provide for constant monitoring of body temperature by rectal, esophageal, tympanic membrane, or axillary probes.
B. To assist in maintenance of total blood volume through replacement of fluid and blood loss as needed	1. Total blood volume of infants is considerably less than that of older children and adults, especially when considered in relation to total body mass. 2. Accurate fluid loss must be calculated and replaced in minute quantities as needed. 3. Loss of fluids is not tolerated well in infants and children and can result in dehydration, whereas too much fluid replacement can result in lung congestion. 4. Blood components, rather than whole blood, are normally transfused because of small volumes needed; this provides child with product actually needed while controlling volume administered. 5. Blood and fluid replacement can be anticipated as follows: a. Loss of 10% total blood volume: normally intravenous fluid replacement with possibility of blood being used.	1. Calculate estimated total blood volume using formula of 85 to 90 ml per kilogram of body weight, if total blood volume has not been determined by laboratory tests. 2. Provide gram scales for weighing used sponges as discarded from the operative field; 1 gm added weight = 1 ml loss (Chapter 4). 3. Provide suction units with reservoirs that measure loss in 5- or 10-ml increments. 4. Measure and record quantity of irrigating fluid usage when computing loss figure. 5. Provide intravenous fluids and equipment as follows: a. For children 2 years of age and under: 250-ml containers. b. For older children: 500-ml containers. c. Attach volume control measuring sets to all intravenous lines. 6. Provide blood transfusion equipment as follows: a. Volume control transfusion set. b. Blood-warming unit with coil.

Continued

Table 5. Nursing goals, considerations, and actions in pediatric surgery—cont'd

Goals	Considerations	Nursing actions
	b. Loss of 15% total blood volume: probable replacement with blood or blood product, depending on status or progress of procedure. c. Loss of 20% total blood volume: transfusion necessary.	c. Add 10-ml syringe and three-way stopcock to transfusion set to provide milliliter-for-milliliter replacement on small child. 7. Record blood drawn for laboratory tests during procedure and add to loss figure. 8. Add 25% of measured loss figure to compensate for blood and fluid loss on drapes, gowns, etc.
C. To facilitate placement of intravenous and/or monitoring lines	1. A child's veins are small and often fragile; previous lines may have been inserted, thereby reducing number of available vessels. 2. Flexible cannulas rather than rigid shaft needles should be used to lessen the danger of penetrating opposite wall of vein. 3. It may be necessary to perform venous cutdown. 4. Lines may be needed for monitoring arterial pressure, central venous pressure, and electrocardiogram, as well as for infusions and transfusions.	1. Consult with anesthesiologist to determine monitoring needs. 2. Provide flexible cannulas in sizes 18 to 24 Fr and in varying lengths. 3. Have venous cutdown equipment in operating room for use if needed. 4. Set up and have readily available intravenous "keep-open" fluids for connecting as soon as line is in place.
D. To place cautery pad (indifferent electrode) so as not to interfere with the operative site, yet facilitate effective hemostasis while providing an electrically safe environment	1. Electrosurgery is an effective means of hemostasis and of expediting procedure, which helps reduce anesthesia time. 2. Infants and small children have less body mass than older children and adults; therefore area of sufficient mass for proper conduction is often difficult to obtain; bony structures are to be avoided. 3. Grounding pad should not interfere with measures applied to control body temperature. 4. Grounding pad must not interfere with operative site. 5. Grounding pad must be protected during preparation to prevent it from becoming wet with prepping solution. 6. Excessive pressure when applying an adhesive type of pad can result in skin irritation or abrasion when pad is removed.	1. Select appropriate size of adhesive grounding pad that can be molded to fit body contour and provide sufficient body mass coverage for proper conduction. 2. Place pad on shoulder, buttocks, thigh, or lengthwise on arm or leg. 3. Apply pad with firm but gentle pressure in area as close as possible to operative site, but positioned so that current will not pass through heart muscle. 4. Place pad so that child does not lie on cord/pad connector.
E. To select positioning, preparation, and draping techniques that expedite the procedures and provide for patient safety	1. Operative site often necessitates total or near total body exposure for preparation of newborns and small children. 2. Body supports of operating table are not normally suited for anatomical configuration of infants and children. 3. Regular armboards and patient restraint straps are not normally used. 4. Headrests and foot rests may be removed to provide closer access to the child.	1. Incorporate temperature control measures into procedures. 2. Plan to have two-person team do prep to expedite procedure when extensive preparation is required. 3. Do not permit prepping solution to pool under child. 4. Make body supports, to conform to size of child, from rolled diapers, towels, or sheets or small, flexible sandbags or foam

Table 5—cont'd

Goals	Considerations	Nursing actions
	5. Weight of drapes can place some infants in compromised position. 6. Many infants and small children are allergic to adhesive mast, so care must be exercised when using self-adhering drapes or adhesive tape to better expose operative site. 7. Skin preparation seldom includes shaving, except for cranial surgery.	rolls. Use inflatable bag or rolled sheet in place of kidney rest; use rolled towel for neck or shoulder support. 5. Provide flexible ether screen to permit better visualization of operative field for anesthesiologist. 6. Provide infant armboards or use padded tongue depressors to stabilize limbs containing intravenous lines. 7. Position Mayo stand over child's legs and lower part of table to help support drapes and prevent accidental leaning on patient. 8. Use nonwoven drapes, where possible, to reduce drape weight. 9. Have available nonallergenic or paper tape for use as needed.

INSTRUMENTS AND SUPPLIES

Basically, the same type of instruments are used in pediatric surgery as in adult surgery. However, the instruments are normally shorter, have more delicate or less pronounced curves, and are lighter in weight. A complete range of sizes of instruments is necessary so that the appropriate size for each child is available. Fewer instruments are normally required because of shorter length and decreased depth of the incision. Basic instrument sets, based on types of surgeries performed, aid in facilitating instrument counts. These sets are easily adapted to meet the patient's needs, as well as conform to the surgeon's preferences, yet eliminate unnecessary instruments from the sterile field.

The following sets are examples of basic instrumentation used in pediatric surgery. The *minor set* is useful when minimal instrumentation is required. The *basic set* is sufficient for a herniorrhaphy, appendectomy, pyloromyotomy, anoplasty, or comparable procedure; it can also be used in conjunction with specialty instruments for basic dissection and clamping needs. The *abdominal set* is used for major abdominal procedures either alone or in conjunction with special instruments.

Smaller and larger instruments should be packaged separately and opened only when needed.

MINOR SET

Cutting instruments

2 Knife handles no. 3 with nos. 10 and 15 blades
1 Lahey scissors, delicate, curved, 5¾ inches
1 Dissecting scissors, straight, 5½ inches, blunt tips
1 Iridectomy scissors, curved, sharp, 4 inches

Holding instruments

4 Towel clamps, 3 inches
1 Dressing forceps, delicate, serrated tip, 5 inches
1 Dressing forceps, delicate, teeth, 5 inches
1 Adson forcep, serrated tip, 4¾ inches
2 Allis forceps, 4 × 5 teeth, 6 inches
2 Babcock forceps, 6¼ inches

Clamping instruments

8 Mosquito forceps, curved, 5 inches
4 Mosquito forceps, straight, 5 inches
4 Crile hemostats, curved, 5½ inches
1 Rochester-Pean forcep, curved, 7¼ inches

Retractors

2 Cushing vein retractors
2 Senn retractors

Suturing items

2 Crile-Wood needle holders, light, 6 inches

Accessory items

2 Medicine cups, stainless steel

BASIC SET

Cutting instruments

2 Knife handles no. 3 with nos. 10 and 15 blades
1 Metzenbaum scissors, 5½ inches
1 Dissecting scissors, straight, 5½ inches, blunt tips
1 Lahey scissors, 6 inches

Holding instruments

4 Towel clamps, 3 inches
2 Dressing forceps, delicate, serrated tip, 5 inches

1 Dressing forceps, delicate, 1 × 2 teeth, 5 inches
1 Adson forcep, serrated tip, 4¾ inches
2 Adson forceps, 1 × 2 mouse tooth, 4¾ inches
1 Tuttle tissue forcep
4 Allis forceps, 4 × 5 teeth, 6 inches
2 Babcock forceps, 6¼ inches
1 Sponge-holding forceps, 8 inches

Clamping instruments

16 Mosquito forceps, curved, 5 inches
6 Mosquito forceps, straight, 5 inches
6 Crile hemostats, curved, 5½ inches
2 Rochester-Pean forceps, curved, 7¼ inches
2 Mixters, right angle, delicate, 7 inches

Retractors

2 Richardson retractors, 9½ inches, ¾ × 1–inch blade
2 Richardson retractors, 9½ inches, 1 × 1¼–inch blade
2 Cushing vein retractors
2 Love retractors

Suturing items

2 Sarot needle holders, delicate, 7¼ inches
2 Mayo-Hegar needle holders, 6 inches

Accessory items

1 Poole suction tube, infant
3 Medicine cups, stainless steel

ABDOMINAL SET

Cutting instruments

2 Knife handles no. 3
2 Knife blades no. 10
2 Knife blades no. 15
1 Knife blade no.11
1 Metzenbaum scissors, curved, 7 inches
1 Lahey scissors, curved, 6½ inches
1 Mayo suture scissors, 5½ inches

Holding instruments

6 Towel clamps, 3 inches
2 DeBakey pickup forceps, 5 inches
2 Dressing forceps with teeth, 5½ inches
2 Dressing forceps without teeth, 5½ inches
2 Adson forceps, 1× 2 teeth, 4¾ inches
2 Adson forceps, serrated tip, 4¾ inches
1 Cushing forceps, 1 × 2 teeth, 7 inches
1 Cushing forceps, serrated tip, 7 inches
2 Tuttle forceps
2 Sponge-holding forceps, straight, 8 inches
2 Babcock forceps, 6¼ inches
6 Allis forceps, 4 × 5 teeth, 6 inches
2 Intestinal forceps, 8½ inches

Clamping instruments

24 Mosquito forceps, curved, 5 inches
8 Mosquito forceps, straight, 5 inches
8 Crile Hemostats, curved, 5½ inches
2 Rochester-Pean forceps, curved, 7¼ inches
4 Munions, curved
6 Mixters, delicate, right angle
4 Mixters, regular, right angle
2 Oschner forceps, straight, 7¼ inches

Retractors

3 Richardson retractors, 9½ inches long: 1 × ¾–inch, 1 × 1¼–inch, and 1½ × 1½–inch blades
2 Cushing vein retractors
3 Malleable retractors, ½, ⅝, and ¾ × 9 inches
2 Deaver retractors, ⅞ and 1 inch wide

Suturing items

2 Sarot needle holders, delicate, 7¼ inches
2 Mayo needle holders, 8 inches
2 Mayo needle holders, 6 inches

Accessory items

1 Poole suction tube, regular
1 Poole suction tube, infant
3 Medicine cups, stainless steel

Sutures

The smaller sizes of both absorbable and nonabsorbable sutures are used. Large-diameter sutures are not normally required or appropriate for the more delicate or fragile tissue of the infant or child. Sutures should have attached needles (atraumatic) to reduce tissue damage. The most common sizes are nos. 000 to 5-0 with ½- and ⅜-circle curved needles. Staples, both pediatric and regular sizes, are often used internally. Many skin incisions are closed with subcutaneous suture, using a subcuticular method, followed by application of paper adhesive dressing strips or collodion.

Sponges

All gauze, 4 × 4 inches, 16 ply x-ray detectable
Laparotomy pads, 12 × 12 inches, x-ray detectable, prewashed
Kittner or peanut sponges

Catheters

Indwelling, retention type:
6 and 8 Fr with 3-cc bag
8 through 14 Fr with 5-cc bag
Ureteral: 4 and 5 Fr with connectors for attaching to closed ureteral drainage systems

OPERATIONS

Several surgical procedures that may be designated pediatric have been presented in previous chapters of this book under particular specialty headings. Following are several other frequently encountered procedures.

Venous cutdown

Definition. Exposure and cannulation of a vein to administer intravenous fluids or blood, infuse vasoactive drugs, measure central venous or right atrial pressure, or administer parenteral venous alimentation.

Considerations. The small size of children's veins and their location in subcutaneous tissue make venipuncture difficult. Direct placement of the catheter ensures proper infusion and decreases the possibility of infiltration. Venous cutdown may be done preoperatively or in conjunction with surgery after induction. Veins frequently used for cutdowns in infants are the saphenous, antecubital, and external and internal jugular.

Setup and preparation of the patient. The area is prepped in the manner previously described and draped with four towels. The instrument tray includes the following:

1 Knife handle no. 3 with nos. 11 and 15 blades
6 Mosquito forceps, 3 curved and 3 straight
2 Adson forceps, 1 plain and 1 with teeth
2 Scissors, fine, 1 curved and 1 straight
Plastic catheter
4 Towel clamps
1 Needle holder
1 Suture no. 5-0 on cutting needle
Fine absorbable suture for ties

Operative procedure

1. A 1-cm transverse incision is made through the skin only, anterior and about 1 cm proximal to the medial malleolus.

2. By blunt dissection with a curved mosquito clamp, the vein is isolated, and a fine, absorbable suture is passed around it.

3. While the suture maintains traction on the vein, a V-shaped nick is made in the vein with the scissors. The plastic catheter is threaded into the vein. The distal suture ligates the vein to prevent venous bleeding; the proximal suture ties the catheter in the vein.

4. The external end of the catheter is connected to the infusion set.

5. The skin edges are approximated with interrupted sutures no. 5-0 on a cutting needle, and a firm pressure dressing is applied.

6. Arm or leg restraints may be necessary.

Intravenous alimentation

Considerations. Total intravenous alimentation is performed on infants and children whose lives are threatened because feeding through the gastrointestinal tract is impossible, inadequate, or hazardous. Common conditions for use are bowel fistulas, inadequate intestinal length, chronic diarrhea, and extensive burns.

Although total intravenous alimentation is used to replenish the malnourished child, it may be started prophylactically if prolonged starvation is expected.

The fluids are delivered through a central venous catheter to avoid peripheral venous inflammation and thrombosis. The fluid concentrations are adjusted to the needs of the individual.

Setup and preparation of the patient. Instruments and supplies include the following:

Minor instrument set plus small delicate vascular clamps
Vessel dilator
Catheter introducer
Radiopaque silicone catheter, such as Broviac
2 Skin hooks
Injectable saline solution
Radiographic dye, such as Hypaque
Syringes and needles, assorted sizes
Dextrose, 10% in water, 500 ml, or special formula solution
Infusion pump and infusion tubing set for alimentation fluid
Nonabsorbable sutures (silk, nylon, or Prolene), size 5-0 on cutting needle and for free ties

A disposable warming mattress placed over the x-ray plate before positioning the child helps eliminate excessive moving of the patient when the placement of the catheter is checked during radiography.

More than one type and size of catheter are normally available. It is essential that the nurse consult with the surgeon as to the type and size of catheter as well as insertion site in order to determine positioning. A common insertion site is the right external jugular vein.

The manufacturer's instructions for handling, preparation, and sterilization of the catheter must be followed. The catheter must not come in contact with linty materials, glove powder, or other foreign matter.

The infusion solution, special formula or dextrose 10% in water, must be started as soon as the catheter is secured to prevent air bubbles from entering the circulatory system and clotting the catheter.

Operative procedure

1. The procedure is essentially a venous cutdown of a major vessel for the purpose of inserting and positioning the catheter in the vena cava just above the atrium.

2. Proper position of the catheter must be confirmed by radiography.

3. The catheter is then secured to the skin with a nonabsorbable suture.

4. The skin is closed with interrupted sutures. Antibacterial ointment and dressing are applied to the skin exit site.

5. The infusion pump is connected to the infusing solution before moving the child from the operating suite.

Tracheostomy

Definition. Neck incision into the trachea, normally at the level of the thyroid isthmus, for the purpose of inserting a tracheostomy tube to establish a permanent or semipermanent airway.

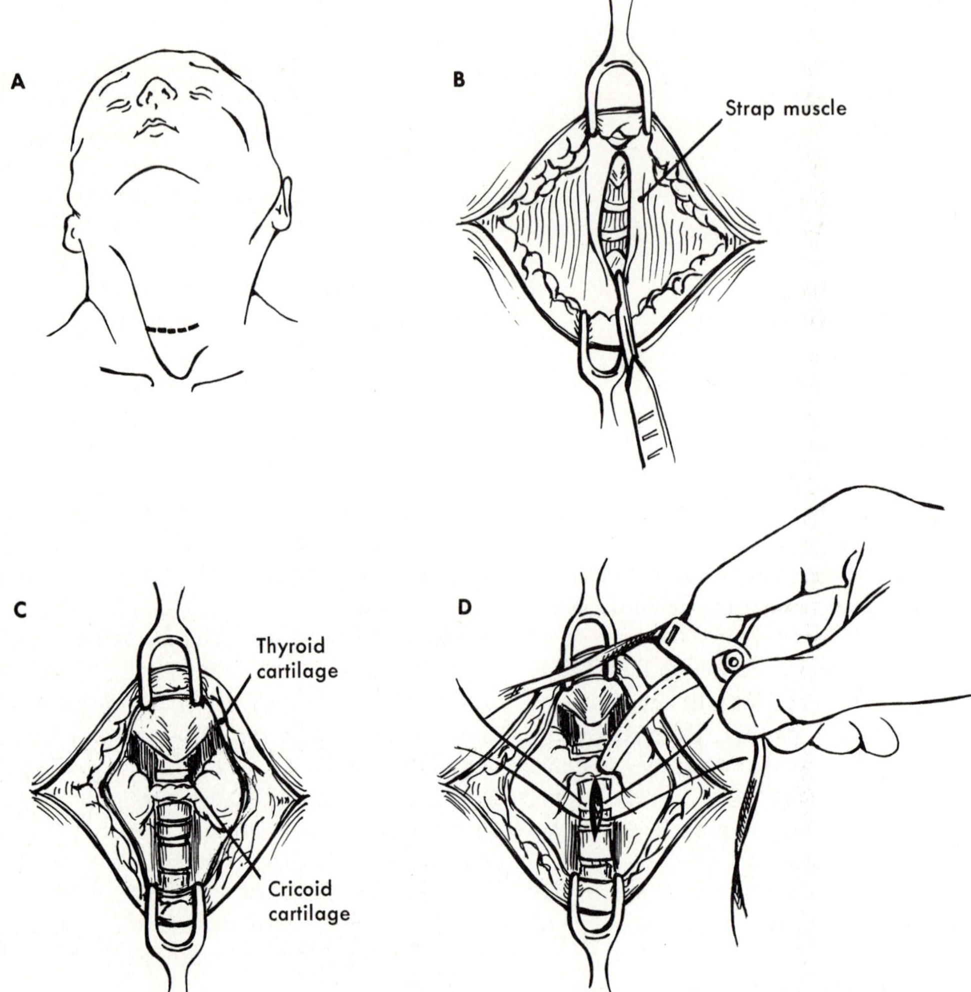

Fig. 25-1. Tracheostomy procedure. **A,** Skin incision. **B,** Isthmus divided. **C,** Incision made, and wound spread. **D,** Tube inserted.

Indications

1. Newborn
   a. Congenital malformations and neoplasms of the upper airway
   b. Long-term ventilatory support for respiratory distress syndrome or chronic neurological conditions
   c. Subglottic stenosis
2. Infants and children
   a. Airway obstruction
   b. Inability to extubate following airway support for croup or epiglottiditis
   c. Long-term ventilatory support problems associated with postoperative respiratory failure or conditions such as Guillain-Barré syndrome

Considerations

1. Is normally an elective procedure when used in conjunction with long-term ventilatory problems to replace an endotracheal airway tube
2. Considered an acute emergency procedure when necessary to provide an airway in acute epiglottiditis or croup
3. May be a secondary procedure when performed in conjunction with other operative procedures, particularly head and neck surgeries
4. Should be performed in the operating suite under general anesthesia

Setup and preparation of the patient. Instrumentation is according to age. A selection of pediatric-sized tubes is provided: the shorter, less curved tube is more appropriate for infants; metal or plastic tubes may be used; cuffed plastic tubes are normally used for long-term mechanical ventilation; and 00 to 6 Fr sizes should be available.

The patient is placed in the supine position with the neck hyperextended. A small roll or sandbag is placed under the shoulders to facilitate palpation of the trachea. The head is maintained in the midline position with sandbags on each side of it.

Operative procedure (Fig. 25-1)

1. The neck is incised (midline) at the level of the thyroid isthmus after the trachea is identified.

2. Hemostasis is maintained during the spreading of strap muscles and dissection of pretracheal fascia and tracheal ring. Long no. 3-0 Prolene stay sutures are used for tracheal cartilage.

3. The tracheostomy tube is inserted in the vertical midline incision of the trachea. Stay sutures are taped to the upper chest and remain in place for approximately a week; lateral traction on stay sutures provides for rapid reinsertion of the tube if it is accidentally dislodged.

4. The tracheostomy tube tie is placed with the knot at the back of the neck so that the infant cannot reach and untie it.

5. The tracheostomy dressing is applied after the tube is connected to ventilation equipment.

Repair of atresia of the esophagus

Definition. Through a right retropleural thoracotomy, closure of the tracheoesophageal fistula and anastomosis of the segments of the esophagus.

Considerations. This congenital anomaly may arise between the third and sixth weeks of fetal life. Four types are recognized, the most common being an upper segment of esophagus ending in a blind pouch and a lower segment of esophagus communicating by a fistula with the trachea. Ideally, this defect is recognized in the first hours of life, but more often the diagnosis is made in the first 36 to 48 hours of life. Prompt surgical intervention allows the child to breathe and eat without the danger of aspirating mucus, saliva, feedings, or stomach contents.

A gastrostomy may be done first to decompress the air-distended stomach, thus facilitating chest movement and ventilation and preventing reflux of stomach contents into the trachea.

Setup and preparation of the patient. The abdominal set is required, plus a pediatric chest tray, which includes the following:

1 Infant rib spreader
2 Sarot needle holders
1 Rongeur
1 Stille elevator
1 Dura elevator
1 Pediatric rib shears
1 Potts-Smith vascular scissors
1 Metzenbaum scissors, 7 inches
1 Scissors, straight, 7 inches
1 DeBakey forceps, 7 inches
2 Potts-Smith forceps, 7 inches
1 Cushing forceps, 7 inches

Accessory items

Small Penrose drain
Umbilical tape
Bone wax
Electrocautery

The infant is positioned for a right thoracotomy. Skin preparation and draping are carried out.

Operative procedure

1. The chest is entered retropleurally, and the fifth rib is resected (Fig. 25-2, *A* and *B*).

2. The pleura is dissected (Fig. 25-2, *C*). A ribbon retractor holds the lung, covered by the pleura, out of the operating field. The azygos vein is divided.

3. Tracheoesophageal fistula is ligated, by tying a silk no. 0 ligature around the fistula.

4. A silk no. 2-0 suture is placed through the muscle of the distal esophagus beyond the former ligature and is sewn to the muscle of the upper pouch, bringing the two portions of esophagus together.

5. The distal esophagus is opened, and a matching opening is made into the upper pouch at its distal end.

Anastomosis is accomplished with interrupted silk no. 3-0 sutures (Fig. 25-2, *D*).

6. The incision is irrigated. A small Penrose drain is inserted close to the anastomosis and is brought out through the lateral corner of the wound.

7. The wound is closed with chromic no. 3-0 sutures. No water-seal drainage is necessary. After surgery a chest x-ray film is obtained in the operating room.

Correction of congenital diaphragmatic hernia

Definition. Replacement of the displaced viscera into the abdominal cavity and surgical correction of the defect (Fig. 25-3).

Considerations. The conventional surgical repair is through the abdomen. The concurrence of intraabdominal abnormalities is somewhat high in babies with diaphragmatic hernia, and the treatment is facilitated with an abdominal approach. It is technically easier to extract the viscera from below than to push them out of the thorax. The abnormal intrathoracic intrusion of the abdominal viscera usually causes severe compromise of intrathoracic pulmonary and vascular activities. Therefore urgent restoration of more normal intrathoracic and intraabdominal relationships is the rule in these newborns.

The lung may be hypoplastic because of prolonged compression in utero by the displaced abdominal viscera. A residual intrapleural space usually remains for a few days after surgery. A chest tube can be inserted and connected to water-seal drainage. Insertion of a gastrostomy tube minimizes postoperative distension and facilitates feeding. Direct suturing of the margins of the defect is usually possible. Insertion of a prosthetic Silastic sheeting is rarely required, but the sheeting should be available.

Setup and preparation of the patient. The abdominal set is required, plus the following:

Electrocautery
Small-sized chest tubes
Umbilical tape
Mushroom catheter
Reinforced Silastic sheeting should be available

Operative procedure

1. A left rectus incision is made. The liver is held to the side with small Deaver or malleable retractors.

2. The viscera are withdrawn from the chest and held downward through the abdominal wound.

3. A small catheter may be inserted into the pleural cavity, and the diaphragm is repaired with a row of fine silk sutures.

4. The flap of the diaphragmatic edge is tacked down over the initial line of sutures with a second row of fine silk sutures.

5. The chest tube is left in place and is brought out through the abdominal wall.

6. The abdomen is closed.

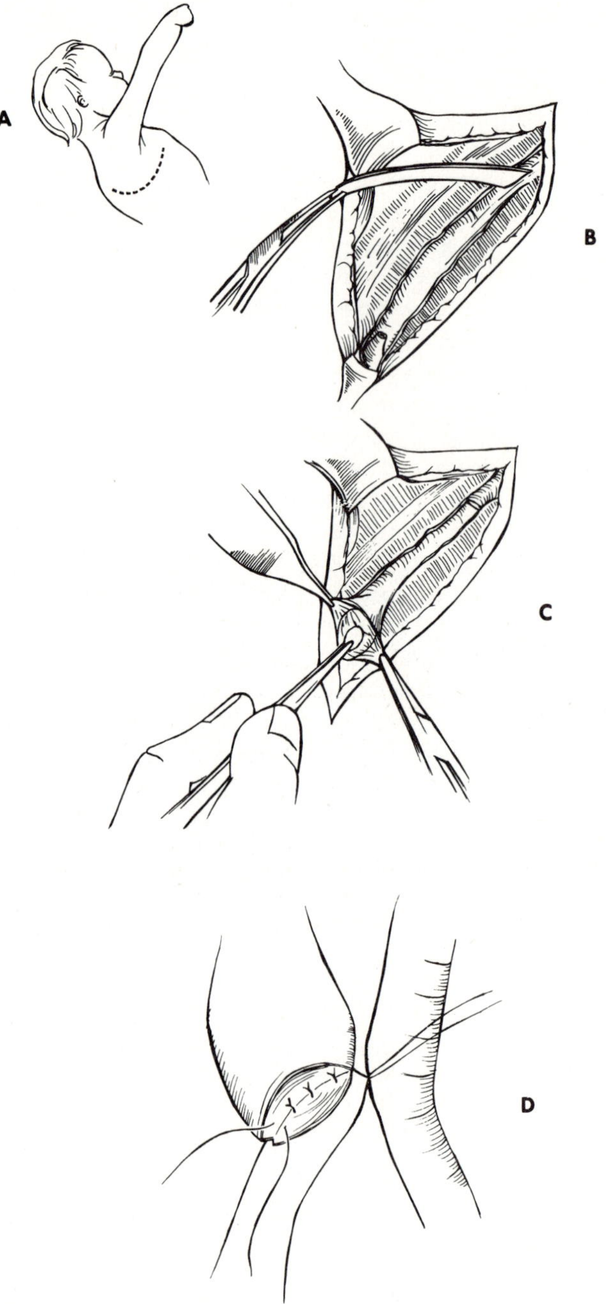

Fig. 25-2. Repair of tracheoesophageal fistula. **A,** Right thoracotomy. **B,** Rib resection. **C,** Pleural separation. **D,** End-to-end anastomosis. (Adapted from Lewis, J.E.: Atlas of infant surgery, St. Louis, The C.V. Mosby Co.)

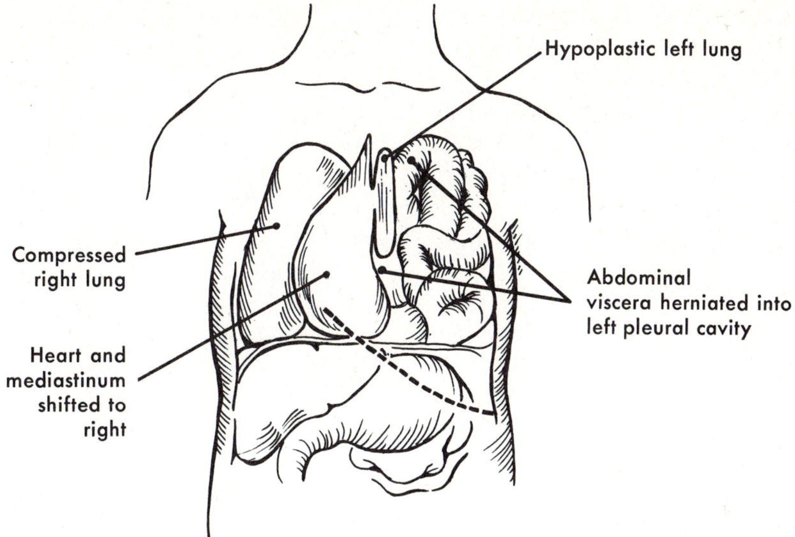

Fig. 25-3. Diaphragmatic hernia.

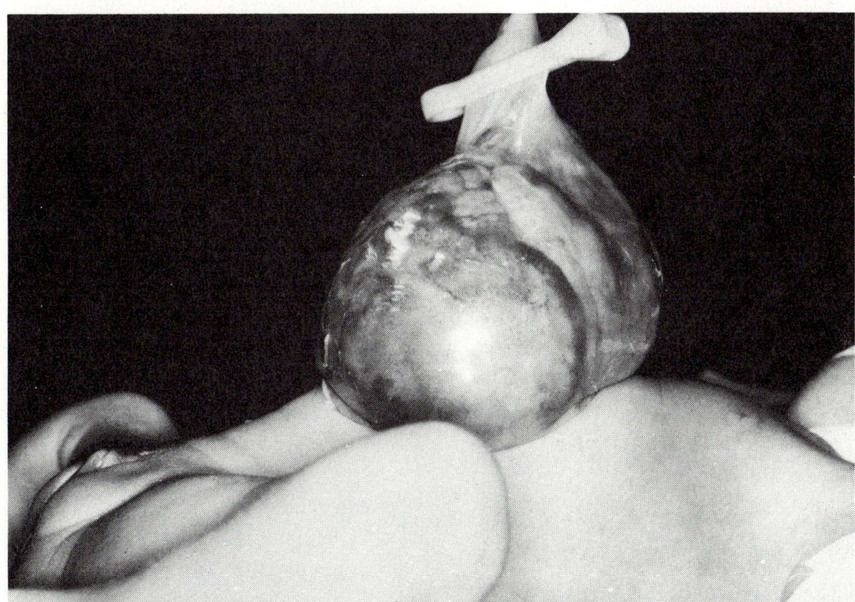

Fig. 25-4. Omphalocele containing liver. (Courtesy John R. Campbell, University of Oregon Health Sciences Center, Portland, Ore.; from Jensen, M.D., Benson, R.C., and Bobak, I.M.: Maternity care: the nurse and the family, ed. 2, St. Louis, 1981, The C.V. Mosby Co.)

Omphalocele repair

Definition. Replacement of the viscera in the abdominal cavity and reconstruction of the abdominal wall.

Considerations. Omphalocele is the protrusion of abdominal viscera outside the abdomen into a sac of amniotic membrane and peritoneum at the base of the umbilical cord (Fig. 25-4). There is no skin covering.

Omphalocele occurs when the viscera fail to withdraw from the exocoelomic position and occupy the peritoneal cavity. Treatment at birth consists of applying warm saline packs on the sac surface and the insertion of a nasogastric tube to prevent distension. Surgical intervention is necessary to prevent rupture of the sac and/or infection. If intrauterine rupture of the sac has occurred, the newly delivered child is kept warm, the bowel is inspected for perforation and torsion, and moist warm dressings are applied.

Setup and preparation of the patient. The infant is prepared as discussed previously. The abdominal set is used.

Operative procedure. The sac is protectively covered, and the abdominal wall integrity is established in one of several ways:

1. In the presence of small defects, the skin edges can be freed, the fascia separated, the sac and contents relocated in the abdomen, and the fascial and skin layers closed.

2. In the presence of larger defects, the skin edges are freed, and flaps are created. These skin flaps are closed over the sac. Reoperation within a few weeks is done to place the viscera within the abdomen under the rectus muscles and fascia.

3. Omphaloceles encompassing most of the abdomen and possibly containing the liver and/or spleen are not easily replaced within the potential abdominal space. Of prime importance is the need for protective covering of the exposed sac and viscera. One technique is the insertion of a sterile Silastic sheeting over the sac and under the skin edges that have been freed. If the defect is too large to allow approximation of the skin edges, the Silastic sheeting may be left exposed. Subsequently, it and the surrounding abdomen are dressed with a 0.5% solution of silver nitrate that inhibits bacterial growth. This does not seem to affect the infant's electrolyte balance. During the ensuing weeks, the exposed sheeting is constricted to slowly return the whole viscera to the abdominal cavity. The abdominal wall is repaired in a later operation.

Another technique for treating large omphaloceles is the painting of the sac and surrounding skin with a 2% solution of merbromin (Mercurochrome) until an eschar forms to add strength to the sac and resist infection, or the sac may be treated with moist 0.5% silver nitrate dressings. The sac membrane gradually contracts, and skin closes the abdominal wall defect. Later surgery then repairs the abdominal musculature.

Umbilical hernia repair

Definition. Repair of protrusion of part of the intestine at the umbilicus. The umbilical hernia is always covered by skin.

Considerations. Small umbilical hernias may be left untreated. They usually close within a few months to a year.

Setup and preparation of the patient. A basic set is required.

The infant is prepared as discussed previously.

Operative procedure

1. An incision is made below the umbilicus through the skin and subcutaneous tissue.

2. Flaps of skin and subcutaneous tissue are mobilized and held back with small retractors to expose the rectus fascia and hernial swelling.

3. Between the rectus sheaths in the midline is the hernial sac, which is completely freed from all surrounding structures.

4. The sac is excised.

5. The peritoneum is closed with a continuous suture.

6. The two edges of the rectus fascia are brought together with interrupted no. 3-0 nonabsorbable sutures.

7. Subcuticular closure of the skin with a continuous, fine, absorbable suture is performed, and a pressure dressing is applied.

Inguinal hernia repair

Definition. Repair of protrusion of a hernial sac, containing the intestine, in the inguinal canal.

Considerations. The testis develops high on the posterior wall of the abdomen. It gradually descends into the scrotum. Before the testis enters the inguinal canal, the processus vaginalis projects downward but retains a communication with the peritoneal cavity. The upper part of the processus does not; the sac remains an indirect inguinal hernia. In the female, a similar hernial sac is contiguous with the round ligament.

Setup and preparation of the patient. A basic set is used.

Routine preparation is done.

Operative procedure

1. A transverse incision is made over the inguinal area in the direction of the skin crease.

2. The subcutaneous tissue is opened, and hemostats are placed on bleeders, which are then ligated.

3. Right-angle retractors are placed inferiorly and medially.

4. The external ring is identified, and the external oblique fascia is cleaned and freed with small Metzenbaum scissors.

5. The external oblique fascia is opened with a no. 15 knife blade, and the upper flap is freed. The lower flap is freed to expose the inguinal ligament.

6. Cord structures are opened at the upper end of the cord. Two pairs of forceps are used to grasp tissues at the same level and separate them.

7. The hernial sac is grasped with a hemostat, and structures of the cord are bluntly peeled downward and away from the sac with forceps until the sac is freed.

8. After the sac is opened and the surgeon's index finger inserted, maintaining upward traction with not more than three hemostats, the sac is pulled upward.

9. The sac is ligated with silk no. 3-0, and excess sac is removed. Repair of the inguinal canal may be done with silk sutures.

10. The subcutaneous tissue is closed with interrupted, fine sutures; closure of the skin is with fine, nonabsorbable subcuticular sutures. Collodion or paper adhesive dressing strips are applied.

Ramstedt-Fredet pyloromyotomy for pyloric stenosis

Definition. Excision of the muscles of the pylorus to treat congenital hypertrophy of the pyloric sphincter obstructing the stomach.

Considerations. Signs and symptoms of high gastrointestinal obstruction appear at about 4 to 6 weeks of age. There is a severe loss of body fluids and electrolytes. The first sign is vomiting in which the vomitus is free of bile.

Setup and preparation of the patient. The stomach is emptied just before induction of anesthesia, and the nasogastric tube is removed to guard against reflux of gastric contents around the tube during induction. A basic set and a pyloric spreader are used.

The patient is prepped in the usual manner.

Operative procedure

1. The abdomen is opened through a right subcostal transverse skin incision. The rectus muscle is split vertically with spreading clamps, and the peritoneum is opened.

2. After the pyloric tumor is delivered into the wound with a small vein retractor, the prepyloric area is grasped and rotated to expose the anterior superior border of the mass. An incision is made in the pyloric mass through the serosa and partially through the circular muscle throughout the length of the tumor (Fig. 25-5, *A*).

3. The circular muscle is spread with the pyloric spreader on the submucosal base, so that all muscle fibers are completely divided (Fig. 25-5, *B*).

4. After completion of the separation, the pyloric end of the stomach is returned to the abdomen, and the peritoneum and posterior rectus sheath are closed by continuous, chromic gut no. 3-0 suture. The anterior rectus sheath is closed with a no. 4-0 absorbable suture.

5. The skin is closed with fine, continuous subcuticular sutures. Small adhesive dressing strips are applied.

Emergency gastrointestinal procedures

Gastrostomy

Definition. Through an abdominal incision, establishment of a temporary or permanent channel from the gastric lumen to the skin to permit gastric emptying, liquid feeding, or retrograde dilatation of an esophageal stricture.

Considerations. A gastrostomy is done often with other surgical procedures to facilitate handling of the infant or child after surgery.

Setup and preparation of the patient. A basic set is required, plus a mushroom (no. 14 or 16 for babies and no. 18, 20, or 22 for older children) or Malecot catheter and a no. 11 knife blade.

Routine prepping of the patient is done.

Operative procedure

1. A short incision is made over the outer border of the left rectus muscle (Fig. 25-6, *A*).

2. The subcutaneous tissues and rectus fascia are exposed with two small retractors (Fig. 25-6, *B*).

3. The anterior rectus fascia is opened, and the rectus muscle is split with clamps, exposing the posterior rectus sheath (Fig. 25-6, *C*).

4. The peritoneum is opened, exposing the liver edge and the greater curvature of the stomach (Fig. 25-6, *D*).

5. The stomach is pulled out through the wound with a Babcock clamp. A circular purse-string stitch of no. 4-0 silk is placed, and in the center of this a stab wound is run through the gastric wall (Fig. 25-6, *E*).

6. A mushroom catheter, often with the tip cut off, is inserted into the stomach, and the purse-string suture is tied (Fig. 25-6, *F*).

7. A second purse-string suture is placed outside the previous one, and the same needle is then taken through the peritoneum and posterior rectus fascia to place the stomach against the peritoneum and thus prevent leaks (Fig. 25-6, *G* and *H*).

8. The catheter is brought out through a left lateral stab wound (Fig. 25-6, *A*).

9. Routine abdominal closure is performed.

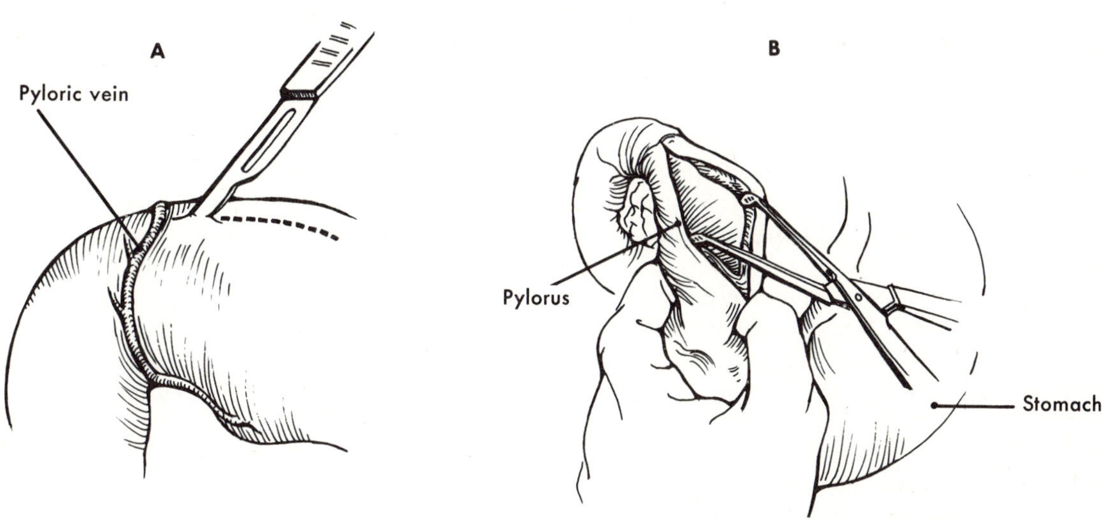

Fig. 25-5. Operative technique for pyloric stenosis. (From Benson, C.D.: Infants' hypertrophic pyloric stenosis. In Mustard, W.T., and others, editors: Pediatric surgery, 2nd edition. Copyright © by Year Book Medical Publishers, Inc., Chicago. Used by permission.)

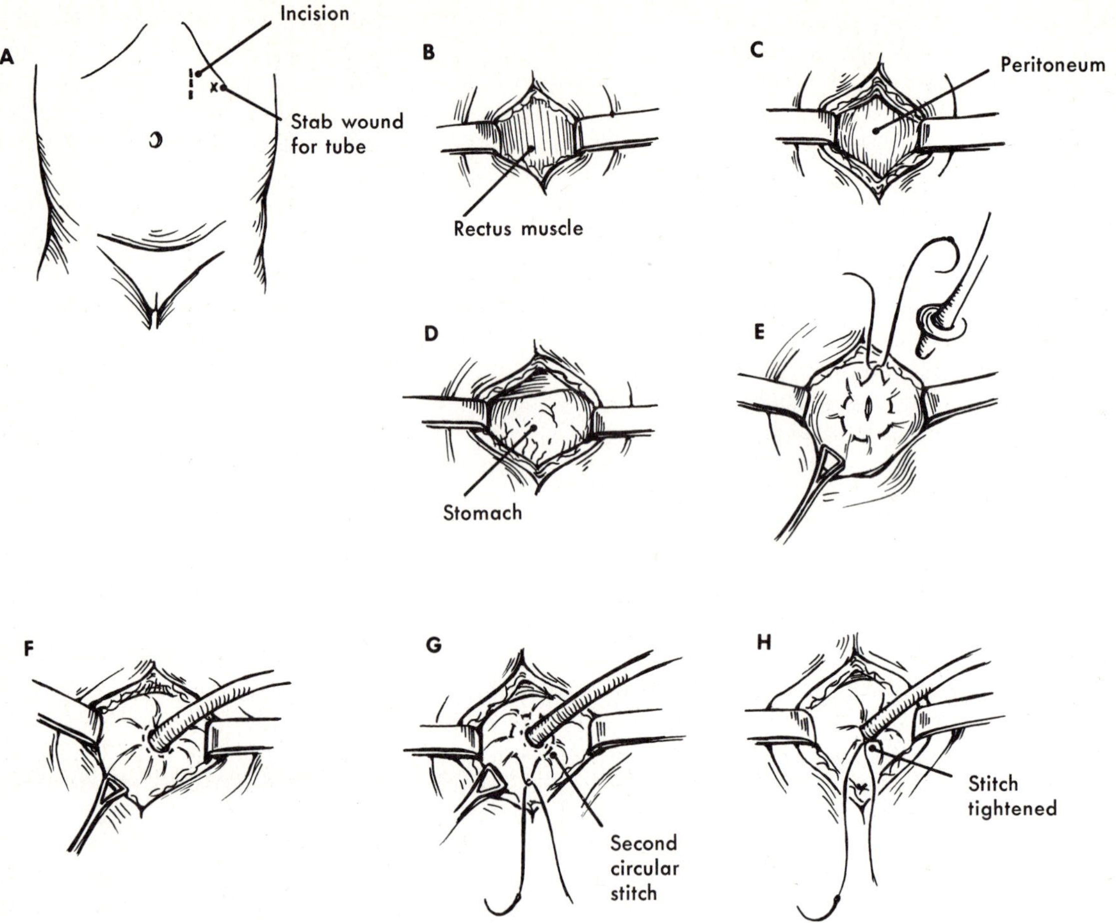

Fig. 25-6. Gastrostomy. **A,** Incision. **B,** Rectus muscle exposed. **C,** Posterior rectus sheath exposed. **D,** Peritoneum opened. **E,** Purse-string stitch placed. **F,** Mushroom catheter inserted. **G,** Second purse-string stitch placed. **H,** Stitch tightened. (Adapted from Gross, R.E.: An atlas of children's surgery, Philadelphia, 1970, W.B. Saunders Co.)

Repair of intestinal obstruction

Definition. (1) Untwisting of a volvulus, (2) division of a congenital band, (3) release of an internal hernia, (4) resection of bowel with anastomosis, or (5) creation of an intestinal stoma.

Considerations. Intestinal obstruction is the most frequent gastrointestinal emergency requiring operation in the newborn. Early recognition is essential. Surgical intervention is usually within the first few hours after birth; delay may increase the risk.

Intestinal obstruction may occur in the infant for a variety of reasons: atresia, stenosis, congenital aganglionosis, meconium ileus, or malrotation. Lesions characterized by complete obliteration of intestinal lumen are classifed as atresia. Those which produce a narrowing or partial obliteration of the lumen are classified as stenosis.

Setup and preparation of the patient. The abdominal set and intestinal instruments are required, plus culture tubes, syringes, and a no. 25 needle.

Usual prepping of the infant or child for surgery is done.

Operative procedure

1. The abdomen is opened through an incision appropriate to the exposure of the particular form of obstruction.

2. Exploration and displacement of the intestines to the abdominal wall helps determine the obstructive lesion. With atresia or stenosis, the entire bowel must be examined to rule out multiple areas of involvement.

3. Detorsion or reduction of bowel decompression or resection is performed when indicated (Chapter 14).

Relief of intussusception

Definition. Reduction of invaginated bowel by the hydrostatic pressure of a barium enema or by laparotomy and manual manipulation.

Considerations. Intussusception is the telescopic invagination of a portion of intestine into an adjacent part with mechanical and vascular impairment. A frequent site is the ileocecal junction. Intussusception in children is most often idiopathic; other causes may include Meckel's diverticulum, polyps, or hematoma of the bowel. Early diagnosis and reduction are essential to bowel viability.

Setup and preparation of the patient. The child is prepared for surgery as described previously. Reduction by barium enema is only attempted with the full cognizance of the radiologist, surgeon, and pediatrician. Should reduction not be accomplished, a laparotomy must be done. The abdominal set is used, with the addition of intestinal instruments.

Operative procedure

1. A transverse or right paramedian incision is made, and the peritoneum is entered (Fig. 25-7, *A*).

2. The cecum and ileum are identified; the intussusception is located and elevated in the fingers of the hand (Fig. 25-7, *B* and *C*).

3. If there is no evidence of bowel compromise, manual reduction is performed by gently milking the intussusceptum out of the intussuscipiens in the same direction as the flow of an enema (Fig. 25-7, *D*). No traction or opposing pull is exerted.

4. Should the viability of the bowel be questioned, a resection is done (Chapter 14).

5. The abdomen is closed in layers, and the wound is dressed.

Colostomy

Definition. Surgical construction of an artificial excretory opening from the colon.

Considerations. Most congenital anomalies that result in colonic obstruction require a temporary colostomy. These include imperforate anus and Hirschsprung's disease. Both conditions ultimately require further pelvic operative procedures, and proper construction of a colostomy is important. In Hirschsprung's disease, the colostomy must be placed in a section of bowel containing ganglia.

Setup and preparation of the patient. A basic set and intestinal clamps are used.

The child is prepped as described previously.

Operative procedure

1. A transverse incision usually is preferred, and the abdomen is entered in the right upper quadrant for a transverse colostomy or the left lower quadrant for a sigmoid colostomy.

2. The loop of colon is freed of peritoneal attachments until it can be brought easily through the abdominal wall without tension.

3. The edges of the mesentery are then sutured to the parietal peritoneum, and the serosa of the colonic loop is sutured with fine chromic to the peritoneum and fascia as well as the skin.

4. The colostomy may be sutured immediately. Some surgeons prefer to close the skin under a colostomy loop; others prefer to suture mucosa directly to skin edges. This decision may depend on the location of the colostomy. An important point is that each layer must be securely attached to the serosa of the colon to prevent evisceration and prolapse. The posterior wall of a loop colostomy may be divided with the cautery several days after surgery.

Resection and pull-through for Hirschsprung's disease

Definition. Removal of the aganglionic portion of the bowel and anastomosis of the normal colon to the anus after multiple biopsies and frozen section of the muscularis of the bowel to determine the presence of normal ganglia.

Considerations. Hirschsprung's disease is characterized by the presence of a segment of colon that lacks ganglia, resulting in an increase of tone and a lack of peristalsis proximally. Colon contents do not pass through the involved segment; thus the proximal normal colon is distended, which causes increasing abdominal distension. The distal colon is more frequently involved, but the disease may encompass the entire colon, with a less favorable prognosis. Prior to definitive surgery, a colostomy is usually made to relieve obstruction and permit function of the normal bowel. Biopsies of the bowel are taken first to establish the level of aganglionosis and which normal ganglia are present.

Several surgical techniques have been devised. Soave's procedure of endorectal pull-through employs internal bypass of the involved segment. The internal sphincter muscle of the anus is retained intact for continence.

Setup and preparation of the patient. The abdominal set, basic set, and intestinal instruments are required. A separate table is needed for the perineal portion of procedure. The setup should include the following:

Mosquito forceps
Metzenbaum scissors, small, curved and straight
Knife handle no. 3 with no. 15 blade
Forceps with and without teeth
Allis forceps
Sponge-holding forceps
Hegar dilators to dilate rectum
Needle holder
Separate suction
Suture no. 3-0 absorbable
Auto sutures (GIA)

The patient is prepped and draped from the nipples to and including the buttocks, genitals, perineal area, and upper thighs to permit positioning for the perineal stage without redraping. (Before preparation, the rectum may be irrigated with warm saline solution.)

A folded towel is placed under the buttocks. The patient is placed in the supine position with knees bent and legs in a modified "ski" position to facilitate abdominal and perineal approaches without redraping. A catheter is inserted to empty the bladder during the operation.

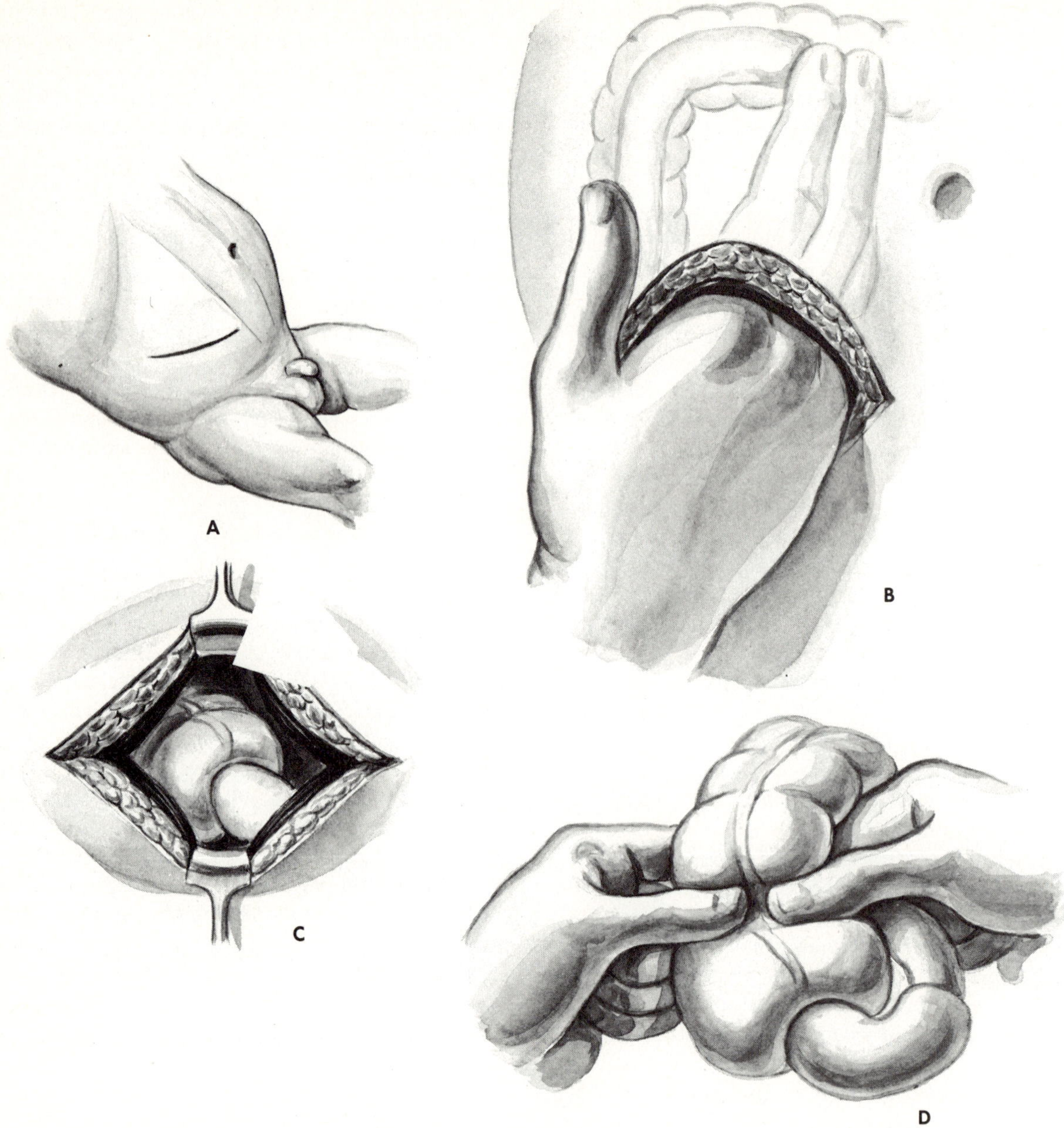

Fig. 25-7. Reduction of intussusception. **A,** Transverse abdominal incision. **B,** Location of intussusception. **C,** Mass delivered into incision. **D,** "Milking" reduction. (From Lewis, J.E.: Atlas of infant surgery, St. Louis, The C.V. Mosby Co.)

Operative procedure

1. A left paramedian incision is made that includes the sigmoid colonic stoma, if one is present.

2. The stoma is freed from the abdominal wall, and the left colon is mobilized. (If there is no sigmoid colonic stoma, the extent of aganglionic intestine is established by biopsy and frozen section, and all involved colon excised. If a stoma is present and the area has already been established as normal, the colon above it constitutes the proximal end of the resection.)

3. The mesocolon and the vessels of the intestine to be resected are divided close to the intestine, with care taken to preserve the blood supply to the rectum (Fig. 25-8, *A*).

4. The mucosal tube is freed from the outer muscular layers by sharp and blunt dissection with Metzenbaum scissors and a gauze-tipped instrument (Fig. 25-8, *B*).

5. A muscular sleeve is transected, and traction sutures of silk no. 4-0 are placed on the distal edge (Fig. 25-8, *C*). The mucosa is stripped down to the anus. The depth of the dissection may be checked by inserting a finger in the anus (Fig. 25-8, *D*).

6. When the mucosa is adequately freed, the perineal phase is started, and the perineal instrument table is used.

7. The anus is dilated and retracted with Allis clamps. A circumferential incision is made, and the mucosal stripping is completed (Fig. 25-8, *E*).

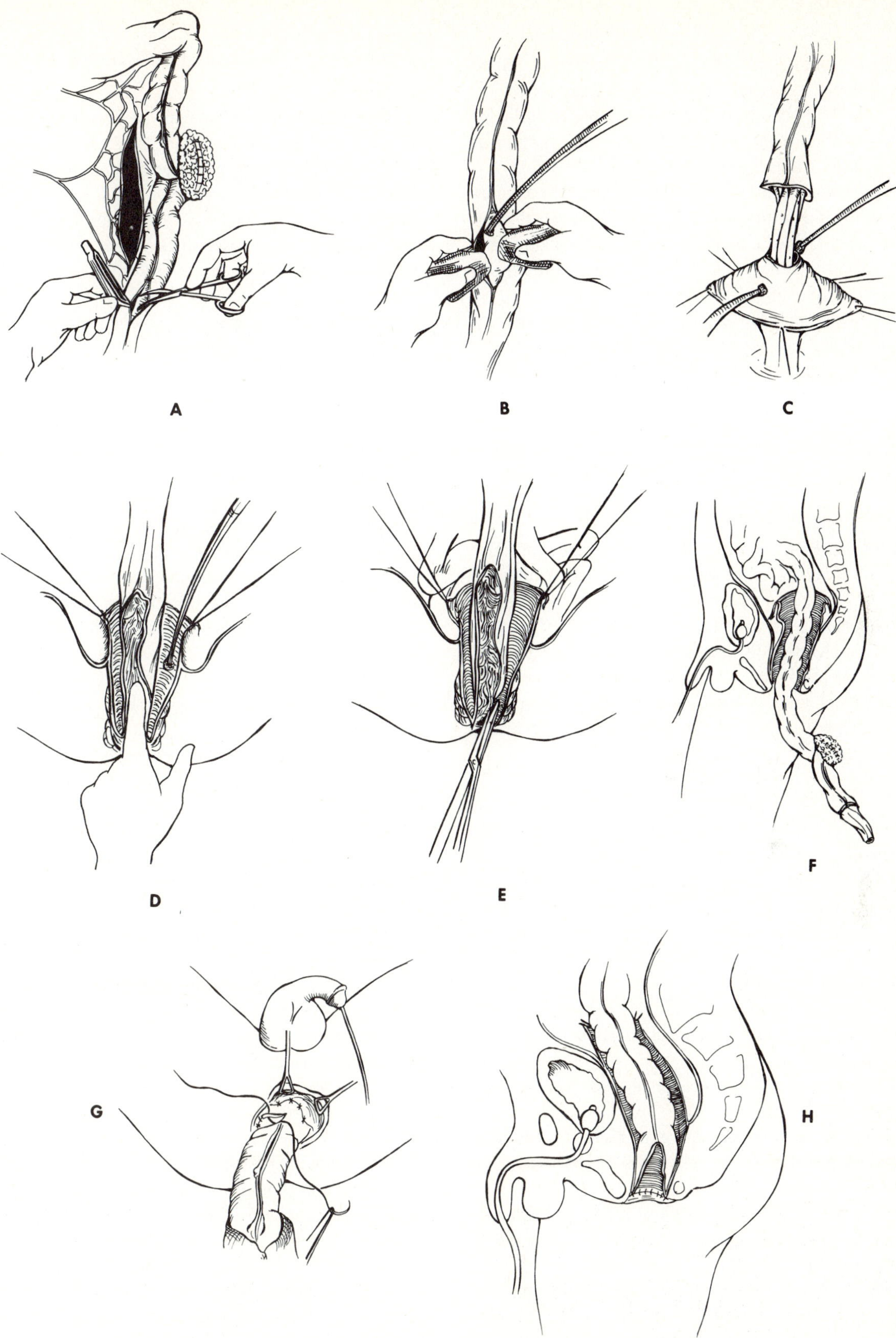

Fig. 25-8. Pull-through for Hirschsprung's disease. **A,** Dissection of mucosal tube begun through longitudinal incision. **B,** Gauze-tipped dissecting instrument used to dissect entire circumference of tube. **C,** Muscular sleeve transected. **D,** Depth of dissection determined by inserting finger in anus. **E,** Circumferential incision made. **F,** Mucosal tube and proximal portion of colon and stoma pulled through rectal muscular cuff. **G,** Anastomosis performed between all layers of colon and anal mucosa. **H,** Anastomosis completed. (Adapted from Boley, S.J.: An endorectal pull-through operation with primary anastomosis for Hirsch-sprung's disease, Surg. Gynecol. Obstet. **127**[2]:353. By permission of *Surgery, Gynecology, and Obstetrics*.)

8. The proximal portion of the intestine is pulled through the rectal muscular sleeve and out the anus (Fig. 25-8, *F*). If the portion of colon to be resected is large, it is excised abdominally before the proximal portion of the intestine is pulled through the anus.

9. Absorbable sutures are used to secure the seromuscular layers of the intussuscepted colon to the rectal muscular cuff. The colon is divided into axial or longitudinal quadrants, and an anastomosis is performed with no. 3-0 absorbable sutures (Fig. 25-8, *G*).

10. Gowns and gloves are changed, and abdominal instruments are used. The abdominal phase of the operation is completed by approximating the proximal edge of the muscular cuff to the seromuscular layer of the colon with silk no. 4-0 sutures (Fig. 25-8, *H*). The abdomen is closed in the routine manner, without drainage.

Repair of imperforate anus

Definition. Establishment of colorectoanal continuity through the external sphincter and closure of fistulas, if present.

Considerations. Imperforate anus may be present in varied forms. A covered anus may be the only defect, in which case surgical incision and repeated dilatation of the sphincter is indicated. A blind rectal pouch with or without genitourinary fistulas is the most prevalent type and the most difficult to repair.

Repair of imperforate anus and rectovaginal fistula

Setup and preparation of the patient. A basic set is required, plus skin hooks, small urethral sounds, and a nerve stimulator.

The patient is positioned and prepped with legs drawn upward.

Operative procedure

1. To identify the tract, a small clamp is inserted into the rectovaginal fistula. A perineal incision is made in the midline.

2. Dissection is carried through the skin and subcutaneous tissues.

3. The fistula is identified and divided. The exterior end is not closed but left open for postoperative drainage.

4. After the rectum is freed on all sides and brought down, the rectoanal repair is begun with chromic gut no. 4-0 sutures.

5. The rectum is opened, and the bowel wall is trimmed back. Traction sutures, usually no. 3-0 chromic gut, are placed through the skin and the full thickness of the bowel.

6. The orifice of the anus should be dilated considerably. It will shrink in a few months.

Sacroabdominoperineal pull-through for imperforate anus

Considerations. Whatever the distinctive malformation, surgical intervention and repair is indicated within 24 to 48 hours. When a sacroabdominoperineal pull-through is indicated, a transverse colostomy may be made during these 24 to 48 hours to irrigate the hiatal lumen and to remove meconium plugs, while allowing proximal colon function. After the colostomy, further diagnostic studies are made, such as cystograms and vaginograms. Definitive surgery is performed when the condition and size of the child permits, usually around 1 year.

Setup and preparation of the patient. The abdominal set is used, as well as Hegar dilators.

Positional changes are required, and supplies should be prepared.

Operative procedure

1. The patient is placed in a prone position with buttocks taped apart; a metal urethral sound is used to mark the urethra in the male or the vagina in the female; a large rubber catheter is threaded into the distal loop of the transverse colostomy to identify the blind rectal pouch.

2. The skin is incised from the coccyx to the projected anal opening (Fig. 25-9, *A*). Dissection is carried out in the midline to expose the blind rectal pouch (Fig. 25-9, *B*) and the puborectal muscle, which is freed from the urethra (or vagina).

3. The perineum is then examined, and the external sphincter is located. A cruciate incision is made over the sphincter, and it is dissected free from overlying skin and subcutaneous tissue. After making an opening through the center of the muscle, it and the puborectal tunnel are joined and dilated by means of Hegar dilators, taking care not to tear either muscle (Fig. 25-9, *C*).

4. A Penrose drain is placed through the tunnel up to the rectal pouch. The sacral incision is closed in layers.

5. After the child is repositioned to a supine position with legs overhanging the table, the abdomen is incised through a left lower quadrant or transverse incision. The pelvic peritoneum is opened, and the rectal pouch is identified.

6. After saline solution is injected into the seromuscular coat of the rectal pouch, the seromuscular layer is circumferentially dissected from the mucosal layer. The mucosa is cross-clamped with two Ochsner forceps and divided. The serosal layer is further stripped from the distal blind pouch, and, as fistulas are identified, they are closed.

7. The proximal bowel is mobilized with preservation of the blood supply to allow length for an adequate pull-through (Fig. 25-9, *D*).

8. A Hegar dilator is inserted through the lumen of the perineal end of the Penrose drain until it reaches the blind rectal pouch. An incision is made through the pouch

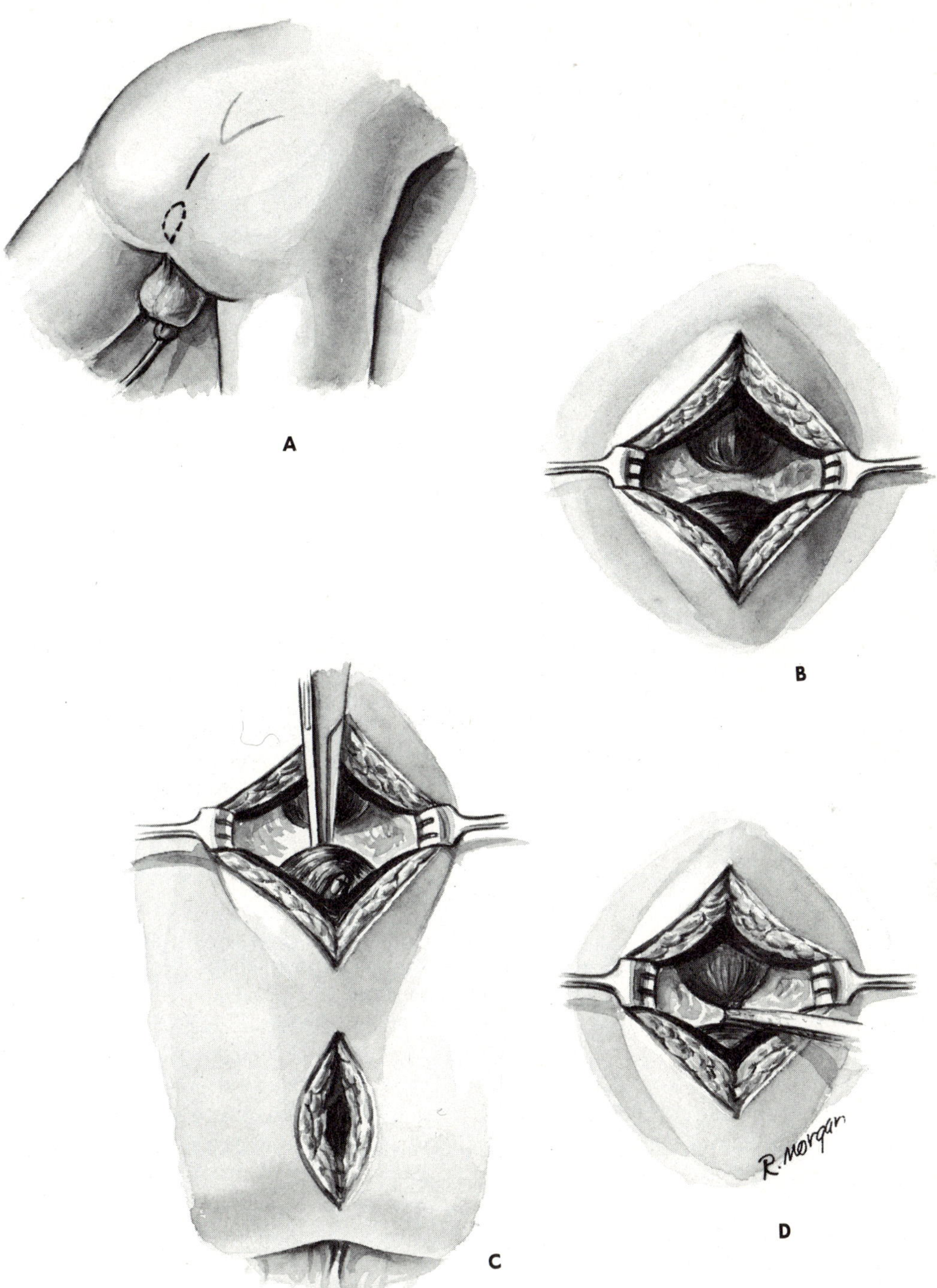

Fig. 25-9. Sacroabdominoperineal pull-through. **A,** Sacral incision. **B,** Dissection exposing rectal pouch and levator muscles. **C,** Elevation of puborectal portion of levator preliminary to dilatation of tunnel. **D,** Mobilization of proximal colon after abdominal incision.

Continued.

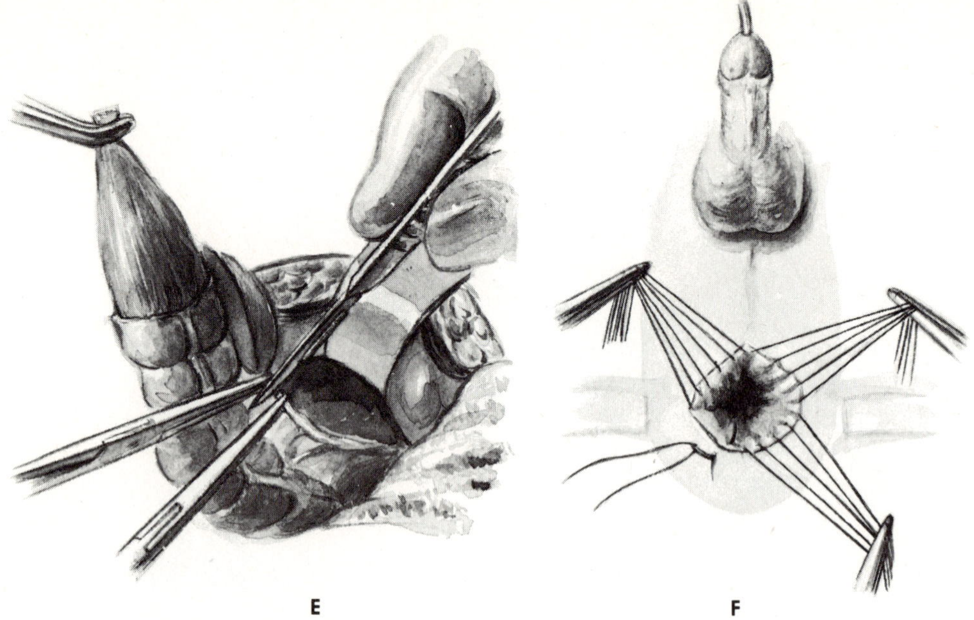

Fig. 25-9, cont'd. E, With forceps, colon is pulled through rectal pouch and sphincter to perineum. **F,** Suturing of colon to anal skin edges. (From Lewis, J.E.: Atlas of infant surgery, St. Louis, The C.V. Mosby Co.)

over the dilator, and it is removed as the Penrose drain is brought into the pouch.

9. Long Allis forceps are passed along the pathway of the Penrose drain, and the edges of the upper segment are grasped and pulled out through the pouch and sphincter onto the perineum. The external sphincter may be incised to accommodate the larger colon (Fig. 25-9, *E*).

10. The anal skin edges are then sewn to the mucosal layer of the pull-through segment with silk sutures no. 4-0 (Fig. 25-9, *F*).

11. The serosal layer is loosely attached to the pull-through segment.

12. The abdomen is closed in the routine manner.

Resection of tumors

Considerations. Tumors occur in children as well as adults. As is always the case with tumors, the therapy administered is dependent on the type of tumor. Examination and judicious investigation of all unusual masses are imperative. Thorough diagnostic workup and prompt definitive treatment may result in cure, even if the tumor is proved malignant. Chemotherapy and radiation therapy are adjuncts to surgical therapy of tumors.

Wilms tumor

Definition. Wilms tumor of the kidney is one of the more common childhood neoplasms. The tumor presents a firm, painless mass whose enlargement may laterally distend the abdomen.

Operative procedure. If the tumor is operable, the following aspects are important:

1. The transabdominal approach, which may be extended to a combined transabdominal-transthoracic approach, is used to inspect abdominal contents and clamp the vessels of the renal pedicle before dissection of the tumor.

2. The opposite kidney should be inspected, and suspicious nodules biopsied to rule out bilateral disease.

3. The extent of the tumor should be marked with hemostatic clips so that the radiation therapy area will be properly designated.

4. The entire primary tumor should be removed, if it does not place the patient in jeopardy.

5. Any residual tumor should be marked with clips.

6. The abdominal cavity and viscera are thoroughly inspected for evidence of tumor extension or metastases. Extensive surgery may include adrenalectomy, partial colectomy, or partial resection of the diaphragm.

Neuroblastoma

Definition. Neuroblastoma is a large retroperitoneal tumor of early childhood. The mass is usually firm, irregular, and nontender. It is a silent tumor in its early stages and metastasizes rapidly.

Considerations. Treatment includes an operation to ligate much of the tumor's blood supply and remove as much of the tumor as possible, as well as chemotherapy and radiation.

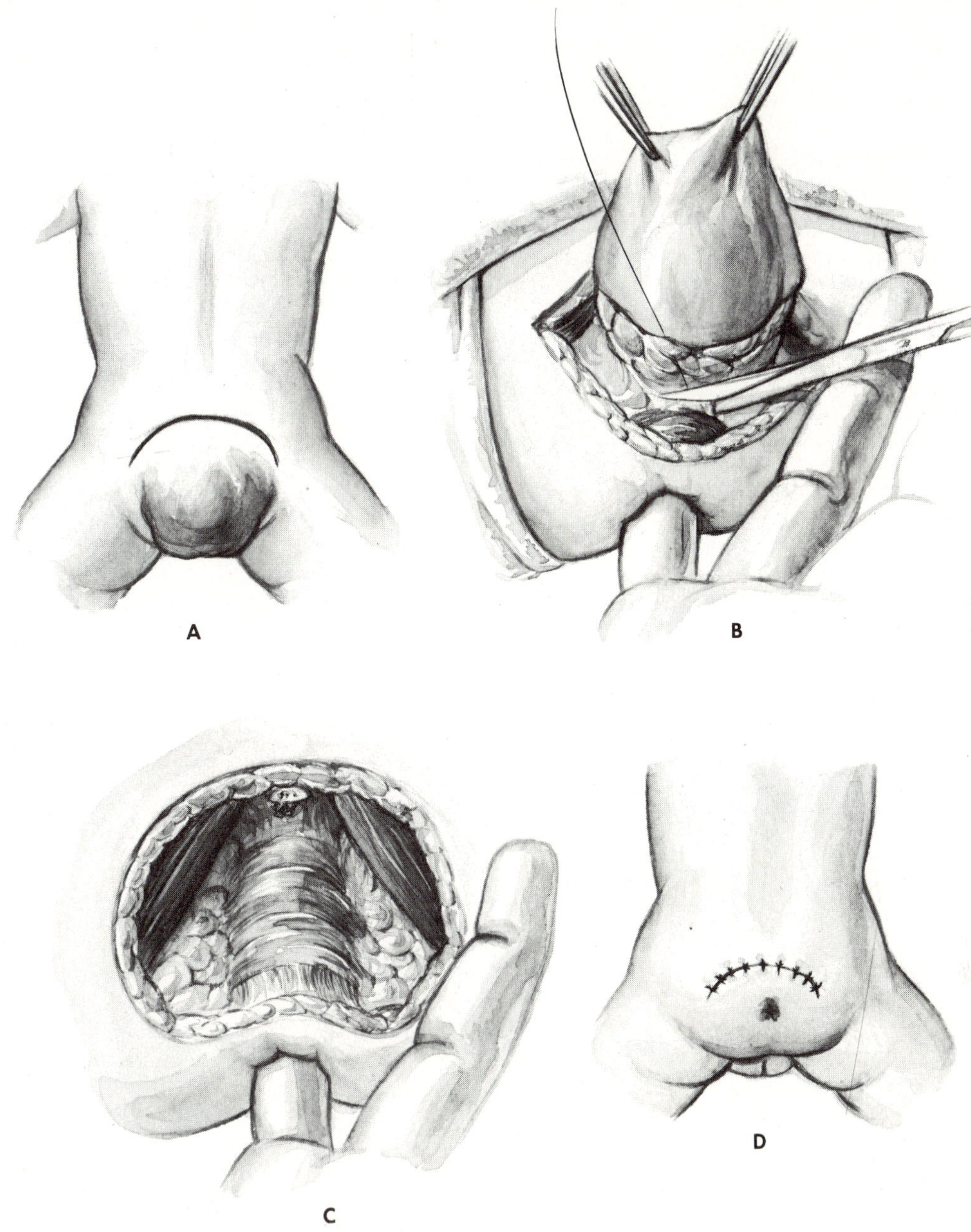

Fig. 25-10. Excision of sacrococcygeal teratoma. **A,** U-shaped incision. **B,** Dissection of teratoma. **C,** Tumor excised while rectum remains intact. **D,** Closed incisional line. (From Lewis, J.E.: Atlas of infant surgery, St. Louis, The C.V. Mosby Co.)

Sacrococcygeal teratoma

The sacrococcygeal teratoma is usually resectable in the newborn but may undergo malignant change if not removed early in life. Tumors resected in the newborn period contain microscopic evidence of malignant cells but have resulted in surgical cure. Early surgical resection is important because these tumors are not sensitive to irradiation and are only temporarily responsive to chemotherapy.

The tumor is in the area of the sacrum and coccyx but may extend into the pelvis or abdomen. Resection is usually feasible by placing the patient in the Kraske position and excising the tumor mass and coccyx en bloc (Fig. 25-10).

SUGGESTED READINGS

Atkinson, L.J., and Kohn, M.L.: Berry and Kohn's introduction to operating room technique, ed. 5, New York, 1978, McGraw-Hill Book Co.

Bell, A.N.: A concept of care for the pediatric patient, AORN J. **19:**623, 1974.

Bell, A.N.: Separating conjoined twins: a care plan, AORN J. **35:**47, 1982.

Bittner, J.S., Freeman, E.L., and Talbert, M.L.: Surgical care of the child: a new challenge for the operating room nurse, AORN J. **9:**37, 1969.

Davis, J.E.: Day surgery: a viable alternative, AORN J. **19:**641, 1974.

Fuller, B.F.: Hemostasis: a balanced system, AORN J. **32:**225, 1981.

Gans, S.L., editor: Surgical pediatrics: non-operative care, ed. 2, New York, 1980, Grune & Stratton, Inc.

Gross, R.E.: An atlas of children's surgery, Philadelphia, 1970, W.B. Saunders Co.

Haller, J.A., Jr., and Talbert, J.L.: Surgical emergencies in the newborn, Philadelphia, 1972, Lea & Febiger.

Harberg, R., and Holt, M.: Surgery for hernia, hydrocele, and undescended testicle, AORN J. **1:**47, 1963.

Ladd, W.E., and Gross, R.E.: Abdominal surgery of infancy and childhood, Philadelphia, 1941, W.B. Saunders Co.

Latham, H.C., and others: Pediatric nursing, ed. 3, St. Louis, 1977, The C.V. Mosby Co.

Lee, R.M.: Day surgery has added benefits for children, AORN J.**19:**632, 1974.

Levin, D.L., Morriss, F.C., and Moore, G.C., editors: A practical guide to pediatric intensive care, St. Louis, 1979, The C.V. Mosby Co.

Levin, R.M.: Pediatric anesthesia handbook, ed. 2, Garden City, N.J., 1980, Medical Examination Publishing Co., Inc.

Lewis, J.E.: Atlas of infant surgery, St. Louis, 1967, The C.V. Mosby Co.

Lipsky, K.: Conjoined twins: psychosocial aspects, AORN J. **35:**58, 1982.

Petrillo, M., and Sanger, S.: Emotional care of hospitalized children: an environmental approach, Philadelphia, 1972, J.B. Lippincott Co.

Raffensperger, J.G., and Primrose, R.B., editors: Pediatric surgery for nurses, Boston, 1968, Little, Brown & Co.

Shipes, E., and Stanley, I.: Necrotizing enterocolitis in premature infants, AORN J. **34:**154, 1981.

Stephen, C.R., Ahlgren, E.W., and Bennett, E.J.: Elements of pediatric anesthesia, ed. 2, Springfield, Ill., 1970, Charles C Thomas, Publisher.

Stewart, D.J.: Manual of pediatric anesthesia—the Hospital for Sick Children, Toronto, New York, 1979, Churchill Livingston, Inc.

Votteler, T.P.: Surgical separation of conjoined twins, AORN J. **35:**35, 1982.

Warden, L.S., and Robinson, M.K.: Osteotomy and intermaxillary fixation, AORN J. **33:**1304, June 1981.

Whaley, L.F., and Wong, D.J.: Nursing care of infants and children, ed. 2, St. Louis, 1983, The C.V. Mosby Co.

White, R.R., editor: Atlas of pediatric surgery, New York, 1965, McGraw-Hill Book Co.

Index

M

W